Textbook of
Sports Medicine

Textbook of Sports Medicine

Basic Science and Clinical Aspects of Sports Injury and Physical Activity

Edited by

Michael Kjær, Michael Krogsgaard
Peter Magnusson, Lars Engebretsen
Harald Roos, Timo Takala
Savio L-Y Woo

Blackwell
Science

© 2003 by Blackwell Science Ltd
a Blackwell Publishing company
Blackwell Science, Inc., 350 Main Street, Malden, Massachusetts 02148-5018, USA
Blackwell Publishing Ltd, 9600 Garsington Road, Oxford, Ox4 2DQ
Blackwell Science Asia Pty Ltd, 550 Swanston Street, Carlton South, Victoria 3053, Australia
Blackwell Wissenschafts Verlag, Kurfürstendamm 57, 10707 Berlin, Germany

First published 2003

ISBN 0-632-06509-5

Catalogue records for this title are available from the British Library and the Library of Congress

Set in 9$\frac{1}{2}$/12 pt Ehrhardt by SNP Best-set Typesetter Ltd., Hong Kong
Printed and bound in India by Thomson Press (India)

Commissioning Editor: Stuart Taylor
Managing Editor: Rupal Malde
Production Editor: Jonathan Rowley
Production Controller: Kate Charman

For further information on Blackwell Science, visit our website:
http://www.blackwellpublishing.com

Contents

Editors and Contributors

Per Aagaard   *Team Denmark Test Center, Sports Medicine Research Unit, University of Copenhagen, Bispebjerg Hospital, Copenhagen, DK-2400N, Denmark*

Steven Abramowitch   *Musculoskeletal Research Center, Department of Orthopaedic Surgery, University of Pittsburgh Medical Center, Pittsburgh, PA 15213, USA*

Lars Bo Anderson   *Institute of Exercise and Sports Science, University of Copenhagen, DK-2200N, Denmark*

Arne Astrup   *Research Department of Human Nutrition, Royal Veterinarian and Agricultural University, DK-2000F, Frederiksberg, Denmark*

Roald Bahr   *The Norwegian University of Sport and Physical Education, Oslo, N-0806, Norway*

Jens Bangsbo   *Laboratory for Human Physiology, August Krogh Institute, University of Copenhagen, DK-2100O, Denmark*

Oded Bar-Or   *Children's Exercise and Nutrition Centre, McMaster University, West Hamilton, Ontario, CAN-L85 4L8, Canada*

Peter Bärtsch   *Division of Sports Medicine, Department of Internal Medicine, University of Heidelberg, DE-69115, Heidelberg, Germany*

Fin Biering-Sørensen   *Clinic for Spinal Cord Injuries, Rigshospitalet, University of Copenhagen, DK-2100O, Denmark*

Leif Bjermer   *Department of Lung Medicine, University Hospital, Norwegian University of Science and Technology, Trondheim, N-7006, Norway*

Per Björntorp   *Department of Heart and Lung Diseases, University of Gothenburg, Sahlgrenska Hospital, SE-416 85, Sweden*

Robert Boushel   *Department of Exercise Science, Concordia University, Montreal, Quebec, CAN-H4B 1R6, Canada*

Stefan Brauth   *Department of Medical Sciences, Uppsala University Hospital, SE-75185, Sweden*

Jens Ivar Brox   *Department of Orthopaedics, Section for Physical Medicine and Rehabilitation, Rikshhospitalet, Oslo, N-0027, Norway*

Nicholas Bruggeman   *Department of Orthopaedic Surgery, Mayo Clinic, Rochester, MN 55905, USA*

William P. Cooney   *Department of Orthopaedic Surgery, Mayo Clinic, Rochester, MN 55905, USA*

Rasmus Damsgaard   *Copenhagen Muscle Research Centre, Rigshospitalet, Copenhagen, DK-2100O, Denmark*

Richard E. Debski   *Musculoskeletal Research Center, University of Pittsburgh Medical Center, Pittsburgh, PA 15213, USA*

Flemming Dela   *Department of Medical Physiology, Panum Institute, University of Copenhagen, DK-2200N, Denmark*

Bjorn Ekblom   *Department of Physiology and Pharmacology, Karolinska Institute, University of Stockholm, SE-11486, Sweden*

Lars Engebretsen   *Department of Orthopaedic Surgery, University of Oslo, Ullevål Hospital, NO-0407, Norway*

Erik Fink Eriksen   *Department of Endocrinology, Aarlus University Hospital, DK-8000C, Denmark*

Ulrich Fredberg   *Department of Medicine, Silkeborg Central Hospital, DK-8600, Denmark*

Jan Fridén   *Department of Hand Surgery, Sahlgrenska University Hospital, SE-41335, Göteborg, Sweden*

Joanna L. Fried   *Department of Obstetrics and Gynaecology, Columbia University, New York, NY 10032, USA*

Göran Friman   *Department of Medical Services, Section of Infectious Diseases, Uppsala University Hospital, SE-75185, Sweden*

Wayne Gibbon   *Department of Sports Medicine, University of Leeds, LS2 9NL, UK*

Leif Hambraeus   *Department of Medical Sciences, Nutrition Unit, Uppsala University, SE-75237, Sweden*

Mark Hargreaves   *Department of Exercise Physiology, School of Health Sciences, Deakin University, Burwood, AUS-3125, Australia*

Steve Harridge   *Department of Physiology, Royal Free & University College Medical School, London, NW3 2PF, UK*

Helge Hebestreit   *Pneumologie/Sportsmedizin, Universitäts-Kinderklinik, Würzburg, DE-97080, Germany*

Heikki Helminen   *Department of Anatomy, University of Kuopio, FIN-70211, Finland*

Jan Henriksson   *Department of Physiology and Pharmacology, Karolinska Institute, University of Stockholm, SE-17177, Sweden*

Nils Hjeltness   *Department of Spinal Cord Injury, Sunnaas Hospital, Nesoddtangen, Norway*

Per Hölmich   *Department of Orthopaedic Surgery, Amager Hospital, University of Copenhagen, DK-2300S, Denmark*

Heikki V. Huikuri   *Department of Medicine, Division of Cardiology, University of Oulo, FIN-90220, Finland*

Kerstin Jensen-Urstad   *Department of Clinical Physiology, Karolinska Hospital, Stockholm, SE-17176, Sweden*

Mats Jensen-Urstad   *Department of Cardiology, Karolinska Hospital, Stockholm, SE-17176, Sweden*

Norman L. Jones   *Department of Medicine, McMaster University, Hamilton, Ontario, CAN-L8N 3Z5, Canada*

Hannu Kalimo   *Department of Pathology, Turko University Hospital, Turko, FIN-20520, Finland*

Pekha Kannus   *Accident and Trauma Research Center, UKK Institute, Tampere, FIN-33500, Finland*

Inge-Lis Kanstrup   *Department of Clinical Physiology, Herlev Hospital, University of Copenhagen, DK-2730, Denmark*

Jon Karlsson   *Department of Orthopaedics, Sahlgrenska University Hospital/Östra, Gothenburg, SE-42685, Sweden*

Albert I. King   *Bioengineering Center, Wayne State University, Detroit, MI 48202, USA*

Michael Kjær   *Sports Medicine Research Center, University of Copenhagen, Bispebjerg Hospital, Copenhagen, DK-2400 NV, Denmark*

Pavo Komi   *Department of Biology of Physical Activity, University of Jyväskylä, FIN-40351, Finland*

Michael Krogsgaard   *Department of Orthopaedic Surgery, Bispebjerg Hospital, University of Copenhagen, DK-2200 NV, Denmark*

Henning Langberg   *Sports Medicine Research Unit, Bispebjerg Hospital, Copenhagen, DK-2400 NV, Denmark*

Robert F. La Prada, *Sports Medicine and Shoulder Divisions, Department of Orthopaedic Surgery, University of Minnesota, MN 55455, USA*

Juhani Leppäluoto   *Department of Physiology, University of Oulo, FIN-90401, Finland*

Ingard Lerein   *Department of Orthopaedic Surgery, Region Hospital of Trondhjem, NO-7006, Norway*

Jack Lens   *Department of Orthopaedic Surgery, University of Minnesota, MN 55455, USA*

Jan Lexell   *Brain Injury Unit, Neuromuscular Research Laboratory, Department of Rehabilitation, Lund University Hospital, SE-22185, Sweden*

Richard L. Lieber   *Department of Orthopaedics and Bioengineering, University of California and V.A. Medical Center, La Jolla, CA 92093-9151, USA*

John C. Loh   *Musculoskeletal Research Center, Department of Orthopaedic Surgery, University of Pittsburgh Medical Center, Pittsburgh, PA 15213, USA*

Stefan Lohmander   *Department of Orthopaedics, University Hospital, Lund, SE-22185, Sweden*

Sverre Mæhlum   *Norsk Idrettsmedisinsk Institutt (NIMI), University of Oslo, NO-0885, Norway*

Peter Magnusson   *Team Denmark Test Center, Sports Medicine Research Unit, University of Copenhagen, Bispebjerg Hospital, Copenhagen, DK-2400 NV, Denmark*

Willem van Mechelen   *Department of Social Medicine, Vreie Universität, Amsterdam, NL-1081, The Netherlands*

Karola Messner   *Department of Neuroscience and Locomotion, Division of Sports Medicine, Faculty of Health Sciences, Linköping, SE-58185, Sweden*

Malachy McHugh   *Nicholas Institute of Sports Medicine and Athletic Trauma, Lenox Hill Hospital, New York, NY 10021, USA*

Frank Moses   *Gastroenterology Service, Walter Reed Army Medical Center, Washington DC, 20307-5001, USA*

Thomas Muellner   *Department of Orthopaedic Surgery, University of Vienna, Austria*

Jørn Müller   *Department of Growth and Reproduction, Rigshospitalet, University of Copenhagen, DK-2100Ø, Denmark*

Pertti Mustajoki   *Department of Medicine, Helsinki University Central Hospital, FIN-00029, Finland*

Bodil Nielsen Johansen   *Institute of Exercise and Sports Science, August Krogh Institute, University of Copenhagen, DK-2100Ø, Denmark*

Rolf Norlin   *Linköping Medical Center, SE-58223, Linköping, Sweden*

Ted Oegena *Department of Orthopaedic Surgery, University of Minnesota, MN 55455, USA*

Sakari Orava *Tohturitalo Hospital, Turka, Fin-20100, Finland*

Bente Klarlund Pedersen *Finsencentret, Department of Infectious Diseases, University of Copenhagen, DK-2100Ø, Denmark*

Hollis Potter *Department of Radiology and Imaging, Hospital for Special Surgery, New York, NY 10021, USA*

Anne Raben *Research Department of Human Nutrition, Centre for Advanced Food Studies, Royal Veterinarian and Agricultural University, DK-2000F, Denmark*

Per Renström *Section of Sports Medicine, Department of Orthopaedics, Karolinska Hospital, Stockholm, SE-17176, Sweden*

Christer Rolf *Centre of Sports Medicine, University of Sheffield, S10 2TA, UK*

Harald Roos *Department of Orthopaedic Surgery, Helsingborg Hospital, Helsingborg, SE-25182, Sweden*

Lena Rydqvist *Linköping Medical Center, SE-58223, Linköping, Sweden*

Kent Sahlin *Department of Physiology and Pharmacology, Karolinska Institute, University of Stockholm, SE-11486, Sweden*

Bengt Saltin *Copenhagen Muscle Research Centre, Rigshospitalet, University of Copenhagen, DK-2100Ø, Denmark*

Tönu Saartok *Section of Sports Medicine, Department of Orthopaedics, Karolinski Hospital, Stockholm, SE 17176, Sweden*

Peter Schwartz *Department of Endocrinology, Rigshospitalet, University of Copenhagen, DK-2200N, Denmark*

Erik Simonsen *Institute for Medical Anatomy, Panum Institute, University of Copenhagen, DK-2200N, Denmark*

Scott Steinman *Department of Orthopaedic Surgery, Mayo Clinic, Rochester, MN 55905, USA*

David Stone *Musculoskeletal Research Center, Department of Orthopaedic Surgery, University of Pittsburgh Medical Center, Pittsburgh, PA 15213, USA*

Sigmund B. Strømme *The Norwegian University of Sport and Physical Education, Oslo, NO-0863, Norway*

Malcolm Sue-Chu *Department of Lung Medicine, University Hospital, Norwegian University of Science and Technology, Trondheim, N-7006, Norway*

Jorun Sundgot-Borgen *Norwegian University of Sport and Physical Education, Oslo, NO-0806, Norway*

Harri Snominen *Department of Health Sciences, University of Jyväskylä, FIN-40351, Finland*

Timo Säppälä *National Public Health Institute, Helsinki, FIN-00300, Finland*

Timo Takala *Department of Biology of Physical Activity, University of Jyväskylä, FIN-40351, Finland*

Rana Tariq *Department of Radiology, Ulleval University Hospital, Oslo, N-0407, Norway*

Kim Thorsen *Department for Sports Medicine, Norrland University Hospital, Umeå University, SE-90185, Sweden*

Alf Thorstensson *Department of Sport and Health Sciences, University College of Physical Education and Sports, Department of Neuroscience, Karolinska Institute, Stockholm, SE-11486, Sweden*

Mikko P. Tulppo   *Merikoski Rehabilitation and Research Centre, University of Oulu, FIN-90100, Finland*

Axel Urhausen   *Institute of Sports and Preventitive Medicine, Department of Clinical Medicine, University of Saarland, D-66041, Saarbruecken, Germany*

Ilkka Vuori   *UKK Institute for Health Promotion Research, Tampere, FIN-33501, Finland*

James H.-C. Wang   *Musculoskeletal Research Center, Department of Orthopaedic Surgery, University of Pittsburgh Medical Center, Pittsburgh, PA 15213, USA*

Michelle Warren   *Department of Obstetrics and Gynaecology, Colombia University, College of Physicians and Surgeons, New York, NY 10032, USA*

Fred Wentort   *Department of Orthopaedic Surgery, University of Minnesota, Minneapolis, MN 55455, USA*

Lars Wesslén   *Department of Medical Sciences, Section of Infectious Diseases, Uppsala University Hospital, Uppsala, Sweden*

Savio L.-Y. Woo   *Musculoskeletal Research Center, Department of Orthopaedic Surgery, University of Pittsburgh Medical Center, Pittsburgh, PA 15213, USA*

King H. Yang   *Bioengineering Center, Wayne State University, Detroit, Michigan, MI 48202, USA*

Hannele Yki-Järvinen   *Department of Medicine, University of Helsinki, FIN-002900, Helsinki, Finland*

Liying Zhang   *Bioengineering Center, Wayne State University, Detroit, Michigan, MI 48202, USA*

Preface

In past decades the number of exercising individuals and the area of sports medicine have grown considerably. Sports medicine has developed both in terms of its clinical importance with appropriate diagnosis and adequate rehabilitation following injury as well as its potential role in the promotion of health and prevention of life-style diseases in individuals of all ages. Furthermore, lately the medical field has gained improved understanding of the use of physical activity as a treatment modality in patients with a variety of chronic diseases and in rehabilitation after disabilities, injuries and diseases. Common to these advancements is the fact that a certain amount of clinical experience has to be coupled with sound research findings, both basic and applied, in order to provide the best possible recommendations and treatments for patients and for the population in general.

There is a tradition in Scandinavia for an interaction between exercise physiology and clinical medicine and surgery, and it is apparent that both areas have hypotheses, inspiration and possible solutions to offer each other. It is therefore apparent that a textbook on sports medicine must attempt to incorporate all of these aspects to be comprehensive. A historical or classical reference has been selected as an introduction to each chapter to reflect the impact that a specific scientific work has had on that field. Having several authors collaborating on each chapter in the book ensures both diversity and a degree of consensus in the text, which will hopefully make the book usable as a reference book, and as a textbook both at the pre- and postgraduate levels. It has been our goal to address each topic within sports medicine in a scientific way, highlighting both where knowledge is well supported by research, as well as areas where the scientific support is minimal or completely lacking. It is the intention that the book will help the people who work clinically within the area of sports medicine in their daily practice, and that it will also provide the basis for further research activity within all areas of sports medicine. Moreover, we wish to highlight where knowledge and methodologies from different, and often distant, areas can interact to create a better understanding of, for example, the mechanisms behind development of tissue injury and its healing.

The editorial group has been delighted that some of the world's leading experts have agreed to participate in this project, and they have all contributed with informative and very comprehensive chapters. I greatly appreciate their contribution and that of the editorial group who worked hard on the completion of the book. Additionally, I wish to acknowledge all other contributors who have helped with the practical procedures of this project. Finally, I hope the reader of this book will share the research dreams, the clinical interest, and the enthusiasm in relation to the sports medicine topics with that of the authors and the entire editorial group.

Michael Kjaer
Copenhagen, September 2002

Introduction

MICHAEL KJÆR

MICHAEL KROGSGAARD

PETER MAGNUSSON

LARS ENGEBRETSEN

HARALD ROOS

TIMO TAKALA

SAVIO L-Y WOO

The exercising human: an integrated machine

Physiological boundaries have fascinated man for a long time, and achievements like climbing up to more than 8800 m above sea level without oxygen supply or diving down to more than 150 m in water without special diving equipment are at the limit of what textbook knowledge tells us should be possible for humans. Likewise, athletes continue to set new standards within sports performance, and patients with chronic diseases master physical tasks of a very challenging nature, like marathon running, that hitherto were thought impossible.

Muscles, tendons and bone are elegantly coupled together to provide an efficient system for movement, and together with joint cartilage and ligaments they allow for physical activity of various kinds. In order to provide energy to contracting muscles, ventilation often rises 20–40-fold and cardiac pump function can increase up to 6-fold during strenuous exercise in well-trained individuals in the attempt to deliver sufficient oxygen to allow for relevant oxidative processes that can be initiated within seconds. In addition, working skeletal muscles can by training achieve substantial increases in their capacity to both store energy and to extract and utilize oxygen. With regards to endurance capacity, humans are still left with the fact that the size of the heart relative to the skeletal muscle is relatively small—even in top-class runners—compared to basically all other animal species.

To drive the human machinery, local as well as distant substrate stores provide fuel for energy combustion, allowing for very prolonged exercise bouts. A controlled interplay between exercise intensity, energy metabolism and regulatory hormones takes place, and intake of different food stores can cause the muscle to adjust its fuel combustion to a large degree. The initiation of signals from motor centers to start voluntary movement and afferent signals from contracting muscle interact to achieve this and several signalling pathways for circulatory and metabolic control are now identified. The brain can make the muscles move, and can at the same time use substances for fuel that are released from muscle. Furthermore, intake of different food sources can cause the muscle to adjust its fuel combustion to a large degree.

Training can cause major tissue and organ adaptation and it is well known that this to a large degree depends upon both genetic and trainable factors (Table 1). More recent studies on identical twins have allowed for a discrimination of these two factors in relation to exercise and have shown that between 30 and 50% of the variation in parameters like maximal oxygen uptake or muscle strength are likely to be attributed to genetic factors. Rather than discourage humans from starting training on this background, it is fascinating to identify factors responsible for training improvements in, for example, muscle tissue. It is evident that contractile force can elicit transcription and translation to produce relevant changes in the amount of contractile or mitochondrial proteins, but the underlying mechanism in both muscle and connective

I

Table 1 The capacity of various tissues and systems, and their ability to adapt to physical activity or inactivity.

Function	Increase during single bout of physical activity ultimate tensile strength	Improvement with training (%)	Time required for adaptation	Decrease in function or maximal load with 3–4 weeks of inactivity (%)
Cardiorespiratory			Months–years	
Ventilation	35-fold	0		
CO	6-fold	90		40
O_2 extraction	2–3-fold	25		30
VO_2	12–18-fold	50–60		40
Muscle metabolism			Weeks–months	
Glycogen/fat stores	–	100		50
Oxidative capacity	–	300		40–100
Connective tissue			Months–years	
Tendon	100 MPa	20		30
Ligament	60–100 MPa	20		30
Bone	50–200 MPa	5–10		30
Cartilage	5–40 MPa	5–10		30
Muscle			Months–years	
Strength	–	100–200		60
Fibre CSA				
Type I	–	40		20
Type II	–	80		30

CO: cardiac output; VO_2: whole body oxygen uptake; CSA: cross-sectional area.

tissue is not understood. Interestingly, substances are now being identified (e.g. mitogenactivated protein kinases) where subtypes are differentially activated by either metabolic stress or by the degree of contractile stress, to cause either increased cell oxidative capacity or muscle cell hypertrophy, respectively. We are therefore at a point where we can begin to master the study of the adaptation of the human body not only to acute exercise, but also to loading and overloading, and this will provide us with prerequisites for study of the ultimate adaptation potential that the human organism achieves, and thereby better describe also on an individual level why tissue becomes overloaded and injured.

The delicate balance between training adaptation and injury—the dilemma of rehabilitation

It is important for the clinician who treats the recreational or elite athlete to have a thorough understanding of the injury, and also the ability of the affected tissue to adapt to immobilization, remobilization and training. One example is the considerable plasticity that skeletal muscle tissue displays. While strength is lost (up to 60%) rapidly within a few weeks of immobilization, it can be regained over the next couple of months, and strength can be augmented up to 2-fold with training for extended periods (months/year). Bone loss also (up to 40%) occurs rapidly within weeks of immobilization and is subsequently regained in the following months of rehabilitation. However, somewhat in contrast to muscle, extended training periods have a relatively modest impact on bone tissue augmentation. Connective tissue loss in tendon is also comparable to muscle and bone; however, in contrast, its slower metabolism requires perhaps up to 12 months or more before complete tissue recovery from an injury and subsequent inactivity. Thus, an injury that demands a limb to be immobilized for a given length of time may require different time periods for the various tissues to return to their preinjury levels.

In this context it is important for the clinician to note that the cardiovascular system recovers the fastest after a period of relative inactivity, which may create a dilemma: the athlete wants to take the rehabilitation and training program to new and challenging levels, but the different tissues may not be able to withstand the associated loads, and re-injury or a new so-called 'overload injury' may result. Thus, a thorough understanding of how tissues adapt to physical activity or lack thereof is paramount for the effective treatment and rehabilitation of the injured person.

While acute injury during exercise may intuitively be somewhat easy to understand, it may be more challenging to grasp the insidious and frequent 'overuse' injuries that occur with training. Some important observations in the field of sports medicine have been made in recent decades that have improved our understanding of these injuries. An awareness of the subject's loading pattern is important, of course. The recreational athlete who runs 5 km/week may subject each lower limb to approximately 2100 landings and take-offs in that time period. In contrast, the long distance runner who runs 100 km/week may subject each lower limb to approximately 38 000 landings and take-offs. Clearly, a certain degree of appropriate tissue adaptation has already taken place to withstand these vastly different loads, but nevertheless, injuries may be sustained by both the recreational and elite athlete and therefore remains an enigma. Interestingly, the weekly loading of tissue induced by sports participation is equivalent to that established by national authorities as the upper limits for what is tolerable for manual labour, suggesting that perhaps there is an inherent tissue limitation to loading.

Disadvantageous alignment, like severe pes planus or genu valgus, for example, may be important factors in determing who can withstand a given loading pattern, although such internal factors cannot entirely explain overuse injury. It has become generally accepted that it takes appreciable time for tissues like connective tissue to adapt to a new or increasing demand, even for the most genetically fortuitous. Therefore, any desired progression or change in a training program should be gradual. However, more detailed information with respect to the training frequency, duration and intensity that is required to avoid an injury is currently lacking, and thus preventative efforts in this respect remain difficult. At the same time, it is becoming increasingly

appreciated that tissues need restitution periods to 'adapt' to the previous bout of physical activity. This is put into practice, for example, by the tri-athlete who loads the cardiovascular system considerably on a daily basis, but stresses the musculo-skeletal system alternately by training either cycling, running or swimming, which may help to avoid injury. It is during the restitution period that tissues are allowed to recover, or further adapt to an increasing demand by either expanding their quantity or improving their quality. It is likely that in years to come researchers will furnish new and improved measurement techniques that will yield important detailed information about tissue adaptation to physical activity and restitution.

Sports injuries and development of treatment: from recreational sports to elite athletes

In many situations the transformation from overload symptoms to a sports injury is poorly defined and understood. Intensified research in anatomy, biochemistry, physiology and mechanisms of tissue adaptation to mechanical loading is needed to provide the basic understanding of overload injury pathogenesis. Although this in itself represents a paramount challenge, it seems even more difficult to understand an individual's disposition for developing symptoms. Why does one individual develop severe Achilles tendon pain in connection with a certain amount of running, while others do not? Why are overhead activities very painful for some athletes but not for others? Why is the functional stability of a cruciate ligament deficient knee or a mechanically unstable ankle joint different between persons despite the same activity level? Obviously it would be essential to identify the weakest link in each individual case, but knowledge of the individual specific factors is very incomplete. Could there be physiologically different levels for initiation of symptoms in different individuals? It is well known that persons with decreased sensory inputs, for example caused by diabetic polyneuropathy, have a high rate of overload injuries like tendonitis or stress fractures, simply because the natural alarm system is out of order. If a physiological difference in, for example, the threshold of sensory inputs exists in otherwise healthy people, the difference between a mechanical load that causes symptoms and one that results in tissue damage would vary from person to person.

Treatment of sports injuries represents major challenges. First, the aim to reduce symptoms is demanded by the athlete, and several pharmacological treatments will work well at rest, but will not provide pain relief when the individual is exercising. Secondly, when surgical treatment is indicated to repair irreversible changes of tissues (e.g. rupture of anterior and posterior cruciate ligaments of the knee) or to change biomechanical inferior or insufficient movement patterns (e.g. multidirectional instability in the shoulder) the procedures need to be minimally invasive in order to leave the remaining tissue as intact as possible and to allow for a quick regeneration process. Thirdly, the rehabilitation procedures and time allowed for recovery will be challenged. This is because athletes are eager to return to their sports. In this aspect, similarities can be drawn to occupational and rehabilitation medicine, which aims towards getting the patient back to the functional level that is required to perform a certain labour task.

In contrast to the little which is known about the individual-based factors, there is increasing knowledge about injury mechanisms in athletic performance. A number of specific pathological entities have been recognized, especially during the past two decades, e.g. secondary impingement and internal impingement of the shoulder in overhead athletes. On the basis of recognizing certain common patterns of injury and understanding their pathogenesis, specific treatments — surgical as well as nonsurgical — have been developed. Probably the first injury to be recognized as a specific lesion connected to sports performance was the Bankart lesion of the shoulder, described in 1923, and the way to repair the lesion was obvious once the pathoanatomical background was established. Similarly, when the SLAP lesion of the labrum in the shoulder was described for the first time about 10 years ago, the surgical treatment options could be defined (for further details see Chapter 6.5).

Arthroscopy, which was introduced for knee disorders back in 1968 and developed for the treatment of shoulder, elbow and ankle disorders in the 1990s, has made direct visualization of joint movement and intra-articular structures possible, and has increased the understanding of many intra-articular sports injuries. For the individual athlete it has resulted in a much more specific diagnosis and treatment, and consequently rehabilitation has become faster and easier than after open surgery. Furthermore, the invention and development of magnetic resonance imaging in the early 1990s, and the refinement and general availability of ultrasound investigation during the late 1990s, has increased the spectrum of diagnostic tools significantly. What still requires specific attention is the relative use of these para-clinical supplements as compared with a good clinical examination and judgement. There is no doubt that the new 'machine-tools', developed to help the sports medicine practitioner, tend to be 'over-used' in the initial phase, which is often followed by a more balanced phase in which it becomes evident that patient history and clinical examination can never be replaced by para-clinical tools, but that the latter provides a fruitful supplement in the process of diagnosis in sports medicine.

The collection of clinical information on symptomatic conditions in athletes can lead to identification of uniform patterns and logically based treatment modalities. Series of treated patients can also give information about the success rate of certain treatments, whereas only randomized studies can identify the best treatment strategy in a specific condition. Unfortunately, there are very few randomized studies in sports medicine and especially within traumatology. This is often due to a high demand for treatment to ensure fast recovery and return to sports participation, and it is unlikely that more than a small part of the surgical and nonsurgical treatment modalities will ever be evaluated by randomized studies. Even though more than 60 000 anterior cruciate ligament (ACL) reconstructions are performed every year in the USA, it is unknown which treatment strategy is the most advantageous. There are different factors influencing the decision to perform ACL reconstruction: the chance to get back to sports, prevention of secondary meniscus and cartilage injury, prevention of giving-way or subluxation episodes, risk for anterior knee pain or other operative complications, or timing of surgery. There is no evidence for how these factors should be weighted, and it is unknown if routine reconstruction in all patients shortly after an ACL injury would reduce the risk of late complications and increase activity level better than a more conservative approach with rehabilitation as primary treatment. It is very important to perform randomized trials at the same time as new treatments are introduced, as it is almost impossible to return to such studies later.

Most rehabilitation programs are based on individual, clinical experience and theoretical principles. Just as with surgical treatment, evidence is still lacking on the effect of a number of general treatment principles. Rehabilitation is very costly, and it is desirable with further development of evidence-based rehabilitation strategies.

New technologies will probably influence the treatment of sports injuries in the near future. Local availability of growth factors may reduce repair and remodelling time after injury or surgery. Scaffolds can be used to introduce a specific architecture. These can be taken over by living tissue, and in combination with controlled gene expression, injured tissue can possibly be restored completely. This will contribute to an avoidance of reconstruction with replacement tissue and accompanying suboptimal recovery, as well as ensure the absence of scar tissue otherwise seen in repair.

In the recreational athlete, many overload conditions are often self-limiting. Nature's alarm system works: overloading of tissues often results in symptoms (pain) long before irreversible changes of the tissue structures happen. With a gradual reduction of activity, symptoms and overloading disappears, and the athlete can resume normal activity again. Tennis elbow is a good example of this mechanism. During one season about 50% of middle-aged persons per-

forming recreational racquet sports will experience symptoms of tennis elbow. The majority of these cases resolve without specific treatment. The interesting phenomenon is, why humans often carry on with exercise despite symptoms and signs of overuse. Interestingly, inflammatory reactions within and around tendons are seen in humans and in a few animal species that are forced to run like race-horses, whereas almost all other species (like mouse, rat or rabbit) do not show signs of tendinitis or peritendinitis despite strenuous activity regimens. Elite athletes can be motivated to continue peak performance despite pain or other symptoms, and it can be difficult or impossible for the natural repair processes to take place. Not enough is known about tissue repair and rehabilitation to define the maximum activity in each individual that is compatible with a full and fast repair.

The boundary between trivial, reversible conditions and irreversible, disabling injuries still has to be defined in many sports. As an example, there is an ongoing discussion about the risk for chronic brain damages in boxing. Furthermore, nearly nothing is known about the long-term effect of continued elite sports activity on degenerative changes in the knee after ACL reconstruction. With this lack of evidence about physical consequences of sports injuries, ethical considerations have a central place in advice and planning. The influence of psychological factors such as competition (matches only take up less than 25% of the active playing time in elite handball, more than 90% of the ACL injuries happen there), self-confidence and acceptance of personal limits have to be acknowledged and further knowledge is warranted.

Table 2 Motivation and needs in different individuals with physical training.

	Performance motivation	Disease-effect motivation	Prevention motivation	Guidelines for training	Tolerable amounts of training
Patient	++ (function)	+++	++	+++	+
Recreational sports	+	–	+++	++	++
Elite athletes	+++ (competition)	–	(+)	+++	+++

The motive for performing physical training can primarily be based upon a wish of increased performance either in sports or in everyday life, or be related to a wish of increased health and disease prevention. All three groups of individuals display an individually varying degree of which for achieving mental well-being in relation to exercise. The tolerable amount of training depends on the ability of the body to withstand loading and varies therefore significantly between athletes and patients, whereas both patients and athletes share a large request for specific guidelines in relation to the training they perform.

Regular physical training: benefits and drawbacks

For more than 5000 years, systematic exercise or sports have been carried out worldwide, and one can easily consider the average individual living today as being much more inactive than they were in the past. It is becoming more and more scientifically documented that physical inactivity is a major risk factor for disease and premature death, and that the magnitude of this lies on the level of other risk factors like smoking, obesity or drinking. Studies have uniformly concluded that being active or beginning physical activity even at an advanced age, will positively influence risk factors for development of inactivity-associated diseases. In spite of the fact that acute training is associated with a transient increased risk of cardiac arrest, taken in the population as a group, as well as the costly treatment of sports injuries, socio-economic calculation has found that, for the recreational athlete, these drawbacks are far outweighed by the cost-saving benefits of physical training such as lower incidence of diseases, faster hospital recovery after disease in general, as well as a lower frequency of infection and time away from work due to sickness. The field of sports medicine is therefore facing a major challenge in improving the level of physical activity in the general population, and for setting up overall guidelines.

Physical training and patients with chronic diseases

Acute and chronic diseases are associated with both organ specific manifestations as well as by more general disturbances in function due to physical inactivity and sometimes even additional hormonal and cytokine-related catabolism. In general, physical training can counteract the general functional disturbances, and maybe even affect or prevent the primary manifestations of disease. It is important to note that the motivational aspects, as well as the requirements for supervision and guidelines, in the patient with a present disease differ markedly from healthy exercising individuals (Table 2).

In principle, most diseases can be combined with a certain degree of physical activity, but the amount of restrictions put upon the patient differs considerably between diseases (Table 3). Certain diseases have been shown to be influenced greatly from physical activity

Table 3 Effects of physical training upon different diseases.

Diseases in which physical training will act preventively in disease development and positively upon primary disease manifestations
Ischemic heart disease
Recovery phase of acute myocardial infarction
Hypertension
Type-2 diabetes
Obesity (most pronounced with respect to prevention)
Osteoporosis
Age-related loss of muscle mass (sarcopenia)
Osteoarthritis (most likely only the prevention)
Back pain
Cancer (prevention of colon and breast cancer)
Depression and disturbed sleep pattern
Infectious diseases (prevention of upper respiratory tract infection)

Diseases in which moderate or no direct effect can be demonstrated upon the primary disease manifestations, but where exercise will positively affect both health associated risk factors and the general disturbances in overall body function
Peripheral vascular diseases (arterial insufficiency)
Type-1 diabetes
Bronchial asthma
Chronic obstructive lung disease
Chronic kidney disease
Most forms of cancer
Most acute and chronic liver diseases
Rheumatoid arthritis
Organ transplanted individuals
Spinal cord injured individuals
Most neurological and mental diseases

Diseases in which much caution has to be taken or where exercise is to be discouraged, and where physical training often can have a worsening effect upon primary disease manifestations or may lead to complications
Myocarditis or perimyocarditis
Acute heart conditions (e.g. unstable angina, acute AMI, uncontrolled arrhythmia or third degree AV-block)
Acute infectious diseases associated with fever (e.g. upper respiratory tract infection)
Mononucleosis with manifest splenomegaly
Aorta stenosis (chronic effect)
Acute severe condition of many diseases mentioned above (e.g. severe hypertension, ketoacidosis in diabetes)
Acute episodes of joint swelling (e.g. rheumatoid arthritis) or severe muscle disease (e.g. myositis)

(e.g. ischemic heart disease, type-2 diabetes), whereas other diseases are known to be relatively insensitive to exercise when it comes to primary disease manifestations (e.g. chronic lung disease, type-1 diabetes). In the later group of diseases, it should, however, be noted that physical training can still have a beneficial effect on health-related parameters that can be achieved by individuals in general. This effect is achievable even in the absence of any worsening of the primary chronic disease. This emphasizes the importance of also encouraging individuals with chronic (and not necessarily fatal) diseases to train on a regular basis from a general health perspective. In addition, almost all diseased individuals can exercise in order to counteract the general loss in function that their disease-related inactivity has caused. In very few cases, extreme caution has to be taken when performing exercise (e.g. acute infectious diseases) (Table 3).

In spite of current knowledge of the effect of physical training on diseases, the exact mechanisms behind this are still only partially described. To find such bio-chemical and physiological pathways will be important not only for addressing which type and dose of physical training should be prescribed for the individual patient, but also for identifying more general 'health-pathways' by which muscular contractions can influence the health status of the individual. Especially in relation to disease, the influence of training on such pathways either by itself or in combination with pharmaceutical drugs will potentially play a role in treatment of disease and maintenance of health into old age. Specific identification of health-related pathways in our genes will furthermore provide insight into the genetic polymorphism and help to explain the interindividual variation in training responses and health-related outcome of these. Evidently, this will also open possibilities for genetic treatment of inherited disorders with regards to tissue and organ adaptability to training, and at the same time inadvertently provide opportunities for misuse of gene therapy in relation to doping, a question that will challenge the sports medicine field ethically.

Part 1
Basic Science of Physical Activity and Sports Injuries: Principles of Training

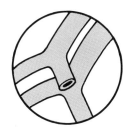

Chapter 1.1
Cardiovascular and Respiratory Aspects of Exercise — Endurance Training

SIGMUND B. STRØMME, ROBERT BOUSHEL,
BJØRN EKBLOM, HEIKKI HUIKURI,
MIKKO P. TULPPO & NORMAN L. JONES

Classical reference

Krogh, A, Lindhard, J The regulation of respiration
and circulation during the initial stages of muscular
work. *J Physiol (Lond)* 1913; **47**: 112–136.

This paper demonstrated changes in respiration and
heart rate with the transition from rest to bicycle exercise. The investigators did experiments on themselves,
and Fig. 1.1.1 shows the changes in tidal air and heart
rate at the onset of exercise. As will be noted, a very
rapid increase in both ventilation and heart rate was
observed, and this led to the conclusion that motor
center activity in parallel with activation of skeletal
muscle caused an increased stimulation of respiratory
centers as well as the heart. This was called cortical
irradiation, and has later been referred to as central
command or feed-forward, and has become an important topic in the discussion of respiratory, circulatory,
and hormonal changes during exercise.

Cardiovascular adaptation

Cardiac output

The pumping capacity of the heart is a critical determinant of endurance performance in exercise events
such as running, cycling, rowing, swimming, etc.,
where a large fraction of total body muscle mass is contracting dynamically. Because of the large dependence
on oxidative metabolism for the total energy turnover
in exercise activities sustained for longer than 3 min,

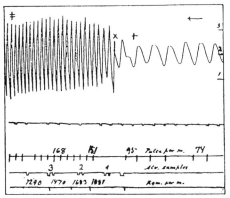

Fig. 1. J. L. Transition from rest to work. Exp. X. Scale in liters. Time in $\frac{1}{15}$ minutes. + Ready, × Begin, ⊕ Stop.

Fig. 1.1.1 A recording of the tidal air on a spirometer
(constructed by Krogh) at rest and at the beginning of exercise.

performance level is, as will be discussed later, largely
dependent on the capacity for O_2 delivery, and thus on
the magnitude of maximal cardiac output.

Maximal aerobic power ($\dot{V}_{O_{2\,max}}$) is a classic measure of the capacity to perform endurance exercise, and
may be described physiologically as the product of
cardiac output and the extraction of O_2 by muscle. For
almost a century it has been recognized that a linear
relationship exists between maximal oxygen uptake
and cardiac output, and this relationship is also
observed in other species [1–3]. It is estimated that
70–85% of the interindividual difference in $\dot{V}_{O_{2\,max}}$ is

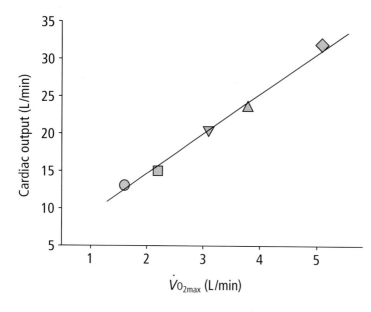

Fig. 1.1.2 Relationship between increases in cardiac output and maximal oxygen uptake in heart failure patients (circles), healthy males after 20 days' bedrest (squares), the same subjects before bedrest (inverted triangle), the same subjects after endurance training (upright triangle), and endurance athletes (diamonds).

attributable to the level of maximal cardiac output [4]. Looked at another way, during whole body exercise, only ~60–80% of maximal mitochondrial respiratory capacity is exploited because of the limits of O_2 delivery [5–7]. Endurance training augments skeletal muscle oxidative capacity and O_2 extraction, but the principal variant for improvements in $\dot{V}_{O_2\,max}$ is maximal cardiac output [8–10] (Fig. 1.1.2).

On the other hand, differences in athletic performance amongst competitive athletes with similar $\dot{V}_{O_2\,max}$ are linked to peripheral mechanisms [11], such as running economy. The basic question as to what limits maximal aerobic power ($\dot{V}_{O_2\,max}$) will be discussed later in this chapter.

Cardiac structure

The increase in maximal cardiac output (Q_{max}) following endurance training results from a larger cardiac stroke volume (SV), whereas maximal heart rate (HR_{max}) is unchanged or even slightly reduced. While heart size is a function of total body size as well as genetic factors, the higher SV achieved by endurance training is attributed to enlargement of cardiac chamber size and to expansion of total blood volume [12]. On the basis of cross-sectional studies in both

female and male endurance-trained athletes, total heart volume is generally 15–25% larger than sedentary size-matched controls, with morphologic differences seen in both the ventricles and the atria [13]. Chamber enlargement is also observed in endurance-trained paraplegics compared to sedentary matched controls [14].

There is a close relationship between cardiac volume and physical performance [12]. However, the cardiac hypertrophy is dependent on the type of sport carried out. There are two main types of myocardial hypertrophy. In weight lifters and other strength-training athletes heart wall thickness is increased, with only minor increases in heart cavity diameters, while endurance athletes have increased heart volume and cavity diameter with a proportional increase in wall muscle thickness [15]. The ratio of wall thickness to cavity diameter is unchanged in the endurance-trained individual but increased as a result of strength training [16].

The left ventricular hypertrophy in the endurance-trained individual is due to volume overload ('eccentric' hypertrophy), while the hypertrophy due to strength training develops as a consequence of pressure overload ('concentric' hypertrophy). Rowing, for instance, represents a mixture of volume and pressure overloading. In the former sarcomeres are added in series to increase cavity diameter, while in the latter sarcomeres are mainly added in parallel, causing wall thickening [17]. Both these are reversible processes since deconditioning from elite sport reduces cardiac size and volume towards what is normal for age and gender [18]. The cardiac morphology of the female athlete heart is the same as in men but the dimensions are in general smaller [19]. Structural and functional echocardiographic indices characterizing the normal limits of the athletic heart are shown in Table 1.1.1.

Whether or not cardiac hypertrophy ('athlete's heart') predisposes the athlete to future cardiac problems has been discussed for many years [20,21]. However, the number and severity of cardiac arrhythmias seem to be the same in young athletes compared to untrained individuals of the same age and gender [22], but increased in active elderly athletes [23]. However, a fast regression of ventricular hypertrophy through physical inactivity may cause some temporary increase in the number of arrhythmias [24].

Table 1.1.1 The upper normal healthy limits of cardiac dimensions associated with exercise training. From Urhausen & Kindermann, *Sports Med* 1999; **288**: 237–44.

	Men	Women
Heart volume (mL/kg)	20	19
Heart weight (g/kg)	7.5	7
LV muscle mass (g/m^2)	170	135
LV mass/$\dot{V}o_{2\,max}$ (g.min/L)	80	80
LVED diameter (mm)	63 (67a)	60 (63a)
Septum, LV post wall thickness	13	12
Septum/LV post wall thickness	1.4	1.3
Hypertrophic index (%)*	48	45
Fractional shortening (%)	>(22-) 27; ↑ exercise	>(22-) 27; ↑ exercise
Early/late transmitral flow velocity	>1.0	>1.0
Left atrium thickness (mm)	43 (47a)	43 (45a)

*Hypertrophic index (%) = septum + LV thickness (mm)/LVED diameter (mm).

Functional adaptations

In addition to structural adaptations, endurance training produces functional improvements in cardiac performance during exercise [25]. Most notable is a more rapid early and peak ventricular filling rate during diastole. An enlarged blood volume, together with greater ventricular compliance and distensibility, and a faster and more complete ventricular relaxation are important factors allowing stroke volume to increase even at high heart rates during exercise [9,26]. Improved myocardial relaxation allows for a more rapid lowering of ventricular pressure, optimizing the left atrial/ventricular pressure gradient for enhanced filling [27]. At the same time, the cardiac output is distributed more selectively to activated regions of skeletal muscle, from where the muscle pump facilitates venous return. As a result of an enlarged end-diastolic volume, left ventricular systolic performance is improved mainly by way of the Frank–Starling mechanism [28].

During submaximal exercise, myocardial work and O_2 consumption are reduced in those who are endurance trained due to a lower heart rate at a given cardiac output as well as a reduced afterload attributable to lower peripheral resistance [29]. The enhanced diastolic filling and reduced afterload ensure that stroke volume is maintained or even progressively increased from submaximal to maximal exercise [9], as compared to the sedentary person whose stroke volume plateaus at submaximal intensities and may fall as maximal exertion is approached [30].

Myocardial vascularization and perfusion

In a comparison of the cross-sectional area of proximal coronary arteries from endurance-trained and sedentary humans it has been suggested that coronary vascular volume may be increased by training [31]. It remains unresolved whether in humans endurance training increases coronary vascular dimensions beyond the vascular proliferation that accompanies normal training-induced cardiac hypertrophy. On the basis of studies in rats, endurance training has been shown to increase myocardial capillary density expressed as capillary/fiber ratio [32]. However, in larger animals, there is little evidence for increased capillary proliferation per fiber, nor is there evidence for proli-

feration of collateral coronary vessels in the healthy
non-ischemic heart.

Commensurate with the reduction in myocardial
work and O_2 consumption at rest and during submaximal exercise after endurance training, coronary blood
flow per unit myocardial mass is reduced [33]. However, studies in animals have shown that endurance
training can increase maximal coronary perfusion per
unit mass of the myocardium [34]. There are only
modest increases in myocardial O_2 extraction from rest
to maximal exercise since extraction is very high even
in the untrained state. However, there is evidence that
exercise training elicits changes in vascular tone leading to an optimized distribution of blood flow, whereby
more capillaries are recruited without a change in capillary density [34,35]. This is probably due to specific
endothelium-mediated vasodilatation. Results from
animal studies suggest that increased endothelial cell
nitric oxide synthase, an enzyme that synthesizes
nitric oxide from L-arginine, contributes to such an
adaptation [36,37].

Heart rate

At the beginning of dynamic exercise, heart rate increases rapidly due to the inhibition of parasympathetic tone. If the exercise is light (heart rate < 100
beats/min), the sympathetic activity applied to the
heart and the vasculature does not increase and tachycardia occurs solely due to the reduction in parasympathetic tone [38]. As the workload increases, heart rate
increases due to further vagal withdrawal and concomitant sympathetic activation (Fig. 1.1.3) [39].

The increase in sympathetic activation may be due
to arterial baroreflex resetting, the muscle metaboreflex or muscle mechanoreceptor activation [40]. During heavy exercise, parasympathetic activity wanes and
sympathetic activity increases in such a way that, at a
workload corresponding to maximal oxygen consumption, little or no parasympathetic tone remains [39].

The analysis of heart rate variability (HRV) has become a frequently used tool for providing information
on cardiovascular autonomic regulation at various
phases of exercise, and also on the effects of physical
training on cardiovascular autonomic regulation. The
most commonly used HRV methods are time and
frequency domain analysis techniques. The standard
deviation of all normal-to-normal R–R intervals over

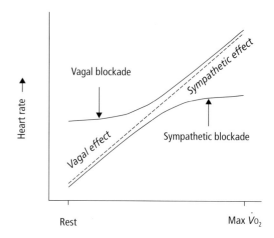

Fig. 1.1.3 Schematic diagram showing the relative
contributions of the sympathetic and parasympathetic systems
to cardioacceleration at various levels of exercise. Comparisons
are between the control state (broken line) and parasympathetic
or sympathetic blockade. (Modified from [138].)

an entire recording (SDNN) is a simple time domain
method. This variable is considered to reflect both
parasympathetic and sympathetic influences on the
heart. The power spectrum of R–R intervals reflects
the amplitude of heart rate fluctuations present at
different oscillation frequencies. The different power
spectral bands reveal different physiologic regulatory
mechanisms; e.g. an efferent vagal activity is a major
contributor to the high frequency component (see Fig.
1.1.4).

A distinct cardiovascular adaptation to endurance
training is a lowering of the heart rate at rest and
during submaximal exercise. Maximal heart rate is
unchanged or in some cases may be slightly reduced.
The lowering of resting and submaximal heart rate is
mediated by alterations in the autonomic nervous system, and by changes in the intrinsic automaticity of the
sinus node and right atrial myocytes [41,42].

Both cross-sectional and longitudinal studies
involving pharmacologic autonomic blockade and
analysis of HRV indicate that increases in cardiac
parasympathetic (vagal) tone make an important contribution to resting bradycardia [41,43]. The chronic
increase in parasympathetic tone occurs within a few
weeks after beginning regular training and this occurs
independently of a lower intrinsic heart rate. In cross-
sectional studies, aerobic fitness and/or long-term

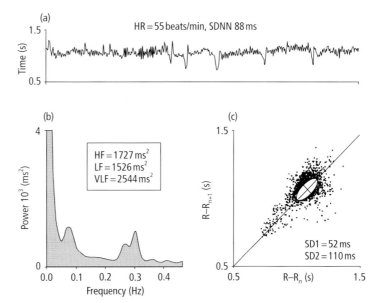

Fig. 1.1.4 Representative examples of R–R interval tachogram (a) and corresponding power spectra (b) and two-dimensional vector analyses of Poincaré plot (c) at rest (30 min recording).

aerobic training have been suggested to be associated with increased HRV, especially with vagally mediated respiratory sinus arrhythmia, at rest [44,45]. Some studies, however, have failed to show such an association [46,47]. The results from most longitudinal studies reveal decreased resting heart rate and increased vagal activity at rest after aerobic training [48,49].

During exercise in the trained, a given increase in cardiac output requires less increase in heart rate due to the maintenance of a larger stroke volume. Studies focusing on autonomic and endocrine responses to training indicate that heart rate is reduced during submaximal exercise (absolute load) in the trained due to a lower intrinsic heart rate, a reduction in sympathetic activity and circulating catecholamines, and a greater parasympathetic influence [41,42,50]. Tulppo and colleagues [50] found that higher levels of physical fitness were associated with an augmentation of cardiac vagal function during exercise, whereas aging resulted in more evident impairment of vagal function at rest. The lower sympathetic activity to the heart at a given submaximal work rate stems in part from diminished reflex signals originating from skeletal muscle due to less metabolite accumulation and attenuated discharge of metaboreceptors [51].

The mechanisms underlying the training-induced increase in vagal tone are thought to be greater activation of the cardiac baroreceptors in response to the enlargement of blood volume and ventricular filling [28,52], as well as changes in opioid [53] and dopaminergic modulation of parasympathetic activity [54]. It is not fully resolved whether a lowering of intrinsic heart rate is a true adaptation to endurance training, but it appears that an intensive and lengthy training period may be necessary for this adaptation [55]. Primates with larger hearts have lower intrinsic heart rates and it has therefore been hypothesized that training-induced cardiac enlargement accounts for the lower intrinsic heart rate with training. A plausible mechanism for reduced intrinsic heart rate is that atrial enlargement reduces the stretch–depolarization stimulus, and thereby alters resting automaticity.

Blood pressure

There is general agreement that endurance training elicits small reductions in resting blood pressure [56,57]. In addition, long-term exercise training has the beneficial effect of preventing the normal age-related increase in blood pressure. A pressure-lowering effect of endurance training has been shown to occur within 6 days after initiating an exercise

program [58]. Reduced adrenal medullary catecholamine output during exercise at a given absolute
work rate may be of importance for the blood pressure
lowering effect of training, as well as changes in sympathetic and renal dopaminergic activity.

The reduction in resting diastolic blood pressure
with training is significantly related to the increase in
exercise capacity, which suggests that high-intensity
training may be important. Attention is currently focused on determining the effectiveness of various
training regimens which induce both reductions in
resting blood pressure and significant improvements
in functional capacity. During exercise at a given submaximal load, blood pressure and vascular resistance
are reduced after endurance training. This adaptation
is associated with reduced sympathetic activation and
lower circulating catecholamines. At high exercise intensities and at maximal exercise, blood pressure is
generally similar before and after training. Yet a given
blood pressure is achieved by a lower vascular resistance and a higher cardiac output in the endurance
trained.

Blood volume

Blood volume (BV) is kept remarkably constant in
many different situations and hyper- and hypovolemia
are corrected fairly rapidly through the mechanism of
renal absorption of sodium. Cross-sectional studies
show that there is a close relationship between $\dot{V}o_{2\,max}$
on the one hand and BV and total amount of hemoglo-
bin (but not the hemoglobin concentration [Hb]) on
the other. Exercise training increases blood volume.
Plasma volume usually increases after a few days of
training, while the expansion of erythrocyte volume
takes longer [59].

The central venous compartment of blood volume
is an important factor for cardiac output. The increased blood volume with physical training is
regarded as a requisite for increased Q_{max}, although it
may be that the blood volume increases in parallel with
the increased $\dot{V}o_{2\,max}$.

Acute plasma volume expansion (using
Macrodex®) increases SV during submaximal and
maximal exercise in well-trained individuals [60,61].
The explanation is that the enhanced BV causes an
enhanced diastolic filling pressure (preload), which
through a direct Frank–Starling mechanism increases

end-diastolic volume. End-systolic volume remains
unchanged or decreases. Consequently SV is increased
[62]. Since peak HR also remains unchanged, Q_{max} is
increased. This increase in the well-trained athletes is
just about enough to compensate for the reduced [Hb]
and arterial oxygen content (C_aO_2), so that the $\dot{V}o_{2\,max}$ is
mainly unchanged compared to control experiments.
However, in untrained or moderately trained individuals a corresponding plasma volume expansion may
increase Q_{max} by a greater amount than that needed to
compensate for the reduction of [Hb] during maximal
exercise and, thus, increase $\dot{V}o_{2\,max}$ [60].

Peripheral vascular adaptations

Regular physical activity results in peripheral vascular
adaptations which enhance perfusion and flow capacity. Thus it has been shown that total leg blood flow
during strenuous exercise increases in parallel with the
rise in maximal aerobic power. In addition, the muscle
arteriovenous oxygen difference is significantly
greater after conditioning. Such adaptations may arise
from structural modifications of the vasculature and
alterations in the control of vascular tone [64,65].

The increase in capillary density of the muscle
seems to be the major factor responsible for the rise in
maximal oxygen extraction. Both cross-sectional and
longitudinal studies have shown greater muscle capillary density in trained than in untrained individuals,
and that physical inactivity is associated with reduced
capillary density [64,66,]. Both capillary density and
blood flow seem to increase in proportion with the rise
in maximal aerobic power during long-term physical
conditioning [66,67].

The rise in peak muscle blood flow appears to be
achieved by enhanced endothelium-dependent
dilatation (EDD) in the muscle which increases its
vasodilator capacity in parallel with expanded oxidative capacity. Accordingly, the rise in cardiac output
can occur without any rise in arterial pressure. An enhanced peak hyperemic blood flow appears to be an
early adaptation to regular exercise [68,69]. A near
70% increase in flow-mediated EDD of the brachial
artery after 10 weeks of aerobic and anaerobic training
was shown by Clarkson *et al.* [70]. Furthermore, a high
correlation between maximal aerobic power and
peripheral vasodilator capacity, measured by vascular
conductance, has been demonstrated [71,72]. King-

well *et al.* [73] found a near 30% greater reduction in forearm vascular resistance to an endothelium-dependent stimulus in endurance athletes as compared to sedentary subjects. This reduction was directly related to maximal aerobic power. In endurance-trained older people a significantly greater EDD, as compared with age-matched sedentary subjects, has also been observed [74]. Additionally, Rinder *et al.* [75] found that abnormal EDD discovered in older, otherwise healthy individuals could be improved with long-term endurance training. They also noted a significant and reasonably good correlation between maximal aerobic power and EDD.

The mechanisms behind the enhanced endothelial function associated with physical training may involve exercise-induced increases in shear stress and pulsatile flow. According to Niebaur and Cooke [76] chronic increases in blood flow induced by training may exert their effect on EDD by modulating the expression of endothelial cell nitric oxide synthase (NOS). It has been shown that endothelium-derived nitric oxide (NO) may influence vascular tone in the periods between exercise bouts. In animal studies, reactivity to stimuli which mediate their effects via NO is increased by training in coronary circulation, as mentioned previously in this chapter [36,37]. Human studies have produced evidence for a role of NO in the regulation of muscle blood flow [77,78]. NOS exists in several isoforms. Consequently, endothelial NOS is named eNOS. Another isoform, called neuronal NOS (nNOS), is located in the sarcolemma and cytosol of human skeletal muscle fibers, in apparent association with mitochondria [79]. Frandsen and coworkers [80] have shown that endurance training may increase the amount of eNOS in parallel with an increase in capillaries in human muscle, while the nNOS levels remain unaltered.

Respiratory adaptation

As there are many variables that contribute to the achievement of $\dot{V}o_{2\,max}$, it may be difficult to identify which mechanism is 'limiting'. This applies particularly to respiratory responses, which are generally considered as non-limiting or 'submaximal' during maximal exercise. Ventilation at maximal exercise is not as high as the maximal achievable ventilation (MAV), but MAV (or maximal breathing capacity,

MBC) is usually measured over 15–20 s, and falls progressively by about 30% after 3–4 min. Thus whilst some athletes may achieve an MAV of 200–220 L/min, their sustainable maximal ventilation is 140–150 L/min, a value frequently achieved during maximal exercise. Of course, such values are accompanied by severe dyspnea, and it may be more helpful to understand factors contributing to limiting dyspnea, than to judge whether a 'limiting' ventilation has been reached. Trained individuals experience much less dyspnea than the untrained. Indeed, early in their experience of exercise, athletes may sense that they are able to exercise with much less dyspnea than their struggling peers, leading them to take up their sport in a serious way.

The study and quantitative measurement of the intensity of dyspnea had to wait firstly for the introduction of the field of psychophysics by Stevens [81], and secondly for the development of appropriate psychophysical techniques by Borg and Noble [82]. The application of these techniques has allowed the assessment of the separate contributions of many factors to dyspnea during exercise in health and disease, and provided some answers as to why the sense of effort in breathing is so much less in trained than in untrained individuals.

Studies employing neurophysiologic techniques have suggested that the sense of dyspnea represents the conscious appreciation of the central outgoing command to the respiratory muscles [83]. Thus, consideration of all the factors contributing to the sensation spans the metabolic demands for ventilation; mechanical capacity to meet the demand; adopted patterns of breathing; pulmonary gas exchange efficiency; central control of breathing; respiratory muscle function; and sensory mechanisms by which the effort of breathing is appreciated. Furthermore, all these physiologic links are interdependent and capable of adaptation, apparently with the overall objective of minimizing discomfort and thereby enhancing performance.

Ventilatory demands of exercise

The major demand on ventilation is CO_2 production ($\dot{V}co_2$); although this is closely related to metabolic oxygen consumption and pulmonary intake, many studies have dissociated the two and shown close corre-

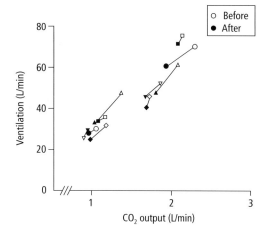

Fig. 1.1.5 Reductions in ventilation at two power outputs in five subjects, before and after training; reductions in VE are closely related to reductions in $\dot{V}CO_2$ (there was no change in $\dot{V}O_2$ at either power output) [86]. Open and filled symbols denote before and after training, respectively.

lation between $\dot{V}CO_2$ and ventilation (VE). At a given power or ATP turnover, $\dot{V}CO_2$ is quantitatively related to the balance between fat and carbohydrate as fuels, and the amount of lactate accumulating in the blood; increases in fat oxidation [84] and reductions in lactate accumulation [85,86] may account for as much as a halving of VE at a given power in trained as against untrained subjects. Higher activities of fat metabolizing enzymes [87], greater mitochondrial surface area [88] and more efficient oxygen delivery mechanisms [89] all contribute to the metabolic changes.

Training-related reductions in VE closely parallel reductions in both $\dot{V}CO_2$ (Fig. 1.1.5) and plasma lactate concentrations [85,86,90]. Thus, at a given power output, an increase of 25% in fat utilization will reduce ventilation by approximately 7%, and a reduction in plasma lactate concentration of 5 mmol/L will be accompanied by a further, up to 30%, reduction. In some athletes changes may be much larger; moreover, when accompanied by the other changes described below, such small effects are magnified, so that ventilation in some athletes may be half that observed in untrained subjects exercising at comparable power [91].

Ventilatory capacity

In terms of dimensions, the maximal breathing capacity is a function of the total lung volume and the maxi-

mal flow rates in inspiration and expiration; volume is related to thoracic volume, and flow rates to airway cross-sectional area. For a given stature and weight both volume and maximal flow tend to be larger in athletes, but studies in twins suggest that this has a genetic basis, and that training has little influence [92]. Within these constraints, athletes employ a larger volume, by being able to achieve both a smaller end-expiratory and larger end-inspiratory volume. They also employ larger flow rates in both inspiration and expiration; indeed some athletes are capable of using virtually all their maximal flow-volume loop during exercise [93,94]. It seems likely that this is because of stronger and more fatigue-resistant respiratory muscles (see below). In older subjects there is a loss of elastic recoil; this reduces flow at low lung volumes and prevents them from achieving a reduction in end-expiratory volume, and contributes to an increase in respiratory effort in older athletes [95].

Pulmonary gas exchange

Pulmonary gas exchange efficiency is broadly related to ventilation–perfusion (V/Q) matching in the lungs, and to diffusion across the alveolar capillary membrane. In general, in healthy subjects larger lungs imply greater alveolar volume and surface area and larger pulmonary capillary volume. The range of V/Q ratios extends from zero (representing anatomic pathways between the right and left sides of the heart, or 'shunt') to infinity (representing anatomic airway dead space); areas in the lungs with a low V/Q ratio contribute to the alveolar–arterial Po_2 difference (A–a Do_2), and those with high V/Q to physiologic dead space (V_D/V_T). Both A–a Do_2 and V_D/V_T are minimized by increases in tidal volume. However, healthy untrained subjects as well as athletes appear to reach similar minimal values for both, and at higher levels of $\dot{V}O_2$ there is no further reduction [94,96].

This phenomenon has been carefully studied, especially for A–a Do_2; in some athletes very wide A–a Do_2 have been observed, leading to arterial Po_2 values as low as 65 mmHg (Fig. 1.1.6) [96].

When associated with a 'rightward shift' of the oxygen dissociation curve due to low arterial pH, such low P_aO_2 values translate into arterial O_2 saturations of 85% or less. The cause of this 'arterial desaturation' and 'failure of gas exchange' has been debated, but

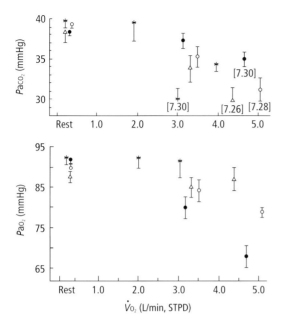

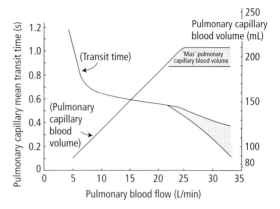

Fig. 1.1.7 Increasing exercise is associated with progressive increases in pulmonary blood flow; pulmonary capillary blood volume increases to a maximum of 200 mL. Capillary mean transit time falls, and at maximum exercise approaches values as short as 0.1 s. From Dempsey [97].

Fig. 1.1.6 Arterial blood gases and pH at rest and during submaximal and maximal treadmill exercise in a group of untrained [*] and three groups of trained subjects. One group of trained subjects (l) showed a significant fall in arterial P_{O_2}, associated with higher P_{CO_2} at maximal exercise. From Dempsey [97].

remains unresolved [97]. There is no doubt that it occurs especially in elite athletes exercising at high $\dot{V}_{O_2}$, leading to theories that include relatively high venous P_{CO_2}, low venous O_2 contents and very short pulmonary capillary transit times (Fig. 1.1.7) contributing to incomplete O_2 diffusion. Interstitial pulmonary edema occurs in animal models of exercise but has never been shown in humans.

Other possible factors include incomplete equilibration for CO_2 in blood traversing the lung [98] combined with low blood pH, leading to incomplete oxygenation of hemoglobin. The limiting process in CO_2 equilibration appears to be the erythrocyte chloride exchanger which has a half-equilibration time that is in excess of pulmonary capillary transit time in heavy exercise [98,99].

Pattern of breathing

Athletes breathe more slowly and deeply than non-athletes, and a slower breathing rate is one of the effects of training. The volumes and flows determine the tidal volume and frequency of breathing during exercise; all other matters being equal, larger tidal volumes and slower frequencies lead to greater efficiency in breathing with lower values for the V_D/V_T ratio. Some subjects entrain breathing frequency with their pedaling or running cadence [100], but there is scope for wide variation in such responses (4 strides/breath vs. 3 strides/breath, for example), so that the entrainment never dominates the pattern. Although the use of a given pattern of breathing is often assumed to be a self-optimizing response to minimize the oxygen cost of breathing, it seems more likely that patterns are adopted consciously or unconsciously to minimize the sense of effort in breathing [101].

Control of breathing

Whilst the mechanisms responsible for the control of breathing during exercise remain a topic of continuing research [102] beyond the scope of the present chapter, there is general agreement that increases in ventilation are a closely related function of the body's CO_2 production.

Many have studied the ventilatory responses to increases in arterial P_{CO_2} (VE/P_{CO_2}), in athletes and untrained subjects. The findings may be summarized as follows.

1 There is a wide range in both VE/P_{CO_2} (1.0–8.0 L/mmHg) and VE/V_{CO_2}(15–50 L/L) in trained and untrained individuals [103,104].
2 There is a relationship between the two indices: low responders to P_{CO_2} have a low response to exercise [105].
3 There is a strong genetic component determining VE/P_{CO_2} [106].
4 Training does not seem to change either VE/V_{CO_2} or VE/P_{CO_2} [86,103].

One might interpret these findings as indicating no influence of ventilatory control on performance. However, the effect of the variations in VE/V_{CO_2} is substantial, even when associated with the normal range of variation in arterial P_{CO_2}. At an exercise power accompanied by a V_{CO_2} of 2.0 L/min, ventilation may range from 35 to 90 L/min in normal subjects [107], with a corresponding variation in breathing effort. A child taking up competitive swimming is presumably more likely to persist if she experiences little breathlessness compared to her panting friends.

The ventilatory responses to hypoxia and P_{CO_2} are closely correlated [108]; this fact may contribute to the lack of response to a falling P_{O_2}, but also may be important in athletes at high altitude. A low ventilatory responsiveness might be seen to predispose to dangerous hypoxia; however, what has emerged from studies simulating the ascent of Mount Everest is that low responders are more likely to reach the summit and are less likely to suffer the deleterious cerebral and pulmonary effects of altitude [109]; these effects appear to be mediated by reductions in arterial P_{CO_2} and associated alkalosis. In athletes who because of their sport have to breath hold for long periods of time, such as synchronized swimmers, the ventilatory response to hypoxia is blunted and breath hold times prolonged [110].

The respiratory muscles

As first systematically studied by Ringqvist [111], the respiratory muscles show considerable variation in strength and endurance, in relation to stature, age and sex, with fairly obvious implications for the capacity to achieve and maintain ventilation during exercise [112], and also for the sense of effort experienced in breathing. Subjects with stronger respiratory muscles achieve higher tidal volumes (and thus lower breathing

frequencies), and experience less dyspnea than those with weaker muscles [113].

The actions of the respiratory muscles differ; expiratory flow is mainly dependent on the elastic recoil of the respiratory system with only a minor contribution from expiratory muscle contraction until very high expiratory flows are recruited. Expiratory muscle contraction mainly acts to reduce end-expiratory lung volume and thus recruit the inspiratory recoil of the thorax and increase the precontraction length of the inspiratory muscles; in this way, they tend to 'unload' the inspiratory muscles [114]. The latter have to generate inspiratory flow against the lung recoil pressure, and thus carry the major responsibility for ventilatory work. Inspiratory muscle training mainly accompanies other aspects of endurance training, but resistive training is known to improve inspiratory muscle strength and endurance [115]. These considerations have important implications in aging athletes in whom there is the normal decline in lung elasticity; end-expiratory lung volume cannot be reduced to the same extent as in the young, forcing the inspiratory muscle to carry a greater proportion of the respiratory work during exercise [116]. Johnson *et al.* [95] found that reductions in elastic recoil and increases in end-expiratory volume paralleled reductions in $\dot{V}_{O_2 max}$ in a group of older (69 ± 1 years) people; such subjects are likely to have been limited by dyspnea.

Sensation of dyspnea

Respiratory muscle oxygen consumption was once thought to increase disproportionately at high levels of ventilation, and thus contribute to a limitation of maximal oxygen intake, but more recent estimates suggest that patterns of breathing are adopted mainly to minimize dyspnea [101].

Because exercise is a voluntary activity, conscious humans stop exercise when the sensation of excessive effort and weakness in exercising muscle or of dyspnea becomes intolerable. A number of sensations related to breathing can be discriminated and scaled [102], including inspiratory muscle tension and displacement, a sense of 'satiety' or appropriateness related to increases in arterial P_{CO_2} [102,117], and a sense of effort related mainly to central outgoing command [118] (Fig. 1.1.8).

Both effort and dyspnea are less in trained compared

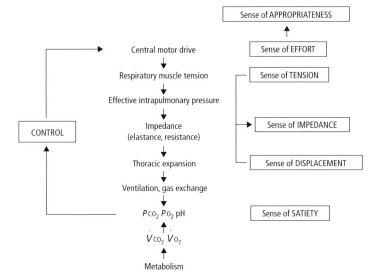

Fig. 1.1.8 Mechanisms contributing to sensations related to breathing during exercise. Whilst the changes in tension developed and displacement of inspiratory muscles can be discriminated and scaled, contributors to the sense of effort include difficulty in breathing (sense of impedance), sufficiency of the ventilatory response ('satiety'), and the outgoing central motor command [102].

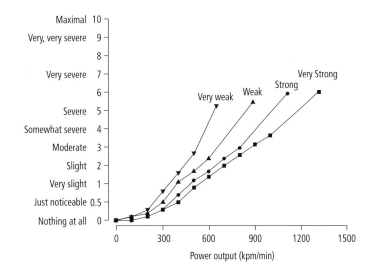

Fig. 1.1.9 Sense of dyspnea during exercise in healthy subjects, grouped according to strength of inspiratory muscles (measured as maximal inspiratory pressure, MIP), into four groups: very weak, MIP < 80% predicted; weak, 80–100%; strong, 100–120%; very strong, > 120%. From Hamilton *et al.* [113].

to untrained individuals, enabling them to maintain higher power for longer. The factors accounting for these differences are numerous and interactive. For dyspnea the reasons are mainly that the pressure generated by the respiratory muscles is relatively less in subjects with large lungs (due to lower elastance and resistance), and strong respiratory muscles (Fig. 1.1.9).

Dyspnea is minimized in trained individuals chiefly through:

1 minimizing V_{CO_2}, through utilization of fat and reduction in lactate production;
2 maximizing P_{CO_2}, through lower VE/V_{CO_2};
3 reducing V_D/V_T, by increasing V_T, a function of lung volume; and
4 increasing inspiratory muscle strength.

At an oxygen consumption of $2\,L/min$, the first three factors could theoretically account for a difference in ventilation from $90\,L/min$ in an unfit individual to $36\,L/min$ in an elite endurance runner. As the sustained ventilatory capacity might be as low as 100 L/min in the former, and as high as 160 L/min in the latter, the percentage of breathing capacity being used might be as high as 90% in the untrained and as low as 25% in the athlete. The associated intensity of dyspnea may thus differ by as much as five-fold [113]. This example also emphasizes that there is great potential for a reduction in the sense of dyspnea by training, with important implications for elite performers, particularly in distance events.

Maximal aerobic power

In elite athletes from endurance sports values for maximal aerobic power ($\dot{V}o_{2\,max}$) of >6.5 L/min or >90 mL/min/kg body weight are frequently obtained. These extremely high values are primarily due to a large maximal cardiac output (Q_{max}). Values of more than 40 L/min have been measured [8]. Since the arteriovenous oxygen difference (a-v$o_{2\,diff}$) during maximal exercise in these well-trained athletes does not differ from that in less trained individuals but is somewhat larger than in untrained individuals, the main cause for the high Q_{max} and, thus, $\dot{V}o_{2\,max}$ in the well-trained athlete is the large stroke volume (SV); values exceeding 200 mL during maximal exercise are reported [8].

In well-trained athletes the hemoglobin concentration [Hb] at rest and during exercise is not different from that obtained in untrained individuals of the same sex and age [8]. Although regular physical training can reduce the oxygen content of the mixed venous blood during maximal exercise in previous untrained individuals [119], the [Hb] obviously sets the upper limits of the a-v$o_{2\,diff}$ during maximal exercise. Therefore, any changes in [Hb] during exercise will have a direct influence on $\dot{V}o_{2\,peak}$, $\dot{V}o_{2\,max}$ and physical performance.

Oxygen transport and utilization includes a series of steps. In the following discussion the different steps of the oxygen cascade from lungs to mitochondria are considered in relation to the basic question: 'What limits $\dot{V}o_{2\,max}$?'

During maximal exercise pulmonary ventilation ($\dot{V}_e$) in untrained or moderately trained individuals reaches 120–150 L/min. Athletes from endurance events with high $\dot{V}o_{2\,max}$ can reach a maximal $\dot{V}_e$ of 200 L/min and over. In maximal voluntary ventilation

tests at rest (MVV_{40}), when the individual is breathing as much as possible with a fixed breathing frequency (40 breaths/min) for 15–20 s, the untrained individual may be able to ventilate 150–180 and athletes up to 220–240 L/min. These volumes far exceed what is used during a maximal exercise test, although they can hardly be maintained for any longer period of time. In addition, most individuals are able to voluntarily increase pulmonary ventilation during a maximal running or cycling test above what is obtained in the test. Furthermore, specific training of the respiratory muscles does not increase either $\dot{V}o_{2\,max}$ or arterial oxygen saturation (S_ao_2) during maximal exercise above pretraining values [120].

The oxygen diffusion capacity of the lung ($D_{L}o_2$) depends on many different factors. If $D_{L}o_2$ limits $\dot{V}o_{2\,max}$ then arterial oxygen pressure (P_ao_2) and S_ao_2 during maximal exercise will fall, unless alveolar ventilation is increased (to increase P_ao_2). However, during heavy exercise both P_ao_2 and S_ao_2 are mainly maintained unchanged or only slightly reduced compared to rest or submaximal exercise in both elite athletes and untrained individuals [8,97]. It should be noted that a certain arterial hypoxemia (desaturation) compared to rest has been observed in some well-trained athletes [121,122]. Whether this is due to hypoventilation, exercise-developed pulmonary edema, insufficient pulmonary capillary transit time, increased blood flow in arterial–venous anastomosis during heavy exercise or other factors is not known [123].

Another important point in this discussion is related to effects of changes in [Hb] during heavy exercise. If $D_{L}o_2$ and/or V_e limit $\dot{V}o_{2\,max}$, then an increase in [Hb] would have no or very little effect. However, both an acute increase of [Hb] through 'blood doping' [62,124] and a more 'chronic' increase of [Hb] through administration of erythropoietin [63] do increase $\dot{V}o_{2\,max}$. This speaks against a functional limitation of $\dot{V}o_{2\,max}$ at the pulmonary level.

Arguments have been put forward that factors related to the peripheral blood circulation (such as capillary density), oxygen utilization in the muscle cells (such as mitochondrial mass and enzyme concentrations) and other factors might limit $\dot{V}o_{2\,max}$. This is certainly true during heavy exercise carried out with small muscle groups, such as isolated dynamic arm work. In this situation the 'peripheral factors' are of utmost importance for, and certainly do limit, the aerobic energy turnover, performance and endurance [125]. However, during exercise with large muscle groups, such as running uphill and combined arm and leg exercise, there are several reasons supporting the idea that the 'periphery' does not limit $\dot{V}_{O_{2\,max}}$.

1 When a maximal rate of work performed by the legs only is divided into a combination of arm and leg work, neither $\dot{V}_{O_{2\,max}}$ [126,127] nor Q_{max} and arterial blood pressure [128] are different from those obtained when using legs only. However, time to exhaustion is much longer when working with arms and legs compared to maximal leg work. For instance, there might be an increase in time to exhaustion from 3 to 6 min. This means that during the combined arm and leg work, when the 'double product' (HR · BP) is the same as during the work with legs only, the heart has been working for 3 min beyond the point when the individual would have had to stop the work with legs only. Thus, the endurance capacity of the heart when working with legs only does not limit cardiac performance as has been suggested [129].

2 When comparing trained and untrained individuals there is no relation between $\dot{V}_{O_{2\,max}}$ and different markers of the peripheral energy turnover such as enzyme activity [130,131]. Furthermore, endurance training may increase and inactivity reduces mitochondria enzyme concentrations considerably without any or only minor changes in $\dot{V}_{O_{2\,max}}$ [132,133].

3 If 'central' (central circulation) and 'peripheral' factors (muscle enzyme concentration and mitochondrial volume) are matched, then aerobic energy turnover for a small muscle group would be of the same order of magnitude as that obtained at $\dot{V}_{O_{2\,max}}$ at the pulmonary level. Measurements of the a-v $_{O_{2\,diff}}$ and blood flow over a well-defined muscle group (musculus quadriceps femoris) during maximal exercise and consequent calculations of the maximal aerobic energy turnover for this muscle group show that estimated $\dot{V}_{O_{2\,peak}}$ per kilo muscle mass far exceeds that of the pulmonary $\dot{V}_{O_{2\,max}}$ per kg muscle mass when working with large muscle groups [134,135]. Thus, the local muscle capacity for aerobic energy turnover exceeds that which can be maximally obtained as $\dot{V}_{O_{2\,max}}$ during heavy exercise using large muscle groups.

4 Changes in $C_{a}O_2$ and arterial oxygen availability will ultimately cause corresponding changes in $\dot{V}_{O_{2\,max}}$ and muscle performance. Reductions of $C_{a}O_2$ through carbon monoxide loading, venesections or hypobaric hypoxia reduce $\dot{V}_{O_{2\,max}}$; this, however, could be due to both central and peripheral limiting factors. But, as previously mentioned, both an 'acute' [62,124] and more 'chronic' [63] increase in $C_{a}O_2$ will increase $\dot{V}_{O_{2\,max}}$ and physical performance more or less in proportion to the induced changes in $C_{a}O_2$.

It seems obvious from these data that the central circulation—mainly the heart function including the blood (BV and [Hb])—have important roles for both limiting and establishing high values of $\dot{V}_{O_{2\,max}}$. Consequently, the next question is: 'What limits the functional capacity of the heart?'.

Since HR_{max} and $C_{a}O_2$ do not increase with physical training, the only structural factor that can explain individual differences in $\dot{V}_{O_{2\,max}}$ is the stroke volume (SV). There is a small increase in SV during transition from rest to light submaximal exercise. SV is well maintained or even increased [9] during maximal exercise, indicating that the oxygen supply to the heart is adequate. The main cause for the increased SV during exercise is an enlarged end-diastolic volume (EDV) caused by augmented venous 'filling' pressure. As mentioned earlier in this chapter, this has been shown in experiments using plasma expanders during exercise. Such plasma expansion increases EDV, and thereby SV and Q_{max} as compared with peak values obtained before plasma expansion [60,61]. Although the plasma expansion reduces [Hb], normal peak O_2 uptake can still be obtained due to the increased SV and Q_{max} [60].

Hammond *et al.* [136] tested the hypothesis that the pericardium restricts heart size and thus limits SV and Q_{max}. They studied exercising pigs before and after pericardiectomy. During maximal treadmill running Q_{max} increased by 29% and $\dot{V}_{O_{2\,max}}$ by 31% due to an estimated 33% increase in EDV. This suggests that the EDV, restricted by the pericardium, sets the upper limit for SV during exercise and thus limits Q_{max}.

With advanced age $\dot{V}_{O_{2\,max}}$ declines due to both reduced Q_{max} and some reduction in a-v $_{O_{2\,diff}}$. The reason for the former is a reduced peak HR, SV being mainly unchanged. Regarding the a-v $_{O_{2\,diff}}$, there is an increase in oxygen content of mixed venous blood in the elderly, probably due to an inability to shunt blood to active muscles [137], thus reducing a-v $O_{2\,diff}$. The effect of regular physical training in the elderly is essentially the same as in young persons; however, the magnitude is generally smaller.

In conclusion, during exercise engaging large muscle groups (running uphill, simultaneous arm and leg work) the $\dot{V}O_{2\,max}$ is limited by the central circulation. Since HR_{max} and C_aO_2 are practically unchanged by physical training, the $\dot{V}O_{2\,max}$ is basically limited by SV. Thus, the principal variant for improvements in $\dot{V}O_{2\,max}$ is maximal cardiac output.

Summary

The pumping capacity of the heart is a critical determinant of endurance performance. The increased maximal cardiac output following endurance training results from a larger cardiac stroke volume, whereas maximal heart rate is unchanged or even slightly reduced. The higher stroke volume is due to enlargement of cardiac chamber size and to expansion of total blood volume. Plasma volume increases usually after a few days of training while the expansion of erythrocyte volume takes a longer time.

Functional improvements in cardiac performance include a more rapid early and peak ventricular filling rate during diastole. The enlarged blood volume, together with greater ventricular compliance and distensibility, and a faster and more complete ventricular relaxation allow stroke volume to increase even at high heart rates. At the same time, the cardiac output is distributed more selectively to activated regions of skeletal muscle, from where the muscle pump facilitates venous return. Endurance training elicits small reductions in resting blood pressure. It remains unresolved whether endurance training increases coronary vascular dimensions beyond the vascular proliferation that accompanies normal training-induced cardiac hypertrophy.

Endurance training results in peripheral vascular adaptations, which enhance perfusion and flow capacity in parallel with rise in maximal aerobic power. These adaptations are caused by an increase in capillary density, and alterations in the control of vascular tone. The rise in peak muscle blood flow appears to be achieved by enhanced endothelium-dependent dilatation in parallel with expanded oxidative capacity. Endothelium-derived nitric oxide (NO), synthesized by nitric oxide synthase (NOS), may contribute to this adaptation.

Training-related reductions in ventilation closely parallel reductions in both $\dot{V}CO_2$ and plasma lactate concentrations. Although largely genetically determined, a larger volume is exploited by athletes as they are able to achieve a smaller end-expiratory and larger end-inspiratory volume, mainly due to stronger and more fatigue-resistant respiratory muscles. Resistive training improves inspiratory muscle strength and endurance. Subjects with stronger respiratory muscles achieve higher tidal volumes (and thus lower breathing frequencies), and experience less dyspnea than those with weaker muscles, thus enabling them to maintain higher power for longer.

The central circulation—mainly the heart function, including the blood volume and hemoglobin concentration—plays an important role in both limiting and establishing high values of maximal aerobic power. During exercise engaging large muscle groups (running uphill, simultaneous arm and leg work) the maximal aerobic power is limited by the central circulation. Since maximal heart rate and arterial oxygen content are practically unchanged by physical training, the maximal aerobic power is basically limited by the stroke volume. Thus, the principal variant for improvements in maximal aerobic power is maximal cardiac output.

Multiple choice questions

1 *Which of the following parameters does not increase appreciably as a response to endurance training:*
a maximal cardiac output
b left ventricular end-diastolic volume
c diastolic filling rate
d left ventricular end-systolic volume
e stroke volume
f maximal heart rate.

2 *What is the relationship between cardiac output (CO), total peripheral resistance (TPR) and arterial pressure (BP):*
a CO=BP/TPR
b BP=TPR/CO
c CO=BP·TPR
d TPR=CO/BP
e BP=CO·TPR
f TPR=BP/CO.

3 *Differences in athletic performance amongst athletes with similar* $\dot{V}o_{2\,max}$ *are linked to:*

a pulmonary gas exchange

b hemoglobin concentration

c total blood volume

d diastolic filling pressure (preload)

e work economy

f heart rate variability.

4 *Physical training results in peripheral vascular adaptations which improve perfusion and blood flow capacity. Such adaptations may arise from:*

a increased capillary density

b decreased resting heart rate

c increased mitochondrial mass

d enhanced endothelium–dependent dilatation

e changes in endothelium–derived nitric oxide concentration

f decreased neuronal nitric oxide synthase.

5 *The sensation of dyspnea is minimized in trained individuals through:*

a shift of the oxygen dissociation curve to the right

b decreased anatomic dead space

c minimization of $\dot{V}co_2$, through utilization of fat and reduction in lactate production

d increased vital capacity

e maximizing Pco_2, through lower $\dot{V}E/\dot{V}co_2$

f increased pulmonary capillary transit time.

References

1 Hill AV, Long CNH, Lupton H. Muscular exercise, lactic acid, and the supply and utilization of oxygen. *Parts VII–VIII Proc Royal Soc London* 1924; **97**: 155–76.

2 Jones JH, Longworth KE, Lindhol A *et al.* Oxygen transport during exercise in large mammals. I. Adaptive variation in oxygen demand. *J Appl Physiol* 1989; **67**: 862–70.

3 Lindhard J. Ueber das minutenvolum des herzens bei ruhe und die muskelarbeit. *Pflüg Arch ges Physiol* 1915; **clxi**: 233–383.

4 Prampero PE. Metabolic and circulatory limitations to $\dot{V}o_{2\,max}$ at the whole animal level. *J Exp Biol* 1985; **115**: 319–32.

5 Hoppeler H, Weibel ER. Structural and functional limits for oxygen supply to muscles. *Acta Physiol Scand* 2000; **168**: 445–56.

6 Rasmussen UF, Rasmussen HN. Human skeletal muscle mitochondrial capacity. *Acta Physiol Scand* 2000; **168**: 473–80.

7 Saltin B. Hemodynamic adaptions to exercise. *Am J Cardiol* 1985; **55**: 42D–47D.

8 Ekblom B, Hermansen L. Cardiac output in athletes. *J Appl Physiol* 1968; **25**: 619–25.

9 Gledhill N, Cox D, Jamnik R. Endurance athletes' stroke volume does not plateau: major advantage is diastolic function. *Med Sci Sports Exerc* 1994; **26**: 1116–21.

10 Saltin B, Blomqvist G, Mitchell JH, Johnson RL Jr, Wildenthal K, Chapmann CB. Response to exercise after bedrest and after training. *Circulation Suppl* 1968; **7**: 1–78.

11 Coyle EF. Physiological determinants of endurance exercise performance. *J Sci Med Sport* 1999; **2**: 181–9.

12 Pelliccia A, Marron BJ, Spataro A *et al.* The upper limit of physiologic cardiac hypertrophy in highly trained elite athletes. *N Engl J Med* 1991; **324**: 295–301.

13 Stolt A, Karjalainen J, Heinonen OJ, Kujala UM. Left ventricular mass, geometry and filling in elite female and male endurance athletes. *Scand J Med Sci Sports* 2000; **10**: 28–32.

14 Huonker M, Schmid A, Sorichter S, Schmidt-Trucksab A, Mrosek P, Keul J. Cardiovascular differences between sedentary and wheelchair-trained subjects with paraplegia. *Med Sci Sports Exerc* 1998; **30**: 609–13.

15 Huston TP, Puffer JC, MacMillan R. The athletic heart syndrome. *N Engl J Med* 1985; **313**: 24–32.

16 Morganroth J, Maron BJ, Henry WL, Epstein SE. Comparative left ventricular dimensions in trained athletes. *Ann Intern Med* 1975; **82**: 521–4.

17 Grossman W, Jones D, McLaurin LP. Wall strength and patterns of hypertrophy of the human left ventricle. *J Clin Invest* 1975; **56**: 56–64.

18 Maron BJ, Pellicia A, Spataro A, Granata M. Reduction in left ventricular wall thickness after deconditioning in highly trained Olympic athletes. *Br Heart J* 1993; **69**: 125–8.

19 Pellicia A, Maron BJ, Culasso F, Spataro A, Caselli G. Athlete's heart in women. Echocardiographic characterization of highly trained elite female athletes. *J Am Med Assoc* 1996; **276**: 211–5.

20 Messerli FH. Pathophysiology of left ventricular hypertrophy. In: Messerli FH, ed. *Left Ventricular Hypertrophy and its Regression*. London: Science Press, 1996: 21–15.

21 Moritz F. Grösse und Form des Herzens bei Meistern in Sport. *Deutsche Archiv für Klinische Medizin* 1934; **176**: 455–66.

22 Palatini P, Maraglino G, Sperti G *et al.* Prevalence and possible mechanisms of ventricular arrhythmias in athletes. *Am Heart J* 1985; **110**: 560–7.

23 Jensen-Urstad K, Bouvier F, Saltin B, Jensen-Urstad M. High prevalence of arrhythmias in elderly male athletes with a lifelong history of regular strenuous exercise. *Heart* 1998; **2**: 161–9.

24 Pavlik G, Bachl N, Wollein W, Lángfy Gy Prokop L. Resting electrocadiographic parameters after cessation of regular endurance training. *Int J Sports Med* 1986; **7**: 226–31.

25 Hardy PS, Maresh CM, Abbott RD. A comparison of myocardial function in former athletes and non-athletes. *Med Sci Sports Exerc* 1976; **8**: 26–30.

26 Bevegard S, Holmgren A, Johnsson B. Circulatory studies in well trained athletes at rest and during heavy exercise with special reference to stroke volume and the influence of body position. *Acta Physiol Scand* 1963; **57**: 26–33.

27 Brandao MUP, Wajngarten M, Rondon E, Giorgi CP, Hironaka F, Negrao CE. Left ventricular function during dynamic exercise in untrained and moderately trained subjects. *J Appl Physiol* 1993; **75**: 1989–95.

28 Levine B. Regulation of central blood volume and cardiac filling in endurance athletes: the Frank–Starling mechanism as a determinant of orthostatic tolerance. *Med Sci Sports Exerc* 1993; **23**: 727–32.

29 Clausen JP, Klausen K, Rasmussen B, Trap-Jensen J. Central and peripheral changes after training of the arms or legs. *Am J Physiol* 1973; **225**: 675–82.

30 Spina RJ, Ogawa T, Martin WH III, Coggan AR, Holloszy J, Ehsani AA. Exercise training prevents decline in stroke volume during exercise in young healthy subjects. *J Appl Physiol* 1992; **72**: 2458–62.

31 Haskell WL, Sims CS, Myll J, Bortz WM, St Goar FG, Alderman EL. Coronary artery size and dilating capacity in ultra-distance runners. *Circulation* 1993; **87**: 1076–82.

32 Bell RD, Rasmussen RL. Exercise and the myocardial capillary–fiber ratio during growth. *Growth* 1974; **38**: 237–44.

33 Barnard RJ, Duncan HW, Baldwin KM, Grimditch G, Buckberg GD. Effects of intensive exercise training on myocardial performance and coronary blood flow. *J Appl Physiol* 1980; **49**: 444–9.

34 Laughlin MH, Overholser KA, Bhatte M. Exercise training increases coronary transport reserve in miniature swine. *J Appl Physiol* 1989; **67**: 1140–9.

35 Heiss HW, Barmeyer J, Wink K *et al.* Studies on the regulation of myocardial blood flow in man. I. Training effects on blood flow and metabolism of the healthy heart at rest and during standardized heavy exercise. *Basic Res Cardiol* 1976; **6**: 658–75.

36 Sessa WC, Pritchard K, Seyedi N, Wang J, Hintze TH. Chronic exercise in dogs increases coronary vascular nitric oxide production and endothelial cell nitric oxide synthase gene expression. *Circulation Res* 1994; **74**: 349–53.

37 Woodman CR, Muller JM, Laughlin MH, Price EM. Induction of nitric oxide synthase mRNA in coronary resistance arteries isolated from exercise-trained pigs. *Am J Physiol* 1997; **273** (*Heart Circulation Physiol*): H2575–9.

38 Victor RG, Seals DR, Mark AL. Differential control of heart rate and sympathetic nerve activity during dynamic exercise. *J Clin Invest* 1987; **79**: 508–16.

39 Tulppo MP, Mäkikallio TH, Takala TES, Seppänen T, Huikuri HV. Quantitative beat-to-beat analysis of heart rate dynamics during exercise. *Am J Physiol* 1996; **271**: H244–52.

40 O'Leary DS, Seamans DP. Effect of exercise on autonomic mechanisms of baroreflex control of heart rate. *J Appl Physiol* 1993; **75**: 2251–7.

41 Ekblom B, Kilbom Å, Soltysiak J. Physical training, bradycardia, and autonomic nervous system. *Scand J Clin Lab Invest* 1973; **32**: 251–6.

42 Lewis SF, Nylander E, Gad P, Areskog NH. Non-autonomic component in bradycardia of endurance-trained men at rest and during exercise. *Acta Physiol Scand* 1980; **109**: 297–305.

43 Dixon EM, Kamath MV, McCartney N, Fallen EL. Neural regulation of heart rate variability in endurance athletes and sedentary controls. *Cardiovascular Res* 1992; **26**: 713–9.

44 Jensen-Urstad K, Saltin B, Ericson M, Storck N, Jensen-Urstad M. Pronounced resting bradycardia in male elite runners is associated with high heart rate variability. *Scand J Med Sci Sports* 1997; **7**: 274–8.

45 Yataco AR, Fleisher LA, Katzel LI. Heart rate variability and cardiovascular fitness in senior athletes. *Am J Cardiol* 1997; **80**: 1389–91.

46 Byrne EA, Fleg JL, Vaitkevicius PV, Wright J, Porges SW. Role of aerobic capacity and body mass index in the age-associated decline in heart rate variability. *J Appl Physiol* 1996; **81**: 743–50.

47 Lazoglu AH, Glace B, Gleim GW, Coplan NL. Exercise and heart rate variability. *Am Heart J* 1996; **131**: 825–7.

48 Levy WC, Cerqueira MD, Harp GD *et al.* Effect of endurance exercise training on heart rate variability at rest in healthy young and older men. *Am J Cardiol* 1998; **82**: 1236–41.

49 Stein PK, Ehsani AA, Domitrovich PP, Kleiger RE, Rottman JN. Effect of exercise training on heart rate variability in older adults. *Am Heart J* 1999; **138**: 567–76.

50 Tulppo MP, Makikallio TH, Seppanen T, Laukkanen RT, Huikuri HV. Vagal modulation of heart rate during exercise: effects of age and physical fitness. *Am J Physiol* 1998; **274**: H424–9.

51 Mostoufi-Moab S, Widmaier EJ, Cornett JA, Gray K, Sinoway LI. Forearm training reduces the exercise pressor reflex during ischemic rhythmic handgrip. *J Appl Physiol* 1998; **84**: 277–83.

52 Convertino VA, Mack GA, Nadel ER. Elevated central venous pressure. a consequence of exercise training-induced hypervolemia. *Am J Physiol* 1991; **29**: R273–7.

53 Angelopoulos TJ, Denys BG, Weikart C, Dasilva SG, Michael TJ, Robertson RJ. Endogenous opioids may modulate catecholamine secretion during high intensity exercise. *Eur J Appl Physiol* 1995; **70**: 195–9.

54 Slavik K, LaPointe DJ. Involvement of inhibitory dopamine-2 receptors in resting bradycardia in exercise-conditioned rats. *J Appl Physiol* 1993; **74**: 2086–91.

55 Bonaduce D, Petretta M, Cavallaro V *et al.* Intensive training and cardiac autonomic control in high level athletes. *Med Sci Sports Exerc* 1998; **30**: 691–6.

56 Fagard RH. The role of exercise in blood pressure control: supportive evidence. *J Hypertension* 1995; **13**:1223–7.

57 Kelley G, Tran ZV. Aerobic exercise and normotensive adults: a meta-analysis. *Med Sci Sports Exerc* 1995; **27**: 1371–7.

58 Meredith IT, Friberg P, Jennings GL *et al.* Time-course of the anti-hypertensive effects of regular endurance exercise in human subjects. *J Hypertension* 1990; **8**: 859–66.

59 Harrison MH. Effect of thermal stress and exercise on blood volume in humans. *Physiol Rev* 1985; **65**: 149–209.

60 Kanstrup I-L, Ekblom B. Acute hypervolemia, cardiac performance and aerobic power during exercise. *J Appl Physiol* 1982; **52**: 1186–91.

61 Krip B, Gledhill N, Jamnik V, Warburton D. Effect of alterations in blood volume on cardiac function during maximal exercise. *Med Sci Sports Exerc* 1997; **29**: 1469–76.

62 Gledhill N. The influence of altered blood volume and oxygen-transport capacity on aerobic performance. *Exerc Sport Sci Rev* 1985; **13**: 75–93.

63 Ekblom B, Berglund B. Effect of erythropoietin administration on maximal aerobic power in man. *Med Sci Sports Exerc* 1991; **1**: 125–30.

64 Ingjer F. Capillary supply and mitochondrial content of different skeletal muscle fiber types in untrained and endurance-trained men. A histochemical and ultrastructural study. *Eur J Appl Physiol* 1979; **40**: 197–209.

65 Kingwell BA, Jennings GL. The role of aerobic training in the regulation of vascular tone. *Nutr Metab Cardiovasc Dis* 1998; **8**: 173–83.

66 Hepple RT. Skeletal muscle: microcirculatory adaptation to metabolic demand. *Med Sci Sports Exerc* 2000; **32**: 117–23.

67 Ingjer F. Maximal aerobic power related to the capillary supply of the quadriceps femoris muscle in man. *Acta Physiol Scand* 1978; **104**: 238–40.

68 Laughlin MH. Endothelium-mediated control of coronary vascular tone after chronic exercise-training. *Med Sci Sports Exerc* 1995; **8**: 1135–44.

69 Sinoway LI, Shenberger J, Wilson J, McLaughlin D, Musch TI, Zelis R. A 30-day forearm work protocol increases maximal forearm blood flow. *J Appl Physiol* 1987; **62**: 1063–7.

70 Clarkson P, Montgomery H, Donald A *et al.* Exercise training enhances endothelial function in young men. *J Am College Cardiol* 1996; **27** (Suppl.): 288A.

71 Martin WH, Kohrt WM, Malley MT, Korte E, Stoltz S. Exercise training enhances leg vasodilatory capacity of 65-year-old men and women. *J Appl Physiol* 1990; **69**: 1804–9.

72 Snell PG, Martin WH, Buckey JC, Blomquist CG. Maximal vascular leg conductance in trained and untrained men. *J Appl Physiol* 1987; **62**: 606–10.

73 Kingwell BA, Tran B, Cameron JD, Jennings GJ, Dart AM. Enhanced vasodilatation to acetylcholine in athletes is associated with lower plasma cholesterol. *Am J Physiol* 1996; **270** (*Heart Circulation Physiol* 39): H2008–13.

74 Rywik TM, Blackman MR, Yataco AR *et al.* Enhanced endothelial vasoreactivity in endurance-trained older men. *J Appl Physiol* 1999; **87**: 2136–42.

75 Rinder MR, Spina RJ, Ehsani AA. Enhanced endothelium-dependent vasodilation in older endurance-trained men. *J Appl Physiol* 2000; **88**: 761–6.

76 Niebaur J, Cooke JP. Cardiovascular effects of exercise role of endothelial shear stress. *J Am College Cardiol* 1996; **28**: 1652–60.

77 Duffy SJ, Tran BT, Harper RW, Meredith IT. Relative contribution of vasodilator prostanoids and NO to metabolic vasodilation in the human forearm. *Am J Physiol* 1999; **276** (*Heart Circulation Physiol*): H663–70.

78 Rådegran G, Saltin B. Nitric oxide in the regulation of vasomotor tone in human skeletal muscle. *Am J Physiol* 1999; **276** (*Heart Circulation Physiol*): H1951–60.

79 Frandsen U, Lopez-Figueroa MO, Hellsten Y. Localization of nitric oxide synthase in human skeletal muscle. *Biochem Biophys Res Comm* 1996; **227**: 88–93.

80 Frandsen U, Höffner L, Betak A, Saltin B, Bangsbo J, Hellsten Y. Endurance training does not alter the level of neuronal nitric oxide synthase in human skeletal muscle. *J Appl Physiol* 2000; **89**: 1033–8.

81 Stevens SS. *Psychophysics. Introduction to its Perceptual, Neural, and Social Prospects.* John Wiley & Sons Inc, New York 1975.

82 Borg GAV, Noble B. Perceived exertion. In: Wilmore JH, ed. *Exercise and Sports Sciences Reviews*, Vol. 2. New York: Academic Press, 1974: 131–53.

83 Gandevia SC. Neural control in human muscle fatigue. changes in muscle afferents, motoneurons and motocortical drive. *Acta Physiol Scand* 1998; **162**: 275–83.

84 Coggan AR, Habash DL, Mendenhall LA, Swanson SC, Kien CL. Isotopic estimation of CO_2 production during exercise before and after endurance training. *J Appl Physiol* 1993; **75**: 70–5.

85 Casaburi R. Mechanisms of the reduced ventilatory requirement as a result of exercise training. *Eur Respiratory Rev* 1995; **5**: 42–6.

86 Taylor R, Jones NL. The reduction by training of CO_2 output during exercise. *Eur J Cardiol* 1979; **9**: 53–62.

87 Gollnick PD, Armstrong RB, Saubert IVCW, Piehl K, Saltin B. Enzyme activity and fiber composition in skeletal muscle of untrained and trained men. *J Appl Physiol* 1972; **33**: 312–9.

88 Hoppeler H, Luthi P, Claassen H, Weibel ER, Howald H. The ultrastructure of the normal human skeletal muscle: a morphometric analysis on untrained men, women and well-trained orienteers. *Pflügers Archiv für des Gesamte Physiologie* 1973; **344**: 217–32.

89 Saltin B, Rowell LB. Functional adaptation to physical activity and inactivity. *Fed Proc* 1980; **39**: 1506–13.

90 Casaburi R, Storer TW, Wasserman K. Mediation of reduced ventilatory response to exercise after endurance training. *J Appl Physiol* 1987; **63**: 1533–8.

91 Edwards RHT, Jones NL, Oppenheimer EA, Hughes RL, Knill-Jones RP. Interrelation of responses during progressive exercise in trained and untrained subjects. *Q J Exp Physiol* 1969; **54**: 394–403.

92 Weber G, Kartodihardjo W, Klissouras V. Growth and physical training with reference to heredity. *J Appl Physiol* 1976; **40**: 211–5.

93 Grimby G, Saltin B, Wilhelmsen L. Pulmonary flow-volume and pressure-volume relationship during submaximal and maximal exercise in young well trained men. *Bull Eur Physiopathol Respiration* 1971; **7**: 157–72.

94 Johnson BD, Saupe KW, Seow KC, Dempsey JA. Mechanical constraints on exercise hyperpnea in athletes. *Am Rev Respiratory Dis* 1990; **141**: A122.

95 Johnson BD, Reddan WG, Seow KC, Dempsey JA. Mechanical constraints on exercise hyperpnea in a fit aging population. *Am Rev Respiratory Dis* 1991; **143**: 968–77.

96 Dempsey JA, Vidruk EH, Mitchell GS. Pulmonary control systems in exercise: update. *Fed Proc* 1985; **44**: 2260–70.

97 Dempsey JA. Is the lung built for exercise ? *Med Sci Sports Exerc* 1986; **18**: 143–55.

98 Jones NL, Heigenhauser GJF. Getting rid of carbon dioxide during exercise. *Clin Sci* 1996; **90**: 323–35.

99 Klocke RA. Velocity of CO_2 exchange in blood. *Annu Rev Physiol* 1988; **50**: 625–37.

100 Bechbache RR, Duffin J. The entrainment of breathing frequency by exercise rhythm. *J Physiol (Lond)* 1977; **272**: 553–61.

101 Casan P, Villafranca CC, Kearon MC, Campbell EJM, Killian KJ. Contribution of respiratory muscle oxygen consumption to breathing limitation and dyspnea. *Can Respiratory J* 1997; **4**: 101–7.

102 Killian KJ, Jones NL, Campbell EJM. Control of breathing during exercise. In: Altose MD, Kawakami Y, eds. *Control of Breathing in Health and Disease*. New York: Marcel Dekker, Inc, 1999: 137–62.

103 Akiyama Y, Kawakami Y. Clinical assessment of the respiratory control system. In: Altose MD, Kawakami Y, eds. *Control of Breathing in Health and Disease*. New York: Marcel Dekker, Inc, 1999: 251–87.

104 Jones NL. Use of exercise in testing respiratory control mechanisms. *Chest* 1976; **70**: 169s–73s.

105 Rebuck AS, Jones NL, Campbell EJM. Ventilatory response to exercise and to CO_2 rebreathing in normal subjects. *Clin Sci* 1972; **43**: 861–7.

106 Saunders NA, Leeder SR, Rebuck AS. Ventilatory response to carbon dioxide in youth athletes: a family study. *Am Rev Respiratory Dis* 1976; **113**: 497–502.

107 Hughes RL, Clode M, Edwards RHT, Goodwin TJ, Jones NL. Effect of inspired O_2 on cardiopulmonary and metabolic responses to exercise in man. *J Appl Physiol* 1968; **24**: 336–47.

108 Rebuck AS, Campbell EJM. A clinical method for assessing the ventilatory response to hypoxia. *Am Rev Respiratory Dis* 1974; **109**: 345–50.

109 Dempsey JA, Schoene RB. Pulmonary system adaptations to high altitude. In: Bone RC, ed. *Pulmonary and Critical Care Medicine.* St Louis: Mosby, 1994: 1–22.

110 Bjurstrom RL, Schoene RB. Control of ventilation in elite synchronized swimmers. *J Appl Physiol* 1987; **63**: 1019–24.

111 Ringqvist T. The ventilatory capacity in healthy subjects. An analysis of the causal factors with special reference to the respiratory forces. *Scand J Clin Lab Invest* (Suppl. 88) 1966; **18**: 1–179.

112 Freedman S. Sustained maximum voluntary ventilation. *Respiratory Physiol* 1970; **8**: 230–44.

113 Hamilton AL, Killian KJ, Summers E, Jones NL. Muscle strength, symptom intensity, and exercise capacity in patients with cardiorespiratory disorders. *Am J Respiratory Crit Care Med* 1995; **152**: 2021–31.

114 Leblanc P, Summers E, Inman MD, Jones NL, Campbell EJM, Killian KJ. Inspiratory muscles during exercise. a problem of supply and demand. *J Appl Physiol* 1988; **64**: 2482–9.

115 Pardy RL, Rivington RN, Despas PJ, Macklem PT. The effects of inspiratory muscle training on exercise performance in chronic airflow limitation. *Am Rev Respiratory Dis* 1981; **123**: 426–33.

116 Johnson BD, Reddan WG, Pegelow DF, Seow KC, Dempsey JA. Flow limitation and regulation of functional residual capacity during exercise in a physically active aging population. *Am Rev Respiratory Dis* 1991; **143**: 960–7.

117 Manning HL, Schwartzstein RM. Dyspnea and the control of breathing. In: Altose MD, Kawakami Y, eds. *Control of Breathing in Health and Disease*. New York: Marcel Dekker, Inc, 1999: 105–35.

118 Gandevia SC, Killian KJ, McKenzie DK, Crawford M, Allen GM, Gorman RB *et al*. Respiratory sensations, cardiovascular control, kinaesthesia and transcranial stimulation during paralysis in humans. *J Physiol (Lond)* 1993; **470**: 85–107.

119 Ekblom B, Åstrand P-O, Saltin B, Stenberg J, Wallström BM. Effect of training on circulatory response to exercise. *J Appl Physiol* 1968; **24**: 518–28.

120 Inbar O, Weiner P, Azgad Y, Rotstein A, Weinstein Y. Specific inspiratory muscle training in well-trained endurance athletes. *Med Sci Sports Exerc* 2000; **32**: 1233–7.

121 Dempsey JA, Wagner PD. Exercise-induced arterial hypoxemia. *J Appl Physiol* 2000; **87**: 1997–2006.

122 Powers SK, Lawler J, Dempsey JA, Dodd S, Landry G. Effects of incomplete pulmonary gas exchange of $\dot{V}_{O_2 max}$. *J Appl Physiol* 1989; **66**: 2491–5.

123 Prefaut C, Durand F, Mucci P, Caillaud C. Exercise-induced arterial hypoxaemia in athletes. *Sports Med* 2000; **30**: 47–61.

124 Celsing F, Svedenhag J, Pihlstedt P, Ekblom B. Effect of anaemia and stepwise-induced polycythaemia on maximal aerobic power in individuals with high and low hemoglobin concentration. *Acta Physiol Scand* 1987; **129**: 47–54.

125 Saltin B, Nazar K, Costill DLE, Stein E, Jansson B, Essén Gollnick PD. The nature of the training response; peripheral and central adaptations to one-legged exercise. *Acta Physiol Scand* 1976; **96**: 289–305.

126 Bergh U, Kanstrup-Jensen I-L, Ekblom B. Maximal oxygen uptake during exercise with various combinations of arm and leg work. *J Appl Physiol* 1976; **41**: 191–6.

127 Åstrand P-O, Saltin B. Maximal oxygen uptake and heart rate in various types of maximal exercise. *J Appl Physiol* 1961; **16**: 977–81.

128 Stenberg J, Åstrand P-O, Ekblom B, Royce J, Saltin B. Hemodynamic response to work with different muscle groups, sitting and supine. *J Appl Physiol* 1967; **22**: 61–70.

129 Noakes TD. Challenging beliefs: ex Africa semper aliquid novi. *Med Sci Sports Exerc* 1997; **29**: 571–90.

130 Hollozy JO. Biochemical adaptations to exercise. Aerobic metabolism. *Exerc Sport Sci Rev* 1973; **1**: 45–71.

131 Saltin B, Henriksson J, Nygaard E, Andersen P. Fiber types and metabolic potentials of skeletal muscle in sedentary men and endurance runners. *Ann New York Acad Sci* 1977; **301**: 3–29.

132 Henriksson J, Reitman JS. Time course of changes in human skeletal muscle succinate dehydrogenase and cytochrome oxidase activities and maximal oxygen uptake with physical activity and inactivity. *Acta Physiol Scand* 1977; **99**: 91–7.

133 Örlander J, Kiessling KH, Ekblom B. Time course of adaptation to low intensity training in sedentary men: dissociation of central and local effects. *Acta Physiol Scand* 1980; **108**: 85–90.

134 Andersen P, Saltin B. Maximal perfusion of skeletal muscles in man. *J Physiol (Lond)* 1985; **366**: 233–49.

135 Rådegran G, Blomstrand E, Saltin B. Peak muscle perfusion and oxygen uptake in humans: importance of precise estimates of muscle mass. *J Appl Physiol* 1999; **87**: 2375–80.

136 Hammond KK, White FC, Bhargava V, Shabetai R. Heart size and maximal cardiac output are limited by the pericardium. *Am J Physiol* 1992; **263**: 1675–81.

137 Gerstenblith G, Lakatta EG, Wiesfelt ML. Age changed in myocardial function and exercise response. *Prog Cardiovascular Dis* 1976; **19**: 1–21.

138 Robinson BF *et al. Circulation Res* 1966; **XIX**: 400–11.

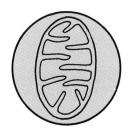

Chapter 1.2
Metabolism during Exercise — Energy Expenditure and Hormonal Changes

JAN HENRIKSSON & KENT SAHLIN

Classical references

Hohwü Christensen E, Hedman R, Holmdahl I. The influence of rest pauses on mechanical efficiency.

Åstrand I, Åstrand P-O, Hohwü Christensen E, Hedman R. Intermittent muscular work.

Åstrand I, Åstrand P-O, Hohwü Christensen E, Hedman R. Myohemoglobin as an oxygen-store in man. *Acta Physiol Scand* 1960; **48**: 443–460.

In this series of three papers, the authors describe the energy expenditure and metabolism resulting from different application of work and rest periods while working on light and heavy workloads. The papers have had a large impact because they were the first, following the initial observations of Karrasch and Müller (*Arbeitsphysiologie* 1951; **14**: 369–382), to attract interest to the physiology and metabolism of intermittent work.

In the first paper, data are given to support the fact that the energy cost per kJ of work is the same or practically the same whether the work is performed continuously for 1 h with an easy load or discontinuously with heavier loads. The results disputed the hypothesis of Müller and coworkers that pauses would significantly increase the oxygen demand for a subsequent work period. In the second paper, the authors showed that an extremely heavy workload, when split into short periods of work and rest, was transformed to a submaximal load on circulation and respiration. To explain the low lactate concentrations after intermittent work (work periods of 10–15 s), the authors proposed two alternative hypotheses: (i) that the rate of formation of lactic acid during a heavy workload is the same, independent of the length of the work period, but that lactic acid during the short periods of rest is eliminated almost at the same rate; and (ii) that the formation of lactic acid during the short work periods is reduced to a minimum because it can take place almost aerobically. From the results in the third paper, the authors dismiss the first hypothesis and conclude that approximately 0.43 L O_2 must have been available in the working muscles at the beginning of each new work period. It is proposed that this amount of oxygen is bound to myohemoglobin (myoglobin) in the muscles and is being 'reloaded' during the pauses to constitute approximately half of the amount of oxygen used during a 10-s work period.

Biochemical pathways of ATP generation

Hydrolysis of ATP is the immediate energy source for almost all energy-requiring processes in the cell:

$$ATP + H_2O \rightarrow ADP + Pi + energy \qquad (1)$$

The store of ATP is limited and must therefore be continuously replenished. Regeneration of ATP occurs through aerobic and anaerobic processes by which energy-rich chemical substances (carbohydrates, fat and phosphocreatine) are transformed into compounds with less stored energy (lactate, H_2O, CO_2 and creatine). This is achieved by sequences of chemical reactions by which part of the change in free energy is used for the synthesis of ATP through a reversal of reaction (1). The ATP–ADP cycle constitutes a basic feature of energy metabolism in all cells and is an intermediate between energy-utilizing and energy-consuming processes.

Skeletal muscle is a unique tissue in terms of the large variation in energy turnover. Transition from rest to exercise involves a drastic increase in energy demand and the rate of ATP utilization can increase more than 100 times. This corresponds to a utilization of the whole muscle store of ATP in about 2–3 s. To maintain a constant muscle ATP concentration, which is necessary for cellular homeostasis, the rate of ATP regeneration must equal the rate of ATP utilization. To meet the energy requirements skeletal muscle is faced with intricate problems related to supply of fuels and oxygen as well as control of the energetic processes. Adjustment of the rate of ATP regeneration to energy requirements is very precise and involves both feed-forward and feedback control mechanisms. A detailed discussion of the control of energy metabolism is outside the scope of this chapter and the reader is referred to other reviews or textbooks.

Aerobic processes of ATP generation

The ultimate process of ATP formation is oxidative phosphorylation during which various substrates are oxidized with oxygen in the mitochondrion. The process is rather complex and will be described only briefly. The fuels for the aerobic processes are mainly pyruvate (derived from carbohydrates) and fatty acids (derived from triglycerides). These fuels are degraded by separate routes to acetyl-CoA within the mitochondrion. The acetyl group of acetyl-CoA is catabolized to CO_2 in the TCA cycle (tricarboxylic acid cycle) by which electrons are transferred from the substrates to coenzymes (mainly NAD^+). The electrons are transferred from the reduced coenzyme (NADH) to the electron transport chain with oxygen being the final electron acceptor. When electrons pass through the electron transport chain their energy level decreases and part of the energy is used to transfer protons through the mitochondrial membrane. When protons diffuse back through the membrane protein (ATP synthase) ADP is phosphorylated to ATP; the whole process is called oxidative phosphorylation. The efficiency of the aerobic processes in terms of oxygen, i.e. the amount of ATP produced per consumed oxygen (P/O_2) is under debate. In textbooks, P/O_2 ratio is often considered to be 6 when carbohydrate (CHO) is oxidized, whereas with free fatty acids (FFA) the P/O_2 ratio is about 10% less. The lower yield of ATP per

oxygen consumed may contribute to the lower power of this process. In this chapter we have used a P/O_2 ratio of 6 to estimate the power and capacity of oxidative phosphorylation. This is probably an overestimate since evidence exists that some of the proton gradient is dissipated by leakage of protons through the inner mitochondrial membrane[1]. The extent of this leakage during exercise is uncertain.

The efficiency in transforming stored chemical energy into work can be calculated from O_2 utilization and performed work. The mechanical efficiency during cycling is about 24% when calculated from the exercise-induced increase in whole-body O_2 uptake and about 34% when calculated from the O_2 uptake by the leg muscles [2]. In contrast, during static contraction the mechanical efficiency is zero, since no external work is performed. Since more than 75% of the released energy is transformed to heat, the maintenance of a constant body temperature is a challenge for whole-body homeostasis during exercise.

Anaerobic processes of ATP generation

Although the aerobic processes dominate during sustained exercise regeneration of ATP can also occur through anaerobic processes. Three different ATP-generating anaerobic processes exist:

Breakdown of PCr: $ADP + PCr + H^+ \rightarrow ATP + creatine$

Glycolysis from glycogen: $3ADP + 3Pi + glucosyl\ unit \rightarrow 3ATP + 2lactate + 2H^+$

ADP fusion: $ADP + ADP \rightarrow ATP + AMP$

Breakdown of PCr

PCr is a high-energy phosphate compound stored in muscle tissue at a concentration three times that of ATP. Creatine kinase (CK) is a highly active enzyme and catalyzes an equilibrium reaction:

$$ADP + PCr + H^+ \leftrightarrow ATP + creatine \qquad (2)$$

During exercise there is an increase in ADP, which by a mass action effect stimulates a shift of the reaction to the right (phosphorylation of ADP to ATP at the expense of PCr). During sustained exercise ADP remains elevated and PCr therefore remains low throughout the exercise period. The degree of PCr depletion at a steady state is related to the exercise intensity. PCr decreases even with low-intensity exercise. At a work rate of 50% of $\dot{V}o_{2max}$ PCr is reduced to 79% of the initial level and at a work rate of 80% of $\dot{V}o_{2max}$ PCr is reduced to 32% of the initial level [3]. During recovery from exercise ADP decreases and the reaction is shifted back to the left. The half-time for PCr resynthesis is about 30 s and after 2–4 min recovery PCr is restored to the initial level. An overshoot in PCr above the pre-exercise level has been observed in fast-twitch muscle fibers after high-intensity exercise [4] and in slow-twitch fibers after prolonged exercise at moderate intensity [5]. The mechanism for this overshoot is not known. The combination of reaction (1) (ATP hydrolysis) and (2) (PCr breakdown) results in increased levels of creatine and P_i. An increase in P_i is considered to interact with the contraction process and is a potential factor in fatigue (see below).

After the original discovery by Harris *et al.*[6] that supplementation with creatine can augment the muscle store of Cr and PCr by about 20% there has been great interest in exploring the role of creatine supplementation as an ergogenic aid. Many but not all studies have shown that creatine increases performance during high-intensity exercise especially when it is performed intermittently, whereas there is no documented effect during prolonged exercise. The mechanism for this ergogenic effect is probably related to an increased availability of high-energy phosphates (augmented store of PCr and increased rate of PCr resynthesis) [7].

Since breakdown of PCr involves uptake of protons the CK reaction has acid–base implications. At the onset of exercise when PCr breakdown is the dominant process an alkalinization of the order of 0.1 pH units has been observed, whereas during sustained high-intensity exercise the CK reaction is an important buffer process by which the acidosis incurred by lactate accumulation is counteracted. It has been estimated that the CK reaction accounts for about 40% of the total intracellular buffer capacity [8].

Lactate formation

During glycolysis muscle glycogen or blood-borne glucose are partially degraded to pyruvate or lactate in about 10 well-defined enzymatic steps. Glycolysis from glycogen results in a higher yield of ATP (3 moles of ATP per mole of glucosyl unit) than glycolysis from glucose (2 moles ATP per mole glucose). Glycolysis to pyruvate precedes the aerobic combustion of CHO in the mitochondrion and is therefore named aerobic glycolysis. Pyruvate can be transferred to lactate, which is a dead-end metabolite. Glycolysis to lactate is named anaerobic glycolysis, since the process does not require oxygen. However, formation of lactate may also occur in the presence of oxygen. The mechanism of lactate formation during submaximal exercise has been extensively discussed over a number of years and remains a controversial issue. However, it is accepted that lactate is formed by a mass action effect through the near-equilibrium reaction catalyzed by lactate dehydrogenase (LDH) and that increases in pyruvate, NADH/NAD$^+$ ratio or H$^+$ are metabolic changes in the cytosol that will promote lactate formation. Activation of glycolysis in excess of pyruvate oxidation and NADH influx to mitochondria will cause cytosolic increases in pyruvate and NADH and will therefore also lead to lactate formation. Factors such as oxygen deficiency, increased recruitment of fast-twitch fibers and low aerobic training status of the muscle (i.e. low mitochondrial and capillary density) are likely to be of importance for this imbalance.

Lactate formation is associated with release of protons and when lactate accumulates the tissue becomes acidotic. Since acidosis may interfere with both the energetic processes and the contraction process lactate formation has become a major interest in exercise physiology.

ADP fusion

The adenine nucleotides (AN) are related to each other through an equilibrium reaction catalyzed by adenylate kinase.

$$ADP + ADP \leftrightarrow ATP + AMP \qquad (3)$$

During conditions of energetic deficiency muscle ADP concentration increases and reaction (3) is shifted to the right. The AN pool can be degraded further through irreversible deamination of AMP to inosine monophosphate (IMP) and ammonia (NH$_3$).

$$AMP \rightarrow IMP + NH_3 \qquad (4)$$

Deamination of AMP enables a further shift of reaction (3) to the right. The combined effect of ATP hydrolysis, ADP fusion and AMP deamination will lead to a net decrease in the AN pool corresponding to an

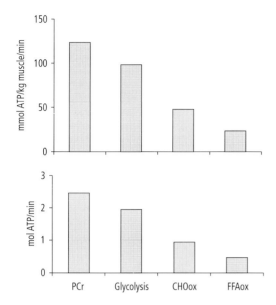

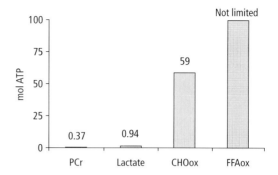

Fig. 1.2.2 Capacity of the energy-yielding processes in human skeletal muscle. Capacity values have been derived from the following assumptions: the whole store of muscle PCr (20 mmol/kg w.wt) is utilized; maximal muscle lactate formation during exercise at 100% $\dot{V}_{O_2\,max}$ is 30 mmol/kg w.wt including efflux to blood of 17%; muscle glycogen content of 80 mmol/kg w.wt; a working muscle of 20 kg. Amount of ATP that can be produced from oxidation of FFA is not limited; hence staple bar is cut off.

Fig. 1.2.1 Power of the energy-yielding processes in human skeletal muscle. Power values are based on reported experimental values in humans under the following conditions: PCr breakdown: 1.3 s electrical stimulation [10]; glycolysis: 10 s cycling [9]; CHO oxidation: calculated from the following assumptions—O_2 utilization by the leg muscles during two-leg cycling is 72% of $\dot{V}_{O_2\,max}$ (5 L/min) [2], working muscle mass 20 kg, 6 mol of ATP per mole of O_2; FFA oxidation: assumed to be 50% of that of CHO oxidation (see text).

energy equivalent of 2 moles of ATP per mole of AN. However, the amount of ATP that can be derived by this process is limited (1–4 mmol ATP/kg muscle or about 1–5% of total anaerobic energy release) and is therefore usually neglected as an energetic process during exercise.

Power and capacity of energetic processes

There are two inherent limits to the energetic processes: the maximum rate (power) and the amount (capacity) of ATP that can be produced. The power and capacity vary drastically between different energetic processes and will also vary between individuals. Peak values of power and capacity in humans, observed in experimental studies, are shown in Figs 1.2.1 and 1.2.2. Factors such as muscle mass, muscle fiber type composition, training status and nutritional factors

will be important determinants of the individual profile of power and capacity.

The limitations of the energetic processes will set an upper limit for energy production and will consequently be a determinant of exercise capacity. The maximal intensity of the exercise is limited by the combined maximal power of the energetic processes. From the data in Fig. 1.2.1 one can calculate that the combined power of PCr breakdown, glycolysis and CHO oxidation is 5.9 mol ATP/min of which anaerobic power contributes 75% or 4.4 mol ATP/min. Estimates of maximal power during a 10-s sprint, using a completely different approach (Fig. 1.2.3), give an ATP turnover of 3.4 mol/min. The difference is expected since the maximal power of oxidative phosphorylation can only be reached after some minutes of delay. Estimated maximal power of energetic processes is very similar to anaerobic energy utilization observed during 10 s of sprint cycling (3.30 mol/min; recalculated by assuming 20 kg of active muscles) [9].

The duration of exercise is limited by the capacity of the recruited energetic processes. For instance with the data shown in Fig. 1.2.2 oxidative combustion of the whole store of muscle glycogen would result in a total gain of 59 moles of ATP. During exercise at 100%

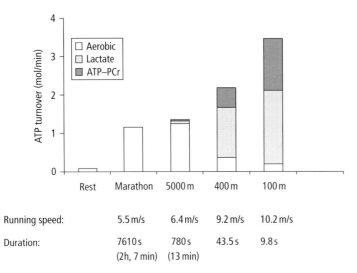

Running speed: 5.5 m/s   6.4 m/s   9.2 m/s   10.2 m/s

Duration: 7610 s   780 s   43.5 s   9.8 s
                      (2h, 7 min) (13 min)

Fig. 1.2.3 ATP turnover at rest and during maximal running of different distances. ATP turnover over 5000 m has been estimated from an assumed $\dot{V}_{O_{2\,max}}$ of 5 L/min and 6 mol of ATP per O_2. ATP turnover over other distances has been estimated from the speed of running (assuming that mechanical efficiency remains constant) and the energy required to accelerate to this speed (assumed efficiency of 25%). Relative recruitment of aerobic processes is from Newsholme *et al.* [73]. Relative contributions of ATP-PCr and lactate to energy turnover: 100-m values are from 10 s cycling [9]; 400 and 5000 m anaerobic ATP formation has been assumed to be limited by the capacity shown in Fig. 1.2.2.

$\dot{V}_{O_{2\,max}}$ (5 L/min), maximal rate of CHO oxidation is 0.96 mol ATP/min (Fig. 1.2.1). Assuming that the whole energy demand is covered solely by oxidation of CHO the duration of exercise would be 61 min (59/0.96). However, exercise at 100% $\dot{V}_{O_{2\,max}}$ is not limited by muscle glycogen level but by other factors such as accumulation of lactic acid and hence exercise is terminated after 5–10 min, long before muscle glycogen depletion. Experiments in humans have shown that exercise at 75% of $\dot{V}_{O_{2\,max}}$ results in glycogen depletion after about 60–90 min, coinciding with muscle fatigue, and is in a reasonable agreement with the estimates in Figs 1.2.1 and 1.2.2.

Breakdown of PCr

Breakdown of PCr is the energy source that can sustain the highest rate of ATP production. The maximum rate of PCr breakdown presented in Fig. 1.2.1 (120 mmol ATP/kg muscle/min) was observed during short-term (1.3 s) electrical stimulation of the quadriceps femoris muscle during isometric conditions [10]. The maximum value is close to V_{max} of myosin ATPase activity measured *in vitro*. It is therefore possible that power during the first few seconds of exercise is limited by the ability to utilize ATP rather than by the rate of ATP regeneration.

The amount of energy that can be produced from PCr is limited by the amount of PCr stored. In human skeletal muscle the concentration of PCr is about 20 mmol/kg w.wt with about a 20% higher concentration in fast-twitch fibers than in slow-twitch fibers. With the maximal rate of PCr breakdown shown in Fig. 1.2.1 complete depletion of the PCr store within about 10 s would be expected. However contribution of ATP from other energy sources and decreased energy expenditure (fatigue) will prolong this time. From thermodynamic considerations the maximal rate of PCr breakdown would be expected to decrease when the PCr content of the muscle decreases. Availability of PCr may therefore be a limiting factor of power output even before the muscle content of PCr is totally depleted.

It is well established that due to its high power and rapid recruitment PCr breakdown is an important energy source during high-intensity exercise and at the onset of exercise. However, there is evidence that the CK reaction also has a role in aerobic metabolism. CK is located both in the intermembrane space of the mitochondria (CKmit) and at sites of ATP utilization in the cytosol. During exercise PCr will regenerate ATP at the site of ATP utilization and creatine will diffuse to mitochondria. PCr is then regenerated by CKmit and diffuses back to the sites of ATP utilization. Through the action of this creatine shuttle the concentration of ADP in the vicinity of mitochondria will be high and oxidative phosphorylation will be stimulated. Experiments with permeabilized fibers have shown that creatine is an important activator of mitochondrial respiration in cardiac tissue and slow-twitch fibers of skeletal muscle [11], and recently creatine supplementation was shown to enhance aerobic metabolism during low-intensity exercise in humans [12].

Glycolysis

The maximum power of glycolysis in human muscle (98 mmol ATP/kg muscle/min, Fig. 1.2.1) was obtained from a study of maximal cycling over 10 s [9]. Glycogen is the major source of lactate, since the rate of glycolysis of blood-borne glucose is much slower than that of glycogen. The rate of glucose utilization is limited by muscle glucose uptake and by inhibition of glucose phosphorylation by hexose phosphates. During high-intensity exercise muscle glucose uptake increases but increases in hexose phosphates will limit utilization of glucose, which will accumulate in the working muscle [13]. Intense exercise results in a massive increase in lactate concentration both in muscle tissue and in blood. During cycling to fatigue at 100% of $\dot{V}O_{2\,max}$ muscle lactate increased more than 20-fold (to 26 mmol/kg w. wt) and muscle pH decreased from 7.1 at rest to 6.6 at fatigue [14]. Part of the formed lactate is exported to blood, (about 17% of total lactate production during this type of exercise [15]), resulting in increased lactate and decreased pH in blood.

The main control of glycogenolysis and glycolysis is exerted by glycogen phosphorylase and phosphofructokinase (PFK), respectively. These enzymes catalyze non-equilibrium reactions and exhibit a complex and diverse mode of control [16]. The V_{max} of glycogen phosphorylase and PFK is close to the observed maximum rate of glycolysis *in vivo* (for references see Connett & Sahlin [16]) and may therefore determine the limit of maximum glycolytic power. The activities of PFK and glycogen phosphorylase are reduced by acidosis. The product of glycolysis (lactic acid) can therefore reduce the rate of glycolysis through feedback inhibition and may be regarded as a safety mechanism, by which cellular damage due to excessive lactic acid accumulation is prevented. Both the power and the capacity of glycolysis (i.e. amount of produced lactate) may therefore be limited by product accumulation (i.e. H^+). Factors such as muscle buffering capacity and export of lactic acid are likely to modulate the response.

Aerobic processes

During two-leg exercise, muscle O_2 utilization may increase 50-fold and with a $\dot{V}O_{2\,max}$ of 5 L/min the rate of ATP generation (assuming a P/O_2 ratio of 6) will be 46 mmol/kg muscle/min (Fig. 1.2.1). It is generally agreed that the major determinant of whole-body maximal aerobic power ($\dot{V}O_{2\,max}$) is cardiac output, which sets an upper limit on O_2 delivery. It has been estimated that exercise with a muscle mass of 10 kg is sufficient to tax the maximal cardiac output in a sedentary subject [17]. The maximal aerobic power of the muscle tissue is therefore not utilized during two-leg exercise where the working muscle mass is about 20 kg or more. However, during exercise with small muscle groups the rate of aerobic energy production may be limited by peripheral factors (e.g. mitochondrial density or O_2 diffusion). During one-leg knee extension the estimated working muscle mass is only about 3 kg and measured O_2 utilization can increase 100-fold (to 300 mL/min/kg muscle [17]). This corresponds to a power of 79 mmol ATP/kg muscle/min, which is 80% of the maximum power of glycolysis.

Several lines of evidence suggest that oxidation of fatty acids cannot proceed at the same rate as for carbohydrate (CHO) oxidation. First, it has been shown that isolated mitochondria have a lower maximal rate of respiration and at a given energy state (ATP/ADP ratio) a lower submaximal rate of respiration with palmitate compared with pyruvate [18]. Secondly, it is known that ultradistance running, which results in a depletion of the body storage of carbohydrates and a switch to fat oxidation [19], causes a decline in the power output to about 50% of $\dot{V}O_{2\,max}$. The reason for the lower rate of aerobic ATP formation from fat is under debate. Oxidation of FFA provides an approximately 10% lower yield of ATP per consumed oxygen compared with CHO and will be one significant factor. Combustion of fatty acids may also be limited by the rate of acetyl-CoA formation where one or several links in the chain may limit the process (fuel transport from the fat depots into the muscle fiber; transport of FFA into mitochondria; rate of β-oxidation). In addition, it has long been recognized that CHO availability may be necessary for optimal function of aerobic energy transduction: 'fat burns in the glow of carbohydrates' (Albert Szent-Györgyi). The basis for this may be that the function of the tricarboxylic acid (TCA) cycle depends on pyruvate-dependent anaplerosis (expansion of TCA cycle intermediates). This hypothesis is supported by the finding that (i) prolonged exercise results in glycogen depletion and reduced levels of TCA cycle intermediates [20] and (ii) TCA cycle intermediates remained low in McArdle patients where glycogen utilization is blocked [3]. However, the hypothesis that the level of TCA cycle intermediates may limit maximal TCA cycle flux has recently been questioned [21]. During prolonged one-legged knee extension exercise it was shown that TCA cycle intermediates decreased but that TCA cycle flux was maintained and PCr increased, and this was considered inconsistent with the hypothesis [21].

The CHO stores limit the amount of energy that can be produced by CHO oxidation. Cycling or running at intensities of between 60 and 80% of $\dot{V}_{O_2 max}$ can normally proceed for 1–2 h before exhaustion and coincide with depletion of the glycogen store in the working muscle. During exercise at low intensities the energy demand is low and can be met by fat oxidation. Since fat is present abundantly the capacity of fat oxidation is very large and metabolic factors will not limit exercise duration.

Influence of muscle mass on power and capacity of whole-body energy production

The power of anaerobic energy production appears to be limited by the activities of key enzymes such as myosin ATPase, creatine kinase and PFK. On a whole-body level an increased working muscle mass will result in a proportional increase in the total enzyme activities and therefore an increased anaerobic energy production ability. However, aerobic power is largely limited by cardiac output and will not therefore be influenced by the working muscle mass. The capacity of both aerobic and anaerobic energy production is limited by intrinsic muscular factors such as amount of glycogen, amount of PCr, and the volume available to distribute inhibitory metabolic end-products. An increased working muscle mass will increase the total available amount of glycogen and PCr and will therefore increase the amount of energy that can be produced by these processes. An increased working muscle mass, achieved either by training-induced hypertrophy or by increased recruitment of fast-twitch muscle fibers, will therefore be of advantage

during high-intensity exercise, since both power and capacity of anaerobic processes increase. However, during endurance running an increased muscle mass will be of disadvantage since energy expenditure will increase due to the increase in body weight. The difference in body composition between sprinters and endurance runners is an obvious sign of this basic concept.

Energetics during exercise

Estimated whole-body ATP turnover increases from about 0.08 mol ATP/min at rest to 1–4 mol ATP/min during running. The ATP turnover during 100 m running is 3 times higher than that during marathon running, whereas ATP turnover during the 5000 m is only 16% higher than that during a marathon. The difference in energy demand is reflected by a large difference in the energetic processes used. A mixture of the described energetic processes is normally used but the relative contribution varies considerably. The intensity of exercise is an important factor in determining the relative recruitment of the energy processes. Another factor is the time taken to activate an energetic process. PCr breakdown is instantaneous and is therefore considered to buffer the ATP level both temporally and spatially within the cell. Therefore the first few seconds of exercise always involve PCr utilization. Although most reports demonstrate that glycolysis contributes to ATP generation from the onset of exercise there appears to be a lag of a couple of seconds before maximum rate of glycolysis is achieved [10]. Aerobic processes reach maximal power ($\dot{V}_{O_2 max}$) after 3–5 min. The delayed onset of aerobic metabolism is the basis for the incurred O_2 deficit during steady-state exercise.

In addition to exercise intensity and duration of exercise other factors such as availability of oxygen and fuels, environmental factors and hormonal changes will modify the extent to which the energetic processes are recruited. In Fig. 1.2.3 the ATP turnover and the estimated contribution of various energetic processes during different running events are shown. The figure does not discriminate between different phases of the exercise (onset of exercise, middle of exercise and spurt) during which both ATP turnover and recruitment will differ from the average values shown.

The energetic challenge during exercise will be different during different running distances. Over 100 m the time is too short for recruitment of aerobic processes and the muscles rely almost solely on anaerobic processes, which also have the high power required to meet the energy demand. At the end of 100 m running, muscle PCr will be reduced to about 50% of the initial level [9] and will reduce the power of this energy process. Muscle lactate will accumulate and reach about 50% of maximal values [9] and muscle pH will decrease. Energetic power will for these reasons be reduced and this may explain why speed often decreases at the end of 100 m.

Over 400 m, the required power exceeds that of the aerobic processes and the duration is too short to reach maximal rates of oxidative energy production. The capacity of the anaerobic processes is insufficient to cover the whole energy demand during 400 m. The challenge is to maximize the aerobic contribution but to avoid too high a lactate concentration early in the race, which could otherwise impair energetic processes and reduce mechanical efficiency. This metabolic strategy is achieved by a rapid acceleration of speed (which will accelerate oxidative energy release), submaximal running during the middle of the race and a maximal spurt. When the distance is completed the whole energetic capacity of both PCr breakdown and glycolysis should have been used. Normally, the speed decreases at the end of the distance and this is probably related to a reduced power of anaerobic energy release.

Over 5000 m, oxidative processes are sufficient to cover the energy requirements. During the race utilization of aerobic processes should be maximized without accumulation of inhibiting amounts of lactate. The high power of anaerobic processes should be saved for the spurt. At the end of the race muscle lactate levels will be high and PCr depleted but due to the high total energy expenditure the relative contribution of anaerobic processes will be low (about 5%).

During the marathon CHO stores are insufficient to cover the energy demand and at the same time the power of FFA oxidation is insufficient. The strategy is to: (i) maximize the CHO stores prior to exercise by CHO loading; (ii) avoid lactate formation since this would rapidly deplete the CHO stores; and (iii) optimize oxidation of FFA. Ideally the glycogen stores should be depleted at the end of the race.

Muscle fatigue and metabolism

The cause of muscle fatigue (i.e. inability to maintain a defined exercise intensity) is considered to be multifactorial. The classic hypothesis is that muscle fatigue is caused by failure of the energetic processes to generate ATP at a sufficient rate. The evidence for this hypothesis is that interventions which increase the power (i.e. aerobic training, hyperoxia, blood doping) or capacity (i.e. CHO loading, creatine supplementation, glucose supplementation) of the energetic processes result in increased performance and delayed onset of fatigue. Similarly, factors that impair the energetic processes (i.e. depletion of muscle glycogen, intracellular acidosis, hypoxic conditions, reduced muscle blood flow) have a negative influence on performance. The evidence is, however, circumstantial and a direct cause and effect relationship remains to be established.

It has been argued that since muscle ATP remains almost unchanged during exhaustive exercise it is unlikely that energetic failure is a cause of fatigue. This line of argument may, however, be too simplistic since temporal and spatial gradients of adenine nucleotides may exist in the contracting muscle. Furthermore, the mechanism may be related to increases in the products of ATP hydrolysis (i.e. ADP, AMP or P_i) rather than to decreases in ATP *per se*. A small decrease in ATP will cause large relative increases in ADP and AMP, due to much lower concentrations of these compounds. Muscle fatigue is generally associated with increased catabolism of adenine nucleotides, which signifies a condition of energetic stress [22]. This lends further support to the hypothesis that muscle fatigue under many conditions is caused by energetic deficiency. Decrease in PCr is another hallmark of energetic deficiency and is paralleled by a similar increase in P_i. There is evidence that increases in P_i will interfere with the contraction process and it is considered to be one of the major factors for the decrease in force [23].

Metabolic factors are likely to play an important role in fatigue and performance during exercise but there is no doubt that conditions exist where fatigue cannot be explained by metabolic changes. Considering the diversity and complexity of exercise this is to be expected.

Energy expenditure and metabolism

Energy expenditure during exercise

Energy expenditure during exercise varies over a large range. From a basal metabolic rate (BMR) of approximately 290–340 kJ/h in men and 240–260 kJ/h in women energy expenditure may increase to 4–5000 kJ/h during heavy exercise. Assuming a mechanical efficiency of around 20%, this permits 1000 kJ/h of work to be performed [24]. During a 10-s bout of exercise more than 10 kJ of work may be performed by a highly trained athlete and during a 1-min bout 40 kJ [25].

The total energy expenditure (TEE) of an adult person averages 10 000–13 000 kJ/24 h. Individuals with physically very demanding occupations may reach values of 17 000–19 000 kJ/24 h. The TEE is made up of three components: the BMR, the dietary-induced thermogenesis (DIT) and the activity-dependent energy expenditure (Table 1.2.1). The BMR is normally the largest component of TEE, averaging 7000–8200 kJ/24 h in men and 5800–6200 kJ/24 h in women. The DIT, which is defined as the extra energy consumption resulting from a meal, normally accounts for one tenth of the TEE. DIT is largest after a protein meal, where it amounts to 18–25% of the energy contained in the meal, but considerably smaller for meals containing carbohydrates (4–7%) and fat (2–4%) [24]. The remaining part of the TEE is the activity-dependent energy expenditure (AEE), which can be calculated based on the 19.7 and 21.2 kJ of energy released for each liter of oxygen consumed during fat and carbohydrate oxidation, respectively (for further discussion, see below). When the oxygen uptake is unknown, different approximations are often used to assess the activity-dependent energy consumption, e.g. quiet sitting corresponding to an energy consumption of about 1.2×BMR, office work 1.3–1.6×BMR, standing 1.4×BMR, cycling 4–6×BMR and various sports activities of the order of 10–20×BMR (Table 1.2.1) [24]. The energy cost of running is independent of running speed and of the order of 4 kJ/km/kg body weight. For walking at a pace of 4.5–5 km/h, the corresponding figure is 3 kJ/km/kg body weight [26]. This means, for example, that the energy content of 100 g fat (3900 kJ) for a 70-kg person covers the energy demand of running approximately 14 km or

Table 1.2.1 Energy expenditure in adult men and women, given as the total energy expenditure/24 h as a multiple of BMR (equal to the physical activity level, PAL). Data from [72].

BMR = basal metabolic rate (kJ/24 h)
DIT = diet-induced thermogenesis (kJ/24 h)
AEE = activity-induced energy expenditure (kJ/24 h)
TEE = total energy expenditure = BMR + DIT + AEE
PAL = physical activity level (includes DIT) = TEE/BMR

BMR	18–29 years	30–39 years	40–64 years
Males	7500	8200	7000
Females	6200	6000	5800

PAL over 24 h with different living conditions

Chair- or bedbound	1.2
Seated work, low leisure time activity	1.4–1.5
Seated work with moving around, low leisure time activity	1.6–1.7
Standing work, low leisure time activity	1.8–1.9*
Strenuous leisure time activity (30–60 min, ≥4 times/week)	+0.3†
Strenuous work or high activity in leisure time	2.0–2.4‡

* For example, 8 h sleeping (0.95), 4 h sitting (1.2), 12 h walking around (2.5).
† Up to a maximal value of 2.0.
‡ 2.4 is considered to be the highest PAL that can be tolerated other than for short periods of e.g. very intensive training.

walking 18 km. It is evident that complex nervous and hormonal regulation is required in order to control the utilization of the different energy substrates during exercise with large variations in energy demand.

Exercise metabolism

Exercise metabolism is focused on the utilization of biologic energy in order to perform work. Biologic energy is found in the oxidizable substrates in the body, namely glucose, free fatty acids and amino acids, and also lactate and glycerol (and under some circumstances ethanol and ketone bodies). In addition to aerobic oxidation, energy is released during the anaerobic degradation of glycogen to lactate. This is the major energy source in some cells and tissues devoid of mitochondria, such as the red blood cells and the kidney tubules, and also in skeletal muscle during short-term, high-intensity exercise. An important issue in metabolic regulation at rest and during exercise is that, under non-starving conditions, the central nervous system (as well as the red blood cells and the kidney tubules) is limited to the use of glucose as the sole energy substrate. The supply of glucose to these tissues is therefore highly prioritized. The skeletal muscle cells store energy in the form of glycogen, triglycerides, ATP and phosphocreatine (PCr). Biologic energy can also be delivered to the muscle in the form of blood-borne energy substrates directly originating from the alimentary tract following a meal or, between meals, in the form of blood-borne substrates released from the storage organs, mainly the liver and the adipose tissue. In the previous part of this chapter, a detailed description was given of the biochemical pathways involved in these processes.

The energy expenditure during exercise originates from aerobic and anaerobic biochemical processes. The energy expenditure originating from the aerobic combustion of nutrients can be determined with great precision by measuring the oxygen uptake of an individual. Each liter of oxygen consumed corresponds to the release of 19.7–21.2 kJ of energy, depending on the relative proportions of carbohydrates or fat being oxidized. These proportions can be determined from the respiratory quotient (*RQ*, the ratio between the amount of CO_2 exhaled and the amount of O_2 taken up). The energy expenditure originating from the anaerobic processes, i.e. glycogen degradation to lactic acid and breakdown of PCr and ATP, can, on the other hand, only be roughly estimated (e.g. based on measurement of the total work performed with subtraction of the aerobic energy delivery). While maximal aerobic power can reach 120 kJ/min in endurance athletes, athletes in events of 1–2 min duration can reach a maximal total anaerobic energy release of 200 kJ. For an untrained person, aerobic power may reach 60 kJ/min and maximal total anaerobic energy release 100 kJ, the former value being limited by the capacity of the heart to eject oxygenated blood into the arterial system and the latter by the total muscle mass that can be recruited in the specific exercise [26]. During maximal work, anaerobic processes dominate when exercise durations are less than approximately 2 min, with longer exercise durations aerobic processes will yield the majority of the energy delivery.

Energy sources at rest and during exercise

Energy sources at rest

At rest, under postabsorptive conditions, fatty acids constitute the primary energy source, accounting for approximately 60% of energy requirements, leaving about 20% for carbohydrates and proteins, respectively. Postabsorptive conditions are said to be present when no nutrients are entering the blood from the intestinal tract. The energy liberated per gram of nutrient combusted is 17 kJ for carbohydrates and proteins and 39 kJ for fat. Therefore, the demand for fat combustion at rest can be covered by the adipose tissue liberating 5 g of fatty acids per hour, of which 1.5 g is taken up by the liver and 2 g by skeletal muscle. The carbohydrates are provided by the liver, which releases 7.5 g/h of glucose, of which 4.5 g is derived from glycogenolysis and 3 g from gluconeogenesis. This covers mainly the 6 g/h of glucose which is used

Table 1.2.2 Typical changes in energy source (g/h) when an individual exercises at successively higher intensity (postabsorptive state) [24,31].

	Rest	Exercise 100 W	Exercise 200 W	Exercise 250 W
Glucose, from liver store	4.5	16	25	40
Glucose, from liver glucose neoformation	3	4	5	5
Glucose, from muscle store	–	40–45	100	150
Fat, from adipose tissue or muscle	5	18	26	22

Values are given in g/h and refer to the postabsorptive state. Exercise metabolism during the absorptive state will vary with meal composition and the time following the meal. Generally, however, more energy will be derived from the blood (glucose, fatty acids, triglycerides) and less from the substrate stores in skeletal muscle and adipose tissue.

by the central nervous system and the red blood cells. Liver glycogenolysis is made possible by the liver store of glycogen (about 75 g in the fed state), whereas substrates for gluconeogenesis are lactate, glycerol and amino acids taken up by the liver from the blood. The amino acids used for gluconeogenesis derive mainly from net proteolysis in skeletal muscle, which releases around 4.5 g amino acids/h. The latter also constitute an important energy substrate for the intestines and the liver [24].

Absorptive conditions prevail for several hours following each meal, with most nutrients being taken up by the body during the first 2–3 h. If it is assumed that the main absorption phase takes place during the first 2.5 hours following each meal, with three meals a day, absorptive conditions will prevail for 7.5 h/24 h, whereas the body during the remaining 17.5 h per day is closer to a postabsorptive state. In the absorptive state, the metabolic situation is different in that now carbohydrate oxidation dominates, normally covering three-quarters of total substrate oxidation, while the substrate stores of the body are refilled rather than used. If 10 500 kJ/24 h is covered by three meals of 3500 kJ each, containing 50% carbohydrates, 35% fat and 15% protein, 100 g glucose, 30 g fatty acids and 30 g amino acids will be made available to the body during the absorptive period after each meal. Due to the shift from predominantly fat to predominantly carbohydrate oxidation during this period, around 50 g of the 100 g of carbohydrates taken up by the body will be oxidized, whereas the remaining 50 g will be used to refill the liver glycogen store (25 g) and the glycogen store in skeletal muscles (25–30 g during non-glycogen-depleted conditions) [24]. The 30 g of fatty acids from each meal enters the blood in the form of a special lipoprotein, the chylomicron. The chylomicron triglycerides (TGs) are degraded by the enzyme lipoprotein lipase (LPL), which is localized in capillary endothelial cells in most organs of the body, but with especially high levels in adipose tissue, myocardium and skeletal muscles. The fate of the enzyme-liberated fatty acids is mainly storage in adipose tissue, but also uptake in liver and skeletal muscle [27]. In muscle tissue the fatty acids are oxidized and/or used for the restoration of muscle TG stores reduced by exercise [28]. In the liver, the chylomicron remnants are taken up and fatty acids resynthesized to triglycerides, which are incorporated into very low density lipopro-

tein, exported and finally also stored in adipose tissue. The 30 g amino acids from each meal are added to the 400–500 g of amino acids being formed per 24 h mainly from the degradation of protein stores of skeletal muscle and liver. Of these amino acids, 300–400 g are used for synthesis and approximately 80 g are used for oxidation in the intestines and the liver [24].

Energy sources during exercise in the postabsorptive state

During exercise, the energy consumption may be increased by 20-fold. The primary factor determining whether carbohydrates or fat are preferentially used during exercise is the exercise intensity, the proportion of energy derived from carbohydrates growing progressively larger with increasing intensity. At a moderate exercise level of 100 W, demanding an oxygen uptake of around 1.5 L/min, equalling an energy expenditure of 1800 kJ/h, the proportions might typically change to 60% carbohydrates and 40% fat. In this situation, the demand for carbohydrates (65 g glucose/h, i.e. 1080 kJ) is met by glycogenolysis (around 40–45 g/h) and glucose uptake (around 20 g/h), whereas the demand for fat is met by lipolysis in adipose tissue and muscle, supplying 18 g fatty acids (i.e. 720 kJ). Under normal circumstances, protein is not an important metabolic fuel during exercise, and it is considered unlikely that, even during prolonged exercise, protein oxidation can cover more than 10% of the energy demand of the exercising body [29]. In spite of this, activation of protein metabolism is an integral part of the acute metabolic response of the body to exercise [30].

To roughly estimate the *RQ* during exercise and therefore the relative demand for carbohydrates and fat, Dill and coworkers used an equation, empirically derived from their data:

Respiratory quotient during exercise
$= 0.81 + 0.04 \cdot$ oxygen uptake in L/min [31].

Although obviously not generally applicable, the equation can be used here to illustrate the increasing demand for carbohydrates at increasing exercise intensities. When the exercise intensity is increased to 200 W (oxygen uptake = 2.8 L/min), this formula indicates an *RQ* value of 0.92 (indicating 70% carbohydrate and 30% fat oxidation). This corresponds to a combustion of 134 g carbohydrates and 26 g fatty acids.

Similarly, exercise at 250 W can be calculated to demand combustion of 192 g carbohydrates and 22 g fatty acids. It is therefore evident that fat combustion will level off with increasing exercise intensities, when simultaneously carbohydrate oxidation, as well as hepatic and muscular glycogenolysis and muscle glucose uptake, increases exponentially (above the 'lactate threshold').

When exercise is prolonged, fat combustion increases. This change is most likely secondary to a continuing depletion of the body's carbohydrate stores. During prolonged exercise at 40% of $\dot{V}_{O_2 max}$ in overnight fasted untrained subjects, plasma free fatty acids contributed to 60% of the fuel demand during the fourth hour of exercise compared to only 30% during the first hour [32]. Asmussen and Christensen describe two subjects being able to work at intensities demanding oxygen uptakes of 2.3 and 2.7 L/min (165–190 W) for 3 h [31]. During the first hour, the subjects combusted 94 g carbohydrates and 35 g fatty acids; during the third hour the corresponding figures were 65 g carbohydrates and 48 g fatty acids.

Endogenous glycogen is the dominant fuel during the initial period of moderate to severe exercise, and during sustained exercise at work rates corresponding to 60–80% of $\dot{V}_{O_2 max}$, fatigue coincides with the depletion of muscle glycogen [33,34]. With the continuous depletion of endogenous glycogen, the utilization of plasma-derived glucose increases and has, during prolonged exercise, been reported to cover up to 75–90% of the estimated carbohydrate oxidation by muscle [35]. The increased glucose uptake by skeletal muscle during heavy exercise must be balanced by a glucose release from the liver of the same magnitude. Because there are only limited possibilities for increasing gluconeogenesis in liver (from 3 to 5 g/h [36], mainly secondary to increased availability of glycerol due to the increased lipolysis in adipose tissue), the majority of the increased glucose output from the liver has to be derived from glycogenolysis. With liver glycogenolytic rates of 25 g/h during heavy and 60 g/h during very heavy exercise, the liver glycogen supply of around 75 g will be rapidly depleted. However, fatigue due to hypoglycemia can be postponed by the ingestion of glucose. Although it may be difficult to ingest large amounts of glucose during exercise, it has been reported that as much as 60 g/h of ingested glucose may be taken up by the body [37] during heavy exer-

cise of long duration. It has been observed that the total amount of carbohydrate used during a marathon race was higher than could be accounted for by the endogenous glycogen stores in the working muscles and the liver. From this, it was concluded that glycogen reserves in inactive muscle and other tissues must also have been mobilized [38]. Glycogenolysis with net lactate release from inactive muscle has been demonstrated during exercise [39].

Relatively little is known about endogenous triglycerides as a potential source of energy for the contracting muscle, but it seems likely to be an important fuel during exercise. During 1.5 h of cycle ergometer exercise to exhaustion, it was found that the decrease in thigh muscle triglyceride concentration averaged 25% [40]. The authors calculated that 70% of total oxidized fatty acids originated from endogenous triglycerides, whereas 30% came from plasma-derived free fatty acids, and that the energy contribution of endogenous triglycerides was 70% of that of glycogen. During the Swedish 7-h Wasa ski race, it was calculated that the decrease in muscle triglycerides corresponded to twice as much energy as the decrease in muscle glycogen [41]. See also the data by Hurley *et al.* [42], which are discussed in the section on training below.

Energy sources during exercise in the absorptive state

When exercise is performed in the absorptive state, less energy will be derived from the substrate stores in skeletal muscle and adipose tissue, and more from glucose, fatty acids and triglycerides in blood, although plasma free fatty acids will be less important as an energy fuel than in the postabsorptive state [43]. In an experimental study, metabolism during 60 min of forearm exercise after an overnight fast was compared with the same exercise 3 h following a meal [44]. In the postabsorptive state, the exercise was fueled by glucose uptake from blood (40%) and by intramuscular depots (60%). Following the meal, the contribution to exercise metabolism from plasma glucose was similar to that in the postabsorptive state, but the muscular uptake of plasma triglycerides was markedly increased and, if oxidized, could cover around 40% of the energy demand. This indicates that, following a meal, the contribution of plasma triglycerides to exercise metabolism may be considerably higher than previously realized. Due to the high blood flow during exercise, arteriovenous differences for VLDL-triglycerides (VLDL-TG) are very difficult to detect accurately, but it has been estimated that, if oxidized, plasma triacylglycerol could cover half of muscle triacylglycerol oxidation during exercise [45]. However, their slow turnover argues against VLDL-TG as an important fuel for the working muscle. It is likely that muscle lipoprotein lipase may be more active towards chylomicron-TG than VLDL-TG [46] and the idea that chylomicron-TG may serve as a fuel for the exercising muscle is further suggested by the fact that postprandial lipidemia is diminished during and after exercise [47]. There is evidence that physical training, by increasing skeletal muscle lipoprotein lipase activity, while reducing that of adipose tissue, causes a redirection of circulating lipid from storage in adipose tissue to oxidation in muscle.

Energy sources during exercise in the trained state

One factor counteracting the low fat combustion at high exercise intensities is the effect of training. It has been convincingly shown that, at a certain exercise intensity, a trained individual uses more fat than an untrained individual. This effect is quite strong and occurs after relatively short periods of training. One group of subjects was studied after 5 and 31 days of training for 2 h daily at a moderately high exercise intensity (60% of the pretraining $\dot{V}_{O_{2\,max}}$) [48]. Following 5 days of training, the total fat oxidation at this intensity had increased by 10% and after 31 days of training, the increase was as high as 70%. The oxidation of carbohydrates during the exercise bout showed the opposite pattern. It is therefore obvious that a good physical fitness level makes it much easier to maintain a high degree of fat combustion during intense exercise [49].

The source of the increased fat usage during exercise in endurance-trained subjects has been debated, however, since the plasma levels of free fatty acids during exercise are often lower than in untrained individuals [50]. This is likely to be secondary to the lower sympathoadrenal activation after training [51] which, unopposed, would lead to decreased lipolysis of not only adipose tissue, but also intramuscular triglycerides. When male subjects exercised at the same absolute intensity (64% of the pretraining $\dot{V}_{O_{2\,max}}$)

before and after a 12-week programme of endurance training, plasma free fatty acid and glycerol concentrations were found to be lower in the trained than in the untrained state [42]. In spite of this, the respiratory exchange ratio was reduced after training, indicating a greater reliance on fat oxidation. Muscle triglyceride utilization was found to be twice as great and muscle glycogen utilization to be 40% lower after, as opposed to before, training. It was concluded that the greater utilization of fat in the trained than in the untrained state was fueled by increased lipolysis of intramuscular triglycerides. This conclusion was supported by a study showing a lower turnover of plasma free fatty acids in the trained state [52]. In fact, Jansson and Kaijser [53] also concluded that the reduced reliance on carbohydrate metabolism in their trained, as compared to their untrained, individuals would have been covered by intramuscular triglycerides. They based this conclusion on the finding of no difference between trained and untrained individuals in the ratio of plasma free fatty acid extraction to O_2 extraction by the working legs.

It is known that increased fat oxidation with training is a local effect since after one-leg training it occurs in the trained leg only [54,55]. Underlying this training response is an increased mitochondrial density and an increased content of mitochondrial enzymes in aerobically trained muscle, accompanied by increases in the enzymes involved in activation, transfer into the mitochondria and β-oxidation of fatty acids [56–58]. Holloszy and coworkers have formulated a hypothetical biochemical mechanism whereby a large concentration of mitochondrial oxidative enzymes in trained muscle would lead to a greater reliance on fat metabolism, a lower rate of lactate formation and sparing of muscle glycogen during exercise [57]. These adaptations in trained skeletal muscle would, at a given exercise intensity, permit the rate of fatty acid oxidation to be higher in the trained than in the untrained muscle, even in the presence of a lower intracellular fatty acid concentration in the trained state.

Exercise and weight regulation

Effect of exercise on body weight
Weight balance implies that food intake equals food oxidation and most probably also that the oxidation

of carbohydrates, fat and protein equals the intake of these nutrients. It has therefore been concluded that the quotient between the intake of carbohydrates and fat (described as the food quotient, *FQ*, i.e. the ratio of carbon dioxide produced to oxygen utilized for the oxidation of the food) over the long term must equal the average *RQ* over 24 h (*RQ*-24 h) for the individual to maintain weight balance [59,60]. Most individuals are in weight balance, where their weight only fluctuates by 1–2%. If unusually little food is taken in on a particular day, the *RQ* will be lowered due to inhibition of glucose oxidation, and fat oxidation will be increased to cover the negative energy balance. Conversely, if more food than usual is taken in during one day, carbohydrate oxidation will be increased (and fat consumption passively decreased to achieve energy balance that day) [59]. Thus, if the intake decreases it will be covered by stored fat; thereafter all of the lost fat is replenished due to an increased carbohydrate oxidation with high intakes. There seems to be no direct regulatory mechanism whereby fat oxidation is increased with a higher fat intake. However if, over the long term, fat intake is increased, fat oxidation must also be increased in order to achieve weight balance. This may be achieved by expansion of the adipose tissue mass, which increases fat oxidation more than carbohydrate oxidation. However, an increase in 24 h fat oxidation (i.e. decrease in *RQ*-24 h) may also be achieved by exercise [60]. Therefore, exercise allows weight maintenance to be achieved with less body fat in physically active individuals, where exercise substitutes for an enlarged fat mass in bringing about rates of fat oxidation corresponding with fat intake. This is one conceivable mechanism by which regular exercise tends to keep the fat depots down [60]. In a meta-analysis by Ballor and Keesey [61] based on 500 scientific studies, it was reported that training reduces the fat mass on average by 0.1 kg per week, and to the same extent in men and women.

Hormonal mechanisms at rest and during exercise

Hormonal regulation of resting metabolism

At rest, insulin and glucagon are the major hormones regulating whether energy fuels are liberated from the storage sites or, conversely, channelled for storage. In the postabsorptive state, the insulin/glucagon concentration ratio is around 2, which allows a normal hepatic release of glucose into the blood. Following a carbohydrate-containing meal insulin increases substantially, which in concert with a slight decrease in glucagon concentration causes the insulin/glucagon ratio to increase by more than 10-fold. This increase is necessary in order to direct glucose for storage in skeletal muscle and liver. With a carbohydrate-poor meal, the rise in insulin will be small, whereas plasma glucagon concentration clearly increases. The resulting decrease in the insulin/glucagon ratio serves to maintain a sufficient hepatic release of glucose in order to cover the needs of the central nervous system and erythrocytes in spite of a carbohydrate-poor meal [32] (Fig. 1.2.4).

Insulin stimulates glycogen synthesis in the liver and also promotes liver glucose uptake, but only at an elevated portal vein glucose concentration. Glycogen synthesis in the liver is also directly stimulated by increased vagal nerve activity. Glucagon, on the other hand, stimulates hepatic glycogenolysis as well as lipolysis in adipose tissue. In addition, glucagon stimulates the liver capacity for gluconeogenesis. The effect of glucagon on adipose tissue lipolysis is, however, secondary to the more powerful stimulation by the sympathetic nervous system, cortisol and growth hormone. Several other factors may stimulate hepatic glycogenolysis, including α- and β-adrenergic stimulation and vasoactive intestinal polypeptide, whereas hepatic gluconeogenesis is stimulated by increased precursor (lactate, pyruvate, amino acids, glycerol) availability, secondary to skeletal muscle glycolysis, skeletal muscle proteolysis and adipose tissue lipolysis. During exercise all these processes are stimulated, as well as hepatic extraction of these precursors and gluconeogenetic efficiency [25].

Hormonal changes with exercise

During exercise, several hormonal systems are activated and increases are seen in plasma concentrations of adrenaline/noradrenaline (epinephrine/norepinephrine), adrenocorticotrophic hormone (ACTH), cortisol, β-endorphin, growth hormone, renin, testosterone, thyroid hormone and several gastrointestinal hormones (Fig. 1.2.4). Arterial levels of glucagon are unchanged or only marginally increased

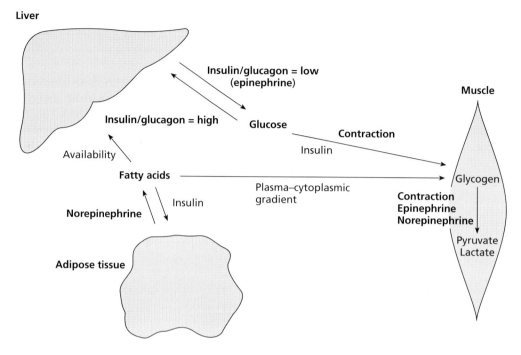

Fig. 1.2.4 Schematic illustration of the quantitatively most important hormonal mechanisms in the regulation of carbohydrate and fatty acid metabolism at rest and during exercise. Mechanisms important during exercise are in bold. A low insulin/glucagon ratio is around 2, a high ratio may be 20 or higher [32,62,63,65–68].

by exercise, whereas insulin is decreased [62]. The decrease in plasma insulin concentration can be quite marked during exercise (< 50% of values at rest) and is thought to be mediated by an increased activity in sympathetic nerves and by small decreases in the blood glucose concentration during exercise. The latter fact explains why the insulin decrease may be attenuated, and even reversed, by voluntary intake of glucose solutions during exercise. Both insulin and glucagon exert a large part of their effect on the liver and this effect will be underestimated based on hormone concentrations in peripheral arteries, because concentrations in the portal vein, which is the relevant concentration for the liver, are considerably higher. Therefore, it is likely that, although peripheral levels may stay unchanged, the glucagon concentration in the portal vein is increased by exercise [63].

The catecholamines in plasma increase with exercise intensity in an exponential manner. The source of circulating epinephrine is the adrenal medulla and the increase with exercise reflects an increased (sympathetic) nerve stimulation of this organ. Norepinephrine also originates to some extent from the adrenal medulla, but the increased norepinephrine concentration in arterial plasma is mainly considered to reflect overflow from postsynaptic sympathetic nerve endings mainly in the heart, but also in the liver and the adipose tissue. The mechanism behind the large sympathetic activation with exercise is not clear, but one important variable is likely to be a decrease in the portal glucose concentration. The two hormones differ in that the plasma concentration of norepinephrine starts to increase at lower rates of exercise and also increases more steeply with increased exercise intensity. At high exercise intensities, or long exercise durations, these hormones may be increased by 10–20-fold. Following exercise, norepinephrine often remains increased for several hours, whereas plasma concentrations of epinephrine return to basal levels within minutes [62,64].

Hormonal regulation of carbohydrate metabolism during exercise

Changes in insulin and glucagon have been reported to account for practically all of the increase in hepatic glucose output with exercise [65,66]. It is believed that the decrease in insulin concentration with exercise makes the liver more sensitive to the stimulation by glucagon. Sympathetic nervous stimulation seems to have no role in stimulating hepatic glucose output during exercise in humans, whereas epinephrine has a stimulating effect, additional to that of glucagon, during prolonged exercise, when epinephrine levels are at their highest. In addition, cortisol has an indirect effect on hepatic gluconeogenesis, by increasing the enzymatic potential for this pathway. The catecholamines are important in 'sensitizing' skeletal muscle glycogenolysis to the stimulating effect of contraction. With exercise leading to hypoglycemia, the compensatory increase in hepatic glucose output is mainly triggered by epinephrine [32].

Hormonal regulation of fat metabolism during exercise

The mobilization of free fatty acids from the adipose tissue during exercise is stimulated by catecholamines, mainly norepinephrine synthetized from sympathetic nerves, and inhibited by insulin. In adipose tissue, degradation of triglycerides into glycerol and free fatty acids is to some degree balanced by reesterification of fatty acids, using acyl-CoA and glycolysis-derived glycerol-3-phosphate. This reesterification has been found to be 20% of the lipolytic rate at rest, but only 12% during exercise, a decrease that makes more free fatty acids available to the working muscle during exercise [67,68].

Effect of training on the hormonal response to exercise

In trained individuals, the hormonal responses to exercise are generally decreased. This is true for the increases in norepinephrine, epinephrine, growth hormone, ACTH and glucagon, as well as for the decrease in insulin. This adaptation is especially marked with regard to the sympathoadrenal activation with exercise and occurs rapidly, within the first 2 weeks of training [51]. The mechanism behind this change is not fully established, but hormonal activation secondary to other stressful stimuli, e.g. hypoxia or hypoglycemia is in fact increased in the trained state and it is well known that the secretory capacity of the adrenal medulla is increased by endurance training: 'sports adrenal medulla' [62]. Trained individuals display lower insulin concentrations in plasma, during both basal and glucose-stimulated conditions, secondary to a decreased pancreatic insulin secretory rate [32] and an increased peripheral insulin sensitivity [69]. Training augments the lipolytic capacity of the adipocyte, which serves to maintain a sufficient lipolytic rate in a trained individual, in spite of a reduced sympathetic activation during exercise at a given intensity [70]. Endurance training also increases the oxidative capacity of the liver as well as the hepatic capacity for gluconeogenesis, although the glucose demand during exercise is clearly decreased in the trained state, as discussed above. This decreased demand is sensed by the body and as little as 10 days of endurance training has been shown to decrease the hepatic glucose output during 2 h of exercise by as much as 25% [71].

Summary

During exercise, energy consumption may be increased by 20-fold. The primary factor determining whether carbohydrates or fat are preferentially used during exercise is the exercise intensity, the proportion of energy derived from carbohydrates growing progressively larger with increasing intensity. When exercise is performed in the absorptive state, less energy will be derived from the substrate stores in skeletal muscle and adipose tissue, and more from glucose, fatty acids and triglycerides in blood. A high level of physical fitness results in a higher degree of fat combustion during intense exercise. In addition, regular exercise allows weight maintenance to be achieved with less body fat in physically active individuals. Changes in insulin and glucagon have been reported to account for practically all of the increase in hepatic glucose output with exercise. The mobilization of free fatty acids from adipose tissue during exercise is stimulated by catecholamines, mainly norepinephrine synthesized from sympathetic nerves, and inhibited by insulin.

Hydrolysis of ATP is the immediate energy source for practically all energy-requiring processes in the cell. The ultimate process of ATP formation is oxidative phosphorylation during which different substrates are oxidized with oxygen in the mitochondrion. In addition, regeneration of ATP can also occur through anaerobic processes (breakdown of PCr, glycolysis from glycogen and ADP fusion). There are two inherent limits to the energetic processes: the maximum rate (power) and the amount of ATP (capacity) that can be produced. Factors such as muscle mass and fiber type composition, training status and nutritional factors are important determinants of the individual profile of power and capacity. Several lines of evidence suggest that oxidation of fatty acids cannot proceed at the same rate as for carbohydrate oxidation. On a whole-body level an increased working muscle mass will result in a proportional increase in the capacity for anaerobic energy production. In contrast, during two-legged exercise, aerobic power is largely limited by cardiac output and not limited by the working muscle mass.

Multiple choice questions

1 *What is the body's demand for fatty acids in the postabsorptive state (at rest, $Vo_2 = 0.3 L/min$):*

a   0.5 g/h

b   1 g/h

c   5 g/h

d   10 g/h

e   15 g/h.

2 *The hepatic glucose output is of the order of 7.5 g/h at rest and 20–60 g/h during heavy exercise. This is covered by the liver glycogen store of approximately 75 g and by the synthesis of new glucose in the liver (gluconeogenesis). What is the maximal capacity of the liver for gluconeogenesis during exercise:*

a   5 g/h

b   10 g/h

c   15 g/h

d   20 g/h

e   25 g/h.

3 *Which of the following hormones are considered to be the most important in the control of hepatic glucose output during exercise:*

a   epinephrine

b   cortisol

c   glucagon

d   insulin

e   norepinephrine.

4 *Breakdown of phosphocreatine in skeletal muscle causes:*

a   pH decrease

b   buffering of protons

c   pH increase

d   release of inorganic phosphate

e   ADP fusion.

5 *Oxidation of fatty acids cannot proceed at the same rate as for carbohydrate oxidation. This can be explained by:*

a   lower oxygen demand

b   high rate of acetyl-CoA formation

c   low β-oxidation capacity

d   low TCA cycle capacity

e   low carnitine-palmityl transferase capacity.

References

1   Brand MD, Chien LF, Ainscow EK, Rolfe DF, Porter RK. The causes and functions of mitochondrial proton leak. *Biochim Biophys Acta* 1994; **1187**: 132–9.

2   Jorfeldt L, Wahren J. Leg blood flow during exercise in man. *Clin Sci* 1971; **41**: 459–73.

3   Sahlin K, Jorfeldt L, Henriksson KG, Lewis SF, Haller RG. Tricarboxylic acid cycle intermediates during incremental exercise in healthy subjects and in patients with McArdle's disease. *Clin Sci (Colchester)* 1995; **88**: 687–93.

4   Söderlund K, Hultman E. ATP and phosphocreatine changes in single human muscle fibers after intense electrical stimulation. *Am J Physiol* 1991; **261**: E737–41.

5   Sahlin K, Söderlund K, Tonkonogi M, Hirakoba K. Phosphocreatine content in single fibers of human muscle after sustained submaximal exercise. *Am J Physiol* 1997; **273**: C172–8.

6   Harris RC, Söderlund K, Hultman E. Elevation of creatine in resting and exercised muscle of normal subjects by creatine supplementation. *Clin Sci (Colchester)* 1992; **83**: 367–74.

7   Greenhaff PL, Bodin K, Söderlund K, Hultman E. Effect of oral creatine supplementation on skeletal muscle phosphocreatine resynthesis. *Am J Physiol* 1994; **266**: E725–30.

8   Sahlin K. Intracellular pH and energy metabolism in skeletal muscle of man with special reference to exercise. *Acta Physiol Scand Suppl* 1978; **455**: 1–56.

9   Bogdanis GC, Nevill ME, Lakomy HK, Boobis LH. Power output and muscle metabolism during and following recovery from 10 and 20 s of maximal sprint exercise in humans. *Acta Physiol Scand* 1998; **163**: 261–72.

10 Hultman E, Sjöholm H. Substrate availability. In: Knuttgen HG, Vogel JM, Poortmans JR, eds. *Biochemistry of Exercise.* Champaign, Illinois: Human Kinetics, 1983 pp. 63–75.

11 Kuznetsov AV, Tiivel T, Sikk P, Kaambre T, Kay L, Daneshrad Z *et al.* Striking differences between the kinetics

of regulation of respiration by ADP in slow-twitch and fast-twitch muscles *in vivo*. *Eur J Biochem* 1996; **241**: 909–15.

12 Rico-Sanz J. Creatine reduces human muscle PCr and pH decrements and Pi accumulation during low-intensity exercise. *J Appl Physiol* 2000; **88**: 1181–91.

13 Katz A, Broberg S, Sahlin K, Wahren J. Leg glucose uptake during maximal dynamic exercise in humans. *Am J Physiol* 1986; **251**: E65–70.

14 Sahlin K, Harris RC, Nylind B, Hultman E. Lactate content and pH in muscle obtained after dynamic exercise. *Pflügers Arch* 1976; **367**: 143–9.

15 Katz A, Broberg S, Sahlin K, Wahren J. Muscle ammonia and amino acid metabolism during dynamic exercise in man. *Clin Physiol* 1986; **6**: 365–79.

16 Connett RJ, Sahlin K. Control of glycolysis and glycogen metabolism. In: Rowell LB, Shepherd JT, eds. *Handbook of Physiology: Integration of Motor, Circulatory, Respiratory and Metabolic Control During Exercise*. Bethesda: The American Physiological Society, 1996: 870–910.

17 Andersen P, Adams RP, Sjogaard G, Thorboe A, Saltin B. Dynamic knee extension as model for study of isolated exercising muscle in humans. *J Appl Physiol* 1985; **59**: 1647–53.

18 Willis WT, Jackman MR. Mitochondrial function during heavy exercise. *Med Sci Sports Exerc* 1994; **26**: 1347–53.

19 Davies CT, Thompson MW. Aerobic performance of female marathon and male ultramarathon athletes. *Eur J Appl Physiol Occup Physiol* 1979; **41**: 233–45.

20 Sahlin K, Katz A, Broberg S. Tricarboxylic acid cycle intermediates in human muscle during prolonged exercise. *Am J Physiol* 1990; **259**: C834–41.

21 Gibala MJ, Young ME, Taegtmeyer H. Anaplerosis of the citric acid cycle: role in energy metabolism of heart and skeletal muscle. *Acta Physiol Scand* 2000; **168**: 657–65.

22 Sahlin K, Broberg S. Adenine nucleotide depletion in human muscle during exercise. Causality and significance of AMP deamination. *Int J Sports Med* 1990; **11** (Suppl. 2): S62–7.

23 Westerblad H, Allen DG, Bruton JD, Andrade FH, Lannergren J. Mechanisms underlying the reduction of isometric force in skeletal muscle fatigue. *Acta Physiol Scand* 1998; **162**: 253–60.

24 Jungermann K, Barth CA. Energy metabolism and nutrition. In: Greger R, Windhorst U, eds. *Comprehensive Human Physiology: from Cellular Mechanisms to Integration*, 1st edn. Berlin: Springer Verlag, 1996: 1425–57.

25 Guyton AC, Hall JE. *Textbook of Medical Physiology*, 10th edn. Philadelphia: Saunders, 2000.

26 Åstrand P-O, Rodahl K. *Textbook of Work Physiology. Physiological Bases of Exercise*, 3rd edn. New York: McGraw-Hill, 1986.

27 Van der Vusse GJ, Reneman RS. Lipid metabolism in muscle. In: Rowell LB, Shepherd JT, eds. *Handbook of Physiology: Integration of Motor, Circulatory, Respiratory and Metabolic Control During Exercise*. Bethesda: The American Physiological Society, 1996: 952–94.

28 Oscai LB, Essig DA, Palmer WK. Lipase regulation of muscle triglyceride hydrolysis. *J Appl Physiol* 1990; **69**: 1571–7.

29 Wagenmakers AJ. Protein and amino acid metabolism in human muscle. *Adv Exp Med Biol* 1998; **441**: 307–19.

30 Henriksson J. Effect of exercise on amino acid concentrations in skeletal muscle and plasma. *J Exp Biol* 1991; **160**: 149–65.

31 Asmussen E, Christensen EH. *Kompendium i Legemsövelsernes Specielle Teori*. Copenhagen: Köbenhavns Universitets Fond til Tilvejebringelse af Laeremidler, 1967.

32 Wasserman DH, Cherrington AD. Regulation of extramuscular fuel sources during exercise. In: Rowell LB, Shepherd JT, eds. *Handbook of Physiology: Integration of Motor, Circulatory, Respiratory and Metabolic Control During Exercise*. Bethesda: The American Physiological Society, 1996: 1036–74.

33 Bergstrom J, Hermansen L, Hultman E, Saltin B. Diet, muscle glycogen and physical performance. *Acta Physiol Scand* 1967; **71**: 140–50.

34 Sherman WM, Costill DL. The marathon: dietary manipulation to optimize performance. *Am J Sports Med* 1984; **12**: 44–51.

35 Wahren J, Felig P, Ahlborg G, Jorfeldt L. Glucose metabolism during leg exercise in man. *J Clin Invest* 1971; **50**: 2715–25.

36 Bergman BC, Horning MA, Casazza GA, Wolfel EE, Butterfield GE, Brooks GA. Endurance training increases gluconeogenesis during rest and exercise in men. *Am J Physiol (Endocrinol Metabolism)* 2000; **278**: E244–51.

37 Jeukendrup AE, Jentjens R. Oxidation of carbohydrate feedings during prolonged exercise: current thoughts, guidelines and directions for future research. *Sports Med* 2000; **29**: 407–24.

38 O'Brien MJ, Viguie CA, Mazzeo RS, Brooks GA. Carbohydrate dependence during marathon running. *Med Sci Sports Exerc* 1993; **25**: 1009–17.

39 Ahlborg G, Wahren J, Felig P. Splanchnic and peripheral glucose and lactate metabolism during and after prolonged arm exercise. *J Clin Invest* 1986; **77**: 690–9.

40 Carlson LA, Ekelund LG, Fröberg SO. Concentration of triglycerides, phospholipids and glycogen in skeletal muscle and of free fatty acids and beta-hydroxybutyric acid in blood in man in response to exercise. *Eur J Clin Invest* 1971; **1**: 248–54.

41 Fröberg SO, Mossfeldt F. Effect of prolonged strenuous exercise on the concentration of triglycerides, phospholipids and glycogen in muscle of man. *Acta Physiol Scand* 1971; **82**: 167–71.

42 Hurley BF, Nemeth PM, Martin WH, Hagberg JM, Dalsky GP, Holloszy JO. Muscle triglyceride utilization during exercise: effect of training. *J Appl Physiol* 1986; **60**: 562–7.

43 Havel RJ, Naimark A, Borchgrevink CF. Turnover rate and oxidation of free fatty acids of blood plasma in man during exercise: studies during continuous infusion of palmitate-1-14C. *J Clin Invest* 1963; **42**: 1054–63.

44 Griffiths AJ, Humphreys SM, Clark ML, Frayn KN. Forearm substrate utilization during exercise after a meal containing both fat and carbohydrate. *Clin Sci* 1994; **86**: 169–75.

45 Kiens B, Essén-Gustavsson B, Christensen NJ, Saltin B. Skeletal muscle substrate utilization during submaximal exercise in man: effect of endurance training. *J Physiol (Lond)* 1993; **469**: 459–78.

46 Potts JL, Fisher RM, Humphreys SM, Coppack SW, Gibbons GF, Frayn KN. Peripheral triacylglycerol extraction in the fasting and post-prandial states. *Clin Sci* 1991; **81**: 621–6.

47 Hardman AE, Aldred HE. Walking during the postprandial period decreases alimentary lipaemia. *J Cardiovascular Risk* 1995; **2**: 71–8.

48 Phillips SM, Green HJ, Tarnopolsky MA, Heigenhauser GF, Hill RE, Grant SM. Effects of training duration on substrate turnover and oxidation during exercise. *J Appl Physiol* 1996; **81**: 2182–91.

49 Henriksson J. Muscle fuel selection: effect of exercise and training. *Proc Nutr Soc* 1995; **54**: 125–38.

50 Holloszy JO. Metabolic consequences of endurance training. In: Horton ES, Terjung RL, eds. *Exercise, Nutrition and Energy Metabolism.* New York: Macmillan, 1988: 116.

51 Winder WW, Hagberg JM, Hickson RC, Ehsani AA, McLane JA. Time course of sympathoadrenal adaptation to endurance exercise training in man. *J Appl Physiol* 1978; **45**: 370–4.

52 Martin WH, Dalsky GP, Hurley BF, Matthews DE, Bier DM, Hagberg JM et al. Effect of endurance training on plasma free fatty acid turnover and oxidation during exercise. *Am J Physiol* 1993; **265**: E708–14.

53 Jansson E, Kaijser L. Substrate utilization and enzymes in skeletal muscle of extremely endurance-trained men. *J Appl Physiol* 1987; **62**: 999–1005.

54 Henriksson J. Training induced adaptation of skeletal muscle and metabolism during submaximal exercise. *J Physiol* 1977; **270**: 661–75.

55 Kiens B, Essen-Gustavsson B, Christensen NJ, Saltin B. Skeletal muscle substrate utilization during submaximal exercise in man: effect of endurance training. *J Physiol* 1993; **469**: 459–78.

56 Henriksson J, Hickner RC. Adaptations in skeletal muscle in response to endurance training. In: Harries M, Williams C, Stanish WD, Micheli LJ, eds. *Oxford Textbook of Sports Medicine,* 2nd edn. Oxford: Oxford University Press, 1998: 45–69.

57 Holloszy JO, Booth FW. Biochemical adaptations to endurance exercise in muscle. *Annu Rev Physiol* 1976; **38**: 273–91.

58 Saltin B, Gollnick PD. Skeletal muscle adaptability. significance for metabolism and performance. In: Peachey L, Adrian RH, eds. *Handbook of Physiology.* Bethesda: The American Physiological Society, 1983: 555–631.

59 Flatt JP. Body composition, respiratory quotient, and weight maintenance. *Am J Clin Nutr* 1995; **62**: 1107S–1117S.

60 Flatt JP. Integration of the overall response to exercise. *Int J Obes Rel Metab Disord* 1995; **19** (Suppl. 4): S31–40.

61 Ballor DL, Keesey RE. A meta-analysis of the factors affecting exercise-induced changes in body mass, fat mass and fat-free mass in males and females. *Int J Obes* 1991; **15**: 717–26.

62 Galbo H. *Hormonal and Metabolic Adaptation to Exercise.* New York: Thieme-Stratton, 1983.

63 Wasserman DH, Lacy DB, Bracy DP. Relationship between arterial and portal vein immunoreactive glucagon during exercise. *J Appl Physiol* 1993; **75**: 724–9.

64 Christensen NJ, Galbo H, Hansen JF, Hesse B, Richter EA, Trap-Jensen J. Catecholamines and exercise. *Diabetes* 1979; **28** (Suppl. 1): 58–62.

65 Wasserman DH, Lickley HL, Vranic M. Interactions between glucagon and other counterregulatory hormones during normoglycemic and hypoglycemic exercise in dogs. *J Clin Invest* 1984; **74**: 1404–13.

66 Wasserman DH, Williams PE, Lacy DB, Goldstein RE, Cherrington AD. Exercise-induced fall in insulin and hepatic carbohydrate metabolism during muscular work. *Am J Physiol* 1989; **256**: E500–9.

67 Horowitz JF, Klein S. Lipid metabolism during endurance exercise. *Am J Clin Nutr* 2000; **72**: 558S–63S.

68 Jeukendrup AE, Saris WH, Wagenmakers AJ. Fat metabolism during exercise: a review. Part I. Fatty acid mobilization and muscle metabolism. *Int J Sports Med* 1998; **19**: 231–44.

69 Henriksson J. Influence of exercise on insulin sensitivity. *J Cardiovascular Risk* 1995; **2**: 303–9.

70 Kjaer M, Bangsbo J, Lortie G, Galbo H. Hormonal response to exercise in humans: influence of hypoxia and physical training. *Am J Physiol* 1988; **254**: R197–203.

71 Mendenhall LA, Swanson SC, Habash DL, Coggan AR. Ten days of exercise training reduces glucose production and utilization during moderate-intensity exercise. *Am J Physiol* 1994; **266**: E136–43.

72 Black AE, Coward WA, Cole TJ, Prentice AM. Human energy expenditure in affluent societies: an analysis of 574 doubly-labelled water measurements. *Eur J Clin Nutr* 1996; **50**: 72–92.

73 Newsholme E, Leech T, Duester G. *Keep on Running.* Chichester: John Wiley & Sons Ltd, 1993.

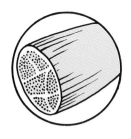

Chapter 1.3
Skeletal Muscle: Physiology, Training and Repair After Injury

MICHAEL KJÆR, HANNU KALIMO &
BENGT SALTIN

Classical reference

Gollnick PD, Armstrong RB, Saltin B, Saubert CW, Sembrowich WL, Shepherd RE. Effect of training on enzyme activity and fiber composition of human skeletal muscle. *J Appl Physiol* 1973; **34**: 107–111.
This reference was the first to report an enhancing effect of endurance training on muscle oxidative enzymes and fiber types in humans. Individuals trained aerobically for 5 months performing 1 h bicycling, 4 days a week at 75% (in the early stage) to 85–90% $\dot{V}o_{2\,max}$ (at the late stage). A significant increase was found in peak pulmonary oxygen uptake rate and this was accompanied by a marked increase in oxidative and glycolytic enzymes (Table 1.3.1). Fiber type distribution of type I (ST) and type II (FT) was not altered significantly by training, but in this study no further subdivision into types IIa or IIb was performed. The study demonstrated a marked ability in skeletal muscle to adapt to physical training with regard to metabolic activity.

Table 1.3.1

	Before	After	Improvement
Oxygen uptake (Vo_{2max}) (L/min)	3.81	4.40	13%
Oxidative enzyme (SDH) (μmol/g)	4.65	9.10	95%
Glycolytic enzyme (PFK) (μmol/g)	28.5	59.0	117%

PFK, phosphofructokinase; SDH, succinate dehydrogenase.

Introduction

Skeletal muscle is composed of two main components: specialized contracting cells, myofibers, and a connective tissue framework formed by fibroblasts. Myofibers are long ribbon-shaped cells of various subtypes with different functional properties. They are surrounded by a distinct basal lamina. Each myofiber is ensheathed by a thin layer of collagenous connective tissue named endomysium. A group of myofibers (from a few tens to a couple of hundred) are bound together by another connective tissue sheath named perimysium and form bundles or fascicles of myofibers. Finally a variable number of bundles are ensheathed by a strong epimysium, which forms the bounding fascia for individual muscles and which continues at the ends of muscles into tendons by which the muscles are attached to the surrounding connective tissue. In addition, motor nerve branches penetrate into the muscle and ultimately divide into axon terminals to innervate each individual myofiber. Sensory nerve fibers enter muscle spindles and convey information about the contraction state of the muscle. Nutrients for the active metabolism of muscle are supplied by an abundant vascular network branching into a rich capillary network around individual myofibers.

The structural organization of human skeletal muscle and its contractile capacity ensure limb stabilization and weight bearing over joints, and allow for active movement of the body[1,2]. Around 40% of total body weight is accounted for by skeletal muscle in an adult human. Skeletal muscle has an amazing ability to adapt to varying workloads, whether increased due to regular physical training, or decreased due to inactivity during injury or disease [3].

Morphology

Muscle cells are derived from mesodermal cells in the somites, which migrate from the parasagittal region into the future sites of individual muscles. These myogenic precursor cells differentiate into myoblasts and begin to synthesize muscle-specific proteins. Important regulators of this process of myogenic differentiation are muscle-specific transcription factors of the myoD family (e.g. MyoD, myogenin and Myf-4) [11a]. Myoblasts fuse into multinuclear myotubes, which form a basal lamina around themselves and begin to synthesize proteins of the contractile apparatus, which will occupy most of the sarcoplasm. Finally, the nuclei move to the periphery of these elongated cells which then display the morphology of fully differentiated myofibers [4] (Fig. 1.3.1).

It is of great importance that some of the myogenic precursor cells do not differentiate, but become localized between the plasma membrane and basal lamina of the myofibers as so-called satellite cells. These serve as reserve cells and are recruited when growth and/or regeneration after injury of myofibers is needed, controlled by mitogenic factors released during growth or upon muscle cell injury [5].

Early in development the motor nerves migrate from the anterior horn cells in the spinal cord to regions where muscle tissue is under formation; this migration is dominated by a high degree of specificity although the details are not fully known. When the developed myofiber and axon terminals meet, acetylcholine receptors spread along the sarcolemma are aggregated into the region of the nerve contact and develop further into the motor endplate or neuromuscular junction (NMJ). In fetal life, axons from several motoneurons can form NMJs on a single myofiber, but later on only one single NMJ remains on each muscle fiber, while the other NMJs undergo degeneration after birth [4].

One motoneuron and the myofibers innervated by its axon terminals form a motor unit, in which myofibers are contracted simultaneously. The number of myofibers which each motoneuron innervates varies considerably depending on the accuracy of movement required. In muscles performing coarse movements like the quadriceps femoris, the number of myofibers per motoneuron is up to 2000, whereas in

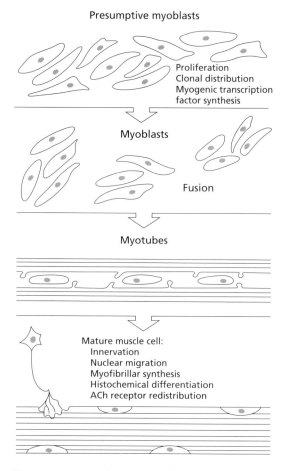

Fig. 1.3.1 Embryonic development and maturation of skeletal muscle cell. Lines illustrate myofibrils, sarcolemma and basal membrane. Nuclei are located intracellularly. Satellite cells are not depicted, but are located outside the sarcolemma and within the basal lamina.

ocular muscles the number is only about 20 per motoneuron. All muscle fibers within a certain motor unit are of the same fiber type (for the properties of different types of fibers, see below). How this differentiation occurs is only partly understood. In mature myofibers, the firing pattern of the innervating motoneuron is traditionally considered to play an important role in fiber type determination [6]. It has been demonstrated that cross-innervation of skeletal muscle (i.e. motoneuron axons from a motor unit containing slow contracting muscle fibers transposed to motor units with fast fibers or vice versa) leads to a change in the fiber type characteristics towards the innervating nerve type. On the other hand, in human fetal muscle fiber types have not yet reached a differentiation level that allows classical fiber type classification. However, more recent molecular biological techniques have demonstrated that even in fetal muscle different types of myoblasts and myotubes exist and thus it is likely that myofibers have already begun their differentiation into fiber types by this stage. These studies demonstrate that during muscle development a selective initial innervation of muscle fibers from specific axons does occur. It is possible that fiber type-specific transmembrane proteins in the sarcolemma can direct axons from spinal motoneurons to muscle cells predisposed to become fast or slow type fibers [7].

Mature muscle cells, which are specialized in the production of force and movement, account for more than 80% of skeletal muscle volume. Muscle cells are elongated and ribbon-shaped, i.e. myofibers, with a diameter of 10–100 μm and a variable length of up to 300 mm. Myofibers are multinucleated due to their formation by fusion of myoblasts, the nuclei of which persist in the mature myofibers and become distributed subsarcolemmally along the whole fiber length. Although this indicates that a high degree of internuclear signaling is needed to allow homogenous cell development, experiments have indicated that muscle cell adaptations to, for example, mechanical loading can vary along the length of the muscle cell. These findings suggest that the individual myonuclei have a certain degree of autonomy.

The cytoplasm of skeletal myofibers, sarcoplasm, contains — as in other eukaryotic cells — the normal set of organelles but in unusually large numbers reflecting the function of the myofiber as a contractile cell. Most of the sarcoplasm is occupied by cytoskeletal proteins organized into regular sarcomeric structures, which extend the whole length of myofibers and which are composed of the two main contractile filaments myosin and actin and their binding and regulatory proteins (for details see [29]). The number of ribosomes, the key organelle of protein synthesis, is relatively low compared with the large amount of proteins present in myofibers, which suggests low turnover rates for many muscle proteins. On the other hand, because muscle cells primarily produce proteins which are used locally,

rough endoplasmic reticulum is also a minor component of the sarcoplasm.

As the mitochondria are responsible for the major (aerobic) part of energy production in myofibers, they contain the enzymes needed for oxidation of substrates and production of ATP. Because active myofibers consume large amounts of energy mitochondria are numerous, although their size and number can vary substantially during the adaptation of a muscle cell to an altered loading pattern, e.g. at the onset of physical training. Mitochondria can transform from single oval organelles into an almost reticular network along the capillaries in physically very well trained individuals. This contributes to an optimal usage of the delivered oxygen in relation to energy production. In extreme situations in highly oxidative fibers the mitochondria can account for more than 10% of the total cell volume [8]. In addition to the aerobic metabolism of substrates, the cytoplasm contains enzymes necessary for the anaerobic formation of ATP from glycogen. Glycogen is stored in abundance in the muscle cell, primarily between myofibrils and adjacent to the sarcoplasmic reticulum [9]. In addition, small lipid droplets are present in sarcoplasm, most abundantly in fiber types with a high oxidative capacity.

Different regions of the sarcomere are named according to their appearance under the microscope. The region that contains myosin is called the A-band (anisotropic appearance in light display) whereas the actin region is called the I-band (isotropic). The region of the A-band where no actin–myosin overlap is present is called the H-band ('helle' means 'light' in German), the thin band, which divides the I-band into two parts, is called the Z-band ('zwischen' means 'in between' in German), and the small band dividing the A-band into two is called the M-band. The sarcomere length is defined as the distance from one Z-band to the next, and serially connected sarcomeres comprise the myofibrils of the muscle, which are arranged in parallel to form the muscle fiber [10,11] (Fig. 1.3.2).

The architecture of the muscle is important for the development of force and for flexibility, in that the muscle force is proportional to the physiologic cross-sectional area of the muscle fibers, whereas the contraction velocity of the muscle is proportional to the muscle length. A more exact description of the

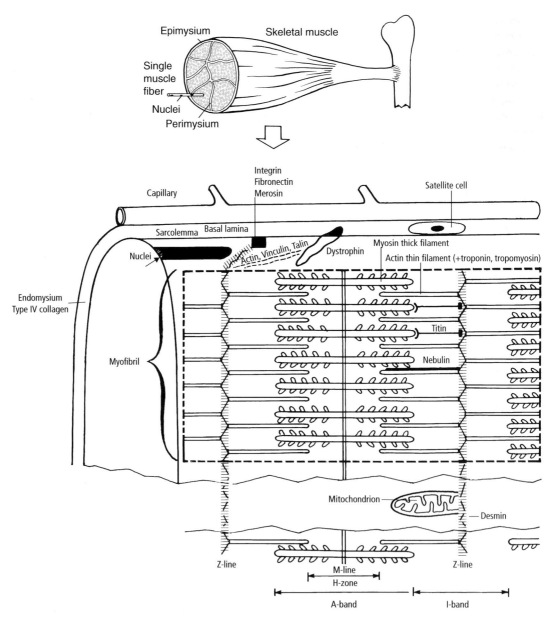

Fig. 1.3.2 Schematic representation of a muscle cell with its cellular structures. Actin and myosin filaments are depicted in detail to illustrate the basis for the contraction process.

relationship between the cross-sectional area and force development requires consideration of the muscle fiber angle compared to the axis for force development (pennation angle). It is evident that fibers that run in the direction of contraction contribute maximal force to the movement, whereas fibers that are at an angle to the work direction will perform a smaller force. However, it has to be taken into account that by angling of the fibers, more fibers are placed within the same muscle bulk, and a larger physiologic cross-sectional area is thereby reached. This means, for example, that the quadriceps and foot plantar flexors have a high physiologic cross-sectional area, with short fibers, and are thereby well suited for large development of force, whereas the hamstring and dorsal flexors of the foot with long muscle fibers and a smaller cross-sectional area are more suited for large movements and ranges of motion. In addition muscles with high pennation angles often experience smaller increases in intramuscular pressure than other muscles (Fig. 1.3.3).

Apart from connecting the muscle to bone, tendon structures are important as energy absorbers, improve the functional movement range of the muscle–tendon complex, and are of importance for the release of elastic energy in explosive movements [1,2]. In skeletal musculature up to 10% of the total content is collagen tissue, and although studies have demonstrated increased turnover of collagen in response to training, the relative amount or even the total content of collagen does not seem to be influenced. The connective tissue in muscle displays passive resistance to stretching, and human models for evaluation of tendon stiffness and stretch-related energy absorption as well as viscoelastic stress relaxation during the static phase have been developed. Repeated stretching of human hamstring muscles results in a shortlived decrease in tissue stiffness. Furthermore, daily stretching exercises over several weeks leads to no change in biomechanical tissue characteristics, but results in an increased range of movement, most likely due to an increased pain tolerance, whereas strength training increases the passive stiffness of the muscle–tendon unit. The load-bearing structures in skeletal muscle during passive stretch are not well defined, and the force transmission is more complicated than previously thought. In addition to the obvious force transmission that occurs in series of muscle–tendon structures, elements of the cytoskeleton are thought to mediate a substantial amount of force transduction in the lateral direction. In support of such a role, individual muscle fibers have been shown not to equal the length of the whole muscle.

Proteins and their function

Muscle proteins can be separated into sarcomeric/ myofibrillar, mitochondrial and cytosolic proteins (Table 1.3.2). The endosarcomeric proteins are dominated by actin-associated (including both actin and troponin and tropomyosin), myosin heavy chain (MHC) and myosin light chain proteins.

These form the two types of contractile filaments. Myosin is an asymmetric molecule with a long twisted root at one end and a more circular arrangement at the other end, and each myosin molecule consists of two heavy and four light chains. Myosin proteins are arranged antiparallel and the molecules are rotated approximately 60 degrees to each other. This results in the characteristic feather-like structure, with parts of the heavy chains sticking out at the ends. It is at this location that the actin binding regions are found, and the myosin heavy chains (MHC) are used for characterization either with immunohistochemistry or via *in situ* hybridization. Actin filaments are thinner than myosin and constructed of actin monomers arranged in an α-helix. Because of this arrangement, a longitudinal cleavage will occur in the filament, in which the regulating protein tropomyosin is located. In addition, the protein troponin is arranged along the actin filament and is responsible for the initiation of the contraction process. Actin and myosin work together during the contraction process, and the filaments are regularly arranged, allowing for some overlap between

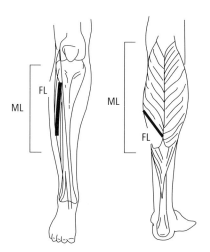

Fig. 1.3.3 Muscle architecture in the lower limb. Whereas dorsiflexors (tibialis anterior) have a high fiber length (FL) to muscle length (ML) ratio and thus are suited for high excursions and velocity, plantar flexors (triceps surae) favor large force production due to their low FL : ML ratio.

Table 1.3.2 Proteins, enzymes and growth/transcription factors in skeletal muscle with tonic stimulation or endurance training.

Gene	Protein	mRNA
Sarcomeric contractile proteins		
Myosin heavy chains		
IIb to IIx to IIa to I	+	+
I to IIa to IIx to IIb	–	–
Myosin light chains		
Fast to slow isoforms	+	+
Actin	?	?
Troponin subunit TnT, TnI, TnC		
Fast to slow isoforms	+	+
Sarcomeric contractile-associated proteins		
Myosin-associated (titin, myomesin, creatine kinase)		
Actin-associated (nebulin, tropomodulin, actinin)		
Z-line-associated (paranemin, synemin, plectin)		
Exosarcomeric cytoskeletal proteins		
Intermediate filaments (desmin, skelemin, vimentin)		
Cytoskeletal anchor proteins (ankyrin, desmin, dystrophin, integrins, syntrophin, talin, vinculin)		
Mitochondrial proteins and enzymes		
TCA cycle enzymes (CS, SDH, MDH)	+	+
Respiratory chain		
nuclear-encoded (cyt-c, NADH/cyt-c)	+	+
mitochondrial-encoded (cyt-ox III, cyt-b)		+
Mitochondrial membrane phospholipid (cardiolipin)	+/–	
Cytosolic proteins and enzymes		
Glycolytic enzymes (HKII, PFK, LDH)	+/–	+/–
Glycogen metabolism (phosphorylase, GS)	– ?	
Fatty acid metabolism (HAD, CAT)	+	
Amino acid metabolism (aminotransferase)	+	+
Myoglobin	+	+
Fatty acid binding protein	+	+
Parvalbumin	+	+
Sarcoplasmic reticulum Ca^{2+}-ATPase (fast to slow isoform)	+/–	+/–
Surface receptors, enzymes and transporters		
N-cadherin	–/+	
Acetylcholine receptor	+	+
Ciliary neurotrophic factor receptor	+	
Beta-adrenergic receptor	+	+
Adenylate cyclase	+	
Insulin-sensitive glucose transporter (GLUT-4)	+	+
Transcription factors and peptide growth factors		
Early response genes (*c-fos, c-jun, egr-1*)	+	+
Myogenic growth factors (MyoD, myogenin)	+	+
Fibroblast growth factors	+	

cyt-ox III, cytochrome oxidase III; CAT, carnitine acyltransferase; CS, citrate synthase; cyt-b, cytochrome-b; cyt-c, cytochrome-c; GS, glycogen synthase; HAD, β-hydroxyacyl coA dehydrogenase; HKII, hexokinase II; LDH, lactate dehydrogenase; MDH, malate dehydrogenase; NADH/cyt-c, nicotinamide adenine dinucleotide (reduced)/cytochrome-c ratio; PFK, phosphofructokinase; SDH, succinate dehydrogenase.

structures, in order for actin and myosin to form cross-bridges and create a contraction [10–12].

A short contraction—a twitch—is initiated via stimuli from motoric centers via myelinated α-motoneurons to the motoric endplate, which ultimately leads to muscle contraction—altogether called exitation–contraction coupling [13]. When the action potential reaches the neuromuscular junction, local calcium channels are opened, enabling potassium-associated initiation of fusion of acetylcholine-filled vesicles with the presynaptic junction cleft, triggering release of transmitter molecules. Other membrane-related proteins such as synapsin and synaptophysin also stimulate vesicle transport and transmitter release. When acetylcholine binds to the receptor on the sarcoplasmic reticulum, several processes are initiated, that all lead to a release of calcium from the sarcoplasmic reticulum, which binds to troponin and results in a cyclic interaction between actin and myosin leading to muscle contraction. The degree of muscle contraction is controlled by the number of motor units activated, and in addition to this the stimulation frequency is modulated and afferent signals from tendon and muscle modify the motoric activity, so that the desired amount of force is achieved [6]. The activation of a muscle fiber via propagation of the action potential does not occur exclusively on the fiber surface, but also across the fiber due to the t-tubuli system. Subsequent activation occurs via recently identified dehydropyridine receptors, which upon activation produce a transmitter substance which enables the sarcoplasmic reticulum system to release Ca^{2+}.

In addition to the contractile myofibrillar proteins, sarcomeric and exosarcomeric muscle proteins exist, including cytoskeletal proteins either as intermediate filaments or as cytoskeletal anchor proteins, which are believed to play an important role in force transmission. Models in which gene expression for some of these proteins is missing will often display decreased muscle function.

Eccentric movements exert high loading forces on the muscle tissue compared with concentric contractions and it is generally accepted that this leads to muscle injury, soreness and elevated serum enzyme levels. Using eccentric exercise on a motor-driven ergometer in humans or eccentric exercise models in animals, it was demonstrated that ultrastructural abnormalities within the myofibrils occurred. These included broadening, smearing or even total disruption of Z-discs, and disorganization of the adjacent A-bands [14] (Fig. 1.3.2).

There is growing evidence that the cytoskeletal protein titin is involved in these ultrastructural changes. Titin is a long elastic molecule which connects M-bands to Z-bands and plays an important stabilizing role for the contractile machinery of skeletal muscle as it is responsible for returning extended sarcomeres to their original length. Another cytoskeletal protein which is damaged by eccentric exercise is desmin, which is responsible for keeping myofibrils in register by connecting neighboring myofibrils at their Z-bands. It has been shown that after only a few minutes of loading desmin immunolabeling is lost in many muscle fibers—preferentially type II fibers. The relative role of cytoskeletal proteins in force transmission during muscle contraction is still debated but dystrophin, titin and desmin are three major proteins that have all been shown to be important (Fig. 1.3.2). The time pattern of morphological changes following eccentric exercise showed that in addition to the loss of desmin staining, fibronectin positive cells (indicative of sarcolemmal disruption) were demonstrated after a few hours. After 3 days some fibers had developed extreme sizes and abnormal shapes and were often invaded by inflammatory cells. In some cases also fibers expressing fetal myosin were found as a sign of regeneration, i.e. the injury had activated satellite cells and these had produced 'new sarcoplasm' where embryonic myosin isoforms were expressed [15,16].

Eccentric loading leads to a reduced capacity of the muscle to perform tetanic contraction, and the muscle strength can be reduced by more than 50% after damaging exercise. The lowest value is obtained either immediately or 1–2 days after exercise, and the muscle gradually recovers strength over 7–14 days [17]. Interestingly, this decrease in force is not related to pain as electrically stimulated contraction is also reduced. Furthermore it has been demonstrated that initial force reduction and especially recovery time is markedly reduced after training or even a few accustomizing bouts of exercise. The fact that some studies demonstrate a further loss in force for up to 2 days after exercise indicates that contraction triggers events that further decrease muscle performance. Muscle shortening and thus reduction in the range of motion can also accompany eccentric exercise, most likely related to abnormally high levels of Ca^{2+} in the sarcoplasma, and may be complicated by increased water content. In addition to this, the eccentric exercise results in delayed-onset muscle soreness (DOMS) which reaches a maximum 1–2 days after exercise, and is described as a dull, aching pain combined with tenderness and stiffness. The tenderness is frequently localized in the region of the distal myotendinous junction, but can also be generalized throughout the muscle. Although there is an inflammatory response with macrophage accumulation and prostaglandin release, and thus sensitizing type III and IV pain afferents, the true explanation for DOMS remains undiscovered.

Mitochondrial proteins are crucial for oxidative capacity of the muscle (see Chapter 1.2) and whereas in endurance training gene expression and protein formation for the different enzymes roughly corresponds to the number of mitochondria, during muscle hypertrophy in response to resistance training the relative content of mitochondrial enzymes either remains constant or decreases. Studies have indicated that tonic contractile activity stimulates expression of protein-coding genes, and interestingly, several mitochondrial complexes require a coordinated expression of genes within both the nuclear and mitochondrial compartments.

Cytosolic proteins are important not only for anaerobic fuel combustion but also for transportation of oxygen and the contraction process. Physical activity is shown to increase gene expression for enzymes involved in both lipid and amino acid metabolism. Glycolytic enzyme gene expression is shown to decrease in animal models, whereas enzyme activity can be shown to increase in human models. GLUT-4 exists both in the cytosol and located in the surface membrane and rises with contraction, and likewise gene expression for several surface receptors increases with activity. Myogenic transcription factors that are important during development and regeneration have also been shown to be activated in relation to mechanical loading of muscle.

Using gene expression and protein formation as markers for adaptive responses to loading, it is important to note that transcription and translational processes are influenced by several factors (Fig. 1.3.4). Firstly, an increase in protein synthesis may be due to and preceded by an increase in mRNA levels. However, it has to be noted that mRNA is subject to degradation as well as processing. Secondly, if the translational efficiency increases, protein formation can increase disproportionately to changes in mRNA. Whereas the levels of mRNA and protein can be determined for several of the factors discussed, the detailed transcriptional processes prior to mRNA formation, and especially the translational steps involved, have only been described to a minor degree for enzymes, proteins and other factors involved in adaptive responses to exercise.

The messengers and signal transduction pathways involved in exercise are complex. Changes in intracellular Ca^{2+} concentration activate or repress signaling pathways for a variety of cellular responses. Changes in energy charges or phosphorylation potential may initiate changes in gene expression, and—though less well investigated—the redox state may also prove important in this process.

Mechanical stretch is well known to cause a hypertrophic response in cardiac muscle, mediated via autocrine and paracrine effects of peptide hormones. In myotubes stretch is found to change Na^+/K^+-ATPase

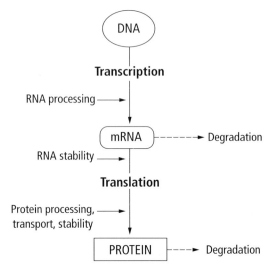

Fig. 1.3.4 Schematic representation of protein synthesis to illustrate events occurring in skeletal muscle and steps at which gene expression can be controlled.

and phospholipase activity and activate growth factors, but MHC slow isoforms have also been shown to be induced by stretching.

During force development under isometric conditions, the maximal force is dependent upon the sarcomere length, so that optimal force is achieved when optimal contact and thus overlap between actin and myosin is reached (length–tension relationship) [18]. In addition, a relationship between magnitude of force and contraction speed exists (force–velocity relationship) (Fig. 1.3.5).

When the muscle is activated to overcome a resistance smaller that its maximal tetanic force, the muscle will shorten under the occurrence of a concentric contraction. The relationship between force and velocity follows a steep rectangular hyperbolic curve, indicating that force decreases markedly with increasing velocity [19].

This is related to the force by which cross-bridges between actin and myosin can be coupled and uncoupled. The higher the velocity in a contraction, the more myosin heads are in a state in which they are not tightly bound to actin, and thus cannot contribute to the development of large muscle force. The speed in which a certain force can be developed is trainable, and this may have great importance in rehabilitation and in patients with reduced muscle force, since it is not only the maximal force that an individual can produce which is crucial, but also the speed at which a certain force can be achieved. The higher the contraction speed, the more myosin heads will not reach an actin and thus will not develop the required force.

Muscle contractions that result in shortening of the muscle are concentric, whereas contractions of muscle accompanied by lengthening are eccentric in nature. The magnitude of external resistance to movement vs. the development of torque produced by a muscle will determine whether there is a change in velocity during the movement and thus whether there is going to be a positive acceleration (speed increase) or a negative acceleration (deceleration or braking of the movement) independently of whether the contraction is concentric or eccentric. Interestingly, it can be debated whether isometric muscle contraction in fact is in accordance with the definition that no change in muscle length has occurred. As isometric or static contraction is normally defined by lack of change in external movement (e.g. over a joint), the fact that connective tissue of tendons is elastic will allow for a shortening of the muscle, and thus a concentric contraction, in the absence of any detectable external movement. Eccentric exercise is not only an important part of normal locomotion, but attracts special attention as this work mode results in the most dramatic changes in muscle with regard to factors such as absorption of power, both in relation to training and with injury.

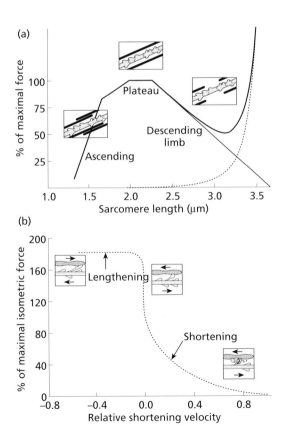

Fig. 1.3.5 Relationship between (a) sarcomere length and contraction force and (b) force–velocity relationship during different types of muscular contractions.

Fiber types

Within the individual motor units muscle fibers with specific characteristics exist with regard to contractile, histochemical and metabolic activity. Furthermore, muscle fibers from a given motor unit are known to be located over a relatively large area of the cross-sectional area of the muscle (up to 25%), indicating that within a given small muscle region all fibers represented in the muscle will be present. Two main categories of motor unit exist, one of which possesses a relatively slow timewise development of maximal force (slow twitch) and the other a fast development of maximal force (fast twitch) [10a, 20,21] (Fig. 1.3.6). With the use of histochemical characterization of skeletal musculature, determining myofibrillar AT-Pase activity and incubating at varying pH levels, three main fiber types were originally described: type I, type IIa and type IIb (now known to be identical to myosin heavy chain classification IIx, which will be used in the rest of this chapter). These are distinctly different from each other with regard to contractility, morphology and metabolic characteristics. Type I fibers are slow contracting, are more red in appearance, and are well equipped for oxidative metabolism, with regard to both enzyme and substrate content. In contrast type II fibers are fast contracting and more white in colour and contain more glycolytic enzymes and fewer oxidative enzymes than type I fibers [22–24].

More recent techniques have allowed refinement of our characterization of muscle fibers and determination of the myosin heavy chain (MHC) isoforms has allowed the demonstration of type I β-slow, type IIa and type IIx as well as several muscle fibers coexpressing two or all three of these isoforms [25]. The MHC-IIb isoform has been demonstrated in species other than humans, and for practical purposes the MHC type IIx is equivalent to the ATPase-stained type IIb fiber (Fig. 1.3.7).

During physical activity, activation of the different muscle fibers is known to depend on the intensity and duration of the work. Intense short-lasting activities involve mainly the type IIx fibers, whereas low-intensity prolonged exercise primarily activates type I fibers and type II fibers are first involved at a later time point when type I fibers have depleted their carbohydrate stores. The distribution of fiber types varies between individual muscles in both the upper and lower extremities, and some muscles are dominated by slow-twitch type I fibers (e.g. the soleus) whereas others possess up to 80% fast-twitch type II fibers (e.g. the

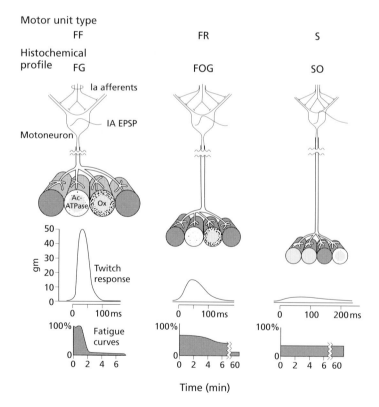

Fig. 1.3.6 Three types of muscle fibers representative of separate motor units in the cat. The different motor units are characterized by recruitment pattern, metabolism, twitch characteristics and fatiguability. FF, fast-fatiguable; FR, fast-resistible; S, slow; FG, fast-glycolytic; FOG, fast-oxidative-glycolytic; SO, slow-oxidative.

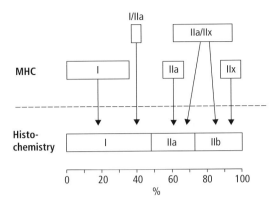

Fig. 1.3.7 Comparison of the fiber type composition in sedentary individuals determined by single-fiber analysis of myosin heavy chain (MHC) composition and myofibrillar ATPase histochemistry in biceps brachii muscle.

Table 1.3.3 Contraction speed (in sarcomere length units per second) of single fibers from human muscle with varying degrees of slow vs. fast fibers (Harridge, personal communication).

	Soleus	Vastus lateralis	Triceps brachii
Type I	0.27	0.29	0.27
Type I/IIa	–	0.67	0.64
Type IIa	1.25	1.10	1.20
Type IIa/IIx	–	1.83	1.73
Type IIx	–	2.24	2.31

triceps brachii). Within a single muscle the relative distribution of the fiber types can vary, but probably not by more than 10–15% between regions. The interindividual variation in muscle fiber type distribution is primarily genetically determined, and studies of mono- and dizygotic twins have shown a close to similar fiber type distribution in monozygotic (r^2 around 0.9), but not in dizygotic twins.

Furthermore, a certain fiber type (e.g. type I) from human musculature displays similar contractile patterns independent of the anatomic position (Table 1.3.3). This indicates that the characteristics of a human muscle are dependent on the relative contribution of the different fiber types rather than on variations in characteristics within a certain muscle fiber type. Although this thight correlation exists for isolated muscle fibers it cannot be extrapolated to whole muscle. However, use of the muscle plays a major role. It has been shown that the specific tension of the muscle fiber is reduced after, say, 42 days of bedrest. Surprisingly, a reduction in specific tension has also been demonstrated after monotonous use of the muscle at a low intensity, as occurs in extreme endurance training.

Muscle fiber plasticity

The plasticity of muscle can in general be classified according to the ability to change either (i) the quantity (i.e. hypertrophy) or (ii) the type of protein (i.e. isoform or phenotype) of the different cellular components of the muscle cell. The muscle cell may respond to loading by increasing the cross-sectional area with no change in the proportion of the different muscle proteins and their expression, and will in this case increase its maximal force but maintain its other inherent functional properties such as contractile speed or endurance [26]. If on the other hand the training results in altered expression in the type of protein (e.g. altered expression of MHC isoforms of the myofibrils) the muscle may also change its intrinsic contractile properties. In real life, responses to training may often be a combination of a change in the amount of protein and the type of protein isoform it expresses. A change in isoforms of proteins means in this situation a slight variation in the amino acid composition, whereby structure, function or enzymatic properties are influenced [3,27,28].

To allow for muscle plasticity to occur, both the protein turnover and the protein synthesis rate have to be taken into account, and the protein half-life will be the important determinant of the time needed to achieve an alteration in muscle plasticity. Whereas some proteins have a relatively long half-life and therefore turnover time, others have a short half-life and thus allow a more rapid adaptation in response to training (e.g. days for glycolytic enzymes). Evidently, a rapid adaptation requires not only a short half-life for the protein but also a high protein synthesis rate in order to allow for synthesis to match or even surpass protein degradation. Furthermore, the time frame for muscle adaptation to training will be fully dependent on the different steps of gene expression, and pretranslational, translational and post-translational regulation often occurs at different time intervals dependent

Table 1.3.4 Muscle fiber characteristics into functional units (based on myosin heavy chain isoforms).

Properties	I	IIa	IIx
Myofibrillar ATPase	Low	Moderately high	High
SR Ca^{2+}-ATPase	Low	Moderately high	High
Glycolytic enzymes	Moderately high	Moderately high	High
ATP buffering enzymes	Moderately high	Moderately high	Moderately high
High-energy phosphate levels	High	High	Very high
Oxidative enzymes	High	High	Moderately high
Blood flow	High	High	Moderately high
Fatiguability	Low	Moderate	Moderate
Contractile speed	Slow	Moderately fast	Fast

on the stimulus and the protein involved (Table 1.3.4).

The mechanisms behind mechanical loading resulting in altered gene expression and thus altered protein content are not clear. Several potential messengers generated within contracting skeletal myofibers are illustrated in Table 1.3.2. The acetylcholine released from the motor nerve binding to its receptor, and the subsequent release of Ca^{2+} from the SR and resulting myofiber contraction can either itself or by generating other intracellular messengers activate signals for altered gene expression in response to mechanical loading. These additional messengers can either be linked to receptor-linked pathways or stretch-dependent pathways, or be a part of the metabolic changes associated with the contraction. What has been shown so far is that resistance training decreases the Ca^{2+} concentration needed to elicit 50% of maximal tension, decreases MHC IIx gene expression, and increases contractile proteins in parallel, all of which together allows greater absolute workloads to be moved [29,30].

Furthermore, serum response element 1 of the skeletal α-actin promoter has been identified as part of the mechanotransduction pathway involved in enhancing actin gene transcription, which results in muscle enlargement (Table 1.3.2). Endurance training, on the other hand, increases and decreases the maximal shortening velocity of individual slow and fast fibers, respectively, both changes contributing to improved endurance performance. Expression of several genes is increased with training, and a complex interaction with and between modulators such as nerves,

cytokines, autocrine/paracrine substances, hormones, temperature, circulatory changes and fluid shifts within muscle takes place and is far from understood in relation to training of skeletal muscle [29,30].

With the use of immunohistochemical and molecular biological techniques for determination of MHC isoforms and thus characterization of fiber types, it has been demonstrated that endurance training can cause a fiber type shift from type IIx to IIa. Although animal studies using long-term low-frequency electrical stimulation of muscle have been able to demonstrate a fiber type shift from II to I, it is more questionable to what degree such a shift can occur in human skeletal musculature in relation to training. It is most likely that such a transformation can occur in humans, as is indicated by findings from long-term electrical stimulation of paralyzed muscle and observations on translocated muscle used for cardiomyoplasty, but obviously extremely long-term loading is required. Thus, it must still be concluded that a high relative content of type I fibers in an endurance athlete is due to genetic rather than training-induced factors.

Termination of training or inactivity rapidly reverses the described training-induced changes in skeletal muscle. Loss of enzymes occurs most rapidly, followed by loss in muscle mass and finally a shift in muscle fiber type towards IIx. At extreme degrees of long-term inactivation (e.g. in spinal cord patients) a complete fiber type shift occurs from type I and IIa to type IIx. Inactivity leads to a loss in muscle mass initially due to both increased degradation and decreased synthesis of myofibrillar protein, followed by a period dominated by increased degradation, and only after 30 days of inactivity is a new and lower steady-state level for protein turnover reached. The degree of muscle atrophy with inactivity depends upon the relative reduction in activity [31]. Thus, antigravity muscles undergo a more pronounced degree of atrophy than other muscles. If muscle is rehabilitated after inactivity the morphology and characteristics of the muscle can be restored relatively fast in comparison with other structures like tendon and bone [32].

Endurance training markedly improves oxidative mitochondrial enzyme content and activity, which is important for both fatty acid oxidation, the TCA cycle and the respiratory chain. Values for oxidative enzyme content of 3–4 times normal as well as reticulum-formed mitochondria can be obtained in elite endurance athletes [8,33–36]. Whereas maximal training effects of type I fibers can be obtained with low and moderate workloads, a somewhat higher training intensity is required to obtain training adaptation of type II fibers (e.g. interval training). Whereas oxidative enzyme level can alter with training independent of fiber type specific myofibrillar isoforms, the fiber type composition in the individual muscle is of major importance for the content of glycolytic enzymes. The time course for adaptation of metabolic enzymes is shorter than for phenotypic changes of skeletal muscle [33,34].

Physical loading of muscle can be achieved either by passive stretching or by development of voluntary or electrically induced muscle force. Depending upon which loading the muscle is subjected to, an adaptation will occur in the form of either increased muscle mass, increased metabolic capacity or alteration in fiber types. In order to differentiate between different types of training they are mainly categorized into either endurance (low resistance, many repetitions) or resistance (high load, few repetitions) training or combinations of the two, which is typically what is seen within different sports events. Changes in muscle force are in general achieved with workloads that exceed 50–60% of the maximal strength expressed either as maximal voluntary contraction (MVC) in isometric exercise or the performance of one maximal bout of dynamic contraction (1 RM = repetition of maximum). In addition, the determination of maximal force developed at a certain angle-speed is used during isokinetic exercise. Although this latter form of contraction does not

fully reproduce the force produced during normal movements, it often correlates with maximal movement performed during functional activities and sports. The connection between the number of repetitions (in dynamic work) or holding time (in static work) and the relative workload varies extensively from muscle to muscle dependent upon the fiber type composition, in that a larger number of type I fibers will shift the curve to the right. For more practical reasons the curve can be used to conclude that a resistance that can be performed dynamically 10–15 times before fatigue develops or a static resistance that can be maintained for less than a minute corresponds to around 70% relative workload.

Whereas changes in the nervous activation of the musculature can improve the performance of the muscle, changes in the muscle tissue force are primarily due to a muscle fiber hypertrophy. Although occasional reports have suggested that strength training can cause hyperplasia, the increase in muscle force is due to an increased muscle cross-sectional area (Fig. 1.3.8). In addition to this it has to be acknowledged that determination of anatomical cross-sectional area in many muscles may underestimate the increase in physiologic cross-sectional area due to the altered pennation angle of the muscle fibers after a training period (see Chapter 1.4 for details). Furthermore, it has been demonstrated that contractile proteins (e.g. myosin light chains) may also alter composition and thus contribute to the fact that training can result in increased contractility force of single muscle fibers in excess of what can be explained by fiber hypertrophy. By determination of maximal muscle force and electromyography the relative contribution in general of fiber hypertrophy and increased neural activation of the muscle can be determined. This principle is used for estimation of maximal contraction force in patients who cannot develop maximal voluntary force due to fatigue or pain. Short-lasting electrical contractions (twitches) on top of voluntary activation can be used for estimation of the true maximal muscle force in an individual. By stimulation at different degrees of voluntary contraction it is possible to estimate the maximal muscle strength, and, for example in elderly individuals, a marked portion of the interindividual variability in maximal voluntary strength can in fact be ascribed to variation in ability to contract the muscle voluntarily.

At the onset of strength training, the dominant factor in strength improvement is an increased neural activation, which causes activation of more motor units and thereby recruitment of more muscle fibers. In addition to this, a more synchronized recruitment of motor units occurs. The neural improvement with training is most pronounced in the first 4–6 weeks of a training period, and interestingly, this effect is evident also in the contralateral extremity, whereas no crossover effect is observed with regard to structural muscle tissue adaptation [37].

Muscle fiber hypertrophy is first evident and measurable after 4–6 weeks, but data indicate that rates of transcription and formation of contractile proteins begin increasing within days into a training period. Muscle strength can be improved markedly over a short period of time (around 1% per day within the first 10–12 weeks). With static training the development of maximal force seems to play a more important role than the number of repetitions for the training effect achieved. Similarly, in dynamic exercise the most pronounced effects are evident with resistance training programs containing six or fewer repetitions per training series prior to fatigue (Table 1.3.5). These findings obviously have to be matched to the initial capacity of the individual prior to training, and thus the realistic possibilities of carrying out high-intensity training. Interestingly, muscle strength training can be carried out even at an advanced age, and it is quantitative rather than qualitative differences that are characteristic of the training responses seen in elderly as compared to young individuals. In general it is believed that the cross-sectional area of type I muscles can improve ~50% with training whereas type II fibers enlarge by 100% of their initial area. More and more evidence points towards the satellite cells being involved in providing genetic material for myofibrillar protein formation and thus the development of hypertrophy.

If training is carried out with low resistance but with a high number of repetitions, no marked strength improvement will be found, whereas muscle endurance will be improved markedly. Muscle strength training decreases mitochondrial and capillary density in the muscle due to a marked increase in the amount of contractile proteins. Furthermore, whereas strength training will not influence concentrations of glycolytic

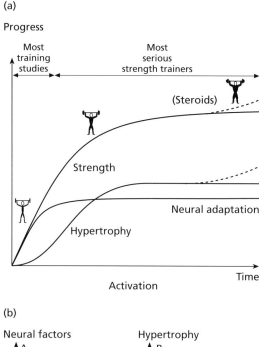

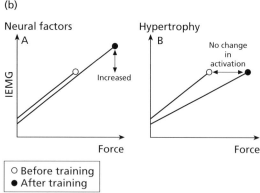

Fig. 1.3.8　(a) Response of muscle force to intensive training. (b) The difference in neural improvement or muscle hypertrophy.

enzymes and only slightly increases the amount of enzymes catalysing energy-rich phosphate compounds, muscle endurance training will markedly increase the capillary density, the number of mitochondria and the amount of glycolytic enzymes. The training effects are specific, and depend on the type of training program, and the transfer value is limited. This concept is important in rehabilitation, where movement patterns and contraction types should be tailored specifically to the functional aim.

Table 1.3.5 Improvements in performance following 10 weeks of dynamic or isometric training in humans.

Muscle endurance training (% improvement) Testing	Static (60%, 5 s, 10–150/day, 35 days)		Dynamic (60%, 10–150/day, 35 days)
Static force	4–11		0
Static endurance	84–122		0
Dynamic force	2–6		29
Dynamic endurance	41–92		630–5040
Strength training (% improvement) Type of training	Program	Static force	Dynamic force
Static	100%, 5 s,×20, 45 days	35	0
Dynamic	50–80%, 6×10, 30 days	0	370

Injury and repair

Skeletal muscle injuries can be divided into two basic types.

1 In a less severe *in situ* necrosis type of injury only the myofibers are damaged, whereas the basal lamina and the mysial sheaths are not breached. In its mildest form such an injury occurs in eccentric exercise and more extensive *in situ* necrosis can be caused for example by ischemia as seen in compartment syndrome or after injection of local anesthetic (e.g. bupivacaine). Repair after *in situ* necrosis can be virtually complete.

2 In a shearing type of injury not only are the myofibers breached but their connective tissue sheaths and intramuscular blood vessels are also torn to a variable extent. Healing after a shearing injury is complicated by the scar formation and complete restoration of the muscle is usually not possible [38,39].

Following muscle damage several proteins are released into serum. One of the most commonly used markers of muscle injury is creatine kinase (CK) which is generally detectable 1–2 days post injury and can remain elevated for 5–6 days after prolonged strenuous exercise. Most of the measured CK is caused by the muscle-specific isoenzyme CK-MM. Carbonic anhydrase III (CA-III) and myoglobin (Mb) are more specific to muscle than total CK is, and the profile differs. CA-III is present in type I fibers only and Mb peaks immediately after long-distance running, making them suitable for markers of acute events. It must be acknowledged that a large variability exists with regard to interindividual differences in responses of

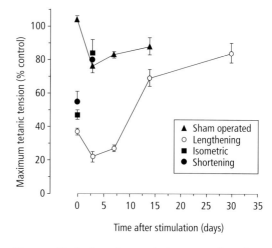

Fig. 1.3.9 Decline in performance in the recovery phase after isometric, dynamic contraction and lengthening contraction.

these muscle damage markers, and that only an indicative relationship between degree of muscle damage and serum markers can be demonstrated.

The exact mechanism behind the cascade of changes associated with eccentric exercise is not clear, but free oxygen radicals and inflammatory processes are suggested to play a role. Two major hypotheses have been proposed to explain damage to skeletal muscle associated especially with eccentric exercise. The first emphasizes metabolic overload, where the ATP demand surpasses the production, leading to a vicious cycle of Ca^{2+} overloading of the cell and further decrease in ATP production. Intracellular calcium activates phospholipase which in turn is involved in a subsequent breakdown of the cell membrane—explaining the fiber necrosis occurring days later—and causes an activation of the arachidonic acid cascade and the production of prostaglandins. The other hypothesis stresses mechanical factors as a cause of exercise-induced muscle damage, pointing out the relatively low metabolic cost but the high mechanical strain per muscle fiber during eccentric exercise. In support of the latter, mechanical disruption of the sarcolemma has been demonstrated immediately after exercise. It has been found that training of a specific muscle group diminishes the structural changes, strength reduction and clinical manifestations associated with eccentric exercise (Fig. 1.3.9). With regard to the cause of muscle injury in eccentric exercise, more recent data have suggested that the decline in force after eccentric contraction is related more to the magnitude of muscle strain than to the stress imposed upon the fibers. Putting this finding into perspective, it is likely that strain results in muscle fiber membrane disruption and subsequent proteolysis or conformational changes of the cytoskeletal network. A candidate could be the calcium-activated protease calpain which uses desmin as a substrate, and is activated by increased intracellular Ca^{2+} concentration. It can be hypothesized that muscle fiber strain increases calcium influx and intracellular Ca^{2+} via stretch-activated channels or disruption of t-tubuli or sarcoplasmic reticulum.

In more extensive *in situ* necrosis type of injuries, as in the compartment syndrome, the myofibers become necrotized within their intact basal lamina over a variable length, in the most severe cases the entire length of the myofiber. Both the basal lamina and the connective tissue framework of different mysial sheath remain intact. The satellite cells are remarkably resistant to different types of injury, including ischemia, and they become activated after the insult has subsided and the regeneration process has been initiated. The basal lamina provides the scaffold within which the regeneration can proceed without major disturbing effects. The production of new myofiber to replace the necrotized part follows in general the same sequence as the formation of skeletal muscle during development (see above). The myoblasts fuse into myotubes which are also able to fuse with the surviving parts of the injured

myofiber and thereby restitution of the entire myofibers and bridging over the entire necrotized segment may occur [15,16,39].

A shearing type of muscle injury may be caused by a strain, contusion, laceration or incision, in which myofibers together with their basal membrane, and their mysial sheaths are ruptured to a variable degree, and thus the functional continuity of the tendon–muscle–tendon complexes is disrupted. In these injuries the spontaneous contraction of the transected myofibers results in the formation of a gap between the stumps of the ruptured fibers, which forms the central zone (CZ) of the injury (Fig. 1.3.10). Due to the rich vascularization of skeletal muscle, hemorrhage from the torn vessels fills up the gap and this hematoma is later replaced by a connective tissue scar.

The injury breaches the plasma membrane of the myofibers and thus exposes sarcoplasm to the extracellular space, initiating necrosis in the injured myofibers inside the preserved though ruptured original basal lamina. The extension of the necrosis along the ruptured myofiber must be halted to prevent destruction of the entire fiber. This is implemented by condensation of cytoskeletal material, which forms a so-called contraction band at a distance of approximately 1–2 mm from the rupture. This band acts as a barrier in the protection of which a demarcation membrane, i.e. a new plasma membrane, is formed and thereby the integrity of the myofiber, though divided into two parts, is restored. The necrotized part will be regenerated, i.e. it forms the regeneration zone (RZ) of the injury, which is delineated from the survival zone (SZ), where myofibers survive with certain reactive changes [15,16].

Blood-derived inflammatory cells gain immediate access to the injury site and substances released from the necrotized area serve as chemoattractants for further extravasation of inflammatory cells. Polymorphonuclear leukocytes of the acute phase are soon followed by monocytes, which are transformed into macrophages and begin to phagocytose the necrotic debris both in the RZ within the original basal lamina cylinders and in the CZ.

The regeneration pattern after shearing muscle injury follows a remarkably uniform scheme. Satellite cells become activated by mitogenic factors derived from the necrotic tissue and by growth factors secreted

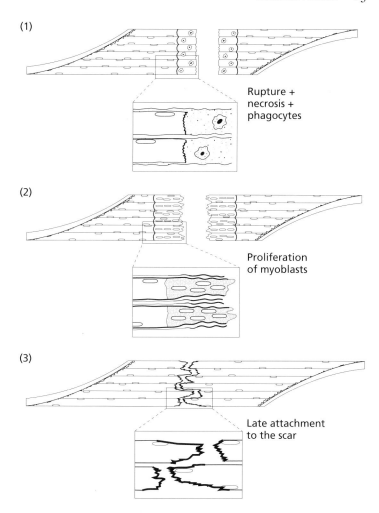

(1)

Rupture +
necrosis +
phagocytes

(2)

Proliferation
of myoblasts

(3)

Late attachment
to the scar

Fig. 1.3.10 Responses to a laceration
trauma in rat muscle. See text for further
explanation.

by macrophages. Experimental studies have suggested that sarcolemmal contact exerts a preventive effect upon satellite cell proliferation. This could explain why only the damaged parts of a fiber with injured sarcolemma respond with regeneration. On the other hand, it has been suggested that satellite cells from the surviving part are also recruited to the RZ. Several growth factors, including insulin-like growth factor I (IGF-I), transforming growth factor β (TGF-β) and basic fibroblast growth factor (bFGF), affect regeneration by either stimulation or inhibition of proliferation, and differentiation of satellite cells depending on the stage of regeneration. For example, bFGF response is coupled to plasma membrane wounding and occurs early in the regeneration, whereas IGF-1

released from the satellite cell itself is thought to stimulate differentiation, which is followed by TGF-β-mediated inhibition of the differentiation process. However, it has to be acknowledged that most data on the involvement of growth factors in the regeneration process after muscle injury, derive from *in vitro* experiments, while results in humans are still almost non-existent.

The activated satellite cells begin to proliferate at about 24 h post injury within the preserved basal lamina in the RZ. The satellite cells differentiate into myoblasts. This is associated — in not only developing but also regenerating muscle — with expression of myogenic transcription factors of the *myoD* gene family (MyoD, myogenin, Myf5, Myf6), which determine the differentiation of the precursor cells along the myogenic lineage by inducing the production of muscle-specific proteins. Myoblasts fuse with each other into multinucleated myotubes. The regenerated muscle cells fill the original basal lamina cylinder of the RZ by approximately day 5, whereafter they extend out of the opening of this basal lamina into the connective tissue of CZ (see below). Proximally the myotubes fuse with the preserved myofibers of the SZ. The regenerating myofibers gradually acquire their mature form with bundles of myofilaments which become organized into regular sarcomeres thereby giving the myofiber its cross-striated appearance. Furthermore, myonuclei assume their normal subsarcolemmal localization [15,16].

The early phase of the regeneration process after shearing injury up until about day 5 is almost identical to that seen after *in situ* necrosis, because it occurs within the basal lamina scaffold. Thereafter, the ends of the regenerating fibers need to enter the connective tissue scar of CZ. This creates a situation in which regeneration of the injured myofibers and formation of the connective scar tissue between the stumps are two simultaneous processes which are at the same time dependent upon but also at odds with each other. On the one hand, the scar is needed to keep the stumps together and it provides the connective tissue with which the ends of the regenerating myofibers can re-establish the firm myofiber to extracellular matrix (ECM) attachment. On the other hand, if the connective tissue scar formation between the stumps is excessive it may impede regeneration of myofibers and reinnervation of the so-called abjunctional stumps (see below).

Within the first day after muscle injury the hematoma between the ruptured myofibers is invaded by inflammatory cells including phagocytes which begin disposal of the blood clot. Blood-derived fibrin and fibronectin cross link to form a primary matrix, which acts as a scaffold and anchorage site for the invading fibroblasts and gives the initial strength to the scar to withstand the forces applied on it. Fibroblasts begin to synthesize both proteins and proteoglycans of the ECM. Fibronectin, collagen type III and tenascin are among the first ECM proteins to be expressed, followed later by production of type I collagen which remains elevated for several weeks. Parallel to the deposition of ECM proteins, the tensile strength of the scar increases. Biomechanical tests have shown that upon pulling, regenerating muscle ruptures at the scar between the stumps until day 10. Thereafter the scar is stronger than the muscle tissue and the rupture occurs within myofibers close to their ends, at the site where the rupture most often occurs also in healthy muscle.

The ends of the regenerating fibers attempt to pierce through the scar tissue from day 5 onwards and maintain a growth cone appearance until about day 10–14. During this active growth period the regenerating fibers reinforce their integrin-mediated adhesion to the ECM (Fig. 1.3.10) on their lateral surfaces in both the intact (SZ) and the regenerating (RZ) parts of the myofibers. This lateral adhesion reduces movements of the stumps and the pull on the still fragile scar, and thus apparently reduces the risk of rerupture. Furthermore, lateral adhesion allows for the use of the injured muscle before complete healing has been achieved. Interestingly, reinforcement of lateral adhesion does not occur if muscle is immobilized after injury, indicating that signals of mechanical stress must be transduced from the surrounding ECM to induce this reinforcement. On the other hand, integrins appear to transduce signals of mechanical stress, which affect the synthesis of ECM proteins in the connective tissue cells, thereby regulating the composition of the surrounding ECM. It is likely that integrin-transduced signals are essential also in regulating various cellular functions in regenerating myofibers. Thus, the increased expression of integrins is more important for enhanced signal transduction in the drastically altered mechanical stress situation in ruptured myofibers than for adhesion as such. These molecular findings support the importance of early mobilization during rehabilitation after muscle injuries.

Around day 14 new myotendinous junctions are formed at the end of regenerating myofibers with clustering of integrin- and dystrophin-associated molecules. Having re-established firm terminal adhesion, myofibers no longer require reinforced lateral adhesion, and integrin and vinculin on the lateral sarcolemma decrease whereas immunoreactivity for dystrophin-associated molecules increases. Thus, these two complexes of adhesion molecules seem to have complementary roles in myofiber–ECM adhesion. Gradually the imposed scar diminishes in size, bringing the stumps closer to each other, and finally myofibers become interlaced. However, full fusion of the stumps does not occur, as indicated from high levels of integrins, for up to 9 months after the injury. Thus it appears that injuries resulting in the division of a muscle into two halves will result in persisting interposed scar tissue in the muscle. The volume of the interposed scar also appears to have significance for reinnervation, and the myogenically denervated abjunctional stumps are reinnervated by axons sprouting from nerves in the adjunctional stumps on the contralateral side of the scar. These thin axons are able to pierce through the scar and induce formation of new neuromuscular junctions on the abjunctional stumps. If the interposed scar is too dense or voluminous the sprouts may be unable to penetrate through it and the abjunctional stumps remain denervated, undergo neurogenic atrophy and are replaced by connective tissue. The processes occurring during regeneration are influenced by mobilization. As an example, adhesion protein complexes have been shown to respond after just a single bout of exercise with regard to transcription and mRNA formation, whereas the protein synthesis rate increases after repetitive exercise bouts only [15,16,40].

Muscle ruptures due to a sports injury can also be complicated by rupture of intramuscular nerve branches, which leaves parts of the muscle denervated. Because in such an injury the nerve itself is damaged, the denervation and consequent atrophy of myofibers is neurogenic. In shearing injury parts of the ruptured myofibers may also become myogenically denervated. This occurs because each myofiber is innervated at a single neuromuscular junction located within the middle third of the myofiber, and the transection of the fiber often leaves the neuromuscular junction on one of the muscle fiber stumps.

Finally, it has been shown that myoblasts grown in a non-moving culture system proliferated with random orientation, whereas cells which were cyclically lengthened and shortened became aligned and synthesized more protein [41]. This indicates that mechanical stress or at least strain has a pronounced effect on the myoblast maturation process, and demonstrates the importance of lengthening–shortening activity in rehabilitation after injury.

Summary

Skeletal muscle represents a unique tissue with multinuclear cells and a variety of proteins responsible for mechanical function and energy supply, allowing stability and active movement. Muscle possesses an enormous ability to adapt to various types of mechanical loading and training. Increased loading results in enhanced protein turnover and in a higher net synthesis of both myofibrillar and mitochondrial components, and hypertrophy of the individual muscle cell occurs. Furthermore, muscle fiber types can alter with mechanical loading, favoring a more oxidative fiber type. Conversely, inactivity causes rapid loss of muscle tissue and oxidative capacity in a reversible fashion. Muscle fibers depend on cytoskeletal and extracellular matrix proteins present within and around muscle fibers in order to optimally transmit force, and overloading can result in both cytoskeletal damage and muscle cell rupture damage. Satellite cells play an important role in regeneration of muscle tissue, under the influence of mechanical stretching and active loading. Complex cellular and molecular regulation lies behind the response of muscle proteins to changes in contractile activity, and responses are modulated by factors as nerves, growth factors, hormones, temperature, circulation and fluid shifts. Such signaling pathways are just beginning to be identified.

Multiple choice questions

1 *Prolonged endurance training results in increased oxidative capacity of the muscle and in:*
a a fiber type shift from type I to type II
b no shift at all
c a fiber type shift from type IIb/IIx to type IIa
d a fiber type shift from type II to type I.

2 *The primary function of the satellite cells involves:*
a synthesis of oxidative enzymes
b connection of motor nerves to the sarcolemma
c acting as a reservoir for formation of myoblasts and myofibrillar structure in injury and supplying genetic material for myofibrillar protein formation in strength training
d formation of extracellular matrix proteins.

3 *Tropomyosin is important for:*
a enabling motoneuron excitation
b blocking of calcium uptake by the mitochondria

c inhibition of actin and myosin interaction

d stimulation of cross-bridge shortening.

4 *Resistance training results in the following adaptation(s) in skeletal muscle:*

a hyperplasia and hypertrophy

b increased levels of oxidative enzymes and hypertrophy

c hypertrophy

d fiber type I formation and hypertrophy.

References

1 Lieber RL, Leonard ME, Brown-Maupin CG. Effects of muscle contraction on the load-strain properties of frog aponeurosis and tendon. *Cell Tissues Organs* 2000; **166**: 48–54.

2 Trestik CL, Lieber RL. Relationship between Achilles tendon mechanical properties and gastrocnemius muscle function. *J Biomechan Eng* 1993; **115**: 225–30.

3 Saltin B, Gollnick PD. Skeletal muscle adaptability. significance for metabolism and performance. In: Peachey LD, ed. *Handbook of Physiology*. Bethesda: American Physiological Society, 1983: 539–54.

4 Jansen JKS, Fladby T. The perinatal reorganization of the innervation of skeletal muscle in mammals. *Prog Neurobiol* 1990; **34**: 39–90.

5 Bischoff R. Interaction between satellite cells and skeletal muscle fibers. *Development* 1990; **109**: 943–52.

6 Milner-Brown HS, Stein RB, Yemm R. The contractile properties of human motor units during voluntary isometric contractions. *J Physiol* 1973; **228**: 285–306.

7 Miller JB, Stockdale FE. Developmental origins of skeletal muscle fibers; clonal analysis of myogenic cell lineages based on expression of fast and slow myosin heavy chains. *Proc Natl Acad Sci* 1986; **83**: 3860–4.

8 Kirkwood SP, Munn EA, Brooks GA. Mitochondrial reticulum in limb skeletal muscle. *Am J Physiol* 1986; **251**: C395–C402.

9 Hultman E. Physiological role of muscle glycogen in man, with special reference to exercise. *Circulation Res* 1967; **21**: 99–112.

10 Huxley AF, Niedergerke R. Structural changes in muscle during contraction. Interference microscopy of living muscle fibers. *Nature* 1954; **173**: 971–3.

10a Edgerton VR, Smith JL, Simpson DR. Muscle fibre type populations of human leg muscles. *Histochem J* 1975; **7**: 259–66.

11 Huxley HE, Hanson J. Changes in the cross-striations of muscle during contraction and stretch, and their structural interpretation. *Nature* 1954; **173**: 973–6.

11a Eftimie E, Brenner HR, Buonanno A. Myogenin and MyoD join a family of skeletal muscle genes regulated by electrical activity. *Proc Natl Acad Sci* 1991; **88**: 1349–53.

12 Dominguez R, Freyson Y, Trybus KM, Cohen C. Evidence that myosin neck bending is taking place during muscular contraction. *Cell* 1998; **94**: 559–71.

13 Hill AV. The heat of shortening and the dynamic constants of muscle. *Proc Royal Soc London* 1938; **126**: 136–95.

14 Friden J, Sjöström M, Ekblom B. Myofibrillar changes following intense eccentric exercise in man. *Int J Sports Med* 1983; **4**: 170–6.

15 Kääriäinen M, Kääriäinen J, Järvinen TLN, Sievänen H, Kalimo H, Järvinen M. Correlation between biomechanical and structural changes during the regeneration after laceration injury of skeletal muscle. *J Orth Res* 1998; **16**: 197–206.

16 Kääriäinen M, Kääriäinen J, Järvinen TLN, Nissinen L, Heino J, Järvinen M, Kalimo H. Integrin and dystrophin associated adhesion protein complexes during regeneration of shearing type muscle injury. *Neuromusc Disord* 2000; **10**: 121–32.

17 McCully KK, Faulkner JA. Injury to skeletal muscle fibers of mice following lengthening contractions. *J Appl Physiol* 1985; **59**: 119–26.

18 Gordon AM, Huxley AF, Julian FJ. The variation in isometric tension with sarcomere length in vertebrate muscle fibers. *J Physiol* 1966; **184**: 170–92.

19 Katz B. The relation between force and speed in muscular contractions. *J Physiol* 1939; **96**: 45–64.

20 Bodine SC, Roy RR, Eldred E, Edgerton VR. Maximal force as a function of anatomical features of motor units in the cat tibialis anterior. *J Neurophysiol* 1987; **6**: 1730–45.

21 Burke RE. Motor unit types of cat triceps surae muscle. *J Physiol* 1967; **193**: 141–60.

22 Buchthal F, Schmalbruch H. Spectrum of contraction times of different fibre bundles in the brachial biceps and triceps muscle of man. *Nature* 1969; **22**: 89–91.

23 Peter JB, Barnard RJ, Edgerton VR, Gillespie CA, Stempel KE. Metabolic profiles on three fiber types of skeletal muscle in guinea pigs and rabbits. *Biochemistry* 1972; **11**: 2627–733.

24 Thompson WJ, Sutton LA, Riley DA. Fibre type composition of single motor units during synapse elimination in neonatal rat soleus muscle. *Nature* 1984; **309**: 709–11.

25 Schiaffino S, Gorza L, Sartore S, Saggin L, Ausoni S, Vianello M, Gundersen K, Lomö T. Three myosin heavy chains isoforms in type 2 skeletal muscle fibres. *J Musc Res Cell Motil* 1989; **10**: 197–205.

26 Chahine KG, Baracchini E, Goldman D. Coupling muscle electrical activity to gene expression via cAMP-dependent second messenger system. *J Biol Chem* 1993; **268**: 2893–8.

27 Baldwin KM, Klinkerfuss GH, Terjung RL, Mole PA, Holloszy JO. Respiratory capacity of white, red and intermediate muscle, adaptive response to exercise. *Am J Physiol* 1972; **222**: 373–8.

28 Salmons S, Henriksson J. The adaptive response of skeletal muscle to increased use. *Muscle Nerve* 1981; **4**: 94–105.

29 Booth FW, Baldwin KM. Muscle plasticity: energy demand and supply processes. In: Rowell LB, Shepherd JT, eds. *Handbook of Physiology*, Section 12. Oxford: American Physiological Society, 1996: 1075–123.

30 Williams RS, Neufer PD. Regulation of gene expression in skeletal muscle by contractile activity. In: Rowell LB, Shepherd JT, eds. *Handbook of Physiology*, Section 12. Oxford: American Physiological Society, 1996: 1125–50.

31 Williams P, Goldspink G. Change in sarcomere length and physiological properties in immobilized muscle. *J Anat* 1978; **127**: 459–68.

32 Thomason DB, Herrick RE, Surdyka D, Baldwin KM. Time course of soleus muscle myosin expression during hindlimb suspension and recovery. *J Appl Physiol* 1987; **63**: 130–7.

33 Gollnick PD, Armstrong R, Saubert C, Piehl K, Saltin B. Enzyme activity and fiber composition in skeletal muscle of untrained and trained men. *J Appl Physiol* 1972; **333**: 312–9.

34 Gollnick PD, Armstrong RB, Saltin B, Saubert CW, Sembrowich WL, Shepherd RE. Effect of training on enzyme activity and fiber composition of human skeletal muscle. *J Appl Physiol* 1973; **34**: 107–11.

35 Henriksson J, Reitman J. Time course of changes in human skeletal muscle succinate dehydrogenase and cytochrome oxidase activities and maximal oxygen uptake with physical activity and inactivity. *Acta Physiol Scand* 1977; **99**: 91–7.

36 Henriksson J. Training induced adaptation of skeletal muscle and metabolism during submaximal exercise. *J Physiol* 1977; **270**: 677–90.

37 Moritani T, Devries HA. Neural factors versus hypertrophy in the time course of muscle strength gain. *Am J Phys Med* 1979; **58**: 115–30.

38 Hurme T, Kalimo H, Sandberg M, Lehto M, Vuorio E. Localization of type I and III collagen and fibronectin production in injured gastrocnemius muscle. *Lab Invest* 1991; **64**: 76–84.

39 Hurme T, Kalimo H. Adhesion in skeletal muscle during regeneration. *Muscle Nerve* 1992; **15**: 482–9.

40 Henry MD, Campbell KP. A role for dystroglycan in basement membrane assembly. *Cell* 1998; **11**: 859–70.

41 Vandenburg HH. Dynamic mechanical orientation of skeletal myofibers in vitro. *Dev Biol* 1982; **93**: 438–43.

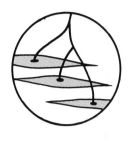

Chapter 1.4
Neuromuscular Aspects of Exercise — Adaptive Responses Evoked by Strength Training

PER AAGAARD & ALF THORSTENSSON

Classical reference

Ikai M, Steinhaus AH. Some factors modifying the expression of human strength. *J Appl Physiol* 1961; **16**: 157–163.

Heavy-resistance strength training generally results in both neural and muscular adaptations. Muscle hypertrophy was already recognized in the late 1800s and has since then been extensively documented at whole-muscle, muscle-fiber and muscle subcellular levels. About the same time it was observed that substantial gains in muscle strength could occur without any detectable changes in the muscle itself, particularly in the early stages of the training regime. (Recent methodologic developments have, however, demonstrated early changes to occur in RNA translation and transcription.) The logical conclusion was that the improvements in strength had to be accounted for by neural adaptations. This assumption required there to be a margin, or force reserve, in the muscle that would not be accessible with a normal maximal voluntary effort due to neural inhibitory mechanisms. Another assumption would be that these mechanisms could be overcome, disinhibited, by adaptations in the nervous system occurring as a result of strength training.

Ikai and Steinhaus reported one of the first convincing demonstrations of the existence of such a muscular reserve of force inherent to the muscle, and thus the presence of inhibitory mechanisms. They showed that the static strength of the arm flexor muscles could be substantially increased above that voluntarily achievable 'by a loud noise, by the subject's own outcry, by certain pharmacologic agents, and by hypnosis'. In Fig. 1.4.1 (original figure) the strength output during repeated maximal voluntary efforts, is shown with and without a preceding gunshot or shout. Similar effects on strength were seen with the other interventions. The authors conclude that all their observations 'support the thesis that the expression of human strength is generally limited by psychologically induced inhibitions' and that the interventions decreased these inhibitions. They also emphasize the large variation between subjects in response to the interventions. They particularly point out one subject who showed no increase in strength under hypnosis. This subject was an 'experienced weight-lifter' and the interpreta-

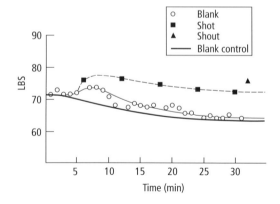

Fig. 1.4.1 Strength output, expressed in pounds (LBS), measured by Ikai & Steinhaus during repeated static contractions of the arm flexors [1].

tion was that 'he was able, probably because of long training, to approximate his physiological limit in the waking state', thus suggesting a trainability of this neural phenomenon.

The existence of a margin for improvement in strength by neural adaptations has since been convincingly demonstrated by other methods, such as electrical stimulation applied directly onto the muscle or to the nerve supplying it. By similar means, a smaller margin has been noted in trained athletes. In addition to the accumulation of indirect evidence for neural adaptations, particularly in the initial phase of a training program, more direct evidence for such adaptations has also emerged. Perhaps the most thought-provoking evidence has been obtained in experiments where the contractions have been only intended, and no activation of the muscles has actually occurred, as verified by electromyographic recordings[1a]. Still, significant improvements in strength were seen (the hypothenar muscles of the hand were investigated) of a magnitude similar to that obtained with conventional 'effortful' contractions. The authors conclude: 'These force gains appear to result from practice effects on central motor programming or planning'. Strength gains were also detected for the corresponding muscles of the opposite hand. Such transfer of training effects, presumably of neural origin, has been frequently documented in the literature. Obviously, these findings have interesting implications for rehabilitative training of unilateral neuromuscular injuries.

Introduction

The assessment of maximal muscle strength

For more than seven decades the contractile strength of human skeletal muscle *in vivo* has been evaluated by use of various types of dynamometers. Early mechanical devices allowed muscle contraction strength to be determined during isometric (static) contraction conditions. In addition, *in vivo* mechanical muscle performance was assessed in dynamic contractions using sophisticated flywheel methodology [2,3]. With the evolution of motor-driven dynamometers it became possible to obtain maximal muscle strength during concentric (shortening) and eccentric (lengthening) muscle contractions. Both isokinetic and non-

isokinetic dynamometers have been used to evaluate the dynamic strength properties of human muscle *in vivo*. While the isokinetic dynamometer is designed to keep joint angular velocity constant, non-isokinetic dynamometers allow acceleration and speed to vary freely throughout the movement. Non-isokinetic dynamometers have been used mainly to examine the strength capacity of the elbow flexors [4,5] and knee extensors [6–8]. These muscles have also been extensively investigated by use of isokinetic dynamometry [9–12] in addition to a large number of other human skeletal muscles [13,14].

The descriptive and clinical relevance of assessing maximal muscle strength by use of isokinetic dynamometry may not seem obvious at first hand. Even though the term 'isokinetic' denotes that joint angular velocity is kept constant (which may itself not always be true) [15], this does not imply that any constancy should exist for the linear velocity of muscle shortening or lengthening. Furthermore, due to the variation in muscle lever arm length(s) throughout the range of joint movement, the recorded moment may not resemble the actual contractile force generated by the muscle [15]. In addition, neuromuscular activation may be reduced under certain loading conditions (e.g. eccentric contractions) and a coactivation of antagonist muscles can also occur. This applies to isokinetic dynamometry as well as to all other types of strength measurements. In result, inconsistent and conflicting moment–velocity relationships may be found in the literature with marked differences observed between studies and muscles examined [14] as well as between subject groups of different training status [16]. Nevertheless, isokinetic dynamometry does appear useful for evaluating the expression of maximal voluntary muscle strength *in vivo*. Firstly, joint angular velocity and movement range can be reproduced with reasonable accuracy. In the experimental set-up this means that multiple trials can be performed and compared successively until reaching a given selection criterion. Secondly, the fact that joint movements are accurately reproduced ensures that the change in muscle strength induced by specific interventions (training, detraining) can be evaluated in a reliable way. Thus, it is important to recognize that a change in maximal isokinetic strength may be a valid indication of the underlying change in maximal muscle force, as for a given subject the relation between joint angular velocity and muscle contraction velocity or between the measured muscle moment and the underlying muscle force is not likely to change. Thirdly, and perhaps most importantly, modern isokinetic dynamometers allow for a standardized and well-controlled evaluation of maximal eccentric muscle strength. This aspect of *in vivo* muscle function deserves special attention as it not only appears to comprise unique mechanisms of neuromuscular activation and inhibition but also involves factors of importance for dynamic joint stability and stiffness.

A hyperbolic relationship exists between the contractile force and velocity of shortening of isolated muscle *in vitro* [17,18] (Fig. 1.4.2). Similar hyperbolic force–velocity relationships may be observed during *in vivo* contraction of human skeletal muscle [4,5,12]. However, force–velocity relations that were clearly non-hyperbolic have been reported as well [11,14,19]. Beyond any doubt the quadriceps femoris has been most extensively used to investigate the maximal contractile strength (moment of force) generated by human skeletal muscle, *in vivo*. The appearance of isokinetic (i.e. constant velocity) dynamometers has allowed maximal dynamic muscle strength to be obtained during standardized and easily reproducible experimental conditions (see above). While some studies obtained the peak moment of force ('torque') exerted within the total range of movement [20–24] others have recorded the moment of force at a specific knee joint angle [11,19,25] or performed both types

of measurements [12,26–28]. Concentric isokinetic quadriceps peak moment occurs at gradually more extended knee joint positions with increasing joint angular velocity [12,14,29]. Accordingly, the corresponding moment–velocity relationship consists of moment values obtained at different parts of the quadriceps length–tension curve. Nevertheless, the moment–velocity pattern based on angle-specific moment appears to deviate most markedly from a hyperbolic curvature at least when obtained in untrained subjects, as reflected by a levelling-off ('plateauing') of moment at low angular velocities [11,14,19,25,26,28,30–32] (see Fig. 1.4.3). A similar plateauing of moment of force during slow concentric contraction has been reported for other muscle groups than the quadriceps, e.g. the arm flexors [9,33]. Interestingly, maximal arm flexor and extensor moments plateaued in subjects of low maximal muscle strength, whereas no plateauing could be demonstrated in subjects of high strength [33] suggesting that this phenomenon can be modulated by strength training. This plateauing in slow concentric muscle strength has previously been hypothesized to arise from a force inhibiting neural mechanism, reducing the level of neural efferent motor drive [11,19].

Maximal eccentric contraction strength is equal to or up to about 40% higher than maximal isometric strength when recorded in the human quadriceps muscle, *in vivo* [26,27,34–36]. In contrast, maximal eccentric contraction force is 50–100% greater than

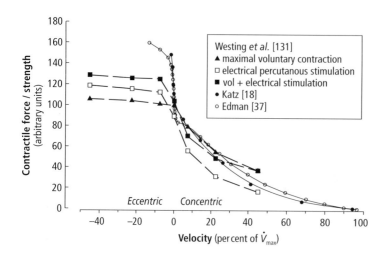

Fig. 1.4.2 Contractile force – velocity relationships obtained for shortening (concentric) and lengthening (eccentric) contractions in isolated *in vitro* preparations of whole muscle [18] and single muscle fibers [37] obtained from the frog. Superimposed curves show muscle strength measured *in vivo* during maximal voluntary activation and/or when percutaneous electrical stimulation was applied to the quadriceps femoris muscle [131].

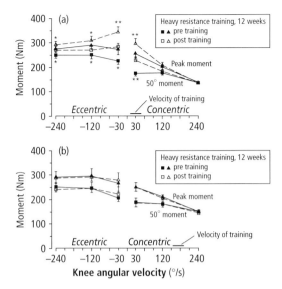

Fig. 1.4.3 Maximal concentric and eccentric quadriceps muscle strength obtained as isokinetic peak moment (triangles) and angle-specifc moment generated at 50° knee joint angle (squares) before and after 12 weeks of (a) heavy resisitance strength training; and (b) low-resistance, high-velocity strength training using concentric contraction alone. Closed and open symbols denote pre- and post-training values, respectively. Adapted from [26].

isometric or slow concentric force when obtained in isolated muscle preparations [18,37] (see Fig. 1.4.2). Reduced levels of neuromuscular activation are one likely reason for this apparent deficit in maximal eccentric muscle strength, *in vivo*. Consistent findings of a marked increase in maximal eccentric muscle strength following heavy-resistance strength training strongly suggest this mechanism of suppressed neural activation to be modifiable with training.

Changes in maximal muscle strength in response to strength training

The influence of strength training on the maximal contraction strength of human muscle *in vivo* has been extensively investigated for the concentric part of the moment–velocity curve [10,20,23,26,30,39,40]. Also, data exist for the training-induced change in maximal eccentric muscle strength [26,39–46].

Following concentric strength training, maximal muscle strength and power have been reported to increase at the specific velocity employed during training

[4,6,7,10,30]. These and similar observations have been taken to indicate a specificity of training velocity and training load. However, it is questionable whether a generalized concept of training specificity should exist, since muscle strength has been reported to increase also at velocities lower than the actual velocity of training [20,23,47,48] as well as at higher velocity [6,39,48]. The conflicting findings of specific as well as non-specific training adaptations probably arise, at least partly, due to a varying influence of learning [49]. While training and data collection have often been performed on the same dynamometer, other studies have emphasized the use of different training and measuring devices. The latter approach is intended to reduce the influence of learning, in order to obtain a more valid measure of the neuromuscular adaptations induced by strength training.

The levelling-off (plateauing) in muscle strength observed during slow concentric contraction has been reported to disappear in response to heavy-resistance strength training [26,30] (see Fig. 1.4.3). These findings point to the existence of a neural force-inhibiting mechanism, which can be modulated by training. Interestingly, strength training using lower loads and higher speeds appears to have no effect [26] (see Fig. 1.4.3), suggesting that heavy training loads should be employed when intending to remove this force-inhibiting mechanism.

Marked increases in maximal eccentric muscle strength have been observed following heavy-resistance strength training [26,39–46,50–52]. Eccentric or coupled concentric–eccentric training seems to evoke greater strength gains than concentric training alone [39,41–43,51]. Importantly, maximal eccentric strength appears to remain unchanged after low-resistance strength training [26,51] (see Fig. 1.4.3). Thus, the exertion of very large muscle forces during training is probably a major prerequisite for any change in maximal eccentric muscle strength to take place.

Neuromuscular adaptations evoked by strength training

The adaptive changes observed in the neuromuscular system in response to specific types of strength training may be differentiated into neural and muscular factors. Thus, it is well known that changes in contractile properties, i.e. increases in maximal contraction force and power as well as in the maximal rate of force development, can occur not only due to alterations in muscle morphology [53] but also as a result of changes in the nervous system [54,55].

Neural adaptation mechanisms may involve changes in motoneuron recruitment and/or rate coding, more synchronized motoneuron firing patterns within the muscle itself as well as between muscle synergists, changes in spinal motoneuron excitability, and altered coactivation of antagonist muscles [54–57]. Early evidence, indicating neural mechanisms to play a significant role, was based on the findings that muscle strength increased more than could be accounted for by increases in muscle size alone [58] and that strength gains were observed with no detectable muscle hypertrophy [20,59–62]. More direct evidence has been provided with the use of electromyography (EMG), although inherent methodologic limitations may exist with the recording of surface EMG during voluntary muscle contraction. To overcome these problems, measurements of evoked spinal responses (H-reflex, V-wave) can be used to examine various aspects of neural adaptation evoked by strength training. In terms of muscle morphology, single muscle fiber area and whole-muscle area and volume have been demonstrated to increase following prolonged regimes of strength training [63]. In addition, based on the refinement of various *in vivo* muscle imaging techniques (MRI, ultrasonography), recent evidence suggests that muscle architecture in terms of muscle fiber pennation angle may also be altered, in turn contributing to the increase in physiologic muscle fiber area and contractile force generation with strength training [207]. The evaluation of muscle myosin heavy chain (MHC) content by use of electrophoretic analysis or immunochemical methods has provided a sensitive measure of the change in myosin isoform composition evoked by strength training. The emergence and evolvement of these methods have allowed an intensified focus on the change in muscle fiber composition induced by strength training and its impact on mechanical muscle performance.

During static as well as dynamic contraction conditions, active muscle stiffness is determined by the total number of attached acto-myosin cross-bridges [64] while also being strongly influenced by the pattern of neural activation [65]. Thus, the increase in muscle size and/or neural innervation observed following strength training, in turn causing more cross-bridges to be attached during contraction, will have a strong positive effect on the ability to achieve high levels of muscle stiffness. In functional terms this effect would be beneficial over the whole movement spectrum, from athletes performing rapid and forceful movements to elderly individuals compensating for unexpected postural perturbations.

The present chapter presents the involvement of various mechanisms and aspects of importance for the neuromuscular adaptation to strength training.

Adaptive changes in neural drive evaluated by electromyography

EMG signal amplitude

The electromyography (EMG) signal is constituted by the composite sum of all the muscle fiber action potentials present within the pick-up volume of the recording electrode(s). At the same time, this overall interference signal is modified by a multitude of intracellular and extracellular factors, which all exert a significant influence on the pattern of spatial and temporal summation of the single action potentials [66,67]. Acceptable test–retest reliability has been demonstrated for the EMG amplitude and power frequency obtained by use of surface electrodes [68]. Data based on intraclass correlation (ICC) analysis indicate that most of the variance in assessing reliability is among subjects rather than between days or trials [68]. For the human quadriceps femoris muscle, acceptable reproducibility was observed for the EMG recorded during static as well as dynamic contraction, including isokinetic knee extension [61,69,70,71]. Thus, with proper recording conditions and validated signal processing techniques, the surface electromyogram appears to be a useful tool for both clinical evaluation and research [68].

From a physiologic perspective the EMG signal can be seen as a complex combination of (i) motor unit recruitment, (ii) variation in firing frequency (rate coding), and (iii) synchronization between firing patterns of individual motoneurons [56]. EMG recording (Figs 1.4.4 and 1.4.18) has been widely used to quantify the neural changes evoked by strength training. A majority of studies has demonstrated increased EMG

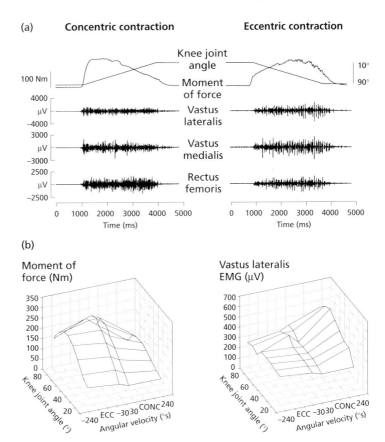

Fig. 1.4.4 (a) Raw tracings of isokinetic knee joint moment and electromyography (EMG) signals obtained in an untrained male subject during maximal concentric (left) and eccentric (right) contraction of the quadriceps femoris muscle. (b) Maximal concentric and eccentric quadriceps muscle strength (left) and vastus lateralis EMG (right) measured in 15 untrained male subjects and displayed as a function of knee joint angle and joint angular velocity. Negative and positive velocities denote eccentric and concentric muscle contraction, respectively [50].

signal amplitude after strength training, indicating a rise in the neural efferent drive to the muscle fibers [43,45,50,61,72–78,86,242,243]. Importantly, neural drive has been found to increase not only in previously untrained subjects but also in highly trained strength athletes [76]. Thus, EMG increased when strength athletes used heavy training loads (above 80% of maximum), but decreased when training was performed at lower loads (70–80% of maximum) [76]. These findings suggest that heavy training loads should be used when seeking optimal neural enhancement.

It is important to notice that the increase in surface EMG amplitude observed following strength training does not provide any conclusive evidence *per se* of the differential change in motoneuron recruitment, firing frequency or synchronization. In addition, it has not always been possible to demonstrate increases in EMG with strength training [79–82]. It should be recognized

therefore that electrode positions as well as skin and muscle tissue properties (i.e. subcutaneous fat layer, muscle fiber pennation angle, etc.) may vary from one recording session to another despite careful measuring procedures. Moreover, the compound surface EMG signal can constitute a summation of several thousand action potentials, causing a significant portion of the signal to be inherently stochastic [67]. Consequently, the sensitivity of the EMG signal as a measure of training effects depends highly on the EMG processing routines used, i.e. sampling rate, filtering algorithms, cut-off frequencies, etc. However, many of the problems inherent with surface EMG can be reduced or even eliminated by use of more sophisticated EMG techniques (recording of intramuscular EMG using indwelling needle or wire electrodes, H-reflex and V-wave measurements, evoked cortical potentials, etc.) as described elsewhere in this chapter.

Motoneuron firing frequency

Two basic questions can be raised: is motoneuron firing frequency influenced by strength training; and if that is the case, what is the functional significance?

To address the latter question first, motor unit discharge rates have been recorded at much higher frequencies than needed to achieve full tetanic fusion in force. Thus, transient firing frequencies of 60–200 Hz were reported in brief bursts of activity during maximal voluntary contraction of human muscles *in vivo* [83–86]. Muscle innervation frequency influences not only the magnitude of contractile tension but also the rate of tension rise (i.e. rate of force development: RFD = Δforce/Δtime), as observed for whole muscle *in situ* [87], single muscle fibers [88,89] and human muscle *in vivo* [90–92]. When individual motor units were examined in the neonatal rat [93] it was noticed that RFD continued to increase at stimulation rates higher than the stimulation rate at which maximum tetanic tension was achieved [92] (Fig.1.4.5). Similar findings have been reported for whole-muscle preparations [87]. Corresponding results have been obtained for human musculature *in vivo*, as stimulation rates of 100 Hz were able to produce greater RFD, but not a greater peak isometric force, than 50 Hz stimulation rates [90]. Thus, the appearance of very high (i.e. supramaximal) firing frequencies likely serves to increase maximal RFD rather than increasing maximal contraction force *per se* [55,56] thereby causing a significant rise in contractile force in the initial phase of contraction (0–250 ms). Importantly, at the onset of contraction the occurrence of discharge doublets in the firing pattern of single motoneurons (interspike interval <5–10 ms, firing frequency >100–200 Hz) cause a marked increase in contractile force and/or RFD [87,91,94]. Thus, muscle force was markedly increased by addition of an extra discharge pulse ('doublet') as demonstrated during constant frequency stimulation of single motor units and whole isolated muscle [94,95] as well as in intact human muscle [96]. This phenomenon has been referred to as the catch-like property of skeletal muscle [95–97]. Interestingly, the occurrence of discharge doublets in the firing pattern of individual motor units was found to increase six-fold (from 5.2% to 32.7%) following ballistic resistance training [86] (see Training for 'explosive' muscle strength, Fig. 1.4.20 below).

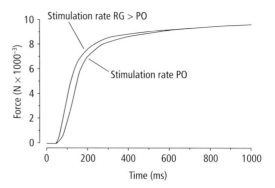

Fig. 1.4.5 Single force–time curves recorded in isolated motor units in the rat soleus muscle using an innervation frequency that elicited maximal tetanic fusion and maximal contraction force (PO) compared to when even greater (i.e. supramaximal) innervation frequencies were used (RG) which also elicited maximal tetanic fusion, however at an elevated rate of force development. Adapted from [92].

The maximal firing frequency of human muscle *in vivo* has been examined by use of intramuscular EMG recording techniques, which allow the firing pattern of single motor units to be identified. Based on such techniques, the maximal firing frequency obtained in the rectus femoris muscle during maximal voluntary contraction (MVC) was 20% greater in trained elderly weight lifters compared to age-matched untrained individuals [98]. Furthermore, using a longitudinal study design maximal firing frequency has been found to increase after strength training of selected hand muscles [99] and leg muscles (vastus lateralis [100], tibialis anterior [86]). Following 12 weeks of ballistic-type resistance training Van Cutsem and coworkers reported a dramatic rise in the firing frequency of single motor units recorded in the tibialis muscle at the onset of maximal, forceful contraction. Mean firing frequencies of 98.0, 75.1 and 58.0 Hz were observed in the first three interspike intervals, respectively, which increased to 182.1, 127.9 and 130.3 Hz following the period of training [86] (Fig. 1.4.6). Interestingly, training-induced increases in maximal motoneuron firing frequency appear to occur in both young and elderly individuals. Although elderly subjects initially demonstrated a lower maximal discharge rate than young subjects, no difference could be observed after strength training [99,100]. These data

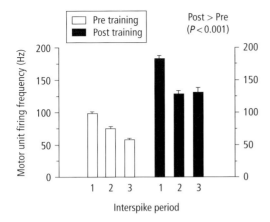

Fig. 1.4.6 Motoneuron firing frequency at the onset of contraction, obtained in the tibialis anterior muscle before and after a period of strength training. A marked increase in instantaneous firing frequency was observed following training, as all post-training values were greater than pre-training values ($P<0.001$). Data adapted from [86].

show that maximal motoneuron firing frequency can be increased in response to strength training, and that this adaptation may overrule the age-related decline in maximal discharge rate.

As depicted from the S-shaped relationship between firing frequency and contraction force [101], an increase in maximal firing frequency can result in a relatively greater increase in surface EMG amplitude compared to the corresponding increase in maximal contractile force [67]. In consequence, training-induced increases in EMG may exceed the increase in maximal muscle strength [45,50], although this is not always a consistent finding [41,43]. Obviously, such disproportionate changes in EMG and force with training do not provide any conclusive evidence for an increase in motoneuron firing frequency, as similar effects would be caused by more synchronized patterns of motoneuron firing (see below).

Motoneuron synchronization

Synchronization in the firing patterns of different motoneurons has been examined by use of EMG cross-correlation analysis techniques, to quantify the degree of temporal association between the discharge signals [102]. Based on such techniques, studies have shown

that the synchronization of motoneuron firing can be altered by learning [101], which suggests that changes in synchronization may also occur as an adaptive response to strength training.

Even though an increased incidence of synchronization between the firing patterns of different motor units within the muscle may occur with strength training [103], the advantage of such intramuscular synchronization, if any, remains unsolved [56]. Studies using artificial nerve stimulation have shown that at submaximal contraction intensity, muscle force is greater with asynchronous than synchronous stimulation [104,105]. In addition, RFD in brief maximal contractions was higher during voluntary (i.e. asynchronous) contractions as compared to evoked tetanic (i.e. synchronous) contractions [91]. However, synchronous stimulation may not adequately mimic *in vivo* muscle contraction, where the occurrence of discharge doublets at the onset of contraction may yield a marked increase in RFD (see above).

Milner-Brown and coworkers [103] found that the discharge patterns of single motor units were more synchronized to the overall interference signal recorded by surface EMG following 6 weeks of strength training. As derived from single motor unit recording, observations of more synchronized firing patterns in weight lifters compared to skill-trained and untrained individuals [106] support the notion that motor unit synchronization can be altered by strength training. Moreover, a longitudinal increase in synchronization between synergistic muscle pairs has been observed following ballistic strength training [57], suggesting that intermuscular synchronization may also change as an adaptive response to strength training.

An increase in motor unit synchronization induced by training is likely to result in a disproportionate increase in EMG amplitude, due to increased superposition of action potentials whose amplitudes are in phase and reduced summation of out-of-phase action potentials. Consequently, the peak-to-peak amplitude of the compound EMG signal is increased along with a decrease in median power frequency (MPF) [57,106a].

Motoneuron properties, evoked reflex responses

Only a few studies have employed measurements of evoked spinal motoneuron responses to examine

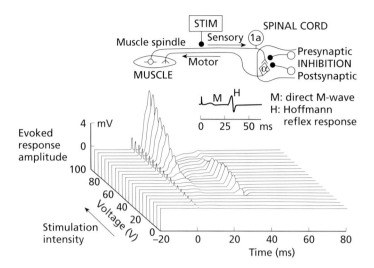

Fig. 1.4.7 Evoked spinal motoneuron properties examined by use of the Hoffman reflex. Adapted from [96,213a].

spinal and supraspinal mechanisms of importance for the training-induced change in maximal muscle strength. The Hoffmann (H) reflex [107,108] may be useful for the assessment of motoneuron excitability *in vivo*, although also reflecting the degree of presynaptic inhibition present for the Ia afferent synapses [109,110]. When the peripheral nerve is electrically stimulated, the H-reflex amplitude is seen to increase and then gradually decrease with rise in stimulation intensity, to become completely suppressed at stimulation intensities, which elicit a maximal M-response (Fig. 1.4.7). This suppression in H-reflex amplitude at maximum stimulation intensity occurs due to an increased collision between (i) antidromic nerve impulses in the motor axon (i.e. action potentials propagating backwards towards the spinal cord) and (ii) ortodromic nerve impulses caused by the Ia afferent reflex volley (i.e. action potentials propagating from the spinal cord to the muscle fibers). When the peripheral nerve is maximally stimulated during ongoing voluntary muscle contraction, the H-reflex response reappears (now denoted a V-wave) since the antidromic impulses are removed ('cleared') as a result of collision with efferent nerve impulses generated by the voluntary effort [111,112] (Fig. 1.4.8a). Thus, an increased descending motor drive causes more motoneuron axons to be cleared for passage of the evoked reflex response, which is directly reflected by an increase in V-wave amplitude [112]. At the same time, any increase in spinal motoneuron excitability and/or enhanced Ia synaptic

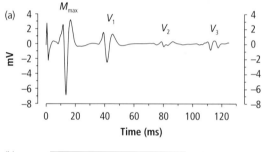

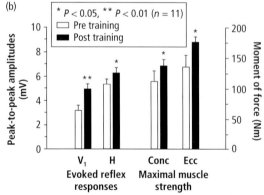

Fig. 1.4.8 (a) Raw EMG signal (sampling frequency 10 kHz) showing maximal M-wave and V-wave responses evoked in the soleus muscle by supramaximal stimulation of the tibial nerve during maximal isometric muscle contraction. (b) Mean V-wave and H-reflex amplitudes, obtained pre- and post-14 weeks of heavy-resistance strength training. The increases observed in V-wave and H-reflex amplitudes suggest an enhanced descending motor drive and/or increased excitability of spinal motoneurons and/or decreased Ia afferent presynaptic inhibition following the period of strength training [119].

transmission efficiency would contribute to the increase in V-wave amplitude as well. Thus, V-wave and H-reflex measurements may be used to quantify the overall change in central descending motor drive, spinal motoneuron excitability and/or presynaptic inhibition induced by strength training [103,112–115, 119]. It is noticeable that the potential problem of invariant recording conditions with repeated measurements of surface EMG is eliminated with this particular type of evoked EMG recording, as the H-reflex and V-wave amplitude are both expressed relative to the peak-to-peak amplitude of the maximal M-response (M_{max}) recorded during supramaximal stimulation of the motor nerve.

Somewhat surprisingly, the H-reflex amplitude recorded in the soleus muscle during resting conditions (determined as H_{max}/M_{max}) was higher in endurance athletes than in power and sprint athletes [116,116a,116b]. However, it could not be excluded that this finding occurred as a result of differences in muscle fiber composition between the two subject groups, since at low stimulation intensities the Ia afferent volley mainly excites the smaller motoneurons in the spinal cord which typically innervate the population of slow-twitch type I muscle fibers. In addition, it may be difficult to interpret differences in H_{max}/M_{max} between subject groups unless the shape of the H–M recruitment curve is identical in the groups examined. Otherwise the H-reflex would be elicited at different relative stimulation intensities, thereby evoking different amounts of antidromic clearing which would cause the H-reflex amplitude to differ. Although more time consuming, the H-reflex can alternatively be recorded using a stimulation intensity that evokes an M-response of a fixed percentage of the maximal direct M-response (e.g. 20% M_{max}) [108,117,119].

Ballet dancers demonstrate lower H-reflex amplitudes in the soleus muscle than physical education students, presumably due to increased presynaptic inhibition in the dancers [110]. In contrast, Mynark and Koceja [118] observed no difference in soleus H-reflex amplitude between trained dancers and controls during standing or prone rest. However, H-reflex gain (ratio of H-reflex to background EMG) was lower in the dancers during isometric contractions at 10, 20 and 30% MVC performed in a standing position, suggesting that the gating of spinal excitatory and in-

hibitory pathways can be modulated to adapt to the contraction-related demands placed upon the system during standing posture [118].

As previously described, the V-wave can be evoked when supramaximal H-reflex stimulation is superimposed onto maximal voluntary muscle contraction. Due to the supramaximal level of nerve stimulation, which excites all Ia afferent axons in the peripheral nerve, the V-wave response comprises all the spinal motoneurons, including the largest type II motor units. V-wave amplitudes recorded in the hand and lower limb muscles of sprinters and weight lifters were elevated relative to untrained control subjects [103,114,115]. Using a longitudinal study design an ~50% increase in V-wave amplitude was observed (recorded as V_1/M_{max}) following 9–21 weeks of strength training [113], indicating an enhanced neural drive in descending corticospinal pathways, elevated motoneuron excitability and/or alterations in presynaptic inhibition. Recent results have verified these findings, demonstrating a 55% increase in V-wave amplitude (V_1/M_{max}) in response to 14 weeks of heavy-resistance strength training [119] (Fig. 1.4.8). Likewise, the H-reflex amplitude recorded during maximal contraction was found to increase after the period of training [119]. Interestingly, it appears difficult to elicit adaptive V-wave changes in certain hand muscles [113]. This finding suggests that the range of neural adaptation may differ between muscles involved in grasping tasks and muscles responsible for propulsive force generation, respectively. Collectively, the data based on measurement of evoked V-wave and H-reflex responses strongly support the notion that neural adaptation can occur both at spinal and supraspinal levels, involving increased motoneuron excitability (and/or changes in presynaptic Ia afferent inhibition) and enhanced central descending motor drive.

Eccentric muscle contraction

It has been suggested that eccentric muscle contractions require unique activation strategies by the nervous system [121]. Indications of a preferential activation of high-threshold motor units have been demonstrated during eccentric muscle contraction of submaximal intensity [122,123], which was suggested to originate from an increased presynaptic inhibition of Ia afferents synapsing onto the low-threshold motoneurons [123,124]. Measurements based on the H-reflex technique (see above) have shown that the modulation of spinal motoneuron excitability and/or presynaptic inhibition may differ between eccentric and concentric contractions of submaximal intensity [125]. Unique and distinct motor patterns could also exist during *maximal* eccentric contraction. Thus, raw EMG tracings obtained in the quadriceps femoris muscle demonstrate large EMG spikes dispersed by short interspike periods of low or absent EMG activity (Fig. 1.4.4). However, EMG mean or median power frequency (MPF) does not seem to differ between maximal concentric and eccentric quadriceps contractions [50,126,127]. More than anything, these contrasting findings probably reflect the insensitivity of surface EMG spectral analysis for detection of subtle changes in motoneuron recruitment. Thus, the possibility exists that even if type II motor units were selectively activated during eccentric contraction, the corresponding increase in MPF due to their high firing frequency could be masked by a relative increase in synchronization as the result of their large unit size (i.e. many muscle fibers being innervated by the same motoneuron) and the appearance of temporal 'on–off' activation patterns, both causing MPF to decrease. In consequence, recording of muscle EMG by use of intramuscular wire or needle electrodes could perhaps clarify this point, as it may allow the recruitment and firing pattern of single motor units to be identified. However, even when employing intramuscular techniques, it is difficult to discriminate signals from individual motor units during contractions of high intensity. Another experimental approach has been taken by use of muscle biopsy sampling, which demonstrated a clear pattern of selective glycogen depletion for histochemically stained type IIb fibers obtained in the vastus lateralis muscle acutely following bouts of maximal eccentric cycle sprint [129]. Although this finding suggests the presence of selective type II muscle fiber recruitment, it could also, at least in part, be explained by a greater glycogen breakdown rate in the type II fibers compared to type I fibers.

Electrical transcutaneous stimulation of passive vs. active muscles has also been used to address the issue of neural activation during eccentric muscle contraction. For the quadriceps femoris and triceps surae muscles

eccentric contraction strength was higher than isometric strength during contractions evoked by electrical stimulation, but not during maximal voluntary muscle contractions [34,36,130,131] (Fig. 1.4.2). Moreover, with artificial activation the normalized moment–velocity relationship of human muscle *in situ* appears to have a more similar shape to that of isolated muscle *in vitro*, during both eccentric and concentric contractions [34,130,131] (Fig. 1.4.2). Quadriceps muscle strength is elevated during eccentric but not concentric contractions when electrical transcutaneous stimulation is superimposed onto maximal voluntary contractions [131,132] (see Fig. 1.4.2). Interestingly, this evoked increase in eccentric contraction strength is seen only in sedentary subjects and not in strength-trained athletes [132], suggesting that the apparent deficit in eccentric muscle strength disappears as an adaptive response to strength training.

More direct evidence exists to suggest that neuromuscular activation is in fact suppressed during eccentric contraction, as the EMG recorded in the quadriceps femoris muscle during maximal eccentric contraction was markedly less than that of maximal concentric contraction, particularly at high speeds [35,41,50,126,132–136] (Fig. 1.4.9). Hence, a neural regulatory mechanism that limits the recruitment and/or discharge rate of motor units during maximal voluntary eccentric muscle contraction has been proposed [35,50,131,137]. The precise mechanisms responsible for such an inhibition in motoneuron activation during eccentric contraction are not known. Although evidence of a preferential recruitment of type II motor units and derecruitment of type I units has been reported for submaximal eccentric muscle contraction *in vivo* [122,123], this could not be verified for maximal eccentric contraction as examined by surface EMG spectral analysis (MPF) [50,126–128]. Unfortunately, no data are available on the recruitment and firing pattern of single motor units during maximal eccentric contraction.

Recent results suggest that the apparent suppression in motoneuron activation during maximal eccentric contraction may be partly or fully removed following intense regimes of heavy-resistance strength training [50]. Thus, maximal eccentric muscle strength was seen to increase in parallel with a partial (lateral and medial vastii) or complete (rectus femoris)

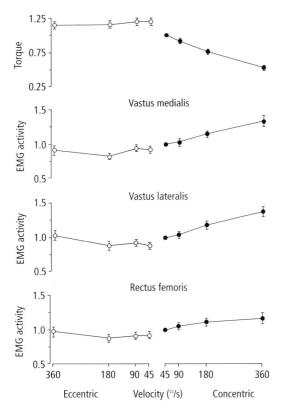

Fig. 1.4.9 Maximal muscle strength (isokinetic moment of force) and EMG-velocity relationships determined during maximal voluntary eccentric and concentric contraction of the quadriceps femoris muscle. A significant suppression in quadriceps EMG was observed during slow concentric as well as in slow and fast eccentric contraction compared to fast concentric contraction. Data from [136].

removal of suppressed EMG signal amplitudes following 14 weeks of strength training, which involved multiple exercise types (squat and leg press and knee extension) using heavy external loads (6–10 RM) [50] (Fig. 1.4.10). On the other hand, quadriceps EMG remained suppressed during maximal eccentric contraction, with no signs of a partial removal, when strength training was performed using a single type of exercise (i.e. maximal isokinetic knee extension) for a moderate period of time (10 weeks) [135]. Based on these findings, the possibility exists that the removal of neural inhibition during maximal eccentric muscle contraction requires heavy-resistance strength training

regimes of long duration and/or a large total work load (number of exercises · number of sets · kg or Nm lifted or exerted in each set).

The finding of a rapid and selective decrease in eccentric but not concentric muscle strength following 14 days of *detraining* in highly trained strength athletes [138] further emphasizes the important effect of strength training not only for achieving but also for retaining optimal neural activation patterns during maximal eccentric muscle contraction.

The specific mechanisms responsible for the adaptation in motoneuron activation during eccentric contraction are so far unidentified. During maximal voluntary muscle contraction afferent motor output is regulated not only via central descending pathways but also through sensory reflex pathways, including group Ib afferents from Golgi organs and group Ia and group II afferents from muscle spindles. Thus, the apparent suppression in motoneuron activation during maximal eccentric muscle contraction may be caused by inhibitory feedback from sensory group I and II afferents. Sensory Ib afferents from Golgi organs located in the muscle–tendon unit converge onto the entire motoneuron pool together with Ia and group II afferents from muscle spindles [139]. The Golgi Ib afferents excite inhibitory interneurons in the spinal cord, which in turn are influenced by higher central nervous system (CNS) centers through descending corticospinal pathways [139,140] (see Fig. 1.4.12 below). It is possible that the removal of motoneuron inhibition, and the resulting increase in maximal eccentric muscle strength observed following heavy-resistance strength training, appears as a result of reduced inhibitory interneuron activity mediated via central descending pathways. Alternatively, reduced presynaptic inhibition of the Ia afferent inflow from muscle spindles would be expected to augment the excitatory spinal inflow during eccentric contraction as well.

Significant increases in maximal eccentric muscle strength have been reported following heavy-resistance strength training [26,39,41–45,50–52], whereas training using low resistance and faster speeds does not seem to have any effect [26,51] (Fig. 1.4.3). Generally, greater gains in eccentric strength have been observed following eccentric or coupled eccentric–concentric training as compared to concentric training [39,41–43,51] although not always a

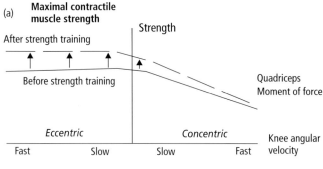

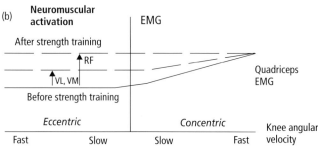

Fig. 1.4.10 (a) Heavy resistance strength training has consistently been shown to result in a significant increase in maximal eccentric and slow concentric strength of the quadriceps femoris muscle (VL, VM, RF). (b) Following 3 months of heavy resistance training the suppression of motoneuron activation was fully (RF) or partially (VL, VM) removed, in parallel with a marked increase in maximal eccentric muscle strength. Data from [50].

consistent finding [40,46]. Also, it should be recognized that concentric heavy-resistance strength training might elicit substantial gains in maximal eccentric [26,40,46,52] and coupled eccentric–concentric [33] muscle strength.

Eccentric strength training may evoke specific adaptive changes in the nervous system. Thus, recordings of surface EMG have demonstrated neural activation to dominantly increase in eccentric contraction conditions following eccentric training, while neural activation during concentric contraction mainly increased following concentric training [41–43]. These findings of training-specific neural adaptations are not surprising, given the fact that all training and strength evaluation tests were carried out in the same dynamometer [41–43]. Nonetheless, neural activation during maximal eccentric contraction also increased when different test and training devices were used [50] (Fig. 1.4.10). In addition, neural contralateral effects, so-called cross-education [141], may be more pronounced with eccentric training, as indicated by a greater relative increase in strength reported for the non-trained limb following eccentric compared to concentric single-limb training [142]. A similar trend was reported by Seger & Thorstensson [135] who also found contraction type

and speed specificity in the transfer of strength gain from the trained to the contralateral, untrained, leg after both eccentric and concentric training.

Bilateral strength deficit

Motoneuron activation and force generation may be significantly reduced in maximal bilateral compared to unilateral muscle contraction. Thus, less EMG and strength have been recorded from each limb during simultaneous contraction of the muscles in both limbs than measured during single limb contractions [143–145] although not present in all studies [146]. Interestingly, strength training involving bilateral muscle contractions appears to reduce or fully abolish the bilateral strength deficit [47]. Since the bilateral deficit in EMG and force can be observed in both maximal isometric and rapid dynamic contractions [145], it has been suggested that the mechanism may act at higher centers involved in programming of the movement [54].

During volitional muscle contraction EEG potentials, defined as movement-related cortical potentials (MRCPs), generated by neural circuits involved in motor preparation and initiation can be obtained from the left (C3) and right (C4) motor cortex areas [96]. In

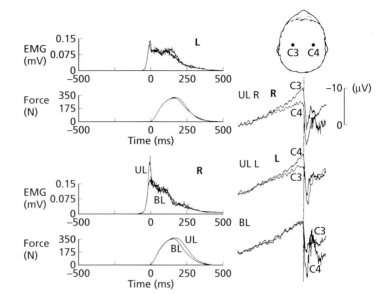

Fig. 1.4.11 Averaged movement-related cortical potentials recorded from the left and right motor cortex area (C3 and C4) and rectified EMG and isometric handgrip force obtained during maximal unilateral (UL) and bilateral (BL) contractions of right and left hand muscles in right-handed subjects. Data from [96].

maximal unilateral muscle contraction, MRCP amplitudes were significantly greater on the contralateral hemisphere [96,143] (Fig. 1.4.11). This contralateral asymmetry of large cortical MRCPs disappeared during maximal bilateral contractions, in which symmetric and MRCPs were observed at both hemispheres (Fig. 1.4.11). The bilateral deficit in force and EMG associated with reduced MRCPs suggests the involvement of an interhemispheric inhibition mediated by commissural nerve fibers in the corpus callosum [96]. Thus, the removal of the bilateral strength deficit, as observed following bilateral strength training, could be the result of adaptive changes in interhemispheric inhibition.

Antagonist muscle coactivation

Coactivation of antagonist muscles is involved in many types of joint movements [147,148]. Antagonist muscle coactivation could be important for several reasons: to protect ligaments at the end-range of joint motion [149,150], to ensure a homogeneous distribution of compression forces over the articular surfaces of the joint [151], and to increase joint stiffness thereby providing protection against external impact forces as well as enhancing the stiffness of the entire limb [152]. In addition, maximal antagonist muscle strength may play an important role in the execution of fast, ballistic

limb movements. Thus, high eccentric antagonist strength allows for a shortened phase of limb deceleration, thereby increasing the time available for limb acceleration, with a resulting rise in maximal movement velocity [153].

Coactivation is elevated during either of two states: when uncertainty exists in the required task, or during anticipation of compensatory muscle forces [147]. During maximal coactivation, the monosynaptic excitatory pathway (Ia) as well as the disynaptic reciprocal inhibitory pathway (Ib) are exposed to spinal inhibition via descending supraspinal pathways [154,155]. The increase in muscle and joint stiffness mainly results from a direct activation from the CNS with the cerebellum playing an important role in switching from reciprocal activation to coactivation [147,156].

It is not well known whether strength training *per se* may induce altered patterns of antagonist coactivation. Intuitively, a decrease in antagonist coactivation would seem desirable, as this would cause net joint moment (agonist joint moment minus antagonist joint moment) to increase. However, as implied above a decrease antagonist muscle coactivation may not be optimal for the integrity of the joint. Antagonist coactivation has been reported to decrease [77a,158], increase [151] or remain unchanged [43,50,76a,77a,135,157,159,

160] in response to strength training. Häkkinen and coworkers [77a] found that coactivation of the lateral hamstring muscle during maximal isometric contraction of the quadriceps femoris was elevated in old subjects (70 years) compared to middle-aged subjects (40 years). However, after 6 months of heavy resistance-training coactivation decreased in the old subjects to reach a level similar to that recorded for the middle-aged subjects, which in turn did not change during the course of training [77a]. Given that antagonist coactivation is markedly elevated when uncertainty exists in the motor task, subjects may occasionally demonstrate very high levels of coactivation during the initial round of experiments. This may, at least in part, explain the decrease in antagonist coactivation that has been observed with training. To minimize this potential problem, conditioning tests could be conducted prior to the round of actual pretraining testing.

Interestingly, a differential change in antagonist motor pattern in terms of a selective decrease in medial (semitendinosus) but unchanged lateral (biceps femoris) hamstring EMG activity was observed in maximal isolated knee extension in response to 14 weeks of heavy-resistance training, involving isolated knee extension and squat exercises [157]. This adaptation indicates an important aspect of motor reprogramming, as it potentially counteracts excessive internal tibia rotation which otherwise may give rise to elevated stress forces in the anterior cruciate ligament (ACL) during active knee extension [150,161].

To obtain a valid measure of antagonist muscle coactivation it is crucial to ensure that the antagonist EMG signal is not contaminated by the EMG activity of adjacent agonist muscles, as a result of EMG cross-talk between electrode pairs [162,163]. The amount of cross-talk between two given EMG signals can be quantified by use of cross-correlation analysis [66,102]. Using a wide range of time phase shifts (i.e. from $\tau=0$ to $\tau=\pm 50$ ms) and long record lengths (>1500 data points), the peak cross-correlation coefficient raised to the second power, $R_{xy}(\tau)^2$, may be taken to represent the percentage cross-talk between electrode sites [102]. Based on this methodology low levels of EMG cross-talk (4–6%) were demonstrated between adjacent quadriceps (agonist) and hamstring (antagonist) muscles in maximal isolated knee extension [164], although substantially higher values have

also been reported [162]. Importantly, the level of cross-talk will depend strictly on the specific measuring set-up used, with electrode size and distance between electrodes being the most critical factors. The above findings therefore indicate that it may be possible, with careful experimental procedures, to minimize the magnitude of EMG cross-talk between antagonist and agonist muscles.

Neural inhibitory mechanisms

Numerous pathways in the nervous system could be responsible for exerting an inhibitory synaptic drive onto the spinal pool of α-motoneurons. As an important feature, these pathways allow for an integration of spinal and supraspinal inputs. It appears therefore that changes in the spinal neural circuitry induced by training, including alterations in synaptic gating, may emerge as a result of adaptive changes at both spinal and supraspinal levels. Consequently, considerable plasticity can be expected for the neural adaptation to specific types of activity and training. For example, inhibition of various inhibitory pathways as a result of strength training would yield an increase in the net excitatory drive to the motoneuron pool.

Ib afferent inflow from Golgi organs

Negative feedback via force-sensing afferents from the Golgi organs arises through the action of inhibitory Ib interneurons, which project to the motoneurons that control the muscle fibers affecting the Golgi organ (Fig. 1.4.12). Golgi organs are primarily located within the muscle, at the site of muscle fiber attachment to the aponeurosis or other tendinous structures (>90%), rather than at the actual tendon (<10%) [139]. Golgi organs respond not only to large but also to small increments in force and the widespread distribution of Golgi organs allows each motor unit to be monitored by at least one to three Golgi organs [139]. Consequently, active and passive muscle forces can be accurately monitored in every portion of the muscle [139]. Importantly, the Ib inhibitory interneurons are influenced by descending corticospinal pathways (i.e. rubrospinal and reticulospinal tracts) [139,140] (see Fig. 1.4.12). Conversely, information from Golgi organs reaches the cerebellum and cerebral sensory cortex through dorsal spinocerebral tracts, suggesting that Ib afferent feedback contributes to conscious

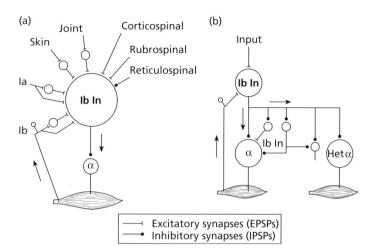

Fig. 1.4.12 (a) Negative feedback via force-sensing neural Ib afferents from Golgi organs arises through the action of inhibitory neurons (Ib In) which project to α-motoneurons that, in turn, control the muscle fibres that affect the Golgi organs. (b) Ib interneurons not only inhibit motoneurons that innervate their parent muscles, but also motoneurons controlling many other muscles (Het α).From [140].

sensations of contractile and passive muscle stress [139]. It is also noticeable that various sensory cutaneous afferents and joint afferents converge onto the pool of inhibitory Ib interneurons, in turn facilitating Ib inhibitory effects (Fig. 1.4.12). Interestingly, this includes the posterior articular nerve (PAN) of the knee joint, which contains sensory axons from the ACL, posterior cruciate ligament (PCL) and joint capsule [165,166]. The facilitary inflow to the Ib inhibitory interneurons from skin and joint sensory afferents not only constitutes a safety mechanism, causing muscle force to be suppressed during joint injury; it probably also contributes to the (re)programming of motor patterns when adapting to specific types of training or when rehabilitating from joint or ligament injury. It should be noted, however, that recent experimental evidence obtained in animal preparations suggest that in certain situations (e.g. quiet standing, specific phases of locomotion) the Golgi organs may exert a common excitatory feedback drive onto the motoneurons of antigravity muscles crossing the same joint [167]. Thus, the Ib afferent pathway appears to be highly complex, and also in humans the possibility exists that reflex reversal mechanisms are functioning at different levels of the CNS to facilitate motor function during standing and locomotion.

It is plausible that the removal of motoneuron suppression and the resulting increase in maximal eccentric muscle strength observed following heavy-resistance strength training (Fig. 1.4.10) is the result of a down-regulation in spinal Ib inhibitory interneuron activity (i.e. 'disinhibition') mediated via central descending pathways.

Renshaw inhibition

In the spinal cord Renshaw cells may serve as a variable gain regulator at the motoneuronal level, controlling the relationship between synaptic input and efferent axonal output. Recurrent inhibition, by which the motoneuron exerts an autoinhibitory influence on itself, is mediated via Renshaw cells (Fig. 1.4.13). Recurrent Renshaw inhibition has been considered as a factor limiting motoneuron discharge frequency, and also to have a regulating influence on the reciprocal Ia inhibitory pathway [111,168]. Animal experiments have shown that Renshaw cells are submitted to several types of supraspinal control that can enhance as well as depress the recurrent pathway [168,169]. Thus, with facilitation of Renshaw cells the input–output relationship of the motoneuron becomes impaired, whereas inhibition of the Renshaw cells causes the input–output relationship to be enhanced (Fig. 1.4.13). As compared to tonic contractions, Renshaw cell activity appears to be more inhibited in maximal phasic contractions, resulting in a reduced level of recurrent inhibition [168]. This could indicate that 'explosive' types of heavy-resistance strength training, aimed at maximizing the contractile rate of force

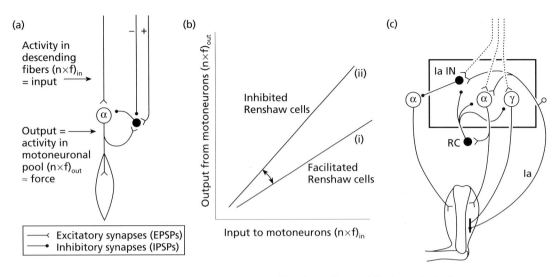

Fig. 1.4.13 (a) Input and output connections of α-motoneurons and Renshaw cells, a specialized type of spinal interneuron. Excitatory and inhibitory synapses are shown. Note that the Renshaw cells themselves receive both excitatory and inhibitory synaptic inputs, from spinal as well as higher centers in the CNS. (b) Simplified diagram of input–output relations of a motoneuron pool involving two different situations: (i) with a facilitation of Renshaw cells, the efferent motoneuron output is diminished for a given neuronal input; (ii) conversely, the inhibition of Renshaw cells causes an overall disinhibition of the α-motoneuron pool, with a resulting rise in efferent motor output for a given synaptic input. The presence of recurrent inhibition provides a basis which allows the input–output relationship of the motoneuron pool to be dynamically modulated. (c) Concept of the motoneuron stage. Neurons constituting the efferent output are indicated by thick lines. RC, Renshaw cell; Ia IN, Ia inhibitory neuron. From [169].

development, should be superior in evoking neural changes as compared to other types of strength training (i.e. low-resistance training, body building).

Adaptive changes in muscle morphology

MHC isoform composition, fiber type conversion

When a nerve impulse reaches the muscle fiber, the muscle membrane is depolarized and calcium is released to the interior of the cell from specialized intracellular organelles (sarcoplasmatic reticulum), in turn triggering a transient process of cyclic attachment and detachment of cross-bridges between actin and myosin molecules within the muscle fiber. As a result of this cross-bridge cycling, the actin and myosin filaments perform a sliding movement relative to each other while generating contractile force. In human skeletal muscle, the myosin molecule is constituted of three major types of polypeptide chains: the myosin heavy chain (MHC, molecular weight approx. 200 kDa) and two distinct types of light myosin chains

(alkali, regulatory chain and DTBN chain, each approx. 20 kDa) [63,170,171]. Recent techniques, such as sodium dodecyl sulfate polyacrylamide gel electrophoresis (SDS-PAGE), have identified distinctly different myosin isoforms within the single muscle fiber as well as in muscle homogenate samples. Using SDS-PAGE three different MHC bands have been separated in adult human skeletal muscle, reflecting differences in molecular density. These bands correspond to the MHC-I, MHC-IIa and MHC-IIx isoforms [8] (Fig. 1.4.14). The fiber type distribution determined by conventional myosin ATPase histochemistry relates closely to the MHC isoform content [172–176]. Although 50–85% of the variance was accounted for (r^2, r-values of 0.7–0.9 observed), the remaining 15–40% reflects that the SDS-PAGE analysis provides a more sensitive and consistent picture of MHC coexpression, i.e. the presence of two or more MHC isoforms within the muscle fiber [8,177].

The term MHC-IIx has found increasing use to denote the fastest contracting MHC isoform found in human skeletal muscle, due to a consistent homology

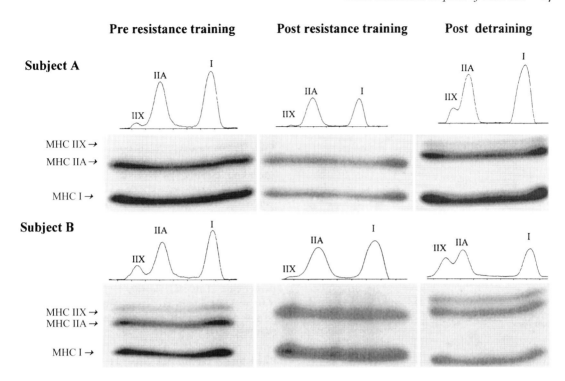

Fig. 1.4.14 SDS-PAGE gel separations showing MHC bands from two subjects before and after 90 days of heavy-resistance strength training followed by 90 days of detraining. Densitometric scans are shown above each of the lanes. Data from [173].

in genome expression between this fast human isoform and the MHC-IIx isoform in the rat [178,179]. Although the MHC-IIb encoding gene has been found in the human genome [180,181], evidence for its expression at the protein level is lacking [182]. It appears, however, that the MHC-IIb isoform is dominantly expressed in certain specialized muscles of the larynx and the eye [182a].

The distribution into various distinct MHC isoforms, as well as its responsiveness to change with training, has significant implications for *in vivo* mechanical muscle function and the adaptation to given physiologic demands [63,183]. For example, a positive relationship has been found between the percentage of fast MHC-II isoforms determined by gel electrophoresis and the ability to produce high muscle force during fast concentric contraction [184,185]. Similar findings have been reported when assessing myosin composition by use of conventional myosin ATPase histochemistry [12,31,186,187].

In human skeletal muscle shifts in fast myosin iso-

form composition, i.e. MHC-IIa→IIx or MHC-IIx→IIa, appear to be readily evoked by training or detraining, respectively [172,173,176,177,188–190]. However, it remains a matter of controversy whether training within a realistic physiologic range can induce transformation between slow and fast myosin isoforms, i.e. MHC-I→II or MHC-II→I [183,191,192]. The finding of an extremely large proportion of IIa and IIx fibers in the quadriceps muscle of long-term spinal cord-injured subjects (>99% vs. 50% in age-matched healthy subjects) led Andersen and coworkers to suggest that the expression of the MHC-IIx isoform represents a default setting, which is overruled with any chronic increase in muscle activity [188]. Interestingly, a marked decrease in MHC-IIx and corresponding increases in type IIa and type I MHC were observed in spinal cord-injured subjects after 6 months of cycle training using functional electrical stimulation (FES) [188].

Not only endurance training but also resistance training appears to effectively suppress the expression of MHC-IIx. Thus, few muscle contractions performed against heavy external loads two or three times per week can reduce MHC-IIx almost completely, with a corresponding increase in MHC-IIa [172,173,175–177,189,190,193]. This indicates that the total number of contractions or nerve impulses is not the only factor which influences the down-regulation of MHC-IIx with resistance training, as otherwise suggested with prolonged endurance training [194]. Rather, the magnitude of contractile force exerted by the muscle fibers appears to be a governing factor as well. Intense muscle contractions may lead to structural deformation of the sarcolemma and the cytoskeleton, thereby activating mechanosensitive or stretch-sensitive signaling pathways affecting gene regulation of the nucleus [195]. Furthermore, exercise-induced changes in gene expression are accelerated by activation of gene-encoding transcription factors such as the myogenic regulatory factor family (MyoD, myogenin, Myf5, MRF4) [196]. The mechanical stress load exerted on the muscle fiber probably acts through similar intracellular pathways to switch off or down-regulate the MHC-IIx gene, while up-regulating the MHC-IIa gene. Also, exercise-induced activation of specific intracellular kinases, which controls the rate of RNA transcription/translation, thereby regulating protein synthesis rate, appears to be involved in the hypertrophic response to resistance training. For example, a strong positive relationship between the activation (i.e. phosphorylation) of $p70^{S6k}$, a 70-kDa S6 protein kinase, and the long-term increase in muscle mass with resistance training was recently reported in the rat, suggesting that this protein kinase plays an important role in the intracellular signaling cascade related to training-induced growth of skeletal muscle [197]. Data obtained in humans suggest that in the initial phase of resistance training (1–2 weeks), the increased rate of myofibrillar protein synthesis is mediated mainly by a more efficient translation of mRNA [198]. On the other hand, the finding that intense bouts of resistance exercise can induce rapid changes in mRNA (0–72 h) which precede changes in MHC content (3–5 weeks) [198a], indicate that resistance training may exert a strong and immediate modulatory effect on gene encoding as well. Similar findings have been reported following high-intensity endurance exercise [199]. In addition, the mismatch between the

expression of specific MHC isoforms and their respective mRNA isoforms observed with resistance training (and detraining) suggests that differentiated adaptive responses may exist for the pre- and post-translational mechanisms related to gene expression [200].

Muscle fiber size

As a result of differences in spinal α-motoneuron cell soma size, the small low-threshold motor units are preferentially recruited in low-level isometric muscle contraction, whereas with increase in muscle force there is an additional and progressive recruitment of large high-threshold motor units, cf. 'Henneman's size principle' [201]. Thus, heavy-resistance strength training will activate both low-threshold and high-threshold motor units, thereby involving slow type I as well as fast type II muscle fibers. Consequently, heavy-resistance strength training can induce significant alterations in muscle fiber morphology as manifested by an increase in type I and type II muscle fiber cross-sectional area [77,78,193,202] (Fig. 1.4.15). A majority of studies, however, have found a preferential or more pronounced hypertrophy of the type II muscle fibers [43,173,176,189,190,203–205] (Fig. 1.4.15). Altogether these findings suggest that type II muscle fibers possess a greater adaptive capacity for hypertrophy compared to type I fibers.

Muscle fiber hypertrophy occurs primarily due to an accumulation of contractile proteins (i.e. myosin and actin) as reflected by an increase in the size and number of myofibrils within the muscle cell, leaving the total number of muscle fibers basically unaltered [206]. Seen in this perspective, individuals genetically predisposed to have a large number of muscle fibers in a given muscle would appear to have the greatest potential for overall muscle hypertrophy in response to training. There is a possibility that neoformation of muscle fibers (hyperplasia) may occur as an effect of intensive resistance training, although for human skeletal muscle its existence remains questionable [63]. The muscle fiber hypertrophy induced by resistance training is often accompanied by an increase in the cross-sectional area or total volume of the muscle obtained by magnetic resonance imaging (MRI) or computed tomography (CT) scanning. Although at first hand a conflicting finding, disproportionate changes in

(a)

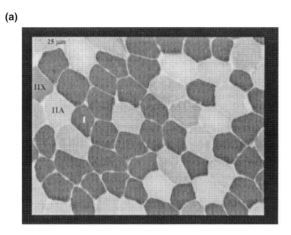

(b)

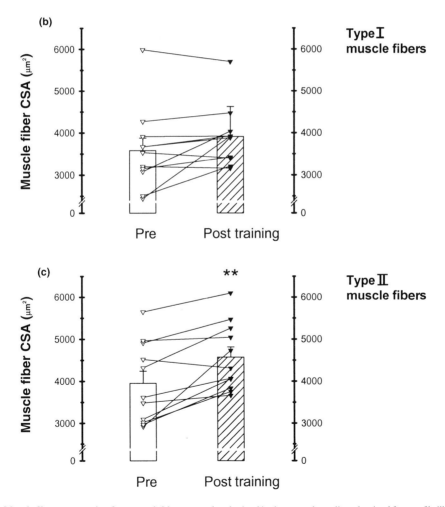

Pre   Post training

Type I
muscle fibers

(c)

∗∗

Pre   Post training

Type II
muscle fibers

Fig. 1.4.15 Muscle fiber cross-section from muscle biopsy samples obtained in the vastus lateralis and stained for myofibrillar ATPase after pre-incubation at pH 4.6 (a). (b–c) Muscle fiber cross-sectional area (CSA) with fiber types IIA and IIX collapsed, before and after 14 weeks of heavy resistance strength training ($n = 11$). Note the increase in type II muscle fiber with training. A trend towards increased type I fiber area was also observed with training [173].

MRI muscle cross-sectional area (CSA) and single muscle fiber CSA may occur with resistance training. Thus, mid-thigh quadriceps CSA as well as total quadriceps volume increased ~25%, whereas single-fiber CSA increased ~25% following 14 weeks of resistance training [77,207,208]. In studies using combined muscle biopsy sampling and muscle imaging (MRI, CT) the increase in muscle fiber CSA induced by resistance training generally appeared to exceed the increase in whole-muscle CSA [77,207–209]. These findings are not explainable by an altered ratio of non-contractile to contractile tissue, which appears to remain unchanged with resistance training in animal models [210] as well as in humans [204,211]. Rather, the disproportionate alteration in fiber CSA and whole-muscle CSA appears to be caused by training-induced alterations in muscle architecture. Thus, muscle fiber pennation angle may increase in response to prolonged heavy-resistance strength training, a change that allows physiologic muscle CSA (muscle fiber CSA) to increase more than anatomic muscle CSA (see 'Changes in muscle architecture', below).

An upper limit seems to exist to the increase in muscle fiber size induced by resistance training [212]. Most likely this limit is closely linked to the genetic endowment of the individual. Because the myonuclei of adult muscle fibers are not capable of mitosis and therefore unable to divide, the nuclear/cytoplasmic ratio would approach zero with unlimited increase in muscle fiber size. Obviously, this would dilute the amount of mRNA in the cell, at some point causing net protein synthesis to cease. Interestingly, satellite cells may play an important role for the maintenance of a constant nuclear/cytoplasmic ratio during cellular hypertrophy. Satellite cells are located dormant under the muscle cell basal membrane. During normal muscle growth, satellite cells contribute nuclei to the muscle cell by proliferating, differentiating and fusing to existing myofibers [213,214]. The satellite cell-derived myonuclei are no longer capable of dividing, but begin to produce muscle-specific proteins that add to the increase in myofiber size [213,214]. The proliferation and differentiation of satellite cells are stimulated by endogenous growth factors such as testosterone, insulin-like growth factor I (IGF-I),

growth hormone, insulin and interleukin-6 [213]. In addition, data exist which suggest that satellite cell activation may be enhanced by anabolic steroid use. Thus, high-level power lifters reporting several years of high-dose anabolic steroid usage (average 9 years) demonstrated ~15% and ~25% elevated myonuclei number in their type IIa and I muscle fibers, respectively, together with a ~35% larger mean muscle fiber area compared to age-matched power lifters that did not use steroids [215]. Interestingly, type I muscle fibers have a lower nucleus/cytoplasm ratio than type II fibers [216]. Thus, the type I fibers would be expected to respond most markedly to anabolic steroid usage, as in fact supported by recent experimental evidence [217].

Opposite to that observed with resistance training, a reduction in muscle fiber CSA (atrophy) may be seen following intensive endurance training [193,218–220]. From a muscle perfusion perspective this adaptation is very important, since it results in an elevated capillary to muscle fiber CSA ratio, which in turn facilitates O_2 delivery and free fatty acid (FFA) uptake into the muscle cell due to the reduced diffusion distance. The elevated FFA uptake results in a reduced rate of glycogen breakdown to yield an enhanced endurance performance (prolonged time to exhaustion). Thus, regimes of concurrent strength and endurance training appear to involve stimuli for cellular hypertrophy as well as atrophy. As a functional consequence, no (or only minor) muscle fiber hypertrophy and no signs of a reduction in capillary density have been observed when strength and endurance training are combined [221–223].

With regard to muscle metabolism and endurance, it is noteworthy that the number of capillaries per fiber appears to either increase [189,202,224] or remain unchanged [225,226] following prolonged (months) resistance training. Likewise, capillary density (cap/mm^2) seems to remain unchanged [189,202,224]. Thus, the capacity for capillary perfusion does not seem markedly impaired by resistance training, at least when performed for 8–16 weeks. On the other hand, previous findings of a reduced capillary density in experienced weight lifters and power lifters [227] but not in body builders [228] suggest that the specific type of resistance exercise could play an important role for this parameter.

Muscle cross-sectional area and volume

During recent years there has been a progressively growing interest in the use of non-invasive imaging techniques such as magnetic resonance imaging (MRI), computed tomography (CT) and ultrasonog- raphy to address the alteration in macroscopic muscle dimensions evoked by resistance training (Fig. 1.4.16).

An accurate estimate of the total volume of a given muscle can be provided by the recording of successive axial MR images along the entire length of the limb.

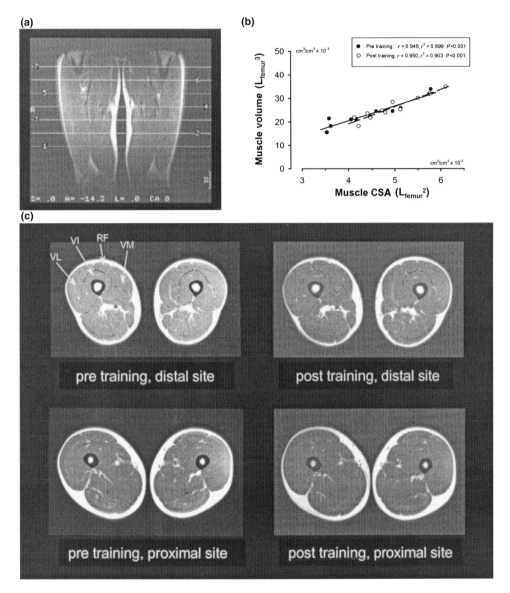

Fig. 1.4.16 (a) Coronal MRI scan of m. quadriceps femoris. (b) The relationship between quadriceps muscle CSA and total quadriceps volume. Pre- and post-training values are shown by closed and open symbols, respectively. (c) Axial MRI images of the thigh obtained at 50% femur length (proximal site) and 30% femur length (distal site) before and after 14 weeks of heavy-resistance strength training. Data adapted from [207 and 229].

The determination of muscle volume can be quite time consuming and costly in terms of time spent in the MR scanner. It is therefore interesting to note that in the quadriceps femoris muscle, which is the muscle that has been most frequently used to examine the effects of resistance training, a strong relationship can be found between muscle CSA obtained at 50% segment length and total muscle volume determined by recording of multiple axial images [229] (Fig. 1.4.16b). Thus, training-induced changes in muscle volume may be well represented by changes in single-site CSA, at least when evaluating large subject groups.

Anatomic muscle CSA obtained by use of MRI or CT has been reported to increase 5–15% in response to prolonged heavy-resistance strength training [41,45,77,77a,81,207–209,230]. Corresponding increases have been found for total quadriceps volume [45,81,207]. Using MRI some researchers have been able to identify the perimeter of the different quadriceps femoris muscles in successive axial images obtained along the length of the femur, to report differentiated hypertrophic response of each muscle compartment (i.e. vastus lateralis, medialis, intermedius and rectus femoris) following resistance training [45,81]. However, such differentiation is not always possible, since substantial fusion may exist between adjacent vastii. Based on cadaver data, 57 of 75 dissected quadriceps muscles showed fusion between the lateral and deep vastii at more than 50% of the entire length of the muscle [231]. In addition, axial MR scans typically show a lack of distinct fascial boundaries between the lateral and deep vastii (posterolaterally) and between the medial and deep vastii (anteromedially) when obtained proximally [207] (Fig. 1.4.16c). Obviously, such fusion of adjacent muscle compartments will have important implications for the interpretation of MRI-based muscle CSA data.

Resistance training involving eccentric alone or coupled eccentric–concentric muscle contractions seems to result in more pronounced morphologic changes than concentric training alone. Accelerated muscle hypertrophy was found after eccentric or coupled eccentric–concentric training compared to concentric training alone, as reflected by a greater increase in single muscle fiber CSA obtained by biopsy sampling [43,78,189] although not confirmed by all studies [39,40]. Likewise, a greater increase in

anatomic muscle CSA obtained by use of MRI or anthropometric measures has been observed following eccentric strength training in most [40,41,232] but not all studies [58]. Furthermore, muscle fiber area remained above pretraining values following detraining from eccentric but not concentric resistance training [189], indicating that the hypertrophic response to eccentric training is more long lasting. The above disparities are likely to be related to differences in training duration between studies. With sufficient duration therefore, eccentric resistance training appears to be more effective for inducing muscle fiber hypertrophy and overall muscle growth than concentric training alone.

Muscle architecture

Many, if not most, skeletal muscles are characterized by a pennate arrangement of the muscle fibers relative to their insertion at the aponeurosis or tendon. This allows physiologic muscle cross-sectional area (equivalent to the muscle fiber area perpendicular to the longitudinal axis of the individual muscle fibers) to greatly exceed the anatomic muscle cross-sectional area measured in a plane perpendicular to the longitudinal axis of the whole muscle. The maximal force-generating capacity of a given muscle is determined by its physiologic CSA, as this represents the maximal number of acto-myosin crossbridges that can be activated during contraction. For a given volume of muscle, physiologic CSA and thereby maximal contractile muscle force is progressively increased at more steep muscle fiber pennation angles, to reach an upper limit at a pennation angle of 45° [230,233]. Consequently, pennate muscles are able to exert very large contractile force compared to non-pennate muscles.

Muscle fiber pennation angle was previously estimated from dissection of cadaver specimens. However, more adequate and accurate measuring techniques have emerged, based on the appearance of high-resolution ultrasonography techniques (Fig.1.4.17). This has allowed fiber pennation angle to be measured at specific muscle lengths (joint angles) and at specific levels of muscle tension. Ultrasound imaging has been increasingly used to investigate the strain and stress forces generated in human tendon and aponeurosis *in vivo* [234–236]. In addition, ultrasonography

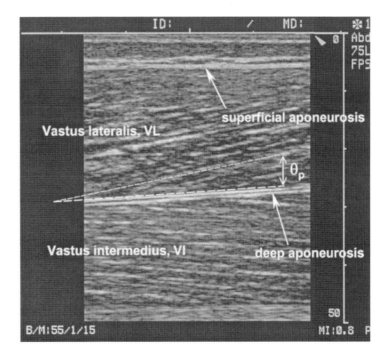

Fig. 1.4.17 Sagittal plane ultrasound image obtained in the relaxed quadriceps femoris muscle at 50% femur length. Muscle fiber pennation angle (θ_p) in vastus lateralis was measured as the angle between VL muscle fibre fascicles and the deep aponeurosis.

has been used to address the more chronic change in muscle fiber pennation angle induced by resistance training.

Findings of steeper muscle fiber pennation angles and greater anatomic muscle CSA in the triceps brachii muscle of body builders compared to untrained subjects [237] suggest that the muscle hypertrophy induced by resistance training could be associated with an increase in fiber pennation angle. This notion was confirmed by longitudinal data demonstrating a significant increase in muscle fiber pennation angle from 16.5° to 21.3° in the triceps brachii muscle following 16 weeks of resistance training [238]. Likewise, an increase in fiber pennation angle from 8.0 to 10.7° was reported for the vastus lateralis muscle after 14 weeks of intense heavy-resistance strength training [207]. In contrast, Rutherford and Jones found an unchanged fiber pennation angle in the lateral and medial vastii after 12 weeks of resistance training, despite a 5% and 13% increase in anatomic CSA and maximal isometric strength, respectively [230]. These conflicting results were probably caused by differences in total training load, which differed by a factor of three. Thus, a change in muscle

architecture evoked by resistance training appears to require considerable effort and time.

The training-induced increase in muscle fiber pennation angle was suggested to allow muscle fiber CSA and thereby maximal force-generating capacity to increase significantly more (16%) than whole-muscle CSA and volume (10%) [207]. Thus, the disproportionate change in macroscopic versus microscopic morphometry observed with strength training [77,207–209] implies that muscle CSA or volume obtained by MRI or CT (i.e. reflecting changes in anatomic CSA) cannot replace the information obtained by measurements of single muscle fiber area in biopsy samples (i.e. reflecting changes in physiologic CSA), or *vice versa*. Clearly, the adaptation in muscle fiber pennation angle should be taken into account when examining training-induced changes in maximal muscle strength, *in vivo*.

Functional aspects

Training for 'explosive' muscle strength

'Explosive' muscle strength can be defined as the rate of force development (RFD = Δforce/Δtime) exerted

(a)

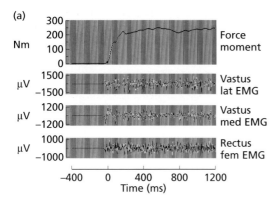

(b)

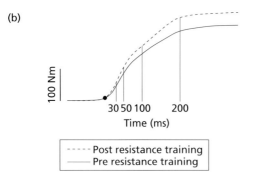

- - - - Post resistance training
——— Pre resistance training

Fig. 1.4.18 EMG and muscle moment of force vs. time: Raw tracings (a), average force-time curve pre post resistance training (b) [242].

within the very initial phase of contraction (0–200 ms) (Fig. 1.4.18). The ability to generate very steep increases in muscle force at the onset of contraction has important functional significance for the force and power generated during rapid, forceful movements. Thus, contraction times of 50–250 ms can be observed in many types of fast movement (e.g. sprint running, long jump take-off, karate, boxing). In contrast, it takes about 300–400 ms to reach maximal force in the human quadriceps femoris muscle [82,242] (Fig. 1.4.18). Consequently, contractile RFD is a major determinant of the maximal force and velocity that can be achieved in very fast movements.

In isometric contraction conditions, RFD is determined by the level of neural activation (efferent motor drive), muscle size (muscle CSA and volume) and fiber type composition (MHC isoforms) while also influenced by the length–tension characteristics of the muscle. During dynamic contraction, the RFD will

also be influenced by the force–velocity characteristics of the muscle. Acutely, a rise in RFD is seen with increasing motoneuron firing frequency [90] and overall neural drive. In terms of muscle morphology, a large CSA will also result in a large absolute RFD. Maximal cross-bridge cycle transition rate appears to be the major limiting factor for the maximal intrinsic RFD of mammalian muscle fiber [239]. Thus, a predominance of type II MHC isoforms results in a high RFD [240], due to their elevated rate of cross-bridge cycling [88]. In consequence, the maximal muscle force that can be reached in situations of short contraction times (i.e. <250 ms) is positively related to the proportion of type II MHC [184].

Based on electromyography (EMG) recordings (Figs 1.4.4 and 1.4.18a), efferent neural drive to the muscle fibers has been found to increase in response to strength training [43,45,50,61,76a,72–78,77a,86,242, 243]. Because a 'parallelism' of the rate of EMG and force development may exist [241], concurrent adaptations in neural drive and contractile RFD can be expected following resistance training. In line with these expectations, RFD and neural efferent drive have both been reported to increase in response to strength training [72,74,75,77a,86,242,243] (Fig. 1.4.19). Interestingly, Schmidtbleicher and Buerhle [243] found that 'power training' at lower loads and fast contraction velocities had no strong effect on these parameters. Duchateau and Hainaut [244] used electrically evoked tetanic contractions to address changes in intrinsic muscle properties, and found that peak RFD was augmented to a greater extent by fast ballistic training than isometric training (31% vs. 18%) in the adductor pollicis muscle. This latter finding suggests that not only heavy-resistance strength training but also maximal ballistic training using lower loads could have an important effect on the increase in RFD. Comparing dynamic and isometric ballistic training (i.e. at high RFD), Behm and Sale observed the increase in RFD to be similar with both these types of training regimes, during evoked as well as voluntary contraction conditions [245]. Thus, the involvement of an intended ballistic effort may be more important for inducing increases in RFD than the type of contraction actually performed.

The marked increase observed in neural drive suggests that the increase in contractile RFD is mainly caused by neural adaptation. In particular the finding

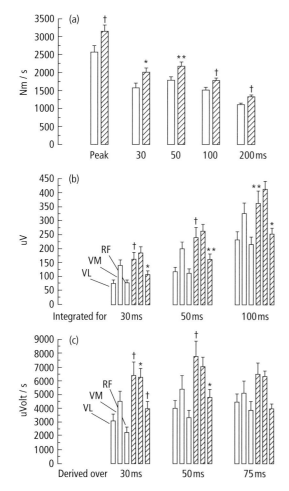

Fig. 1.4.19 Changes in RFD and neural drive pre- and post-14 weeks heavy resistance training. Error bars denote SEM. (a) Rate of force moment of development during maximal isometric contraction of the quadriceps femoris muscle calculated in time intervals from the onset of contraction. (b) Neural drive calculated as the mean integrated EMG divided by integration time. (c) Neural drive quantified as the rate of EMG rise [242].

[242]. Muscle fiber hypertrophy could also have contributed to the increase in RFD, as evidenced by an increase in type II muscle fiber CSA following training (19%) [173]. Recently, Duchateau and colleagues reported increased contractile RFD together with an increase in firing frequency as well as a six-fold increased occurrence of 'discharge doublets' in the firing pattern of single motor units following ballistic-type resistance training [86] (Fig. 1.4.20). This increased incidence of 'discharge doublets' may be particularly important for the training-induced increase in RFD, by taking increasing advantage of the catch-like property of skeletal muscle (See Adaptive changes in neural drive: motoneuron firing frequency).

Collectively, the above findings suggest that the (see Adaptive changes in neural drive: motoneuron firing frequency) major stimulus for training-induced increases in RFD may reside in the high-frequency motor unit firing pattern associated with an intended ballistic movement [245]. For this purpose training probably should involve heavy-resistance strength training combined with a more ballistic type of training using somewhat lower loads. Based on the training experience accumulated in top-level track and field athletics and power lifting, the most optimal training stimulus perhaps can be achieved when heavy-resistance strength exercises executed in an 'explosive' manner (i.e. emphasis on acceleration of the load) are combined with specific ballistic-type exercises using lower loads.

There is no doubt that the increase seen in contractile RFD is one of the single most important functional benefits associated with resistance training. Very fast movements are characterized by muscle contraction times of 80–200 ms, which is considerably less than the time it takes to reach maximal force (Fig. 1.4.18). Consequently, increases in RFD evoked by resistance training may greatly enhance the maximal force and velocity that can be achieved during very fast movements. In support of this notion, maximal muscle force and power were markedly elevated during very fast movement speeds following heavy-resistance strength training [6]. Likewise, the increase in contractile RFD likely is responsible for the increase in maximal unloaded movement speed reported following heavy-resistance strength training [246]. It is important to notice that training-induced changes in contractile RFD will have important functional consequences,

of disproportionately large increases in EMG amplitude (18–132%) and rate of EMG rise (39–106%) compared to RFD (18–26%) and maximal muscle strength (16%) (Fig. 1.4.19) suggests that an increase in motoneuron firing frequency may be responsible for the training-induced rise in contractile RFD [67]. This notion was further supported by the finding that RFD normalized to MVC, i.e. expressed as % MVC/s, increased in the initial phase of contraction (0–1/6 MVC, corresponding to the initial 30–50 ms)

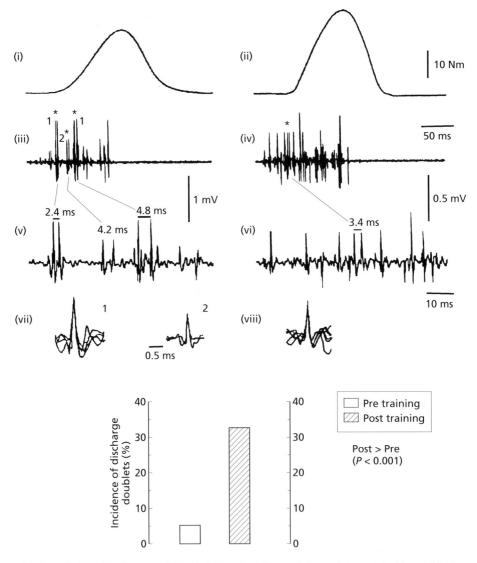

Fig. 1.4.20 Discharge doublets, Van Cutsem 1998 [86], their Fig. 4 (top). Bar graph (bottom) shows the incidence of discharge doublets before and after a period of strength training.

not only in athletes, but also in non-athletic subjects. For example, in the elderly individual, high muscular RFD may play an important role for the ability to rapidly regain postural balance and thereby avoid falls.

Training for optimal neural and morphologic adaptation

From the findings presented in this chapter strength training appears effective for evoking significant adap-

tive changes within the nervous system as well as in the muscle itself (Fig. 1.4.21). Training with heavy loads (1–8 RM) seems to emphasize various aspects of neural adaptation, in turn causing significant increases in contractile RFD [247] and maximal eccentric strength [50]. The use of moderate to heavy training loads (6–12 RM) may be more optimal for the development of muscle hypertrophy [247] and may also prove more effective for inducing alterations in muscle

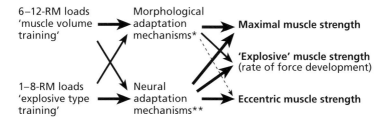

Fig. 1.4.21 Diagram summarizing neural and morphological effects evoked by resistance training. *↑ Muscle cross-sectional area (CSA); ↑ CSA type II muscle fibers (type II MHC isoforms). Changes in muscle architecture (↑ fiber pennation angle). ** ↑ Neural drive to muscle fibers (↑ iEMG); ↑ motoneuron excitability; ↓ motoneuron inhibition.

architecture. It should be noted, however, that the adaptation evoked by resistance training involves a mixture of neural and morphologic mechanisms that often cannot be separated from each other.

As described above, the increase in maximal muscle strength can be the result of changes in muscle size or muscle architecture (angle of fiber pennation), and/or of neural changes, i.e. enhanced efferent motor outflow to the muscle fibers. The increase in contractile RFD is caused by an increased neural drive, especially within the initial 0–100 ms of contraction. In addition, there may be a significant contribution from muscle fiber hypertrophy. The functional outcome is that movements can be performed more rapidly and that muscle force and power generated during fast movements will be enhanced. Eccentric muscle strength is increased mainly due to neural adaptation mechanisms, which likely include a reduced inhibition of the motoneurons during maximal eccentric contraction. However, muscle fiber hypertrophy will contribute as well. These adaptations cause muscle force and power to be enhanced in functional situations, such as during rapid limb acceleration and deceleration, and in forceful stretch–shortening cycle activities, e.g. jumping and sprinting. Moreover, an increase in the maximal eccentric strength of antagonist muscles has been suggested to be of importance for the magnitude of dynamic joint stabilization provided by antagonist coactivation [16,26,248]. In consequence, the increase in eccentric antagonist muscle strength may be expected to result in a reduced incidence of joint injury. Another important aspect that is often overlooked, is that regular resistance training may allow the individual to tolerate better a higher intensity of training which, in turn, will improve performance.

Summary

Strength training induces marked increases in maximal concentric, eccentric and isometric muscle strength as well as in the contractile rate of muscle force development. Adaptive changes occur both in the nervous system and within the muscle itself. Experimental data obtained by electromyography have indicated several mechanisms for neural adaptation, including increase in efferent motor drive, increased motor unit firing frequency, enhanced intramuscular and intermuscular motor unit synchronization, increased motoneuron excitability and decreased presynaptic inhibition of spinal α-motoneurons. Down-regulation of inhibitory pathways, at either the supraspinal or spinal level, e.g. of Ib Golgi afferents and Renshaw recurrent inhibition, may contribute to the increase in maximal muscle strength in response to heavy-resistance strength training, particularly during eccentric muscle contractions. Adaptations in muscle morphology include increase in muscle fiber cross-sectional area (CSA), whole-muscle CSA and volume, and changes in muscle architecture in terms of an increased angle of muscle fiber pennation, as demonstrated by histochemical, magnetic resonance and ultrasonographic techniques, respectively. Using modern gel electrophoresis and antibody classification methods, effects of strength training have also been demonstrated at the subcellular level, e.g. as shifts in myosin heavy chain isoforms, mainly between MHC-IIa and IIx. The enhancement of neuromuscular function induced by strength training will have significant benefits for the performance and ability to endure intense training in most sports as well as for carrying out many activities in everyday life, not least in the elderly. Training with moderate to heavy loads and eccentric, concentric and isometric contractions, should be integral parts of preventive and rehabilitative training for muskuloskeletal injuries.

Multiple choice questions

1 *Which of the following statements about isokinetic strength measurements is correct?*
a 'Isokinetic' implies that the muscle contraction velocity is kept constant over the whole range of motion.
b Under true isokinetic conditions the measured moment of force equals the net muscle strength produced around the joint investigated.
c Since the muscle lever arm changes with joint angle over the range of motion, the muscle force has to change accordingly to keep the torque constant.
d Under eccentric isokinetic measurements the dynamometer has to produce a torque that is lower than the net torque produced by the muscles.
e During isokinetic strength measurement the joint angular velocity is constant over the entire range of motion.

2 *Which of the following neural adaptations is least likely to occur after heavy-resistance strength training?*
a Increased efferent drive from higher neural centers to the agonist motoneuron pool.
b Increased firing frequency of agonist α-motoneurons.
c Decreased presynaptic inhibition of Ia afferents onto homonymous motoneurons.
d Increased activation from supraspinal centers onto the Renshaw cells innervating the agonist motoneurons.
e Decreased inhibition from Ib afferents on agonist motoneurons.

3 *Which of the following muscular adaptations is the least likely to occur after heavy-resistance strength training?*
a A shift from myosin isoform MHC-IIx to MHC-IIa.
b A larger relative area of type II as compared to type I muscle fibers.
c A higher number of capillaries per muscle fiber.
d A larger angle of pennation.
e An increased number of type IIb muscle fibers.

4 *Which of the following statements about eccentric (lengthening) muscle contractions is false?*
a In eccentric muscle contractions the force produced per unit of muscle activation is larger than in concentric muscle contractions.
b In eccentric muscle contractions the EMG required to produce a certain muscle force is lower than in concentric muscle contractions.
c The effect of slow vs. fast movement velocity on maximal voluntary muscle strength is smaller in eccentric than in concentric muscle contractions.
d Combining eccentric and concentric contractions in strength training gives a larger strength gain than concentric training alone.
e The potential gain in maximal voluntary strength by disinhibition of inhibitory pathways is smaller in eccentric than in concentric muscle contractions.

5 *Which of the following statements about neural adaptations to strength training is false?*
a Training of each limb separately will decrease the difference in strength between summed unilateral and bilateral contractions, respectively (the so-called bilateral strength deficit).
b Training of one limb can increase the strength of the other, so called cross-education.
c Training with ballistic movements can lead to an increased occurrence of so-called discharge doublets, which, in turn, may lead to a higher rate of force development (RFD).
d The intention and effort to develop force quickly during heavy-resistance strength training can lead to an increased ability to produce force at high speeds.
e Strength training of agonist muscles does not necessarily result in a decreased coactivation of antagonist muscles.

References

1 Ikai M, Steinhaus AH. Some factors modifying the expression of human strength. *J Appl Physiol* 1961; **16**: 157–63.
1a Yue G, Cole KJ. Strength increases from the motor program: comparison of training with maximal voluntary and imagined muscle contractions. *J Neurophysiol* 1992; **67**: 1114–23.
2 Hansen TE, Linhard J. On the maximum work of human muscles especially the flexors of the elbow. *J Physiol* 1923; **57**: 287–300.
3 Hill AV. The maximum work and mechanical efficiency of human muscles, and their most economical speed. *J Physiol* 1922; **56**: 19–41.

4 Kaneko M, Fuchimoto T, Toji H, Suei K. Training effect of different loads on the force–velocity relationship and mechanical power output in human muscle. *Scand J Sports Sci* 1983; **5**(2): 50–5.

5 Wilkie DR. The relation between force and velocity in human muscle. *J Physiol* 1950; **110**: 249–80.

6 Aagaard P, Simonsen EB, Trolle M, Bangsbo J, Klausen K. Effects of different strength training regimes on moment and power generation during dynamic knee extension. *Eur J Appl Physiol* 1994; **69**: 382–6.

7 Kanehisa H, Miyashita M. Effects of isometric and isokinetic training on static strength and dynamic power. *Eur J Appl Physiol* 1983; **50**: 365–71.

8 Klitgaard H, Bergman O, Betto R, Salviati G, Clausen T, Saltin B. Co-existence of myosin heavy chain I and IIa isoforms in human skeletal muscle fibres with endurance training. *Pflügers Arch* 1990; **416**: 470–2.

9 De Koning FL, Blinkhorst RA, Vos JA, Van't Hof MA. The force–velocity relationship of arm flexion in untrained males and females and arm-trained athletes. *Eur J Appl Physiol* 1985; **54**: 89–94.

10 Moffroid M, Whipple R. Specificity of speed of exercise. *Phys Ther* 1970; **50**: 692–1700.

11 Perrine JJ, Edgerton VR. Muscle force–velocity and power–velocity relationship under isokinetic loading. *Med Sci Sports* 1978; **10**: 159–66.

12 Thorstensson A, Grimby G, Karlsson J. Force–velocity relations and fiber composition in human knee extensor muscles. *J Appl Physiol* 1976; **40**: 12–6.

13 Perrin DH. *Isokinetic Exercise and Assessment.* Champaign, IL.: Human Kinetics Publishers, 1993.

14 Taylor NA, Cotter JD, Stanley SN, Marshall RN. Functional torque-velocity and power-velocity characteristics of elite athletes. *Eur J Appl Physiol* 1991; **62**: 116–21.

15 Marshall RN, Mazur SM, Taylor NA. Three-dimensional surfaces for human muscle kinetics. *Eur J Appl Physiol* 1990; **61**: 263–70.

16 Aagaard P, Simonsen EB, Larsson B, Beyer N, Magnusson P, Kjær M. Isokinetic muscle strength and capacity for muscular knee joint stabilization in elite sailors. *Int J Sports Med* 1997; **18**: 521–5.

17 Hill AV. The heat of shortening and the dynamic constants of muscle. *Proc Royal Soc London Series B* 1938; **126**: 136–95.

18 Katz B. The relation between force and speed in muscular contraction. *J Physiol* 1939; **96**: 45–64.

19 Wickiewicz TL, Roy RR, Powell PL, Perrine JJ, Edgerton VR. Muscle architecture and force–velocity relationships in humans. *J Appl Physiol* 1984; **57**(2): 435–43.

20 Costill DL, Coyle EF, Fink WF, Lesmes GR, Witzman A. Adaptations in skeletal muscle following strength training. *J Appl Physiol* 1979; **46**: 96–9.

21 Coyle EF, Costill DL, Lesmes GR. Leg extension power and muscle fiber composition. *Med Sci Sports* 1979; **11**: 12–5.

22 Ivy JL, Withers RT, Brose G, Maxwell BD, Costill DL. Isokinetic contractile properties of the quadriceps with relation to fiber type. *Eur J Appl Physiol* 1981; **47**: 247–55.

23 Lesmes GR, Costill DL, Coyle EF, Fink WJ. Muscle strength and power changes during maximal isokinetic training. *Med Sci Sports* 1978; **10**: 256–60.

24 Ryushi T, Fukunaga T. Influence of subtypes of fast-twitch fibres on isokinetic strength in untrained men. *Int J Sports Med* 1986; **7**: 250–3.

25 Prietto CA, Caiozzo VJ. The *in vivo* force–velocity relationship of the knee flexors and extensors. *Am J Sports Med* 1989; **17**: 607–11.

26 Aagaard P, Simonsen EB, Trolle M, Bangsbo J, Klausen K. Specificity of training velocity and training load on gains in isokinetic knee joint strength. *Acta Physiol Scand* 1996; **156**: 123–9.

27 Westing SH, Seger JY, Karlson E, Ekblom B. Eccentric and concentric torque-velocity characteristics of the quadriceps femoris in man. *Eur Appl Physiol* 1988; **58**: 100–4.

28 Yates JW, Kamon E. A comparison of peak and constant angle torque-velocity curves in fast and slow-twitch populations. *Eur J Appl Physiol* 1983; **51**: 67–74.

29 Aagaard P, Simonsen EB, Trolle M, Bangsbo J, Klausen K. Isokinetic hamstring/quadriceps strength ratio: influence from joint angular velocity, gravity correction and contraction mode. *Acta Physiol Scand* 1995; **154**: 421–7.

30 Caiozzo VJ, Perrine JJ, Edgerton VR. Training induced alterations of the in vivo force–velocity relationship in human muscle. *J Appl Physiol* 1981; **51**: 750–4.

31 Froese EA, Houston ME. Torque-velocity characteristics and muscle fiber type in human vastus lateralis. *J Appl Physiol* 1985; **59**: 309–14.

32 Fuglevand AJ. Resultant muscle torque, angular velocity and joint angle relationships and activation patterns in maximal knee extension. In: Jonsson B, ed. *Biomechanics X-A.* Champaign, Illinois: Human Kinetics, 1987: 559–65.

33 Hortobagyi T, Katch FI. Eccentric and concentric torque-velocity relationships during arm flexion and extension. *Eur J Appl Physiol* 1990; **60**: 395–401.

34 Dudley GA, Harris RT, Duvoisin MR, Hather BM, Buchanan P. Effect of voluntary vs. artificial activation on the relationship of muscle torque to speed. *J Appl Physiol* 1990; **69**: 2215–21.

35 Seger JY, Thorstensson A. Muscle strength and myoelectric activity in prepubertal and adult males and females. *Eur J Appl Physiol* 1994; **69**: 81–7.

36 Seger JY, Thorstensson A. Electrically evoked eccentric and concentric torque-velocity relationships in human knee extensor muscles. *Acta Physiol Scand* 2000; **169**: 63–9.

37 Edman KAP. Double-hyperbolic force–velocity relation in frog muscle fibres. *J Physiol* 1988; **404**: 301–21.

38 Caiozzo VJ, Haddad F, Baker MJ, Baldwin KM. Influence of mechanical loading on myosin heavy-chain protein and mRNA isoform expression. *J Appl Physiol* 1996; **80**: 1503–12.

39 Colliander EB, Tesch PA. Effects of eccentric and concentric muscle actions in resistance training. *Acta Physiol Scand* 1990; **140**: 31–9.

40 Seger JY, Arvidson B, Thorstensson A. Specific effects of eccentric and concentric training on muscle strength and morphology in humans. *Eur J Appl Physiol* 1998; **79**: 49–57.

41 Higbie EJ, Cureton KJ, Warren GL, Prior BM. Effects of concentric and eccentric training on muscle strength, cross-sectional area and neural activation. *J Appl Physiol* 1996; **81**: 2173–81.

42 Hortobagyi T, Barrier J, Beard B, Braspennincx J, Koens P, Devita P, Dempsey L, Lambert J. Greater initial adaptations to submaximal muscle lengthening than maximal shortening. *J Appl Physiol* 1996; **81**: 1677–82.

43 Hortobagyi T, Hill JP, Houmard JA, Fraser DD, Lambert NJ, Israel RG. Adaptive responses to muscle lengthening and shortening in humans. *J Appl Physiol* 1996; **80**: 765–72.

44 Komi PV, Buskirk ER. Effect of eccentric and concentric muscle conditioning on tension and electrical activity of human muscle. *Ergonomics* 1972; **15**: 417–34.

45 Narici MV, Roig S, Landomi L, Minetti AE, Cerretelli P. Changes in force, cross-sectional area and neural activation during strength training and detraining of the human quadriceps. *Eur J Appl Physiol* 1989; **59**: 310–9.

46 Spurway NC, Watson H, McMillan K, Connolly G. The effect of strength training on the apparent inhibition of eccentric force production in voluntary activated human quadriceps. *Eur J Appl Physiol* 2000; **82**: 374–80.

47 Coyle EF, Feiring DC, Rotkis TC, Cote RW III, Roby FB, Lee W, Wilmore JH. Specificity of power improvements through slow and fast isokinetic training. *J Appl Physiol* 1981; **51**: 1437–42.

48 Housh DJ, Housh TJ. The effects of unilateral velocity-specific concentric strength training. *J Orth Sports Phys Ther* 1993; **17**: 252–6.

49 Rutherford OM, Jones DA. The role of learning and coordination in strength training. *Eur J Appl Physiol* 1986; **55**: 100–5.

50 Aagaard P, Simonsen EB, Andersen JL, Magnusson P, Halkjær-Kristensen J, Dyhre-Poulsen P. Neural inhibition during maximal eccentric and concentric quadriceps contraction: effects of resistance training. *J Appl Physiol* 2000; **89**: 2249–57.

51 Duncan PW, Chandler JM, Cavanaugh DK, Johnson KR, Buehler AG. Mode and speed specificity of eccentric and concentric exercise training. *J Orth Sports Phys Ther* 1989; **11**: 70–5.

52 Petersen S, Wessel J, Bagnall K, Wilkins H, Quinney A, Wenger H. Influence of concentric resistance training on concentric and eccentric strength. *Arch Phys Med Rehab* 1990; **71**: 101–5.

53 Goldberg AL, Etlinger JD, Goldspink DF, Jablecki C. Mechanism of work induced hypertrophy of skeletal muscle. *Med Sci Sports Exerc* 1975; **7**: 248–61.

54 Sale DG. Neural adaption to resistance training. *Med Sci Sports Exerc* 1988; **20**(5): S135–S145.

55 Sale DG. Neural adaption to strength training. In: Komi PV, ed. *Strength and Power in Sports*. The IOC Encyclopaedia of Sports Medicine, Vol. III. Oxford: Blackwell Scientific Publications, 1992: 249–65.

56 Behm DG. Neuromuscular implications and applications of resistance training. *J Strength Cond Res* 1995; **9**: 264–74.

57 Moritani T. Neuromuscular adaptations during the acquisition of muscle strength, power and motor tasks. *J Biomech* 1993; **26** (Suppl. 1): 95–107.

58 Jones DA, Rutherford OM. Human muscle strength training. the effects of three different regimes and the nature for the resultant changes. *J Physiol* 1987; **391**: 1–11.

59 Dons B, Bollerup K, Bonde-Petersen F, Hancke S. The effect of weight-lifting exercise related to muscle fiber composition and muscle cross-sectional area in humans. *Eur J Appl Physiol* 1979; **40**: 95–106.

60 Komi PV, Viiytasalo JT, Rauramaa R, Vihko V. Effect of isometric strength training on mechanical, electrical and metabolic aspects of muscle function. *Eur J Appl Physiol* 1978; **40**: 45–55.

61 Moritani T, deVries HA. Neural factors versus hypertrophy in the time course of muscle strength gain. *Am J Phys Med Rehabil* 1979; **58**: 115–30.

62 Thorstensson A. Observations on strength training and detraining. *Acta Physiol Scand* 1977; **100**: 491–3.

63 Kraemer WJ, Fleck SJ, Evans WJ. Strength and power training. physiological mechanisms of adaptation. In: Holloszy JO, ed. *Exercise and Sports Science Reviews*, 24. Baltimore: Williams & Wilkins, 1996: 363–97.

64 Walmsley B, Proske U. Comparison of stiffness of soleus and medial gastrocnemius muscle in cats. *J Neurophysiol* 1981; **46**: 250–9.

65 Joyce GC, Rack PM, Westbury DR. The mechanical properties of cat soleus muscle during controlled lengthening and shortening movements. *J Physiol* 1969; **204**: 461–74.

66 Basmajian JV, DeLuca CJ. *Muscles Alive: Their Functions Revealed by Electromyography*. Baltimore: Williams & Wilkins, 1985.

67 DeLuca CJ. The use of surface electromyography in biomechanics. *J Appl Biomech* 1997; **13**: 135–63.

68 Kamen G, Caldwell GE. Physiology and interpretation of the electromyogram. *J Clin Neurophysiol* 1996; **13**: 366–84.

69 Viitasalo JT, Saukkonen S, Komi PV. Force-time characteristics and fiber composition in human leg extensor muscles. *Electromyogr Clin Neurophysiol* 1980; **20**: 487–501.

70 Sleivert GG, Wenger HA. Reliability of measuring isometric and isokinetic peak torque, rate of torque development, integrated electromyography, and tibial nerve conduction velocity. *Arch Phys Med Rehab* 1994; **75**: 1315–21.

71 Yang JF, Winter DA. Electromyography reliability in maximal and submaximal isometric contractions. *Arch Phys Med Rehab* 1983; **64**: 417–20.

72 Häkkinen K, Alén M, Komi PV. Changes in isometric force

and relaxation time, EMG and muscle fiber characteristics of human skeletal muscle during training and detraining. *Acta Physiol Scand* 1985; **125**: 573–85.

73 Häkkinen K, Komi PV. Electromyographic changes during strength training and detraining. *Med Sci Sports Exerc* 1983; **15**: 455–60.

74 Häkkinen K, Komi PV. Training induced changes in neuromuscular performance under voluntary and reflex conditions. *Eur J Appl Physiol* 1986; **55**: 147–55.

75 Häkkinen K, Komi PV, Alén M. Effect of explosive type strength training on isometric force- and relaxation-time, electromyographic and muscle fiber characteristics of leg extensor muscles. *Acta Physiol Scand* 1985; **125**: 587–600.

76 Häkkinen K, Komi OV, Alén M, Kauhanen H. EMG, muscle fiber and force production characteristics during a 1 year training period in elite lifters. *Eur J Appl Physiol* 1987; **56**: 419–27.

76a Häkkinen K, Alén M, Kallinen M, Newton RU, Kraemer WJ. Neuromuscular adaptation during prolonged strength training, detraining and re-strength training in middle-aged and elderly people. *Eur J Appl Physiol* 2000; **83**: 51–62.

77 Häkkinen K, Newton RU, Gordon SE, McCormick M, Volek JS, Nindl BC, Gotshalk LA, Campbell WW, Evans WJ, Häkkinen A, Humphries BJ, Kraemer WJ. Changes in muscle morphology, electromyographic activity, and force production characteristics during progressive strength training in young and older men. *J Gerontol Biol Sci Med Sci* 1998; **53**: B415–23.

77a Häkkinen K, Kallinen M, Izquierdo M, Jokelainen K, Lassila H, Mälkiä E, Kraemer WJ, Newton RU, Allén M. Changes in agonist–antagonist EMG, Muscle CSA, and fore during strength training in middle-aged and older people. *J Appl Physiol* 1998; **84** 1341–9.

78 Hortobagyi T, Dempsey L, Fraser D, Zheng D, Hamilton G, Lambert J, Dohm L. Changes in muscle strength, muscle fiber size and myofibrillar gene expression after immobilization and retraining in humans. *J Physiol* 2000; **524**(1): 293–304.

79 Cannon G, Cafarelli E. Neuromuscular adaptations to strength training. *J Appl Physiol* 1987; **63**: 2396–402.

80 Garfinkel S, Cafarelli E. Relative changes in maximal force, EMG, and muscle cross-sectional area after isometric training. *Med Sci Sports Exerc* 1992; **24**: 1220–7.

81 Narici MV, Hoppeler H, Kayser B, Landoni L, Claassen H, Gavardi C, Conti M, Cerretelli P. Human quadriceps cross-sectional area, torque and neural activation during 6 months strength training. *Acta Physiol Scand* 1996; **157**: 175–86.

82 Thorstensson A, Karlsson J, Viitasalo JHT, Luhtanen P, Komi PV. Effect of strength training on EMG of human skeletal muscle. *Acta Physiol Scand* 1976; **98**: 232–6.

83 Desmedt JE, Godaux E. Ballistic contractions in man: characteristic recruitment pattern of single motor units of the tibialis anterior muscle. *J Physiol* 1977; **264**: 673–93.

84 Grimby L, Hannerz J. Firing rate and recruitment order of toe extensor motor units in different modes of voluntary contraction. *J Physiol* 1977; **264**: 865–79.

85 Marsden CD, Meadows JC, Merton PA. Isolated single motor units in human muscle and their rate of discharge during maximal voluntary effort. *J Physiol* 1971; **217**: P12–3.

86 Van Cutsem M, Duchateau J, Hainaut K. Changes in single motor unit behavior contribute to the increase in contraction speed after dynamic training in humans. *J Physiol* 1998; **513**(1): 295–305.

87 Buller AJ, Lewis DM. The rate of tension development in isometric contractions of mammalian fast and slow skeletal muscle. *J Physiol* 1965; **176**: 337–54.

88 Metzger JM, Moss RL. Calcium-sensitive cross-bridge transitions in mammalian fast and slow skeletal muscle fibres. *Science* 1990; **247**: 1088–90.

89 Metzger JM, Moss RL. pH modulation of the kinetics of a Ca^{2+}-sensitive cross-bridge state transition in mammalian single skeletal muscle fibres. *J Physiol* 1990; **428**: 751–64.

90 Grimby L, Hannerz J, Hedman B. The fatigue and voluntary discharge properties of single motor units in man. *J Physiol* 1981; **316**: 545–54.

91 Miller RG, Mirka A, Maxfield M. Rate of tension development in isometric contractions of a human hand muscle. *Exp Neurol* 1981; **73**: 267–85.

92 Nelson AG. Supramaximal activation increases motor unit velocity of unloaded shortening. *J Appl Biomech* 1996; **12**: 285–91.

93 Nelson AG, Thompson WJ. Contractile properties and myosin phenotype of single motor units from neonatal rats. *Am J Physiol* 1994; **266**: C919–C924.

94 Burke RE, Rundomin P, Zajack FE. The effect of activation history on tension production by individual muscle units. *Brain Res* 1976; **18**: 515–29.

95 Burke RE, Rundomin P, Zajack FE. Catch property in single mammalian motor units. *Science* 1970; **168**: 112–24.

96 Moritani T, Yoshitake Y. The use of electromyography in applied physiology. *J Electromyogr Kinesiol* 1998; **8**: 363–81.

97 Binder-Macleod SA. Variable-frequency stimulation patterns for the optimization of force during muscle fatigue. Muscle wisdom and catch-like properties. *Adv Exp Med Biol* 1995; **384**: 227–40.

98 Leong B, Kamen G, Patten C, Burke J. Maximal motor unit discharge rates in the quadriceps muscles of older weight lifters. *Med Sports Exerc* 1999; **31**: 1638–44.

99 Patten C. Age and training related influences on motor unit control properties. In: *Proc XVIIth Int Soc Biomech Cong.* (abstract) Calgary, Canada, 1999: 246.

100 Kamen G, Knight CA, Laroche DP, Asermely DG. Resistance training increases vastus lateralis motor unit firing rates in young and old adults. *Med Sci Sports Exerc* 1998; **30**(5) (Suppl.): S337 (abstract).

101 Enoka RM. Morphological features and activation patterns of motor units. *J Clin Neurophysiol* 1995; **12**: 538–59.

102 Winter DA, Fuglevand AJ, Archer SE. Crosstalk in surface electromyography: theoretical and practical estimates. *J Electromyogr Kinesiol* 1994; **4**(1): 15–26.

103 Milner-Brown HS, Stein RB, Lee RG. Synchronization of human motor units: possible role of exercise and supraspinal reflexes. *Electroenceph Clin Neurophysiol* 1975; **38**: 245–54.

104 Lind AR, Petrofsky JS. Isometric tension from rotary stimulation of fast and slow cat muscles. *Muscle Nerve* 1978; **1**: 21–8.

105 Rack PM, Westbury DR. The effects of length and stimulus rate on tension in the rat soleus muscle. *J Physiol* 1969; **204**: 443–60.

106 Semmler JG, Nordstrom MA. Motor unit discharge and force tremor in skill- and strength-trained individuals. *Exp Brain Res* 1998; **119**: 27–38.

106a Yao W, Fuglevand, AJ, Euoka RM. Motor-unit synchronization increases EMG amplitude and decreases force steadiness of simulated contractions. *J Neurophysiol* 2000; **83**: 441–52.

107 Hugon M. Methodology of the Hoffmann reflex in man. In: Desmedt JE, ed. *New Developments in Electromyography and Clinical Neurophysiology*, Vol. 3. Basel: Karger, 1973: 277–93.

108 Schieppati M. The Hoffmann reflex: a means for assessing spinal reflex excitability and its descending control in man. *Prog Neurobiol* 1987; **28**: 345–76.

109 Hultborn H, Meunier S, Pierrot-Deseilligny E, Shindo M. Changes in presynaptic inhibition of Ia fibres at the onset of voluntary contraction in man. *J Physiol* 1987; **389**: 757–72.

110 Nielsen J, Crone C, Hultborn H. H-reflexes are smaller in dancers from the royal Danish ballet than in well-trained athletes. *Eur J Appl Physiol* 1993; **66**: 116–21.

111 Hultborn H, Pierrot-Deseilligny, E. Changes in recurrent inhibition during voluntary soleus contractions in man studies by an H-reflex technique. *J Physiol* 1979; **297**: 229–51.

112 Upton ARM, McComas AJ, Sica REP. Potentation of 'late' responses evoked in muscles during effort. *J Neurol Neurosurg Psychiat* 1971; **34**: 699–711.

113 Sale DG, MacDougall JD, Upton A, McComas A. Effect of strength training upon motoneuron excitability in man. *Med Sci Sports Exerc* 1983; **15**: 57–62.

114 Sale DG, Upton A, McComas A, MacDougall JD. Neuromuscular function in weight-trainers. *Exp Neurol* 1983; **82**: 521–31.

115 Upton ARM, Radford PF. Motorneuron excitability in elite sprinters. In: Komi PV, ed. *Biomechanics V-A. International Series on Biomechanics*, Vol. 1A. University Park Press, Baltimore, 1975: 82–7.

116 Casabona A, Polizzi MC, Perciavalle V. Differences in H-reflex between athletes trained for explosive contractions and non-trained subjects. *Eur J Appl Physiol* 1990; **61**: 26–32.

116a Rochcougar P, Dassonville J, Le Bars R. Modification of the Hoffmann reflex in function of athletic training. *Eur J Appl Physiol* 1979; **40**: 165–70.

116b Maffiuletti NA, Martin A, Babault N, Pensini M, Lucas B, Schieppati M. Electrical and mechanical H$_{max}$-to-M$_{max}$ ratio in power and endurance-trained athletes. *J Appl Physiol* 2001; **90**: 3–9.

117 Dyhre-Poulsen P, Simonsen EB, Voigt M. Dynamic control of muscle stiffness and H reflex modulation during hopping and jumping in man. *J Physiol* 1991; **437**: 287–304.

118 Mynark RG, Koceja DM. Comparison of soleus H-reflex gain from prone to standing in dancers and controls. *Electroenceph Clin Neurophysiol* 1997; **105**: 135–40.

119 Aagaard P, Simonsen EB, Andersen JL, Magnusson P, Dyhre-Poulsen P. Neural adaptation to resistance training: changes in evoked V-wave and H-reflex responses. *J Appl Physiol* 2002; **92**: 2309–18.

120 Aagaard P, Simonsen EB, Andersen JL, Magnusson P, Halkjær-Kristensen J, Dyhre-Poulsen P. Neural adaptation to strength training in man: spinal and supraspinal mechanisms. In: Bangsbo J *et al.*, eds. *Proceedings of the 2nd Annual Congress of the European College of Sports Science I*, 1997: 336 (abstract).

121 Enoka RM. Eccentric contractions require unique activation strategies by the nervous system. *J Appl Physiol* 1996; **81**: 2339–46.

122 Howell N, Fuglevand AJ, Walsh ML, Bigland-Ritchie B. Motor unit activity during isometric and concentric-eccentric contractions of the human first dorsal interosseus muscle. *J Neurophysiol* 1995; **74**: 901–4.

123 Nardone A, Romanò C, Schieppati M. Selective recruitment of high-threshold human motor units during voluntary isotonic lengthening of active muscles. *J Physiol* 1989; **409**: 451–74.

124 Nardone A, Schieppati M. Shift of activity from slow to fast muscle during voluntary lengthening contractions of the triceps surae muscle in humans. *J Physiol* 1988; **395**: 363–81.

125 Ròmano C, Schieppati M. Reflex excitability of human soleus motoneurons during voluntary shortening or lengthening contractions. *J Physiol* 1987; **390**: 271–84.

126 Tesch PA, Dudley GA, Duvoisin MR, Hather BM, Harris RT. Force and EMG signal patterns during repeated bouts of concentric and eccentric muscle actions. *Acta Physiol Scand* 1990; **138**: 263–71.

127 Tyler TF, McHugh MP, Nicholas SJ, Gleim GW. Evidence for preferential type II fiber recruitment in maximum eccentric contraction is lacking in frequency analysis of the EMG (abstract). In: Bangsbo J *et al.*, eds. *Proceedings of the 2nd Annual Congress of the European College of Sports Science I*, 1997: 388 (abstract).

128 McHugh MP, Tyler TF, Greenberg SC, Gleim GW. Differences in activation pattern between eccentric and concentric quadriceps contractions. *J Sports Sci* 2002; **20**: 83–91.

129 Fridén J, Sjöström M, Ekblom B. Myofibrillar damage fol-

lowing intense eccentric exercise in man. *Int J Sports Med* 1983; **4**: 170–6.

130 Pinniger GJ, Steele JR, Thorstensson A, Cresswell AG. Tension regulation during lengthening and shortening actions of the human soleus muscle. *Eur J Appl Physiol* 2000; **81**: 375–83.

131 Westing SH, Seger JY, Thorstensson A. Effects of electrical stimulation on eccentric and concentric torque-velocity relationships during knee extension in man. *Acta Physiol Scand* 1990; **140**: 17–22.

132 Amiridis IG, Martin A, Morlon B, Martin L, Cometti G, Pousson M, van Hoecke J. Co-activation and tension-regulating phenomena during isokinetic knee extension in sedentary and highly skilled humans. *Eur J Appl Physiol* 1996; **73**: 149–56.

133 Bobbert M, Harlaar J. Evaluation of moment–angle curves in isokinetic knee extension. *Med Sci Sports Exerc* 1992; **25**: 251–9.

134 Kellis E, Baltzopoulos V. Muscle activation differences between eccentric and concentric isokinetic exercise. *Med Sci Sports Exerc* 1998; **30**: 1616–23.

135 Seger JY, Thorstensson A. Effects of eccentric and concentric isokinetic training on EMG and electromechanical efficiency. In: *Neuromuscular aspects of eccentric knee extensor actions – effects of electrical stimulation, age, gender and training.* Doctoral dissertation, Department of Neuroscience, Karolinska Institute, Stockholm, Sweden, 1998.

136 Westing SH, Cresswell AG, Thorstensson A. Muscle activation during maximal voluntary eccentric and concentric knee extension. *Eur J Appl Physiol* 1991; **62**: 104–8.

137 Webber S, Kriellaars D. Neuromuscular factors contributing to in vivo eccentric moment generation. *J Appl Physiol* 1997; **83**: 40–5.

138 Hortobagyi T, Houmard JA, Stevenson JR, Fraser DD, Johns RA, Israel RG. The effects of detraining on power athletes. *Med Sci Sports Exerc* 1993; **25**: 929–35.

139 Jami L. Golgi tendon organs in mammalian skeletal muscle: functional properties and central actions. *Physiol Rev* 1992; **72**: 623–66.

140 Loeb GE. Neural control of locomotion. *Bioscience* 1989; **39**: 800–4.

141 Enoka RM. Muscle strength and its development: new perspectives. *Sports Med* 1988; **6**: 146–68.

142 Hortobagyi T, Lambert NJ, Hill JP. Greater cross-education following training with muscle lengthening than shortening. *Med Sci Sports Exerc* 1997; **19**: 107–12.

143 Oda S, Moritani T. Movement-related cortical potentials during handgrip contractions with special reference to force and electromyogram bilateral deficit. *Eur J Appl Physiol* 1995; **72**: 1–5.

144 Otsuki T. Decrease in voluntary isometric arm strength induced by simultanous bilateral exertion. *Behav Brain Res* 1983; **7**: 165–78.

145 Vandervoort AA, Sale DG, Moroz J. Comparison of motor unit activation during unilateral and bilateral leg extension. *J Appl Physiol* 1984; **56**: 46–57.

146 Jakobi JM, Cafarelli E. Neuromuscular drive and force production are not altered during bilateral contractions. *J Appl Physiol* 1998; **84**: 200–6.

147 DeLuca CJ, Mambrito B. Voluntary control of motor units in human antagonist muscles: coactivation and reciprocal activation. *J Neurophysiol* 1987; **58**: 525–42.

148 Smith AM. The coactivation of antagonist muscles. *Can J Physiol Pharmacol* 1981; **59**: 733–47.

149 Draganich LF, Vahey JW. An in vitro study of anterior cruciate ligament strain induced by quadriceps and hamstring forces. *J Orth Res* 1990; **8**: 57–63.

150 More RC, Karras BT, Neiman R, Fritschy D, Woo SL, Daniel DM. Hamstrings—an anterior cruciate ligament protagonist. *Am J Sports Med* 1993; **21**: 231–7.

151 Baratta R, Solomonow M, Zhou BH, Letson D, Chuinard R, D'Ambrosia R. Muscular coactivation. The role of the antagonist musculature in maintaining knee stability. *Am J Sports Med* 1988; **16**: 83–7.

152 Milner TE, Cloutier C. Compensation for mechanically unstable loading in voluntary wrist movement. *Exp Brain Res* 1993; **94**: 522–32.

153 Jaric S, Ropret R, Kukolj M, Ilic DB. Role of antagonist and antagonist muscle strength in performance of rapid movements. *Eur J Appl Physiol* 1995; **71**: 464–8.

154 Nielsen J, Kagamihara Y. The regulation of disynaptic reciprocal Ia inhibition during co-contraction of antagonist muscles in man. *J Physiol* 1992; **456**: 373–91.

155 Nielsen J, Kagamihara Y. The regulation of presynaptic inhibition during co-contraction of antagonist muscles in man. *J Physiol* 1993; **464**: 575–93.

156 Nielsen J. *Co-contraction of antagonist muscles in man.* Doctoral dissertation, Department of Neurophysiology, Institute of Medical Physiology, Panum Institute, University of Copenhagen, 1998.

157 Aagaard P, Simonsen EB, Andersen JL, Magnusson SP, Dyhre-Poulsen P. Changes in antagonist muscle coactivation pattern during maximal knee extension following heavy-resistance strength training. *J Physiol* 2001; **531**: 62.

158 Carolan B, Cafarelli E. Adaptations in co-activation in response to isometric resistance training. *J Appl Physiol* 1992; **73**: 911–7.

159 Colson S, Pousson M, Martin A, Van Hoecke J. Isokinetic elbow flexion and coactivation following eccentric training. *J Electromyogr Kinesiol* 1999; **9**: 13–20.

160 Valkeinen H, Alen M, Häkkinen A, Hannonen P, Häkkinen K. Changes in unilateral knee extension and flexion force and agonist-antagonist EMG during strength training in fibromyalgia women and healthy women. In: *Proceedings of the 5th Annual Congress of the European College of Sports Science II*, 2000: 764 (abstract).

161 Hirokawa S, Solomonow M, Lu Y, Lou Z, D'Ambrosia R. Anterior-posterior and rotational displacement of the tibia

elicited by quadriceps contraction. *Am J Sports Med* 1992; **20**: 299–306.

162 Koh TJ, Grabiner MD. Cross talk in surface electromyograms of human hamstring muscles. *J Orth Res* 1992; **10**: 701–9.

163 Koh TJ, Grabiner MD. Evaluation of methods to minimize crosstalk in surface electromyography. *J Biomech* 1993; **26** (Suppl. 1): 151–7.

164 Aagaard P, Simonsen EB, Andersen JL, Magnusson P, Bojsen-Møller F, Dyhre-Poulsen P. Antagonist muscle coactivation during isokinetic knee extension. *Scand J Med Sci Sports* 2000; **10**: 58–67.

165 Lundberg A, Malmgren K, Schomburg ED. Convergence from Ib, cutaneous and joint afferents in reflex pathways to motoneurons. *Brain Res* 1975; **87**: 81–4.

166 Lundberg A, Malmgren K, Schomburg ED. Role of joint afferents in motor control exemplified by effects on reflex pathways from Ib afferents. *J Physiol* 1978; **265**: 763–80.

167 Pearson KG. Proprioceptive regulation of locomotion. *Curr Opin Neurobiol* 1995; **5**: 786–91.

168 Pierrot-Deseilligny E, Morin C. Evidence for supraspinal influences on Renshaw inhibition during motor activity in man. In: Desmedt JE, ed. *Spinal and Supraspinal Mechanisms of Voluntary Motor Control and Locomotion. Prog. Clin. Neurophysiol*, Vol. 8. Basel: Karger, 1980: 142–69.

169 Hultborn H, Lindström S, Wigström H. On the function of recurrent inhibition in the spinal cord. *Exp Brain Res* 1979; **37**: 399–403.

170 Schiaffino S, Reggiani C. Molecular diversity of myofibrillar proteins: gene regulation and functional significance. *Physiol Rev* 1994; **76**: 371–423.

171 Staron RS, Johnson P. Myosin polymorphism and differential expression in adult human skeletal muscle. *Comp Biochem Physiol* 1993; **106B**: 463–75.

172 Adams GR, Hather BM, Baldwin KM, Dudley GA. Skeletal muscle myosin heavy chain composition and resistance training. *J Appl Physiol* 1993; **74**: 911–5.

173 Andersen JL, Aagaard P. Myosin heavy chain IIX overshooting in human skeletal muscle. *Muscle Nerve* 2000; **23**: 1095–104.

174 Fry AC, Allemeier CA, Staron RS. Correlation between percentage fiber type area and myosin heavy chain content in human skeletal muscle. *Eur J Appl Physiol* 1994; **68**: 246–51.

175 Staron RS, Karapondo DL, Kraemer WJ, Fry AC, Gordon SE, Falkel JE, Hagerman FC, Hikida RS. Skeletal muscle adaptations during early phase of heavy-resistance training in men and women. *J Appl Physiol* 1994; **76**: 1247–55.

176 Staron RS, Leonardi MJ, Karapondo DL, Malicky ES, Falkel JE, Hagerman FC, Hikida RS. Strength and skeletal muscle adaptations in heavy-resistance trained women after detraining and retraining. *J Appl Physiol* 1991; **70**: 631–40.

177 Andersen JL, Klitgaard K, Saltin B. Myosin heavy chain isoforms in single fibres from m. vastus lateralis of sprinters: influence of training. *Acta Physiol Scand* 1994; **151**: 135–42.

178 Ennion S, Sant'ana Pereira JAAA, Sargeant AJ, Young A, Goldspink G. Characterization of human skeletal muscle fibres according to the myosin heavy chains they express. *J Musc Res Cell Motil* 1995; **16**: 35–43.

179 Smerdu V, Karsch-Mizrachi I, Campione M, Leinwand LA, Schiaffino S. Type IIx myosin heavy chain transcripts are expressed in type IIb fibers of human skeletal muscle. *Am J Physiol* 1994; **267**: C1723–C1728.

180 Weiss A, McDonough D, Wertman B, Acakpo-Satchivi L, Montgomery K, Kucherlapati R, Leinwand L, Krauter K. Organization of human and mouse skeletal myosin heavy chain gene clusters is highly conserved. *Proc Natl Acad Sci USA* 1999; **96**: 2958–63.

181 Weiss A, Schiaffino S, Leinwand L. Comparative sequence analysis of the complete human sarcomeric myosin heavy chain family: implications for functional diversity. *J Mol Biol* 1999; **290**: 61–75.

182 Baldwin KM, Haddad F. Invited review. Effects of different activity and inactivity paradigms on myosin heavy chain gene expression in striated muscle. *J Appl Physiol* 2001; **90**: 345–57.

182a Andersen JC, Weiss A, Sandri C, Schjerling P, Thornell LE, Pedrosa-Domellof F, Leinwand L, Schiaffino S. The 2B myosin heavy chain gene is expressed in human skeletal muscle. *J Physiol* 2002; **539**: 29–30.

183 Pette D, Staron RS. Cellular and molecular diversities of mammalian skeletal muscle fibers. *Rev Physiol Biochem Pharmacol* 1990; **166**: 1–76.

184 Aagaard P, Andersen JL. Correlation between contractile strength and myosin heavy chain isoform composition in human skeletal muscle. *Med Sci Sports Exerc* 1998; **30**: 1217–22.

185 Harridge SDR, White MJ, Carrington CA, Goodman M, Cummings P. Electrically evoked torque-velocity characteristics and isomyosin composition of the triceps surae in young and elderly men. *Acta Physiol Scand* 1995; **154**: 469–77.

186 Gregor RJ, Edgerton VR, Perrine JJ, Campion DS, DeBus C. Torque-velocity relationships and muscle fiber composition in elite female athletes. *J Appl Physiol* 1979; **47**: 388–92.

187 Johansson C, Lorentzon R, Sjöström M, Fagerlund M, Fugl-Meyer AR. Sprinters and marathon runners. Does isokinetic knee extensor performance reflect muscle size and structure? *Acta Physiol Scand* 1987; **130**: 663–9.

188 Andersen JL, Mohr T, Biering-Sørensen F, Galbo H, Kjaer M. Myosin heavy chain isoform transformation in single fibers from m. vastus lateralis in spinal cord injured individuals: effects of long term functional electrical stimulation (FES). *Pflügers Arch* 1996; **431**: 513–8.

189 Hather BM, Tesch P, Buchanan P, Dudley GA. Influence of eccentric actions on skeletal muscle adaptations to resistance training. *Acta Physiol Scand* 1991; **143**: 177–85.

190 Staron RS, Malicky ES, Leonardi MJ, Falkel JE,

Hagerman FC, Dudley GD. Muscle hypertrophy and fast fiber type conversion in heavy resistance-trained women. *Eur J Appl Physiol* 1990; **60**: 71–9.

191 Fitts RH, Widrick JJ. Muscle mechanics: adaptations with exercise-training. *Exerc Sports Sci Rev* 1996; **24**: 427–73.

192 Harridge SDR. The muscle contractile system and its adaptation to training. In: Marconnet P, Saltin B, Komi PV, Poortmans J, eds. *Human Muscular Function During Dynamic Exercise*. Basel: Karger, 1996: 82–94.

193 Kraemer WJ, Patton JF, Gordon SE, Harman EA, Deschenes MR, Reynolds K, Newton RU, Triplet NT, Dziados JE. Compatibility of high-intensity strength and endurance training on hormonal and skeletal muscle adaptations. *J Appl Physiol* 1995; **78**: 976–89.

194 Howald H, Hoppeler H, Claasen H, Mathieu O, Staub R. Influences of endurance training on the ultrastructural composition of different muscle fiber types in humans. *Pflügers Arch* 1985; **403**: 369–76.

195 Williams RS, Neufer PD. Regulation of gene expression in skeletal muscle by contractile activity. In: Rowell LB, Shephard JT, eds. *Handbook of Physiology, Exercise: Regulation and Integration of Multiple Systems*. New York: Oxford University Press, 1996: 1124–50.

196 Cox DM, Quinn ZA, McDermott JC. Cell signaling and the regulation of muscle-specific gene expression by myocyte enhancer-binding factor 2. *Exerc Sports Sci Rev* 2000; **28**: 33–8.

197 Barr K, Esser K. Phosphorylation of p70^{S6k} correlates with increased skeletal muscle mass following resistance training. *Am J Physiol* 1999; **276**: C120–C127.

198 Welle S, Bhatt K, Thornton CA. Stimulation of myofibrillar synthesis by exercise is mediated by more efficient translation of mRNA. *J Appl Physiol* 1999; **86**: 1220–5.

198a Caiozzo VJ, Haddad F, Baker MJ, Baldwin KM. Influence of mechanical loading on myosin heavy-chain protein and mRNA isoform expression. *J Appl Physiol* 1996; **80**: 1503–12.

199 O'Neill DS, Zheng DA, Anderson WK, Dohm GL, Houmard JA. Effect of endurance exercise on myosin heavy chain gene regulation in human skeletal muscle. *Am J Physiol* 1999; **276**: R414–R419.

200 Andersen JL, Schiaffino S. Mismatch between myosin heavy chain mRNA and protein distribution in human skeletal muscle fibers. *Am J Physiol* 1997; **272**: C1881–9.

201 Henneman E. Relation between size of neurons and their susceptibility to discharge. *Science* 1957; **126**: 1345–7.

202 McCall GE, Byrnes WC, Dickinson A, Pattany PM, Fleck SJ. Muscle fiber hypertrophy, hyperplasia, and capillary density in college men after resistance training. *J Appl Physiol* 1996; **81**: 2004–12.

203 MacDougall JD, Ward GR, Sale DG, Sutton JR. Biochemical adaptation of human skeletal muscle to heavy-resistance training and immobilization. *J Appl Physiol* 1997; **43**: 700–3.

204 Roman WJ, Fleckenstein J, Stray-Gundersen J, Alway SE, Pesock R, Gonyea WJ. Adaptations in the elbow flexors of elderly males after heavy-resistance training. *J Appl Physiol* 1993; **74**: 750–4.

205 Thorstensson A, Hultén B, v Döbeln W, Karlsson J. Effect of strength training on enzyme activities and fiber characteristics in human skeletal muscle. *Acta Physiol Scand* 1976; **96**: 392–8.

206 Goldspink DF. Cellular and molecular aspects of adaptation in skeletal muscle. In: Komi PV, ed. *Strength and Power in Sports*. The IOC Encyclopaedia of Sports Medicine, Vol. III. Oxford: Blackwell Scientific Publications, 1992: 211–29.

207 Aagaard P, Andersen JL, Leffers AM, Wagner Å, Magnusson SP, Halkjær-Kristensen J, Dyhre-Poulsen P, Simonsen EB. A mechanism for increased contractile strength of human pennate muscle in response to strength training: changes in muscle architecture. *J Physiol* 2001; **534**: 613–23.

208 Esmarck B, Andersen JL, Olsen S, Mizuno M, Kjaer M. Timing of protein intake after resistance exercise bouts is paramount for muscle hypertrophy over a 12-week training period in elderly humans. *J Physiol* 2001 (abstract).

209 Frontera WR, Meredith CN, O'Reilly KP, Knuttgen HG, Evans WJ. Strength conditioning in older men: skeletal muscle hypertrophy and improved function. *J Appl Physiol* 1988; **64**: 1038–44.

210 Mikesky AE, Giddings CJ, Matthews W, Gonyea WJ. Changes in muscle fiber size and composition in response to heavy-resistance exercise. *Med Sci Sports Exerc* 1991; **9**: 1042–9.

211 Wang N, Hikida RS, Straon RS, Simoneau JA. Muscle fiber types of women after resistance training — quantitative ultrastructure and enzyme activity. *Pflügers Arch* 1993; **424**: 494–502.

212 Alway SE, Grumbt WH, Stray-Gundersen J, Gonyea WJ. Effects of resistance training on elbow flexors of highly competitive bodybuilders. *J Appl Physiol* 1992; **72**: 1512–21.

213 Vierck J, O'Reilly B, Hossner K, Antonio J, Byrne K, Bucci L, Dodson M. Satellite cell regulation following myotrauma caused by resistance exercise. *Cell Biol Int* 2000; **24**: 263–72.

213a Stein RB, Capaday C. The modulation of human reflexes during functional motor tasks. *Trends Neurosci* 1988; **11**: 328–32.

214 Yan Z. Skeletal muscle adaptation and cell cycle regulation. *Exerc Sports Sci Rev* 2000; **28**(1): 24–6.

215 Kadi F, Eriksson A, Holmner S, Thornell LE. Effects of anabolic steroids on the muscle cells of strength trained athletes. *Med Sci Sports Exerc* 1999; **31**: 1528–34.

216 Tseng BS, Kasper CE, Edgerton VR. Cytoplasm-to-myonucleus ratios and succinate dehydrogenase activities in adult rat slow and fast muscle fibers. *Cell Tissue Res* 1994; **275**: 39–49.

217 Kadi F. Adaptation of human skeletal muscle to training and anabolic steroids. *Acta Physiol Scand Suppl* 2000; **646**: 5–47.

218 Klausen K, Anderson LB, Pelle I. Adaptive changes in

work capacity, skeletal muscle capillarization and enzyme levels during training and detraining. *Acta Physiol Scand* 1981; **113**: 9–16.

219 Ratzin Jackson C, Dickinson AL, Ringel SP. Skeletal muscle fiber area alterations in two opposing modes of resistance-exercise training in the same individual. *Eur J Appl Physiol* 1990; **61**: 37–41.

220 Terados N, Melichna J, Sylven C, Jansson E. Decrease in skeletal muscle myoglobin with intensive training in man. *Acta Physiol Scand* 1986; **128**: 651–2.

221 Bell GJ, Syrotuik D, Martin TP, Burnham R, Quinney HA. Effect of concurrent strength and endurance training on skeletal muscle properties and hormone concentrations in humans. *Eur J Appl Physiol* 2000; **81**: 418–27.

222 Hickson RC, Dvorak BA, Gorostiaga EM, Kurowski TT, Foster C. Potential for strength and endurance training to amplify endurance performance. *J Appl Physiol* 1988; **65**: 2285–90.

223 Tanaka H, Swensen T. Impact of resistance training on endurance performance. *Sports Med* 1998; **25**: 191–200.

224 Green H, Goreham C, Ouyang J, Ball-Burnett M, Ranney D. Regulation of fiber size, oxidative potential, and capillarization in human muscle by resistance training. *Am J Physiol* 1998; **276**: R591–R596.

225 Luhti JM, Howald H, Claasen H, Rosler K, Vock P, Hoppeler H. Structural changes in skeletal muscle tissue with heavy-resistance exercise. *Int J Sports Med* 1986; **7**: 123–7.

226 Tesch PA, Thorson A, Colliander EB. Effects of eccentric and concentric resistance training on skeletal muscle substrates, enzyme activities and capillary supply. *Acta Physiol Scand* 1990; **140**: 575–80.

227 Tesch PA, Thorsson A, Kaiser P. Muscle capillary supply and fiber type characteristics in weight and power lifters. *J Appl Physiol* 1984; **56**: 35–8.

228 Schantz P. Capillary supply in hypertrophied human skeletal muscle. *Acta Physiol Scand* 1982; **114**: 635–7.

229 Aagaard P, Simonsen EBEB, Andersen JL, Leffers AM, Wagner Å, Magnusson SP, Halkjær-Kristensen J, Dyhre-Poulsen P. MRI assessment of quadriceps muscle size before and after resistance training. Determination of volume vs single-site CSA. *Med Sci Sports Exerc* 2001; **33**(5) (Suppl.): 147.

230 Rutherford OM, Jones DA. Measurement of fiber pennation using ultrasound in the human quadriceps in vivo. *Eur J Appl Physiol* 1992; **65**: 433–7.

231 Willan PLT, Mahon M, Goland JA. Morphological variations of the human vastus lateralis muscle. *J Morph* 1990; **169**: 235–9.

232 Walker PM, Brunotte F, Rouhier-Marcer I, Cottin Y, Casillas JM, Gras P, Didier JP. Nuclear magnetic resonance evidence of different muscular adaptations after resistance training. *Arch Phys Med Rehab* 1998; **79**: 1391–8.

233 Alexander RMcN, Vernon A. The dimensions of knee and ankle muscles and the forces they exert. *J Hum Mov Stud* 1975; **1**: 115–23.

234 Herbert RD, Gandevia SC. Changes in pennation with joint angle and muscle torque: in vivo measurements in human brachialis muscle. *J Physiol* 1995; **484**: 523–32.

235 Magnusson SP, Aagaard P, Rosager S, Dyhre-Poulsen P, Kjaer M. Load-displacement properties of the human triceps surae aponeurosis in vivo. *J Physiol* 2001; **531**: 277–88.

236 Narici MV, Binzoni T, Hiltbrand E, Fasel J, Terrier F, Cerretelli P. In vivo human gastrocnemius architecture with changing joint angle at rest and during graded isometric contraction. *J Physiol* 1996; **496**: 287–97.

237 Kawakami Y, Abe T, Fukunaga T. Muscle-fiber pennation angles are greater in hypertrophied than in normal muscles. *J Appl Physiol* 1993; **74**: 2740–4.

238 Kawakami Y, Abe T, Kuno S, Fukunaga T. Training induced changes in muscle architecture and specific tension. *Eur J Appl Physiol* 1995; **72**: 37–43.

239 Fitts RH, McDonald KS, Schluter JM. The determinants of skeletal muscle force and power: their adaptability with changes in activation pattern. *J Biomech* 1991; **24** (Suppl. 1): 111–22.

240 Harridge SDR, Bottinelli R, Canepari M, Pellegrino MA, Reggiani C, Esbjörnsson M, Saltin B. Whole-muscle and single-fiber contractile properties and myosin heavy chain isoforms in humans. *Pflügers Arch* 1996; **432**: 913–20.

241 Komi PV. Training of muscle strength and power: interaction of neuromotoric, hypertrophic and mechanical factors. *Int J Sports Med* 1986; **7** (Suppl.): 10–6.

242 Aagaard P, Simonsen EB, Andersen JL, Magnusson SP, Halkjær-Kristensen J, Dyhre-Poulsen P. Increased contractile RFD and neuromuscular activation induced by heavy-resistance strength training. *Med Sci Sports Exerc* 1999; **31**(5) (Suppl.): S115 (abstract).

243 Schmidtbleicher D, Buehrle M. Neuronal adaptation and increase of cross-sectional area studying different strength training methods. In: Johnson B, ed. *Biomechanics X-B*. Champaign, Illinois: Human Kinetics Publishers, 1987: 615–20.

244 Duchateau J, Hainaut K. Isometric or dynamic training: differential effects on mechanical properties of a human muscle. *J Appl Physiol* 1984; **56**: 296–301.

245 Behm DG, Sale DG. Intended rather than actual movement velocity determines velocity-specific training response. *J Appl Physiol* 1993; **74**: 359–68.

246 Schmidtbleicher D, Haralambie G. Changes in contractile properties of muscle after strength training in man. *Eur J Appl Physiol* 1981; **46**: 221–8.

247 Schmidtbleicher D. Training for power events. In: Komi PV, ed. *Strength and Power in Sports*. The IOC Encyclopaedia of Sports Medicine, Vol. III. Oxford: Blackwell Scientific Publications, 1992: 381–95.

248 Aagaard P, Simonsen EB, Magnusson P, Larsson B, Dyhre-Poulsen P. A new concept for isokinetic hamstring/quadriceps strength ratio. *Am J Sports Med* 1998; **26**: 231–7.

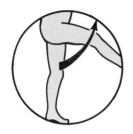

Chapter 1.5
Biomechanics of Locomotion

ERIK B. SIMONSEN & PAAVO V. KOMI

Classical reference

Winter D. A. *Biomechanics and Motor Control of Human Movement*. New York: John Wiley & Sons, Inc., 1990.

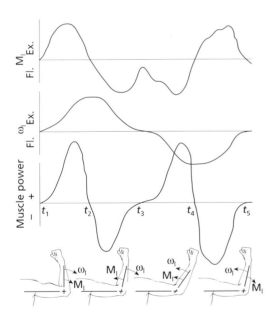

Fig. 1.5.1 Kinetic analysis of a continuous flexion/extension of the elbow joint. The top panel shows the net joint moment calculated by inverse dynamics. Extensor dominance is here defined as positive values. The middle panel shows the angular velocity; extension is positive. The lower panel shows the muscle power obtained by multiplication of joint moment and angular velocity; positive power indicates concentric contraction and negative power eccentric contraction of the dominating muscle group at a given point during the movement. Adapted from Winter [25].

Introduction

Biomechanics is a scientific interdiscipline combining physics, anatomy and physiology. Within sports medicine biomechanics is useful for measuring loadings of anatomic structures in general and for evaluating function before and after some sort of intervention such as rehabilitation and/or surgery.

In this chapter space does not permit a wide-ranging presentation of biomechanical analyses of a great number of sporting events. The purpose of the chapter is therefore to present the most commonly used methods of biomechanics to readers, who are assumed to be only remotely familiar with biomechanics. After the methodological part a few examples of biomechanical movement analysis are presented. It is hoped that by the end of the chapter the reader will appreciate the possibilities of biomechanics in relation to sports medicine.

Biomechanical equipment

Video cameras

A major part of all biomechanical research is concerned with movement analysis, which requires some sort of recording of the actual movements. In the early days of biomechanics and up until recently, 16-mm cine-film was widely used for this purpose. One advantage of film was that it could easily be recorded at various frequencies, up to several thousands of frames per second if necessary during very fast movements. The major disadvantages were that the media were expensive and the development process often took days. The use of video cameras provides instant recordings but normally at slow sampling frequencies like 50 or 60 Hz, which is sufficient for walking but not for faster movements. Also, the resolution of video recordings is much poorer than that of film and with high-speed video cameras poorer still. However, the technology is constantly improving and high-speed video has started to appear in less expensive versions with increasingly high resolution.

A *high-speed shutter* is a common facility, which should not be confused with high-speed video recordings. *Shutter* refers to the duration of the exposure of each frame. During recordings of fast movements it is normally necessary to use a shuttertime of 1/500 or 1/1000 of a second to 'freeze' the movement, otherwise fast-moving markers will appear blurred on the video recordings.

When using several video cameras it is often convenient to ensure that they operate synchronously. This can easily be accomplished through a standard *genlock* facility, which allows one camera (master) to control exposure of the other cameras (slaves). Cameras with a built-in video recorder (camcorders) cannot be genlocked. Using several cameras will normally also require some sort of *event synchronization,* which means that one frame corresponding to a certain time position of a recording can be identified on all cameras. A simple way to perform event synchronization is to flash a light in the field of view from a position visible to all cameras.

Force platforms

A force platform is a device designed to measure external reaction forces, which are often termed *ground reaction forces.* A force platform can normally measure forces in three orthogonal directions together with torsional moments about three orthogonal axes. The latter are used for calculations of *center of pressure,* which is the location on the force platform where the resultant force is applied. During dynamic movement the center of pressure changes location continuously (Fig. 1.5.2) and it may be used to find the point of application of force on the foot during e.g. running, which is required to calculate joint moments by inverse dynamics (see later). The center of pressure on a force platform may also be used as a biomechanical parameter itself representing projections of the whole-body center of mass (postural sway) during standing.

A force platform needs to be of a particular size if it is to record reliable forces during human movement.

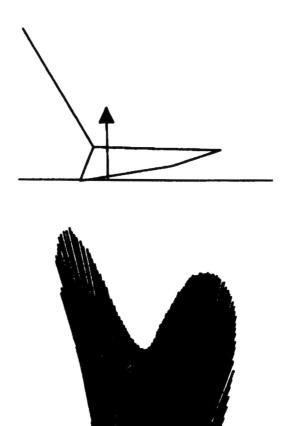

Fig. 1.5.2 Top: the resulting vector of the ground reaction forces must be aligned to the foot to calculate joint moments by inverse dynamics. The point of force application called the center of pressure changes continuously during e.g. the stance phase of walking, as demonstrated in the lower panel.

Most platforms are about 50×50×5 cm, which gives the construction a resonance frequency of about 500 Hz. This is sufficient to ensure that vibrations are not created by forces originating from human movements. Hitting the platform with a hammer will start a vibration of the natural frequency.

Biomechanical laboratories for the investigation of, for example, gait have been designed in various ways.

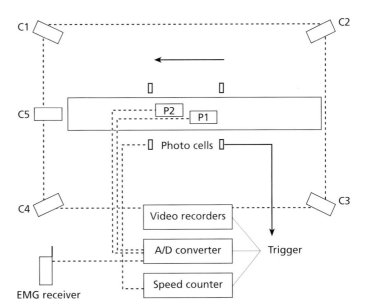

Fig. 1.5.3 Schematic drawing of a gait lab with five cameras (C1–5), two force platforms (P1 and P2) and photocells to record the gait velocity during experiments.

One approach is to use a motor-driven treadmill with a number of cameras placed around it. The use of a treadmill has both advantages and disadvantages. The advantages are that it may reduce the space requirements considerably and that the gait velocity can be strictly controlled. The major disadvantage is that investigation of kinematics is limited. To calculate net joint moments by inverse dynamics in two dimensions both the vertical and the horizontal ground reaction force need to be measured and the center of pressure aligned to the spatial positions of the foot. Therefore, the majority of gaitlabs consist of some sort of walkway containing one or two force platforms (Fig. 1.5.3).

In vivo tendon and ligament force measurements in humans

Information on the forces produced by individual skeletal muscles, tendons and ligaments is important to the understanding of muscle mechanics, muscle physiology, musculoskeletal mechanics, neurophysiology and motor control. The methods applied to produce these forces have been both direct and indirect. Indirect estimation can refer to such methods as the mathematical solution of the actual muscle force in the indeterminate musculoskeletal system. Electromyography (EMG) has been used as an indirect predictive measure of individual muscle torques. Both of these estimates are subject to error, the magnitude of which may vary considerably. For example, the main problem in the use of EMG is its sensitivity to varying conditions of muscle action types, velocity of shortening or lengthening, fatigue, training and detraining.

Recent developments in technology and surgical implantation procedures have made it possible to measure forces of the muscle–tendon unit (and ligaments) quite successfully. Since Salmons [1] introduced a version of the buckle transducer for recording tendon forces in animals, a number of experiments have been performed, especially investigating cat locomotion. These important developments then led to application of this direct *in vivo* technique in human locomotion [2], primarily for studying the loading of the Achilles tendon (AT) during normal activities such as walking, running, hopping and jumping [3–7]. The buckle transducer in human experiments is shown schematically in Fig. 1.5.4. The transducer consists of a main frame, two strain gauges, and a center bar placed across the frame. The size of the frame and bending of the cross-bar varies depending on the size of the AT in question. Final selection of the frame and cross-bar is done during surgical operation, which is performed under local anesthesia. To provide normal propriocep-

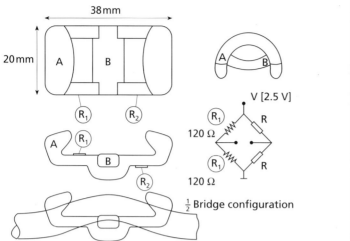
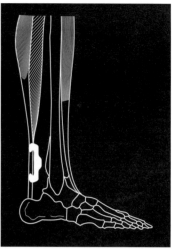

Fig. 1.5.4 (a) Schematic presentation of the 'buckle'-type transducer designed for experiments in which human subjects can perform even maximal activities, e.g. in running and jumping. A, Main buckle frame; B, cross-bar. R_1 and R_2 are resistors of the $\frac{1}{2}$ Wheatstone bridge configuration. The lower part demonstrates schematically (and with slight exaggeration) the bending of the Achilles tendon when the transducer is *in situ*. (b) Schematic presentation of the buckle transducer implanted around the Achilles tendon [3].

tion, lidocaine is not injected into the tendon or muscle tissues. The operation usually lasts 15–20 min while the subject is in a prone position on the operating table. The cable containing the wires from the strain gauges is threaded under the skin and brought to the exterior approximately 10 cm above the transducer. After the cut has been sutured and carefully covered with sterile tapes, the cable of the transducer is connected to an amplifying unit for immediate check-up. Calibration of the transducer is usually performed immediately before the experiments. In contrast to the animal experiments, a slightly more indirect approach must be used to calibrate the AT transducer in human subjects. Experiments can then be performed for approximately 2–3 h, depending on the quantity of local anesthesia applied, and measurements can vary from slow walking to maximal jumping.

Use of the buckle transducer in the study of AT force measurements produces important parameters such as peak-to-peak force and rate of force development which can then be used to describe the loading characteristics of the tendon under normal locomotion. When these parameters are combined with other external measurements, such as cinematography for calculation of muscle–tendon complex length

changes, the important concepts of muscle mechanics, such as instantaneous length–tension and force–velocity relationships can be examined in natural situations such as stretch–shortening cycle (SSC) activities [4,8]. Simultaneous recording of EMG activity can add to the understanding of the force potentiation mechanism during SSC-type movement.

The major advantage of direct *in vivo* measurement is that continuous recording of AT force is possible, which is immediately available for inspection. The second important feature of this measurement approach is the fact that several experiments can be performed in one session and the movements are truly natural. The section on p. 125 gives examples of the AT force recordings during different locomotion tasks performed with the buckle transducer.

The buckle transducer method is naturally quite invasive, and may raise objections from the ethical committee in question. Due to the relatively large size of the buckle there are not many tendons which can be selected for measurements. The AT is, however, an ideal one due to large space between the tendon and bony structures within the Karger triangle. Other restrictions in the use of this method are difficulties in the calibration procedure, and problems in the applica-

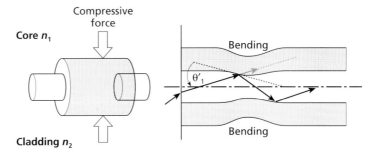

Fig. 1.5.5 Basic demonstration of how compression on the optic fiber (left) causes microbending (right) and less light through the core–cladding interface. (From Alt *et al.* [15].)

tion of the technique when long-term and repeated implantation may be of interest. As is the case in animal experiments the buckle transducer method cannot isolate the forces of the contractile tissue from the tendon tissues. The method can therefore only be used to demonstrate the loading characteristics of the entire muscle–tendon complex.

Optic fiber technique

In order to overcome some of the disadvantages of the buckle transducer technique, an alternative method has recently been developed. As was the case for the buckle method this new optic fiber technique was first applied to animal tendons [9]. However, it had already been successfully used as a pressure transducer in sensitive skin application [10] and for measurement of foot pressure in different phases of cross-country skiing [11]. The measurement is based on light intensity modulation by mechanical modification of the geometric properties of the plastic fiber. The structure of optical fibers used in animal and human experiments [9,12–14] consists of two-layered cylinders of polymers with small diameters. When the fiber is bent or compressed the light can be reduced linearly with pressure, and the sensitivity depends on fiber index, fiber stiffness and/or bending radius characteristics. Figure 1.5.5 demonstrates the principle of the light modulation in the two-layer (cladding and core) fiber when the fiber diameter is compressed by external force. The core and cladding will be deformed and a certain amount of light is transferred through the core–cladding interface. In order to avoid the pure effect of bending of the fiber, when the fiber is inserted through the tendon (Fig. 1.5.6) it must have a loop large enough to exceed the so-called critical bending radius.

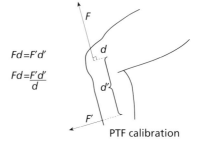

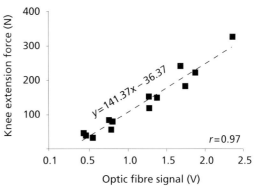

Fig. 1.5.6 Measured forces and moment arms for the calibration of patellar tendon force (PTF). The optic fiber output was related to the muscle force (F) that had been converted from the external force output (F') using equation $Fd = F'd'$, where d is moment arm of tendon force and d' is moment arm of the foot or leg [14].

Figure 1.5.7 demonstrates how the optic fiber is inserted through the tendon. A hollow 19-gauge needle is first passed through the tendon (a). The sterile optic fiber is then passed through the needle; the needle is removed and the fiber remains *in situ* (b). Both ends of the fiber are then attached to the transmitter–receiver unit and the system is ready for measurement (c). The

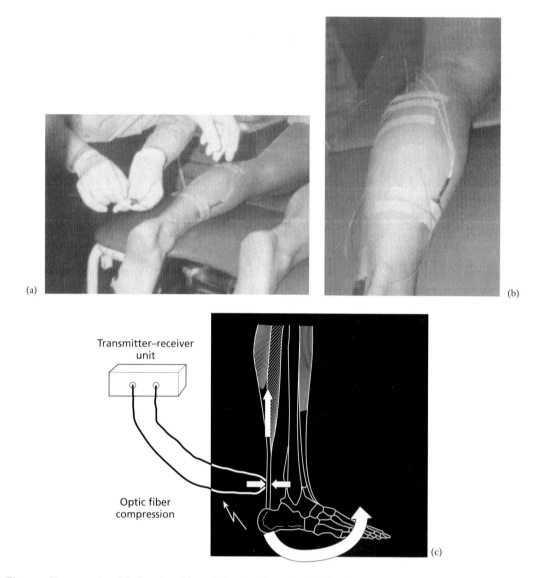

Fig. 1.5.7 Demonstration of the insertion of the optic fiber into the tendon. (a) After the 19-gauge needle has been inserted through the tendon, the 0.5 mm thick optic fiber is threaded through the needle. The needle is then removed and the optic fiber remains *in situ* inside the tendon (b), and both ends of the fiber are connected to the transmitter–receiver unit (c). In real measurement situations this unit is much smaller and can be fastened onto the skin of the calf muscles.

calibration procedure usually provides a good linear relationship between external force and optic fiber signal. Figure 1.5.6 gives a representative example of such a relationship for the patella tendon measurements.

Although the optic fiber method may not be more accurate than the buckle transducer method, it has several unique advantages. First of all it is much less invasive and can be reapplied to the same tendon after a few days of rest. In addition, almost any tendon can be studied provided that the critical bending radius is not exceeded. The optic fiber technique can also be used to measure the loading of the various ligaments. In the hands of an experienced surgeon the optic fiber can be inserted through even deeper ligaments such as the anterior talofibular ligament [15]. In such a case, however, special care must be taken to ensure that the optic fiber is in contact with the ligament only and that contact with other soft tissue structures is prevented by catheters.

Foot pressure transducers

Force platforms as described above can be used to measure both static and dynamic plantar forces provided that the platform is capable of producing independent measures of both vertical and shear forces. In many applications, both clinical and athletic, it is desirable to have a continuous recording of the pressure distribution under the foot. Forces acting under the foot in various foot pathologies such as diabetic neuropathy, leprosies, injury and deformation are naturally different from these measured in healthy athletes. Post-operative follow-up of corrective surgery such as free flap reconstruction of severe tibial factures can be performed by measuring plantar pressures under the foot [16].

The behavior of the foot–shoe interface cannot usually be detected with force plates or even with pedopadographs. For this reason discrete in-shoe transducers have been developed. In the basic design a number of pressure-sensitive transducers are implanted in the shoe insole. The sensors can be of different types, such as capacitive, conductive polymer, sensitive ink or various forms of piezoelectric resistors. For technical details the reader is referred to the thorough review article of Cabb and Claremont [17]. The number of sensors per insole varies depending on the manufacturer. In some cases there can be close to 1000 discrete sensors or as few as 16 in one insole. The common rule is that the smaller the number of sensors, the more carefully the sensor locations must be planned in order to match the important anatomic loading sites of the foot.

In athletic activities it is desirable to use devices which allow continuous recording for several minutes. In the author's (Komi) laboratory considerable experience has been gained from the use of a portable, in-shoe pressure data acquisition system (Paromed-system®, GmBH, Germany) (Fig. 1.5.8), which

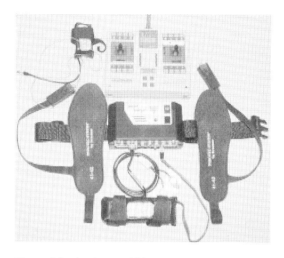

Fig. 1.5.8 In-shoe data acquisition system (Paromed-system®, GmBH, Germany) widely used in measurements of plantar pressures during different activities. Both insoles have 16 piezoelectric microsensors embedded into water-filled hydrocells.

measures simultaneously plantar pressure distribution and EMG activities. The system has in each insole 16 piezoelectric microsensors embedded into water-filled hydrocells. The insoles (32 in total) and EMG cables (from muscles) are connected to the 'Data Logger' which is fixed by a belt to the subject's back. The sampling frequency for the plantar pressures is 200 Hz. The analysis produces continuous records from each channel and the computer software produces (also continuous) contour curves during the entire contact phase on the ground. Figure 1.5.9 gives an example of the pressure contours from a patient who had clear asymmetry due to femur length discrepancy.

As with any biomechanical method, plantar pressures provide only partial information on locomotion and loading characteristics. For this reason it is very desirable to combine plantar pressure recordings with other parameters obtained from e.g. video cameras and EMG amplifiers. Figure 1.5.10 is an example of such an arrangement, where ski-jumping take-off is studied using a variety of different measuring techniques [18]. In addition to plantar pressure measurements, the forces can also be recorded from a 9-m force plate placed under the take-off table [19] or from the smaller force plates implanted into the ski bindings (Pelkonen *et al.* in progress).

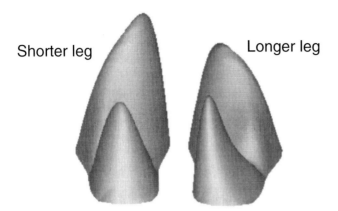

Shorter leg   Longer leg

Fig. 1.5.9 Example of the plantar pressure contour curves during the contact phase of walking in a patient with considerable leg length discrepancy [48].

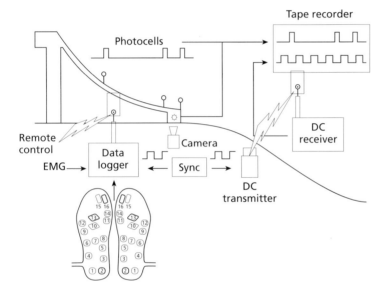

Fig. 1.5.10 Schematic presentation of how plantar pressure measurements can be combined with other biomechanical parameters in the study of ski-jumping [18].

Goniometers and accelerometers

An electrogoniometer is an analog device used to record joint angles. A simple type of goniometer consists of a potentiometer with two rods, which can be aligned and attached to, for example, the thigh and the shank to measure the knee-joint angle. The potentiometer type of goniometer has to be aligned so that the axis of rotation of the potentiometer is more or less identical to the joint's axis of rotation. Another type of goniometer is based on strain gauge technology as it measures the bending of a spring. This type has the advantage that it does not need to be aligned to the joint's axis of rotation and it is available for measurements in two perpendicular planes, e.g. for flexion/extension and abduction/adduction at the shoulder joint. Three-dimensional goniometers, which also include inward/outward rotation, exist but they are rare. A typical example of the use of goniometers is in the measurement of muscle strength parameters in isokinetic devices. Compression of soft tissues usually dislocates the joint's axis of rotation with respect to the axis of rotation of the lever arm, resulting in inaccurate data on joint position (Fig. 1.5.11) [20].

Accelerometers are small lightweight transducers

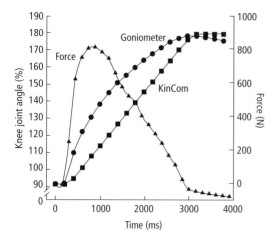

Fig. 1.5.11 Knee joint angle and force vs. time measured during a concentric contraction at 30°/s. The curves labeled 'KinCom' and 'Goniometer' are angle measurements from the KinCom machine and the knee-mounted goniometer, respectively ('180 deg.' denotes full extension). The goniometer signal shows the correct knee joint angle because the center of the knee joint becomes misaligned with the machine's axis of rotation during the maximal contraction [20].

capable of measuring acceleration. Like force transducers they can be based on strain gauge or piezoelectric technology. The latter transducers can only measure dynamic events, while an accelerometer based on strain gauges is capable of measuring the gravitational acceleration, when for example lying on a table. Major problems with the use of accelerometers are that they are difficult to 'mount' on a human being and that they measure the acceleration in only one direction. One solution is to use three accelerometers mounted perpendicular to each other and then compute the 'resulting' acceleration. This gives an accurate value but the direction of the acceleration is largely unknown. The reader is referred to Winter *et al.* [21] and Dyhre-Poulsen *et al.* [22] for examples of the use of accelerometers.

Electromyography

Electrical potentials from active muscle fibers may be recorded by intramuscular needle or wire electrodes or on the skin by surface electrodes. During dynamic movement needle electrodes are considered too inconvenient. Wire electrodes are useful for recording from

'deep' muscles as surface electrodes have a pick-up depth of only a few mm. Very thin wires ($\approx$50 μm) are used to record from single motor units but wires of about 250 μm in diameter inserted a few cm apart largely resemble the EMG from surface electrodes. Wire electrodes are difficult to work with, but in some cases there are no alternatives as, for example, with the iliopsoas muscle [23,24].

To obtain high-quality EMG signals from the skin it is necessary to remove hair and dead cells to reduce skin resistance. Ag/AgCl adhesive electrodes with a lead-off area of $\approx$10 mm^2 with some sort of electrolytic gel are normally placed about 2 cm apart along the estimated muscle fiber direction. A bipolar set-up means that the two electrodes will measure the potentials relative to a reference electrode, preferably placed over bony tissue. The surface EMG is an AC signal, which oscillates between negative and positive values some 80–100 times per second. It is, however, a compound signal made of many interfering action potentials from single motor units. Therefore, the surface EMG contains frequency components from about 10 to 500 Hz. Normally, a sampling frequency of 1000 Hz is sufficient to obtain an acceptable digital representation of a raw surface EMG. When used for biomechanical movement analysis EMG signals are often full wave rectified and lowpass filtered with a cut-off frequency of about 10–15 Hz (Fig. 1.5.12). This representation is called a 'linear envelope' and it is convenient for quantification in terms of amplitude, integrated EMG and duration. The integrated EMG is the area under the linear envelope.

Recordings of EMG during dynamic movement are often contaminated by so-called *movement artefacts*, which are low-frequency components of the recordings originating from movements of the electrodes rather than being a part of the EMG. In the recording phase such artefacts can be more or less abolished by the use of preamplifiers positioned close to the recording electrodes, because these preamplifiers not only amplify the signal but also lower the impedance before 'transportation' through wires to the main amplifier. It is possible to remove movement artefacts further subsequently by application of a highpass filter with a cut-off frequency of 10–20 Hz.

Electromyography is very useful when combined

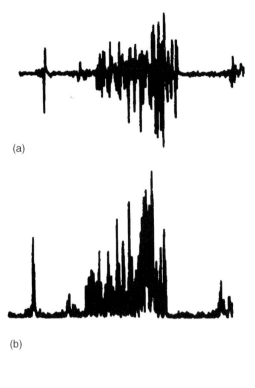

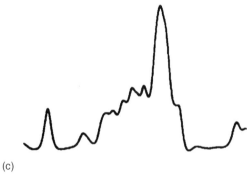

(a)

(b)

(c)

Fig. 1.5.12 (a) A so-called 'raw' EMG recording of the soleus muscle during walking. In (b) the signal is rectified and all negative values are made positive and in (c) the rectified signal has been lowpass filtered with a cut-off frequency of 10 Hz to form a linear envelope.

with biomechanical movement analysis. Calculation of net joint moments by inverse dynamics gives only the net result of the muscle contractions about the joint. Information about cocontraction cannot be provided without simultaneous EMG recordings.

Biomechanical analysis

Offline/online digitization

Computer systems for biomechanical movement analysis can be divided into offline and online systems. The latter may use active or passive markers. Active markers emit light or sound or other signals which are registered by a receiver unit several times per second. Passive markers most often reflect infrared light, which is flashed by special video cameras. The video signal is looped through a special electronic device, which will extract only the light of infrared intensity. The center of each marker is then calculated and x,y-coordinates are transferred to a computer. This whole process runs on line, i.e. 50–200 times per second for up to six cameras. As a consequence the visible video pictures are lost and only the coordinates of the small markers placed at anatomic landmarks on the subject are left in a computer. If anything goes wrong, for example if markers passing close by each other get mixed or if a marker cannot be 'seen' by at least two cameras at any time, it is often difficult to correct the errors. However, when such systems work perfectly, they can provide almost instant results. Online systems are typically limited to permanent laboratories.

Offline systems are based on video recordings. Normally, analog video signals are stored on tape and later sampled by a computer with a so-called frame-grabber. Video recordings from digital cameras can also be input to a computer by commercial interface devices. Once the video sequences exist in digital form in a computer, they can be processed frame by frame by specially dedicated software. Usually contrasting markers are placed at anatomic landmarks on the subject and these can then be digitized manually or semiautomatically to obtain x,y-coordinates from each frame. If the software can identify a large number of markers on most of the frames the process of offline digitization may be fairly fast, meaning for example 30–40 min for 400 frames corresponding to a gait cycle of 80 frames per camera and five cameras.

A major advantage of offline video analysis is that field events can easily be recorded and analysed even from sports competitions without markers on the subjects.

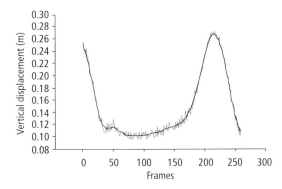

Fig. 1.5.13 Vertical displacement of an ankle joint marker during a normal walking cycle. The noisy curve is raw data from digitization while the smooth curve represents the same signal lowpass filtered with a cut-off frequency of 5 Hz (the film was recorded at 200 frames/s).

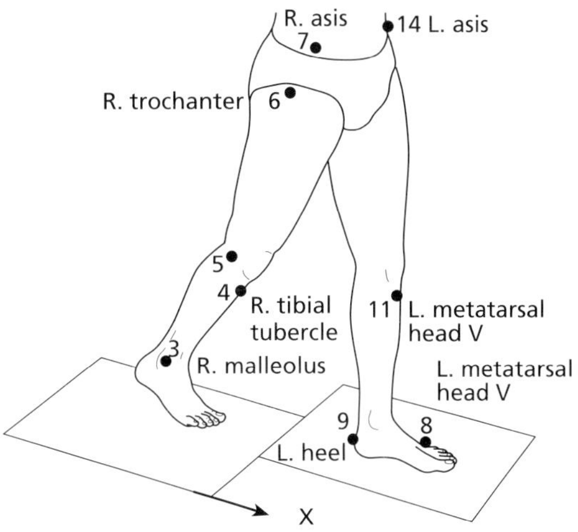

Fig. 1.5.14 Marker placement on a three-dimensional link segment model [33].

Noise reduction/filtering

In every process of digitization of markers placed on a subject small errors will be present. A marker placed on the skin will move with the skin, but most importantly it is impossible for either a computer or a human being to digitize exactly the center of a marker. These errors represent a kind of noise component superimposed on the pure movement signal (Fig. 1.5.13). It can be shown that the noise is of a random character but of an absolute amplitude [25]. This amplitude may be 2–3 mm on a scale of 2 m. The result of a digitization is so-called time–position data and the noisy component seems to affect the time–position data only to a certain degree. However, when the first derivative is taken (differentiation) to obtain velocity data, the noise becomes more evident, and with the second derivative it becomes clear that something has to be done to reduce the errors from digitization. Various types of digital smoothing or filtering can be applied to time–position data to reduce the noise, but most often a so-called 4th order lowpass Butterworth filter is used to remove frequency components above e.g. 5 Hz. However, this implies that both the noise and some fraction of the real movement signal are attenuated and it follows that movement data will never be accurate when originally obtained as time–position data. After filtering, velocity and acceleration can be calculated so that clear signals are obtained, and provided the same

cut-off frequency is used throughout an experiment the error component can be assumed to be of a constant and systematic nature (Fig. 1.5.13).

Link-segment models

In a biomechanical analysis of movement the human body is normally converted into a model consisting of rigid body segments connected by hinge joints (two dimensional) or spherical joints (three dimensional) (Fig. 1.5.14). The segments are most often assumed to be rigid, each segment mass is set to a certain fraction of the whole body and the segment center of mass is assumed to be located at a certain proportional distance along. The anthropometric data used to establish a link-segment model are normally based on Dempster [26] and the model is therefore confined to data from a limited number of Caucasian cadavers. Biomechanics worldwide is in great need of additional anthropometric data relating to ethnic differences. It is obvious that a link-segment model is basically inaccurate in many aspects. However, it is reasonable to assume that the inaccuracies of a model represent a systematic error, which allows the investigator to compare results on the same subject in various situations. Several mechanisms may be studied with link-segment models, while absolute values can never be accurate.

Kinematics

A kinematic analysis of a movement usually includes calculation of joint angles. An anatomic joint angle is an angle between two segments while a so-called segment angle is between a segment and the vertical or the horizontal plane. Joint angular velocity obtained by time differentiation of angle data is also often considered part of a kinematic analysis, because this parameter can be expressed as, for example, flexion and extension indicated by positive and negative angular velocity, respectively (see Fig. 1.5.1 above). All positions and velocities are in principle kinematic parameters. Segmental mechanical energy in terms of potential, kinetic and rotational energy also belongs to kinematics, because accelerations are not needed for these calculations.

Kinetics

Kinetic parameters are acceleration, force and moment (torque). The most common kinetic parameter is so-called net joint moments calculated by *inverse dynamics*. These moments provide information as to which muscle group is exerting the strongest force on a joint and how strongly these muscles are pulling on the bones. When no external forces are acting on the body segments of interest, as occurs e.g. during kicking or throwing, the calculation of inverse dynamics is fairly simple. Continuous extension and flexion of the elbow joint represents a situation with no external forces. A calculation of joint moments by inverse dynamics shows that this movement is fairly complicated with regard to muscle action and contraction mode (see Fig. 3.5.1).

It can be seen that a positive moment in this case indicates extensor muscle dominance while a negative moment indicates flexor dominance. A counter-clockwise pulling direction is normally defined as positive. The term *dominance* refers to the fact that both flexors and extensors may be active simultaneously (cocontraction) and as a consequence a zero moment could theoretically be the result of intensive cocontraction. It is further seen from Fig. 3.5.1 that flexion and extension are 'out of phase' with the joint moment in certain time periods. However, this could merely mean that, for example, the flexor muscles decelerate the last part of the extension and then turn the movement directly into flexion. Multiplication of angular velocity and joint moment yields power and it is seen that negative power means eccentric muscle work and positive power concentric work (Fig. 3.5.1). It is considered an important feature of inverse dynamics that the method can provide information about the contraction mode of the muscles.

During jumping, walking and running external reaction forces are applied to the most distal segment, the foot. These forces have to be measured by a force platform together with the center of pressure on the platform, so that the point of force application on the foot can be found on every frame. This method of inverse dynamics is also called *the free body segment method*, because the calculations are performed on one segment at a time. The calculation includes joint reaction forces acting on both ends of the segment, inertial properties and the influence of the moment from the previous segment (Fig. 1.5.15).

The joints of the lower extremities are positioned so that a positive moment about the ankle joint is a dorsi-flexor moment, a positive moment about the knee joint is an extensor moment and a positive moment about the hip joint a flexor moment. The example of walking shows that the ankle joint is plantar–flexor dominated during the stance phase, the knee joint shows short flexor, extensor, flexor and extensor dominance while the hip joint is extensor dominated in the first half of the stance phase and flexor dominated in the last part of the stance phase (Fig. 1.5.16). The reason why walking with flexor dominance about the knee joint is possible without collapsing is that the movement is dynamic and that the three joints of the leg operate together. The moments of the ankle, knee and hip joint are often added to form a so-called support moment representing the action of the whole leg. Doing so requires extensor moments to be considered as positive during the calculation (Fig. 1.5.16). If the support moment is positive, the leg will not collapse.

Bone-on-bone forces can be calculated as the sum of all forces acting about a joint. After calculation of the net joint moment it is necessary to compute an estimated internal moment arm for the dominating muscle group to obtain the muscle force. Bone-on-bone forces are often confused with joint reaction forces, which are a part of the inverse dynamics calculation (see Fig. 1.5.15). Cocontraction about the actual joint will cause the bone-on-bone forces to be underesti-

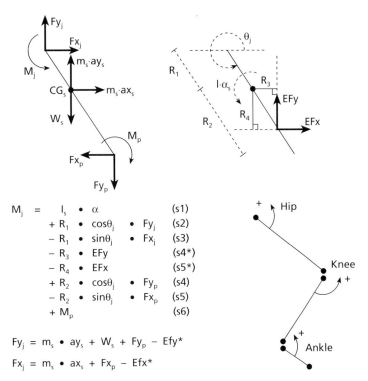

Fig. 1.5.15 Free body diagram showing the calculation of inverse dynamics in two dimensions. M denotes a moment; F, joint reaction force; EF, external reaction force; I, moment of inertia; α, angular acceleration; m, segment mass; W, m×g of a segment; R a, distance to segment mass center; a, linear acceleration of segment mass center; θ, segment angle with respect to the horizontal plane. Suffix j denotes the joint of interest and the proximal end of the segment; p refers to parameters transferred from the previous segment and acting on the distal end of the segment; x, horizontal direction; y, vertical direction.

$$
\begin{aligned}
M_j \;=\; & I_s \cdot \alpha && (s1) \\
 & + R_1 \cdot \cos\theta_j \cdot Fy_j && (s2) \\
 & - R_1 \cdot \sin\theta_j \cdot Fx_j && (s3) \\
 & - R_3 \cdot EFy && (s4*) \\
 & - R_4 \cdot EFx && (s5*) \\
 & + R_2 \cdot \cos\theta_j \cdot Fy_p && (s4) \\
 & - R_2 \cdot \sin\theta_j \cdot Fx_p && (s5) \\
 & + M_p && (s6)
\end{aligned}
$$

$$Fy_j = m_s \cdot ay_s + W_s + Fy_p - Efy*$$

$$Fx_j = m_s \cdot ax_s + Fx_p - Efx*$$

mated; it is therefore considered ideal to record an EMG simultaneously. The reader is referred to Scott and Winter [27] and Simonsen *et al.* [28] for examples of bone-on-bone forces during locomotion.

Muscle–tendon unit models

As mentioned above it is possible to deduce from inverse dynamics whether the muscles contract eccentrically or concentrically. However, this applies to muscles spanning only one joint. Several muscles are bi-articular and their length changes depend on the motion of the two joints they cross. On the basis of cadaver studies [29,30] it is possible to model a number of muscles in the lower extremities all working in the sagittal plane with flexion or extension. Models of the soleus and the gastrocnemius muscles are seen in Fig. 1.5.17. The length of a muscle–tendon unit is in this case calculated from origin to insertion. Since the muscle fibers are normally only a few cm long and connected in series with the aponeurosis and tendons it is not possible to separate the length changes of the muscle fibers and the tendinous structures, respectively.

Three-dimensional analysis

Using only one camera for a movement analysis limits the calculations to two dimensions (2D). This is not necessarily considered a disadvantage since many movements take place primarily in the sagittal plane and a 2D analysis is much easier to perform than a three-dimensional (3D) one [31].

A 3D set-up requires that each marker of interest is visible to at least two cameras at any point during the movement. Most systems require some sort of calibration cube to be filmed by all cameras. Digitizing markers on the cube with known coordinates in 3D makes it possible to calculate the exact position of the cameras and to calculate further the third dimension of each marker by so-called *direct linear transformation* [32].

Three-dimensional kinetics

The complexity of calculating joint moments by inverse dynamics increases almost exponentially when advancing from 2D to 3D. In 3D it is necessary to compute joint centers, but the biomechanical commu-

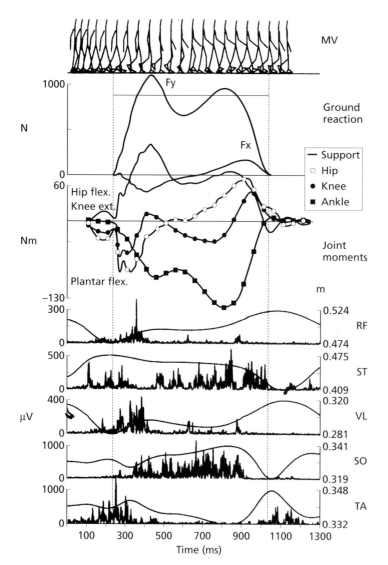

Fig. 1.5.16 A complete two-dimensional analysis of one walking cycle consisting of recordings from film, force platform and EMG. From top to bottom: stick-diagram of the movement, ground reaction forces (the horizontal line represents body mass), net joint moments of ankle, knee and hip joint and the total support moment of the leg, rectified EMGs from the rectus femoris, semitendinosus, vastus lateralis, soleus and tibialis anterior muscles with changes in muscle–tendon lengths superimposed on the EMGs (inflection denotes lengthening of the muscle–tendon unit).

nity suffers from the lack of anthropometric data for this purpose. The formulas published by Vaughan *et al.* [33] are often used, but these formulas are only based on X-ray data from one subject and alternative formulas are mostly substantiated. Another complication with 3D is that calculation of joint centers is closely related to specific marker set-ups. It is necessary to place three markers on each segment in order to calculate the segment's attitude, which again allows for calculation of joint moments about anatomic axes. This means that, for example, a hip flexor moment can

be recognized irrespective of how the subject turns in space during the recorded movement. A major drawback of the 3D approach is that only few joints are spherical joints. For example, it seems nonsensical to calculate abduction/adduction moments about the knee joint. Nevertheless relatively large moments of abduction/adduction about this joint appear from a 3D kinetic analysis of walking or running [33]. Moments of internal/external rotation must also be considered very uncertain due to small movements of segment rotation about a longitudinal axis.

(a)

(b)

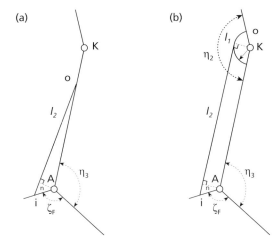

Fig. 1.5.17 Trigonometric models of (a) the soleus and (b) gastrocnemius muscles (the two heads are lumped). K, knee joint; A, ankle joint; i, insertion; o, origin; η_2, knee joint angle; η_3, ankle joint angle; l_2, length of the soleus muscle–tendon unit; $l_1 + l_2$, length of the gastrocnemius muscle–tendon unit; ζ_F is an angle taken from Frigo and Pedotti[29].

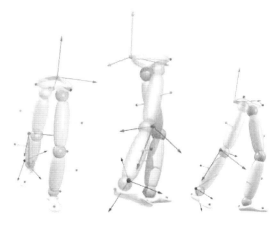

Fig. 1.5.18 Illustration of a three-dimensional link-segment model consisting of pelvis, thigh, shank and foot segments connected by spherical joints. The markers used for digitization are shown; in this case the Helen Hays marker set-up was used, which includes some of the markers on wands sticking out from the segments. To calculate joint moments representing anatomic flexion/extension, abduction/adduction and inward/outward rotation no matter how the subject is oriented in space, it is necessary to define local segment coordinate systems, which are related to the global reference coordinate system of the laboratory. (Adopted from Arial Dynamics Inc.)

Fig. 1.5.19 The top flow diagram illustrates the process of inverse dynamics. However, the position data are not coordinates of markers but a joint angle calculated using marker coordinates. The lower panel shows the process of forward dynamics (simulation), where you start with muscle force and end with movement. θ is a joint angle, ω angular velocity, α angular acceleration, I moment of inertia, τ muscle moment, λ internal moment arm, F muscle force and Δt a time constant.

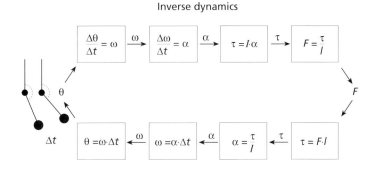

Inverse dynamics

Forward dynamics (simulation)

Simulation

Calculation of net joint moments by inverse dynamics is called *inverse* because one actually works in the opposite direction to nature when measuring the movements and the external forces used to calculate the muscle forces that generated the movement. Using *forward dynamics* represents a method which simulates biology in the sense that you build a link-segment

model in a computer with muscles attached to the segments (Figs 1.5.18–1.5.20). The muscles possess anatomic and physiologic properties like fiber length, tendon length, tendon compliance, internal moment arms of the muscles, force–velocity relationship and length–tension relationship. The computer is then programmed to activate the muscles in random order until the desired movement is accomplished, which

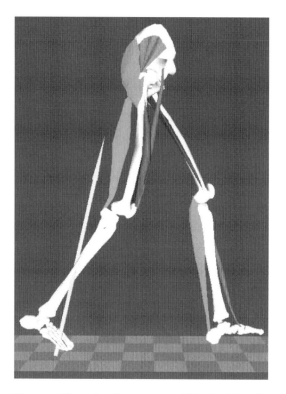

Fig. 1.5.20 Illustration of a computer model for simulation of walking. (Adopted from Musculographics Inc.)

may take weeks or months. *Optimization* of a simulation model is accomplished with a so-called *cost function*, which signifies the target of the simulation or rather the criteria of success. *Performance optimization* is, for example, the length of a long jump calculated theoretically from the vertical and horizontal velocities of a long jump model at take-off, but the same movement may be optimized by *tracking* the joint displacements or the ground reaction forces produced by a real long-jumper. For a review see van den Bogert [34].

It is often necessary to perform experiments with inverse dynamics to verify the behavior of a model. However, once a simulation model moves realistically it is possible to 'ask' the model questions, which cannot easily be investigated experimentally with real subjects. Examples of such questions or rather manipulations are to make certain muscles stronger or weaker or to move the insertion point of a muscle. It is also possible to apply perturbations to a moving model.

Gerritsen *et al.* [35] found that a simulation model of human walking driven by simulated muscles could recover from a sudden perturbation while a model driven by 'mechanical' joint moments lost balance and fell to the floor.

Examples of biomechanical investigations

Different movement strategies in vertical jumping

Vertical jumping is often used as a standard test for dynamic strength in the lower extremities. Three types of vertical jumps prevail in the literature: (i) drop jump, in which the subject starts by jumping downward from a box onto the floor and performs a vertical jump immediately after the landing: this is a typical SSC (stretch–shortening cycle) type of exercise; (ii) countermovement jump, which is also an SSC exercise but with less eccentric loading; and (iii) squat jump (Figs 1.5.21 and 1.5.22), where the subject starts from a static squatting position, i.e. a movement ideally consisting of pure concentric contractions.

Direct *in vivo* tendon forces during normal locomotion

Normal locomotion and/or muscle function usually refers to stretch–shortening cycles [2], where the active muscle is first stretched (eccentric action) prior to shortening (concentric action). The purpose of SSC is to make the performance more efficient as compared to isolated forms of either isometric or concentric actions. Figure 1.5.23 is a typical example of how the buckle transducer technique, which can be used to characterize the loading of the triceps surae muscle–tendon complex, is combined with simultaneous EMG recordings. The figure shows several important features of the loading characteristics in this example of moderate-speed running. First, the changes in the muscle–tendon length (segment length) are very small (6–7%) during the stretching phase. This suggests that the conditions favor the potential utilization of short-range elastic stiffness (SRES) [36] in the muscle. Various length changes are reported in the literature demonstrating that the effective range of SRES in *in vitro* preparations is 1–4% [37,38]. In the intact muscle tendon, *in vivo*, this value is increased because series

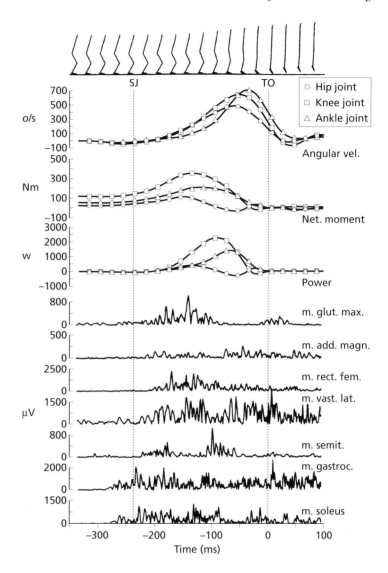

Fig. 1.5.21 A squat jump performed with a simultaneous strategy. From top to bottom: stick diagram showing a subset of the frames, which were recorded at 500 Hz; angular velocity of extension; net joint moments; net joint power; and rectified EMG from seven muscles. Extensor-dominated moments are all positive and positive power indicates concentric contractions. SJ is start of the jump and TO is toe-off.

elasticity and fiber geometry must be taken into account. This could then increase the muscle–tendon lengthening to 6–8%. When measurements are made at the muscle fiber level the values could be naturally smaller, as shown by Roberts *et al.* [39] in turkeys running on level ground.

Achilles tendon force (ATF) curves similar to the one shown in Fig. 1.5.23 can then be used to plot both the peak-to-peak ATF and the rate of ATF development during ground contact against the running velocity. This presentation is from a subject who was

able to run at different velocities (ranging from 3 to 9 m/s) with the buckle transducer around his AT.

The figure shows that the maximum ATF seems to have reached its highest value by a speed of 6 m/s, in which case the value was 9 kN corresponding to 12.5 body weight (BW). As the cross-sectional area of the tendon was 0.81 cm², the peak force for this subject was 11.1 kN/cm², a value which is well above the range of the single load ultimate tensile strength [40]. The qualitative presentation shows that the maximum rates of ATF development, measured during the sharp

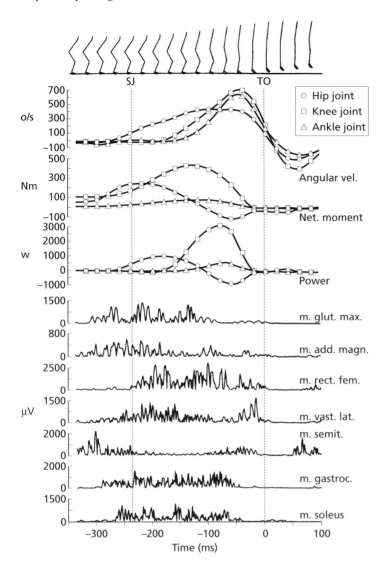

Fig. 1.5.22 A squat jump performed with a sequential strategy. From top to bottom: stick diagram showing a subset of the frames, which were recorded at 500 Hz; angular velocity of extension; net joint moments; net joint power; and rectified EMG from seven muscles. Extensor-dominated moments are all positive and positive power indicates concentric contractions. SJ is start of the jump and TO is toe-off.

rising phase after the contact, increased linearly with the increase in running velocity during contact. This information is important, because it suggests that the rate of force development rather than the peak-to-peak force may be more relevant for characterizing biological tissue loading during locomotion.

It is well known from basic muscle physiology that the force–velocity (F–V) relationship [41] describes the fundamental mechanical properties of human muscle. This Hill curve differs, however, in one fundamental respect from the natural situation: the forces are measured during constant (maximal) activities. In natural and normal locomotion, such as SSC of Fig. 1.5.23, the EMG activity is variable and not constant in any parts of the cycle. Thus the instantaneous force–velocity curves measured for the functional contact phase are consequently very different from the classical curve obtained for pure concentric actions with isolated preparations [41] or with human forearm flexors [42,43].

Figure 1.5.25 gives examples of the instantaneous F–V curves for running (a) and hopping (b). The

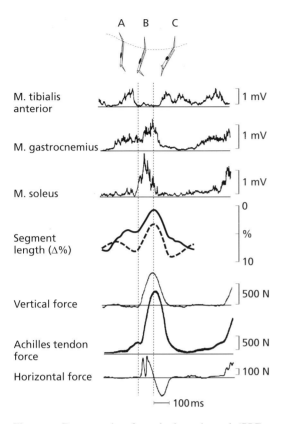

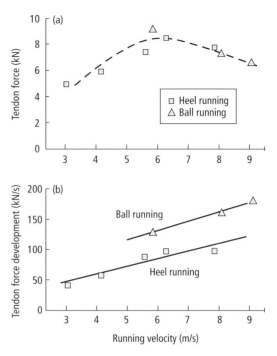

Fig. 1.5.24 Peak Achilles tendon forces (a) and peak rates of tendon force development (b) for one subject running at different velocities. The buckle transducer was implanted around the subject's Achilles tendon [49].

Fig. 1.5.23 Demonstration of stretch–shortening cycle (SSC) for the triceps surae muscle during the (functional) ground contact phase of human running. Top: Schematic position representing the three phases of SSC (preactivation (A), eccentric (B) and concentric (C)). The rest of the curves represent parameters in the following order (from top to bottom): rectified surface EMG records of the tibialis anterior, gastrocnemius and soleus muscles; segmental length changes of the two plantar flexor muscles; vertical ground reaction force; directly recorded Achilles tendon force; and the horizontal ground reaction force. The vertical lines signify, respectively, the beginning of the foot (ball) contact on the force plate and the end of the eccentric phase. The subject was running at moderate speed [49].

buckle experiments (left) did not include comparative records obtained in a classical way, but the form of the FV curves suggests considerable force potentiation in the concentric phase. Our recent experiments with the optic fiber technique, although not yet performed at high running speeds, suggest similar potentiation. The right side of Fig. 1.5.25 shows simultaneous plots for both patella and AT forces during hopping. The

data signify that in short contact hopping the triceps surae muscle behaves in a bouncing ball-type fashion (see also [6,44]). When the hopping intensity is increased or changed to countermovement-type jumps, the patella tendon force increases and the AT force may decrease [13]. The classical type of curve obtained with constant maximal activation for an isolated concentric action is also superimposed with the AT force in the same graph (Fig. 1.5.25, right). The shaded area between the two AT curves suggests a remarkable force potentiation for this submaximal effort.

The direct *in vivo* technique reliably measures the forces in the tendon (and ligament), but the results and relationships obtained cannot, however, be used to generate simultaneous information about: (i) the change in length of the muscle fibers; (ii) the change in the fiber orientation with the line of force application; or (iii) the change in length of the tendinous compartment. Thus the force–velocity curves presented in Fig. 1.5.25 must be interpreted more correctly as referring

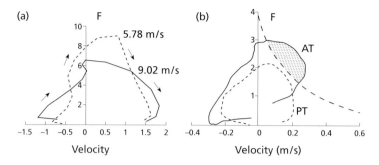

Fig. 1.5.25 Examples of instantaneous force–velocity curves measured in (a) human running and (b) hopping. The records on the left were obtained with the buckle transducer [49] and those on the right with the optic fiber [13]. Each record is for a functional (contact) phase on the ground. In each curve the upward deflection signifies stretching (eccentric actions) and the downward deflection shortening (concentric action) of the muscle tendon complex during ground contact. The velocity axis has been derived from segmental length changes according to Grieve *et al.* [30].

to the function of the muscle–tendon as one entity. However, experiments are currently in progress to utilize a relatively high resolution and frame rate (>60 Hz) ultrasound technique to capture the movements in the fascicle compartment during SSC actions in combination with the optic fiber and EMG recordings for both triceps surae and quadriceps femoris muscles.

Plantar pressures during sporting activities

The basic methodology of plantar pressure recording was introduced above on p. 113. The experimental set-up shown schematically in Fig. 1.5.25 was successfully used in actual ski-jumping. Figure 1.5.26 gives examples of how this methodology produced results from the various plantar pressure sensors and from the EMG activities recorded from selected muscles. It is clear from simple observation of Fig. 1.5.26 that the jumper ML had a clearly unbalanced take-off as shown by dramatic bilateral differences in the pressure contours at the moment of take-off. These results also demonstrate that during the run-in and take-off, the locations which detect the pressures are primarily points 1 and 2 (heel area) and 15 and 16 (toe area). Figure 1.5.27, on the other hand, gives a unique demonstration of the plantar pressures of selected insole points and EMG activities throughout the entire ski-jumping performance, including not only the take-off but also the entire run-in, flight and landing.

While ski-jumping take-off represents an explosive

type muscle action with relatively small impact loading, the triple jump is an activity where the impact loads on muscle, joint and bones are probably the highest of all sporting activities (Figs 1.5.29–1.5.31). Figure 1.5.28 gives an example of the ground reaction forces and plantar pressures (one sensor only) during the contact phases of the hop, step and jump. In these situations the maximal vertical force (F_z) can exceed 10 000 kN in the braking phase, being slightly higher on the 'step' contact as compared to 'hop' or 'jump' of the triple jump. In relative units these values represent 5–7 times the body weight. When compared with normal walking, for example, the triple jump loading, as measured with F_z ground reaction forces, is almost 10 times greater.

Modeling anterior cruciate ligament loadings at the knee joint

A side-cutting maneuver is an important and common movement in many sports events, especially ball-games. The purpose of the maneuver is to pass a defending player by faking the direction opposite to the intended movement. Normally, the player will approach the defending player head on, touch down on the left foot, brake the forward velocity and step to the right side. During the braking action, the quadriceps femoris muscle contracts eccentrically causing an anterior shear force on the tibia that stresses the anterior cruciate ligament (ACL) of the knee joint (Fig. 1.5.32). The peak knee joint moment (239 Nm) calcu-

Run-in

Take-off

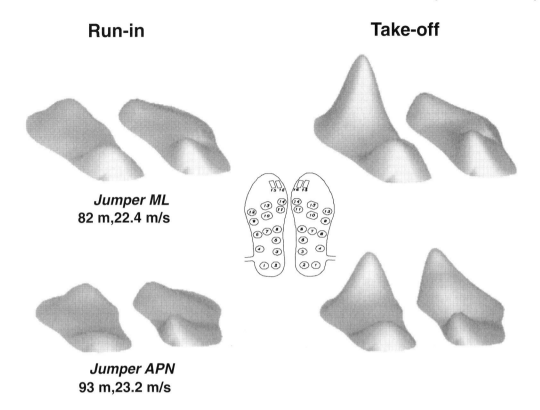

Jumper ML
82 m, 22.4 m/s

Jumper APN
93 m, 23.2 m/s

Fig. 1.5.26 Examples of the pressure contours from two different ski jumpers (ML and APN) during the run-in and take-off phases. Sensor locations of the pressure insoles are shown as well [50].

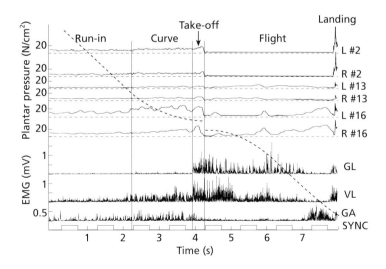

Fig. 1.5.27 An example of the selected pressure, EMG (GL, gluteus; VL, vastus lateralis; GA, gastrocnemius) and sync pulse curves from one ski-jump with run-in speed of 23.2 m/s and length of jump 93 m [50].

lated by inverse dynamics was found to occur during the braking action at a knee joint angle of 126° (average of six subjects). The model then showed an average shear force on the ACL of 520N (range 215–673N) (Fig. 1.5.33). The ACL has been shown to have a maximum strength of 2000N in young people [45]. Therefore, the side-cutting maneuver cannot directly cause a rupture of a normal ACL [46].

The hamstring muscles have frequently been sug-

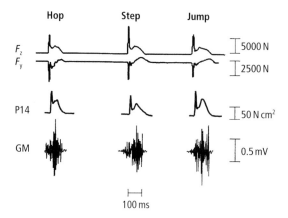

Fig. 1.5.28 Example of the two-dimensional ground reaction forces, plantar pressure distribution of the forefoot sensor (P14), and raw EMG signal of the gluteus maximus (GM) in the triple jump. The length of jump was 15.24m [16].

gested to be able to lower the loadings on the ACL. However, an EMG analysis showed that these muscles were only moderately activated during the braking action of the side-cutting maneuver. The peak amplitudes of the medial and lateral hamstrings were 34 and 39% of maximum EMG, respectively (Figs 1.5.33 & 1.5.34). In comparison the vasti were activated close to 100%. Estimates of shortening and/or lengthening velocities were calculated by muscle models based on cadaver data from Frigo and Pedotti [29] and expressed as percentage muscle fiber length per second using cadaver data from Wickiewicz *et al.* [47]. These calculations showed that the hamstring muscles shortened during the braking action and that the shortening velocity was up to about 400% fiber length per second, which strongly indicates that the muscles cannot produce force of any significance in this situation. Thus the hamstring muscles cannot reduce ACL loadings during a side-cutting maneuver [46].

Summary

Biomechanics is an interdiscipline mostly concerned with movement analysis. The laws of physics are used to calculate strain applied to anatomic structures during movement. Movements are recorded by video cameras, and small markers or sensors are placed on the subject at anatomic landmarks. The video signals

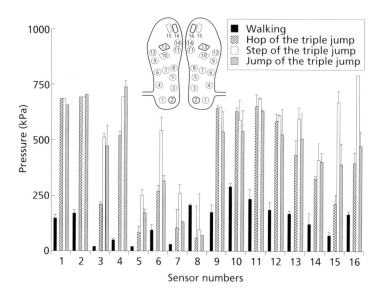

Fig. 1.5.29 Example of the peak pressures of the various sensors for one male jumper measured during the hop, step and jump phases of the triple jump and during walking. The missing standard deviation bars indicate that the signals exceeded the range of sensors [16].

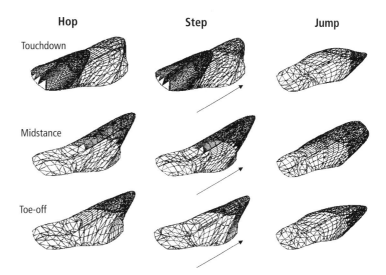

Fig. 1.5.30 The contour curves of the plantar pressures measured 20 ms after touchdown, in the middle of the stance phase and the toe-off. The arrows indicate jumping direction [16].

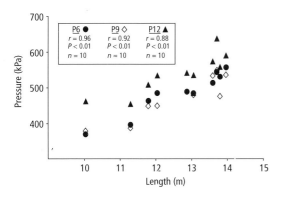

Fig. 1.5.31 Relationship between the length of the triple jump and the peak plantar pressures of the lateral forefoot (sensors 6, 9 and 12) of one experienced male jumper measured during the hop, step and jump.

are analysed by computer in real time or off line depending on the specific equipment. The coordinates of the markers are used to calculate velocities and accelerations and joint angles, and when combined with measurements of external forces acting on the body, net joint moments or muscle forces can be calculated by a method called *inverse dynamics*. Movement analysis in three dimensions requires the use of several video cameras recording from different views. The third dimension is then calculated by *direct linear transfor-*

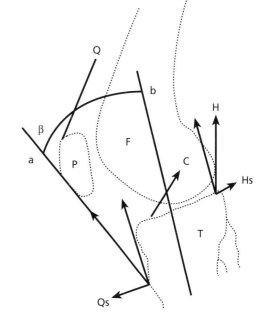

Fig. 1.5.32 A biomechanical model of the knee joint intended to evaluate stress applied to the anterior cruciate ligament during movement. Abbreviations: F, femur; T, tibia; P, patella; C, force acting on the anterior cruciate ligament; Q, quadriceps femoris muscle; H, hamstring muscles; Qs, quadriceps shear force; Hs, hamstring shear force; and β, the angle between a and b signifying the angle of the patellar ligament relative to tibia, which changes with the position of the knee joint.

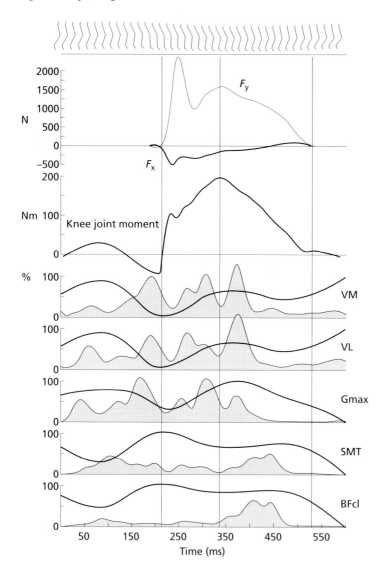

Fig. 1.5.33 One subject performing a side-cutting maneuver. From top: stick diagram of the left leg during a side-cutting maneuver; the vertical (Fy) and the horizontal (Fx) ground reaction force; the net knee joint moment; EMG from five leg muscles. The EMGs are linear envelopes and expressed relative to a maximum EMG measured during isometric conditions. The curves superimposed on the EMGs are estimates of muscle–tendon unit length changes. Inflection indicates lengthening. Abbreviations: VM, vastus medialis; VL, vastus lateralis; Gmax, gluteus maximus; SMT, semitendinosus and semimembranosus muscles, BFcl, biceps femoris caput longum muscle.

mation. External reaction forces are most often measured by force platforms, but a detailed pressure distribution of the plantar surface of the foot can also be measured using special devices mounted inside a shoe. Power generated by the muscles during movement may be calculated using net joint moments and angular velocity. Muscle power then provides detailed information about the muscle activity with regard to eccentric and concentric contractions.

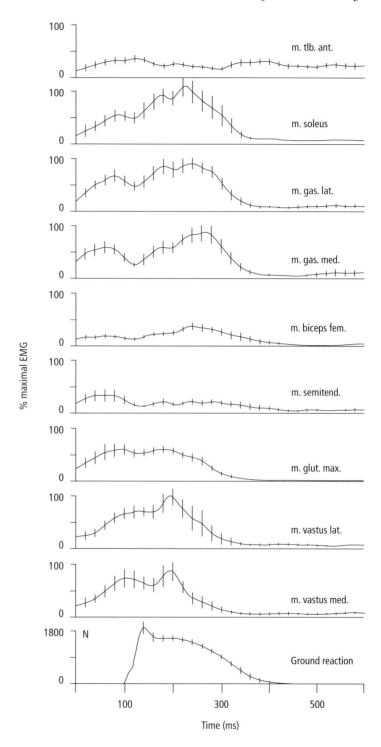

Fig. 1.5.34 Linear envelope EMGs from seven leg muscles recorded during a side-cutting maneuver. The bottom panel is the vertical ground reaction force. The data represent an average of 10 trials across six subjects and are expressed relative to maximum EMG. Error bars are standard error of the mean.

Multiple choice questions

1 *Noisy movement data are filtered with a:*

a highpass filter

b bandpass filter

c lowpass filter.

2 *Inverse dynamics is a method used to calculate:*

a joint moments

b joint angles

c angular acceleration.

3 *A goniometer measures:*

a acceleration

b velocity

c angles.

4 *Center of pressure is measured on:*

a a force platform

b the floor

c the foot.

5 *Tendon forces may be measured using:*

a a force platform

b optic fibers

c EMG.

References

1 Salmons S. The 8th International Conference on Medical and Biomechanical Engineering—meeting report. *Bio Med Eng* 1969; **4**: 467–74.

2 Komi PV. Physiological and biomechanical correlates of muscle function: Effects of muscle structure and stretch-shortening cycle on force and speed. *Exerc Sport Sci Rev/ACSM* 1984; **12**: 81–121.

3 Komi PV, Salonen M, Järvinen M, Kokko O. *In vivo* registration of Achilles tendon forces in man. I. Methodological development. *Int J Sports Med* 1987; **8**: 3–8.

4 Komi PV. Relevance of *in vivo* force measurements to human biomechanics. *J Biomech* 1990; **23** (Suppl. 1): 23–34.

5 Gregor RJ, Komi PV, Browing RC, Järvinen M. A comparison of the triceps surae and residual muscle moments at the ankle during cycling. *J Biomech* 1991; **24**: 287–97.

6 Fukashiro S, Komi PV, Järvinen M, Miyashita M. Comparison between the directly measured Achilles tendon force and the tendon force calculated from the ankle joint moment during vertical jumps. *Clin Biomech* 1993; **8**: 25–30.

7 Voigt M, Dyhre-Poulsen P, Simonsen EB. Stretch-reflex control during human hopping. *Acta Physiol Scand* 1998; **163**(2): 181–94.

8 Komi PV. Stretch-shortening cycle: a powerful model to study normal and fatigued muscle. *J Biomech* 2000; **33**: 1197–206.

9 Komi PV, Belli A, Huttunen V, Bonnefoy R, Geyssant A, Lacour JR. Optic fiber as a transducer of tendomuscular forces. *Eur J Appl Physiol* 1996; **72**: 278–80.

10 Bocquet J-C, Noel J. Sensitive skin-pressure and strain sensor with optical fibres. In: *Proceedings of 2nd Congress on Structural Mechanics of Optical Systems*, 13–15 January 1987, Los Angeles, California, USA.

11 Candau R, Belli A, Chatard JC, Carrez J-P, Lacour J-R. Stretch shortening cycle in the skating technique of cross country skiing. *Sci Motricité* 1993; **22**: 252–6.

12 Arndt AN, Komi PV, Brüggemann G-P, Lukkariniemi J. Individual muscle contributions to the *in vivo* Achilles tendon force. *Clin Biomech* 1998; **13**: 532–41.

13 Finni T, Komi PV, Lepola V. *In vivo* muscle dynamics during jumping. In: *Third Annual Congress of the European College of Sport Science*, 15–18 July 1998, Manchester, UK.

14 Finni T, Komi PV, Lepola V. *In vivo* human triceps surae and quadriceps femoris muscle function in a squat jump and counter movement jump. *Eur J Appl Physiol* 2000; **83**: 416–26.

15 Alt W, Lohrer H, Gollhofer A, Komi P. Estimation of ankle ligament load using a fiber optic transducer *in vivo*. 2002; in press.

16 Perttunen JR, Nieminen H, Tukiainen E, Kuokkanen H, Asko-Seljavaara S, Komi PV. Asymmetry of gait after free flap reconstruction of severe tibial fractures with extensive soft-tissue damage. *Scand J Plastic Reconst Surg Hand Surg* 2000; **34**(3): 237–43.

17 Cabb J, Claremont DJ. Transducers for foot pressure measurement: survey of recent developments. *Med Biol Eng Computing* 1995; **33**: 525–32.

18 Komi PV, Virmavirta M. Ski jumping take-off performance: determining factors and methodological advances. In: Müller E, ed. *Science and Skiing*. Cambridge: Chapman & Hall, Cambridge University Press, 1997: 3–36.

19 Virmavirta M, Avela J, Komi PV. A comparison of different methods to determine the take-off velocity in vertical jumps. In: Häkkinen K, Keskinen KL, Komi PV, Mero A, eds. *Book of Abstracts. XVth International Congress of Biomechanics*, 1995: 972–3.

20 Sørensen H, Zacho M, Simonsen EB, Dyhre-Poulsen P, Klausen K. Joint angle errors in the use of isokinetic dynamometers. *Isokinetics Exerc Sci* 1998; **7**: 129–33.

21 Winter DA, Wells RP, Orr GW. Errors in the use of isokinetic dynamometer. *Eur J Appl Physiol Occup Physiol* 1981; **46**: 397–408.

22 Dyhre-Poulsen P, Laursen AM. Programmed electromyographic activity and negative incremental muscle stiffness in monkeys jumping down. *J Physiol* 1984; **350**: 121–36.

23 Dorge HC, Andersen TB, Sørensen H, Simonsen EB, Aagaard H, Dyhre-Poulsen P, Klausen K. EMG activity of the iliopsoas muscle and leg kinetics during the soccer place kick. *Scand J Med Sci Sports* 1999; **9**(4): 195–200.

24 Andersson EA, Nilsson J, Thorstensson A. Intramuscular EMG from the hip flexor muscles during human locomotion. *Acta Physiol Scand* 1997; **161**(3): 361–70.

25 Winter DA. *Biomechanics and Motor Control of Human Movement*. New York: John Wiley & Sons, Inc., 1990.

26 Dempster WT. *Space Requirements of the Seated Operator*.

WADC Technical Report. Ohio: Wright Patterson Airforce Base, 1955: 55–159.

27 Scott SH, Winter DA. Internal forces at chronic running injury sites. *Med Sci Sports Exerc* 1990; **22**(3): 357–69.

28 Simonsen EB, Dyhre-Poulsen P, Voigt M, Aagaard P, Sjøgaard G, Bojsen-Møller F. Bone-on-bone forces during loaded and unloaded walking. *Acta Anat* 1995; **152**: 133–42.

29 Frigo C, Pedotti A. Determination of muscle length during locomotion. In: Asmussen E, Jørgensen K, eds. *International Series of Biomechanics VI-A* 1978: 355–360. University Park Press, Baltimore.

30 Grieve DW, Pheasant S, Cavanagh PR. Predictions of gastrocnemius length from knee and ankle joint posture. In: Asmussen E, Jorgensen K, eds. *Biomechanics VI-A*. Baltimore: University Park Press, 1978: 405–12.

31 Alkjær T, Simonsen EB, Dyhre-Poulsen P. Comparison of inverse dynamics calculated by two- and three-dimensional models during walking. *Gait Posture* 2002; in press.

32 Miller NR, Shapiro R, McLaughlin TM. A technique for obtaining spatial kinematic parameters of segments of biomechanical systems from cinematographical data. *J Biomech* 1980; **13**: 535–47.

33 Vaughan CL, Davis BL, O'Connor JC. *Dynamics of Human Gait*. Leeds, UK: Human Kinetic Publishers, 1992: 1–137.

34 van den Bogert AJ. Analysis and simulation of mechanical loads on the human musculoskeletal system: a methodological overview. *Exerc Sports Sci Rev* 1994; **22**: 23–51.

35 Gerritsen KG, van den Bogert AJ, Hulliger M, Zernicke RF. Intrinsic muscle properties facilitate locomotor control—a computer simulation study. *Motor Control* 1998; **2**: 206–20.

36 Rack PMH, Westbury DR. The short range stiffness of active mammalian muscle and its effect on mechanical properties. *J Physiol* 1974; **240**: 331–50.

37 Ford LE, Huxley AF, Simmons RM. Tension responses to sudden length change in stimulated frog muscle fibres near slack length. *J Physiol* 1978; **269**: 441–515.

38 Huxley AF, Simmons RM. Proposed mechanism of force generation in striated muscle. *Nature* 1971; **233**: 533–8.

39 Roberts TJ, Marsch RL, Weyand PG, Taylor CR. Muscular force in running turkeys. the economy of minimizing work. *Science* 1997; **275**: 1113–15.

40 Butler DL, Grood ES, Noyes FR. *et al.* Effects of structure and strain measurement technique on the material properties of young human tendons and fascia. *J Biomech* 1984; **17**: 579–96.

41 Hill AV. The heat and shortening of the dynamic constant of muscle. *Proc Royal Soc London, B* 1938; **126**: 136–95.

42 Wilkie DR. The relation between force and velocity in human muscle. *J Physiol* 1950; **110**: 249.

43 Komi PV. Measurement of the force–velocity relationship in human muscle under concentric and eccentric contraction. In: Jokl E, ed. *Medicine and Sport, Biomechanics III*, Vol. 8. Basel: Karger, 1973: 224–9.

44 Fukashiro S, Komi PV. Joint moment and mechanical power flow of the lower limb during vertical jump. *Int J Sports Med* 1987; **8**: 15–21.

45 Woo SL, Hollis JM, Adams DJ, Lyon RM, Takai S. Tensile properties of the human femur–anterior cruciate ligament–tibia complex. The effects of specimen age and orientation. *Am J Sports Med* 1991; **19**: 217–25.

46 Simonsen EB, Magnusson SP, Bencke J, Næsborg H, Havkrog M, Ebstrup JF, Sørensen H. Can the hamstring muscles protect the anterior cruciate ligament during a side-cutting maneuver. *Scand J Med Sci Sports* 2000; **10**: 78–84.

47 Wickiewicz TL, Roy RR, Powell PL, Edgerton VR. Muscle architecture of the human lower limb. *Clin Orth Rel Res* 1983; **179**: 275–83.

48 Perttunen JR, Kyröläinen H, Komi PV, Heinonen A. Biomechanical loading in the triple jump. *J Sports Sci* 2000; **18**: 363–70.

49 Komi PV. Stretch–shortening cycle. In: Komi PV, ed. *Strength and Power in Sport*. The IOC Encyclopaedia of Sports Medicine, Vol. III. Oxford: Blackwell Scientific Publications 1992: 169–79.

50 Virmavirta M, Komi PV. Plantar pressures during ski jumping take-off. *J Appl Biomechan* 2000; **16**(3): 320–6.

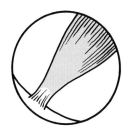

Chapter 1.6
Connective Tissue in Ligaments, Tendon and Muscle: Physiology and Repair, and Musculoskeletal Flexibility

PETER MAGNUSSON, TIMO TAKALA,
STEVEN D. ABRAMOWITCH,
JOHN C. LOH & SAVIO L-Y. WOO

Classical reference

Woo S.L-Y. *et al.* Mechanical properties of tendons and ligaments II. The relationships of immobilization and exercise on tissue remodeling. *Biorheology* 1982; **19**: 397–408.

Considering the enormity of problems related to injuries to tendons and ligaments, relatively little used to be known about the stress-related remodeling of these soft tissues. Tipton, Akeson, Noyes and Woo are credited with demonstrating the deleterious effects of immobilization on tendons and ligaments around the knee, including joint stiffness and significant weakening of the biomechanical properties of ligaments. On the other hand, studies were also performed to reveal the positive, but limited, effects of exercise on the properties of tendons and ligaments. It was then possible to establish a non-linear relationship between increased or decreased stress and motion, and the homeostasis of soft tissues. Whether these processes cause changes in the mechanical properties or changes in the mass of these tissues, or both, was the subject addressed in the paper by Woo and coworkers.

Using a rabbit model, femur–medial collateral ligament–tibia complexes (FMTC) were tensile tested after 9 and 12 weeks of immobilization, and after 9 weeks of immobilization followed by 9 weeks of remobilization. It was found that the 9- and 12-week immobilized groups had failure loads of only 31% and 29%, respectively, of the contralateral controls ($P<0.01$) with all specimens failing by tibial avulsion. In the remobilized groups, the mechanical properties of the FMTC remained inferior to the controls and the mode of failure was still tibial avulsion.

The effects of short-term (3 months) and long-term (12 months) exercise in the swine digital extensor and flexor tendons were also compared. Animals were exercised by running at a speed of 6–8 km/h for a total of 40 km/week. In the extensor tendon of the forepaw, exercise had no significant effects on mechanical properties in the short term, but long-term increases in cross-sectional area and tensile strength over those of age-matched, non-exercised controls were observed. On the other hand, in the flexor tendon, there were no significant effects on mechanical properties nor cross-sectional area of the tissue substance, but there was a 19% increase in ultimate load which could be attributed to an increase in strength of the tendon–bone junction.

As a result of the data obtained in this study, together with those published by Noyes, Tipton and Laros, a hypothetical curve was drawn to represent the homeostatic response of soft tissues in response to stresses and motion, depicting a highly non-linear relationship (Fig. 1.6.1). Immobilization can significantly compro-

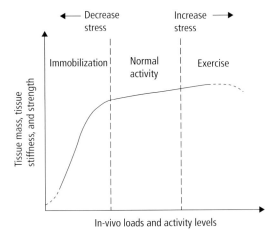

Fig. 1.6.1 Hypothetical response of ligaments to levels of stress.

mise both the structural properties of the bone–ligament–bone complex and the mechanical properties of the ligament, with weakening more pronounced at the insertion sites. The effects of exercise or increased tension are much less pronounced, as the gains are minimal even with a substantial duration of exercise.

Biochemical composition of muscle extracellular matrix: the effect of loading

Extracellular matrix

Multicellular organisms are formed of specialized cells that are assembled in tissues. The extracellular matrix (ECM) outside the cells is a complex and dynamic meshwork that contains collagens, non-collagenous glycoproteins, proteoglycans and elastin. The extracellular matrix supports the cellular elements and maintains the structural integrity of multicellular organisms. Further, it helps cells to bind together and regulates various cellular processes, such as cell growth, proliferation, differentiation, migration and adhesion.

Skeletal muscle collagen

Collagen is the most abundant protein of the ECM and constitutes about 20–25% of all protein in the body [1]. To date 19 distinct collagen types have

been identified in vertebrates [2]. They are usually divided into two subgroups on the basis of their supramolecular structures: fibrillar-forming and non-fibrillar-forming collagens. In skeletal muscle, collagen is mainly present in three fibrillar-forming forms, collagen types I, III and V, and one non-fibrillar-forming collagen, type IV of basement membranes [3,4]. Of these, types I and III are the most abundant. In addition, collagen types II, XI, XIII, XIV, XV and XVIII have been found in skeletal muscle and type VI in cardiac muscle [5–9]. In epimysium and perimysium collagen type I and III are present, with the former dominating, while all major collagen types have been observed in the endomysium [10,11]. It has been shown that slow-twitch muscles contain more collagen than fast-twitch muscles [12–14], and that the concentration of endomysial collagen is higher around slow than fast skeletal muscle fibers in rats [13].

Post-translational processing of collagen

In skeletal muscle collagen is produced principally by fibroblasts on the membrane-bound ribosomes of the rough endoplasmic reticulum. Collagen biosynthesis is characterized by the presence of an extensive number of co- and post-translational modifications of the polypeptide chains, which contribute to the quality and stability of the collagen molecule [15] (Fig. 1.6.2a). The polypeptide chains form triple-helical procollagen molecules that are secreted into the extracellular space by exocytosis. Procollagens contain amino-terminal and carboxy-terminal extension peptides at the respective ends of the collagen molecule, and after secretion, the amino-propeptides are cleaved by specific proteinases and the collagens self-assemble into fibrils or other supramolecular structures.

The three polypeptide chains, which form the triple-helical structure, are called α-chains. The molecular organization of the different collagen types differs so that type I collagen is a heterotrimer of two identical α1(I) chains and one α2(I) chain, type III collagen is a homotrimer with α1(III) chains. The most common form of type IV collagen consists of two α1(IV) chains and one α2(IV) chain, although other forms also exist. The α-chains are composed of repeating amino acid sequences Gly-X-Y, where the glycine residue in every third position enables the three α-chains to coil around one another. Proline and

(a)

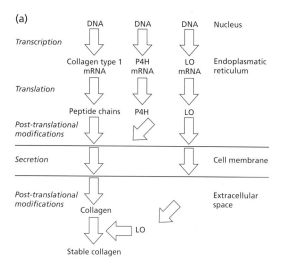

(b)

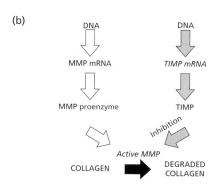

Fig. 1.6.2 (a) Collagen expression. Scheme of pre- and post-translational events in collagen expression (P4H, prolyl 4-hydroxylase; LO, lysyl oxidase). P4H activity correlates with collagen synthesis. LO activity is required for formation of pyridinoline cross-linked stable collagen. (b) Collagen degradation. Matrix metalloproteinases (MMPs) and their inhibitors (TIMPs) regulate the degradation of collagen.

4-hydroxyproline residues appear frequently at the X- and Y-positions, respectively, and promote the formation of intermolecular cross-links [16]. The stability and quality of the collagen molecule are largely based on the intra- and intermolecular cross-links. The 4-hydroxyproline as a part of the polypeptide chain is an almost unique feature of collagen, and its assay is therefore suitable for evaluating collagen content [17]. The formation of 4-hydroxyproline is catalyzed by

prolyl 4-hydroxylase (PH). The levels of PH activity generally increase and decrease with the rates of collagen biosynthesis, and assays of the enzyme activity have been used for estimating changes in the rate of collagen biosynthesis in many experimental and physiologic conditions [15,18–30]. The activity of galactosylhydroxylysyl glucosyltransferase (GGT), another post-translational enzyme of collagen synthesis, also reflects the rate of collagen biosynthesis, although the changes in GGT activity are usually less pronounced and occur more slowly than in the case of PH [15,22,23,25–29]. Total collagen concentration is 40–50% higher in slow-twitch than in fast-twitch muscle [14]. The concentration is higher both around individual type I fibers than type II fibers, and in the endomysium and perimysium of slow-twitch muscle than fast-twitch muscle [31]. Muscle is attached to its tendon at the end of the fibers, where the collagen fibrils of muscle fuse or interdigitate with the collagen fibrils of the tendon [32]. Collagen degradation is initiated by matrix metalloproteinases (MMPs), which are present in tissues mostly as latent proMMPs. Tissue inhibitors of MMPs (TIMPs) inhibit their activation. The scheme of collagen degradation is presented in Fig. 1.6.2(b).

Functions of collagen in skeletal muscle

The connective tissue network of skeletal muscle has a dynamic role during muscle differentiation and normal muscle growth and it serves as a supportive structure in skeletal muscle and tendon [3,4,33,34]. Collagen forms the linkages between the muscle and its associated collagenous tissues such as tendon or fascia, and is also the fibrillar component of the cell-to-cell connections both between individual muscle cells and between the muscle cells and neighboring small blood vessels and nerves. It gives coherence and mechanical strength and also functions as an elastic, stress-tolerant system as well as distributing the forces of muscular contractions in both muscle and tendon. The tensile strength is based on intra- and intermolecular cross-links, and the orientation and density of the fibrils and fibers. In addition, collagen like the other ECM compounds conforms to the microenvironment around single muscle fibers and participates in the growth of cells and tissue regeneration after damage [35].

Effects of immobilization on collagen in skeletal muscle synthesis and degradation

The metabolism of muscular and tendinous collagen and the connective tissue network is known to respond to altered levels of physical activity. Cast immobilization of rat hind limb leads to a decrease in the enzyme activities of collagen biosynthesis in both skeletal muscle and tendon [25,27], which suggests that the biosynthesis of the collagen network decreases as a result of reduced muscular and tendinous activity. The rate of total collagen synthesis depends mostly on the overall protein balance of the tissue [30], but it seems to be positively affected by stretch in both muscle and tendon [25,27]. Changes in the total collagen content of muscle, measured as hydroxyproline content, are usually small or absent during immobilization lasting for a few weeks, which probably reflects the slow turnover of collagen [25], but increased collagen contents have also been observed [36].

Collagen expression during immobilization has been shown to be at least partially down-regulated at the pretranslational level [19]. The mRNA for the α-subunit of PH had already decreased after 1 day of immobilization. The mRNAs for type I (Fig. 1.6.3a) and III collagens were also decreased after 3 days of immobilization. Stretch seems to counteract this decrease [37].

Breakdown of ECM compounds like collagens is initiated by MMPs. Immobilization leads to an increase in proMMP-2 expression at both pre- and post-translational levels suggesting accelerated collagen breakdown. It is of interest that stretch partially prevents this phenomenon also [38].

Effects of denervation and reinnervation on collagen in skeletal muscle

The responses in muscular collagen biosynthesis differ between denervation and disuse atrophies [27]. Denervation atrophy is associated with an increase in the activities of PH and GGT and muscular collagen concentration suggesting development of fibrosis of the muscle tissue. Thus denervation seems to 'uncouple' the regulation of the adaptive responses of muscular collagen biosynthesis from the atrophy process of the whole muscle [27]. Perimysial collagen accumulation occurs also in muscle of spinal cord-injured individuals [39]. During reinnervation both the PH and

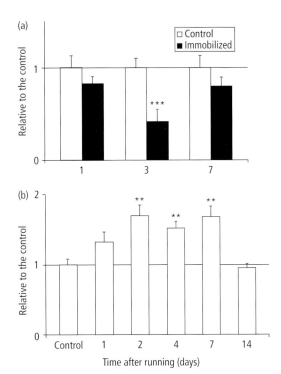

Fig. 1.6.3 (a) Type I collagen mRNA level in cast-immobilized soleus muscle. The results indicate a rapid pretranslational down-regulation of type I collagen expression during immobilization. (b) Prolyl 4-hydroxylase (P4H) after a single bout of prolonged exercise in rat quadriceps femoris muscle (MQF). The results suggest accelerated collagen synthesis.

GGT enzyme activities and the hydroxyproline (Hyp) concentration decreased to the control level in spite of accelerated muscular growth [40].

Effects of increased physical activity on collagen in skeletal muscle

The specific activities of PH and GGT, as well as Hyp concentration, are known to be greater in the antigravity soleus muscle than in the dorsiflexor tibialis anterior which is not tonically active [26,41]. Skeletal muscle is known to respond to increased loading caused by endurance training [14,28,42], acute exercise [24] (Fig. 1.6.3b) or experimental compensatory hypertrophy [30,43] by increased collagen synthesis and/or accumulation in the muscle. Strenuous exercise, especially acute weight-bearing exercise that contains eccentric components, is known to cause muscle damage [44]. Up-regulation of collagen synthesis may be a part of the repair process but may also occur without any evidence of muscle damage [20]. Acceleration of collagen biosynthesis after exercise may thus reflect both physiologic adaptation and repair of the damage. Exercise training before exhaustive running has been shown to partially prevent the increase in collagen-synthesizing enzymes [24]. (Pro)MMP-2 is up-regulated at both pre- and post-translational levels after a single bout of exercise, suggesting an increase in the capacity of collagen degradation.

Tendon injury

Tendons serve to transmit force from the contractile unit to the bone in order to produce movement. In contrast to the muscle, the cross-sectional area of the tendon is relatively small, and thus, the stress (force/area) imposed on the tendon is substantial during physical activities. However, tendons are remarkably strong and can withstand stresses that far exceed those transmitted during daily activities, including sports. Nevertheless, tendon injuries as a result of physical activity remain a substantial clinical problem, and the reasons for these injuries remain an enigma. Moreover, it is particularly puzzling that these patients are often relatively well-trained individuals. Consequently, appropriate and effective treatments, and possible preventive efforts, based on scientific evidence are currently lacking. Many tendon injuries are thought to be caused by 'overloading' of the tendon with a gradual onset of symptoms and a presumed associated inflammatory response and structural changes. However, a large portion of the existing knowledge on connective tissue properties and metabolism has been limited to animal models and some cadaver studies with respect to tendon mechanical properties. While such studies have contributed important information to our understanding of connective tissue they also draw attention to the limited conclusive evidence available on *in vivo* changes in the physically active human body. One problem with animal studies has been the difficulty in establishing a model that could reproducibly mimic an 'overload' time course of events. Moreover, there has been a lack of techniques that allow for the continuous sampling of tissue variables during exercise, which may prove useful in studying potential contributory factors for 'overload' reactions. However, some recent *in vivo* human models have been developed that can monitor metabolism, blood flow and inflammatory activity and collagen turnover during exercise. These methods, together with the recently developed method of ultrasound determination of the mechanical properties of human tendon during muscular contraction, may prove valuable in future research efforts to understand tendon adaptation to physical activity.

Collagen metabolism and tendon loading

It is commonly believed that, if not inert, tendon is metabolically relatively inactive. However, animal studies suggest that tensile strength, stiffness, cross-sectional area and collagen content are augmented with increases in physical activity, which suggests that the tendon is metabolically active. In contrast, decreased physical activity and immobilization down-regulate collagen biosynthesis [25,27]. Collagen synthesis depends on overall protein synthesis, but appears to also be affected by tensile loading [25,27]. Interestingly, in an animal model it has been demonstrated that cell metabolism and matrix turnover is not necessarily uniform throughout the whole tendon tissue (deep vs. superficial) [45]. Therefore, the possibility cannot be excluded that intratendinous connective tissue turnover is multicompartmental, with 'rapid' and slow turnover compartments, rather than involving just a single compartment. Ultimately, such intratendinous differences may have a profound effect on the corresponding mechanical properties. Recently the microdialysis technique was used for *in vivo* determination of indirect markers of collagen turnover in the peritendinous tissue about the Achilles tendon [46,47]. It was shown that both a single bout of exercise and chronic (11 weeks') exercise appear to stimulate human type I collagen synthesis [47,48] (Fig. 1.6.4). Furthermore, collagen degradation seems to be transiently elevated initially, but with time a net synthesis takes place [48]. Whether the synthesis results in macroscopically increased tendon mass, and thereby increased strength and stiffness, remains unknown. However, it was recently shown that well-trained runners had a markedly greater Achilles tendon cross-sectional area than age-matched sedentary controls (Magnusson *et al.*, unpublished) (Fig. 1.6.5). These data suggest that the human tendon is metabolically active and that it is affected by physical activity. How-

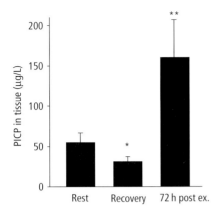

Fig. 1.6.4 Carboxy-terminal propeptides of type I collagen (PICP) measured as a marker for collagen synthesis during rest, immediately after (recovery) and 72 h after a 36-km run.

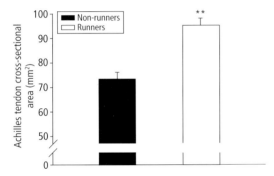

Fig. 1.6.5 The cross-sectional area of the Achilles tendon in well-trained runners (>80 km/week) and controls (Magnusson *et al.*, unpublished).

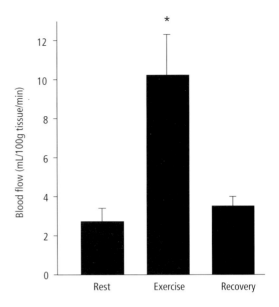

Fig. 1.6.6 Mean blood flow values as determined with the ^{133}Xe washout technique in the peritendinous space 5 cm proximal to the insertion of the human Achilles tendon, *in vivo*. Note that blood flow increases 3–4-fold with intermittent static exercise.

ever, it remains unknown exactly how degradation and synthesis are affected by the time course of events (loading/restitution) and to what extent various forms of loading affect their interrelationship.

Blood supply and inflammatory reaction

It is widely believed that the Achilles tendon is injury prone secondary to a compromised blood supply 2–5 cm proximal to the insertion onto the calcaneus. Using a xenon washout technique it was recently shown that blood flow in the peritendinous region of the human Achilles tendon rose up to 3–7 times during resisted plantar flexion, which parallels the augmented flow to the muscle [49,50] (Fig. 1.6.6). Further, the

simultaneous use of near-infrared spectroscopy indicates that vasodilatation and tissue oxygenation are coupled during exercise [51]. These data suggest that blood flow is not necessarily compromised in the region of the Achilles tendon, although its role in tendon pathology remains unknown. Moreover, exactly how and what factors contribute to the regulation of blood flow in the tendon region remains to be addressed. Bradykinin plays a role in both vasodilatation and nociception, and is therefore particularly interesting as a potentially important regulator in tendon tissue. For human mesenchymal tendon cells in cultures, it has been demonstrated that repeated stretches lead to an increase in prostaglandin production that can be blocked by endomethacin [52]. A system has recently been developed that allows cells to be grown in microgrooves instead of substrates with smooth culture surfaces [53]. In this new culture system, tendon fibroblasts were found to become elongated in shape and aligned in the direction of microgrooves with and without stretching, and therefore the shape and alignment of the tendon fibroblasts and their loading conditions are similar to those *in vivo* (Fig. 1.6.7). Furthermore, preliminary data revealed

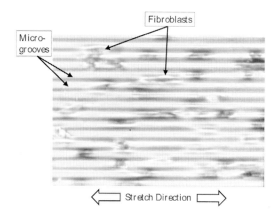

Fig. 1.6.7 Fibroblasts grown in silicon microgrooves and aligned along the direction of stretch.

that cyclic stretching of the tendon fibroblasts induced the production of PGE2 in a stretching-magnitude-dependent manner. Specifically, at 4% stretching the PGE2 production was not increased; however, at 8% and 12% the PGE2 levels were increased about 1.7- and 2.2-fold, respectively, compared with the unstretched cells. Since PGE2 is a known inflammatory mediator, the results of this study suggest that tendon overuse injury may involve the release of PGE2 from overstretching of tendon fibroblasts *in vivo*, and this may subsequently result in the tendon inflammation and pain often seen in the clinical setting. Moreover, in a human model it has also been shown that exercise is associated with peritendinous release of prostaglandin [46,47]. That is, inflammatory mediators are released in response to tensile loading of the human tendon, but to what extent this response is related to collagen synthesis/degradation and hence tissue strength and quality, and thus ability to withstand repetitive tensile loading remains unknown.

While it is generally believed that repetitive loading leads to microscopic failure of collagen structures and an inflammatory process followed by symptomatic pain, the exact etiology remains to be established. Animal models have been developed in an effort to examine the initiating factors of tendon overuse injuries. One such representative model of tendon injury was created by injection of bacterial collagenase into Achilles tendons of horses and rabbits [54,55]. Microscopic examination revealed degenerative

changes in the tendons and increased numbers of capillaries. However, according to current standards for evaluating tendon disorders, these models appear to represent tendinosis rather than tendon overuse injury, which is associated with tendon inflammation. Recently, our research center developed an animal model of tendon overuse injury [56] by means of the use of cell activating factors (a combination of various cytokines). When injected into rabbit patellar tendons, the cytokines produced biologic and biomechanical changes in the tendons. These include increased cellularity at and around the injection site (Fig. 1.6.8), and decreased failure load of the tendon (Fig. 1.6.9). Thus, this model offers an opportunity to study tendinitis, but whether this model represents tendon overuse injury induced by repetitive loading remains to be verified.

Tendon strain and regional differences

The tendon stress during muscular contraction is associated with a given tendon strain (% elongation). Although unsubstantiated, it is commonly believed that the magnitude of tendon strain may be associated with microtears of the tendon and subsequent clinical symptoms. Investigations of human tendon behavior have largely been limited to biomechanical testing of isolated cadaver tissue specimens. However, the recent advance of using real-time ultrasonography has provided a useful method for studying human aponeurosis and tendon tissue behavior during contraction, *in vivo*. Using such a method it was recently shown that the mechanical properties of the human Achilles tendon and aponeurosis, *in vivo*, exceeded those mechanical properties previously reported for the human tibialis anterior tendon, *in vivo*, but were similar to those obtained for various human and mammalian tendons during isolated biomechanical testing procedures [57] (Fig. 1.6.10). It remains unexplored whether the mechanical properties of the tendon are altered in response to various types of exercise.

The tendon has a complex anatomic hierarchy and whether there are regional differences in the stress–strain distribution throughout the tendon is also unknown at present. It has been shown that strain of the collagen fibril is less than that of the whole tendon [58]. Such a discrepancy in fibril and tendon strain suggests that some structural gliding may develop

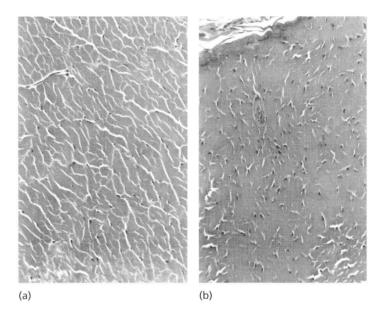

Fig. 1.6.8 Saline solution injection causes minimal cellularity at the injection site (a). In contrast, cytokine injection increases cellularity at 4 weeks (b). The matrix appears unchanged.

(a)   (b)

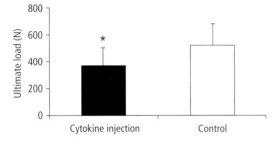

Fig. 1.6.9 Cytokine-injected tendons in rabbits had significantly lower ultimate load (*$P < 0.05$) at 16 weeks after injection compared with the control group injected with saline. Data are adapted from Stone *et al.* 1999 [56].

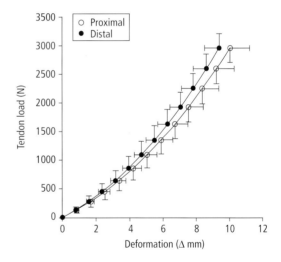

Fig. 1.6.10 The estimated stress–strain for the proximal and distal human Achilles tendon and aponeurosis after correction for small amounts of ankle joint rotation and antagonist coactivation.

within the tendon. Whether such an intratendon differential strain (shear) plays a role in mechanical signaling for tendon metabolism, or if it is a potential mechanism for 'microtear' and subsequent inflammatory reactions and clinical symptoms is unresearched. Further, intra- and intermolecular cross-links are formed that promote stability of the collagen molecule and collagen fibril, respectively. Pyridinoline is an important component of cross-links of the mature collagen fiber, and it has been shown that the ratio of pyridinoline to collagen is particularly high in tendon and ligament compared to bone [59]. Therefore, cross-link formation probably plays an integral role in tissues that are subjected to tensile stress. Nevertheless, it re-

mains unknown whether various aspects of physical activity (contraction mode, intensity, duration and restitution time) have any effect on these cross-link formations and subsequent tendon properties.

Animal models have shown that there is an inverse relationship between type III and type I collagen fibril diameter during development: type III collagen fibril number declines with maturation and larger type I fibrils increase [60], which may reflect a change to a larger and more stress-resistant fibril. However, region-specific observations of fibril morphology have not been made in a human tendon model, nor has it been investigated whether the different regions within a tendon vary in their mechanical properties.

Biomechanics of human skeletal muscle–tendon flexibility

Physical activity is important to maintain good health, and human movement is not possible without some degree of the fitness component commonly called musculoskeletal flexibility. Flexibility training is thought to be an important and effective training stimulus for maintenance and augmentation of flexibility. Clearly the demands of participation in sports require a certain sport-specific musculoskeletal flexibility. In sports such as gymnastics the necessity for immense flexibility is obvious; however, reaching for a ball in soccer, clearing a hurdle or performing a tennis serve may also require a certain sport-specific flexibility, which may be achieved by specifically designed flexibility training programs. However, it should also be kept in mind that an individual's existing flexibility may be an inherent characteristic or a sport-specific adaptation, and not just the result of flexibility training [109]. Although there is presently no universally accepted definition of flexibility it is most commonly defined as maximal joint range of motion across a joint or series of joints. Flexibility has also been defined as the length–tension relationship of the muscle–tendon unit. However, the former appears to be a more clinically useful definition since it can easily be measured with a goniometer. It should be noted that a goniometer endpoint measurement is subjective in nature and therefore provides no information about the resistance the muscle provides throughout the range of motion; thus the 'stiffness' or 'compliance' of the muscle cannot be evaluated. The following section will consider the biomechanics of stretching of the muscle–tendon unit, and it should be kept in mind that it does not cover stretching of the injured or immobilized muscle–tendon unit, complex issues like flexibility and injury risk.

Mechanisms for flexibility improvement

It is indisputable that increases in musculoskeletal flexibility can be achieved by flexibility training. However, the mechanisms for both the short- and long-term changes in flexibility as a result of flexibility training have until recently been largely unclear. The immediate or short-term response to stretching has previously been attributed to either neurophysiologic [110] or mechanical factors [111]. The neurophysiologic explanation suggests that the limiting factor during stretching is muscular resistance attributed to reflex activity, as measured by electromyography (EMG). Thus, the aim of stretching would be to inhibit the reflex activity, which in turn would reduce resistance and thereby allow for further increases in joint range of motion [110]. Paradoxically, the particular stretching techniques most effective in increasing joint range of motion have been associated with an elevated EMG response [112]. At the same time, it has been shown that during a 90-s static stretch resistance declines by ~30% in the absence of any measurable EMG response [113]. Therefore, contractile reflex activity does not appear to significantly contribute to resistance to stretch. The other common explanation for the effects of stretching includes an altered mechanical property of the muscle [111]. Yet a third mechanism was recently suggested, where improvement in joint range of motion was attributed to an amplified stretch tolerance, rather than a change in EMG activity or mechanical properties [114,115].

Biomechanical response to stretch

The relationship between the force and the deformation (expressed as the slope of the line, $\Delta F/\Delta L$) is the stiffness of the structure [116]. That is, the increase in deformation is proportional to the applied force (Hooke's law), such that a stiffer structure will deform less for a given applied external load. The reciprocal of stiffness ($\Delta L/\Delta F$) is termed compliance. The area under the curve is the energy absorbed by the structure that can potentially be returned when the load is removed. The application of an external applied tensile force will be opposed by the internal bonds of the structure. This tensile stress can be defined as the internal force divided by the cross-sectional area of the material (F/area). The stress will cause the structure to change in shape, or deform, which is called tensile strain. Tensile strain can be defined as the change in length divided by the original length (($\Delta L/L_0$), which is a dimensionless unit, but often expressed as a percentage of the original length. The relationship between stress and strain (Δ*stress*/Δ*strain*) is the elastic modulus of the material, sometimes referred to as Young's modulus.

Biological materials are viscoelastic and do not respond to external loading in a way that can be described in simple linear mechanical terms. Viscoelastic behavior has been described in rheological models where the relationship between force and deformation is dependent on time. Linear elasticity is a load-dependent response and linear viscosity is a rate-dependent response [117]. Typically tissues will respond in a non-linear fashion with an initial 'toe-region' followed by an approximately linear region during *dynamic loading* on account of its viscoelastic properties. If the tissue is held fixed at some new length, *static loading*, the tension will decline in a non-linear fashion with time, which is termed viscoelastic stress relaxation (Fig. 1.6.12). These are the two phases that a muscle–tendon undergoes during a static stretch.

A single static stretch

In the animal models it is known that materials respond in a non-linear fashion during the dynamic and static loading phase of a stretch, indicating viscoelastic behavior [111,116,118]. Recently it was also shown in a human model that the muscle–tendon unit behaves in a similar fashion during stretching [113–115,119–121]. That is, the muscle displays viscoelastic properties in the absence of any measurable EMG response from the target muscle being stretched (Fig. 1.6.12). During the dynamic loading phase there is a non-linear increase in resistance to stretch, and during the static loading phase there is a non-linear decline in resistance to stretch, a viscoelastic stress relaxation response. The viscoelastic stress relaxation response is most pronounced in the initial 10–15 s, but continues to significantly abate for approximately 45 s. During a 90-s static stretch resistance declines by about 30% altogether. Although there is significant viscoelastic stress relaxation during a 45-s static stretch there is no measurable effect on the subsequent immediate stretch [122]. This means that resistance to stretch diminishes during the static phase of a stretch, but has no lasting effect on the viscoelastic properties.

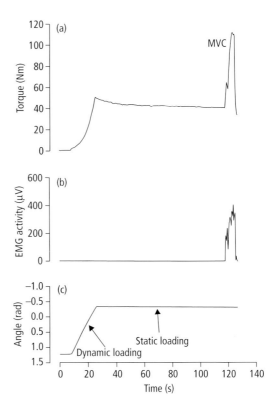

Fig. 1.6.12 A static stretch of the hamstring muscle group for one individual. (a) The passive torque about the knee joint that corresponds to the tension in the hamstring muscles during the passive static stretch procedure is shown. A maximal voluntary contraction (MVC) is performed at the end of the stretch. (b) The corresponding EMG amplitudes. Note the absence of EMG activity in the hamstring muscles despite the increase in torque in the dynamic loading phase, and the decline in torque in the static loading phase (viscoelastic stress relaxation). (c) The angle (negative value indicates greater angle of stretch) of the mechanical lever arm that passively stretches the hamstring muscles at 0.0875 rad/s (5°/s) during the dynamic loading phase. During the static loading phase the lever arm remains stationary.

Repeated stretches — short-term effect

Animal data demonstrate that if the target tissue is stretched repeatedly, resistance to stretch, in both the dynamic and the static portion, will decline with each subsequent stretch [117]. Therefore, stretching of a muscle group in the sports arena or rehabilitation setting is typically not performed once as described above, but is repeated several times. In the human muscle–tendon complex the effect of five consecutive

90-s static stretches has been examined [120]. To see if any effect was lasting in nature the resistance to stretch was re-examined 1 h later. In the last of the five stretches both passive energy (the area under the curve of the dynamic loading phase) (30%) and stiffness (13%) declined. However, surprisingly, the observed decline in the viscoelastic properties was transient since they had returned to baseline values when measured 1 h later. In contrast to a single 45-s stretch, the 90-s stretch had an effect on the subsequent stretch; however, again the effect on the viscoelastic properties was transient (>1 h).

Although stretching procedures places tensile load on several structures it remains unknown what their relative contributions are to the stress relaxation response. The transmission of tension in passively stretched muscle is complex and may engage several structures, including titin, intramuscular connective tissue and tendon. Passive stretch in a physiologic range results in 2% strain of tendon, but 8% strain of the muscle–tendon junction [123], demonstrating differential viscoelastic properties in various regions of the muscle–tendon unit, and that tendon is less likely to deform during loading.

Repeated stretches — long-term effect

While earlier literature attributed short-term changes in flexibility to neurophysiologic events, it commonly ascribed long-term improvements in flexibility to changes in the passive properties [124]. In a recent study static stretching exercises for the human hamstring muscle group were performed in the morning (5×45 s) and in the afternoon (5×45 s) on one leg while the opposite side served as control [115]. After 3 weeks the resistance to stretch for a given angle was unchanged on both sides (Fig. 1.6.13). However, when stretched to a maximal tolerated joint angle the stretch side could be extended further after training, i.e. the subjects became more flexible. This increase in angle was accompanied by a comparable increase in peak torque and energy (without any change in EMG activity). Therefore, increases in flexibility, i.e. maximal range of motion, can be achieved from stretch training as a consequence of increased tolerance to tensile load, rather than through a change in the viscoelastic properties of the muscle. On the basis of these results, and since the change in the viscoelastic behav-

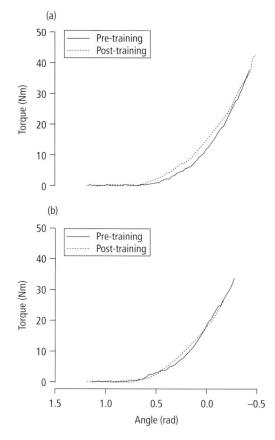

Fig. 1.6.13 Maximal torque-angle data for one subject in the dynamic loading phase of a static stretch before and after 3 weeks of flexibility training twice a day. (a) The training side. Note that after training the subject reached a greater knee joint angle prior to the onset of discomfort with an accompanying increase in torque. It should also be noted that the pre- and post-training slope is similar. That is, the muscle–tendon unit did not change its passive properties (slope), but the subject's tolerance to stretch was enhanced after training. (b) The control side: The slope and the endpoint do not differ over the training period.

ior is transient in nature and reverses within 1 h (see above), it is questionable if stretching, as it is commonly performed by athletes, can permanently change the passive properties of a muscle.

The mechanism for an altered stretch tolerance is presently unknown. However, the increased tolerance on the training side and lack thereof on the control side suggests that peripheral mechanisms, such as afferent information from muscle, tendon and joint receptors, may play a role. However, the possibility cannot be excluded that central factors may be involved as well. Finally, from a clinical standpoint it is important to point out that although the passive properties do not appear to be altered as a result of flexibility training it does lead to improvements in joint range of motion. Therefore, to meet sport-specific flexibility demands it may be desirable to perform flexibility training. Finally, the possibility cannot at present be ruled out that stretching in a skeletally immature person may have a long-lasting effect on the viscoelastic properties of the muscle–tendon unit, nor is it known whether such changes are advantageous or not.

Determinants of flexibility

Unquestionably people exhibit differences in musculoskeletal flexibility. A component of a person's existing flexibility may be inherited, a sport-specific adaptation (loading history) or achieved by flexibility training. Previous investigations on human flexibility have measured maximal joint range of motion, but not the passive properties of the muscle–tendon unit. At the same time, it has been shown that tolerance to tensile load plays an important role in short-term and long-term gains in flexibility (see above) rather than the passive properties of the muscle. To address whether tolerance also contributed to differences in flexibility endurance athletes were classified as tight (inflexible) and normal based on a simple toe-touch test. It was observed that both passive properties (stiffness) of the hamstring muscle group and stretch tolerance explained the difference in flexibility [119]. That is, 'tight' athletes had a muscle–tendon unit with greater stiffness than athletes with normal flexibility for a given common angle (Fig. 1.6.14a). However, the athletes with normal flexibility achieved a greater maximal joint angle (muscle length) and accompanying maximal tensile stress, and thus had a greater tolerance to tensile loading. When the tensions in the individual muscles were analysed it was observed that a combination of a more extended knee joint angle, i.e. a reduced moment arm, and a greater external moment explained the substantial differences in stress between the tight and flexible subjects at a maximal joint angle (Fig. 1.6.14b). Towards the extremes of motion, as in hurdling, considerable passive tension is probably generated and may therefore play a role in the deceleration

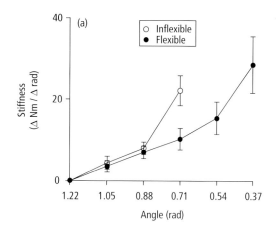

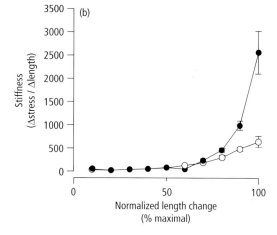

Fig. 1.6.14 (a) Absolute biceps femoris moment stiffness data (mean±s.e.m.) for *angles common to all subjects* in the flexible and tight groups (*$P<0.05$). The moment stiffness followed an exponential curve and elevated earlier during knee extension in the tight than in the flexible subjects. Thus, after 0.71 rad the stiffness reached 22 and 10 ΔNm/Δrad for the respective groups. However, the flexible subjects reached a greater maximal angle of stretch, and had at that angle a greater stiffness than the flexible subjects (tolerance). (b) Muscle stiffness (Δ*stress*/Δ*length*) for the biceps femoris muscle as a function of normalized length change. Significantly different from inflexible, *$P<0.05$, **$P<0.01$.

of the leg in the terminal swing phase. The material properties of skeletal muscle are thought to be related to the amount of collagen [41], and perhaps collagen content or the number of cross-links contributed to the observed difference in stiffness.

It is well known that stiffness of connective tissue increases with aging, in part due to an increase in cross-links. Interestingly, when we examined the musculoskeletal passive properties on a cross-sectional basis in a very narrow age range, younger athletes (15–21 years) had a muscle–tendon unit with greater stiffness than slightly 'older' athletes (26–32 years) for a given common angle. Such differences may be related to age-related changes in connective tissue [118]. However, the younger athletes also achieved a greater maximal joint angle (muscle length) and accompanying maximal tensile stress, and thus had a greater tolerance. Therefore, it appears that material properties and tolerance to tensile load play a role both in determining differences in flexibility and in age-related changes in flexibility.

Warm-up and stretching

Warming up prior to participation in sport is commonly believed to aid performance and reduce injury risk, and because the muscle–tendon unit is thought to exhibit temperature-dependent viscoelastic behavior, it is recommended that warm-up precedes stretching exercises [125]. Although there is limited scientific evidence in a human model for such a tenet it was recently investigated whether the passive energy absorption of the human muscle–tendon unit would decrease after a brief (10-min) warm-up exercise bout, and sustained (30-min) exercise [121]. It was clearly demonstrated that a 10-min warm-up procedure and 30 min of continuous running elevated intramuscular temperature significantly (from 35.0 °C to 38.8 °C), but did not affect the passive energy absorption of the hamstring muscle–tendon unit. When static stretching exercises were added to the regimen after the 10-min warm-up period the passive energy absorption declined immediately; however, this reduction in passive energy absorption was not sustained after an additional 30 min of continuous running. It is well known that continuous exercise rapidly results in an equilibrium between heat production and heat dissipation. In the above experiment about 80% of the temperature increase occurred in the initial 10 min of work, which confirms that increased tissue temperature can be achieved relatively soon after initiation of exercise, and that 10 min of warm-up exercise may be sufficient preparation for muscle performance [126]. Temperature-dependent viscoelastic behavior of biological tissue has previously been shown in temperature ranges

that far exceed those achieved during a warm-up procedure in human skeletal muscle [127]. However, it appears that despite the repeated mechanical loading during 40 min of running, and its associated increase in intramuscular temperature, the passive energy absorption of the muscle–tendon unit remains unchanged. It has been suggested that elastic recoil may play a role in energy expenditure during locomotion [128,129], and although this is speculative, the temperature and repetitive load insensitive passive energy behavior may serve to maintain passive elastic energy return during locomotion.

Ligaments: physiology and repair

Athletic activities can result in a wide variety of joint injuries through either direct trauma or repetitive stress [61]. Although the predilection for specific injuries varies with the sport (e.g. elbow instability in baseball players, shoulder dislocations in football players and wrestlers, knee injuries in basketball players), all injuries can be debilitating and often involve ligamentous structures. Ligaments are structures that are known to play an important role in mediating normal joint mechanics. These parallel-fibered, dense connective tissues share the transmission of forces with other periarticular tissues to provide joint stability [62].

In the knee, a common injury site is the medial collateral ligament (MCL). Injuries to this structure may be isolated to the superficial MCL or extend to include the deep capsular and posterior oblique ligaments [63–65]. Laboratory studies using animal models have shown that a ruptured MCL can heal spontaneously without surgical intervention. However, the healed tissue remains mechanically, structurally and materially inferior to normal ligaments [66–68]. Nevertheless, the ability of the MCL to heal offers an opportunity for the examination of the mechanism of ligament healing. In addition, anatomically, the MCL is a broad, flat ligament with a good aspect ratio (length to width) and relatively uniform cross-sectional area making it well suited for biomechanical studies. Understanding healing in the MCL provides a good foundation for understanding the healing processes of other ligaments. In this section ligament healing and repair using the MCL as a model will be presented. Also, current and future approaches towards enhancing the quality of the healed ligament, namely functional tissue engineering that includes the use of growth factors, gene transfer technology, cell therapy, tissue scaffolding and other mechanical factors, will be examined.

Natural history of MCL injury

Healing of the MCL has been found to be a long and complex process that is subject to local and external influences. Generally, the process involves several discrete but overlapping phases: the acute inflammatory or reactive response phase, the repair phase, and finally the tissue remodeling phase. In the acute inflammatory phase, the cellular and tissue responses to injury occur within approximately the first 72 h following a given insult. Capillary damage results in enhanced permeability of local blood vessels, allowing inflammatory cells to migrate into the tissue defect. Fibroblastic proliferation and the formation of scar matrix consisting of randomly aligned collagen and amorphous ground substance occurs simultaneously [66].

The repair phase encompasses those cellular and tissue processes occurring from 48–72 h until roughly 6 weeks post injury. This time period marks the gradual subsiding of inflammation together with the active commencement of the healing process. Grossly, highly vascular granulation tissue fills the tissue defect, covering the free ends of torn or ruptured tissue [66,69]. Fibroblasts become the predominant cell type and continue to actively synthesize extracellular matrix. This matrix becomes progressively more organized with time, yet collagen fibrils remain relatively disorganized.

The remodeling phase is also marked by tissue remodeling, lasting months and years after the initial injury. It should be noted that an injured MCL never regains the properties of the normal MCL [66–68]. The healed ligaments have elevated numbers of vessels, fat cells and voids and increased water content. The diameter of collagen fibers is smaller with fewer numbers of stable collagen cross-links. The healing MCL also contains elevated type III and V collagens, along with an elevated number of proteoglycans (PG).

Biomechanical properties

Biomechanical characterization of the MCL can be done via (i) functional testing, which involves deter-

mining its contribution to knee kinematics as well as the *in situ* forces in the MCL in response to an external load, and (ii) uniaxial tensile testing, which provides an assessment of the structural properties of the femur–MCL–tibia complex (FMTC) and mechanical properties of the ligament substance. Readers are encouraged to study Chapter 2 of *The Orthopedic Basic Science Book* (published by the American Academy of Orthopedic Surgery) for details [69].

Functional testing provides insight into the kinematics or motion of the knee joint which is governed by a combination of joint geometry and tensile properties of ligaments. Each joint has six degrees of freedom (DOF): three translations and three rotations. For the knee joint, there are three axes that can be defined: the femoral shaft axis, the epicondylar axis, and a floating anterior–posterior axis perpendicular to these two axes. Translation along these three axes will lead to distraction/compression, medial–lateral translation, and anterior–posterior translation, respectively. Rotations about these three axes will lead to internal–external rotation, flexion–extension, and varus–valgus rotation, respectively.

Structural properties of the FMTC are extrinsic measures of performance of the overall structure in response to a uniaxial tensile test. These properties are obtained from the resulting load–elongation curve (Fig. 1.6.11a). The stiffness, in N/mm, is the slope of the curve between two defined limits of elongation. The ultimate load, in N, is the highest load placed on the complex before failure and the ultimate elongation, in mm, is the maximum elongation of the complex. Finally, the energy absorbed at failure, in N-mm, is the area under the entire load–elongation curve. These data are a reflection of the overall properties of the complex spanning from insertion to insertion.

Mechanical properties of the ligament's midsubstance are intrinsic measures of the local tensile properties as represented by a stress–strain curve (Fig. 1.6.11b). Stress is defined as force per unit cross-sectional area, while strain in the MCL is typically defined as the ratio of the difference between the initial length and current length to the initial length. The modulus, in MPa, is obtained from the linear slope of the stress–strain curve between two limits of strain. The tensile strength, in MPa, is the maximum stress achieved; while the ultimate strain (percentage) is the

(a)

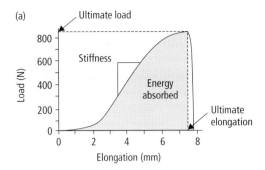

(b)

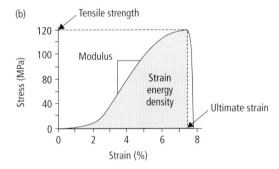

Fig. 1.6.11 (a) Typical load–elongation curve of a bone–ligament–bone complex. (b) Typical stress–strain curve describing the mechanical properties of the ligament substance.

strain at failure. Finally, the strain energy density, in MPa, is the area under the stress–strain curve. A system for tracking markers that strategically delineates the midsubstance is necessary to measure local strain. Video analysis techniques have assisted the tracking of stain markers deployed in one- or two-dimensional patterns on the ligament's surface. In addition, stress is determined from the gross load-cell readings normalized by the specimen's cross-sectional area.

Using the skeletally mature New Zealand white rabbit as a model, the structural properties of the healing FMTC and the mechanical properties of the healing MCL have been demonstrated to remain inferior to those of the intact ligament up to 1 year after injury [70]. Structural properties of the FMTC, including stiffness and ultimate load to failure improved during the early stages of healing (i.e. from 6 to 12 weeks), but remained inferior to controls. After 52 weeks of healing, only the stiffness of the FMTC returned to near normal levels, while the ultimate load was still significantly lower than the controls. Further,

the modulus and tensile strength of the healing MCLs at all time periods, remained significantly inferior, in spite of increased cross-sectional area. Thus, the healing process involves a larger quantity of poorer quality ligamentous tissue.

Factors influencing ligament healing

There are numerous factors that contribute to the healing response of an injured ligament. Known factors include the site and severity of the injury. In addition to intrinsic factors such as circulation and infection, studies have also shown that treatments such as repair vs. non-repair, rehabilitation and exercise can have significant impact on the process of ligament healing.

Intrinsic factors

There exist a number of intrinsic factors that may contribute to the healing response of the injured ligament. In a study on the healing MCL of hypophysectomized rats, interstitial cell-stimulating hormone (ICSH) and testosterone replacement significantly affected the ultimate load of the repaired ligament, as well as the collagen and glycosaminoglycan synthesis or degradation rates [70]. Any disease that affects endocrine or metabolic homeostasis may also affect ligament healing. For example, diabetes mellitus can result in circulatory abnormalities that may negatively affect ligament healing as insulin deficiency has been shown to alter collagen synthesis and cross-linking [71,72]. Ligament healing can also be affected by local conditions such as poor circulation or infection which hinders the proliferation of cells, thereby prolonging the inflammatory phase of healing.

Surgical repair vs. non-repair

For an isolated MCL injury, animal studies have shown better results with non-operative treatment than surgical repair followed by immobilization [73]. Earlier studies in the canine model and more recent studies using a rabbit model examined the effects of suture repair of the injured MCL [68,69,74]. At 48 weeks, no statistically significant differences could be demonstrated between surgically repaired and non-repaired groups for any biomechanical property, including varus–valgus knee rotation, and structural properties of the FMTC. However, the mechanical properties of the MCL midsubstance, i.e. the quality of the healed tissue, were significantly different from intact MCLs. These findings are in agreement with clinical reports which have reported positive outcomes with non-operative treatment followed by early motion and functional rehabilitation [75]. As a result of scientific studies and clinical experience, it is now generally agreed that the preferred method of treatment for isolated grade III injuries of the MCL [63] is non-operative (conservative).

Immobilization vs. controlled motion and exercise

In the past, immobilization following ligament injury was believed to protect the healing ligament from stress [76]. However, it has been shown in the laboratory that immobilization can result in disorganization of collagen fibrils, decreases in the structural properties of the FMTC, resorption of bone at the ligament insertion sites, and many detrimental effects on the knee joint [77]. Conversely, controlled motion has been shown to be beneficial to the healing ligament [78]. Intermittent passive motion has been reported to improve the longitudinal alignment of cells and collagen at 6 weeks. Improved matrix organization and collagen concentration, together with an increase of up to four times in the ultimate load of the FMTC were demonstrated [77]. Some clinical data exist on the advantages of motion following ligament injury showing that clinical results are better with early motion and functional rehabilitation following isolated MCL injuries at 5-year follow-up [75]. Current clinical recommendations after MCL injuries include an early controlled range of motion exercises as soon as pain subsides [63,75]. However, in an unstable joint, i.e. cases involving multiple ligamentous injuries, motion too early or applied too aggressively may be detrimental to the healing process.

Combined MCL and ACL injuries

Severe knee injuries can involve multiple ligaments, and the prognosis for these combined ligamentous injuries is generally worse regardless of which treatment is selected. For a combined ACL + MCL injury, multiple treatment modalities have been studied clinically,

including combined MCL repair and ACL reconstruction, ACL reconstruction only, or non-operative treatment of both ligaments [79]. No differences in valgus instability or knee function during activities were observed between the three groups studied. The effects of ACL deficiency on the healing of the injured MCL have been studied in our research center using rabbit and canine models [80]. Biomechanical evaluation indicated that following an untreated ACL + MCL injury, there was a significant increase in varus–valgus laxity, a reduction in tissue quality of the healed MCL, and considerable degeneration of the joint. Other animal studies suggest that MCL repair with ACL reconstruction reduces varus–valgus laxity and improves structural properties of the FMTC in the short term (i.e. 12 weeks). After 52 weeks, however, no differences in biomechanical or biochemical properties were observed. Further studies in our research center revealed that non-operative treatment with full weight bearing and mobilization of the MCL injury with reconstruction of the ACL can result in successful MCL healing [81]. This approach also appears to be the preferred method of treatment for many clinicians [82].

Future directions

Functional tissue engineering is a multidisciplinary field that has gained major interest in the scientific community. The ability to produce tissue that replicates or enhances normal functioning tissue is of obvious practical benefit. There are several methods of approach to tissue engineering for ligament healing on the horizon. The use of growth factors, gene transfer technology, cell therapy tissue scaffolding and mechanical factors are all being studied. These new approaches are promising and a brief discussion of each will be presented.

Growth factors

Growth factors are small polypeptides synthesized by a variety of cells that function by binding to specific cell surface receptors which activate complex intracellular signal transduction pathways. Growth factors regulate cell migration, proliferation, differentiation and matrix synthesis and aid in repairing a damaged ligament by regulating cellular behavior and modulating the wound environment [83–92]. At our research center, platelet-derived growth factor BB (PDGF

BB), basic fibroblast growth factor (bFGF) and epidermal growth factor (EGF) have been found to have a stimulatory effect on cell proliferation, while transforming growth factor-β (TGF-β1) promoted matrix synthesis of MCL fibroblasts in a rabbit model suggesting that ligament healing may be promoted with a combination of these factors [87]. A follow-up *in vivo* study demonstrated that high-dose PDGF-BB *in vivo* resulted in an FMTC with higher ultimate load, energy absorbed to failure and ultimate elongation than controls [84]. Additionally, an ongoing *in vitro* study (unpublished) in our laboratory suggests a time-specific response to the addition of TGF-β1. Preliminary data suggest collagen synthesis to injured rabbit MCL fibroblasts increases with the addition of TGF-β1 at day 7, but not at days 3 or 14. To date, only a few growth factors have been studied (TGF-β1, PDGF, EGF, etc.); however, much research is required to identify and delineate the effects of yet undiscovered and unstudied growth factors.

Gene transfer technology

The application of gene transfer technology to ligament healing was examined recently [62]. Both retroviral *in vitro* transfection of the desired genes into the cells followed by the transplantation of genetically modified cells into the host tissue and adenoviral direct delivery of genes into host cells were used in the MCL of rabbit knees [62,83]. Both techniques resulted in expression of the *lacZ* marker gene by fibroblasts. Gene expression lasted for up to 10 days in the retroviral technique and up to 6 weeks in the adenoviral technique [83]. Therapeutic methods for ligament repair using non-viral gene transfer have also been investigated [93]. In one experiment, the HVJ–liposome complex containing an antisense nucleotide for decorin (a proteoglycan) was injected into the healing sites of injured MCLs. Mechanical properties, including ultimate stress, were shown to be significantly improved. Despite these promising results, major obstacles impede practical implementation of gene transfer as a biological intervention in ligament healing [62]. These obstacles include immune response of the viral proteins and transgene-encoded proteins [94], viability of transfected cells *in vivo* after retransplantation, and loss of gene expression of the retrovirus by promoter methylation [95]. Fortunately, it is believed

that ligament healing requires gene expression of the order of weeks, so this strategy is considered very promising.

Stem cell therapy

The principle of stem cell therapy is to provide a source of cells for ligaments or a mechanism to introduce genes for gene transfer [62]. The success of cell therapy for ligament repair relies on the viability of the transplanted cells and the affinity of the cells for the host tissue. Mesenchymal stem cells (MSCs) are considered a candidate for cell therapy. MSCs have been demonstrated to differentiate into various cells that form mesenchymal tissues under different culture conditions *in vitro* [96–99]. Multipotent differentiation of these cells into mesenchymal tissues has also been demonstrated *in vivo* [97,100].

In our research center, nucleated cells obtained from centrifuged bone marrow were used as transplantation donor cells [101–103]. Female transgenic rats were used as donors and recipients, with transgenes introduced into chromosome 4. The nucleated cells were injected into a pocket made around the transected MCL of recipient rats. Preliminary results revealed the survival of donor cells at the healing site of the MCL 3 and 7 days postoperatively. Transplanted donor cells could also be identified in the midsubstance of ligaments at 7 days. This is significant in that the migratory potential of transplanted cells may have been demonstrated. Migration of transplanted cells is an attractive attribute for ligament healing. These early results are encouraging [104].

Tissue scaffolds

Tissue scaffolds are extracellular matrix materials that serve as the structural framework upon which tissue regeneration can occur. A variety of biological and non-biological scaffolding materials have been used [105,106]. The application of small intestinal submucosa (SIS) scaffolding techniques to ligament healing has been investigated in our research center. When a mop-end tear of a rabbit MCL was approximated and covered with SIS, the healed ligament was found to have a larger cross-sectional area with increased stiffness. A number of issues including possible host immunological response, ascertaining the strength properties of scaffold-derived grafts, the degree of incorporation into host tissue, and the long-term viability of tissue remain to be addressed.

Mechanical factors

The effects of mechanical factors on ligament fibroblasts have been studied with a new apparatus developed in our research center. Previous studies have shown that cells grown and stretched on culture dishes with smooth surfaces realign nearly perpendicular to the direction of stretch. This orientation is in contrast with the *in vivo* model where cells align along the collagen fiber direction [107]. Using a cell stretching apparatus whereby cells are grown in an oriented fashion on silicon dishes that contain parallel microgrooves, we are able to align fibroblasts to grow along the direction of stretch (see Fig. 1.6.7). As this model better mimics the *in vivo* environment, future experiments exploring the effects of ligament fibroblasts will be closer to those in the *in vivo* situation.

Discussion

Ligamentous healing is a complicated process that involves multiple factors including extent of injury, vascular supply, time of medical intervention, and the effects of biomechanical and biochemical environments. New technologies like the Robotic/UFS testing system have opened the door to a better understanding of the effects on joint motion on ligament healing [108]. Animal and clinical research at different levels of the healing cascade from growth factors to tissue scaffolds has increased understanding of the healing process. Clearly, advances in the ability to heal ligaments will require future investigators that come from multiple fields including biology, biochemistry, bioengineering, medicine, surgery, and others. It is only with this collaborative approach that valuable information may be derived, such that the successful management of the debilitating effects of ligamentous injuries can become more achievable.

Summary

The extracellular matrix outside the cells is a complex and dynamic meshwork of collagens, non-collagenous glycoproteins, proteoglycans and elastin. The matrix supports the cellular elements and maintains the structural integrity of multicellular organisms. It also binds cells together and regulates various cellular processes, including cell growth, proliferation, differentiation, migration and adhesion. The tensile strength of the matrix is based on intra- and intermolecular cross-links, and the orientation and the density of the fibrils and fibers. The metabolism of collagen and the connective tissue network is known to respond to altered levels of physical activity. Biosynthesis decreases with reduced activity, and changes associated with immobilization can in part be counteracted by stretch. Exercise accelerates biosynthesis, and may reflect both physiologic adaptation and repair of the damage.

Tendon injuries as a result of altered and/or increased physical activity are a considerable clinical problem. What constitutes the most effective treatment and possible preventive efforts is currently unknown. Many tendon injuries are thought to be due to 'overloading' of the tendon with a gradual onset of symptoms and a presumed associated inflammatory response and structural changes. However, a large proportion of the existing knowledge on connective tissue properties and metabolism has been limited to animal models. Nevertheless, some recent *in vivo* human models have been developed that can monitor metabolism, blood flow and inflammatory activity and collagen turnover during exercise. These methods, together with the recently developed method of ultrasound determination of the mechanical properties of human tendon during muscular contraction, may prove valuable in the future research efforts to understand tendon adaptation to physical activity.

Physical activity can result in a wide variety of joint injuries, and often includes the MCL. Although the MCL can heal spontaneously without surgical intervention it remains mechanically, structurally and materially inferior to normal ligaments. Ligamentous healing is a process that involves multiple factors including extent of injury, vascular supply, time of medical intervention, and the effects of biomechanical and biochemical environments. The healing response may be influenced by intrinsic factors, including endocrine and metabolic homeostasis. The current recommended method of treatment for isolated grade III injuries of the MCL is non-operative, including early controlled range of motion exercises. However, functional tissue engineering, including growth factors, gene transfer technology, cell therapy and tissue scaffolding are being studied with respect to ligament healing. Early data show that some growth factors have stimulatory effects on cell proliferation and the mechanical properties of ligaments. Gene transfer as a biological intervention in ligament healing is also a potentially promising treatment strategy.

Stretching is often performed to improve musculoskeletal flexibility, and muscle displays viscoelastic properties in the absence of muscle activity. Resistance to stretch diminishes during a stretch, but has no lasting effect on the viscoelastic properties. Flexibility improvements can be achieved with stretch training due to altered tolerance to tensile load, rather than a change in the viscoelastic properties of the muscle. Physical activity elevates intramuscular temperature, but does not affect the passive properties of the hamstring muscle–tendon unit.

Multiple choice questions

1 *Which of the following is a unit of stiffness:*

a N-mm

b N/mm

c MPa

d mm².

2 *Which phase of ligament healing is marked by inflammation, blood vessel permeability, and early fibroblast proliferation:*

a reactive phase

b repair phase

c remodeling phase

d none of the above.

3 *Which of the following influences a person's musculoskeletal flexibility:*

a tolerance to tensile load

b age

c stiffness

d all of the above

e *a* and *c*.

4 *Which of the following statements are true?*

a All major collagen types have been observed in the endomysium.

b The concentration of endomysial collagen is higher around slow than fast skeletal muscle fibers.

c Proline and 4-hydroxyproline promote the formation of intermolecular cross-links.

d All of the above.

5 *The human Achilles tendon responds to acute tensile loading by:*

a an increased blood flow

b an increased collagen metabolism

c *a* but not *b*

d *a* and *b*.

References

1 Waterlow JC, Garlic PJ, Millward DJ. *Protein Turnover in the Mammalian Tissues and in the Whole Body*. Netherlands: Elsevier/North-Holland Biomedical Press, 1978.

2 Prockop DJ, Kivirikko KI. Collagens: molecular biology, diseases, and potentials for therapy. *Annu Rev Biochem* 1995; **64**: 403–34.

3 Bailey AJ, Shellswell GB, Duance VC. Identification and change of collagen types in differentiating myoblasts and developing chick muscle. *Nature* 1979; **278**: 67–9.

4 Duance VC, Rostall DJ, Beard H, Bourne FJ, Bailey AJ. The location of three collagen types in skeletal muscle. *FEBS Letter* 1977; **79**: 248–52.

5 Bashey RI, Martinez-Hernandez A, Jiminez SA. Isolation, characterization and localization of cardiac collagen type VI, association with other extracellular matrix components. *Circulation Res* 1992; **70**: 1006–17.

6 Kivirikko K, Saarela J, Myers JC, Autio-Harmainen H, Pihlajaniemi T. Distribution of type XV collagen transcripts in human tissue and their production by muscle cells and fibroblasts. *Am J Pathol* 1995; **147**: 1500–9.

7 Saarela J, Ylikärppä R, Rehn M, Purmonen S, Pihlajaniemi T. Complete primary structure of two variant forms of human type XVIII collagen and tissue-specific differences in the expression of the corresponding transcripts. *Matrix Biol* 1998; **16**(6): 319–28.

8 Sandberg M, Tamminen M, Hirvonen H, Vuorio E, Pihlajaniemi T. Expression of mRNAs coding for the α1 chain of type XIII collagen in human fetal tissues: comparison with expression of mRNAs for collagen types I, II and III. *J Cell Biol* 1989; **109**: 1371–9.

9 Wälchli C, Koch M, Chiquet M, Odermatt BF, Trueb B. Tissue-specific expression of the fibril-associated collagens XII and XIV. *J Cell Sci* 1994; **107**: 669–81.

10 Foidart M, Foidart J-M, Engel WK. Collagen localization in normal and fibrotic human skeletal muscle. *Arch Neurol* 1981; **38**: 152–7.

11 Light N, Champion AE. Characterization of muscle epimysium, perimysium and endomysium collagens. *Biochem J* 1984; **219**: 1017–26.

12 Garcia-Bunuel L, Garcia-Bunuel VM. Connective tissue and the pentose phosphate pathway in normal and denervated muscle. *Nature* 1967; **4**: 913–4.

13 Kovanen V, Suominen H, Heikkinen E. Collagen in slow twitch and fast twitch muscle fibres in different types of rat skeletal muscle. *Eur J Appl Physiol* 1984; **52**: 235–42.

14 Kovanen V, Suominen H, Heikkinen E. Connective tissue of 'fast' and 'slow' skeletal muscle in rats—effects of endurance training. *Acta Physiol Scand* 1980; **108**: 173–80.

15 Kivirikko KI, Myllylä R. Post-translational modifications.

In: Weiss JB, Jayson MIV, eds. *Collagen in Health and Disease*. Edinburgh: Churchill Livingstone, 1982: 101–20.

16 Vuorio E, de Crombrugghe B. The family of collagen genes. *Annu Rev Biochem* 1990; **59**: 837–72.

17 Kivirikko KI, Myllylä R. Biosynthesis of the collagen. In: Piez KA, Reddi AH, eds. *Extracellular Matrix Biochemistry*. New York: Elsevier, 1982: 83–118.

18 Han X, Karpakka J, Kainulainen H, Takala TES. Effects of streptozotocin-induced diabetes, physical training and their combination on collagen biosynthesis in rat skeletal muscle. *Acta Physiol Scand* 1995; **155**: 9–16.

19 Han X, Wang W, Myllylä R, Virtanen P, Karpakka J, Takala TES. Immobilization decreases mRNA levels of fibrillar collagen types I and III and α-subunit of prolyl 4-hydroxylase. *J Appl Physiol* 1999; **87**: 90–6.

20 Han X-Y, Wang W, Komulainen J, Koskinen SOA, Kovanen V, Vihko V, Trackman PC, Takala TES. Increased mRNAs for procollagens and key regulating enzymes in rat skeletal muscle following downhill running. *Pflügers Arch* 1999; **437**: 857–64.

21 Kääpä E, Han X, Holm S, Peltonen J, Takala T, Vanharanta H. Collagen synthesis and types I, III, IV, and VI collagens in an animal model of disc degeneration. *Spine* **20**: 59–66.

22 Karpakka J, Väänänen K, Orava S, Takala TE. The effects of preimmobilization training and immobilization on collagen synthesis in rat skeletal muscle. *Int J Sports Med* 1990; **11**: 484–8.

23 Karpakka JA, Pesola MK, Takala TE. The effects of anabolic steroids on collagen synthesis in rat skeletal muscle and tendon. A preliminary report. *Am J Sports Med* 1992; **20**(3): 262–6.

24 Myllylä R, Salminen A, Peltonen L, Takala TES, Vihko V. Collagen metabolism of mouse skeletal muscle during repair of exercise injuries. *Pflugers Arch* 1986; **407**: 647–70.

25 Savolainen J, Komulainen J, Vihko V, Väänänen K, Puranen J, Takala TES. Collagen synthesis and proteolytic activities in rat skeletal muscles: effect of cast-immobilization in the lengthened and shortened positions. *Arch Phys Med Rehab* 1988; **69**(11): 964–9.

26 Savolainen J, Väänänen K, Vihko V, Puranen J, Takala TES. Effect of immobilization on collagen synthesis in rat skeletal muscles. *Am J Physiol* 1987; **252**: R883–R888.

27 Savolainen J, Myllylä V, Myllylä R, Vihko V, Väänänen K, Takala TES. Effects of denervation and immobilization on collagen synthesis in rat skeletal muscle and tendon. *Am J Physiol* 1988; **254**: R897–R902.

28 Takala TES, Myllylä R, Salminen A, Anttinen H, Vihko V. Increased activities of prolyl 4-hydroxylase and galactosyl-hydroxylysyl glucosyltransferase, enzymes of collagen biosynthesis, in skeletal muscle of endurance trained mice. *Pflügers Arch* 1983; **399**: 271–4.

29 Takala TE, Rämö P, Kiviluoma K, Vihko V, Kainulainen H, Kettunen R. Effects of training and anabolic steroids on collagen synthesis in dog heart. *Eur J Appl Physiol* 1991; **62**(1): 1–6.

30 Turto H, Lindy S, Halme J. Protocollagen prolyl hydroxylase activity in work-induced hypertrophy of rat muscle. *Am J Physiol* 1974; **226**: 63–5.

31 Kovanen V. Effects of aging and physical training on rat skeletal muscle (doctoral thesis). *Acta Physiol Scand* 1989; 135 (Suppl. 577).

32 Davison PF. Tendon. In: Weiss B, Jayson MIV, eds. *Collagen in Health and Disease*. London: Churchill Livingstone, 1982: 498–505.

33 Kühl U, Öcalan M, Timpl R, Mayne R, Hay E, von der Mark K. Role of muscle fibroblasts in the deposition of type-IV collagen in the basal lamina of myotubes. *Differentiation* 1984; **28**: 164–72.

34 Mayne R, Sanderson RD. The extracellular matrix of muscle. *Coll Rel Res* 1985; **5**: 449–68.

35 Chiquet M, Matthisson M, Koch M, Tannheimer M, Chiquet-Ehrismann R. Regulation of extracellular matrix synthesis by mechanical stress. *Biochem Cell Biol* 1996; **74**(6): 737–44.

36 Jozsa L, Thoring J, Järvinen M, Kannus P, Lehto M, Kvist M. Quantitative alterations in intramuscular connective tissue following immobilization: an experimental study in the calf muscles. *Exp Mol Pathol* 1988; **49**: 267–78.

37 Ahtikoski AM, Koskinen SOA, Kovanen V, Virtanen P, Takala TES. Regulation of synthesis of type I collagen in skeletal muscle after immobilization: effect of stretch. *Med Sci Sports Exerc* 1997; **29** (5 Suppl.): abstract no. 650.

38 Ahtikoski AM, Koskinen SOA, Virtanen P, Kovanen V, Risteli J, Takala TES. Immobilization and stretch effect on the concentration of type IV collagen and compounds related to its synthesis and degradation in muscles. In: *2nd Annual Congress of the European College of Sport Science*. Copenhagen, Denmark, 1997: 23–25.8.

39 Koskinen SOA, Kjaer M, Mohr T, Biering Sørensen F, Suuronen T, Takala TES. Type IV collagen and its degradation in paralyzed human muscle: effect of functional electrical stimulation. *Muscle Nerve* 2000; **23**: 580–9.

40 Virtanen P, Tolonen U, Savolainen J, Takala TES. Effect of reinnervation on collagen biosynthesis in rat skeletal muscle. *J Appl Physiol* 1992; **72**(6): 2069–74.

41 Kovanen V, Suominen H, Heikkinen E. Mechanical properties of fast and slow skeletal muscle with special reference to collagen and endurance training. *J Biomech* 1984; **17**: 725–35.

42 Kovanen V, Suominen H, Peltonen L. Effects of aging and life-long physical training on collagen in slow and fast skeletal muscle in rats. A morphometric and immunohistochemical study. *Cell Tissue Res* 1987; **248**: 247–55.

43 Williams PE, Goldspink G. Connective tissue changes in surgically overloaded muscle. *Cell Tissue Res* 1981; **221**(2): 465–70.

44 Armstrong RB, Ogilvie RW, Schwane JA. Eccentric exercise-induced injury to rat skeletal muscle. *J Appl Physiol* 1983; **54**: 80–93.

45 Birch L, Bailey AJ, Goodship AE. Macroscopic 'degeneration' of equine superficial digital flexor tendon is accompa-

nied by a change in extracellular matrix composition. *Equine Vet J* 1998; **30**(6): 534–9.

46 Langberg H, Skovgaard D, Karamouzis M, Bulow J, Kjaer M. Metabolism and inflammatory mediators in the peritendinous space measured by microdialysis during intermittent isometric exercise in humans. *J Physiol* 1999; **515**: 919–27.

47 Langberg H, Skovgaard D, Pedersen Bulow J, Kjaer M. Type I collagen turnover in the peritendinous connective tissue after exercise dtermined by microdialysis. *J Physiol* 1999; **521**: 299–306.

48 Langberg H, Rosendal L, Kjaer M. Training induced changes in peritendinous type I collagen turnover determined by microdialysis. *J Physiol* 2002; **534**: 397–402.

49 Boushel R, Langberg H, Green S, Skovgaard D, Bulow J, Kjaer M. Blood flow and oxygenation in peritendinous tissue and calf muscle during dynamic exercise. *J Physiol* 1999; **524**: 305–13.

50 Langberg H, Bulow J, Kjaer M. Standardized intermittent static exercise increases peritendinous blood flow in human leg. *Clin Physiol* 1999; **19**(1): 89–93.

51 Boushel R, Langberg H, Olesen J, Nowak M, Simonsen L, Bulow J, Kjaer M. Regional blood flow during exercise in humans measured by near-infrared spectroscopy and *indocyanine green. J Appl Physiol* 2000; **89**(5): 1868–78.

52 Almekinders I, Banes AJ, Ballanger CA. Effects of repetitive motion on human fibroblasts. *Med Sci Sports Exerc* 1993; **25**: 603–7.

53 Wang JH-C, Grood ES, Florer J, Wenstrup R. Alignment and proliferation of MC3T3–E1 osteoblasts in microgrooved silicone substrate subjected to cyclic stretching. *J Biomech* 2000; **33**(6): 729–35.

54 Silver IA, Brown PN, Goodship AEA. Clinical and experimental study of tendon injury, healing and treatment in the horse. *Vet J* 1983; Suppl. 1: 1–43.

55 Backman C, Boquist L, Friden J, Lorentzon R, Toolanen G. Chronic Achilles paratendonitis: an experimental model in the rabbit. *J Orth Res* 1990; **8**(4): 541–7.

56 Stone D, Green C, Rao U *et al.* Cytokinine-induced tendinitis: a preliminary study in rabbits. *J Orth Res* 1999; **17**(2): 168–77.

57 Magnusson SP, Aagaard P, Rosager S, Dyhre-Poulsen P, Kjaer M. Load-displacement properties of the human triceps surae aponeurosis *in vivo. J Physiol* 2001; **531**: 277–88.

58 Fratzl P, Misof K, Zizak I, Rapp G, Amenittsch H, Bernstorf S. Fibrillar structure and mechanical properties of collagen. *J Struct Biol* 1997; **122**: 119–22.

59 Gineyts E, Cloos PAC, Borel O, Grimaud L, Delmas PD, Garnero P. Racemization and isomerization of type I collagen C-telopeptides in human bone and soft tissues: assessment of tissue turnover. *Biochem J* 2000; **345**: 481–5.

60 Birk DE, Mayne R. Localization of collagen types I, III and V during tendon development. Changes in collagen types I and III are correlated with changes in fibril diameter. *Eur J Cell Biol* 1997; **72**: 352–61.

61 Rettig ME, Dassa GL, Raskin KB, Melone CP Jr. Wrist fractures in the athlete. Distal radius and carpal fractures. *Clin Sports Med* 1998; **17**(3): 469–89.

62 Woo SL, Hildebrand K, Watanabe N, Fenwick JA, Papageorgiou CD, Wang JH. Tissue engineering of ligament and tendon healing. *Clin Orth Rel Res* 1999; **367** (Suppl.): S312–23.

63 Indelicato PA. Non-operative treatment of complete tears of the medial collateral ligament of the knee. *J Bone Joint Surg (Am)* 1983; **65**(3): 323–9.

64 Reider B. Medial collateral ligament injuries in athletes. *Sports Med* 1996; **21**(2): 147–56.

65 Warren LF, Marshall JL. The supporting structures and layers on the medial side of the knee: an anatomical analysis. *J Bone Joint Surg (Am)* 1979; **61**(1): 56–62.

66 Frank C, Woo SL, Amiel D, Harwood F, Gomez M, Akeson W. Medial collateral ligament healing. A multidisciplinary assessment in rabbits. *Am J Sports Med* 1983; **11**(6): 379–89.

67 Niyibizi C, Kavalkovich K, Yamaji T, Woo SL-Y. Type V collagen is increased during rabbit medial collateral ligament healing. *Knee Surg Sports Traumatol Arthrosc* 2000; **8**: 281–5.

68 Weiss JA, Woo SL, Ohland KJ, Horibe S, Newton PO. Evaluation of a new injury model to study medial collateral ligament healing: primary repair versus non-operative treatment. *J Orth Res* 1991; **9**(4): 516–28.

69 Woo SL-Y, An K-N, Frank CB, Livesay GA, Ma CB, Zeminski J, Wayne JS, Myers BS. Anatomy, biology, and biomechanics of tendon and ligament. In: Buckwalter JA, Einhorn TA, Simon SR, eds. *Orthopedic Basic Science Biology and Biomechanics of the Musculoskeletal System.* Rosemont, IL: American Academy of Orthopaedic Surgeons, 2000: 581–616.

70 Tipton CM, Matthes RD, Maynard JA, Carey RA. The influence of physical activity on ligaments and tendons. *Med Sci Sports* 1975; **7**(3): 165–75.

71 Reiser KM, Crouch EC, Chang K, Williamson JR. Lysyl oxidase–mediated crosslinking in granulation tissue collagen in two models of hyperglycemia. *Biochim Biophys Acta* 1991; **1097**(1): 55–61.

72 Sell DR, Monnier VM. End-stage renal disease and diabetes catalyze the formation of a pentose-derived crosslink from aging human collagen. *J Clin Invest* 1990; **85**(2): 380–4.

73 Woo SL, Gomez MA, Inoue M, Akeson WH. New experimental procedures to evaluate the biomechanical properties of healing canine medial collateral ligaments. *J Orth Res* 1987; **5**(3): 425–32.

74 Woo SL, Inoue M, McGurk-Burleson E, Gomez MA. Treatment of the medial collateral ligament injury. II. Structure and function of canine knees in response to differing treatment regimens. *Am J Sports Med* 1987; **15**(1): 22–9.

75 Reider B, Sathy MR, Talkington J, Blyznak N, Kollias S. Treatment of isolated medial collateral ligament injuries in

athletes with early functional rehabilitation. A five-year follow-up study. *Am J Sports Med* 1994; **22**(4): 470–7.

76 Hastings DE. The non-operative management of collateral ligament injuries of the knee joint. *Clin Orth Rel Res* 1980; **147**: 22–8.

77 Woo SL, Gomez MA, Sites TJ, Newton PO, Orlando CA, Akeson WH. The biomechanical and morphological changes in the medial collateral ligament of the rabbit after immobilization and remobilization. *J Bone Joint Surg (Am)* 1987; **69**(8): 1200–11.

78 Tipton CM, James SL, Mergner W, Tcheng TK. Influence of exercise on strength of medial collateral knee ligaments of dogs. *Am J Physiol* 1970; **218**(3): 894–902.

79 Hillard-Sembell D, Daniel DM, Stone ML, Dobson BE, Fithian DC. Combined injuries of the anterior cruciate and medial collateral ligaments of the knee. Effect of treatment on stability and function of the joint. *J Bone Joint Surg (Am)* 1996; **78**(2): 169–76.

80 Woo SL, Young EP, Ohland KJ, Marcin JP, Horibe S, Lin HC. The effects of transection of the anterior cruciate ligament on healing of the medial collateral ligament. A biomechanical study of the knee in dogs. *J Bone Joint Surg (Am)* 1990; **72**(3): 382–92.

81 Yamaji T, Levine RE, Woo C, Niyibizi KW, Kavalkovich, KW. Weaver-Green CM. Medial collateral ligament healing one year after a concurrent medial collateral ligament and anterior cruciate ligament injury: an interdisciplinary study in rabbits. *J Orth Res* 1996; **14**(2): 223–7.

82 Shelbourne KD, Patel DV. Management of combined injuries of the anterior cruciate and medial collateral ligaments. *Instructional Course Lectures* 1996; **45**: 275–80.

83 Hildebrand KA, Deie M, Allen CR, Smith DW, Georgescu HI, Evans CH, Robbins PD, Woo SL. Early expression of marker genes in the rabbit medial collateral and anterior cruciate ligaments: the use of different viral vectors and the effects of injury. *J Orth Res* 1999; **17**(1): 37–42.

84 Hildebrand KA, Woo SL, Smith DW, Allen CR, Deie M, Taylor BJ, Schmidt CC. The effects of platelet-derived growth factor-BB on healing of the rabbit medial collateral ligament. An in vivo study. *Am J Sports Med* 1998; **26**(4): 549–54.

85 Kobayashi D, Kurosaka M, Yoshiya S, Hashimoto J, Saura R, Akamatu T, Mizuno K. The effect of basic fibroblast growth factor on primary healing of the defect in canine anterior cruciate ligaments. *Trans Orthopaed Res Soc* 1995; **20**: 630.

86 Letson AK, Dahners LE. The effect of combinations of growth factors on ligament healing. *Clin Orth Rel Res* 1994; **308**: 207–12.

87 Marui T, Niyibizi C, Georgescu HI, Cao M, Kavalkovich KW, Levine RE, Woo SL. Effect of growth factors on matrix synthesis by ligament fibroblasts. *J Orth Res* 1997; **15**(1): 18–23.

88 Murphy PG, Hart DA. Influence of exogenous growth factors on the expression of plasminogen activators and plasminogen activator inhibitors by cells isolated from normal and healing rabbit ligaments. *J Orth Res* 1994; **12**(4): 564–75.

89 Murphy PG, Hart DA. The cell biology of ligaments and ligament healing. In: Jackson DW, ed. *The Anterior Cruciate Ligament: Current and Future Concepts* 1993; **14**: 165–77.

90 Scherping SC Jr, Schmidt CC, Georgescu HI, Kwoh CK, Evans CH, Woo SL. Effect of growth factors on the proliferation of ligament fibroblasts from skeletally mature rabbits. *Connective Tissue Res* 1997; **36**(1): 1–8.

91 Schmidt CC, Georgescu HI, Kwoh CK, Blomstrom GL, Engle CP, Larkin LA, Evans CH, Woo SL. Effect of growth factors on the proliferation of fibroblasts from the medial collateral and anterior cruciate ligaments. *J Orth Res* 1995; **13**(2): 184–90.

92 Woo SL-Y, Suh J-K, Parsons I, Wang J-H, Watanabe N. Biological intervention in ligament healing effect of growth factors. *Sports Med Arthroscopy Rev* 1998; **6**: 74–82.

93 Nakamura N, Timmermann SA, Hart DA, Kaneda Y, Shrive NG, Shino K, Ochi T, Frank CB. A comparison of *in vivo* gene delivery methods for antisense therapy in ligament healing. *Gene Ther* 1998; **5**(11): 1455–61.

94 Yang Y, Nunes FA, Berencsi K, Furth EE, Gonczol E, Wilson JM. Cellular immunity to viral antigens limits E1-deleted adenoviruses for gene therapy. *Proc Natl Acad Sci USA* 1994; **91**(10): 4407–11.

95 Challita PM, Kohn DB. Lack of expression from a retroviral vector after transduction of murine hematopoietic stem cells is associated with methylation in vivo. *Proc Natl Acad Sci USA* 1994; **91**(7): 2567–71.

96 Caplan AI. Mesenchymal stem cells. *J Orth Res* 1991; **9**(5): 641–50.

97 Ferrari G, Cusella-De Angelis G, Coletta M, Paolucci E, Stornaiuolo A, Cossu G, Mavilio F. Muscle regeneration by bone marrow-derived myogenic progenitors. *Science* 1998; **279**(5356): 1528–30. [Published erratum appears in *Science* 1998; **281**(5379): 923.]

98 Kadiyala S, Young RG, Thiede MA, Bruder SP. Culture expanded canine mesenchymal stem cells possess osteo-chondrogenic potential in vivo and in vitro. *Cell Transplant* 1997; **6**(2): 125–34.

99 Lazarus HM, Haynesworth SE, Gerson SL, Rosenthal NS, Caplan AI. Ex vivo expansion and subsequent infusion of human bone marrow-derived stromal progenitor cells (mesenchymal progenitor cells): implications for therapeutic use. *Bone Marrow Transplant* 1995; **16**(4): 557–64.

100 Wakitani S, Goto T, Young RG, Mansour JM, Goldberg VM, Caplan AI. Repair of large full-thickness articular cartilage defects with allograft articular chondrocytes embedded in a collagen gel. *Tissue Engineering* 1998; **4**(4): 429–44.

101 Caplan AI. The mesengenic process. *Clinics Plastic Surg* 1994; **21**(3): 429–35.

102 Huard J, Goins WF, Glorioso JC. Herpes simplex virus type 1 vector mediated gene transfer to muscle. *Gene Ther* 1995; **2**(6): 385–92.

103 Watanabe N, Woo SL-Y, Papageorgiou C, Wang JH. Potential use of bone marrow cells for medial collateral ligament healing. *Trans Tissue Engineering Workshop* 1999: 208.

104 Awad HA, Butler DL, Boivin GP, Smith FN, Malaviya P, Huibregtse B, Caplan AI. Autologous mesenchymal stem cell-mediated repair of tendon. *Tissue Engineering* 1999; **5**(3): 267–77.

105 Kim SS, Vacanti JP. The current status of tissue engineering as potential therapy. *Semin Pediatric Surg* 1999; **8**(3): 119–23.

106 Zimmerman SD, McCormick RJ, Vadlamudi RK, Thomas DP. Age and training alter collagen characteristics in fast- and slow-twitch rat limb muscle. *J Appl Physiol* 1993; **75**: 1670–4.

107 Wang JH. Substrate deformation determines actin cytoskeleton reorganization: a mathematical modeling and experimental study. *J Theoret Biol* 2000; **202**(1): 33–41.

108 Rudy TW, Livesay GA, Woo SL, Fu FH. A combined robotic/universal force sensor approach to determine in situ forces of knee ligaments. *J Biomech* 1996; **29**(10): 1357–60.

109 Magnusson SP, Gleim GW, Nicholas JA. Shoulder weakness in professional baseball pitchers. *Med Sci Sports Exerc* 1994; **26**: 5–9.

110 Hutton RS. Neuromuscular basis of stretching exercise. In: Komi PV, ed. *Strength and Power in Sports.* The IOC Encyclopaedia of Sports Medicine, Vol. III. Oxford: Blackwell Scientific Publications. 1993: 29–38.

111 Taylor DC, Dalton JD Jr, Seaber AV, Garrett WEJ. Viscoelastic properties of muscle–tendon units. The biomechanical effects of stretching. *Am J Sports Med* 1990; **18**: 300–9.

112 Moore MA, Hutton RS. Electromyographic investigation of muscle stretching techniques. *Med Sci Sports Exerc* 1980; **12**: 322–9.

113 Magnusson SP, Simonsen EB, Dyhre-Poulsen P, Aagaard P, Mohr T, Kjaer M. Viscoelastic stress relaxation during static stretch in human skeletal muscle in the absence of EMG activity. *Scand J Med Sci Sports* 1996; **6**: 323–8.

114 Magnusson SP, Simonsen EB, Aagaard P, Dyhre-Poulsen P, McHugh MP, Kjaer M. Mechanical and physiological responses to stretching with and without preisometric contraction in human skeletal muscle. *Arch Phys Med Rehab* 1996; **77**: 373–8.

115 Magnusson SP, Simonsen EB, Aagaard P, Sorensen H, Kjaer M. A mechansim for altered flexibility in human skeletal muscle. *J Physiol* 1996; **497**: 291–8.

116 Butler DL, Grood ES, Noyes FR. Biomechanics of ligaments and tendons. In: Hutton RS, ed. *Exercise and Sports Sciences Reviews.* Philadelphia: Franklin Institute, 1978: 125–81.

117 Viidik A. Functional properties of collagenous tissues. *Int Rev Connective Tissue Res* 1973; **6**: 127–215.

118 Kovanen V, Suominen H. Effects of age and life-long endurance training on the passive mechanical properties of rat skeletal muscle. *Comp Gerontol* 1988; **2**: 18–23.

119 Magnusson SP, Simonsen EB, Aagaard P, Boesen J, Kjaer M. Determinants of musculoskeletal flexibility: Viscoelastic properties, cross-sectional area, EMG and stretch tolerance. *Scand J Med Sci Sports* 1997; **7**: 195–202.

120 Magnusson SP, Simonsen EB, Aagaard P, Kjaer M. Biomechanical responses to repeated stretches in human hamstring muscle *in vivo. Am J Sports Med* 1996; **24**: 622–8.

121 Magnusson SP, Aaagaard P, Larsson B, Kjaer M. Passive energy absorption by human muscle–tendon unit is unaffected by increase in intramuscular temperature. *J Appl Physiol* 2000; **88**: 1215–20.

122 Magnusson SP, Aagaard P, Nielson JJ. Passive energy return after repeated stretches of the hamstring muscle–tendon unit. *Med Sci Sports Exerc* 2000; **32**: 1160–4.

123 Lieber RL, Leonard ME, Brown CG, Trestik CL. Frog semitendinosis tendon load-strain and stress–strain properties during passive loading. *Am J Physiol* 1991; **261**: C86–C92.

124 Gajdosik RL. Effects of static stretching on the maximal length and resistance to passive stretch of short hamstring muscles. *J Orth Sports Phys Ther* 1991; **14**: 250–5.

125 Garrett WE. Muscle strain injuries: clinical and basic aspects. *Med Sci Sports Exerc* 1990; **22**: 436–43.

126 Astrand PO, Rodahl K. *Textbook of Work Physiology.* New York: McGraw-Hill Co., 1986.

127 Saltin B, Hermansen L. Esophageal, rectal, and muscle temperature during exercise. *J Appl Physiol* 1966; **21**: 1757–62.

128 Alexander RM. Energy-saving mechanisms in walking and running. *J Exp Biol* 1991; **160**: 55–69.

129 Gleim GW, Stachenfeld NS, Nicholas JA. The influence of flexibility on the economy of walking and jogging. *J Orth Res* 1990; **8**: 814–23.

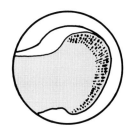

Chapter 1.7
Cartilage Tissue —
Loading and Overloading

KAROLA MESSNER,
JACK LEWIS, TED OEGEMA &
HEIKKI J. HELMINEN

Classical reference

Swanepoel MW, Adams LM. The stiffness of human
    apophyseal articular cartilage as an indicator of
    joint loading. *Proc Inst Mech Eng* 1994; **208**:
    33–43.

Despite the fact that osteoarthrosis is a considerable problem, relatively little is known about the mechanical properties of joints under mechanical loads. The apophyseal joints are of interest because their primary function is to restrict motion and they are subjected to prolonged loading. It has been hypothesized that articular cartilage is mechanically conditioned by the daily amount of stress imposed on it, such that 'soft' cartilage conditioned by low magnitudes of stress is more susceptible to injury by infrequent high magnitudes of stress. Swanepoel and Adams measured the mean thickness and stiffness of the human lumbar apophyseal cartilage in the upper lumbar segments (see Tables 1.7.1 and 1.7.2). The data indicated that there were region-specific differences within the joint. Moreover, compared to previous data in the literature, the data of Swanepoel and Adams suggest that the articular cartilage of human apophyseal joints is softer than the articular cartilage of the ankle, knee and hip joint. Together the results suggest that low daily load conditioning has influenced the mechanical properties of the joint.

Background

Loading is essential for cartilage health and function. Cartilage can sustain loads over a large range of load magnitudes and frequencies and maintain its mechan-ical integrity and biological stability for a lifetime. However, loads that are outside of this range and are too high or too low can stimulate cartilage to remodel, compromising its functional capacity. Also, loads occurring during trauma can lead to cartilage damage and subsequent degeneration. Understanding the response of cartilage to underloading, overloading, impact loading and altered loading is essential in guiding injury prevention and treatment.

The mechanical properties of adult articular cartilage depend on the content of the different extracellular matrix proteins (proteoglycans, collagens, etc.), and their three-dimensional structure and interactions.

Table 1.7.1 Thickness distribution of the cartilage of the superior concave apophyseal surface (mm ± 95% CI). From Table 2 in Swanepoel & Adams.

Area	Anterior	Center	Posterior
Superior	1.20±0.23	1.07±0.18	0.79±0.17
Center	1.13±0.10	1.21±0.10	1.03±0.13
Inferior	0.91±0.12	1.14±0.12	1.09±0.12

Table 1.7.2 Stiffness distribution of the cartilage of the superior concave apophyseal surface (MPa ± 95% CI). From Table 3 in Swanepoel & Adams.

Area	Anterior	Center	Posterior
Superior	2.84±0.64	2.23±0.46	2.21±0.45
Center	2.79±0.30	3.01±0.35	2.51±0.48
Inferior	2.77±0.39	2.92±0.42	2.57±0.63

Cartilage with a high content of glycosaminoglycans (GAGs), attached to the core protein of aggrecan, the main cartilage proteoglycan (PG), is stiffer during compressive tests than cartilage with a lower GAG content [1]. Thus, physiologically high-loaded cartilage regions appear to be stiffer than low-loaded areas within the same joint [2]. Chondrocytes harvested from various regions of adult sheep knees maintain in culture their location-specific production of PGs [3]. Since chondrocytes from newborn lambs do not show similar location-specific variations in matrix production, it is reasonable to suggest that the loading conditions during postnatal development determine this change in chondrocyte phenotype. Thus, each part of a particular joint is optimally adapted to the physiologic loading conditions in adulthood by the characteristics of its cells and the construction of the extracellular matrix. Since cartilage is a tissue with low turnover, it should be noted that this adaptation takes approximately 20 years in humans.

Responses of articular cartilage to cyclic, static and impact loading

Loading models

Two tools that have been used to study cartilage response to load are *in vitro* models of cartilage explant loading and *in vivo* models of cartilage impact loading. In this section, work in these two areas will be reviewed.

These two tools address several issues related to cartilage function. First is the question of what loads are required for healthy cartilage. Too small a load can lead to atrophy, an excessive load can lead to cartilage damage and future degeneration. Second is the question of cartilage response to excessive functional loading, such as might occur during aggressive activity with repetitive loading. Under what loads and conditions might cartilage be damaged, what actually occurs in the cartilage during this injurious loading, how might this be prevented, and how might it be treated if damage does occur? Finally, there is the question of the response of cartilage to traumatic impact loading. Under what conditions is cartilage and the cartilage/bone interface damaged, what is the nature of this damage, and how might it be treated?

Before examining these questions, it is useful to de-scribe what is known of the load environment of articular cartilage. In moderate activities, such as walking, maximum surface pressures in the hip joint have been measured to be of the order of 4–6 MPa [4]. During lifting, pressures rose to nearly 14 MPa [4]. The time history of this loading would be of the order of 1/s for walking, with load rise times of the order of 200 ms [5]. This rise time reduces to approximately 100 ms in jogging [5]. Surface pressures in trauma can rise to and above the failure level of cartilage. These values for joints are not well known, but from *in vitro* tests are estimated to be in the range of 25 MPa [6,7] to 50 MPa, with rise time of a few ms. The *in vivo* environment of cartilage is thus quite dynamic.

Loading of cartilage explants

In vitro models of cartilage response to moderate load have consisted of cartilage explants, subjected to a variety of controlled load environments [8]. These models usually consist of cartilage removed from an animal at slaughter, maintaining the cells in the living state. Cartilage pieces, with or without the bone, are prepared and loaded in a culture environment. The time history of loading is varied, with load frequency, duration and magnitude as variables. Outcome variables have included synthesis rates of PGs and matrix proteins, gene regulation, tissue swelling as a measure of matrix damage, cell viability and mechanical properties of the explant. The numerous studies all differ in test conditions and outcome variables, making precise comparison difficult. However, several general conclusions have emerged from this work. Static compression of unconfined cartilage explants causes a dose-dependent inhibition of PG synthesis [8]. Compressive stress of 1 MPa for 12 h in cow cartilage reduced PG synthesis rates by 50% [9]. Increased stress or duration further depresses synthesis. Ragan *et al.* [10] further found that 24 h of static compression depressed mRNA levels for both aggrecan and the normal type IIa collagen.

Cyclic and static loading

Cyclic or intermittent compression has various effects on cartilage explants, depending on the loading conditions, such as frequency, time between loads and test duration. Cyclic compression generally increases PG synthesis in the short term [8] and alters expression of other matrix proteins [11]. Unconfined compression of cartilage disks at 1 Hz produced an increase of 40% in PG synthesis rate [12]. However increasing both the load magnitude and the duration of loading can reduce PG synthesis [13], and increase release from the matrix and cell death [14]. Cyclic loading also alters the synthesis and retention of fibronectin, with either increases [13] or decreases [14], depending on the loading conditions. Fibronectin is an important molecule in matrix assembly, which increases during remodeling, but is also rapidly up-regulated in response to matrix damage.

The studies discussed so far have focused on cartilage function as influenced by loads within a relatively normal range. Other investigators have specifically explored the upper limits of normal loading and how cartilage explants respond to loads above this limit. Quinn *et al.* [15,16] studied the effect of injurious static compression on cartilage explants. They imposed strains over 60% on bovine cartilage discs 3 mm in diameter by 1 mm thick, leading to grossly visible cracks. They found decrease in tensile strength, increased cell apoptosis and elevated PG turnover, including increased synthesis and loss of the small PGs. Cells also appeared to be slower in response to cell stimulatory factors, such as interleukin 1 (IL-1). How much of this change is due to loss of cells and alteration of remaining viable cells is unknown. Chen *et al.* [17] applied cyclic loads of increasing magnitude and loading rate to cartilage explants. They found that damage to the cartilage required repeated impacts with a peak stress of at least 2.5 MPa and a stress rate of at least 30 MPa/s for 2 min or longer, suggesting that impact damage is cumulative and stress-rate dependent. Explants loaded repetitively at 5 MPa at 0.3 Hz for 2, 20 and 120 min showed increased water content, increased fibronectin synthesis and increased collagen breakdown. The latter observation supported the assumption that increased water content was due to collagen damage in the matrix.

Tests of static and cyclic compression on cartilage explants have shown that load affects chondrocyte metabolism, but it is difficult to understand the relevance of specific values to *in vivo* conditions. At what point will change in chondrocyte biology lead to cartilage damage *in vivo* and how is this damage defined? How are the explant loading and stress conditions related to

in vivo conditions? While it is clear that increasingly severe loading leads to a progressive process of matrix damage, reduced synthesis of matrix structural molecules, increased lytic enzymes and cell death, the load conditions *in vivo* for this process are still poorly defined. These experimental models can be considered useful in the study of cartilage response to loading and damage, but not for simulations of *in vivo* function. This is still an area of active research that must progress further before clinical relevance can be defined.

Impact loading

Impact loading of cartilage explants provides a closer simulation of *in vivo* injurious load conditions than static and cyclic loading conditions. Joint trauma, and cartilage load during that trauma, are due to a single high-magnitude load, that occurs in the order of milliseconds. Although the specific time/load history will not be known, the approximate histories can be reasonably estimated. The outcome variables are also better defined. Immediate and future cell and matrix damage are the main concerns. Several investigators have studied cartilage explants under impact loading. The classic study was performed by Repo and Finlay [18], who loaded cartilage explants with a thin subchondral bone plate with a falling plate, with a displacement stop. They measured cell viability by autoradiography of incorporated radioactive proline, and found that cell death began at about 25 MPa, with fracturing and fissuring occurring simultaneously with cell death. Jeffrey *et al.* [19,20] used a different drop weight system to load cartilage explants with no bone with up to 200 MPa surface stress. They found increased mass due to swelling and decreased cell viability with severity of impact. They also found increased loss of newly synthesized protein and GAG when impacted explants were cultured up to 15 days after impact. Torzilli *et al.* [21] and Borelli *et al.* [22] used a similar impact system to impact 1-mm thick strips of cartilage with stresses ranging from 0.5 MPa to 65 MPa. These authors used a conventional materials test machine to load the tissue at a constant stress rate of 35 MPa/s. They measured PG synthesis by sulfate incorporation, cell viability and death with the fluorescing dyes fluoresceine diacetate and ethidium bromide, and water content. They found stimulated PG synthesis at the lower stress levels (<1.0 MPa), but progressively reduced synthesis with increasing stress level. They also found increased relative water content with impact stress, and decreased cell viability, initially at the surface, but progressively throughout the tissue with increasing load. They estimated a critical stress level above which matrix damage occurred, as measured by water content and cell death, to be 15–20 MPa.

Impacted explants provide another useful experimental model for study of the response of cartilage to injuries. There is still much that is unknown about this response and this is an active area of research, but the work has identified several elements of cartilage damage that can be related to *in vivo* conditions. Although there is still controversy as to how the load conditions relate to *in vivo* loads and stresses, tissue cracking and cell death provide a useful link between the *in vitro* model and *in vivo* conditions. This work will undoubtedly continue to evolve and further our understanding of cartilage response to impact load.

Impact loading of articular cartilage *in situ*

Useful as the impacted explant model is, it still lacks important elements as a simulation of joint trauma. Cellular response probably depends on microenvironmental and loading conditions. Consequently, several investigators have developed *in vivo* models of cartilage and joint trauma. Thompson *et al.* [23,24] used a falling weight on the anesthetized canine patellofemoral joint as a model of joint trauma. This was a closed model, without invasion of the joint. Immediately after impact, there were surface fissures in the patellar cartilage that did not extend to the calcified cartilage and subchondral bone, and also cracks through the calcified cartilage and bone, into the uncalcified cartilage (Fig. 1.7.1). A 'bone bruise' was visible on magnetic resonance imaging (MRI) [24]. At 3 months after impact, loss of PG in the area of damage was evident. At 6 months after impact, there was further loss of PG in the cartilage, fibrillation was increased, and cloning of chondrocytes was evident (Fig. 1.7.2). At 12 months after impact, however, the PG staining had partially returned, and no additional fibrillation was evident (Fig. 1.7.3). The process appeared to have stabilized and bone bruises visualized by MRI had decreased. A model of the response of the cartilage/bone to trauma was proposed, as shown in

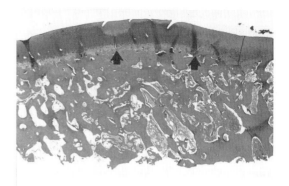

Fig. 1.7.1 Sagittal section of the canine patella 2 weeks after loading. Fractures are seen in the zone of calcified cartilage (arrows), and clefts in the cartilaginous surface are seen above (×15). *J Bone Joint Surg* 1991; **73**-A(7): 994.

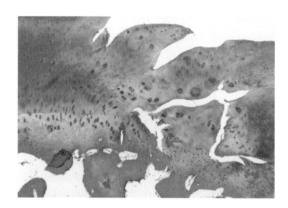

Fig. 1.7.2 Patellar articular cartilage 24 weeks after transarticular loading. There are clefts in the zone of calcified cartilage, more extensive fibrillation, a decrease in safranin-O staining and numerous clones of chondrocytes (safranin-O and fast green staining ×50). *J Bone Joint Surg* 1991; **73**-A(7): 1000.

Fig. 1.7.4 [25]. Whether this process, which still had cartilage fissures and remodeling of fractures in the zone of calcified cartilage, would have remained stable or progressed to further degeneration is unknown. The damage site at the distal pole of the patella was non-weight-bearing, so this may have been a favored position. In a short-term evaluation of this model, Pickvance *et al.* [26] found a variety of cytokines up-regulated in the cartilage during the early phase of proteoglycan loss, but a decline by 6 months.

Subsequent to this work, these authors developed

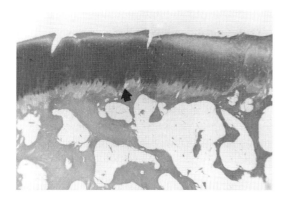

Fig. 1.7.3 Canine patellar articular cartilage 1 year after loading, showing surface clefts extending into the radial zone, with a step-off in the zone of calcified cartilage (arrow) and minimum loss of safranin-O staining of the matrix. There are identifiable clones of cells on the right-hand side of the photomicrograph (safranin-O and fast green staining × 50). *J Bone Joint Surg* 1993; **75-A**(5): 709.

an open model in which the distal femur of the canine was impacted with a spherical or cylindrical indenter and drop-weight mechanism [27]. This allowed more precise control over the impact location, stress level and stress analysis of the impact. Immediately after impact with the spherical indenter at a load condition that would create subchondral cracks and some surface cartilage cracks, the cartilage appeared essentially normal on histology, other than the cracking. There was also essentially normal cell viability, other than some cell loss around the cartilage surface cracks. At 2 weeks after impact with the cylindrical indenter, with the same goals, there was loss of PG, but otherwise no changes. This model was then applied in conjunction with transection of the anterior cruciate ligament (ACL) in an attempt to create an accelerated degenerative model. Contrary to expectations, at 6 months after impact and surgery, there was no difference between impact sites and contralateral leg controls with respect to PG staining, cell viability and cell cloning. There were no apparent degenerative changes due to either the cartilage impact or the ACL transsection over this

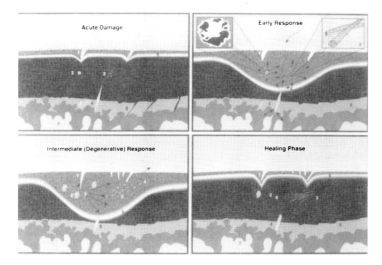

Fig. 1.7.4 Schematic representation of the proposed different phases of the responses of articular cartilage after acute trauma. (a) Acute damage: (1) surface fractures, (2) cell damage, (3) microscopic matrix damage, (4) fractures from zone of calcified cartilage (ZCC) into cartilage, (5) stair-step fracture of ZCC, (6) surface disruption, (7) subchondral bone damage into marrow space. (b) Early response: (1) factors diffuse in from synovium, (2) cell death or repair, (3) matrix damage accelerates, (4) repair of ZCC begins, (5) stair-step fractures begin to heal, (6) factors may diffuse in from subchondral bone. (c) Intermediate (degenerative) response: (1) cracks propagate, (2) cells clone, (3) enhanced matrix damage, (4) cell secretes factors, (5) endochondral repair occurs, (6) increased area of proteoglycan loss. (d) Healing phase: (1) surface cracks stabilize, (2) cell clones stabilize, (3) microdamage stabilizes, (4) crack fills in, (5) step-offs of ZCC are healed, (6) region of proteoglycan depletion is diminished, (7) subchondral bone stabilizes. *Agents Actions* 1993; **40**: 220–3.

time period (unpublished data). Since a cell viability assay, rather than a cell death assay, was used in these studies, it cannot be said with certainty that there was no cell death. However, if there was cell death it was not extensive and the common histologic measures of osteoarthritic cartilage did not show significant changes. The traumatized cartilage was not undergoing degeneration within the period of observation, even with the cut ACL. Again, the impacted cartilage was not in an area of active loading; perhaps this prevented further changes. Also, the cut ACL model of osteoarthritis [28] has been shown to require several years to develop into a clear state of degenerative osteoarthritis, so perhaps this *in vivo* model of open impact would evolve into a degenerative model with more time.

Newberry *et al.* [6,7] used a similar model of patella impact in the Flemish Giant rabbit. They used a closed impact of the joint with a falling weight, with the load parallel to the femur with the joint flexed to 120°. They found consistent surface cracking of patellar cartilage immediately after impact. The cracks ran in the superior–inferior direction and were thought to be due to the shear stress generated as the patella settled deeper into the trochlear groove during the impact. They measured histology and indentation stiffness of the patellar cartilage at various times after impact and found decreases in stiffness near the cracks at 12 months after impact. There was also evidence of histologic changes consistent with cartilage degeneration at 12 months. These were relatively minor changes and whether they would progress to significant degenerative changes is unknown.

It is somewhat remarkable that the rather severe impacts imposed in both the Thompson and Newberry studies [6,7,23,24] did not create a frank degenerative condition. Loads applied were intentionally below that which would create gross bone fracture, but were otherwise quite severe, creating surface stresses in the range of 50 MPa. Because of the major differences in stress state at the contact surface, it is difficult to compare results of the *in vivo* models with those of the impacted explants. Taken together, the *in vitro* and *in vivo* impact models demonstrate the type of injury to the tissue that can occur during trauma, but they have not demonstrated that these changes can progress to symptomatic osteoarthritis. It is not clear if a longer time *in vivo* is required, if some causative factor

in the disease process is being left out, or if the damage is not sufficiently severe. At this time we are still left with the question of what degree and measure of damage is required for progression to a symptomatic disease state after joint trauma.

In spite of this question, there are several points that can be gleaned from the impact experiments on the explants and the *in vivo* models. First, at the same level of tissue damage, the more chondrocytes that survive, the better the chances are for repair. A comparison of the *in vitro* vs. *in vivo* responses of the surviving chondrocytes suggests that the injured joint environment exacerbates the chondrocytic response. The *in vitro* response to impact is a transient up-regulation of molecules seen in repair, such as fibronectin and small proteoglycans like decorin and biglycan, and a rapid decrease in aggrecan. *In vivo*, there is a rapid loss of proteoglycan and up-regulation of cytokines, such as IL-1 and tumor necrosis factor α (TNF-α) around the chondrocyte, which only later gives way to repair. This would suggest that in patients with damaged cartilage as evidenced by bone bruises in areas that are weight-bearing, rehabilitation protocols that provide a gradual return of full use might spare cartilage and improve repair. A second point is that, if chondrocytes die, there is no evidence they can be replaced, so preservation of chondrocytes is important. In cartilage, these cells are responsible for maintaining several hundred to almost a thousand times their own volume of extracellular matrix. While it is true that when they die they cannot be recruited by cytokines or bad biomechanics to degrade their matrix, it is also true that they cannot repair the matrix. This means that after impact, in areas with dead chondrocytes, the toll of everyday wear and tear will slowly cause the tissue to fail.

How to preserve cells in areas of trauma is still unclear, but there are some suggestions. In acute trauma, there are two mechanisms for cell death: necrosis and apoptosis. Acute cell death by necrosis will be hard to eliminate unless the trauma is prevented or the forces of trauma are modified. Apoptosis, programmed cell death, could possibly be prevented if we understood the steps that alter the environment to initiate apoptosis. Likely candidates in a traumatized joint for pushing the cell into apoptosis are altered mechanical environment [29], exposure to inflammatory components [30], or sources of free radicals such as iron from intra-articular blood [31]. Rational treatments that alter these post-traumatic joint changes may improve recovery.

Long-term effects of various loading conditions on articular cartilage

Effects of joint immobilization and remobilization

Experiments with dogs

Immobilization of a joint causes atrophy of the articular cartilage and the adjoining tissues of the joint [32]. Casting of the knee (stifle) joint of beagle dogs in 90° flexion for 11 weeks causes up to 20–48% reduction in GAG concentration of articular cartilage [33]. This is noteworthy because the GAGs bind cations and water which maintain the osmotic swelling property and turgor of cartilage. The GAGs are depleted mainly from the superficial zone of articular cartilage. The immobilized cartilage turns out to be more immature, as shown by an average decrease of the chondroitin 6-sulfate (CS-6)/chondroitin 4-sulfate (CS-4) ratio of the GAG chains. CS-4 isomer is the predominant isomer in the immature cartilage. The total PG synthesis needs not be locally decreased after immobilization [34], even though it usually is. The collagen fibril network, which forms the structural backbone of cartilage and which is able to constrain the swelling property of PGs, shows no significant changes during immobilization. The number of collagen cross-links in cartilage can be lowered, however. The immobilization of the canine knee joint decreases cartilage stiffness (up to 25%) as determined in the form of shear modulus [35]. Under compression, the flow rate of cartilage interstitial fluid, expressed as the retardation time spectrum, increases in the immobilized dogs. In the synovial fluid, concentrations of cartilage metabolism products are reduced. Normal cartilage stiffness remains in the joint surface contact areas, e.g. between the patella and the patellar surface of the femur, probably as a consequence of sustained patellofemoral contact during the 90° immobilization in flexion.

Immobilization-induced atrophic changes of articular cartilage are for the most part restored after remobilization. In early studies with adult dogs, the PG content of articular cartilage was reported to return to the level of the contralateral limb by 3 weeks after removal of the cast [36], whereas a 6-week rigid external fixation, which inhibits normal loading of the joint, effectively prevented recovery [37]. In more recent studies the situation has proved to be more complicated, however. Namely, during remobilization of young beagle dogs for 15 weeks, after a prior 11-week immobilization period, the GAG content of articular cartilage is restored to the control level in the patellofemoral regions and in the condyles of the tibia but not on the summits of femoral condyles where the concentrations remain below the control level [34,35]. Also, in certain cartilage regions the equilibrium shear modulus of cartilage, i.e. cartilage stiffness, remains at a lower level and cartilage permeability at a higher level than in controls. The decreased CS-6/CS-4 ratio that results from immobilization is restored within 15 weeks of remobilization close to the control level. The arrangement of collagen fibrils is not different from controls after remobilization for 15 or 50 weeks. The amount of collagen cross-links of cartilage and the concentration of synovial fluid metabolites are normalized after remobilization. However, even after a remobilization period of 1 year (50 weeks) there are cartilage areas, like the lateral condyle of the tibia, where the PG concentration of the articular cartilage remains low, especially in the superficial zone [34]. In some regions the stiffness of cartilage also stays below the control level [38]. These results indicate that in certain places the atrophic changes of immobilization are slowly and possibly only with difficulty reversible after remobilization (Fig. 1.7.5).

Experiments with rabbits

Response of the rabbit articular cartilage to immobilization depends on whether the knee joint is immobilized in extension or flexion. Immobilization in extension causes compression between the femoral and tibial joint surfaces resulting in injury of the articular cartilage (compression necrosis) at the contact area [39]. Immobilization of the joint in flexion for more than 7 weeks makes the uncalcified cartilage thinner and more cellular, and the matrix shows diminished staining reaction in its ground substance [40]. These are signs of cartilage atrophy. Articular cartilage from joints which are first immobilized and then remobilized for 7–8 weeks still shows a diminu-

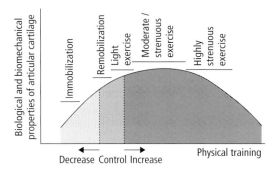

Fig. 1.7.5 Hypothesis as to the effect of intermittent physical exercise on the biologic and biomechanical properties of articular cartilage. It is suggested that atrophy occurs in articular cartilage on account of suboptimal physical stresses, while remobilization after prior immobilization at most places restores the cartilage properties to control level. Light, moderate and strenuous stresses within physiologic limits stimulate the tissue to develop improved biologic properties. Stresses beyond the physiologic limits can harm the cartilage. (Modified from [32]).

tion in the staining reactions of the intercellular matrix. However, the staining pattern is reversed to control intensity when the remobilization is prolonged to 20 weeks [40].

Human studies

When a normal joint experiences prolonged (months or years) or permanent immobilization, the synovial connective tissue encroaches upon the joint cleft and becomes confluent with the unopposed articular surfaces with eventual obliteration of the joint cavity. This process obliterates the space between the cartilage and the synovial membrane, thereby compromising and inhibiting the normal synovial fluid nutrition of the articular cartilage [41,42]. This leads to irreparable cartilage injury called obliterative degeneration of articular cartilage. With prolonged immobilization a gradual resorption of cartilage and replacement by connective tissue takes place. The cartilage-replacing connective tissue will be in contact with the subchondral bone and in some instances communicates with the bone marrow.

In areas where the articular surfaces are in direct opposition to one another, the articular cartilage becomes fibrillated and small cystic defects appear in the superficial and deep zones of uncalcified cartilage. These de-

fects are replaced by reparative, mesenchymal tissue which matures to dense connective tissue and may eventually ossify. With further progression of the condition, there is total replacement of the articular cartilage with intra-articular fibrous tissue. The condition may eventually lead to bony ankylosis [41,42].

Effects of running training

Experiments with dogs

In dogs, light or moderate intensity level training improves the properties of articular cartilage while repetitive, intensive and strenuous training can cause injury to the cartilage. Response of the articular cartilage of young beagle knee (stifle) joint to running training has been studied with three different training programs. Running exercise of 4 km/day on a treadmill, 5 days a week, for 15 weeks increases the thickness and PG content (16–26%) in the femoral cartilage, whereas collagen content is unaltered [35,43]. A slight stiffening of the cartilage takes place in the proximal part of the patellar surface and patellofemoral and tibial cartilages. The rate of cartilage deformation during compression decreases. Using the same model, running exercise of either 20 km/day or 40 km/day for 15 weeks reduces the GAG content in the superficial zone of femoral and tibial condylar cartilages [35,44], increases water content and decreases the concentration of collagen in the cartilage of the lateral femoral condyle. However, the overall PG content of the cartilage does not change significantly during 40 km/day running [45]. Running exercise of 20 km/day does not cause further improvement in the biomechanical properties of articular cartilage over that observed after the 4 km/day program, and more strenuous running exercise (40 km/day) reduces the stiffness of articular cartilage [35]. The long-distance running exercise (40 km/day) decreases (24–34%) the collagen birefringence of the superficial zone cartilage at the weight-bearing sites of femoral and tibial condyles [46]. It is therefore anticipated that a derangement, or even a disorganization, of the superficial collagen network is the reason for this decline of birefringence and simultaneous softening of cartilage. At the same time, histomorphometric parameters of the subchondral bone show marked signs of bone remodeling in all sites examined [47]. The observed peripheral thickening of the cartilage with increased bone remodeling can be hypothesized to represent compensatory and adaptive mechanisms aiming at increasing articular surface area and congruence. Also the centrally observed depletion of GAGs and softening of the cartilage after a 40 km/day running program can serve this purpose instead of simply denoting the appearance of early changes of osteoarthritis. Vigorous running training of dogs on treadmills has given rise to definite injuries of articular cartilage [48].

Few studies have been published on the interrelationship between exercise, aging and cartilage. Importantly, lifelong moderate running of beagle dogs with jackets weighing 130% of their body weight did not produce any evidence of knee articular cartilage injury after 4 km/day exercise on the treadmill, 5 days a week, for a total of 527 weeks [49].

Experiments with horses

There are several reports that indicate that loading has profound effects on the biomechanical properties and PG synthesis in the carpal bone cartilage of horses. This is the site prone to be affected by equine osteoarthritis. When 2-year-old horses underwent a high-intensity treadmill training for 19 weeks and were compared with a group of low-intensity trained horses, the cartilage from strenuously trained horses showed more fibrillation and chondrocyte clusters than cartilage from gently trained horses [50]. Dorsal carpal cartilage is locally significantly softer than the same cartilage from low-intensity trained horses. Cartilage sections from the high-intensity trained animals exhibited reduced superficial toluidine blue staining compared with that from the gently exercised group, indicating reduced concentration of GAGs and PGs in these areas. These sites also exhibited increased fibronectin immunoreactivity which indicates that equine fibronectin is localized at sites of cartilage degeneration [51]. These results suggest that strenuous training of horses can lead to deterioration of cartilage at sites with high clinical incidence of cartilage lesions. Gentle exercise, instead, is followed by increase in cartilage stiffness and reduced fluid permeability. Interestingly, high-intensity training leads to greater calcified, but not uncalcified, cartilage thickness. This response is maximal at sites that withstand high intermittent loads.

Experiments with rats, mice, hamsters, guinea-pigs and rabbits

Rats running on a treadmill between the ages of 6 and 24 months show more severe osteoarthritis in the knee joints than control animals [52]. Also in C57BL mice, lifelong moderate running (1 km/day) on a treadmill between 2 and 18 months of age increases the incidence and severity of osteoarthritis in the knee joints [53]. On the other hand, voluntary running of mice in a running wheel decreases the prevalence of osteoarthritis in mice [54]. Thus, it appears that both the mouse strain and the mode of running training, either forced or voluntary, affect the articular cartilage response. In young hamsters, voluntary running prevents the appearance of osteoarthritic lesions of articular cartilage as compared to a group of sedentary animals [55]. In young adult (28-week) guinea-pigs, an 18-week running program (2500 m/day, 5 days a week) increases the birefringence of the superficial collagen network in femoral and tibial cartilages, indicating either an improved orientation or increased content of collagen fibrils in cartilage (Hyttinen *et al.* unpublished observations). The same training program in adult mature (62-week) guinea-pigs causes an opposite reaction: running reduces significantly the collagen birefringence in the superficial zone suggesting an early derangement or disintegration of the cartilage collagen network. Running training affected the overall prevalence of osteoarthritis in neither the young nor older guinea-pigs.

Gradually started, low-intensity training of young rabbits increased PG content in the knee articular cartilages as deduced from uronic acid assays of PG extracts [56]. The structure of extractable PGs is slightly changed, i.e. chondroitin sulfate chains are more completely sulfated and the keratan sulfate/chondroitin sulfate ratio is elevated as an indication of enhanced cartilage maturation. Another feature of early cartilage maturation is the increased proportion of the non-extractable GAGs after running training. Collagen content is not affected by the low-intensity training.

Human studies

In humans also, it is apparent that cartilage responds in a very site-specific way to joint loading. Thus the differences in magnitudes and types of joint loading, e.g.

shear or weight-bearing, probably explain the site-dependent differences in cartilage response. In contrast to the site-dependent response in articular cartilage, the subchondral bone shows a more general remodeling activity. Early loading effects are probably adaptive responses in both the articular cartilage and subchondral bone and they do not necessarily represent initial signs of cartilage degeneration.

The prevailing view is that light or moderate, or at times even strenuous, physical exercise is beneficial to articular cartilage and joint structures (Fig. 1.7.5). This kind of activity strengthens joint structures, articular cartilage included, having also the capacity to prevent degenerative ailments of the musculoskeletal system, such as osteoarthritis. The high prevalence of knee osteoarthritis in former soccer players and American football players has been attributed to the high incidence of ligament, meniscal and joint injuries. There is some data showing that long-distance runners are prone to acquiring radiographic signs of knee or hip osteoarthritis. Radiographs of athletes may show signs of '*periarthropathie sportive*', i.e. periarticular bone changes and calcification of ligament and tendon insertions, while at the same time the joint space may be normal in weight-bearing radiographic studies. The marginal lips or 'osteophytes' in the radiographs have been considered as being signs of joint and bone remodeling [57,58]. Some studies indicate that former marathon or elite long-distance runners do not show any or show only little increase in osteoarthritis later in life [59,60]. For athletes as well, joint dysplasia, neurological deficits or increased body weight increase the risk of osteoarthritis. It is important to note that repetitive mechanical stress in manual labor, particularly in occupations that involve movements with dynamic joint instability, is associated with development of osteoarthritis [61]. Dynamic joint instability can occur during knee bending and lifting of heavy objects. This emphasizes the importance of correct biomechanical execution of athletic performances for the maintenance of joint health.

Effects of altered weight-bearing

Experiments with dogs

Altered weight-bearing in the joint predisposes the individual to osteoarthritis. Osteotomy through an oper-

ation of a 30° valgus angulation of the young beagle tibia shifts load from the medial to the lateral condyle and causes a slowly progressive osteoarthritis in immature and young adult canine knee (stifle) joints [62]. On account of the altered weight-bearing with local peak loads, early degenerative changes in articular cartilage can be observed 7 months after the operation and the lesions are more severe after 18 months. A striking reduction in the collagen-induced birefringence takes place in the superficial zone of cartilage indicating a failure in the orientation and/or arrangement of the collagen fibrils. An increase of the articular cartilage thickness can also be observed. The most significant changes appear in the lateral compartment of the knee joint. Increased levels of cartilage matrix-degrading metalloproteinase activity and its inhibitor are observed in the synovial fluid. Subchondral bone shows signs of increased remodeling on the operated side.

Increased weight-bearing of a healthy joint has been studied in experiments where the use of one limb has been eliminated by casting, operation or amputation. The untreated contralateral limb then carries more load. This causes microscopic and biochemical changes in the weight-bearing articular cartilage. In the beagle dog knee contralateral to the casted one, the overall content of PGs remains unchanged or increases [33]. The PG structure changes towards the more mature type, e.g. showing increased keratan sulfate/chondroitin sulfate ratio. Interestingly, in the contralateral rabbit knee, focal spots of degenerative change are observed with minor alterations in the cartilage surface [63]. This means that the response to elevated weight-bearing seems to be species dependent.

Human studies

In human amputees, the amputated side shows osteoporotic changes in the bone. It has been suggested that osteoporosis would spare the joints from osteoarthritis through increased compliance during joint loading. In agreement with this, it has been observed that the prevalence of osteoarthritis is low in the hips and knees of poliomyelitis patients [64]. On the amputated side there has been observed reduced thickness of the articular cartilage in many, but not in all, amputees. The reduced thickness appears to correlate with the limb stump length, since the reduction appears regularly in the thigh upper-third amputees but in none of the lower-third amputees. In the lower limb amputees, a significant increase of osteoarthritis has been observed in the knee of the unamputated side [65,66]. It is obvious that after amputation the contralateral side carries surplus load and the biomechanical conditions are altered. This exposes the weight-bearing joint to unphysiologic stresses and peak loads.

Intra-articular injuries

The loading conditions of an individual joint may be changed dramatically in adulthood by an intra-articular injury to, for example, cartilage, ligaments and/or menisci. These injuries have been shown both *in vitro* and *in vivo* to result in permanent changes of joint kinematics as shown below, despite active attempts at treatment [67–69]. Hence, the joint changes which occur as a rule some years after an intra-articular injury and treatment may in part be caused by the inability of adult chondrocytes to adapt sufficiently to the sudden change in joint loading patterns and also by the simultaneous remodeling of the subchondral bone.

Isolated cartilage injury

It has been shown in several experimental studies that an isolated cartilage injury leads eventually to degeneration of the cartilage adjacent to the defect [70]. Also osteophyte formation is common in this situation. These changes may be caused by the abnormally high stresses acting on the rim of the defect [71]. The cartilage surfaces opposing an isolated cartilage injury often show fibrillation [72] probably initiated by the mechanical irritation of the uneven wound surface. As shown experimentally, inflammatory factors associated with hemarthrosis seem to play a decisive role in the initiation of joint changes after an intra-articular injury [73]. It may even be that mechanical factors cause degenerative joint changes at least in part via release of these inflammatory agents. Transforming growth factor β1 (TGF-β1) has been shown to induce the formation of osteophytes and also to influence cartilage metabolism [74]. The concentration of this substance in joint fluid increases after drilling of a full-thickness cartilage defect. It is most probably released from the exposed bone marrow and other blood sources [75]. High concentrations of this factor,

as found physiologically in immature animals, has been associated with the occurrence of more severe cartilage degeneration adjacent to the cartilage wound than lower concentrations, as found to be the rule in older rabbits [75]. Young cartilage also seems to be more sensitive than adult cartilage to IL-1 and iron, which both degrade cartilage and are increased in hemarthrosis [76,77]. The cartilage degeneration adjacent to an artificially created defect is common by 3 months in animal models, but it does not seem to worsen with time [70].

Thus, there is evidence that the cartilage adjacent to an isolated cartilage injury eventually develops signs of degeneration via mechanical and chemical alterations of the environment owing to the trauma and permanent change in joint kinematics. However, it is unclear whether these alterations advance and finally lead to joint destruction.

Ligament injury

Injuries to knee ligaments are very common in sports. Since there is only limited knowledge of the alterations in joint kinematics caused by rupture of the various ligaments (e.g. medial and lateral collateral ligaments, cruciate ligaments), this section concentrates on the changes affecting the anterior cruciate ligament of the knee joint, which has been studied most intensively. The anterior cruciate ligament counteracts specifically the anterior sagittal displacement of the tibia which is provoked by quadriceps action. Sectioning of the anterior cruciate ligament *in vitro* results in an increase of sagittal displacement of the tibia and rotational limits. A combined tear of the anterior cruciate and the medial collateral ligaments results in larger increases in anterior displacement, valgus angulation and internal rotation [78].

Clinically, an anterior cruciate ligament deficient knee shows a higher sagittal displacement during gait than a normal knee, especially during the swing phase of the step [79]. During stair climbing the net amount of sagittal displacement seems not to be affected, but there are signs that the main area of contact between tibia and femur has shifted backward on the tibia [69]. In addition, these altered motion patterns are not corrected by reconstruction of the ligament [69]. In a goat animal model, 1 year after resection of the anterior cruciate ligament and immediate reconstruction with a patellar tendon autograft, the subchondral density maximum of the medial tibial plateau is displaced to the medial edge indicating that an unphysiologic varus stress is acting on the joint though the knee appears stable in the sagittal plane [68]. In animal models, transection of the anterior cruciate ligament has shown to cause severe joint irritation, formation of osteophytes and cartilage degeneration [80]. This demonstrates that a tear of the anterior cruciate ligament leads to a permanent change in knee motion pattern, which in consequence induces joint remodeling. Clinically, in the majority of cases severe cartilage damage can be observed at arthroscopy or radiographic signs of knee osteoarthritis develop after an injury to the anterior cruciate ligament [81].

Meniscus injury and meniscectomy

The convex-shaped knee joint femoral condyles and the relatively flat tibial plateaux fit together by means of the knee joint menisci. In consequence, removal of the menisci leads to an immediate, remarkable reduction of joint contact area and simultaneous increase in contact stresses [82]. Other functions of the menisci are shock absorption [83], joint stabilization [84] and joint lubrication [85].

The peripheral dislocation of the wedge-shaped menisci from the joint during loading is prevented by the central insertions to bone. The insertional ligaments and the circumferential fibres of the menisci are in tension during compressive loading and part of the axial load is transformed into hoop stresses at the meniscal periphery. Even though removal of the menisci leads to a dramatic increase of stresses on the tibial plateau, this immediate effect is soon diminished by the remodeling and adaptation of the condyles which takes place *in vivo* [86]. Signs of this remodeling are flattening of the subchondral bone and ridge formation [87]. However, not only do the shapes of the subchondral region of the knee condyles change after meniscectomy but also the bone density. The bone density at the periphery of the tibial plateau underlying the meniscus in an uninjured knee joint is usually lower than at the central part which is not covered by the meniscus, but in joints lacking a meniscus the subchondral bone density increases at the periphery [88]. Clinically, subchondral sclerosis and a general increase of bone mineral density in the proximal tibia is

common after meniscectomy and simultaneously indicates the beginning of osteoarthrosis [89,90]. The increase in bone mineral density is interpreted as an adaptation of the subchondral bone to the increase in peak stresses and strains in the proximal tibia after meniscectomy [67,82,91]. There is a theory proposing that stiffening of subchondral bone may cause cartilage changes as a secondary phenomenon, and that progression of cartilage lesions requires stiffened subchondral bone [92]. After meniscectomy, the increase in bone mineral density of the proximal tibia may be associated with a stiffening of subchondral bone, which eventually initiates or at least aggravates the cartilage changes after this lesion and operative procedure. Findings in a sheep model indicate that meniscectomy may result in not only a change of stress magnitude but also in a permanent shift of main contact area. Here, the area of highest subchondral bone density in the proximal tibia is shifted to a more posterior and medial location 1 year after meniscectomy [67]. In rabbits, meniscectomy causes cartilage ulceration as early as 3 days after the procedure [93]. Advanced knee joint degeneration with cartilage fibrillation of larger areas and formation of deep clefts, and osteophyte formation occurs during the months following creation of a meniscal rupture or when the meniscus has been removed [94]. In patients, radiographic osteoarthritis is common after clinical meniscectomy [87,89,95]. It was shown that the risk of developing a radiographic knee osteoarthritis was increased 14-fold 21 years after meniscectomy, compared to the control population [95]. Increased uptake of radionuclides in the subchondral bone of knees with a meniscal tear indicates that not only meniscectomy but also a meniscal tear leads to a significant bone remodeling [96].

Summary

Loading is essential for the function and metabolism of articular cartilage, but under- or overloading may be deleterious. Articular cartilage assumes its mechanical properties during the long course of postnatal development. In adulthood, the turnover rate of cartilage is slow, and therefore the response of articular cartilage to changed loading conditions is limited. Cyclic and compressive loading *in vitro* has shown to both increase and decrease the synthesis of matrix proteoglycans (PGs) depending on loading conditions. Injurious loads may lead to cell apoptosis and loss of matrix PGs. Impact damage seems to be cumulative and stress-rate dependent. Impact loading *in vivo* leads to an initial loss of PGs, but the lesion seems more likely to partly recover with time than to develop into symptomatic osteoarthritis. Long-term joint immobilization leads to depletion of cartilage PGs and atrophy, changes which appear to be mostly reversible after remobilization. Running exercise of light or moderate intensity improves the biological properties of articular cartilage while repetitive intensive and strenuous training can cause injury to the cartilage. Altered weight-bearing along with a change in joint alignment, or amputation of one extremity, predisposes joint cartilage to osteoarthritis. Intra-articular injuries to cartilage, ligaments or menisci also predispose to osteoarthritis, probably through the permanent change in size and location of the contact area between the opposing joint surfaces. Although considerable understanding has been gained as to the response of cartilage to particular load and injury conditions, it still is not clear what specific features lead to osteoarthritis: whether it is the initial injury, some feature of continued loading or other pathology after the injury, or some combination of these.

Multiple choice questions

1 *What is the response of cartilage explants to moderately increased cyclic loading:*

a increased collagen synthesis

b increased proteoglycan synthesis

c increased collagen degradation

d increased proteoglycan degradation.

2 *What is the short-term consequence to cartilage of sub-fracture traumatic loading of a joint:*

a degradation of proteoglycans and collagens

b cell cloning, loss of proteoglycans

c chondrocyte death, cracking of cartilage and subchondral bone, release of cytokines

d cartilage thinning, cell cloning, increased subchondral bone thickness.

3 *What are the approximate load rise times and stress magnitudes during joint trauma:*

a 1 s, 50 MPa

b 100 ms, 50 MPa

c 1 ms, 50 MPa

d 100 ms, 5 MPa.

4 *Joint immobilization with unloading for weeks or months:*

a causes atrophy of articular cartilage

b causes necrosis of articular cartilage

c is the main reason for osteoarthritis

d causes mostly reversible changes in articular cartilage

e depletes cartilage of proteoglycans.

5 *With regard to regular joint loading:*

a It has crucial effects on chondrocyte and cartilage metabolism.

b Extracellular matrix proteoglycan changes appear to dominate over the collagen framework alterations.

c It does not affect the biomechanical properties of cartilage.

d Moderate loading has predominantly positive effects on the biological properties of normal articular cartilage.

e Very vigorous and repetitive loading may worsen the biological properties of normal articular cartilage.

6 *Injury to the anterior cruciate ligament:*

a leads to a permanent shift of joint contact area

b does not influence joint kinematics except during strenuous activities

c leads to a permanent change in joint kinematics

d causes changes that are reversible by reconstruction of the anterior cruciate ligament

e does not lead to knee osteoarthritis.

7 *Which of the following are correct? Meniscectomy:*

a causes an increase in joint contact area

b causes a decrease in joint contact area

c causes an increase in stress on the tibial plateau

d causes a decrease in stress on the tibial plateau

e does not cause bone remodeling.

References

1 Kempson GE, Muir H, Freeman M, Swanson S. Correlations between the compressive stiffness and the chemical constituents of human articular cartilage. *Biochim Biophys Acta* 1970; **215**: 70–7.

2 Räsänen T, Messner K. Regional variations of indentation stiffness and thickness of normal rabbit knee articular cartilage. *J Biomed Materials Res* 1996; **31**: 519–24.

3 Little C, Ghosh P. Mechanical loading of articular cartilage is a major determinant of chondrocyte phenotypic expression. *Trans Orthopaed Res Soc* 1994; **19**: 489.

4 Luepongsak N, Krebs DE, Olsson E, Riley PO, Mann RW. Hip stress during lifting with bent and straight knees. *Scand J Rehab Med* 1997; **29**: 57–64.

5 Bergmann G, Graichen F, Rohlmann A. Hip joint loading during walking and running, measured in two patients. *J Biomech* 1993; **26**: 969–90.

6 Newberry WN, Zukosky DK, Haut RC. Subfracture insult to a knee joint causes alterations in the bone and in the functional stiffness of overlying cartilage. *J Orthopaed Res* 1997; **15**: 450–5.

7 Newberry WN, Garcia JJ, Mackenzie CD, Decamp CE, Haut RC. Analysis of acute mechanical insult in an animal model of post-traumatic osteoarthrosis. *J Biomechan Eng* 1998; **120**: 704–9.

8 Guilak F, Sah R, Van Setton LA. Physical regulation of cartilage metabolism. In: Mow VC, Hayes WC, eds. *Basic Orthopaedic Biomechanics*, 2nd edn. Philadelphia: Lippincott-Raven Publishers, 1997: 179–207.

9 Gray ML, Pizzanelli AM, Grodzinsky AJ, Lee RC. Mechanical and physiochemical determinants of the chondrocyte biosynthetic response. *J Orthopaed Res* 1988; **6**: 777–92.

10 Ragan PM, Badger AM, Cook M *et al.* Down-regulation of chondrocyte aggrecan and type-II collagen gene expression correlates with increases in static compression magnitude and duration. *J Orthopaed Res* 1999; **17**: 836–42.

11 Wong M, Siegrist M, Cao X. Cyclic compression of articular cartilage explants is associated with progressive consolidation and altered expression pattern of extracellular matrix proteins. *Matrix Biol* 1999; **18**: 391–9.

12 Sah RL, Grodzinsky AJ, Plaas AHK, Sandy JD. Effects of static and dynamic compression on matrix metabolism in cartilage explants. In: Kuettner KE, Schleyerbach R, Peyron JG, Hascall VC, eds. *Articular Cartilage and Osteoarthritis*. New York: Raven Press, 1992: 373–92.

13 Steinmeyer J, Ackermann B, Raiss RX. Intermittent cyclic loading of cartilage explants modulates fibronectin metabolism. *Osteoarthritis Cartilage* 1997; **5**: 331–41.

14 Steinmeyer J, Ackermann B. The effect of continuously applied cyclic mechanical loading on the fibronectin metabolism of articular cartilage. *Res Exp Med* 1999; **198**: 247–60.

15 Quinn TM, Grodzinsky AJ, Hunziker EB, Sandy JD. Effects of injurious compression on matrix turnover around individual cells in calf articular cartilage explants. *J Orthopaed Res* 1998; **16**: 490–9.

16 Quinn TM, Maung AA, Grodzinsky AJ, Hunziker EB, Sandy JD. Physical and biological regulation of proteoglycan turnover around chondrocytes in cartilage explants. Implications for tissue degradation and repair. *Ann New York Acad Sci* 1999; **878**: 420–41.

17 Chen CT, Burton-Wurster N, Lust G, Bank RA, Tekoppele JM. Compositional and metabolic changes in damaged cartilage are peak-stress, stress-rate, and loading-duration dependent. *J Orthopaed Res* 1999; **17**: 870–9.

18 Repo RU, Finlay JB. Survival of articular cartilage after controlled impact. *J Bone Joint Surg (Am)* 1977; **59**: 1068–76.

19 Jeffrey JE, Gregory DW, Aspden RM. Matrix damage and chondrocyte viability following a single impact load on articular cartilage. *Arch Biochem Biophys* 1995; **322**: 87–96.

20 Jeffrey JE, Thomson LA, Aspden RM. Matrix loss and

synthesis following a single impact load on articular cartilage in vitro. *Biochim Biophys Acta* 1997; **334**: 223–32.

21 Torzilli PA, Grigiene R, Borrelli J Jr, Helfet DL. Effect of impact load on articular cartilage: cell metabolism and viability, and matrix water content. *J Biomechan Eng* 1999; **121**: 433–41.

22 Borrelli J Jr, Torzilli PA, Grigiene R, Helfet DL. Effect of impact load on articular cartilage: development of an intra-articular fracture model. *J Orth Trauma* 1997; **11**: 319–26.

23 Thompson RC Jr, Oegema TR Jr, Lewis JL, Wallace L. Osteoarthrotic changes after acute transarticular load. An animal model. *J Bone Joint Surg (Am)* 1991; **73**: 990–1001.

24 Thompson RC Jr, Vener MJ, Griffiths HJ, Lewis JL, Oegema TR Jr, Wallace L. Scanning electron-microscopic and magnetic resonance-imaging studies of injuries to the patellofemoral joint after acute transarticular loading. *J Bone Joint Surg (Am)* 1993; **75**: 704–13.

25 Oegema TR, Lewis JL, Thompson RC. Role of acute trauma in development of osteoarthritis. *Agents Actions* 1993; **40**: 220–3.

26 Pickvance EA, Oegema TR Jr, Thompson RC Jr. Immunolocalization of selected cytokines and proteases in canine articular cartilage after transarticular loading. *J Orthopaed Res* 1993; **11**: 313–23.

27 Mente PL, Lewis JL, Oegema TR Jr, Thompson RC Jr. Damage after blunt trauma to a joint surface. *Transactions of the Second Combined Orthopaedic Research Societies, San Diego*, 1995: 125.

28 Dedrick DK, Goldstein SA, Brandt KD, O'Connor BL, Goulet RW, Albrecht M. A longitudinal study of subchondral plate and trabecular bone in cruciate-deficient dogs with osteoarthritis followed up for 54 months. *Arthritis Rheumatism* 1993; **36**: 1460–7.

29 Tew SR, Kwan AP, Hann A, Thomson BM, Archer CW. The reactions of articular cartilage to experimental wounding: role of apoptosis. *Arthritis Rheumatism* 2000; **43**: 215–25.

30 Lotz M, Hashimoto S, Kuhn K. Mechanisms of chondrocyte apoptosis. *Osteoarthritis Cartilage* 1999; **7**: 389–91.

31 Kilic BA, Kilic I, Koseoglu MH, Guven C, Demirkan F, Kilinc K. Effects of intra-articular vitamin E and corticosteroid injection in experimental hemarthrosis in rabbits. *Pediatric Hematol Oncol* 1998; **15**: 339–46.

32 Tammi M, Paukkonen K, Kiviranta I, Jurvelin J, Säämänen A-M, Helminen HJ. Joint loading-induced alterations in articular cartilage. In: Helminen HJ, Kiviranta I, Säämänen Tammi M, Paukkonen K, Jurvelin J, eds. *Joint Loading. Biology and Health of Articular Structures*. Bristol: Wright, 1987: 64–88.

33 Kiviranta I, Jurvelin J, Tammi M, Säämänen A-M, Helminen HJ. Weight-bearing controls glycosaminoglycan concentration and articular cartilage thickness in the knee joint of young Beagle dogs. *Arthritis Rheumatism* 1987; **30**: 801–9.

34 Haapala J, Arokoski JPA, Hyttinen MM *et al.* Remobilization does not fully restore immobilization induced articular cartilage atrophy. *Clin Orth Rel Res* 1999; **362**: 218–29.

35 Kiviranta I, Tammi M, Arokoski J *et al.* Effects of mechanical loading and immobilization on the articular cartilage. *Baillière's Clin Orthopaed* 1997; **2**: 109–22.

36 Palmoski M, Perricone E, Brandt KD. Development and reversal of a proteoglycan aggregation defect in normal canine knee cartilage after immobilization. *Arthritis Rheumatism* 1979; **22**: 508–17.

37 Behrens F, Kraft EL, Oegema TR. Biochemical changes in articular cartilage after joint immobilization by casting or external fixation. *J Orthopaed Res* 1989; **7**: 335–43.

38 Haapala J, Arokoski J, Pirttimäki J *et al.* Incomplete restoration of immobilization induced softening of young beagle knee articular cartilage after 50-week remobilization. *Int J Sports Med* 2000; **21**: 76–81.

39 Finsterbush A, Friedman B. Early changes in immobilized rabbits' knee joints. a light and electron microscopic study. *Clin Orth Rel Res* 1973; **92**: 305–19.

40 Sood SC. A study of the effects of experimental immobilization on rabbit articular cartilage. *J Anat* 1971; **108**: 497–507.

41 Enneking WF, Horowitz M. The intra-articular effects of immobilization on the human knee. *J Bone Joint Surg (Am)* 1972; **54**: 973–85.

42 Salter RB. *Textbook of Disorders and Injuries of the Musculoskeletal System*, 3rd edn. Baltimore: Williams & Wilkins, 1999.

43 Säämänen A-M, Tammi M, Kiviranta I, Jurvelin J, Helminen HJ. Levels of chondroitin-6-sulfate and non-aggregating proteoglycans at articular cartilage contact sites in the knees of young dogs subjected to moderate running exercise. *Arthritis Rheumatism* 1989; **32**: 1282–92.

44 Arokoski J, Kiviranta I, Jurvelin J, Tammi M, Helminen HJ. Long-distance running causes site-dependent decrease of the cartilage glycosaminoglycan content in the knee joint of beagle dogs. *Arthritis Rheumatism* 1993; **36**: 1451–9.

45 Visser NA, de Koning MH, Lammi MJ, Hakkinen T, Tammi M, van Kampen GP. Increase of decorin content in articular cartilage following running. *Connective Tissue Res* 1998; **37**: 295–302.

46 Arokoski J, Hyttinen MM, Lapveteläinen T *et al.* Decreased birefringence of the superficial zone collagen network in the canine knee (stifle) articular cartilage after long distance running training, detected by quantitative polarized light microscopy. *Ann Rheumatic Dis* 1996; **55**: 253–64.

47 Oettmeier R, Arokoski J, Roth AJ *et al.* Subchondral bone and articular cartilage responses to long distance running training (40 km per day) in the beagle knee joint. *Eur J Exp Musculoskel Res* 1992; **1**: 145–54.

48 Vasan N. Effects of physical stress on the synthesis and degradation of cartilage matrix. *Connective Tissue Res* 1983; **12**: 49–58.

49 Newton PM, Mow VC, Gardner TR, Buckwalter JA, Albright JP. The effect of lifelong exercise on canine articular cartilage. *Am J Sports Med* 1997; **25**: 282–7.

50 Murray RC, Zhu CF, Goodship AE, Lakhani KH, Agrawal CM, Athanasiou KA. Exercise affects the mechanical properties and histological appearance of equine articular cartilage. *J Orthopaed Res* 1999; **17**: 725–31.

51 Murray RC, Janicke HC, Henson FM, Goodship A. Equine carpal articular cartilage fibronectin distribution associated with training, joint location and cartilage deterioration. *Equine Vet J* 2000; **32**: 47–51.

52 Walker JM. Exercise and its influence on aging in rat knee joints. *J Orth Sports Phys Ther* 1986; **8**: 310–9.

53 Lapveteläinen T, Nevalainen T, Parkkinen JJ *et al.* Lifelong moderate running training increases the incidence and severity of osteoarthritis in the knee joint of C57BL mice. *Anat Record* 1995; **242**: 159–65.

54 Lanier RR. The effects of exercise on the knee-joints of inbred mice. *Anat Record* 1946; **94**: 311–21.

55 Otterness IG, Eskra JD, Bliven ML, Shay AK, Pelletier J-P, Milici AJ. Exercise protects against articular cartilage degeneration in the hamster. *Arthritis Rheumatism* 1998; **41**: 2068–76.

56 Säämänen A-M, Tammi M, Kiviranta I, Helminen HJ. Running exercise as a modulator of proteoglycan matrix in the articular cartilage of young rabbits. *Int J Sports Med* 1988; **9**: 127–32.

57 Adams ID. Osteoarthrosis and sport. *Clinics Rheum Dis* 1976; **2**: 523–41.

58 Cabot JR. Lésions chroniques dans le sport (1) au niveau des extrémités inférieures. *Méd Éducation Phys Sport* 1964; **4**: 277–302.

59 Kujala U, Kaprio J, Sarna S. Osteoarthritis of weight bearing joints of lower limbs in former elite male athletes. *Br Med J* 1994; **308**: 231–4.

60 Puranen J, Alaketola L, Peltokallio P, Saarela. J. Running and primary osteoarthritis of the hip. *Br Med J* 1975; **276**: 424–5.

61 Vingård E, Alfredsson L, Goldie I, Hogstedt C. Occupation and osteoarthrosis of the hip and knee: a register based cohort study. *Int J Epidemiol* 1991; **20**: 1025–31.

62 Panula HE, Helminen HJ, Kiviranta I. Slowly progressive osteoarthritis after tibial valgus osteotomy in young beagle dogs. *Clin Orth Rel Res* 1997; **343**: 192–202.

63 Paukkonen K, Jurvelin J, Helminen HJ. Effects of immobilization on the articular cartilage in young rabbits. A quantitative light microscopic stereological study. *Clin Orth Rel Res* 1986; **206**: 270–80.

64 Glyn JH, Sutherland I, Walker GF, Young AC. Low incidence of osteoarthrosis in hip and knee after anterior poliomyelitis: a late review. *Br Med J* 1966; **2**: 739–42.

65 Benichou C, Wirotius JM. Articular cartilage atrophy in lower limb amputees. *Arthritis Rheumatism* 1982; **25**: 80–2.

66 Burke MJ, Roman V, Wright V. Bone and joint changes in lower limb amputees. *Ann Rheumatic Dis* 1978; **37**: 252–4.

67 Anetzberger H, Metak G, Scherer MA, Putz R, Müller-Gerbl M. Anpassung der subchondralen Knochenplatte nach Meniskektomie als Folge einer Änderung der Spannungsverteilung. *Osteologie* 1995; **4**: 224–32.

68 Müller-Gerbl M, Anetzberger H, Scherer M, Putz R, Blümel G. Pathological subchondral bone density patterns

after successful reconstruction of the ACL. *Trans Orthopaed Res Soc* 1994; **19**: 615.

69 Vergis A. *Sagittal plane knee translation in healthy and ACL deficient subjects. A methodological study in vivo with clinical implications.* Medical dissertation no. 613, Linköping, Sweden, 1999.

70 Wei X, Gao J, Messner K. Maturation-dependent repair of untreated osteochondral defects in the rabbit knee joint. *J Biomed Materials Res* 1997; **34**: 63–72.

71 Brown TD, Pope DF, Hale JE, Buckwalter JA, Brand RA. Effects of osteochondral defect size on cartilage contact stress. *J Orthopaed Res* 1991; **9**: 559–67.

72 Messner K, Gillquist J. Synthetic implants for the repair of osteochondral defects of the medial femoral condyle: a biomechanical and histological evaluation in the rabbit knee. *Biomaterials* 1993; **14**: 513–21.

73 Xie D-I, Homandberg GA. Fibronectin fragments bind to and penetrate cartilage tissue resulting in proteinase expression and cartilage damage. *Biochim Biophys Acta* 1993; **1182**: 189–96.

74 van Beuningen HM, van der Kraan PM, Arntz OJ, van den Berg WB. Transforming growth factor-beta 1 stimulates articular chondrocyte proteoglycan synthesis and induces osteophyte formation in the murine knee joint. *Lab Invest* 1994; **71**: 279–90.

75 Wei X, Messner K. Age- and injury-dependent concentrations of transforming growth factor-β1 and proteoglycan fragments in rabbit knee joint fluid. *Osteoarthritis Cartilage* 1998; **6**: 10–8.

76 Brighton CT, Bigley EC, Smolenski BI. Iron induced arthritis in immature rabbits. *Arthritis Rheumatism* 1970; **13**: 849–57.

77 Hickery MS, Vilim V, Bayliss MT, Hardingham TE. Effect of interleukin-1 and tumor necrosis factor-alpha on the turnover of proteoglycans in human articular cartilage. *Biochem Soc Trans* 1990; **18**: 953–4.

78 Shoemaker SC, Daniel DM. The limits of knee motion. In: Daniel, D *et al.*, eds. *Knee Ligaments.* New York: Raven Press, 1990: 153–61.

79 Marans HJ, Jackson RW, Glossop ND, Young MC. Anterior cruciate ligament insufficiency: a dynamic three-dimensional motion analysis. *Am J Sports Med* 1989; **17**: 325–32.

80 Myers SL, Brandt KD, O'Connor BL, Visco DM, Albrecht ME. Synovitis and osteoarthritic changes in canine articular cartilage after anterior cruciate ligament transection. *Arthritis Rheumatism* 1990; **33**: 1406–15.

81 Maletius W, Messner K. Eighteen to twenty-four-year follow-up after complete rupture of the anterior cruciate ligament. *Am J Sports Med* 1999; **27**: 711–7.

82 Kurosawa H, Fukubayashi T, Nakajima H. Load-bearing mode of the knee joint: physical behavior of the knee joint with or without menisci. *Clin Orth Rel Res* 1980; **149**: 283–90.

83 Voloshin AS, Wosk J. Shock absorption of meniscectomized and painful knees: a comparative in vivo study. *J Biomed Eng* 1983; **5**: 157–61.

84 Allen CR, Wong EK, Livesay GA, Sakane M, Fu FH, Woo L-Y. Importance of the medial meniscus in the anterior cruciate ligament-deficient knee. *J Orthopaed Res* 2000; **18**: 109–15.

85 MacConaill MA. The function of intra-articular fibrocartilages, with special reference to the knee and inferior radio-ulnar joints. *J Anat* 1932; **66**: 210–27.

86 Bylski-Austrow DI, Malumed J, Meade T, Schafer JA, Cummings JF, Grood ES. Effect of medial meniscectomy on joint contact pressure. *Trans Orthopaed Res Soc* 1991; **16**: 581.

87 Fairbank TJ. Knee joint changes after meniscectomy. *J Bone Joint Surg (Brit)* 1948; **30**: 664–70.

88 Noble J, Alexander K. Studies of tibial subchondral bone density and its significance. *J Bone Joint Surg (Am)* 1985; **67**: 295–302.

89 Appel H. Late results after meniscectomy in the knee joint. *Acta Orthop Scand Suppl* 1970; **133**: 1–111.

90 Petersen MM, Olsen C, Lauritzen JB, Lund B, Hede A. Late changes in bone mineral density of the proximal tibia following total or partial medial meniscectomy: a randomized study. *J Orthopaed Res* 1996; **14**: 16–21.

91 Bourne RB, Finlay JB, Papadopoulos P, Andreae P. The effect of medial meniscectomy on strain distribution in the proximal part of the tibia. *J Bone Joint Surg (Am)* 1984; **66**: 1431–7.

92 Radin EL, Rose RM. Role of subchondral bone in the initiation and progression of cartilage disease. *Clin Orth Rel Res* 1986; **213**: 34–40.

93 Caputo CB, Sygowski LA, Patton SP *et al.* Protease inhibitors decrease rabbit cartilage degradation after meniscectomy. *J Orthopaed Res* 1988; **6**: 103–8.

94 Shapiro F, Glimcher MJ. Induction of osteoarthrosis in the rabbit knee joint. *Clin Orth Rel Res* 1980; **147**: 287–95.

95 Roos H, Laurén M, Adalberth T, Roos EM, Jonsson K, Lohmander LS. Knee osteoarthritis after meniscectomy. *Arthritis Rheumatism* 1998; **41**: 687–93.

96 Marymont JV, Lynch MA, Henning CE. Evaluation of meniscus tears of the knee by radionuclide imaging. *Am J Sports Med* 1983; **11**: 432–5.

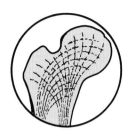

Chapter 1.8
Bone Tissue — Bone Training

PETER SCHWARZ, ERIK FINK ERIKSEN &
KIM THORSEN

Classical reference

Nielsson BE, Westlin NE. Bone density in athletes.
Clin Orth Rel Res 1971; **77**: 179–182.
This paper was one of the first to show that trained individuals within a variety of different sports events in
general had a higher bone mineral density compared to
sedentary age-matched individuals. Furthermore, the
study showed that within sports events that contained
a high workload of the lower extremities the bone mineral density in the distal femur was increased, whereas
swimmers, for example, did not show any changes in
bone mineral density compared to sedentary individuals. Later studies have confirmed these findings,
although the methodologies have been somewhat
more advanced, and the design has become more
sophisticated.

The data from Nielsson & Westlin together with
other data have been put together in an overview
illustration by Drinkwater (Fig. 1.8.1). (Physical
activity, fitness, and osteoporosis. In: Bouchard C,
Shepperd RJ, Stephen T, eds. *Physical activity, Fitness
and Health*. Toronto: Human Kinetics Publishers,
1994: 724–36.)

Introduction

Physical activity has been proposed as one strategy for
improving or maintaining the structural competence
of bone. The intent of this chapter is to present an
overview of the current knowledge on bone biology
and bone mass in relation to mechanical loading and
unloading.

Physical activity transmits loads to the skeleton by at
least two mechanisms: direct impact from weight-
bearing activity and forces imposed on bone from

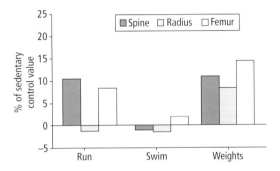

Fig. 1.8.1 Bone density of female athletes compared to
sedentary controls.

muscle pull. Ideally, the stress on bone induced by
physical activity should optimize the anatomic
structure and increase bone strength[1]. It is generally
assumed that a high level of physical activity corresponds to a high level of mechanical loading, with the
exception of a few non-weight-bearing activities, such
as swimming. The classical example of the positive effects of activity on bone in humans are studies demonstrating greater deposition in the dominant playing
arm vs. the non-dominant arm of tennis players across
different age groups [2–4]. Overuse, on the other hand,
may induce fatigue fractures, so-called stress fractures
in bone.

Effects of mechanical
forces on bone cells

Mechanotransduction plays a crucial role in bone
physiology. Mechanotransduction can be divided
into four distinct steps: (i) mechanocoupling; (ii)

biochemical coupling; (iii) transmission of signal; and (iv) effector cell response [5].

Mechanocoupling denotes deformations in bone that stretch bone cells within and lining the bone matrix and create fluid movement within the canaliculae of bone. The loading, which is associated with extracellular fluid flow and the creation of streaming potentials within bone, stimulates new bone formation *in vivo*.

Biochemical coupling denotes the coupling of cell-level mechanical signals into intracellular biochemical signals. It includes force transduction through the integrin–cytoskeleton–nuclear matrix structure and stretch-activated cation channels within the cell membrane.

Transmission of the mechanical signal resulting in altered protein synthesis and cell activity involves G protein-dependent pathways, and linkage between the cytoskeleton and the phospholipase C or phospholipase A pathways. In the transmission of signal, osteoblasts, osteocytes and bone-lining cells act as sensors of mechanical signals and may communicate the signal through cell processes connected by gap junctions. These cells also produce paracrine factors that may signal osteoprogenitors to differentiate into osteoblasts and attach to the bone surface. Insulin-like growth factors (IGFs) and prostaglandins (PGs) are possible candidates for intermediaries in signal transduction.

The cellular response to mechanical loading depends on the magnitude, duration and rate of the applied load. Loading must be cyclic to stimulate new bone formation. Longer duration, lower amplitude loading has the same effect on bone formation as loading with short duration and high amplitude. Aging reduces the osteogenic effects of mechanical loading *in vivo*. Also, some hormones (e.g. estradiol) may interact with local mechanical signals to change the sensitivity of the sensor or effector cells to mechanical load. Generally mechanical strain enhances bone formation and inhibits bone resorption.

In the following sections we will attempt to provide a more detailed review of the effects of mechanical stimuli on bone, and the cellular pathways involved in mechanotransduction.

Effects of mechanical stimuli at the cellular level

The effects of mechanical strain on bone cells involve not only rapid changes in activity, but also longer term changes in cellular recruitment resulting in altered rates of remodeling. It is important to distinguish between effects on quiescent bone areas, where the osteocyte–lining cell complex plays a dominant role, and effects on modeling and remodeling bone where direct effects on osteoclasts and osteoblasts modulated by neighboring osteocytes dominate. Cellular responses to mechanical strain in one area may spread to other areas of bone (e.g. from quiescent to remodeling surfaces) via two systems: (i) gap junctions between osteocytes, lining cells and osteoblasts; and (ii) secretion of paracrine factors (e.g. cytokines, growth factors, nitrogen oxide and PGs).

Strain-sensitive structures in bone cells

Integrins

Bone cells interact with surrounding matrix constituents via binding to integrins on the cell surface. Binding of integrins to various matrix proteins and membrane deformation elicit a cascade of events that results in transduction of the mechanical signal into a cellular response via activation of nuclear transcription factors and activation of neighboring cells via paracrine signals (Fig. 1.8.2). Integrins form dimers consisting of α- and β-subunits. These subunits may combine in a variety of ways to form cellular receptors binding to various matrix constituents. Osteoblasts and osteoclasts display large concentrations of fibronectin and vitronectin receptors on their surface. Upon cellular contact with the bone surface the integrins cluster and activate intracellular pathways, resulting in changes in cellular morphology, cell migration, cell proliferation and cytokine production (Fig. 1.8.2).

Changes and rearrangements within the cytoskeleton of osteoblasts constitute crucial components of the signal transduction in response to mechanical stimulation. In avian osteoblasts mechanical strain increases synthesis and accumulation of the proteins vinculin and fibronectin, as well as the increase in the number and size of stress fibers and focal adhesion complexes [6]. This cytoskeletal reorganization activates

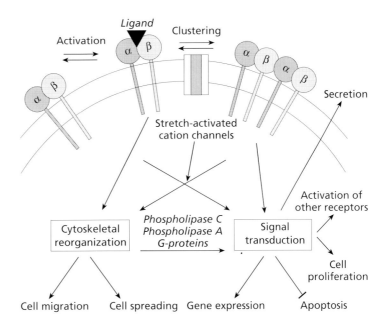

Fig. 1.8.2 Integrins are cellular receptors binding to matrix constituents of bone playing a crucial role in mechanotransduction. Upon binding to ligand (e.g. collagen, vitronectin) the dimers cluster and cause cytoskeletal reorganization as well as stimulation of a variety of signal transduction pathways. These effects cause changes in cell morphology and spreading and activation of intracellular signal transduction via phospholipases and G proteins. Alterations in gene expression due to activation of nuclear transcription factors cause either apoptosis or increased cell proliferation. Stretch-activated calcium channels in the cell membrane may also activate intracellular signal transduction pathways.

so-called focal adhesion kinases that play a key role in transmission of the mechanical signal to the nucleus. Integrins are also involved in increased cell apoptosis in response to mechanical stimuli. During distraction osteogenesis osteoblastic apoptosis has been demonstrated, especially at high strain levels [7].

The non-collagenous matrix protein osteopontin is also involved in the signal transduction. The pathway for mechanical activation of osteopontin depends on the structural integrity of the microfilament component of the cytoskeleton. In contrast, the protein kinase A pathway, which also activates this gene in osteoblasts, acts independently of the cytoskeleton in the transduction of its activity [8].

Calcium and sodium channels

Other important structures involved in the cellular response to mechanical stimuli are stretch-activated calcium channels and sodium channels in the cell membrane. Activation through membrane perturbations results in osteoblastic calcium pulses due to increased transmembrane transport of calcium and liberation of calcium from intracellular stores [9]. Calcium channels are involved in the immediate load response and modulation of intracellular calcium and seem to be important in the early phases of os-

teoblastic responses to loading [10]. In combination, blockers of stretch-activated channels (e.g. gadolinium, Gd^{3+}), and blockers of epithelial-like Na^{2+} channels (e.g. benzamil), abolish the effects of stretching on bone cells. The calcium signal may spread to neighboring cells via gap junctions, but also via liberation of ATP and ADP stimulating purinergic membrane receptors [11].

Nuclear transcription factors involved in the transmission of mechanical signals to the nucleus

Activation of both integrins and stretch-sensitive calcium channels results in increased levels of nuclear transcription factors, mainly MAPKs (mitogen-activated protein kinases) and ERKs (extracellular-related kinases).

Matsuda *et al.* [12] studied the effects of different MAPKs on osteoblastic cells subjected to stimulation with either mechanical strain, stimulation with epidermal growth factor (EGF) or hypoxia. Cell proliferation was promoted in the presence of 10 ng/mL of EGF or in hypoxic conditions (5% O_2), whereas it was inhibited by cyclic stretch (9% strain, 6 cycles/min). The mitogenic response of peridental ligament (PDL) cells to EGF or hypoxia was associated with phosphorylation of ERK, while phosphorylation of c-Jun N-terminal kinase (JNK) was observed in mechanical stretch-loaded cells. Thus, stress-responsive changes in proliferation and osteoblastic differentiation of PDL cells may be mediated by ERK I and II and by JNK, respectively, and the balance between the two pathways may determine the cell fate.

Pathways involved in the spreading of the mechanical signal to neighboring cells

Growth factors
Mechanical strain causes membrane perturbations, stimulation of integrin clustering resulting in increased secretion of growth factors (Fig. 1.8.2). The most important growth factors associated with cellular responses to mechanical stimuli are transforming growth factor β (TGF-β), insulin-like growth factors (IGFs), fibroblast growth factor (FGF) and EGF.

TGF-β, basic FGF, and IGF-I are present in high concentrations during distraction osteogenesis and localized to osteoblastic and a small number of mesenchymal cells. Furthermore, bone distracted at faster rates shows higher concentration of these factors, and the presence of TGF-β corresponds with regions of intramembranous ossification observed [13]. TGF-β1 seems to enhance strain-related suppression of osteoblastic proliferation in MC3T3 cells [14]. Cheng *et al.* reported that strain-related increase in proliferation in reactive oxygen species (ROS) cells was accompanied by a four-fold increase in levels of insulin-like growth factor II (IGF-II), while neither IGF-I nor the IGF-I receptor seemed to be involved [15].

Estradiol and dihydrotestosterone both amplify the response of bone to mechanical stimulation via a mechanism which is independent of prostanoid formation [16]. The mitogenic effects of estrogen and EGF involve the estrogen receptor, whereas those of FGF and the IGFs do not [17]. Thus, antiestrogens like tamoxifen and ICI 182780 prevent osteoblastic proliferative responses to strain, while estradiol enhances strain-induced mitogenesis. The reduced ability to maintain the structural strength of bone after the menopause could be explained by less effective strain-related remodeling when estrogen is absent and/or the estrogen receptor could be downregulated. Recent studies indicate that strain may directly affect estrogen receptor alpha-related stimulation of estrogen response elements [18].

Prostaglandins
Loading stimulates bone formation through prostaglandin (PG)-dependent mechanisms. Mechanical loading of bone explants stimulates prostaglandin E2 (PGE_2) and prostacyclin (PGI_2) release and increases glucose 6-phosphate dehydrogenase (G6PD) activity. This response is blocked by indomethacin and imitated by exogenous prostaglandins. However, only exogenously added PGI_2 is able to mimic the effects in organ cultures — exogenously added PGE_2 is without effects [19,20], and PGI_2 is also the PG showing the most pronounced response after straining of bone cells, where it increases together with IGF-II [21].

Nitric oxide
Physiologic levels of dynamic mechanical strain produce rapid increases in nitric oxide (NO) release from rat ulna explants and primary cultures of osteoblast-like cells and embryonic chick osteocytes. The predominant nitric oxide synthetase in strained bone is the endothelial form (eNOS), while inducible NOS (iNOS) was found to be virtually absent. Furthermore osteocytes produce significantly greater quantities of NO per cell in response to mechanical strain than osteoblast-like cells derived from the same bones [22].

Both NO and PG production have been implicated in the early responses to mechanical stimulation *in vivo*.

While NO or PGE_2 were unaltered after loading of rat calvarial or long bone cells, increased fluid flow induced both PGE_2 and NO production. Increased production of the two mediators was observed in all the osteoblastic populations used but not in rat skin fibroblasts. Fluid flow appeared to act through an increase in wall-shear stress. The authors suggest that mechanical loading of bone is sensed by osteoblastic cells through fluid flow-mediated wall-shear stress rather than by mechanical strain [23].

Gap junctions
Groups of osteoblasts and osteocytes are connected via gap junctions. Changes in intracellular calcium can spread from cell to cell via these junctions, and thus

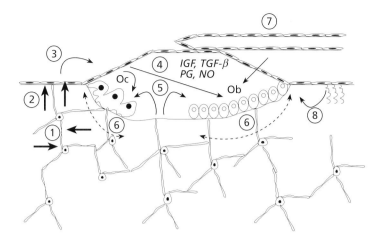

Fig. 1.8.3 Pathways involved in mechanotransduction. The osteocyte network constitutes the principal mechanosensor of bone (1). Osteocytes react to changes in hydrostatic pressure around cellular processes caused by mechanical deformation of bone (1). Probably stretching of membrane-bound stretch-sensitive calcium channels of osteocytes also plays a role (1). Activation of osteocytes by mechanical strain is transmitted to the lining cells layer via intracellular messengers and gap junctions (2), and this process may cause activation of bone remodeling on quiescent bone surfaces (2) or stimulation of osteoclasts and osteoblasts at neighboring remodeling sites (3). The spreading of the mechanical stimulus involves production of growth factors, cytokines, prostaglandins and NO from lining cells (4) and signaling via gap junctions in the lining cell layer. It is also conceivable that some prostaglandins and growth factors (principally TGF-β and IGFs) are liberated by osteocytes at sites where contact with the lining cells layer is interrupted (e.g. at remodeling sites) (5). At remodeling sites membrane deformation in osteoclasts and osteoblasts due to mechanical strain can affect activity of the two cells directly via integrins and stretch-sensitive calcium channels (6). Electromagnetic fields created by deformation-induced piezoelectricity (8) and stretching of blood vessels (7) may also modulate osteoclastic and osteoblastic activity.

affect cell populations some distances away from the actual site for mechanical stimulation (Fig. 1.8.3).

Other factors involved in responses to mechanical stimuli

Electromagnetic fields

Bending and stretching of bone creates electrical fields thought to originate from the apatite crystals (piezoelectricity) (Fig. 1.8.3). Electromagnetic fields generated during mechanical stimulation show distinct effects on bone. As mentioned above they reduce osteoclastic recruitment and increase osteoblastic bone formation. The response is highly frequency dependent, with frequencies below 75 Hz being most effective [24]. Magnetic field exposure inhibits cell growth through a mechanism independent of gap junctional coupling, while the alteration in alkaline phosphatase (AP) activity appears to be stimulated by electric fields independent of gap junctions [25].

Cellular responses to mechanical strain

Osteoclasts

Very little is known about osteoclastic responses to mechanical stimuli. Mechanical strain reduces osteoclast recruitment [26]. All known pathways may be involved in this response (Fig. 1.8.3), but the reduction may also be related to electrical field generation [27].

Osteoblasts

Mechanical stimulation of bone tissue by physical activity stimulates bone formation in normal bone and may attenuate bone loss in osteoporotic patients. Normal bone cells seem to increase proliferation and TGF-β secretion in response to mechanical strain, while osteoporotic cells do not [28]. Osteoblastic cells from different locations in the skeleton react differently to mechanical strain, e.g. cells from calvariae show a much lower response in terms of G6PD activity to strain than cells obtained from ulnae [29].

The first observations demonstrating effects of mechanical stress on bone cells were reported by Glucksmann [30]. Using cultured chick embryo rudiments he demonstrated that increased tension in the rudiments enhanced bone formation, while reduced tension reduced bone formation. Later studies using organ cultures subsequently demonstrated increased DNA and RNA synthesis, increased AP activity and increased glucose consumption.

Pazzaglia *et al.* [31] used the rat bent tail to investigate the effects of mechanical forces on bones and joints. They found that metaphyseal and epiphyseal trabeculae on the compressed side were thicker and denser than those of the distracted part of the vertebrae. No significant differences in osteoclast number between the compressed and distracted sides in two different age groups were reported, suggesting that the response of living bone to altered strain is mediated by osteoblasts.

In another study the authors used fluid forces to investigate the response of osteoblastic cells to strain. When forces were low, neither strain magnitude nor strain rate was correlated with osteopontin expression. Higher magnitude fluid forces, however, significantly increased osteopontin message levels. These data indicate that fluid forces, and not mechanical stretch, influence osteopontin expression in osteoblasts and suggest that fluid forces induced by extracellular fluid flow within the bone matrix may play an important role in bone formation in response to mechanical loading [32].

Kaspar *et al.* applied cyclic strain to human osteoblasts over 2 days (30 min/day) with a frequency of 1 Hz and a strain magnitude of 1000 microstrain. This resulted in increased proliferation (10–48%) and carboxy-terminal (C-terminal) collagen type I propeptide release (7–49%), while alkaline phosphatase activity and osteocalcin release were significantly reduced by up to 25 and 32%, respectively. Thus, cyclic strain at physiologic magnitude leads to increased matrix production while secretion of proteins related to matrix mineralization is decreased [33].

Osteocytes

One of the characteristic features of bone is a population of live cells of the osteoblast lineage distributed both on the surface (lining cells) and throughout the matrix (osteocytes). These cells communicate with one another via gap junctions, and neurotransmitters also seem to be involved. Osteocytes have also been implicated in a variety of functions securing bone integrity. These include: arrest of fatigue cracks; mineral exchange; osteocytic osteolysis; renewed remodeling activity after release by resorption; stimulation and guidance of osteoclastic cutting cones involved in mineral exchange and the repair of microdamage; strain detection; and the control of mechanically related bone modeling/remodeling [34].

Osteocytes seem to be the primary mechanosensory cells of bone, and the lacunocanalicular network constitutes the structure that mediates mechanosensing. Strain-derived flow of interstitial fluid through this network seems to mechanically activate the osteocytes, as well as ensuring transport of cell signaling molecules and nutrients and waste products. This concept allows an explanation of local bone gain and loss, as well as remodeling in response to fatigue damage.

The number of osteocytes and periosteal cells displaying positive reaction for G6PD is increased after mechanical stimulation while enzymes like glyceraldehyde 3-phosphate dehydrogenase (GA3PD) or lactate dehydrogenase (LDH) remain unchanged. These findings suggest that loading increases the activity of the oxidative part of the pentose monophosphate shunt pathway. It is also consistent with stimulation of a synthetic process, such as the production of RNA from ribose 5-phosphate [35].

Many modulators such as parathyroid hormone (PTH), prostanoids and extracellular Ca^{2+} influence osteocytic mechanotransduction. It has been postulated that osteocytes transduce signals of mechanical loading that result in anabolic responses such as the expression of c-fos, IGF-I and osteocalcin. The upregulation of steady-state levels of their mRNA is biphasic, being preceded by cyclooxygenase-2 (COX-2) gene expression. Compared to a typical transient immediate early expression of c-fos, COX-2 shows another distinct peak about 8 h after the initiation of stretching. Second peaks in IGF-I and osteocalcin expression are entirely dependent on the first wave of COX-2 expression. Extracellular Ca^{2+} is also essential to the osteocytic response to stretching [17,36].

Effects of mechanical strain on bone turnover and bone remodeling

Bone remodeling is also affected by mechanical strain. The general trend is decreased bone degradation, possibly caused by reduced osteoclast recruitment as mentioned above. Young recruits subjected to military training display increased bone mass at the heel of 3%, but at the same time bone formation and resorption markers go down by 10–12% [37]. The impact of physical activity on bone turnover may, however, depend on the kind of exercise performed. In dogs immobilization increases bone resorption [34]. Aerobic training causes changes compatible with reduced bone resorption activity, while anaerobic training seems to result in an overall accelerated bone turnover [38].

Exercise may act in synergy with hormones like growth hormone (GH) and IGFs; for example, exercise amplifies periosteal bone formation induced by GH [39]. Exercise also seems to interact with estrogen effects on bone [40]. The changes in bone mass and turnover only occur in the strained parts of the skeleton. No effects in non-weight-bearing parts have been demonstrable [41].

Sows trained on a treadmill 20 min per day for 20 weeks exhibited greater active periosteal surface and greater periosteal and osteonal bone formative activity as reflected in the mineral appositional rate (MAR) than untrained sows [42].

In another study the training group subjected to weight training (three times weekly) displayed significant increases in serum osteocalcin and serum bone-specific AP activity within the first month, and persisting throughout the training period, while there was no significant change in plasma procollagen type I C-terminal concentration. Urinary deoxypyridinoline excretion was transiently suppressed and returned to the initial value but was never stimulated during the 4 months.

Smit and Burger [43] have recently used finite element analysis to simulate strain forces in cortical bone and resorption lacunae during remodeling. This simulation showed reduced deformation in front of and increased strain behind regions of osteoclastic resorption of cortical basic multicellular units (BMUs). A similar simulation of cancellous BMUs revealed higher strains at the bottom of resorption lacunae, where resorption is terminated and osteoblasts are recruited to refill the gap. The authors conclude that strain distributions may regulate coupling between resorption and formation during bone remodeling.

Results obtained using the functionally isolated turkey ulna preparation suggest that adaptive bone remodeling is extremely sensitive to alterations in both the magnitude and distribution of the strain generated within the bone tissue [44]. Furthermore, it appears that a loading regime can only influence bone remodeling when it is dynamic in nature. The full osteogenic potential of its influence is then achieved after only an extremely short exposure to this stimulus. The potency of the stimulus appears to be proportional to the magnitude of the strain engendered. The threshold for induction of adaptive remodeling differs between different areas of the skeleton; strain levels that are common in one location and induce no alteration in bone remodeling may induce adaptive remodeling in others [44].

El Haj *et al.* tested the response of cancellous bone biopsies to mechanical load-bearing [45]. Two cellular responses to mechanical loading were demonstrated: (i) a rise in intracellular G6PD in lining cells immediately after loading; and (ii) an increase in RNA synthesis. Both responses were inhibited by indomethacin.

In the limbs, where the ability to withstand repetitive loading is important, the general form of the bone will be achieved as a result of growth alone, while the remaining characteristics result from adaptive responses to functional load-bearing. It is the adaptive response to the total activity pattern that influences bone modeling and remodeling and so determines the bone's architecture [46].

The effects of physical inactivity and activity on bone mass and bone mineral density in humans

Most studies are observational studies and have focused on relationships between activity patterns, parameters of fitness or athletic status on the one hand, and bone mass on the other.

Nilsson and Westlin [47] and later Dalén and Olsson [48] was among the first to show that training is associated with higher bone mineral density (BMD) compared to controls, evaluated in cross-sectional studies. These two studies documented that in certain leg training activities, there is a relationship between training load and BMD in the distal femur. Swimming, however, was not associated with higher BMD than in controls [49].

Several other cross-sectional studies in the previous decades have correlated physical activity to BMD, most of them confirming that physical training is associated with higher BMD.

Observational studies can be suggestive as to the effect of different kinds of activities on bone mass. However, the study groups are independent samples and therefore a causal relationship between the different variables of interest cannot be established. In addition, the subjects investigated in these studies are highly selected. Individuals with a high muscle mass (and thereby bone mass) are more prone to engage in activities involving resistance training such as weight-lifting, while individuals with a low muscle mass might preferentially choose to participate in endurance training activities like long-distance running.

Although most investigators would prefer prospective studies, only a few of these have been undertaken to investigate the effect of physical activity on the acquisition of bone and the effect of detraining on bone in humans. The main problems with these studies have been difficulty in maintaining sufficient length and intensity of training and lack of compliance.

It has been proposed that loading generates mechanical deformations in the specific bone, inducing an adaptive response to activity. The loading put on bone, by both ground reaction forces as well as muscle-induced strains during activity, contributes to the skeletal adaptation to exercise. These factors are related in many activities and no exercise trial providing information regarding the role of muscle-induced strain alone in the skeletal response in humans has been published.

Development of peak bone mass

Bone mass accumulates during childhood and adolescence and the maximal bone mass, i.e. peak bone mass, is achieved late in the second decade of life. In females, it has been shown that the increment in bone mass is maximal at menarche, 2 years after the peak increment in height [49]. Heredity is an important determinant of peak bone mass, accounting for 60–80% of the observed variance in peak bone mass. Regarding lifestyle factors, physical activity and diet have been proposed

to be of major importance in peak bone mass development. These factors are potentially modifiable but their relative contribution to peak bone mass is mostly uncertain.

Immobilization and inactivity

Immobilization or disuse exerts deleterious effects on bone mineral density and bone integrity. Prolonged bed rest or space flight of long duration is followed by a marked bone loss. Bed rest for 3 weeks in patients with lumbar disc protrusion is associated with a decrease in BMC (bone mineral content) of 0.9% per week [50]. In simulated weightlessness, continuous bed rest for 17 weeks is accompanied by a bone loss that may exceed 0.5% per week [51]. On the 1–6-month MIR space missions, the estimated bone loss was 0.9% per month in the tibial cancellous envelope, despite aerobic physical activity for 2 h twice a week [52]. In microgravity, most bone is lost in locations of the skeleton that are ordinarily exposed to the highest weight-bearing. However, a systemic effect from the weightlessness, mediated by an excessive production of glucocorticoids, cannot be excluded as bone loss has been described in non-weight-bearing parts of the skeleton after a space flight. One explanation for these alterations in bone metabolism may be the selective resistance to the anabolic actions of GH induced by skeletal unloading [53]. In examining bone metabolism during immobilization periods, the striking observation is the uncoupling between bone resorption and bone formation. The exact mechanism by which unloading induces bone loss is not known but a prominent feature is a rapid increase in bone resorption associated with a later more and more sustained subtle decrease in bone formation [53]. Bone loss, even after shorter periods of immobilization in adults, is often partially irreversible, despite full recovery of mobility [3]. It has been shown that a low level of physical activity is an independent risk factor for hip fracture in elderly women [54].

Physical activity and bone mass in the young

Observational studies

A large number of cross-sectional studies on bone mass in athletes and controls have been published. In 1971 Nilsson and Westlin found that athletes had higher bone mass [47]. Female and male athletes

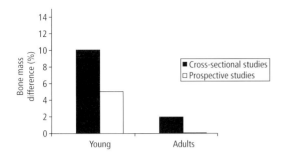

Fig. 1.8.4 The observed difference in bone mass between active and inactive subjects in cross-sectional and prospective studies in young people and adults, respectively.

involved in resistance-training activities such as weight-lifting, tennis, ice hockey, volleyball, soccer, basketball, ballet dancing and badminton all have higher bone mass than do inactive controls. Bone mass in athletes involved in weight-bearing activities has generally been found to be 10–15% higher than in inactive controls [55] (Fig. 1.8.4).

The difference in bone mass between individuals engaged in aerobic activities such as long-distance running, cross-country skiing or swimming and sedentary controls is often subtle [56]. Extreme endurance training is associated with low bone mass in females (see Chapter 4.6) and males [57], primarily caused by decreased endogenous levels of sex hormones.

The starting age of individuals participating in load-bearing activities seems to be of major importance. Preferentially, the activity should be started before puberty to maximize peak bone mass. Haapasalo *et al.*, investigating female tennis and squash players, showed that the players who started their active career before puberty had higher bone mass than players who started after puberty, despite a similar number of years of playing [58].

The response to loading activities seem to be site-specific, implying, for example, that activities such as tennis that put load on one arm increase bone mass in the loaded arm but not in the inactive, non-loaded arm [58].

Prospective studies

In order to provide evidence that physical activity affects the rate of bone accretion, it is necessary to perform controlled prospective, longitudinal, intervention studies in well-defined groups.

Only a few prospective studies have been conducted in prepubertal children. In the study by Morris *et al.* the girls in a high-impact group gained significantly more bone (10% in the femoral neck and 3.5% in the lumbar spine) over the 10-month experimental period than the controls [59]. In prepubertal boys, weight-bearing physical activity for 8 months, for 30 min three times a week was associated with a 100% higher bone accretion rate compared to the rate in the control group [60].

In examining the effect of loading activities in premenopausal women, longitudinal studies often demonstrate rather small increases in bone mass, 1–6% over an 8–24-month period [61]. By contrast, a 3-year study on the effects of moderate strengthening exercises in physically active, non-athletic women aged 30–40 years showed no significant effect on bone mass [62]. Lack of adherence to the determined exercise program and high dropout rates (around 50%) in most long-term studies are of great concern and must surely weaken any conclusion regarding the effect of the physical activity on bone mass and bone mineral density. However, once an increase in bone mass has been obtained secondary to an exercise program, this can be preserved by unsupervised regular weight-bearing activity twice a week [55].

In younger males, it has been shown that intensive physical activity can accelerate bone accretion to a very high extent in as short a period as 14 weeks. The mean increase in tibial bone mass was 7.5% secondary to this extremely demanding military training [56]. However, more than 40% of the subjects discontinued the training program due to stress fractures of the tibia. It was concluded that high stresses put on bone resulted in either massive hypertrophy or fatigue fractures of long bone.

Physical activity and bone mass in adults

Prospective studies in men

Very limited data are available on the effect of exercise on bone in men. Williams *et al.* [63] compared 20 middle-aged men who participated in a long-distance running training program to 10 inactive controls. Runners who were compliant showed greater increases in BMD in the calcaneus than controls. However, men who did not train consistently did not.

In a 2-year follow-up study of men (and women) over the age of 50 Michel *et al.* [64] found a positive correlation between training intensity and training load and BMD at the lumbar spine in both sexes. Furthermore, they showed that a graduated reduction in training intensity and training load led to significant BMD loss, whereas continued training at the high level showed a reduction in age-related BMD loss. However, data on training in men is still so limited that it would not be prudent to draw conclusions about the effects of exercise on bone in the adult male.

Prospective studies in women

Quite a few prospective studies have investigated physical training and BMD in pre- and post-menopausal women. Most studies of premenopausal women show some positive influence of physical training on bone. It appears that higher loads, such as those produced by greater impact, lead to greater bone mass. The activities through which these loads can be achieved need to be identified. Clearly, high-impact gymnastic training is not practical for most women, but a combination of stepping and jumping exercises may prove worthwhile. The data also suggest that it is important to distinguish young adult women from older premenopausal women, since bone may respond better to increased mechanical loads in the earlier years.

The accelerated bone loss in postmenopausal women due to the decrease in reproductive hormones at menopause is a powerful contributor to the observed decrease in bone mass during life in females. Aloia *et al.* [65] were among the first to report bone mass benefits of exercise in postmenopausal women, measuring the total body calcium before and after exercise; an increase from 781 ± 95 g to 801 ± 118 g was reported. Since that time several exercise studies investigating the effect of either moderate training or muscle-building training on BMD have been performed. Most studies of moderate training programs have used non-randomized exercise interventions to investigate the effects with varying results. Krølner *et al.* studied women with a previous distal radius fracture and demonstrated that the BMC of the lumbar spine increased in response to a program of walking, run-

ning, standing and rest [66]. BMC of the forearm was stable in patients as well as in controls. Nelson *et al.* [67] studied the effect of walking on BMD. The program was 50 min of walking four times a week for 1 year and showed varying results by skeletal site. A slight BMD increase of about 0.5% was found in the lumbar spine in the trained women compared to a significant decrease of 7.0% in controls. On the other hand, no difference was found in the femoral neck between volunteers and controls. In a 3-year follow-up study of Smith *et al.* [68] on elderly women (aged 69–95) it was shown that training gave a significant BMD increase compared to age-matched controls. The greatest magnitude of BMD change, an increase of 6.1% after 22 months due to training in postmenopausal women, has been reported by Dalsky *et al.* [69]. They compared women during walking, stair climbing or jogging combined with weight-bearing exercise in the form of rowing to a group of age-matched controls. After 9 and 22 months of training, BMD of the lumbar spine was increased compared to controls although the benefit had flattened out after 22 months of training. Volunteers who dropped out showed a decrease in BMD towards baseline, supporting the view that exercise patterns must be continual to maintain a higher bone mass. Only a few studies have investigated postmenopausal women on hormone replacement therapy in combination with calcium and training, and these three studies are all inconclusive concerning the effect of training on BMD [66,68,70].

Several investigators have attempted to investigate the effects of muscle training programs on bone mass. As studies of moderate training, most of these studies are non-randomized; although they give some evidence for a positive effect of weight-bearing training on loss of bone mass, this effect does not offset the decrease due to reproductive hormone deficiency. In studies investigating the effects of muscle- and strength-building programs on bone [62,71–74], Revel *et al.* [73] reported a negative association between training and BMD, Sinarki *et al.* [62] and Pruitt *et al.* [72] found no changes in their studies whereas Rundgren *et al.* [74] found a slight beneficial BMD effect. However, only Revel *et al.* [73] reported a statistically increased bone mass secondary to exercise.

Perhaps the most interesting information has been

presented by Berard *et al.* [75] who performed a meta-analysis on the effect of physical activity on the bone mass of healthy postmenopausal women, including all published studies of this kind from 1966 to 1996. All studies included were prospective intervention studies, randomized or not, evaluating the effectiveness of an exercise program of any duration, frequency and intensity, with a control group; 217 papers were included. Based on the complete material no beneficial results of training were seen; however, in a subgroup, a significant effect of physical activity was detected on BMD at L2–L4 of the lumbar spine in studies published after 1991. No effect could be seen on forearm and femoral neck. This meta-analysis suggests that exercise programs might be beneficial in preventing spinal bone loss. The findings from different types of studies regarding the relationship of physical activity to BMD are illustrated in Fig. 1.8.4.

Summary

Bone cells and bone organ cultures certainly display a wide variety of distinct responses to mechanical stimulation. Adaptation of bone architecture to mechanical strain requires feedback concerning the relationship between current loading and existing architecture. This feedback is most probably derived from the strain in the bone matrix. The arrangement of the osteocyte network is ideally suited both to detect strain throughout the matrix and to influence adaptive modeling and remodeling in a strain-related manner via the lining cells. The tight interaction between the different subgroups of bone cells suggests that all bone cells may act as mechanosensors and that several different pathways are available for the transduction of mechanical stimuli.

The general response to mechanical stimulation is reduced bone resorption and an increased bone formation. Weight-bearing activities clearly increase bone acquisition rate in children and adolescents and improve peak bone mass. However, the positive changes in bone mass in adults after exercise regimens are limited, but weight-bearing physical activity seems to prevent or decrease the rate of bone loss, including in the elderly. Besides the effect on bone mass, regular physical activity increases muscle strength, improves balance and reduces the risk of falling. Inactivity and immobilization increase bone loss and are associated with an increased fracture risk. However, no prospective study on the effects of regular physical activity on fracture rates has been performed.

In order to increase and preserve bone mass in a specific region, the stress to the area must exceed the accustomed load threshold. The activity should be weight-bearing and dynamic rather than static, inducing high strain rates in bone preferentially in unusual patterns to evoke an osteogenic response. Furthermore, it should be repeated regularly in order to preserve bone mass and, thereby, bone strength. More specific and sensitive methods for bone mass and bone strength measurements in prospective, randomized studies at all ages are needed in order to evaluate the possible positive effect of training on BMD.

Multiple choice questions

1 *How does physical activity affect bone remodeling?*
a It enhances bone formation.
b It inhibits bone resorption.
c It enhances bone formation and has no major effect on bone resorption.
d It inhibits bone resorption and has no major effect on bone formation.
e *a* and *b*.

2 *A skeletal training program can preferentially include:*
a water activities
b cycling
c gymnastics
d walking and jogging
e *a*, *b* and *c*
f *a* and *d*
g *c* and *d*.

3 *The following statements are true:*
a The skeleton adapts to the load put on it.
b Walking increases bone mass in the arms.
c Swimming is associated with increased spine bone mineral density (BMD).
d Bed rest induces a rapid bone loss.
e *a* and *d*.
f *b*, *c* and *d*.
g *a*, *b*, *c* and *d*.

4 *The following statements about mechanotransduction are correct:*
a Mechanotransduction can be divided into four distinct steps.

b Mechanocoupling and mechanotransduction are words for the same process.

c The cellular response step to mechanical loading depends on the magnitude, duration and rate of the applied load.

d *a* and *b*.

e *a* and *c*.

f *a*, *b* and *c*.

5 *The most important growth factors associated with cellular responses to mechanical stimuli are:*

a transforming growth factor β (TGF-β), insulin-like growth factors (IGFs), fibroblast growth factor (FGF) and epidermal growth factor (EGF)

b IGFs, FGF and EGF

c TGF-β, IGFs and FGF.

References

1 Wolff J. *Das Gesetz der Transformation der Knochen*. Berlin: Verlag von August Hirschwald, 1892: 1–152.

2 Huddelston AL, Rockwell D, Kulund DN *et al*. Bone mass in lifetime tennis players. *J Am Med Assoc* 1980; **244**: 1107–9.

3 Kannus P, Haapasalo H, Sievanen P, Oja P, Vuori I. The site-specific effects of long-term unilateral activity on bone mineral density and content. *Bone* 1994; **15**: 279–84.

4 Pirnay F, Bodeux M, Crielaard JM *et al*. Bone mineral content and physical activity. *Int J Sport Med* 1987; **8**: 331–5.

5 Duncan RL, Turner CH. Mechanotransduction and the functional response of bone to mechanical strain. *Calcified Tissue Int* 1995; **57**: 344–58.

6 Meazzini MC, Toma CD, Schaffer JL, Gray ML, Gerstenfeld LC. Osteoblast cytoskeletal modulation in response to mechanical strain in vitro. *J Orth Res* 1998; **16**: 170–80.

7 Meyer T, Meyer U, Stratmann U, Wiesmann HP, Joos U. Identification of apoptotic cell death in distraction osteogenesis. *Cell Biol Int* 1999; **23**: 439–46.

8 Toma CD, Ashkar S, Gray ML, Schaffer JL, Gerstenfeld LC. Signal transduction of mechanical stimuli is dependent on microfilament integrity: identification of osteopontin as a mechanically induced gene in osteoblasts. *J Bone Min Res* 1997; **12**: 1626–36.

9 Tsai JA, Larsson O, Kindmark H. Spontaneous and stimulated transients in cytoplasmic free Ca^{2+} in normal human osteoblast-like cells: aspects of their regulation. *Biochem Biophys Res Comm* 1999; **263**: 206–12.

10 El Haj AJ, Walker LM, Preston MR, Publicover SJ. Mechanotransduction pathways in bone: calcium fluxes and the role of voltage-operated calcium channels. *Med Biol Eng Comp* 1999; **37**: 403–9.

11 Jørgensen NR, Henriksen Z, Brodt C *et al*. Human osteoblastic cells propagate intracellular calcium signals by two different mechanisms. *J Bone Min Res* 2000; **15**: 1024–32.

12 Matsuda N, Morita N, Matsuda K, Watanabe M. Proliferation and differentiation of human osteoblastic cells associated with differential activation of MAP kinases in response to epidermal growth factor, hypoxia, and mechanical stress in vitro. *Biochem Biophys Res Comm* 1998; **249**: 350–4.

13 Farhadieh RD, Dickinson R, Yu Y, Gianoutsos MP, Walsh WR. The role of transforming growth factor-beta, insulin-like growth factor I, and basic fibroblast growth factor in distraction osteogenesis of the mandible. *J Craniofacial Surg* 1999; **10**: 80–6.

14 Gosain AK, Song LS, Santoro T *et al*. Effects of transforming growth factor-beta and mechanical strain on osteoblast cell counts: an in vitro model for distraction osteogenesis. *Plastic Reconstructive Surg* 2000; **105**: 130–6, discussion 137–9.

15 Cheng M, Zaman G, Rawlinson SC, Mohan S, Baylink DJ, Lanyon LE. Mechanical strain stimulates ROS cell proliferation through IGF-II and estrogen through IGF-I. *J Bone Min Res* 1999; **14**: 1742–50.

16 Cheng MZ, Zaman G, Rawlinson SC, Pitsillides AA, Suswillo RF, Lanyon LE. Enhancement by sex hormones of the osteoregulatory effects of mechanical loading and prostaglandins in explants of rat ulnae. *J Bone Min Res* 1997; **12**: 1424–30.

17 Damien E, Price JS, Lanyon LE. The estrogen receptor's involvement in osteoblasts' adaptive response to mechanical strain. *J Bone Min Res* 1998; **13**: 1275–82.

18 Zaman G, Cheng MZ, Jessop HL, White R, Lanyon LE. Mechanical strain activates estrogen response elements in bone cells. *Bone* 2000; **27**: 233–9.

19 Rawlinson SC, el-Haj AJ, Minter SL, Tavares IA, Bennett A, Lanyon LE. Loading-related increases in prostaglandin production in cores of adult canine cancellous bone *in vitro*: a role for prostacyclin in adaptive bone remodelling? *J Bone Min Res* 1991; **6**: 1345–51.

20 Rawlinson SC, Mohan S, Baylink DJ, Lanyon LE. Exogenous prostacyclin, but not prostaglandin E2, produces similar responses in both G6PD activity and RNA production as mechanical loading, and increases IGF-II release, in adult cancellous bone in culture. *Calcified Tissue Int* 1993; **53**: 324–9.

21 Zaman G, Suswillo RF, Cheng MZ, Tavares IA, Lanyon LE. Early responses to dynamic strain change and prostaglandins in bone-derived cells in culture. *J Bone Min Res* 1997; **12**: 769–77.

22 Zaman G, Pitsillides AA, Rawlinson SC, Suswillo RF, Mosley JR, Cheng MZ *et al*. Mechanical strain stimulates nitric oxide production by rapid activation of endothelial nitric oxide synthase in osteocytes. *J Bone Min Res* 1999; **14**: 1123–31.

23 Smalt R, Mitchell FT, Howard RL, Chambers TJ. Induction of NO and prostaglandin E2 in osteoblasts by wall-shear stress but not mechanical strain. *Am J Physiol* 1997; **273**: E751–8.

24 McLeod KJ, Rubin CT. Frequency specific modulation of

bone adaptation by induced electric fields. *J Theoret Biol* 1990; **145**: 385–96.

25 Vander MM, Donahue HJ, Rubin CT, McLeod KJ. Osteoblastic networks with deficient coupling: differential effects of magnetic and electric field exposure. *Bone* 2000; **27**: 227–31.

26 Rubin J, Fan X, Biskobing DM, Taylor WR, Rubin CT. Osteoclastogenesis is repressed by mechanical strain in an *in vitro* model. *J Orth Res* 1999; **17**: 639–45.

27 Rubin J, McLeod KJ, Titus L, Nanes MS, Catherwood BD, Rubin CT. Formation of osteoclast-like cells is suppressed by low frequency, low intensity electric fields. *J Orth Res* 1996; **14**: 7–15.

28 Neidlinger-Wilke C, Stalla I, Claes L, Brand R, Hoellen I, Rubenacker S *et al.* Human osteoblasts from younger normal and osteoporotic donors show differences in proliferation and TGF beta-release in response to cyclic strain. *J Biomech* 1995; **28**: 1411–8.

29 Rawlinson SC, Mosley JR, Suswillo RF, Pitsillides AA, Lanyon LE. Calvarial and limb bone cells in organ and monolayer culture do not show the same early responses to dynamic mechanical strain. *J Bone Min Res* 1995; **10**: 1225–32.

30 Glucksmann A. Studies on bone mechanics *in vitro* II. The role of tension and pressure in chondrogenesis. *Anat Res* 1939; **73**: 39–56.

31 Pazzaglia UE, Andrini L, Di Nucci A. The effects of mechanical forces on bones and joints. Experimental study on the rat tail. *J Bone Joint Surg (Brit)* 1997; **79**: 1024–30.

32 Owan I, Burr DB, Turner CH, Qiu J, Tu Y, Onyia JE *et al.* Mechanotransduction in bone: osteoblasts are more responsive to fluid forces than mechanical strain. *Am J Physiol* 1997; **273**: C810–5.

33 Kaspar D, Seidl W, Neidlinger-Wilke C, Ignatius A, Claes L. Dynamic cell stretching increases human osteoblast proliferation and CICP synthesis but decreases osteocalcin synthesis and alkaline phosphatase activity. *Biomech* 2000; **33**: 45–51.

34 Lanyon LE. Osteocytes, strain detection, bone modeling and remodeling. *Calcified Tissue Int* 1993; **53** (Suppl. 1): S102–6.

35 Skerry TM, Bitensky L, Chayen J, Lanyon LE. Early strain-related changes in enzyme activity in osteocytes following bone loading in vivo. *J Bone Min Res* 1989; **4**: 783–8.

36 Mikuni-Takagaki Y. Mechanical responses and signal transduction pathways in stretched osteocytes. *J Bone Min Res* 1999; **17**: 57–60.

37 Etherington J, Keeling J, Bramley R, Swaminathan R, McCurdie I, Spector TD. The effects of 10 weeks military training on heel ultrasound and bone turnover. *Calcified Tissue Int* 1999; **64**: 389–93.

38 Zorbas YG, Naexu KA, Federenko YF. Mechanisms of osteoporosis development during prolonged restriction of motor activity in dog. *Rev Espan Fisiol* 1994; **50**: 47–54.

39 Oxlund H, Andersen NB, Ortoft G, Orskov H, Andreassen TT. Growth hormone and mild exercise in combination markedly enhance cortical bone formation and strength in old rats. *Endocrinology* 1998; **139**: 1899–904.

40 Westerlind KC, Wronski TJ, Ritman EL, Luo ZP, An KN, Bell NH *et al.* Estrogen regulates the rate of bone turnover but bone balance in ovariectomized rats is modulated by prevailing mechanical strain. *Proc Natl Acad Sci USA* 1997; **94**: 4199–204.

41 Tommerup LJ, Raab DM, Crenshaw TD, Smith EL. Does weight-bearing exercise affect non-weight-bearing bone? *J Bone Min Res* 1993; **8**: 1053–8.

42 Smith EL, Gilligan C. Physical activity effects on bone metabolism. *Calcified Tissue Int* 1991; **49** (Suppl.): S50–4.

43 Smit TH, Burger EH. Is BMU-coupling a strain-regulated phenomenon? A finite element analysis. *J Bone Min Res* 2000; **15**: 301–7.

44 Rubin CT, Lanyon LE. Regulation of bone formation by applied dynamic loads. *J Bone Joint Surg (Am)* 1984; **66**: 397–402.

45 El Haj AJ, Minter SL, Rawlinson SC, Suswillo R, Lanyon LE. Cellular responses to mechanical loading in vitro. *J Bone Min Res* 1990; **5**: 923–32.

46 Lanyon LE. The physiological basis of training the skeleton. The Sir Frederick Smith Memorial Lecture. *Equine Vet J Suppl* 1990; **9**: 8–13.

47 Nilsson BE, Westlin NE. Bone density in athletes. *Clin Orth Rel Res* 1971; **77**: 79–82.

48 Dalen N, Olsson K. Bone mineral content and physical activity. *Acta Orthop Scand* 1974; **45**: 170–4.

49 Cadogan J, Blumsohn A, Barker ME, Eastell R. A longitudinal study of bone gain in pubertal girls: anthropometric and biochemical correlates. *J Bone Min Res* 1998; **13**: 1602–12.

50 Krølner B, Toft B. Vertebral bone loss: an unheeded side effect of therapeutic bed rest. *Clin Sci* 1983; **64**: 537–40.

51 Leblanc AD, Schneider VS, Evans HJ, Engelbretson DA, Krebs JM. Bone mineral loss and recovery after 17 weeks of bed rest. *J Bone Min Res* 1990; **5**: 843–50.

52 Vico L, Collet P, Guignandon A, Lafage-Proust MH *et al.* Effects of long-term microgravity exposure on cancellous and cortical weight-bearing bones of cosmonauts. *Lancet* 2000; **355**: 1607–11.

53 Halloran BP, Bikle DD, Harris J *et al.* Skeletal unloading induces selective resistance to the anabolic actions of growth hormone on bone. *J Bone Min Res* 1995; **10**: 1168–76.

54 Gregg EW, Cauley JA, Seeley DG, Ensrud KE, Bauer DC. Physical activity and osteoporotic fracture risk in older women. Study of Osteoporotic Fractures Research Group. *Ann Intern Med* 1998; **129**: 81–8.

55 Heinonen A, Kannus P, Sievänen H, Pasanen M, Oja P, Vouri I. Good maintenance of high-impact activity-induced bone gain by voluntary, unsupervised exercises: an 8-month follow-up of a randomized controlled trial. *J Bone Min Res* 1999; **14**: 125–8.

56 Margulies JY, Simkin A, Leichter I *et al.* Effect of intensive physical activity on the bone-mineral content in the lower limbs of young adults. *J Bone Joint Surg* 1986; **68-A**: 1090–3.

57 MacDougall JD, Webber CE, Martin J *et al.* Relationship among running milage, bone density, and serum testosterone in male runners. *J Appl Physiol* 1992; **73**: 1165–70.

58 Haapasalo H, Sievänen H, Kannus P, Heinonen A, Oja P, Vuori I. Dimensions and estimated mechanical characteristics of the humerus after long term tennis loading. *J Bone Min Res* 1996; **11**: 864–72.

59 Morris FL, Naughton GA, Gibbs JL, Carlson JS, Wark JD. Prospective ten-month exercise intervention in premenarcheal girls: positive effects on bone and lean mass. *J Bone Min Res* 1997; **12**: 1453–62.

60 Bradney M, Pearce G, Naughton G *et al.* Moderate exercise during growth in prepubertal boys: changes in bone mass, size, volumetric density, and bone strength: a controlled prospective study. *J Bone Min Res* 1998; **13**: 1814–21.

61 Sinaki M, Wahner HW, Offord KP, Hodgson SF. Efficacy of non-loading exercises in prevention of vertebral bone loss in postmenopausal women: a controlled trial. *Mayo Clinic Proc* 1989; **64**: 762–9.

62 Sinaki M, Wahner HW, Bergstrahl EJ *et al.* Three-year controlled, randomized trial of the effect of dose-specified loading and strengthening exercises on bone mineral density of spine and femur in non-athletic, physically active women. *Bone* 1996; **19**: 233–44.

63 Williams JA, Wagner J, Wasnich R, Heilburn L. The effect of long-distance running upon appendicular bone mineral content. *Med Sci Sports Exerc* 1984; **16**: 223–7.

64 Michel BA, Bloch DA, Fries JF. Weight-bearing exercise, over exercise, and lumbar bone density over age fifty. *Arch Intern Med* 1989; **149**: 2325–9.

65 Aloia JF, Cohn SH, Ostuni JA, Cane R, Ellis K. Prevention of involutional bone loss by exercise. *Ann Intern Med* 1978; **89**: 356–8.

66 Krølner B, Toft B, Nielsen SP, Tondevold T. Physical exercise as prophylaxis against involutional vertebral bone loss: a controlled trial. *Clin Sci* 1983; **64**: 541–6.

67 Nelson ME, Fischer EC, Dilmanian FA, Dallal GE, Evans WJ. A 1-year walking program and increased dietary calcium in postmenopausal women: effects on bone. *Am J Nutr* 1991; **53**: 1304–11.

68 Smith EL, Reddan W, Smith PE. Physical activity and calcium modalities for bone mineral increase in aged women. *Med Sci Sports Exerc* 1981; **13**: 60–4.

69 Dalsky GP, Stocke KS, Ehsani AA, Slatopolsky E, Lee WC, Birge SJ. Weight-bearing exercise training and lumbar bone mineral content in postmenopausal women. *Ann Intern Med* 1988; **108**: 824–8.

70 Heikkinen J, Kurtilla-Matero E, Kyllonen E, Vuori J, Takula T, Vaananen HK. Moderate exercise does not enhance the positive effect of estrogen on bone mineral density in postmenopausal women. *Calcified Tissue Int* 1991; **49**: 583–4.

71 Ayalon J, Simkin A, Leichter I, Raifmann S. Dynamic bone loading exercises for postmenopausal women. Effect on the density of the distal radius. *Arch Phys Med Rehab* 1987; **68**: 280–3.

72 Pruitt LA, Jackson RD, Bartells RL, Lehnhard HJ. Weight-training effects on bone mineral density in early post-menopausal women. *J Bone Min Res* 1992; **7**: 179–85.

73 Revel M, Mayoux-Benhamou MA, Rabourdin JP, Bagheri F, Roux C. One-year psoas training can prevent lumbar bone loss in postmenopausal women: a randomized controlled trial. *Calcified Tissue Int* 1993; **53**: 307–11.

74 Rundgren A, Aniansson A, Ljungberg P, Wetterqvist H. Effects of training program for elderly people on mineral content of the heel bone. *Arch Gerontol Geriatr* 1984; **3**: 243–8.

75 Berard A, Bravo G, Gauthier P. Meta-analysis of the effectiveness of physical activity for the prevention of bone loss in postmenopausal women. *Osteoporosis Int* 1997; **7**: 331–7.

Part 2
Aspects of Human Performance

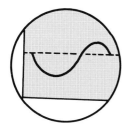

Chapter 2.1
Recovery after Training — Inflammation, Metabolism, Tissue Repair and Overtraining

JAN FRIDÉN, RICHARD L. LIEBER,

MARK HARGREAVES & AXEL URHAUSEN

Classical reference

Fridén J, Lieber RL. Structural and mechanical basis of exercise-induced muscle injury. *Med Sci Sports Exerc* 1992; **24**: 521–530.
The figure illustrates the generalized relationship between muscle length, force and velocity. To achieve a given force 'plane', a variety of sarcomere lengths/ velocity combinations are possible. If this generalized relationship is restricted to constant lengths, a force–velocity curve is obtained (Fig. 2.1.1, right panel). If it is restricted to constant velocities, a length–tension curve is obtained (left panel). Slight differences in length and velocity between adjacent sarcomeres during lengthening, due to the steepness of the lengthening portion of the force–velocity relationship, may make the forces vary considerably. A stress imbalance can lead to distension or disruption of cytoskeletal components interconnecting sarcomeres causing more or less severe myofibrillar disorganization.

Muscle inflammation and repair after exercise-induced injury
Exercise-induced muscle injury is a common problem

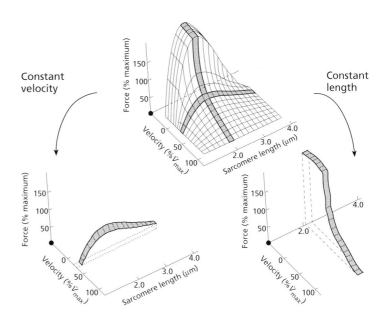

Fig. 2.1.1

in, and can account for, significant disability. Most subjects improve over time, but some develop more long-lasting symptoms. Delayed soreness after unaccustomed exercise is very common. Numerous studies have demonstrated that muscle damage and muscle soreness are more common following exercise involving eccentric contractions (i.e. lengthening of activated muscle) than after isometric or concentric contractions [1–4]. Muscle fiber disruption, of the kind occurring after eccentric exercise, would be expected to provide a significant inflammatory stimulus. However, since the inflammation process, which involves proteolysis by infiltrating neutrophils and macrophages, can itself cause damage in excess of that originally experienced by the tissue, it can be argued that prevention of inflammation would improve muscle status following injury.

How is inflammation involved in muscle injury?

It has been shown that after a bout of eccentric exercise, muscle maximum force generation continues to decline for several days. These data suggest that the initial mechanical events of exercise trigger subsequent events which result in further muscle injury. Tidball summarized in an excellent review the events following muscle injury cells [5]. Mononucleated cells are activated by injury, and then provide the chemotactic signal to circulating inflammatory cells. Three subsequent stages of inflammation were postulated. First, neutrophils rapidly invade the muscle lesion and promote inflammation by releasing cytokines that attract and activate additional inflammatory cells. Neutrophils may further damage the injured muscle by releasing oxygen free radicals that can damage cell membranes. In the next stage, there is an increase in macrophages that phagocytose debris. The final stage is presumed to be an increase of a second subpopulation of macrophages that are associated with muscle regeneration. Tidball concluded that only few of the inflammatory cell subpopulations have been conclusively demonstrated to function in injured muscle *in vivo*.

In a rabbit muscle injury study, a large population of muscle fibers with extreme sizes and abnormal shapes were observed [6]. These fibers were frequently invaded by inflammatory cells and the abnormal fibers

were consistently stained heavily with ATPase at pH 10.3, suggesting that such fibers were of the fast type. Based on the large proportion of very small muscle fibers, 3 days post exercise was the time point when most of the degeneration and regeneration was taking place. A stereotypic topographic distribution of the injuries was seen: the majority of injuries occurred in the superficial muscle region while the deeper regions were relatively spared. Simultaneous to the phagocytosis of the damaged muscle fibers, the satellite cells located within the basal lamina of the original cell undergo activation and begin to proliferate (Fig. 2.1.2). Regenerating myotubes differentiate and produce contractile and cytoskeletal material necessary for the alignment of the sarcomeres [7] (Plate 1, facing p. 192).

A series of reports from the laboratory of Bill Evans have suggested that inflammation plays a major role in the subsequent injury that occurs after eccentric contraction. For example, Cannon *et al.* [8,9] measured an increase in numbers and activity of circulating neutrophils following eccentric contraction and hypothesized that inflammation-mediated events result in a greater muscle damage then would occur if inflammation were inhibited. This, of course, has great implications with regard to the use of anti-inflammatory medications for muscle injury treatment.

Two experiments have tested the role of free radical formation in producing muscle injury. In the first, Zerba and coworkers treated mice with a single intraperitoneal injection of superoxide dismutase (SOD) which is an antioxidant believed to be involved in damaging muscle after eccentric exercise. Zerba *et al.* [10] found that animals treated with SOD produce higher muscle forces 3 days after exercise than untreated animals. This was in spite of the observation that SOD had no effect on animals immediately after the exercise protocol. They concluded that the free radical production and subsequent tissue damage contributed to the injury seen in untreated muscles 3 days after exercise. Use of vitamin E as the antioxidant demonstrated the opposite effect. Since vitamin E attenuates free radical propagation and is particularly effective in stopping initiation and propagation of lipid peroxidation, Warren *et al.* [11] tested the hypothesis that vitamin E supplementation would attenuate soleus muscle injury. They fed a vitamin E-enriched

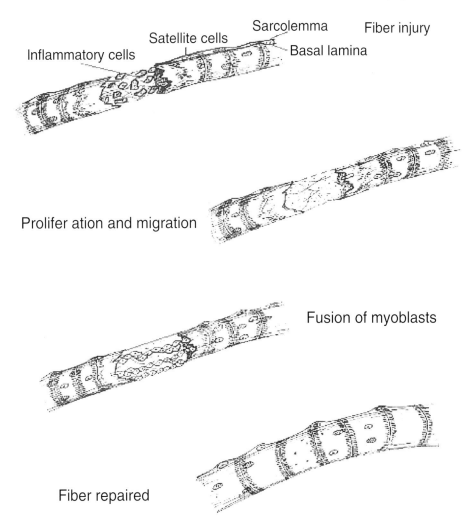

Inflammatory cells   Satellite cells   Sarcolemma   Fiber injury
                                         Basal lamina

Prolifer ation and migration

Fusion of myoblasts

Fiber repaired

Fig. 2.1.2 Muscle cytological events after injury. In the first 2 days after injury leukocytes and macrophages infiltrate into the damaged region. Mononucleated satellite cells fuse together and form newly multinucleated myotubes that further develop to striated myofibers.

diet to exercising rats, and documented a significant increase in muscle vitamin E levels and decreased muscle susceptibility to oxidized stress. However, vitamin E supplementation did not attenuate injury as measured by changes in contractile or metabolic factors. The vitamin E study was performed on a predominantly slow muscle while the SOD study was performed on a predominantly fast muscle. Since muscle injury can predominantly affect specific fiber types [12] these results may reflect a fiber type-specific phenomenon. Ward and coworkers reported that cytokines, interleukin 1 and tumor necrosis factor, released from macrophages have direct stimulatory effects on oxygen radical formation in neutrophils and may 'prime' macrophages for enhanced oxygen radical responses [13].

Non-specific anti-inflammatory (NSAID) drugs may prevent muscle injury

Muscle fiber disruption after exercise would be expected to provide a significant inflammatory stimulus. In addition, the continued tension decrease following

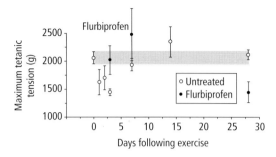

Fig. 2.1.3 Time course of tibialis anterior muscle force change for flurbiprofen-treated (closed circles) and untreated (open circles) muscles. Note the early protective and late detrimental effect of flurbiprofen. Hatched bar represents time period of NSAID administration. Stippled bar represents mean ± SEM of normal tibialis anterior muscle maximum tetanic tension (from [14]).

the initial tension drop (Fig. 2.1.3) suggests that an inflammatory process may be involved after the initial injury. However, since the inflammation process which includes proteolysis by infiltrating neutrophils and macrophages can itself cause damage in excess of that originally experienced by the tissue, it could be argued that prevention of inflammation would improve muscle status following injury. Using a rabbit skeletal muscle model following eccentric contraction-induced muscle injury it was demonstrated that a flurbiprofen-treated group recovered remarkably compared to non-treated, eccentrically exercised muscles after only 3 days and 7 days, but then showed a significant decline in torque generation after 28 days. This represents a short-term benefit but a detriment from a slightly longer term perspective after NSAID treatment. Thus, flurbiprofen-treated muscles demonstrated increased muscle strength at the early time periods but depressed strength after 28 days.

Immunohistochemical changes in muscles subjected to NSAID treatment were significantly different from the non-treated muscles described above. First, NSAID treatment greatly attenuated muscle injury 3 days postexercise as evidenced by a dramatically reduced area fraction of desmin negative. It was obvious that flurbiprofen administration attenuated the inflammatory reaction as evidenced by decreased serum levels of circulating white blood cells, decreased numbers of infiltrating neutrophils and macrophages, and decreased serum levels of creatine kinase—a marker for muscle fiber injury [14].

Metabolism during recovery from exercise

There are a number of important metabolic processes that occur during recovery from exercise. These include the restoration of intramuscular creatine phosphate (CP) and glycogen levels, removal of metabolites such as lactate, and protein synthesis for the repair of muscle damage and/or increased muscle mass.

CP resynthesis

Postexercise CP resynthesis occurs rapidly with a half-time of 50–60 s and is important for the recovery of power-generating capacity following intense exercise [15]. It is critically dependent upon oxygen availability [16,17] and CP resynthesis is faster in individuals with a high muscle oxidative capacity. Dietary creatine supplementation increases muscle CP levels and postexercise CP resynthesis and is associated with enhanced high-intensity exercise performance [18]. For these reasons there has been considerable interest in this compound as an ergogenic aid. The resynthesis of CP and restoration of myoglobin oxygen stores contribute to the elevated oxygen consumption during postexercise recovery. Other potential factors include elevated heart rate and ventilation, increased body temperature, elevated catecholamines, glycogen synthesis and uncoupling of mitochondrial respiration. The long-held view that lactate oxidation contributes to an increase in postexercise oxygen consumption does not appear to be correct [19].

Lactate removal

The major fates of lactate during postexercise are oxidation and conversion to other substrates such as glucose, glycogen and certain amino acids. Contracting skeletal muscle can oxidize lactate, explaining why an active recovery facilitates lactate removal [20]. Lactate removal is enhanced in individuals with high muscle oxidative capacity and capillary density. Although lactate can be converted to glycogen in skeletal muscle, it appears to be a minor substrate and blood glucose is the major glycogenic precursor following intense exercise [21].

Glycogen resynthesis

During the postexercise period, restoration of muscle glycogen reserves is crucial for recovery of exercise

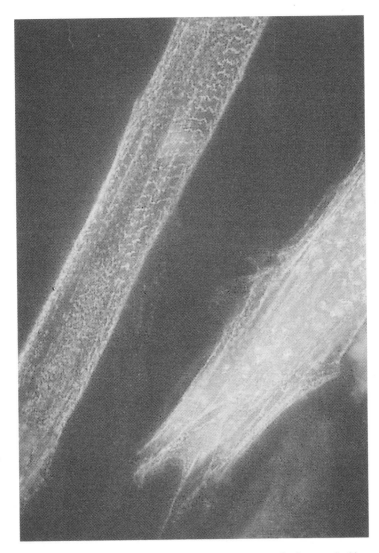

Plate 1 Satellite cell/myotube isolated from normal biceps muscle of a 12-week-old human fetus and cultured for 2 weeks. Stain is against α-actinin. A striated band pattern is seen in the myotube to the left. (Photograph courtesy of Jari Ikaheimonen.)

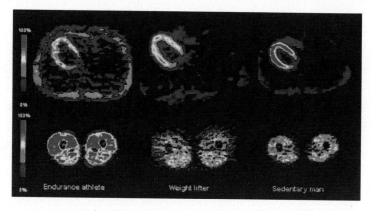

Plate 2 Examples of [18F] FDG images as determined with PET and callibrated to the same counts pixel level. Cross-sections are shown of thoracic region (upper images) and femoral region (lower images).

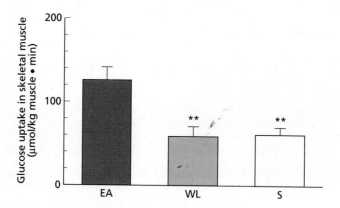

Plate 3 Rate of glucose uptake in skeletal muscle of an endurance athlete (EA), weight lifter (WL) and sedentary person (S) as measured with positron emission tomography (PEG) and 2–deoxy–2–[18F]fluoro–D–glucose (18F]FDG). **$P < 0.01$ vs. EA.

capacity [22,23]. Glucose is the major precursor for glycogenesis and must be supplied in the postexercise period to facilitate muscle glycogen resynthesis. The lowering of muscle glycogen levels during exercise results in activation of the enzyme glycogen synthase [24] and the more extensive the glycogen depletion, the greater the activation of glycogen synthase and glycogen storage [25]. The control of muscle glycogen synthesis is shared between sarcolemmal glucose transport and glycogen synthase [26], and glycogen storage in the immediate postexercise period is positively correlated with both glycogen synthase activity and total GLUT-4 content [27,28]. Complete restoration of muscle glycogen stores following prolonged, strenuous exercise requires ingestion of carbohydrate and usually takes at least 20–24 h. The optimal amount of carbohydrate ingested appears to be about 0.7–1 g/kg body mass/2 h, i.e. 50–70 g every 2 h for a 70-kg person, aiming for a 24-h intake of 500–600 g [29,30]. Glucose and sucrose are better substrates for glycogen storage than fructose [29] and ingestion of high glycemic index (GI) carbohydrates results in a greater 24-h muscle glycogen storage than ingestion of low GI carbohydrates [31]. It has been suggested that the inclusion of protein in a carbohydrate supplement, to enhance insulin secretion, increases glycogen storage in the early postexercise period [32], although this strategy is not supported by other studies [33,34]. In addition, over a 24-h recovery period the overall composition of the diet appears not to have a major influence, provided total carbohydrate intake is adequate [35]. Postexercise muscle glycogen storage is impaired by muscle damage [36,37], which can only partially be overcome by increasing dietary carbohydrate intake [36]. The mechanisms responsible for this are thought to include disruption of the sarcolemma, resulting in impaired insulin signaling and action [38,39], and a decrease in skeletal muscle GLUT-4 [40].

Protein metabolism

Both resistance and endurance exercise have profound effects on postexercise protein metabolism [41]. Although there are conflicting results in the literature, most likely as a consequence of methodologic differences and limitations, it appears that exercise increases both protein degradation and synthesis. Obviously, for muscle growth or repair, there must be a positive net

muscle protein balance such that muscle protein synthesis exceeds degradation. Both processes are increased following exercise and the increased muscle protein synthesis appears critically dependent upon the intramuscular availability of amino acids [41]. Although amino acid ingestion has been shown to enhance postexercise muscle protein synthesis [42], it is premature to recommend specific protein supplementation for the promotion of muscle anabolism [43]. In addition to promoting postexercise muscle glycogen resynthesis, the ingestion of carbohydrate may also contribute to enhanced postexercise protein anabolism [44,45].

Overtraining

The efficiency of physical training essentially depends on the intensity, volume, periodization and modus of the training stimuli. After each bout of physical exercise a catabolic phase exists at first with decreased tolerance of effort, characterized by reversible biochemical, hormonal, immunologic and other changes. During the succeeding anabolic phase, characterized by a higher adaptive capacity and enhanced performance capacity, the next training stimulus can be effective ('supercompensation'). A well-balanced training programme therefore needs to include adequate phases of regeneration and regular assessments of the current individual tolerance of stress.

Overtraining — definitions and symptoms

The expression 'overtraining' means rather the process of overload training, which seems to be necessary to induce a higher level of adaptation. A dysbalance between the overall strain and the actual individual tolerance of stress at first leads to short-term overtraining, called 'overreaching', which can be reversed by a more prolonged (several days up to 2–3 weeks) period of regeneration. More prolonged exposure to the stressors with concomitant deficit of regeneration and/or an individual sensitivity can induce an 'overtraining syndrome' (OTS; synonym 'staleness'). OTS can be defined as a decrease in sports-specific performance and increased fatigue in training and competition without organic disease, accompanied by more or less pronounced vegetative complaints, which occurs despite a maintained or even increased training load and which after regeneration lasts longer than approximately 2–3 weeks. It is important to exclude other causes of a decreased performance, especially infectious diseases—especially mononucleosis and other, usually viral, infections, in some cases even a concomitant endo- or myocarditis; electrolyte disturbances (e.g. an iron-deficiency anaemia); and endocrine (e.g. thyroidal or adrenal) disorders.

The predominantly sympathetic ('basedowoid') form of the OTS is more easily recognized because of more pronounced vegetative complaints including increased heart rate, sleep disorders, emotional instability and organ-related complaints, while the so-called parasympathetic ('addisonoid') form of the OTS is typically associated with less obvious symptoms and a more depressive mood state [46,47]. However, fairly often a mixture of these two forms exists, because the sympathetic type in fact represents an early transient stage shifting to the chronic parasympathetic one.

Even today, the frequent occurrence of this feared 'illness' of the athlete (the term 'malfunction' or 'dysregulation' would be more suitable) is still in stark contrast with the diagnostic tools currently available. It is true that in the literature a great number of parameters, which can be conspicuous in the state of OTS, are mentioned. However these data are frequently based more on anecdotal reports than on experimentally well founded findings.

Causes of overtraining

During exercises performed at intensities well below the aerobic–anaerobic transition, no significant rise in blood lactate levels and only slight stimulation of sympathetic activity is to be expected. In contrast to this, prolonged training performed at intensities exceeding the range of the individual anaerobic threshold is characterized by a disproportionate increase of stress hormone (free epinephrine and norepinephrine) concentration, and thus the frequency of such training sessions should be limited [48]. Repetitive or prolonged training with higher lactate concentrations and thus high adrenergic stimulation without adequate regenerative periods, and the higher stress resulting from repetitive competitions represent the most frequent causes of an OTS. The question as to whether an increase in intensity [49,50], or in volume of training [51] is more likely to induce an OTS seems a theoretical one because both factors are interdependent determi-

nants of the overall training load. For example, an increase in training mileage ('volume') at intensities around the anaerobic threshold in fact represents an increase of the overall training intensity. Another exercise-related factor believed to increase the likelihood of OTS is training monotony [52].

Apart from training and competitions, however, 'external' stressors with regard to professional and social lives as well as diseases and injuries should also be taken into consideration. For example, we are often confronted with an OTS in students during the examination period or after a too short period of recovery after infectious diseases, when coaches or athletes fear that too much training time is being lost, or when advice as to the recommended regeneration period during the week after a training camp is not respected.

Altered mood profile and vegetative complaints

The regular assessment of psychological profiles may be helpful in the estimation of an athlete's current exercise tolerance, provided that a genuine collaboration and positive motivation can be ensured. Studies have shown significantly disturbed psychological profiles in OTS: while large changes in the fatigue and vigour scores of the profile of mood state follow increases in training load, high depression scores represent typical markers in OTS [53]. The self-condition scale according to Nitsch especially reveals altered indices of the capacity to act and fatigue in overreaching, and additionally of mood, in OTS [50]. The slightly elevated subjective rating of perceived exertion during standardized exercise [54] seems rather too insensitive for diagnosis of an OTS in practice.

The predominant subjective symptom during OT seems to be the feeling of 'heavy legs', rather than muscle soreness, not only during unusually low exercise intensities but also during daily routine activities. Furthermore athletes frequently complain about chronic fatigue and sleep disturbances.

Ergometric testing and blood chemistry in overtraining

The objective assessment of the decrease in performance, which should still represent the cardinal symptom of an OTS, is often difficult under laboratory conditions. It requires a specific and standardized testing methodology, the comparison with individual reference values respecting the periodization of training and knowledge with regard to the mechanisms of the limited energy supply during OTS.

The existing findings indicate at least in endurance-trained athletes an impairment of the speed endurance or short-term endurance with impaired anaerobic lactic capacity, which is primarily recognized when reaching the limit of physical exhaustion [47,50,51,55,56]. The maximal blood lactate concentration in these exercises lasting approximately 30 s–30 min is typically reduced in OTS. In a so-called 'stress test'—a short-term endurance exercise test on the cycle ergometer performed at the intensity of 110% of the individual anaerobic threshold—the exercise duration to exhaustion was significantly decreased by 27% during OTS [50]; other authors report a decrease in running time at 18 km/h on the treadmill by 29% [56]. During incremental graded test procedures, however, the maximal power output and the maximal oxygen uptake are not always decreased in overtrained athletes [47,50,51,57]. The anaerobic alactic performance also seems not to be affected systematically.

Although the lactate–performance curve and the anaerobic threshold certainly represent useful tools in the monitoring of training, in the case of an overtrained athlete they may be misleading. In a case report of an Olympic rower presenting himself in a state of OTS [Fig. 2.1.4], the maximal lactate concentration during rowing competition and the corresponding performance were clearly decreased in comparison to his usual values. This could be confirmed in an incremental graded exercise test on the rowing ergometer. However, during submaximal workloads his lactate–performance relationship as well as the corresponding calculation of anaerobic threshold remained unchanged or even slightly shifted towards higher levels of power output. This represents a fairly typical finding in OTS [50,54]. The simple orientation on anaerobic threshold curves would dramatically overestimate the actual exercise tolerance of an overtrained athlete.

Nonetheless, useful information can be obtained from the lactate–performance curve in OTS. In another case report, the blood lactate profile of a female long-distance runner, who presented with decreasing performance as the result of OTS, revealed that she

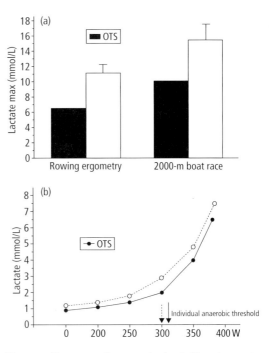

Fig. 2.1.4 Case report of an overtrained male Olympic rower in comparison with his normal values (means and SD). (a) Maximal blood lactate concentrations after incremental graded test on rowing ergometer and 2000 m competition in boat. (b) Lactate–performance relationship during submaximal rowing ergometry (from Urhausen A, Kindermann W. Aktuelle Marker für die Diagnostik von überlastungszuständen in der Training praxis. *Deutsch Z Sportmed* 2000; **51** 226–33).

had usually performed her endurance training with a running velocity up in the sharply sloping section of the lactate curve, exceeding by about 17% the individual anaerobic threshold and therefore situated clearly above the range of maximal lactate steady state. In doing so, her running training was predominantly performed at an intensity leading to a pronounced anaerobic energy yield and sympathetic drive, and thus to increased lactate acidosis [47].

The individual maximal heart rate is often—but only slightly—decreased and confirms the complaint of overtrained athletes that they are not able to train at their usual heart rate level. The described reduction of the respiratory exchange ratio [50,54] can be explained by a shift of the energy delivering processes to an enhanced metabolization of fat subsequent to a reduced supply of carbohydrates without depleted intramuscular glycogen stores [54].

There are no typical changes in blood substrates or enzyme activities in OTS [49–51,56–58]. The substrates (urea, glucose, uric acid, creatinine, ferritin) and enzyme activities (creatine kinase) usually remain within or return to normal ranges. They may, however, be used to differentiate an OTS from other performance-limiting conditions and to prevent an OTS by indicating current overload training characterized by negative nitrogen balance with enhanced gluconeogenesis (urea) or high mechanical muscular strain (creatine kinase).

Pathomechanism and hormonal dysregulation in overtraining

Endogenous hormones are of major importance both in supplying energy during physical exercise and in the adaptations during the subsequent regeneration period. Depending on the duration and intensity of physical exercise, and during periods of intense training or repetitive competitions, changes in the blood concentrations of hormones can be measured, e.g. a decrease of the testosterone/cortisol ratio, which indicate an alteration of the anabolic–catabolic balance and can be reversed by regenerative measures. Some authors even describe correlations to training-induced changes of strength [59]. However, it seems that the testosterone/cortisol ratio reflects more the actual physiological strain of training than an OTS [48,58]. Cortisol concentrations in particular at rest may change in a biphasic way showing an increase during acute overload training and decreasing in chronic OTS.

Hormonal changes also seem to play an essential role with regard to the pathomechanisms involved in OTS, where peripheral and central mechanisms seem to have a synergetic effect. The various (supra)hypo-thalamopituitary–target gland axes are influenced by peripheral stimuli and at the same time they modulate peripheral functions [48,60]. This may even include the synthesis of Na^+/K^+-ATPase and thus the maintenance of the membrane potential which depends on glucocorticoid action (Fig. 2.1.5) [61]. In support of an impaired central regulation theory, a significantly decreased maximum exercise-induced rise of pituitary hormones such as adrenocorticotrophic (ACTH) and growth hormone, and cortisol during OTS in comparison to the normal state has been shown [49]. These re-

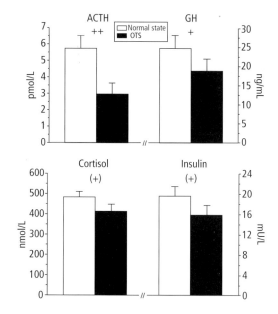

Fig. 2.1.5 Impaired maximal exercise-induced increase of adrenocorticotrophic hormone (ACTH), growth hormone (GH) ($P < 0.01$), cortisol and insulin ($P < 0.1$) after exhaustive short-endurance cycle ergometer test with an intensity of 110% of the individual anaerobic threshold ('stress test') in 15 endurance athletes (means and SD) [61].

sults represent an interesting parallel to the reduced response of ACTH, growth hormone and cortisol to an insulin-induced hypoglycemia in four overtrained marathon runners, in whom the pituitary response to luteinizing hormone (LH) was unaffected [62]. It was concluded that a hypothalamic dysfunction exists in OTS. These impaired hormonal reactions of over-trained athletes contrast with the usually increased levels induced by training.

The sympathoadrenergic system may also be involved in the pathogenesis of OTS [60,63]. The OTS resembles a disturbed autonomic regulation, which in its parasympathicotonic, chronic form presents with a depressed intrinsic sympathetic activity (basal nocturnal urinary excretion) and a diminished maximal exercise-induced secretion of free (nor)epineph-rine leading to an impaired full mobilization of anaerobic lactic reserves [47,51]. In addition a decreased β-adrenoreceptor density indicating a loss of sensitivity of target organs to catecholamines is suggested [60].

Multiple studies indicate that a chronic exposure to

repetitive stress leads to altered neuroendocrine regulation and possibly inhibits the pulsatile hypothalamic hormonal release through the corticotrophin-releasing hormone, opioid and/or serotonic pathways. A popular hypothesis [64] suggests an amino acid imbalance in blood with increased brain tryptophan uptake and transformation to 5-hydroxytryptamin (serotonin) which may cause mood changes and central fatigue. However, modifications of the central serotonergic system by physical activity are very complex [65] and it still remains uncertain whether data mainly derived from prolonged exercise in rats can be transferred to chronically overtrained athletes.

Overall it is suggested that the described hormonal changes represent self-protecting feedback mechanisms preventing the fatigued organism against further stress-related exhaustion. With regard to a 'hormonal monitoring of training', however, the difficult standardization of hormonal measurements in training practice should be taken into consideration.

'Treatment' of overtraining syndrome

The first treatment of overreaching is rest and the removal of external stressors. After several days, however, regenerative to shorter extensive endurance training sessions are suitable, which should not exceed the maximal exercise intensity achievable without an increase of blood lactate (aerobic lactate threshold). It is strongly recommended that the training modalities are varied by including other sports in order to prevent training monotony. Coordinative and pure speed sessions (very short high intensity with long periods of rest) can be allowed as soon as the athlete is able to exercise at an adequate level. It is only after a normal and stable exercise tolerance has been restored, which in OTS takes weeks to—in the worst cases—even months, that the training intensity should reach and finally exceed the range of anaerobic threshold over a longer period of time (intensive endurance, intensive intervals and speed endurance training sessions). Effective treatment of OTS by pharmacologic agents (e.g. antidepressants) or food supplements has not yet been proven.

Summary

Muscle injury after high-load exercise is of varying severity in different muscle types, can be fiber-type specific, primarily due to fiber strain in the acute phase, and is exacerbated by the postinjury inflammation process itself, resulting in an additional delayed injury to the muscle. Mononucleated cells are activated and provide the chemotactic signal to circulating inflammatory cells. Neutrophils invade the muscle lesion and promote inflammation by releasing cytokines that attract and activate additional inflammatory cells. Several important metabolic processes occur during recovery and repair after exercise. These include restoration of intramuscular creatine phosphate (CP) and glycogen levels, removal of metabolites such as lactate, and protein synthesis for the repair of muscle damage and/or increased muscle mass. During the subsequent anabolic phase characterized by a higher adaptive capacity and enhanced performance capacity, the next training stimulus can be very effective ('super-compensation') and a well-balanced training program therefore needs to include adequate phases of regeneration and regular assessments.

Multiple choice questions

1 *Muscle damage and muscle soreness are most common following exercise involving:*
a eccentric muscular activity
b isometric muscular activity
c fatiguing muscular activity
d concentric muscular activity
e regular muscular activity.

2 *The satellite cells are located:*
a within the cytoplasm of the muscle fiber
b at the Z-disk level of the muscle fiber
c underneath the basal lamina of the muscle fiber
d in the endothelial cells
e in the endomysial collagen network.

3 *How long does it take for complete replenishment of glycogen stores after prolonged, strenuous exercise:*
a 20–24 h
b 20–30 min
c 5–7 days
d 7–10 days
e <10 min.

4 *Typical results of blood parameters at rest in studies with overtrained athletes are:*
a decreased glucose
b increased urea
c increased creatine kinase

d increased ammonia

e none of these results is typical.

5 *What are typical results of blood hormone parameters in studies with endurance athletes in a state of chronic overtraining syndrome:*

a decreased testosterone/cortisol ratio at rest

b increased epinephrine at rest and after maximal exercise

c increased growth hormone after maximal exercise

d decreased growth hormone after maximal exercise

e decreased adrenocorticotrophin (ACTH) after maximal exercise.

References

1 Armstrong RB, Ogilvie RW, Schwane JA. Eccentric exercise-induced injury to rat skeletal muscle. *J Appl Physiol* 1983; **54**: 80–93.

2 Evans W, Meredith CN, Cannon JG, Dinarello CA, Frontera WR, Hughes VA, Jones BH, Knuttgen HG. Metabolic changes following eccentric exercise in trained and untrained men. *J Appl Physiol* 1985; **61**: 1864–8.

3 Faulkner JA, Jones DA, Round JM. Injury to skeletal muscles of mice by force lengthening during contractions. *Q J Exp Physiol* 1989; **74**: 661–70.

4 Fridén J. Changes in human skeletal muscle induced by long term eccentric exercise. *Cell Tissue Res* 1984; **236**: 365–72.

5 Tidball JG. Inflammatory cell response to acute muscle injury. *Med Sci Sports Exerc* 1995; **27**: 1022–32.

6 Fridén J, Lieber RL. Segmental muscle fiber lesions after repetitive eccentric contractions. *Cell Tissue Res* 1998; **293**: 165–71.

7 Carlson BM, Faulkner JA. The regeneration of skeletal muscle fibers following injury: a review. *Med Sci Sports Exerc* 1983; **15**: 187–98.

8 Cannon JG, Meydani SN, Fielding RA, Fiatarone MA, Meydani M, Farhangmehr M, Orencole SF, Blumberg JB, Evans WJ. Acute phase response in exercise. II. Associations between vitamin E, cytokines, and muscle proteolysis. *Am J Physiol* 1991; **260**: R1235–R1240.

9 Cannon JG, Orencole SF, Fielding RA, Meydani M, Meydani SN, Fiatarone MA, Blumberg JB, Evans WJ. Acute phase response in exercise. interaction of age and vitamin E on neutrophils and muscle enzyme release. *Am J Physiol* 1990; **259**: R1214–R1219.

10 Zerba E, Komorowski TE, Faulkner JA. Free radical injury to skeletal muscles of young, adult and old mice. *Am J Physiol* 1990; **258**: C429–C435.

11 Warren JA, Jenkins RR, Packer L, Witt EH, Armstrong RB. Elevated muscle vitamin E does not attenuate eccentric exercise-induced muscle injury. *J Appl Physiol* 1992; **72**: 2168–75.

12 Lieber RL, Fridén J. Selective damage of fast glycolytic muscle fibers with eccentric contraction of the rabbit tibialis anterior. *Acta Physiol Scand* 1988; **133**: 587–8.

13 Ward PA, Warren JS, Johnson KJ. Oxygen radicals, inflammation, and tissue injury. *Free Rad Biol Med* 1988; **5**: 403–8.

14 Mishra DK, Fridén J, Schmitz MC, Lieber RL. Antiinflammatory medication after muscle injury. A treatment resulting in short-term improvement but subsequent loss of muscle function. *J Bone Joint Surg (Am)* 1995; **77**: 1510–9.

15 Bogdanis GC, Nevill ME, Boobis LH, Lakomy HKA, Nevill AM. Recovery of power output and muscle metabolites following 30 s of maximal sprint cycling in man. *J Physiol* 1995; **482**: 467–80.

16 Haseler LJ, Hogan MC, Richardson RS. Skeletal muscle phosphocreatine recovery in exercise-trained humans is dependent on O_2 availability. *J Appl Physiol* 1999; **86**: 2013–8.

17 Sahlin K, Harris RC, Hultman E. Resynthesis of creatine phosphate in human muscle after exercise in relation to intramuscular pH and availability of oxygen. *Scand J Clin Lab Invest* 1979; **39**: 551–8.

18 Casey A, Constantin-Teodosiu D, Howell S, Hultman E, Greenhaff PL. Creatine ingestion favorably affects performance and muscle metabolism during maximal exercise in man. *Am J Physiol* 1996; **271**: E31–E37.

19 Roth DA, Stanley WC, Brooks GA. Induced lactacidemia does not affect post-exercise O_2 consumption. *J Appl Physiol* 1988; **65**: 1045–9.

20 Choi D, Cole KJ, Goodpaster BH, Fink WJ, Costill DL. Effect of passive and active recovery on the resynthesis of muscle glycogen. *Med Sci Sports Exerc* 1994; **26**: 992–6.

21 Bangsbo J, Madsen K, Kiens B, Richter EA. Muscle glycogen resynthesis in recovery from intense exercise in humans. *Am J Physiol* 1997; **273**: E416–E424.

22 Brewer J, Williams C, Patton A. The influence of high carbohydrate diets on endurance running performance. *Eur J Appl Physiol* 1988; **57**: 698–706.

23 Fallowfield JL, Williams C. Carbohydrate intake and recovery from prolonged exercise. *Int J Sport Nutr* 1993; **3**: 150–64.

24 Bak JF, Pedersen O. Exercise-enhanced activation of glycogen synthase in human skeletal muscle. *Am J Physiol* 1990; **258**: E957–E963.

25 Zachwieja JJ, Costill DL, Pascoe DD, Robergs RA, Fink WJ. Influence of muscle glycogen depletion on the rate of resynthesis. *Med Sci Sports Exerc* 1991; **23**: 44–8.

26 Azpiazu I, Manchester J, Skurat AV, Roach PJ, Lawrence JC. Control of glycogen synthesis is shared between glucose transport and glycogen synthase in skeletal muscle fibres. *Am J Physiol* 2000; **278**: E234–E243.

27 Hickner RC, Fisher JS, Hansen PA *et al.* Muscle glycogen accumulation after endurance exercise in trained and untrained individuals. *J Appl Physiol* 1997; **83**: 897–903.

28 McCoy M, Proietto J, Hargreaves M. Skeletal muscle GLUT-4 and postexercise muscle glycogen storage in humans. *J Appl Physiol* 1996; **80**: 411–5.

29 Blom PCS, Høstmark AT, Vaage O, Kardel KR, Mæhlum S.

Effect of different post-exercise sugar diets on the rate of muscle glycogen synthesis. *Med Sci Sports Exerc* 1987; **19**: 491–6.

30 Ivy JL, Lee MC, Brozinick JT, Reed MJ. Muscle glycogen storage after different amounts of carbohydrate ingestion. *J Appl Physiol* 1988; **65**: 2018–23.

31 Burke LM, Collier GR, Hargreaves M. Muscle glycogen storage after prolonged exercise. Effect of the glycemic index of carbohydrate feedings. *J Appl Physiol* 1993; **75**: 1019–23.

32 Zawadzki KM, Yaspelkis BB, Ivy JL. Carbohydrate–protein complex increases the rate of muscle glycogen storage after exercise. *J Appl Physiol* 1992; **72**: 1854–9.

33 Carrithers JA, Williamson DL, Gallagher PM, Godard MP, Schulze KE, Trappe SW. Effects of postexercise carbohydrate–protein feedings on muscle glycogen restoration. *J Appl Physiol* 2000; **88**: 1976–82.

34 Van Hall G, Shirreffs SM, Calbet JAL. Muscle glycogen resynthesis during recovery from cycle exercise: no effect of additional protein ingestion. *J Appl Physiol* 2000; **88**: 1631–6.

35 Burke LM, Collier GR, Beasley SK *et al.* Effect of coingestion of fat and protein with carbohydrate feedings on muscle glycogen storage. *J Appl Physiol* 1995; **78**: 2187–92.

36 Costill DL, Pascoe DD, Fink WJ, Robergs RA, Barr SI, Pearson D. Impaired muscle glycogen resynthesis after eccentric exercise. *J Appl Physiol* 1990; **69**: 46–50.

37 O'Reilly KP, Warhol MJ, Fielding RA, Frontera WR, Meredith CN, Evans WJ. Eccentric exercise-induced muscle damage impairs muscle glycogen repletion. *J Appl Physiol* 1987; **63**: 252–6.

38 Del Aguila LF, Krishnan RK, Ulbrecht JS *et al.* Muscle damage impairs insulin stimulation of IRS-1, PI 3-kinase, and Akt-kinase in human skeletal muscle. *Am J Physiol* 2000; **279**: E206–E212.

39 Kirwan JP, Hickner RC, Yarasheski KE, Kohrt WM, Wiethop BV, Holloszy JO. Eccentric exercise induces transient insulin resistance in healthy individuals. *J Appl Physiol* 1992; **72**: 2197–202.

40 Asp S, Daugaard JR, Richter EA. Eccentric exercise decreases glucose transporter GLUT-4 protein in human skeletal muscle. *J Physiol* 1995; **482**: 705–12.

41 Tipton KD, Wolfe RR. Exercise-induced changes in protein metabolism. *Acta Physiol Scand* 1998; **162**: 377–87.

42 Tipton KD, Ferrando AA, Phillips SM, Doyle D, Wolfe RR. Postexercise net protein synthesis in human muscle from orally administered amino acids. *Am J Physiol* 1999; **276**: E628–E634.

43 Wolfe RR. Protein supplements and exercise. *Am J Clin Nutr* 2000; **72**: 551S–557S.

44 Rasmussen BB, Tipton KD, Miller SL, Wolf SE, Wolfe RR. An oral essential amino acid–carbohydrate supplement enhances muscle protein anabolism after resistance exercise. *J Appl Physiol* 2000; **88**: 386–92.

45 Roy BD, Tarnopolsky MA, MacDougall JD, Fowles J, Yarasheski KE. Effect of glucose supplement timing on protein metabolism after resistance training. *J Appl Physiol* 1997; **82**: 1882–8.

46 Israel S. Die Erscheinungsformen des Übertrainings. *Sportmed* 1958; **9**: 207–9.

47 Kindermann W. Overtraining—expression of a disturbed autonomic regulation. *Deutsch Z Sportmed* 1986; **37**: 238–45.

48 Urhausen A, Gabriel H, Kindermann W. Blood hormones as markers of training stress and overtraining. *Sports Med* 1995; **20**: 251–76.

49 Urhausen A, Gabriel H, Kindermann W. Impaired pituitary hormonal response to exhaustive exercise in overtrained endurance athletes. *Med Sci Sports Exerc* 1998; **30**: 407–14.

50 Urhausen A, Gabriel H, Weiler B, Kindermann W. Ergometric and psychological findings during overtraining: a prospective long-term-follow-up study in endurance athletes. *Int J Sports Med* 1998; **19**: 114–20.

51 Lehmann M, Gastmann U, Petersen KG, Bachl N, Seidel A, Khalaf AN, Fischer S, Keul J. Training–overtraining: performance, and hormone levels, after a defined increase in training volume versus intensity in experienced middle- and long-distance runners. *Br J Sports Med* 1992; **26**: 233–42.

52 Foster C. Monitoring training in athletes with reference to an overtraining syndrome. *Med Sci Sports Exerc* 1998; **30**: 1164–8.

53 Morgan WP, Brown DR, Raglin JS, O'Connor PJ, Ellickson KA. Psychological monitoring of overtraining and staleness. *Br J Sports Med* 1987; **21**: 107–14.

54 Snyder AC, Kuipers H, Cheng B, Servais R, Fransen E. Overtraining following intensified training with normal muscle glycogen. *Med Sci Sports Exerc* 1995; **27**: 1063–70.

55 Callister R, Callister RJ, Fleck SJ, Dudley GA. Physiological and performance responses to overtraining in elite judo athletes. *Med Sci Sports Exerc* 1990; **22**: 816–24.

56 Fry RW, Morton AR, Garcia Webb P, Crawford GP, Keast D. Biological responses to overload training in endurance sports. *Eur J Appl Physiol* 1992; **64**: 335–44.

57 Bruin G, Kuipers H, Keizer HA, Vandervuisse GJ. Adaptation and overtraining in horses subjected to increasing training loads. *J Appl Physiol* 1994; **76**: 1908–13.

58 Kirwan JP, Costill DL, Flynn MG, Mitchell JB, Fink WJ, Neufer PD, Houmard JA. Physiological responses to successive days of intense training in competitive swimmers. *Med Sci Sports Exerc* 1988; **20**: 255–9.

59 Häkkinen K, Pakarinen AAI, En M, Kauhanen H, Komi PV. Relationships between training volume, physical performance capacity, and serum hormone concentrations during prolonged training in elite weight lifters. *Int J Sports Med* 1987; **8** (Suppl. 1): 61–5.

60 Lehmann M, Foster C, Dickhuth H-H, Gastmann U. Autonomic imbalance hypothesis and overtraining syndrome. *Med Sci Sports Exerc* 1998; **30**: 1140–5.

61 Viru A. *Hormones in Muscular Activity*, Vol. II. Boca Raton: CRC press, 1985: 51–6.

62 Barron JL, Noakes TD, Levy W, Smith C, Millar RP. Hypo-

thalamic dysfunction in overtrained athletes. *J Clin Endocrinol Metab* 1985; **60**: 803–6.

63 Hooper SL, Mackinnon LT, Gordon RD, Bachmann AW. Hormonal responses of elite swimmers to overtraining. *Med Sci Sports Exerc* 1993; **25**: 741–7.

64 Newsholme EA, Blomstrand E, McAndrew N, Parry-Billings M. Biochemical causes of fatigue and over-training. In: Shephard RJ, Astrand PO, eds. *Endurance in Sport*. The IOC Encyclopaedia of Sports Medicine, Vol. II. Oxford: Blackwell Scientific Publications, 1992: 351–64.

65 Chaouloff F. The serotonin hypothesis. In: Morgan WP, ed. *Physical Activity and Mental Health*. Washington: Taylor & Francis, 1997: 179–98.

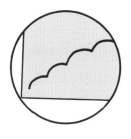

Chapter 2.2
Principles of Rehabilitation Following Sports Injuries: Sports-Specific Performance Testing

MALACHY McHUGH,

JENS BANGSBO &

JAN LEXELL

Classical reference

Wigerstad-Lossing I, Grimby G, Jonsson T, Morelli B, Peterson L, Renstrom P. Effects of electrical muscle stimulation combined with voluntary contractions after knee ligament surgery. *Med Sci Sports Exerc* 1988; **20**: 93–98.
This study compared the effect of electrical muscle stimulation combined with voluntary muscle contractions with a program of voluntary muscle contractions only during immobilization in casts after anterior cruciate ligament surgery. Patients were randomized into two groups: an experimental group and a control group. Postoperatively patients were immobilized for 3 weeks in a full leg cast with the knee flexed at an angle of 20–30° and then in a knee cast for another 3 weeks. Both groups had a standard program of quadriceps muscle contractions. In addition, the experimental group received electrical stimulation of the quadriceps muscle 4×10 min, 3 times a week, at a frequency of 30 Hz. During each stimulation, the patients were requested to contract the quadriceps muscle voluntarily as well. The 6-week period resulted in a significantly larger reduction in the knee extension isometric muscle strength in the control group than in the experimental group. The cross-sectional area of the quadriceps muscle was significantly less reduced during the immobilization period in the experimental

group than in the control group. Both the relative fiber area of type I fibers and the activity of citrate synthase and triphosphate dehydrogenase were significantly reduced in the control group during the immobilization period. These data demonstrate the impressive effects of immobilization on muscle tissue, and that electrical stimulation in combination with simultaneously performed voluntary contractions can limit some of the muscle weakness, muscle wasting and reduction in oxidative and glycolytic muscle enzyme activity during immobilization after knee ligament surgery (Fig. 2.2.1).

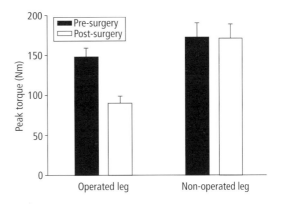

Fig. 2.2.1 Maximal isometric torque for knee extension at 30° before and after 6 weeks of immobilization during which the patients performed voluntary contractions combined with electrical stimulation (from Wigerstad-Lossing *et al.*, table 3.)

Introduction

Physical activity is unquestionably associated with numerous health benefits. However, while both the injury incidence and severity and type of injury may vary from one sport to another, there is clearly some inherent injury risk associated with almost all sports participation. Contact sports are more commonly associated with a greater risk of sudden traumatic injuries, while sports with repetitive, low-impact activity are characteristically linked to so-called overload/overuse injuries. When the injury has in fact been sustained, the optimal management includes formal rehabilitation, which is a currently growing specialty. It should be noted that some of the existing knowledge in the area of rehabilitation is based on tradition, clinical experience and extrapolations from animal models. Nevertheless, over the last decade this specialty has developed and is more and more incorporating science into the clinical decision-making process. While additional research in the area of rehabilitation is clearly needed, there is a growing body of literature that supports the use of active rehabilitation paradigms for decreased pain, reduced neural inhibition and early restoration of range of motion to achieve a fast return of muscle function. Additionally, the early return is usually to a performance at a preinjury level. While there is generally a lack of controlled randomized investigation our basic understanding of the process of tissue healing following injury and surgery, and tissue response to immobilization and inactivation, constitutes an important basis for protocols that currently define the most effective rehabilitation of different injuries.

Principles of rehabilitation of sports injuries

Athletes, athletic demands of various sports, different injuries and many other components contribute to making the rehabilitation of an individual with a specific injury a considerable challenge. Thus, it is difficult, if not impossible, to have a cookbook approach to the rehabilitation process. While specific rehabilitation protocols exist and may indeed be useful they should only serve as guidelines. It is not within the scope of this chapter to provide detailed descriptions of those many detailed rehabilitation protocols, but to provide the reader with some general guidelines to

rehabilitation, evaluation during rehabilitation and performance testing. Because of the multifactorial complexity of the rehabilitation process for a given athlete and injury it is valuable to follow a general framework that has emerged from clinical practice and consists of four principal components: evaluation, planning and intervention, and re-evaluation. The evaluation, which includes a thorough subjective history and objective examination, serves as the important basis for the rehabilitation process. The evaluation will result in a set of identified problems that a careful plan of intervention will try to address. Since the injury status will probably change more or less rapidly with time, it is paramount to re-evaluate the situation on a daily basis. This provides the clinician with important feedback about the progress of the rehabilitation and the effectiveness of the intervention plan. Moreover, it serves to let the clinician know when to progress the patient to the next phase, and finally it can provide the patient with feedback about the rehabilitation process.

A dynamic rehabilitation process is typically divided into three general time phases (see below) with specific goals and plans for each phase. In optimal circumstances the rehabilitation of a sports-related injury can be initiated immediately at the time of injury. This phase is commonly referred to as the acute/subacute phase. Thereafter follows the recovery phase during which the affected tissues are allowed to go through healing and repairing processes. During the recovery phase the clinical signs and symptoms will abate and finally disappear; however, the athlete is still not ready for return to preinjury athletic performance. Therefore, the third phase of the rehabilitation process follows which is referred to as the 'return to sport' phase. This phase involves the preparation for actual return to the preinjury level of sports participation and performance. The length of time for each of these three phases may vary due to numerous factors, such as the athlete's preinjury level of fitness, the severity and type of injury, whether or not surgery was performed, the type of activity that the athlete will return to, etc. Based on these various factors, the athlete's personal goals and the progression of the rehabilitation process the rehabilitation professional determines the advancement from one phase to the next, and thereby ensures the optimal restoration of function in a timely manner. By far the most common error which results in a setback or re-injury is when the athlete returns to sports participation too early. In this context it is paramount to teach the athlete to distinguish between that pain perceived as 'good pain' associated with training, i.e. that which is related to muscular exertion, and the pain which may be associated with too great a loading of the affected tissue which is detrimental to the healing process. Following an injury, general cardiovascular fitness, muscular strength, balance and coordination are affected, and the rehabilitation program should address all of these areas besides the actual injury. Finally, the rehabilitation process following an athletic injury should progress into a training program aimed at maintaining function and preventing re-injury. Prevention of injury is at times particularly important since some injuries, like muscle–tendon strains, are associated with a high re-injury risk. Altogether the rehabilitation process can be seen as a complete functional restoration program that allows the athlete to return to the previous level of performance as soon as possible after the injury. To ensure patient compliance it is necessary to educate the athlete about the rehabilitation process, the injury, tissue healing time, etc. An understanding of the rehabilitation process also helps minimize frustration on the part of the athlete.

Type of injury

Sports-related injuries are commonly categorized into (i) macrotrauma: trauma sustained during a direct sudden event, and (ii) microtrauma: trauma sustained from repetitive, often low-impact, activity. Macrotrauma often occurs in sports involving some form of impact, such as a contact sport (ice hockey or football) or a high-velocity sport (downhill skiing). Knee injuries involving anterior cruciate ligament tear, joint dislocation, rupture of muscle or soft tissue injury are common examples of macrotrauma. Microtrauma is frequently seen in athletes involved in track and field events and racket sports, and result from the inability of tissues like tendon and muscle to adapt to the imposed repetitive loading. Macrotraumas are often categorized as acute injuries, while microtraumas are chronic injuries.

Acute/subacute phase

During this phase, pain, swelling and joint effusion, reduced joint range of motion and muscle activation are common results. Injury to a joint or soft tissue always leads to reduced muscle activation across the injured joint or the joint adjacent to the soft tissue injury. This, in turn, causes atrophy, i.e. reduced muscle mass, which is typically most prominent in the antigravity muscles. As part of the postinjury pain treatment, the athlete is often immobilized, which adds further to the muscle atrophy. Together, this results in reduced muscle strength, which then becomes one of the main functional goals during the subsequent rehabilitation. This reduction in muscle volume stems from a reduction in the size of the individual fibers, with both fiber types being affected to varying degrees. Neurophysiologic factors also play a role in the immobilization-related atrophy and can be seen as a central activation failure, which is the inability to recruit and optimally activate motor units. The main focus during this phase is to alleviate injury signs and symptoms through surgical, medical, pharmacologic and physical modalities, including appropriately prescribed activity (Table 2.2.1). The application of these treatment modalities also promotes tissue healing and recovery by controlling the inflammation process and increasing blood flow. Cold as well as heat are common methods used together with various forms of electrical stimulation, acupuncture and pain medication. Although rest and/or immobilization is commonly prescribed during this phase, it is imperative that appropriate activities are simultaneously prescribed to maintain as much strength and range of motion as possible in the injured extremity, and to retard any decline in general strength and fitness. Criteria for advancement to the next phase include acceptable pain control, adequate pain tissue healing and range of motion. Pain is often used as the fundamental guiding factor by which the rehabilitation is progressed. A rule of thumb is that all activities that do not cause pain are allowed. This may be appropriate in most circumstances, but the rehabilitation professional should be aware of the subjectivity in the presentation of pain, which is commonly monitored on an individual basis on a 10-cm visual analog scale (VAS).

Table 2.2.1 The various phases of rehabilitation.

Acute/subacute phase

Aims
Elimination of injury-provoking activity
Reduction of injury signs and symptoms through appropriate
    treatment

Treatments
Rest and/or immobilization
Physical modalities
Surgery
Medication
Appropriately prescribed activity

Factors that determine advancement to the next phase
Pain
Tissue healing
Range of motion

Recovery phase

Aims
Elimination of indirect tissue dysfunction
Restoration of range of motion in injured limb
Maintenance of general fitness
Improvement of strength

Treatments
Physical methods
Medication
Flexibility, proprioception and neuromuscular control training
Progressive strengthening exercise

Factors that determine advancement to the next phase
Pain
Tissue healing
Range of motion
Flexibility
Strength

Return to sport phase

Aims
Restoration of normal flexibility, proprioception and
    neuromuscular control
Regaining of normal strength and endurance
Return to previous level of sports performance.

Treatments
Specific strength, power and endurance exercise
Sports-related technique-oriented activities

Criteria for return to sport
No pain
Normal flexibility, proprioception and neuromuscular control
Normalized strength and endurance
Appropriate technique and skill for the activity

Recovery phase

The main focus during the recovery phase is to restore function. The repair process of the injured tissue has been accomplished, but the strength and function of the tissue are not completely restored. During this phase, the tissue can be exposed to progressive loads to regain its previous function. An important concept in this phase is that the loading of the affected and adjacent tissue is gradual so that set-backs in the rehabilitation process are avoided. The length of this phase can vary considerably depending on the severity and type of injury, and therefore general and cardiovascular fitness should be maintained through the phase with, for example, aquatic exercises, cycling and strength training of uninjured limbs.

Return to sport phase

This final phase focuses entirely on the return to sports. Flexibility, strength, endurance, proprioception and neuromuscular control should be completely restored. This allows the athlete to gradually increase the demand on sports-specific skills. The aim is to perform exercises that are closely linked to the type of activity that the athlete will return to. Compared to the actual sport, many activities during this phase are submaximal. Hence, the athlete should gradually perform exercises that require maximum power, strength and endurance. Moreover, this phase should also emphasize the prevention part of the rehabilitation process.

Evaluation during rehabilitation

Numerous rehabilitation protocols have been described for the most common sports injuries. Many of these protocols progress patients based on specific evaluations at fixed time points following the injury or surgery. For example, the often cited 'accelerated' rehabilitation protocol following anterior cruciate ligament (ACL) reconstruction, by Shelbourne and Nitz [1], progresses patients to agility drills 5–6 weeks following surgery, if knee extension strength is ≥70% of the non-involved limb. Often the choice of such specific criteria for progression is somewhat arbitrary and based more on clinical experience than controlled research. In fact, the example above was based on the observation that most patients did not comply with a more conservative protocol but still had good outcomes. Progression in rehabilitation should be based on a combination of variables including the nature of the injury and/or surgery, the normal time course of tissue repair and the individual patient's ability to tolerate the progression. For example, following Achilles tendon repair, early full weight-bearing without immobilization is now advocated [2,3]. However, this is dependent on the strength of the repair and the patient's ability to regain motion. Even the strongest repair will be at jeopardy if the patient has not regained sufficient ankle motion and is forced to walk on a dorsiflexed ankle early after repair.

To properly evaluate a patient during rehabilitation it is necessary to know what component to evaluate, when and how to evaluate it and, finally, how to interpret the results. In the majority of cases rehabilitation is directed towards restoring joint range of motion (ROM), muscle function and joint stability, with the goal of returning the patient to sport without a significant risk of re-injury. It follows that most evaluation procedures assess joint motion, muscle function and joint stability during rehabilitation. Additionally performance-related tests are used to assess integrated musculoskeletal function in preparation for return to sports.

Evaluation of joint range of motion

Measurement error in goniometry

The goniometer is the gold standard tool for clinical measures of joint range of motion. These instruments are inexpensive and portable, and require only a basic understanding of anatomy for measurements on most joints. However, measurement sensitivity may preclude detection of clinically relevant effects, which is especially true when factoring in intertester variability. Therefore, it is advisable for the same tester to perform repeated measurements. It is also important for a tester to appreciate their own measurement error in absolute terms for specific motions. This allows the clinician to determine what magnitude of change they can accurately detect. This detection threshold can then be compared with what is thought to be a clinically relevant change for that measurement. Establishing 95% limits of agreement (LOA) according to the Bland–Altman approach [4] is a useful approach to determining absolute error [5]. For example, preoperative loss of passive knee extension is a risk factor for

postoperative motion loss and arthrofibrosis following ACL reconstruction [6]. It has also determined that the actual magnitude of the preoperative extension loss is not important, it is simply the presence or absence of full extension equal to the contralateral leg that identifies risk [7]. Thus, on a case-by-case basis, standard goniometric measurements lack the sensitivity to accurately detect ROM to 1°. Retrospectively measurement error was assessed for the tester in that study by establishing 95% LOA for the preoperative and postoperative measures on the non-involved limb. The non-involved ROM should not vary over time. The LOA was 3°, indicating that 95% of repeated measures were within 3° of the original measurement. Therefore, for knee extension ROM this tester had a detection threshold of 3°. Residual extension loss of >5° following ACL reconstruction is thought to be associated with patellofemoral pain [8]. It is desirable to have a detection threshold that is less than the clinically relevant measure. This approach to measurement error is much more useful than citing a unitless measurement of reliability such as a test–retest correlation or even a specific error in degrees as described by other researchers for a given test.

For many motions, error in goniometric assessment of ROM is primarily due to the subjective nature of assessing the limits of motion. For example, maximum straight leg raise ROM is a standard assessment of hamstring flexibility. Determination of maximum passive ROM is a function of the force applied by the tester and the subject's perception of the discomfort of the stretch. An increase in ROM may be attributed to a change in muscle tension due to a stretching intervention. However, the increased ROM may simply be due to increased force applied by the tester and increased tolerance of the stretch by the subject [9]. However, this issue may be less important in the rehabilitation setting where ROM is often limited by pain and the intervention is geared towards limiting the pain restriction rather than altering the mechanical properties of the tissues surrounding the joint. For example, shoulder flexion ROM may be limited by pain in patients with subacromial impingement. Rehabilitation is aimed at reducing the inflammation causing this pain thereby allowing a greater ROM. In this situation an alteration in tolerance of the stretch is the goal, not a source of measurement error.

Goniometric and alternative measurement techniques

Physical therapists routinely differentiate between passive and active ROM measurements. There are no specific criteria for when to perform one vs. the other, or which is more clinically important. For some motions active ROM may be more accurate because the tester can use both hands to orient the goniometer. For some passive measurements the tester must hold the limb in position while trying to orient the goniometer and this can lead to error. However, active ROM may sometimes be limited by agonist muscle weakness rather than by a restriction of joint motion. Active ROM can also be documented using electrogoniometers. However, these have not gained wide clinical use possibly due to issues of cost. They are most applicable to evaluating functional ROM with specific tasks but measurement error issues remain unresolved [10].

Fluid-based goniometers, working on the principle of a carpenter's level, have also been used to measure joint ROM [11]. While these have not gained popular use, the advent of digital levels in carpentry may provide a new perspective on their use in assessing joint angles.

Some alternative techniques negate the use of a goniometer. For example, internal rotation of the shoulder is frequently measured by noting the maximal vertebral level reached by the patient's thumb [12]. This may be an easier test for the orthopedist to perform than a goniometric measurement. The question of which is more clinically useful remains open to debate and may depend on the specific pathology. Subacromial impingement is associated with a loss of internal rotation and part of the rehabilitation process involves restoring this motion. The loss of internal rotation ROM is thought to be due to tightness in the posterior capsule. In accordance with this assumption, Tyler *et al.* [13] developed a specific measurement of posterior capsule tightness. This measurement involves measuring the height at which the elbow hangs when the arm is held in an abducted position in sidelying. Intratester reliability was good (intraclass correlation coefficient (ICC)=0.92–0.95). Patients with impingement had posterior capsule tightness that was related to the loss of internal rotation ROM [14]. It has yet to be determined if the posterior capsule measurement is more clinically relevant than internal rotation ROM.

Summary

For most orthopedic conditions accurate measurement of joint ROM during rehabilitation is essential for evaluating progress. Standard goniometry is the most accepted and practiced clinical method of assessing ROM. It is important to understand what represents a clinically relevant loss or change in ROM for a given motion and whether the measurement technique can actually detect such a change. To this end the clinician should determine their own threshold of detection for common goniometric assessments.

Evaluation of joint stability

Static joint stability

Most clinical assessments of joint stability involve manual tests that, for the most part, require a high degree of expertise. Furthermore these manual tests are graded according to a subjective assessment of joint motion. The Lachman test for anterior knee instability and the anterior drawer tests for ankle and anterior shoulder instability are common clinical tests. In general the clinician attempts to assess the magnitude of translation and the quality of the ultimate restraint to translation, i.e. 'end feel' or 'endpoint'. These tests are used initially to diagnose injuries and subsequently to assess the quality of repair. The improvement in joint stability with surgical repairs and reconstructions is usually so dramatic that clinical tests are often adequate for demonstrating improvements despite their subjective nature. However, clinicians often have difficulty in discriminating subtle but clinically important changes in joint stability that may occur during rehabilitation in non-surgical or postsurgical patients. One of the largest postoperative patient populations in sports medicine is the ACL reconstruction patient. The Lachman and pivot shift tests are performed routinely following surgery but it is unclear if these tests are sensitive to changes in graft integrity. For example, a change in Lachman grade from grade 1 (0–5 mm) to grade 2 (6–10 mm) may be difficult to detect in a large number of patients.

Various techniques have been developed to increase the sensitivity of clinical tests of joint stability. For example, stress radiography has been used to compare different ankle ligamentous reconstruction procedures [15]. More applicable to the rehabilitation setting is the use of knee arthrometers to assess graft integrity following ACL reconstruction. The KT-1000 is the most widely used arthrometer. It was initially developed to aid in the diagnosis of ACL injuries [16] and was also used to document improvements with surgery [17]. Serial KT-1000 testing is now practiced to assess changes in graft integrity during rehabilitation [1,18]. While this is definitely a useful adjunct to evaluation in rehabilitation there are several issues that must be taken into account when interpreting the results.

1 As with any test it is necessary to establish the measurement error. Robnett *et al.* [19] estimated that the KT-1000 may only be able to detect a 5-mm change from a previous measurement in anterior tibial displacement. While this is probably more sensitive than a manual Lachman test a more sensitive measure is probably needed to detect changes in graft integrity on a case-by-case basis. As previously mentioned with respect to goniometric measurements, it is beneficial for the clinician to get an estimate of their own detection threshold, which is about a 3-mm error for most experienced testers. This detection threshold will allow for detection of clinically relevant changes in graft integrity.

2 The original criteria for interpreting KT-1000 results were based on the ability to detect ACL disruption. A 3-mm or more side-to-side difference in anterior tibial displacement was established as a valid criterion for identifying ACL disruption [16]. However, this criterion clearly does not apply to patients who have had ACL reconstructions. As many as one-third of patients can be expected to have a difference of 3 mm or more following ACL reconstruction with a positive endpoint on Lachman tests and no associated symptoms [1,13]. Postoperatively a difference of less than 3 mm has been categorized as normal, 3–5 mm as loose, and greater than 5 mm as a failure [20]. However, this grading system has not been validated, since the clinical significance of a 3–5 mm difference or greater than 5 mm difference postoperatively has yet to be established. The value of postoperative KT-1000 measures has been questioned [21].

3 Little is known about what factors affect postoperative KT-1000 results. The tension at which the graft is set intraoperatively will impact on arthrometric stability measurements [22,23]. If the graft is set at a tension of 45 N or less patients will have greater postoperative laxity. A tension of 80–90 N results in greater stability. It is of note that preoperative KT-1000 measurements are related to postoperative KT-1000 results ($r = 0.47$, $P < 0.001$) [22]. Patients with greater preoperative side-to-side difference in anterior tibial displacement had greater postoperative laxity. About 10% of our patients have greater than 5 mm side-to-side difference following ACL reconstruction and three-quarters of these patients had greater than 5 mm difference preoperatively. It may not be possible to assess KT-1000 results following surgery without knowing a patient's preoperative scores. Evaluation criteria for following ACL reconstruction should include the side-to-side difference and the improvement from the preoperative measure. A side-to-side difference of greater than 5 mm with an improvement in anterior displacement of 3 mm or more should be regarded as a good surgical result.

The use of arthrometers to evaluate joint stability has been primarily limited to the knee joint. However, some attempts have been made to use a similar approach in documenting anterior shoulder instability [24,25]. The KT-1000 arthrometer has actually been used for this purpose with promising preliminary results [24]. However, the development of a joint-specific arthrometer is required. An ankle arthrometer has been developed for measuring anterior–posterior and inversion–eversion laxity [26]. Preliminary results in subjects without pathology showed good reliability but validity in a patient population has yet to be tested.

Dynamic joint stability

Although many surgical and non-surgical treatments are aimed at improving dynamic joint stability true objective tests of dynamic stability are lacking. Eastlack *et al.* [27] have developed a battery of dynamic hopping tests for ACL-deficient patients in an attempt to identify individuals who will not develop functional instability. These tests are an important adjunct to rehabilitation for the ACL-deficient patient. While the long-term prognosis for the patients identified as 'copers' remains unknown these tests may be useful in identifying patients for whom surgery can be delayed until the end of a season. This provides an opportunity to rehabilitate the patient to return to play within the season of injury, perform postseason surgery and return to play the following season again.

Balance training is an integral part of rehabilitation for ankle instability [28,29]. Surprisingly, a standardized clinical test has not been developed to assess balance in the athletic ankle instability population. Indices of postural sway based on center of pressure distribution on a force plate have been used to assess balance in patients with a history of ankle sprains, but these tests do not lend themselves to wide clinical use [28,30,31].

Proprioception training (often including balance exercises) is also an integral part of most upper and lower extremity rehabilitation programs. Proprioception refers to the combination of sensation of joint movement and sensation of joint position [32]. Ligamentous injuries are thought to result in a loss of proprioception while certain rehabilitation techniques are aimed at restoring proprioception (see [32] for review). The actual measurement of proprioceptive deficits usually involves testing the ability to detect the initiation of passive joint motion (kinesthesia) or the ability to detect when the joint has returned to a previous position (joint position sense). One of the advantages of these tests is that the movement velocities are extremely slow, thereby reducing measurement error. Information with respect to clinical significance of these proprioception deficits and functional carryover of training effects is lacking. A disadvantage of the measurement technique is that neuromuscular proprioceptive feedback is removed by the passive nature of the test movement. Given the potential for neuromuscular input and adaptation during dynamic motions [33] a more integrated approach to the measurement of proprioception may be needed.

Evaluation of muscle function

In sports medicine the restoration of muscle function is by far the largest component of most rehabilitation protocols. It follows that most standard evaluations of progress in rehabilitation primarily involve an assessment of muscle function. This assessment is usually based on some measurement of force-generating capacity. A multitude of factors must be considered when choosing a particular test of muscle function. Typical considerations include:

1 What are the specific muscle groups of interest?

2 Will voluntary or artificially stimulated contractions be evaluated?
3 Is the goal to assess strength, endurance or power?
4 Should the assessment involve concentric, eccentric or isometric contractions?
5 Will the test instrument be an isokinetic dynamometer, a free weight isotonic system, a hand-held dynamometer or some other device?
6 Will measurements be made throughout the range of motion?

The answer to each of these questions will vary depending on such factors as the specific injury, the patient's symptoms, the time post injury or surgery, the functional demands of the particular muscle group to be tested and accessibility of the instrumentation.

Affected muscle groups — linkage

It is often a mistake in rehabilitation to concentrate on the muscle groups surrounding the injured joints and ignore potential deficits in muscle groups along the kinetic chain. The concept of linkage describes how impairments in one area can impact other areas in the musculoskeletal system. This has been best illustrated in ankle pathology where proximal muscle groups may be more affected than the muscles surrounding the injured joint [34]. There is an association between ankle sprains and hip abduction weakness but it is unclear if it is a cause or effect. Furthermore, following ankle injury there is increased reliance on the hip musculature in response to ankle perturbations [35].

The role of neuromuscular stimulation techniques

For the most part muscle function testing will involve voluntary contractions. However, it is often difficult for clinicians to determine the extent to which muscle weakness is due to incomplete activation as opposed to atrophy. This is an important issue since the optimal treatment for reversing atrophy usually involves resistance exercises aimed at overloading the muscle. By contrast, the optimal treatment for improving muscle activation often involves modalities that reduce pain and/or joint effusion or stimulation protocols aimed at 'muscle re-education'. Specific stimulation protocols have been developed to identify the contribution of inhibition to muscle weakness [36]. Stimulation training protocols may be beneficial in conditions where inhibition limits training effects with voluntary contractions. For example, Snyder-Mackler *et al.* [37] demonstrated that electrical stimulation enhanced recovery of quadriceps strength following ACL reconstruction. However, strength recovery was highly dependent on the training contraction intensity which was limited by the patient tolerance of the associated discomfort. The electrically stimulated training intensity ranged from < 10% of the contralateral maximal voluntary contraction (MVC) to 70% of the contralateral MVC. The training dosage involved 15 stimulated contractions three times per week, from the second to the sixth postoperative week. Quadriceps strength was approximately 70% of the uninvolved side following 4 weeks of stimulation compared with approximately 50% in the comparison group. While these results are very encouraging, the question of patient comfort remains a confounding factor. In a similar study Lieber *et al.* [38] found that patients could only tolerate electrical stimulation intensities sufficient to elicit contractions from 15% to 45% of MVC from 1 to 20 weeks following ACL reconstruction. Not surprisingly, electrical stimulation did not prove better than voluntary contractions.

In contrast to electrical stimulation, magnetic stimulation of peripheral nerves represents a relatively painless alternative to electrical stimulation which has a wide application in musculoskeletal rehabilitation. Polkey *et al.* [39] demonstrated that single magnetic pulses to the femoral nerve could be used to objectively assess muscle strength and fatigue in both normal subjects and patients with known muscle weakness. However, they did not quantify contraction intensities elicited from stimulation trains resulting in tetanic contractions. The technology is now available to deliver trains of pulses to peripheral nerves to elicit tetanic contractions for as long as 10 s. This offers the potential to deliver supramaximal contractions to assess strength independently of neural inhibition and to train muscles which cannot be fully activated voluntarily. This technology was recently applied in a group of subjects without pathology [40]. Magnetic stimulation of the femoral nerve elicited torques of 70% MVC with minimal discomfort. The magnitude of torque response was inversely related to the subject's percentage body fat. The primary limitation to eliciting greater torques was related to specifications of the unit

rather than to subject tolerance. With the addition of more booster units, higher frequencies and intensities could be used and should produce even higher torque levels. However, at present this technology is too expensive for wide clinical use and the software applications are not conducive for training protocols.

Strength, endurance and power

A common misconception is that decreased muscle strength (weakness) and decreased muscle endurance (increased fatigability) occur concomitantly following injury and associated disuse. However, muscle strength and endurance are at best unrelated and may in fact be inversely related. Snyder-Mackler *et al.* [41] found that quadriceps weakness following ACL reconstruction was inversely related to reduced fatigue. The rate of torque decline (fatigue) during sustained electrically stimulated submaximal knee extension contractions was markedly less on the involved side compared to the non-involved side 4 weeks following surgery. The results were recently confirmed in the same patient population using voluntary contraction and electromyographic indices of fatigue [42]. Both studies point to the possibility of selective fast-twitch fiber atrophy as a mechanism for the observed effects. The clinical relevance of these findings is that quadriceps endurance exercises are not indicated following ACL reconstruction.

The fact that a weak muscle may be less fatigable can be seen as a functional adaptation to counteract the increased demands placed on it. During repetitive activity a weak muscle will be working at a higher relative intensity than a contralateral normal muscle for a given absolute load. Thus the weak muscle can be expected to fatigue more rapidly because it is working at a higher relative intensity. The fatigue resistance (apparent in the weak muscle when tested at similar relative loads) may help to offset the fatigue induced by working at a higher relative intensity.

Muscle endurance exercise are often used in rehabilitation to prepare patients for the specific demands of their sports. These exercises are an important part of the sport-specific phase of rehabilitation. It is important that the chosen exercises are as sport specific as possible since endurance exercises have been shown to be very task specific with minimal carryover to related tasks [43]. Task specificity [43] and poor measurement reliability (compared with strength tests) [44] may limit the efficacy of standardized endurance tests in rehabilitation.

The disassociation between strength and endurance, apparent in patients following ACL reconstruction, is also apparent in patients with low back pain. In this condition patients present with normal strength but decreased endurance [45]. Thus endurance-type training is indicated for this patient population.

Muscle power is frequently overlooked in rehabilitation. Many dynamic sports require the ability to produce high muscle forces in a minimal amount of time. For these activities performance is dependent on muscle power rather than muscle strength. While high load is optimal for strength training the optimal load for power training is dependent on the force–velocity relationship of the muscles involved. For isolated muscles the relationship of muscle force to the velocity of contractile shortening is an inverse hyperbolic curve. Muscle force is highest during low-velocity movements and lowest during high-velocity movements. In contrast the relationship of muscle force to muscle power is parabolic. Maximum muscle power occurs in the midportion of the force–velocity curve at muscle forces of 30–40% of maximum. Training studies have demonstrated that high-velocity training with loads equal to 30–40% MVC result in the greatest gains in power. Clinically, the force–velocity relationships for single joint movements can be estimated according to the relationship of torque to angular velocity. Based on this relationship a power curve can be calculated from which an optimal training intensity can be set for power training.

Contraction type

The contraction type to be tested is to some extent dependent on the test instrument used. For the most part clinicians can decide between purely concentric, eccentric or isometric tests or reciprocal concentric/eccentric tests. Isokinetic dynamometers provide the greatest freedom of choice in this regard. Measurement error is an important consideration in choosing the appropriate contraction type. However, a definitive statement cannot be made regarding differences in measurement error between each of the three contraction types. Error will be affected by the joint being tested, the muscle group and the chosen contraction velocity. Generally slow-speed concentric and isometric contractions are thought to be the most reproducible [46]. Clinical factors may dictate the choice of contraction type. For example, isometric strength at 30° was used to quantify quadriceps weakness in the early postoperative phase following ACL reconstruction [42]. The potential for pain during testing was reduced by testing in a position of minimal patellofemoral compression. This could have also been achieved by testing concentrically at high speed, but this may be a less reproducible test. High-speed eccentric testing may be more informative in assessing recovery from a muscle strain [47] but may also have increased risk of re-injury. Often concentric testing is preferred because of the low muscle forces relative to eccentric and isometric contractions. There is also less post-test muscle damage with concentric testing. If the goal of a test is to assess fatigability eccentric contractions are not appropriate since eccentric contractions are much more fatigue resistant than concentric and isometric contractions [48,49].

Test instrument

Typically strength can be measured on an isokinetic dynamometer, a free weight isotonic system or a hand-held dynamometer or manually using a clinical grading system. While the latter method is common in physicians' offices or on the sidelines of sports events the other more objective measures are usually available in the rehabilitation setting. The primary disadvantage of isotonic testing using a free weight apparatus is that repeated trials are required to establish a one-repetition maximum. However, this type of testing replicates the training situation for many patients. Although isokinetic dynamometry is regarded as the gold standard for strength assessment, hand-held dynamometers offer a much less expensive, portable alternative. The reliance on tester strength limits the number of motions that can be tested, but hand-held dynamometry has been used effectively to test shoulder abduction [50], shoulder internal–external rotation and scapular-plane elevation [51,52], and hip flexion, abduction and adduction [53]. In fact measurement error was shown to be better for hand-held dynamometry than for isokinetic testing of shoulder abduction strength [50].

Functional range of motion

One of the advantages of isokinetic testing is that it allows maximal force to be generated throughout the full range of motion unlike isotonic or single-angle isometric testing. However, only rarely do clinicians take advantage of this and actually examine strength through the functional range. For example strength loss with aging is associated with a loss of functional range of the muscles [54]. The shape of the length–tension curve (i.e. the ROM–torque curve) may be revealing of functional capacity following injury but has not been studied specifically. A decreased slope on the descending limb of the length–tension curve (i.e. increased force-generating capacity at increased muscle lengths) is thought to protect muscle from exercise-induced damage [55]. It may be useful to examine the ability to generate muscle force at increased muscle lengths in patients recovering from muscle strains.

Summary

Specific tests for assessing joint ROM, joint stability and muscle function encompass most of the types of evaluations performed in rehabilitation. Functional tests, such as the single-limb hop test used in ACL reconstruction rehabilitation, provide an additional picture of general musculoskeletal performance. When such tests are applied they should involve a combination of a sport-specific demand and an injury-specific demand. Using the same example of the single-limb hop test for the ACL reconstruction patient this involves a sport-specific demand for high friction sports such as basketball and soccer but is an inappropriate test for a low friction sport such as ice hockey [56].

Certain general principles apply to evaluations regardless of whether they involve testing ROM, stability or muscle function. The measurement error should be sufficiently low to enable the detection of clinically relevant effects. Clinicians should establish their own detection thresholds for commonly used clinical tests. Interpretations of test results must be based on established criteria validated for the specific patient population. As new tests and new testing equipment are developed to provide more accurate or less expensive assessments, these tests should be validated with the appropriate patient populations.

Fitness training and performance testing

Introduction

In order to understand how to perform fitness training and how to evaluate performance in a sport the physical requirements of the sport have to be understood. Performance in any sport is determined by the athlete's technical, tactical, physiological and psychosocial characteristics (Fig. 2.2.2). These elements are closely linked to each other, e.g. the full technical quality of an athlete may not be exploited if the athlete's physical capacity is low.

The physical demands in a sport are very much related to the activities of the athlete. In some sports continuous exercise is performed with either a very high or moderate intensity during the entire event, such as a 100-m and a marathon run, respectively (Fig. 2.2.3). In other sports like soccer and basketball athletes perform different types of exercise ranging from standing still to maximal running, and the intensity can vary at any time. Under optimal conditions the physical demands of the sport are closely related to the athlete's physical capacity, which can be divided into the following categories: (i) the ability to perform prolonged exercise (endurance); (ii) the ability to exercise at high intensity; (iii) the ability to sprint; and (iv) the ability to develop a high power output (force) in single actions during competition such as kicking in soccer and jumping in basketball (Fig. 2.2.2). The basis for performance within these categories is the characteristics of the cardiovascular system and the muscles, combined with the interplay of the nervous system. These characteristics are to a great extent determined by genetic factors but they can also be developed by training. A number of environmental factors such as temperature and for outdoor sports the weather and the surface of the competition ground also influence the demands on the athletes.

In some sports it is important that the athlete has a very high capacity within at least one of the categories of physical capacity to perform at a top level; for example, a marathon runner needs a high endurance capacity, but not a well-developed ability to produce a high power output. In other sports, such as team sports, an athlete may need an all-round fitness level. In such sports an athlete with a moderate en-

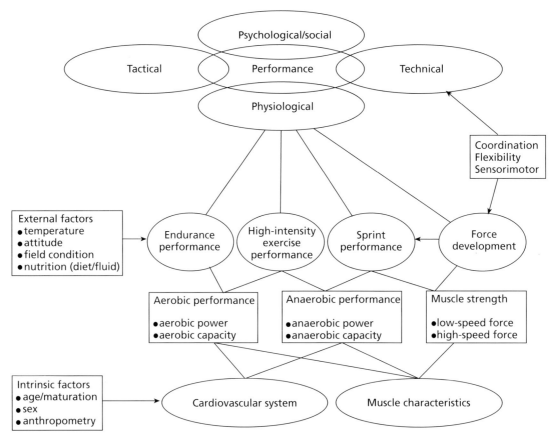

Fig. 2.2.2 Physiologic factors within a holistic model of performance in a sport. Performance is determined by an athlete's tactical, psychological/social, technical and physiologic capacity. These areas overlap and influence each other. The physiologic factors can be divided into several performance abilities (upper part). These are dependent on variables, which in part can be evaluated separately (middle part). Cardiovascular capacity, neural factors and muscle characteristics comprise basic components of physiologic performance that are determined by both intrinsic biologic make-up and training status (lower part). Performance in a sport can also be influenced by various external factors, including environment and nutrition.

durance capacity may to some extent compensate for this weakness by having good capabilities in other areas relevant to the sport, e.g. a high technical standard or good sprinting ability.

In the remainder of this chapter the general principles of training to improve specific aspects of physical performance will be described and the use of tests to evaluate performance of athletes will be discussed.

Physiology of training

Fitness training in any sport has to be focused on the demands of the sport, and in many sports it has to be multifactorial in order to cover the different aspects of

physical performance in the sport. To be able to fulfil these requirements, it is useful to divide fitness training into a number of components related to the purpose of the training (Fig. 2.2.4). The terms aerobic and anaerobic training are based on the energy pathway that dominates during the activity periods of the training session (Fig. 2.2.3). Aerobic and anaerobic training represent exercise intensities below and above the maximum oxygen uptake, respectively. However, in some sports like ball games, in which the ball is used in the fitness training, the exercise intensity for an athlete varies continuously, and some overlap exists between the two categories of training.

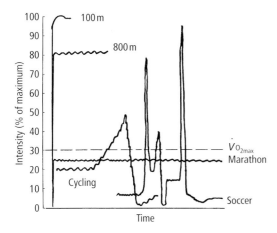

Fig. 2.2.3 Examples of exercise intensities in various sports. Note that the intensity corresponding to the maximum oxygen uptake ($\dot{V}_{O_2\,max}$) is around 30% of maximal intensity, but there are large individual differences.

The separate components within fitness training are briefly described below. They include aerobic, anaerobic and specific muscle training.

Aerobic training

Aerobic training causes changes in central factors such as the heart and blood volume, which result in a higher maximum oxygen uptake [57]. A significant number of peripheral adaptations also occur with this type of training [58]. The training leads to a proliferation of capillaries and an elevation of the content of mitochondrial enzymes, as well as the activity of lactate dehydrogenase 1–2 isozymes (LDH_{1-2}). Furthermore, the mitochondrial volume and the capacity of one of the shuttle systems for NADH are elevated [59]. These changes cause marked alterations in muscle metabolism. The overall effects are an enhanced oxidation of lipids and sparing of glycogen, as well as a lowered lactate production, both at a given and at the same relative work-rate [58].

The optimal way to train central and peripheral factors is not the same. Maximum oxygen uptake is most effectively elevated by exercise intensities of 80–100% of $\dot{V}_{O_2\,max}$ (20–40% of maximal intensity; Fig. 2.2.3). For a muscle adaptation to occur, an extended period of training appears to be essential, and therefore, the mean intensity needs occasionally to be below 80% of $\dot{V}_{O_2\,max}$. This does not imply that high-intensity training does not elevate the number of capillaries and mitochondrial volume in the muscles engaged in the training, but that the duration of this type of training is often too short to obtain optimal adaptations at a local level.

The dissociation between changes in $\dot{V}_{O_2\,max}$ and muscle adaptation by means of training and detraining is illustrated by results from two studies. In one study long-distance runners were kept inactive for 2 weeks (first week with the leg in a cast) which did not result in a change in $\dot{V}_{O_2\,max}$ [60]. On the other hand, the detraining period led to a 25% decrease in performance in an exhaustive run (from about 18–13.5 min) which was associated with a 24% lowering of the activity of the oxidative enzyme succinate dehydrogenase (SDH). During the following 2 weeks of retraining $\dot{V}_{O_2\,max}$ did not change, whereas performance and SDH were still lowered by 10 and 20%, respectively. The level of inactivity does not have to be as extreme as in this study to have a marked effect on performance and muscle respiratory capacity. In another study top-class soccer players abstained from training for 3 weeks [61]. It was found that $\dot{V}_{O_2\,max}$ was unaltered, whereas performance in a field test was lowered by 8%, and there was a reduction in oxidative enzymes of 20–30% (Fig. 2.2.5).

The recovery processes from intense exercise are related both to the oxidative potential and to the number of capillaries in the muscles [62]. Thus, aerobic training not only improves endurance performance of an athlete, but also appears to influence an athlete's ability to repeatedly perform maximal efforts. The overall aim of aerobic training is to increase the work-rate during competition, and also in ball games to minimize a decrease in technical performance as well as lapses in concentration induced by fatigue towards the end of a game. The specific aims of aerobic training are as follows.

• To improve the capacity of the cardiovascular system to transport oxygen. Thus, a larger percentage of the energy required for intense exercise can be supplied aerobically, allowing an athlete to work at higher exercise intensity for prolonged periods of time.

• To improve the capacity of muscles specifically used in the sport to utilize oxygen and to oxidize fat during prolonged periods of exercise. Thereby, the limited store of muscle glycogen is spared and an athlete can

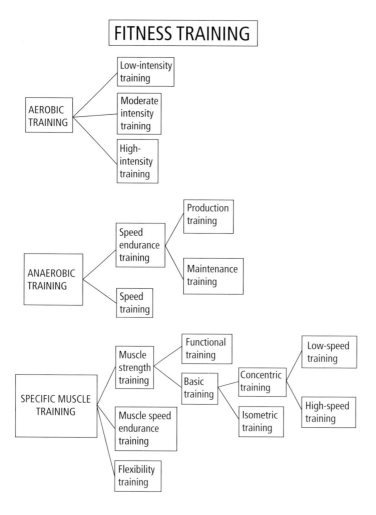

Fig. 2.2.4 Components of fitness training.

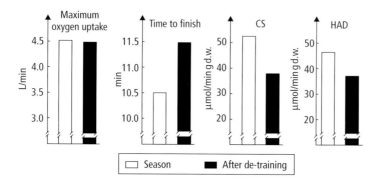

Fig. 2.2.5 Maximum oxygen uptake, performance in a field test, activities of oxidative enzymes citrate synthase (CS) and β–hydroxy–CoA–dehydrogenase (HAD; involved in fat oxidation) of Danish top–class soccer players during the season and after 3 weeks of holiday.

exercise at a higher intensity towards the end of a game.
• In some sports, like team sports, to improve the ability to recover after a period of high-intensity exercise. As a result, an athlete requires less time to recover before being able to perform in a subsequent period of high-intensity exercise.

Components of aerobic training

Aerobic training can be divided into three overlapping components: *aerobic low-intensity training (aerobic$_{LI}$)*, *aerobic moderate-intensity training (aerobic$_{MO}$)* and *aerobic high-intensity training (aerobic$_{HI}$)* (Fig. 2.2.4). Table 2.2.2 illustrates the principles behind the various categories of aerobic training, which take into account the fact that in some sports the training may be performed as a game, and thus the heart rate of the athlete may frequently alternate during the training.

During aerobic$_{LI}$ athletes perform light physical activities, such as jogging and low-intensity games. This type of training may be carried out the day after a competition or the day after a hard training session to help the athlete to return to a normal physical state. Aerobic$_{LI}$ may also be used to avoid athletes getting into a condition known as 'overtraining' in periods involving frequent training sessions (maybe even twice a day) and a busy competitive schedule.

The purpose of aerobic$_{MO}$ is to elevate the capillarization and the oxidative potential in the muscle (peripheral factors). Thus, the functional significance is an optimization of substrate utilization and thereby an improvement in endurance capacity. One of the aims of aerobic$_{HI}$ is to improve central factors such as the pumping capacity of the heart which is closely related to $\dot{V}_{O_{2\,max}}$. These improvements increase an athlete's capability to exercise repeatedly at high intensities for prolonged periods of time.

Anaerobic training

In a number of sports an athlete performs activities that require rapid development of force, such as sprinting, quickly changing direction or jumping. Also, in many sports the lactate-producing energy system (glycolysis) is highly stimulated during periods of competition. Therefore, the capacity to perform high-intensity exercise may specifically have to be trained. This can be achieved through anaerobic training.

Anaerobic training results in an increase in the activity of creatine kinase (CK) and glycolytic enzymes; such an increase implies that a certain change in an activator results in a higher rate of energy production of the anaerobic pathways. Intense training does not appear to influence the total creatine phosphate (CP) pool, but it allows the muscle glycogen concentration to be elevated, which is of importance for performance during repeated high-intensity exercise [63]. The capacity of the muscles to release and neutralize H^+ (buffer capacity) is also increased after a period of anaerobic training [64]. This will lead to a lower reduction in pH for a similar amount of lactate produced during high-intensity exercise. Therefore, the inhibitory effects of H^+ within the muscle cell are smaller, which may be one of the reasons for a better performance in high-intensity tests after a period of anaerobic training. Another important effect of the anaerobic training is an increased activity of the muscle

Table 2.2.2 Principles of aerobic training.

	Heart rate				Oxygen uptake	
	% of HR_{max}		Beats/min		% of $\dot{V}_{O_{2\,max}}$	
	Mean	Range	Mean*	Range*	Mean	Range
Low-intensity training	65	50–80	130	80–160	55	20–70
Moderate-intensity training	80	65–90	160	130–180	70	55–85
High-intensity training	90	80–100	180	160–200	85	70–100

*If HR_{max} is 200 beats/min.

Table 2.2.3 Principles of anaerobic training.

	Duration		Intensity	Number of repetitions
	Exercise	**Rest**	**Intensity**	**Number of repetitions**
Speed training	2–10 s	>10 times the exercise duration	Maximal	2–10
Speed endurance training				
Production	15–40 s	>5 times the exercise duration	Almost maximal	2–10
Maintenance	20–90 s	1–3 times the exercise duration	High	2–10

Na^+/K^+ pumps resulting in a reduced net loss of potassium from the contracting muscles during exercise, which may also lead to increased performance [65].

The overall aim of anaerobic training is to increase an athlete's potential to perform high-intensity exercise. The specific aims of anaerobic training are summarized below.
• To improve the ability to act quickly and to produce power rapidly. Thus, an athlete reduces the time required to react and elevates sprinting performance.
• To improve the capacity to produce power and energy continuously via the anaerobic energy-producing pathways. Thereby, an athlete elevates the ability to perform high-intensity exercise for longer periods of time.
• To improve the ability to recover after a period of high-intensity exercise, which is particularly important in ball games. As a result, an athlete requires less time before being able to perform maximally in a subsequent period of exercise, and in ball games the athlete will therefore be able to perform high-intensity exercise more frequently during a match.

Components of anaerobic training

Anaerobic training can be divided into *speed training* and *speed endurance training* (Fig. 2.2.4). The aim of speed training is to improve an athlete's ability to act quickly in situations where speed is essential. Speed endurance training can be further separated into two subcategories: *production training* and *maintenance training*. The purpose of production training is to improve the ability to perform maximally for a relatively short period of time, whereas the aim of maintenance training is to increase the ability to sustain exercise at a

high intensity. Table 2.2.3 illustrates the principles of the various categories of anaerobic training.

Anaerobic training must be performed according to an interval principle. During speed training the athletes should perform maximally for a short period of time (<10 s). The periods between the exercise bouts should be long enough for the muscles to recover to near-resting conditions, so as to enable an athlete to perform maximally in a subsequent exercise bout. In many sports, speed is not merely dependent on physical factors. It also involves rapid decision-making which must then be translated into quick movements. Therefore, in ball games speed training should mainly be performed with a ball. Speed drills can be designed to promote an athlete's ability to sense and predict situations, and the ability to decide on the opponents' responses in advance.

Through speed endurance training the creatine kinase and glycolytic pathways are highly stimulated. The exercise intensity should be high (>30% of maximal intensity; Fig. 2.2.3), to elicit major adaptations in the enzymes associated with anaerobic metabolism. In *production training* the duration of the exercise bouts should be relatively short (15–40 s), and the rest periods in between the exercise bouts should be comparatively long (2–4 min) in order to maintain a very high intensity during the exercise periods throughout an interval training session. In *maintenance training* the exercise periods should be 20–90 s and the duration of the rest periods should be one to three times longer than the exercise periods, to allow athletes to become progressively fatigued.

The adaptations caused by speed endurance training are mostly localized to the exercising muscles. Thus, it is important that an athlete performs move-

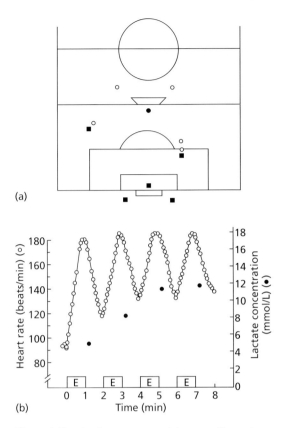

(a)

(b)

Fig. 2.2.6 Speed endurance soccer training game. Two against two with man-to-man marking and two goalkeepers. The players play for 1 min followed by 1 min of rest. Below is shown the heart rate and blood lactate response for a player. The high heart rate towards the end of the exercise periods and the high lactate levels show that the anaerobic system is heavily stimulated.

ments in a manner similar to those used during competition, e.g. an oarsman should train in the boat or on a rowing ergometer. In ball games this can be obtained by performing high-intensity games or drills with a ball. Figure 2.2.6 illustrates a soccer game within the maintenance category of speed endurance training. It also shows heart rate and blood lactate values for a player during the game, illustrating that the game fulfils the criteria for speed endurance training.

Specific muscle training

Specific muscle training involved training of muscles in isolated movements. The aim of this type of training

is to increase performance of a muscle to a higher level than can be attained just by participating in the sport. Specific muscle training can be divided into *muscle strength*, *muscle speed endurance* and *flexibility* training (Fig. 2.2.4). The effect of this form of training is specific to the muscle groups that are engaged, and the adaptation within the muscle is limited to the kind of training performed.

A brief description of muscle strength training is given below. Further information about strength training can be obtained in Chapter 1.4.

Strength training

In many sports there are activities which are forceful and explosive, e.g. high jumping, hiding in boxing and turning in ice hockey. The power output during such activities is related to the strength of the muscles involved in the movements. Thus, it is beneficial for an athlete in such sports to have a high level of muscular strength, which can be obtained by strength training.

Strength training can result in hypertrophy of the muscle, partly through an enlargement of muscle fibers. In addition, training with high resistance can alter the fiber type distribution in favor of fast-twitch fibers [66]. There is also a neuromotor effect of strength training and part of the increase in muscle strength can be attributed to changes in the nervous system. Improvements in muscular strength during isolated movements seem closely related to training speeds. However, significant increases in force development at very high speeds (10–18 rad/s) have also been observed with slow-speed high-resistance training [67].

One essential function of the muscles is to protect and stabilize joints of the skeletal system. Hence, strength training is also of importance in preventing both injuries and reoccurrence of injuries. A prolonged period of inactivity, e.g. during recovery from an injury, will considerably weaken the muscle. Thus, before an athlete returns to training after an injury, a period of strength training is needed. The length of time required to regain strength depends on the duration of the inactivity period but generally several months are needed. In a group of soccer players observed for 2 years after a knee operation, it was found that the average strength of the quadriceps muscle of the injured leg was only 75% of the strength in the other leg [68].

The overall aim of muscle strength training is to develop an athlete's muscular make-up. The specific aims of muscle strength training are:
• to increase muscle power output during explosive activities such as jumping and accelerating;
• to prevent injuries; and
• to regain strength after an injury.

Components of strength training
Strength training can be divided into *functional strength training* and *basic strength training* (Fig. 2.2.4). In functional strength training, movements related to the sport are used. The training can consist of activities in which typical movements are performed under conditions that are physically more stressful that normal. During basic strength training muscle groups are trained in isolated movements. For this training different types of conventional strength training machines and free weights can be used, but the body weight may also be used as resistance. Strength training should be carried out in a manner that resembles activities and movements specific to the sport. Based on the separate muscle actions the basic strength training can be divided into isometric, concentric and eccentric muscle strength training (Fig. 2.2.4). Several principles can be used in concentric strength training. Table 2.2.4 illustrates a principle which is based on determinations of five-repetition maximum (5 RM) and which allows for muscle groups to be trained at both slow and fast speeds.

Common to the two types of strength training is that the exercise should be performed with a maximum effort. After each repetition an athlete should rest a few seconds to allow for a higher force production in the subsequent muscle contraction. The number of repetitions in a set should not exceed 15. During each training session two to four sets should be performed with each muscle group, and rest periods between sets should be longer than 5 minutes. During this time the athletes can exercise with other muscle groups.

Training methods
A major part of fitness training in any sport should be performed in a manner closely related to the activities specific to that sport, e.g. with a ball in basketball, since this ensures that the specific muscle groups used in the sport are trained. In addition, in some sports the athletes will thus develop technical and tactical skills under conditions similar to those encountered during a match. Thirdly, this form of training usually provides greater motivation for the athletes compared to training not focused on the sport.

Individual physical demands must be considered when planning fitness training and a part of the fitness training may, even in team sport, be performed on an individual basis. The training should be focused on improving both the strong and weak abilities of an athlete. It is important to be aware of the fact that, due to hereditary differences, there will always be differences in the physical capacity of athletes, irrespective of training programs.

Table 2.2.4 Principles of muscle strength training.

	Workload	Number of repetitions	Rest between repetitions (s)	Number of sets
Concentric				
Low-speed	5RM*	5	2–5	2–4
High-speed	50% of 5RM	15	1–3	2–4
Isometric				
	85–100% of max maintained for 5–15 s	5–10	5–15	2–4

*RM, repetition maximum.

Evaluation of physical performance

This section will deal with various aspects of evaluation of physical performance and give a number of examples of tests that are relevant and easy to use.

Reasons for testing

Competition naturally provides the best test for an athlete but it is difficult to isolate the various components within the sport and get objective measures of performance. Fitness testing can provide relevant information about specific parts of a sport. Before selecting a test, clear objectives should be defined. There may be a number of reasons for testing an athlete:
- To study the effect of a training program.
- To motivate an athlete to train more.
- To give an athlete objective feedback.
- To make an athlete aware of the aims of the training.
- To evaluate whether an athlete is ready to compete.
- To determine the performance level of an athlete during a rehabilitation period.
- To plan short- and long-term training programs.
- To identify the weaknesses of an athlete.

Choosing a test

To obtain useful information from a test, it is important that the test to be performed is relevant and resembles the conditions of the sport in question. For example, a cycle test is of minor relevance for a swimmer.

There are a number of laboratory tests which evaluate various aspects of performance (Fig. 2.2.2) and are commonly used. These include determination of maximum aerobic power (maximum oxygen uptake) to evaluate the athlete's ability to take up and utilize oxygen as described in Chapter 1.1. A Wingate test consists of 30 s of maximal cycle exercise aiming at determining the maximum anaerobic power and ability to maintain a high power output. Strength measurements in which strength or power of an isolated muscle group is measured during either isometric, concentric or eccentric contractions are other laboratory tests often used. Such tests provide general information about the capacity of an athlete and may separate different performance levels of athletes within a sport. For example, for soccer players the

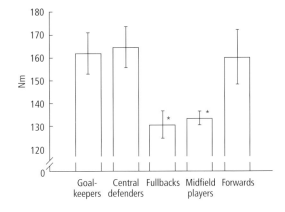

Fig. 2.2.7 Maximum knee extensor torque (Nm) under isokinetic loading at a velocity of 180°/s for Danish top-class soccer players in various positions. Means + SE are given.
* Significantly different from goalkeepers, central defenders and forwards.

strength produced by the knee extensors during an isokinetic movement at a velocity of 180°/s was significantly higher for goalkeepers, defenders and full-backs than for midfield players and forwards (Fig. 2.2.7). In some sport such general tests can provide information as to sport-specific requirements; e.g. to be a top-class cross-country skier a maximum oxygen uptake of higher than 80 mL/min/kg is needed.

Such classical laboratory tests may also be useful for comparisons of performance between various sports. However, they may only to a limited extent express the performance of the athlete during competition. For example, Fig. 2.2.8 shows that for 30 top-class soccer players there was no relationship between peak knee extensor power output and kick performance, suggesting that the strength of the knee extensors alone does not determine the final impact on the ball in a kick. Strength of other muscle groups, such as the hip muscles, may be important and technical skill is also a predominant factor in the soccer kick, which incorporates a complex series of synergistic muscle movements, involving the antagonistic muscles as well.

Being more specific to the sport will increase the validity of a test, i.e. the test result better reflects the performance of the athlete. Below are provided a number of examples of sport-specific tests that are simple to organize; some require special equipment in order to

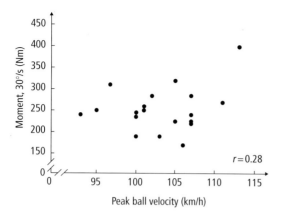

Fig. 2.2.8 Individual relationship between kick performance (peak ball velocity) and maximum knee extensor torque (Nm) under isokinetic loading at a velocity of 30°/s for Danish top-class soccer players.

simulate the activities in the sport and others require only simple materials.

Rowing performance

Rowing is characterized by a certain movement involving muscles of the whole body. A rowing ergometer has been developed in which it is possible to simulate the movement in the boat. Performance can be evaluated by measuring the total work performed within a given time, e.g. 6 min as in some races, or the time to exhaustion at a given external work rate [69]. To obtain further information about the oarsman a number of physiological measurements can be added to the test such as pulmonary oxygen uptake in which the rate of rise of oxygen uptake in the initial phase of exercise and the peak oxygen uptake during the rowing are determined. It is of no doubt that such a test has a high validity for rowing performance on water.

Running tests

One of the most widely used field tests is the Cooper test. In the Cooper test the participants run the furthest possible distance in 12 min. It is simple to perform, but it has the disadvantage that the athletes need to know how to tactically perform the test in order to obtain the best test result. It also requires a course with a distance of at least 200 m. Its popularity probably re-

sults from the fact that it is simple and a correlation between performance and $\dot{V}O_{2\,max}$ has been observed. However, the type of running in the test may only be relevant for track runners and they have the most simple test in any case, namely the competition. Furthermore, the relationship between the test and $\dot{V}O_{2\,max}$ may not be very useful, since in many sports, such as ball games, $\dot{V}O_{2\,max}$ is a poor marker of physical performance during competition.

The 'yo-yo' tests are a series of tests that evaluate various aspects of performance in an easy way [70]. The tests contain running activities that are relevant for many sports. With the tests the physical capacity is evaluated in a fast and simple manner. Two markers are positioned 20 m apart. A CD is placed in a CD player and the test can be performed. The participant runs like a yo-yo back and forth between the markers at given speeds that are controlled by the CD. The speed is regularly increased, and when the individual no longer can maintain the speed, the test is ended. The test result is determined as the distance covered during the test.

It is also possible to perform the tests without exhausting the participants. In this case the test is stopped after a given time and the heart rate is measured to evaluate the development of the cardiovascular system. The lower the heart rate the higher is the capacity of the individual. This type of test is especially useful for athletes that are in a rehabilitation period. The tests can be used by anyone, irrespective of training status, since each of the three tests has two levels. There is a test for untrained and less trained individuals, and one test for well-trained athletes.

There are three yo-yo tests. In one test the participants perform continuous exercise, called the yo-yo endurance test, and in two tests the participants carry out intermittent exercise, namely the yo-yo intermittent endurance test and the yo-yo intermittent recovery test. The principles of the yo-yo intermittent tests are similar to the continuous yo-yo test, except that in the intermittent tests the athletes have a period of active rest between each of the 2×20-m shuttles.

The tests are briefly described below and examples given of sports where each of the tests is relevant. Also provided are examples of how the tests have been used to determine the performance of athletes.

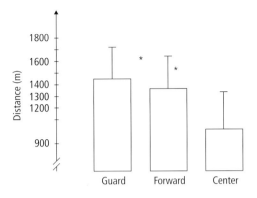

Fig. 2.2.9 Yo-yo intermittent endurance test performance of male top-class basketball players in different positions. * Significantly different from center players.

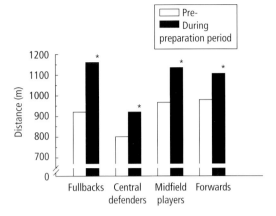

Fig. 2.2.10 Yo-yo intermittent recovery test performance of professional male soccer players in different positions of a team at the start (open bars) and at the end (solid bars) of a 6-week preparation period prior to the season. Means are given. * Significantly different from the start of the preparation period.

Yo-Yo endurance test

The yo-yo endurance test lasts for 5–15 min and is used for the evaluation of the ability to work continuously for a longer period of time. This test is especially useful for individuals that participate in endurance exercise, such as distance running.

Yo-Yo intermittent endurance test

The yo-yo intermittent endurance test lasts 10–20 min and consists of 5–18-s intervals of running interspersed with regular 5-s rest periods. The test evaluates an individual's ability to repeatedly perform intervals over a prolonged period of time. The test is especially useful for the athlete that performs interval sports, such as tennis, team handball, basketball and soccer. Figure 2.2.9 shows the performance of top-class basketball players in different positions.

Yo-Yo intermittent recovery test

The yo-yo intermittent recovery test lasts 2–15 min and focuses on the ability to recover after intense exercise. Between each exercise period (5–15 s) there is a 10-s pause. The test is particularly suitable for sports in which the ability to perform intensive exercise after short recovery periods can be decisive for the outcome of a competition, such as badminton, soccer, basketball, ice hockey and football. The test is able to pick up changes in performance illustrated in Fig. 2.2.10, which shows the performance level of professional

soccer players before and after a preparation period before a new season. All player groups had marked improvements, showing that the test is able to detect significant changes in physical capacity in soccer.

Repeated sprint test

The ability to be able to run fast and to perform repeated sprints can be tested easily by having the athlete sprint a given distance a number of times separated by a period of recovery that allows a decrease in performance. In relation to the latter aspect Balsom *et al.* [71] observed that performance in a 30-m sprint could be maintained when subjects have a recovery period between each sprint of 120 s, but a marked decrease was found when the recovery time was 30 s. This means that in order to evaluate an athlete's ability to recover from intense exercise the rest period between 30-m sprints should be less than 120 s and preferably 30 s. In a test to measure the ability to sprint and at the same time change direction, athletes perform seven sprints each lasting about 6 s, separated by 25-s rest periods. Figure 2.2.11 shows how the performance of 25 professional soccer players changed during a preparation period. The significant decrease in the sprint time shows that the test can be used to detect changes in performance.

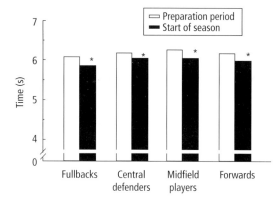

Fig. 2.2.11 Mean time of repeated sprints for professional male soccer players in different positions of a team at the start (open bars) and at the end (solid bars) of a 6-week preparation period prior to the season. Means are given. * Significantly different from the start of the preparation period.

Summary

The performance potential of an athlete can be improved by fitness training, which can be divided into aerobic training, anaerobic training, and specific muscle training. Common to all types of fitness training is the fact that the exercise performed during the training should be as similar as possible to the sport.

There are a number of reasons to use tests to evaluate performance of an individual. It is, however, important that the test chosen is relevant for the activity of the individual, e.g. a cycling test for a cyclist and an intermittent running test for a basketball player. Laboratory tests can provide general information about the fitness level of an individual, but they rarely give an exact measure of performance in a sport. By using a field test a more precise measure of performance will often be obtained.

Multiple choice questions

1 *Standard goniometric measurements:*
a can detect changes in joint range of motion of 1°
b have associated errors that are objective in nature
c have associated errors that are related to the patient's perception of tension
d measure joint range of motion, but not muscle–tendon stiffness
e all of the above.

2 *Immobilization:*
a causes muscle atrophy
b results in a disproportionate loss of muscle endurance and strength
c in the early phase of rehabilitation should focus on local muscle endurance training
d all of the above
e *a* and *b*, but not *c*.

3 *In speed endurance training:*
a changes mainly of central factors are induced
b performance intensities should be 70–80% of $\dot{V}O_{2\,max}$
c the duration of exercise bouts should be relatively short (15–90 s)
d the specific aim is to oxidize fat during prolonged exercise periods
e all of the above.

4 *Strength training:*
a Strength training results in hypertrophy of the muscle fibers and changes in the nervous system.
b In basic strength training muscle groups are not trained in isolated movements.
c High-resistance training can change the fiber type distribution towards fast-twitch fibers.
d The number of repetitions in a set should exceed 15.
e *a* and *c*.
f All of the above.

5 *Relevant for a soccer player:*
a isokinetic strength of the knee extensors
b yo-yo intermittent endurance test
c yo-yo intermittent recovery test
d repeated sprint test
e all of the above.

References

1 Shelbourne KD, Nitz P. Accelerated rehabilitation after anterior cruciate ligament reconstruction. *Am J Sports Med* 1990; **18**: 292–9.

2 Aoki M, Ogiwara N, Ohta T, Nabeta Y. Early active motion and weightbearing after cross-stitch Achilles tendon repair. *Am J Sports Med* 1998; **26**: 794–800.

3 Speck M, Klaue K. Early full weightbearing and functional treatment after surgical repair of acute Achilles tendon rupture. *Am J Sports Med* 1998; **26**: 789–93.

4 Bland JM, Altman DG. Statistical methods for assessing agreement between two methods of clinical measurement. *Lancet* 1986; **1**(8476): 307–10.

5 Atkinson G, Nevill AM. Statistical methods for assessing

measurement error (reliability) in variables relevant to sports medicine. *Sports Med* 1998; **26**: 217–38.

6 Cosgarea AJ, Sebastianelli WJ, DeHaven KE. Prevention of arthrofibrosis after anterior cruciate ligament reconstruction using the central third patellar tendon autograft. *Am J Sports Med* 1995; **23**: 87–92.

7 McHugh MP, Tyler TF, Gleim GW, Nicholas SJ. Preoperative indicators of motion loss and weakness following anterior cruciate ligament reconstruction. *J Orth Sports Phys Ther* 1998; **27**: 407–11.

8 Sachs RA, Daniel DM, Stone ML, Garfein RF. Patellofemoral problems after anterior cruciate ligament reconstruction. *Am J Sports Med* 1989; **17**: 760–5.

9 Magnusson SP, Simonsen EB, Aagaard P, Dyhre-Poulson P, McHugh MP, Kjaer M. Mechanical and physiological responses to stretching with and without pre-isometric contraction in human skeletal muscle. *Arch Phys Med Rehab* 1996; **77**: 373–8.

10 Christensen HW. Precision and accuracy of an electrogoniometer. *J Manipul Phys Ther* 1999; **22**: 10–4.

11 Rheault W, Miller M, Nothnagel P, Straessle J, Urban D. Intertester reliability and concurrent validity of fluid-based and universal goniometers for active knee flexion. *Phys Ther* 1988; **68**: 1676–8.

12 Mallon WJ, Herring CL, Sallay PI, Moorman CT, Crim JR. Use of vertebral levels to measure presumed internal rotation at the shoulder: a radiographic analysis. *J Shoulder Elbow Surg* 1996; **5**: 299–306.

13 Tyler TF, McHugh MP, Gleim GW, Nicholas SJ. Association of KT-1000 measurements with clinical tests of knee stability one year following anterior cruciate ligament reconstruction. *J Orth Sports Phys Ther* 1999; **29(9)**: 540–5.

14 Tyler TF, McHugh MP, Gleim GW, Nicholas SJ. The effect of immediate weight bearing after anterior cruciate ligament reconstruction. *Clin Orth Rel Res* 1998; **357**: 141–8.

15 Liu SH, Baker CL. Comparison of lateral ankle ligamentous reconstruction procedures. *Am J Sports Med* 1994; **22**: 313–7.

16 Daniel DM, Stone ML, Sachs R, Malcom L. Instrumented measurement of anterior laxity in patients with acute anterior cruciate ligament disruption. *Am J Sports Med* 1985; **13**: 401–7.

17 Malcom LL, Daniel DM, Stone ML, Sachs R. The measurement of anterior knee laxity after ACL reconstructive surgery. *Clin Orth* 1985; **196**: 35–41.

18 Barber-Westin SD, Noyes FR, Heckmann TP, Shaffer BL. The effect of exercise and rehabilitation on anterior–posterior knee displacements after anterior cruciate ligament autograft reconstruction. *Am J Sports Med* 1999; **27**: 84–93.

19 Robnett NJ, Riddle DL, Kues JM. Intertester reliability of measurements obtained with the KT-1000 on patients with reconstructed anterior cruciate ligaments. *J Orth Sports Phys Ther* 1995; **21**: 113–9.

20 Aglietti P, Buzzi R, Menchetti PM, Giron F. Arthroscopically assisted semitendinosus and gracilis tendon graft in reconstruction for acute anterior cruciate ligament injuries in athletes. *Am J Sports Med* 1996; **21(6)**: 726–31.

21 Passler JM, Babinski K, Schippinger G. Failure of clinical methods in assessing graft integrity after anterior cruciate ligament reconstruction: an arthroscopic evaluation. *Arthroscopy* 1999; **15**: 27–34.

22 Nicholas SJ, D'Amato MJ, Hershman EB, McHugh MP, Tyler TF, Gleim GW, Kolstad K. *Does* initial graft tension during acl reconstruction affect the restoration of static knee stability. In: *Proceedings of the American Orthopaedic Society for Sports Medicine*. Specialty Day. Orlando FL: The American Orthopaedic Society for Sports Medicine, 18 March 2000: 78–9.

23 Yasuda K, Tsujino J, Tanabe Y, Kaneda K. Effects of initial graft tension on clinical outcome after anterior cruciate ligament reconstruction. *Am J Sports Med* 1997; **25**: 99–106.

24 Pizzari T, Kolt GS, Remedios L. Measurement of anterior-to-posterior translation of the glenohumeral joint using the KT-1000. *J Orth Sports Phys Ther* 1999; **29**: 602–8.

25 Sauers EL, Borsa PA, Herling DE, Stanley RD. Instrumental measurement of glenohumeral joint laxity and its relationship to passive range of motion and generalized joint laxity. *Am J Sports Med* 2001, **29**: 143–50.

26 Kovaleski JE, Gurchiek LR, Heitman RJ, Hollis JM, Pearsall AW. Instrumented measurement of anteroposterior and inversion–eversion laxity of the normal ankle joint complex. *Foot Ankle Int* 1999; **20**: 808–14.

27 Eastlack ME, Axe MJ, Snyder-Mackler L. Laxity, instability, and functional outcome after ACL injury: copers versus non-copers. *Med Sci Sports Exerc* 1999; **31**: 210–5.

28 Holme E, Magnusson SP, Becher K, Bieler T, Aagaard P, Kjaer M. The effect of supervised rehabilitation on strength, postural sway, position sense and re-injury risk after acute ankle ligament sprain. *Scand J Med Sci Sports* 1999; **9**: 104–9.

29 Rozzi SL, Lephart SM, Sterner R, Kuligowski L. Balance training for persons with functionally unstable ankles. *J Orth Sports Phys Ther* 1999; **29**: 478–86.

30 Gauffin H, Tropp H, Odenrick P. Effect of ankle disk training on postural control in patients with functional instability of the ankle joint. *Int J Sports Med* 1988; **9**: 141–4.

31 Leanderson J, Eriksson E, Nilsson C, Wykman A. Proprioception in classical ballet dancers. A prospective study of the influence of an ankle sprain on proprioception in the ankle joint. *Am J Sports Med* 1996; **24**: 370–4.

32 Lephart SM, Pincivero DM, Giraldo JL, Fu FH. The role of proprioception in the management and rehabilitation of athletic injuries. *Am J Sports Med* 1997; **25**: 130–7.

33 Hutton RS, Atwater SW. Acute and chronic adaptations of muscle proprioceptors in response to increased use. *Sports Med* 1992; **14**: 406–21.

34 Nicholas JA, Strizak AM, Veras G. A study of thigh muscle

weakness in different pathological states of the lower extremity. *Am J Sports Med* 1976; **4**: 241–8.

35 Beckman SM, Buchanan TS. Ankle inversion injury and hypermobility: effect on hip and ankle muscle electromyography onset latency. *Arch Phys Med Rehab* 1995; **76**: 1138–43.

36 Manal TJ, Snyder-Mackler L. Failure of voluntary activation of the quadriceps femoris muscle after patellar contusion. *J Orth Sports Phys Ther* 2000; **30**: 655–60.

37 Snyder-Mackler L, Delitto A, Stralka SW, Bailey SL. Use of electrical stimulation to enhance recovery of quadriceps femoris muscle force production in patients following anterior cruciate ligament reconstruction. *Phys Ther* 1994; **74**: 901–7.

38 Lieber RL, Silva PD, Daniel DM. Equal effectiveness of electrical and volitional strength training for quadriceps femoris muscles after ACL surgery. *J Orth Res* 1996; **14**: 131–8.

39 Polkey MI, Kyroussis D, Hamnegard CH, Mills GH, Green M, Moxham J. Quadriceps strength and fatigue assessed by magnetic stimulation of the femoral nerve in man. *Muscle Nerve* 1996; **19**: 549–55.

40 Kremenic I, McHugh M, Ben-Avi S, Leonhardt D. Quadriceps activation via transcutaneous magnetic stimulation of the femoral nerve. In: *Proceedings of the Orthopaedic Research Society 47th Annual Meeting.* San Francisco, CA, 25–28 February 2001.

41 Snyder-Mackler L, Binder-Macleod SA, Williams PR. Fatigability of human quadriceps femoris muscle following ACL reconstruction. *Med Sci Sports Exerc* 1993; **25**: 783–9.

42 McHugh MP, Tyler TF, Nicholas SJ, Browne MG, Gleim GW. Electromyographic analysis of quadriceps fatigue following anterior cruciate ligament reconstruction. *J Sports Phys Ther* 2001; **31**: 25–32.

43 Enoka RM, Stuart DG. Neurobiology of muscle fatigue. *J Appl Physiol* 1992; **72**: 1631–48.

44 Pincivero DM, Lephart SM, Karunakara RA. Reliability and precision of isokinetic strength and muscular endurance for the quadriceps and hamstrings. *Int J Sports Med* 1997; **18**: 113–7.

45 Suzuki N, Endo S. A quantitative study of trunk muscle strength and fatigability in the low back pain syndrome. *Spine* 1983; **8**: 69–74.

46 Sapega AA. Muscle performance evaluation in orthopaedic practice. *J Bone Joint Surg (Am)* 1990; **72**: 1562–74.

47 Jonhagen S, Nemeth G, Eriksson E. Hamstring injuries in sprinters. The role of concentric and eccentric hamstring muscle strength and flexibility. *Am J Sports Med* 1994; **22**: 262–6.

48 Hortobágyi T, Tracy J, Hamilton G, Lambert J. Fatigue effects on muscle excitability. *Int J Sports Med* 1996; **17**: 409–14.

49 Tesch PA, Dudley DA, Duvoisin MR, Hather BM, Harris RT. Force and EMG signal patterns during repeated bouts of eccentric muscle actions. *Acta Physiol Scand* 1990; **138**: 263–71.

50 Magnusson SP, Gleim GW, Nicholas JA. Subject variability of shoulder abduction strength testing. *Am J Sports Med* 1990; **18**: 349–53.

51 Magnusson SP, Constantini NW, McHugh MP, Gleim GW. Strength profiles and performance in Masters' level swimmers. *Am J Sports Med* 1995; **23**: 626–31.

52 Magnusson SP, Gleim GW, Nicholas JA. Shoulder weakness in professional baseball pitchers. *Med Sci Sports Exerc* 1994; **26**: 5–9.

53 McHugh MP, Spitz AL, Lorei MP, Nicholas SJ, Hershman EB, Gleim GW. Effect of anterior cruciate ligament deficiency on the economy of walking and jogging. *J Orth Res* 1994; **12**: 592–7.

54 Brown M, Fisher JS, Salsich G. Stiffness and muscle function with age and reduced muscle use. *J Orth Res* 1999; **17**: 409–14.

55 McHugh MP, Connolly DAJ, Eston RG, Kremenic IJ, Gleim GW. The role of passive muscle stiffness in symptoms of exercise-induced muscle damage. *Am J Sports Med* 1999; **27**: 594–9.

56 Tyler TF, McHugh MP. Neuromuscular rehabilitation of a female olympic ice hockey player following ACL reconstruction. *J Sport Phys Ther* 2001; **31**: 577–87.

57 Ekblom B. Effect of physical training on oxygen transport system in man. *Acta Physiol Scand Suppl* 1969; **328**(5): 45.

58 Henriksson J, Hickner RC. Skeletal muscle adaptation to endurance training. In: Macleod DAD, Maughan RJ, Williams C, Madely CR, Charp JCM, Nutton RW, eds. *Intermittent High Intensity Exercise.* London: E and FN Spon Publication, 1996: 5–26.

59 Schantz P, Sjøberg B. Malate–aspartate and alpha-glycerophosphate shuttle enzyme levels in untrained and endurance trained human skeletal muscle. *Acta Physiol Scand* 1985; **123**: 12A.

60 Houston ME, Bentzen H, Larsen H. Interrelationships between skeletal muscle adaptations and performance as studied by detraining and retraining. *Acta Physiol Scand* 1979; **105**: 163–70.

61 Bangsbo J, Mizuno M. Morphological and metabolic alterations in soccer players with detraining and retraining and their relation to performance. In: Reilly T, Lees H, Murphy WJ, eds. *Science and Football I.* London: E & FN Spon Publication, 1988: 114–24.

62 Tesch PA, Wright JE. Recovery from short-term intense exercise: its relation to capillary supply and blood lactate concentration. *Eur J Appl Physiol* 1983; **52**: 98–103.

63 Reilly T, Bangsbo J. Anaerobic and aerobic training. In: Elliott B, ed. *Applied Sport Science: Training in Sport.* Australia, 1998: 351–409.

64 Pilegaard H, Domino K, Noland T, Juel C, Hellsten Y, Halestrap AP, Bangsbo J. Effect of high intensity exercise training on lactate/H^+ transport capacity in human skeletal muscle. *Am J Physiol* 1999; **276**: E255–E261.

65 Bangsbo J. Physiology of muscle fatigue during intense exercise. *Clin Pharm Sport Exerc* 1997; 123–31.

66 Andersen JL, Klitgaard H, Bangsbo J, Saltin B. Myosin heavy chain isoform in single fibres from m. vastus lateralis of soccer players: effects of strength-training. *Acta Physiol Scand* 1994; **150**: 21–6.

67 Aagaard P, Trolle M, Simonsen EB, Klausen K, Bangsbo J. Moment and power generation during maximal knee extension performed at low and high speed. *Eur J Appl Physiol*, 1994; **69**: 376–81.

68 Ekstrand J. *Soccer injuries and their prevention.* Thesis, Linköping University Medical Dissertation 130, 1982.

69 Bangsbo J, Petersen A, Michalsik L. Accumulated O_2 deficit during intense exercise and muscle characteristics of elite athletes. *Int J Sports Med* 1993; **14**: 207–13.

70 Bangsbo J. *Fitness Training in Football—a Scientific Approach.* Bagsvaerd: HO & Storm, 1994.

71 Balsom PD, Seger JY, Sjödin B, Ekblom B. Physiological responses to maximal intensity intermittent exercise. *Eur J Appl Physiol* 1992; **65**: 144–9.

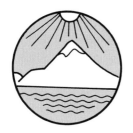

Chapter 2.3
Physical Activity
and Environment

PETER BÄRTSCH,

BODIL NIELSEN JOHANNSEN &

JUHANI LEPPÄLUOTO

Classical reference

Nielsen M. Die Regulation der Körpertemperatur bei
Muskelarbeit. *Skand Arch Physiol* 1938; **79**:
193–230.

The thermal environment has profound effects on performance and health. The maintenance of core temperature at optimal level in a range of environmental temperatures is essential for performance. This is accomplished through the action of the autonomic control centers in the hypothalamus.

The rise in body core temperature during exercise was considered to be the result of a failure in the ability of the organism to dissipate fully the increased heat produced during exercise. Marius Nielsen demonstrated that the rectal temperature increased and after 40–50 min reached a new, higher level, which was maintained until the exercise was stopped. (He had one subject work at constant intensity and rectal temperature for $4\frac{1}{2}$ h.) From his experiments it seemed that the rise in core temperature was only dependent on the exercise intensity. Thus, at ambient temperatures of between 5 and 35 °C, the core temperature level for a given intensity was the same, despite large variations in the contribution of evaporation, convection and radiation to the total heat loss. He concluded from the experiments that the rise in body temperature during exercise was a regulated rise, probably beneficial for performance.

Discussions on the setting of body temperature during exercise have now gone on for more than 60 years. The knowledge of the anatomic organization and function of the temperature centers in the brain inspired discussions as to the validity of rectal temperature as an index of the regulated temperature. Other candidates such as tympanic temperature, supposed to reflect brain temperature, or esophageal temperature, an index of the temperature of the blood leaving the heart were proposed. The latter is today preferred by exercise physiologists for reflecting fast changes in core temperature and signals to the brain centers. The concept of a setting of the temperature at higher levels during exercise has also changed. Now it seems that a mathematical/technical description of the resetting during exercise is rather a reduction in the set point, rendering the 'human thermostat' more sensitive to

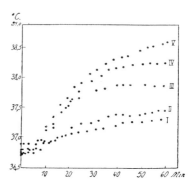

Abb. 2. Die Rektaltemperatur während der Arbeit. Vp. P. J.
I   360 kgm/Min.
II   540   „
III   900   „
IV   1080   „
V   1260   „

Fig. 2.3.1. Rectal temperature during exercise at different intensities. From [4].

an absolute core temperature during work. How the setting of the core temperature during exercise relative to the $\dot{V}O_{2\,max}$ is accomplished is still an open question. The beneficial effect of a high core temperature in endurance sport activities is now also questionable, as discussed in the section on exercise and temperature (p. 236).

Introduction

The first part of this chapter discusses the profound effects thermal environment has on performance and health. The maintenance of core temperature at optimal level for performance is accomplished through the action of the autonomic control centers in the hypothalamus. This is possible within a wide range of environmental temperature conditions, the prescriptive, or thermoneutral zone. The historical figure (Fig. 2.3.1) shows data from the work of M. Nielsen. This paper supports the notion of regulation of body core temperature at an optimal level for performance. The individual's capacity for heat production by shivering and heat loss by sweat evaporation and vasodilatation determines the limits for performance. Proper clothing allows activity in even the coldest climates. However, cold exposure can result in injuries, local tissue damage and hypothermia. The cooling effect of the environmental temperature is strongly influenced by the wind speed. In hot environments the cardiovascular stress is increased, and sweating may result in dehydration. This combination markedly reduces performance, especially in endurance-type events and may lead to heat-related illness. These disorders, heat exhaustion and heat stroke can best be prevented by fluid replacement and by a prior acclimatization to heat.

The second part of this chapter discusses the effects of altitude on physical performance. Reduced air pressure (and consequently reduced partial pressure of oxygen), reduced air density, lower temperature and a lower water content of air may all affect physical performance at high altitude in different ways and degrees depending on the type of exercise. Hypoxia is certainly the factor that has the biggest impact on life at high altitude. Immediate adjustments to maintain adequate oxygen supply to the tissue are an increase of ventilation and cardiac output for a given workload. The major long-term adjustments (acclimatization) con-

sist of a further slow increase of ventilation, increased erythropoiesis and adaptations at the tissue level. Athletes try to profit from altitude acclimatization for sea-level performance by training at high altitude. Because the decrease of performance at altitude may offset benefits from acclimatization, many athletes prefer to 'sleep high and train low'. Most issues regarding different modalities or concepts of high altitude are still rather controversial. Rapid adjustments to hypoxia may not always be very successful. A significant number of individuals develop acute mountain sickness and some even life-threatening illnesses such as high-altitude pulmonary or cerebral edema during the first few days after rapid ascent to altitudes above 2500–3000 m. The prevalence of these acute high-altitude illnesses increases with altitude and rate of ascent. Furthermore, there is a considerable interindividual difference in susceptibility to these illnesses.

Thermal environment

Introduction

Temperature regulation is a good example of a homeostatic mechanism. It keeps the (deep) body temperature within a very narrow range that allows maintenance of bodily functions in almost every climatic condition. Humans with their naked skin and numerous sweat glands are tropical animals, and the capacity of the thermoregulatory system is directed towards heat dissipation rather than heat conservation. Technical developments in clothing and housing have, however, allowed people to inhabit permanently all places on the earth and even in space at temperatures close to absolute zero.

Heat balance

The metabolic processes liberate heat as a waste product. When substrates are metabolized in the human body most of the energy equivalent of the combusted substrate is converted into heat. During exercise some of the energy is transformed to external work, but the efficiency of these processes is usually less than 20–25%.

The efficiency, E, is defined as:

$$E\% = (external\ work \times 100\%)\big/ metabolic\ energy\ cost$$

Therefore, 75–100% of the liberated energy appears as heat in the active muscle tissue. The amount of heat generated in the body must be dissipated to the environment, or else the heat content and the temperature of the body will increase and endanger the homeostatic milieu of the body. The autonomic temperature centers in the hypothalamus control the body core temperature by appropriate activation of, respectively, heat loss or heat conservation processes. In this way the body core temperature is maintained at a constant, regulated level in the face of varying environmental temperatures. This balance can be described by the heat balance equation:

$$M \pm W = \pm C \pm R \pm E \pm S$$

(Heat liberation = heat loss)

where

M is metabolic energy liberation
W is external work (positive when going downhill)
C is heat exchange by convection
R is heat exchange by radiation
E is heat exchange by evaporation and
S is heat storage.
This last term becomes zero when the heat gains and losses are equal.

Physical laws determine the direction and magnitude of the heat exchanges by convection and radiation, i.e. the temperature difference between the body surface and the air temperature, respectively, the mean radiant temperature of the environment. The heat loss by evaporation depends on the water vapor pressure difference between the skin surface and the air[1]. However, physiologic mechanisms influence the skin surface temperature and vapor pressure through the control of skin blood flow and sweating.

The skin surface temperature varies with the temperature in the environment. In cool conditions the difference to the environment is wide, so heat loss by C and R are the main routes for heat loss. The warmer the environmental conditions become, the more the skin surface temperature approaches the environmental temperature, and therefore, the need for evaporative heat loss increases. At an air temperature of about 35 °C skin temperature equals environmental temperature, and the total heat liberation must be dissipated by evaporation of sweat (Fig. 2.3.2). In the diagram the

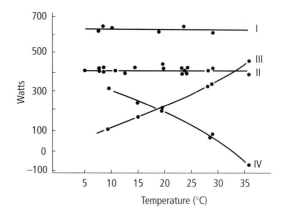

Fig. 2.3.2 Heat exchange during exercise at 150 W for 60 min at different room temperatures in a nude subject. I Total heat production, II heat loss, III evaporative heat loss, IV convective and radiative heat loss (after [4]).

heat lost by convection, radiation and evaporation in an exercising (cycling) person is illustrated for environmental temperatures between 5 °C and 35 °C. During exercise part of the heat production is stored in the body, causing the core temperature to increase.

Core temperature

The core temperature of the body is measured in the deep esophagus or in the rectum. For clinical purposes a less reliable measurement can be obtained by measuring oral temperature or tympanic temperature, the latter by infrared radiation receivers. The body temperature during rest is maintained close to 37 °C, varying in a circadian rhythm. During exercise the body temperature increases to higher levels, proportional to the relative workload, i.e. to the percentage of the maximal aerobic capacity of the individual [2] (Fig. 2.3.3).

This higher temperature is maintained as long as the exercise is continued, and within the prescriptive zone, it is independent of the environmental temperature.

The prescriptive zone

The body core temperature during exercise is uninfluenced by environmental temperature over a wide range of temperatures [3,4] due to the thermoregulatory control of the heat production and heat loss mecha-

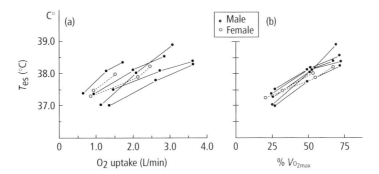

Fig. 2.3.3 Esophageal temperature (T_{es}) at 60-min exercise in seven subjects with different maximal aerobic capacity. (a) T_{es} plotted against absolute oxygen uptake; (b) T_{es} plotted against relative oxygen uptake, $\%\dot{V}_{O_2 max}$ (after [2]).

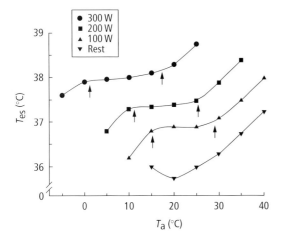

Fig. 2.3.4 Esophageal temperature in one subject after 2 h at rest and cycling at intensities between 100 and 300 W at environmental temperatures between −5 and 40 °C. The thermoneutral zone marked with arrows moves to the left with increasing work and heat production (adapted from Kitzing *et al. Int Z Angew Physiol* 1972; **30**: 119–31).

nisms, i.e. shivering, skin blood flow and sweating. The range of environmental conditions in which the body temperature is independent of these conditions is called the prescriptive zone [4]. Above the *upper critical temperature*, core temperature increases to a higher level than during exercise in thermoneutral conditions, while on the other hand, below the *lower critical temperature* the core temperature falls. The actual range of the prescriptive zone, also called the thermoneutral zone, depends on the rate of heat production and additionally, for the upper limit, on the physiologic capacity for heat dissipation, whereas for the lower critical temperature, on the maximal rate of heat production and vasoconstriction (Fig. 2.3.4).

Physiologic responses to cold exposure

Technical developments have changed the situations in which humans are exposed to cold. The number of people working outdoors in cold conditions is presently declining, while that of people participating in recreational activities, e.g. winter sports is evidently increasing. Physical fitness is important for the thermoregulatory responses to cold. Fit people have a higher metabolic response and a higher skin temperature at the onset of shivering. On the other hand, body fat provides protection against cooling [5].

Cold can be defined as conditions which activate heat conservation responses, and may be experienced in air or water, or in contact with solid materials. Unclothed or clothed parts of the body can be locally exposed to cold (hands, face and legs) or the whole body may be cooled. The duration of the cold exposure may last for seconds to several weeks, and can be recurrent. The effects of cold exposure will therefore depend on these factors.

Many of the cold-induced physiologic responses attenuate physical performance. Low temperature of muscles causes poor efficiency and coordination, and risk of muscle and tendon tears. Shivering muscles make use of energy stores, and shivering may also cause clumsiness. Physiologic mechanisms activated by cold are presented in the box below. Cold-induced skin vasoconstriction leads to increased blood pressure, plasma extravasation (leakage of fluid from the plasma to the interstitium) and diuresis. Increased sympathetic activation and hemoconcentration reduce maximal physical performance. Finally bronchoconstriction in winter athletes is common and may lead to exercise-induced asthma (see Chapter 4.5). A recent study showed that 23% of the Olympic winter sport athletes in the US had exercise-induced bron-choconstriction [6].

Physiologic mechanisms activated by cold

Increased heat production:
• cold sensations activate voluntary movements
• sympathetic nerves become active
• norepinephrine secreted, availability of thyroid hormones increased
• all leading to increased expression of mitochondrial uncoupling proteins for heat production in muscle
• muscle tension increases and shivering starts
• food intake increases.

Decreased heat loss:
• skin blood flow decreases
• horripilation
• behavioral activity, curling up.

Heat production in the cold

Voluntary activity (behavioral thermoregulation)

Unpleasant cold sensations result in behavioral responses (increased motor activity, curling up and searching for warmer places and clothing).

Shivering

The hypothalamic temperature center receives inputs from skin cold receptors and projects them to the motor cortex and finally to the motor nerves. This leads to increased muscle tone and to oscillating contractions of muscles, shivering, that occurs mostly in trunk muscles. Shivering increases metabolic rates by 2–5 times the resting value. Due to the increased metabolic rate shivering should be avoided in winter sports.

Chemical or non-shivering thermogenesis

Chemical thermogenesis is well established in rodents and newborn humans and closely related to uncoupling protein 1 (UCP 1) in brown fat. Cold exposure elicits the release of norepinephrine and thyroid hormones and activates sympathetic nerves that stimulate the expression of UCP 1. It uncouples the normal oxidative phosphorylation in the mitochondria and the production of protons is decreased. Less ATP is formed and more heat is generated (Fig. 2.3.5). The role of UCP 1 in adults is not well established, but recent studies have shown the presence of homologues of UCP 1. UCP 2 is widely expressed in fat, muscles and viscera and stimulated by starving and fatty acids. UCP 3 is abundantly expressed in skeletal muscles and is stimulated by cold. UCP 2 and 3 also regulate the production of ATP and their roles in heat production are under research [7].

Meals increase heat production by a mechanism formerly called specific dynamic action, now diet-induced thermogenesis (DIT). The resting metabolic rate is increased about 10% for 1–2 h after a meal.

Heat loss

In cold environments radiation and convection are the main avenues for heat loss. In winter sports convection dominates the heat transfer, since warm layers of air around the body are rapidly conveyed away from the skin by the air movement produced by the ongoing activity. The so-called wind chill index (WCI) has been constructed in which the combined effects of environmental temperature and wind are converted to a hypothetical temperature in still air, which has the same cooling effect as the actual wind speed and temperature [8,9]. The values calculated are rates of heat loss per m^2 (Fig. 2.3.6). For instance, −10 °C at a wind speed of 9 m/s corresponds to the temperature of −28 °C in still air. Climatic conditions with a WCI of between 1200 and 1400 W/m^2 are very cold, between 1400 and 1600 W/m^2 bitterly cold and between 1600 and 1800 W/m^2 dangerous: exposed flesh will freeze in 1 min. Frostbite begins to occur when WCI is over 1300 W/m^2. The WCI concept was re-examined [8], and the predictions compared with the incidences of finger frostbite. The conclusion was that there is little risk of finger frostbite at temperatures above −10 °C independent of wind velocity, while below −15 °C the

Basal state

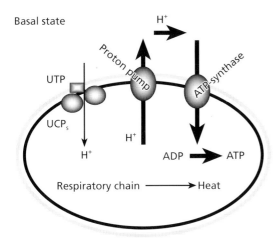

After cold stimulation

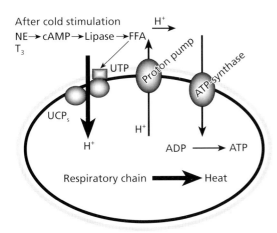

Fig. 2.3.5 Mitochondrial activity in basal state, and after cold stimulation. After cold stimulation the uncoupling protein (UCP) in brown fat allows a shortcut for protons through the mitochondrial membrane, releasing the energy bound in the H^+ as heat. The stimulation is achieved by norepinephrine (NE) or thyroid hormone (T3), which increase the formation of cAMP, lipase and free fatty acids (FFAs). FFA displaces uridine triphosphate (UTP) from the UCP channel (protein allowing protons to enter the mitochondria).

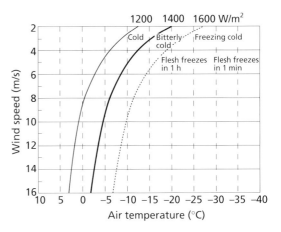

Fig. 2.3.6 Diagram for estimating the combined cooling effect of temperature and wind speed (wind chill index, WCI). The index estimates the effect on exposed, unprotected skin areas (in W/m^2) and the exposure time before freezing. The curves were constructed by using the formula $WCI = (10 \cdot v^2 + 10.45 - v) \cdot (33 - T_a)$, where v is wind velocity and T_a ambient temperature.

effect of wind speed is underestimated. Thus, in skiing competitions or other outdoor mass events special caution has to be paid to the WCI. If the weather conditions show a WCI of more than 1600 W/m^2, sports competitions should be cancelled, and expeditions require special clothing. In the Nordic countries the lower limit is set at −20 °C air temperature for skiing competitions, but wind speed has not been taken into account, which it ought to be. Physicians responsible for medical care in skiing competitions or mass events should be encouraged to use a WCI rather than the simple thermometer reading.

Clothing

In cold weather appropriate clothing is necessary to maintain the proper heat balance. In winter sports such as skiing, biathlon and orienteering heat production is high, and the main emphasis should be placed on the protection of fingers, feet, ears and nose against local cooling and frostbite. An additional problem due to the unavoidable sweating is the transport of the moisture away from the skin and through the clothing. New synthetic fibers allow sweat to pass through the textile, but they are not suitable in events in which heat production is smaller, such as mountaineering or trekking. In cross-country skiing competitions the metabolic rate exceeds 1500 W; in this situation clothing with an insulation value of 1–1.5 clo units is sufficient at the temperature of −20 °C. At the same temperature a resting subject needs an insulation of 5–6 clo units. (The clo unit is defined by the insulation value of traditional indoor clothing; 1 clo = 0.155 $m^2 \cdot °C/W$. See also [9].) This great variation in required insulation between rest and activity is a problem for people who have accidents or get tired during outdoor activities in cold climates. Furthermore, clothing soaked by rain loses its thermal insulation properties and presents a serious thermoregulatory problem in cold and windy conditions [10]. Enough (and dry) clothing must be brought along! The IREQ index [11] makes it possible to calculate the cold protective clothing needed for any combination of activity level and climatic variables.

Acclimatization to cold

Practically no studies exist in which the effects of cold acclimatization on physical performance have been studied. We know from some studies that the unpleasantness of cold sensations becomes reduced or habituated after 1–4 daily cold exposures, and that increased sympathetic activity and shivering is attenuated within a week [12–14]. True cold acclimatization is difficult to induce in humans. Three types of adaptation to cold are described: (i) *metabolic*, where a greater metabolic response to cold stress is developed [15,16]; (ii) *hypothermic*, where core temperature falls (e.g [12]); and (iii) *insulative* [17] with a lowering of the skin to environment gradient and heat loss, and with little change in core temperature and metabolic rate during cold exposure.

Immersion in cold water 5 days per week over 5 weeks has been found to induce the type of adaptation described as insulative [18]: a lowering of resting rectal temperature, a slower rise in metabolic rate (indicating a delay in onset of shivering) and a lower skin temperature. It appears that a repeated fall in core temperature is necessary to induce the sympathetic activation, while a cold skin alone is enough to stimulate the increased vasoconstrictor response obtained after 5 weeks' daily cold water immersions [19]. However, when healthy men were exposed to cold air for 11 days, a hypothermic type of acclimatization was observed instead (i.e. reduced cold sensations, decreased core and increased skin temperature in some places, reduced norepinephrine response, and no changes in metabolic rate or heat debt responses) [13]. It is evident that acclimatization in cold water is different from that in cold air. Moreover, cold water acclimatization increases norepinephrine response and peripheral resistance, and decreases cardiac output [18,19], all of which are *not* beneficial for physical performance.

Therefore, cold air and not cold water acclimatization is perhaps the type of acclimatization that should be used if performance in cold air is to be improved.

It is evident that unacclimatized subjects perform less well than acclimatized, and therefore some kind of cold acclimatization should be obtained before winter sports competitions. It is in the author's knowledge that subjects who are about to participate in the demanding polar expeditions acclimatize by sleeping overnight outdoors for several weeks before their expeditions (see Case story 2.3.1).

Performance in cold conditions

As mentioned in the introduction most of the energy liberated during physical exercise is converted to heat. Depending on the metabolic rate, the prescriptive zone and upper and lower critical temperature shifts (see Fig. 2.3.4) and the physiologic mechanisms for heat loss and heat conservation are taxed to varying degrees, depending on how the heat balance is attained. Therefore, some benefits for exercise and performance are obtained in cooler environments. In submaximal cycling at ambient temperatures of 4, 11, 21 and 31 °C, the time to exhaustion was longest at 11 °C and shortest at 31 °C, demonstrating that the effect of ambient temperature on exercise capacity follows an inverted U-shaped relationship [21]. This study demonstrates that exercise capacity is greater in low suprazero ambient temperatures than at higher temperatures, where the physiologic load on the circulatory system is higher. The ambient temperatures in winter sports are usually below the freezing point and evidently the best conditions for prolonged high intensity physical activity prevail close to but above zero. Optimal performance must therefore be obtained by choosing the proper clothing.

The deleterious effects of cold on performance are manifested on two levels. The more common is the effect of peripheral vasoconstriction and cooling, which lowers the temperature in the tissues, e.g. in hands and feet. The rate of the physiologic and chemical processes is then slowed down, including the rate of muscle contraction and nerve conductivity. Furthermore, stiffness in tendons and connective tissue is increased. This leads to clumsiness and increases the risk for injury (Fig. 2.3.7). Thus, for winter sports competitions warming up is of great importance.

Case story 2.3.1 Instructions to participants in mass events in winter sports

After mass sport events we often read in newspapers that a participant, usually an older man, has succumbed before the finishing line. Several studies on sport-related sudden deaths have been reported and recently reviewed [20]. The incidence of sudden deaths increases after 30–40 years of age and peaks at 50–60 years. Males clearly outnumber females. Deaths are often related to high dynamic loads (tennis, skiing, swimming, cycling). The incidence is higher in cross-country skiing than in jogging/running, indicating that skiing produces a higher cardiovascular load than running. Cold exposure also contributes an increased risk for cardiac deaths. In younger age groups infections or vaccinations are further risk factors. Based on these findings some suggestions for participants in winter sports can be made.

1 Long-term training and cold acclimatization is necessary before demanding mass events in cold climates.

2 Subjects over 40 years should have a cardiac check-up.

3 Ongoing infections and recent vaccinations are absolute risk factors for participation.

4 Finally, the organizers must arrange appropriate medical aid (resuscitation unit with defibrillator) at larger mass events and competitions.

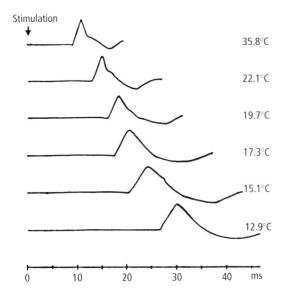

Fig. 2.3.7 The effect of local tissue temperature on muscle action potential. Note the increased latency and the stretched duration of the potential with decreasing temperatures (after Vanggaard *Aviat Space Environ Med* 1975; **46**: 33–6).

The less common effect of cold is when the whole body is cooled, resulting in a fall in core temperature (hypothermia, see below).

Cold injuries

General

The harmful effects of cold on the human body may be a direct effect of the low temperature, e.g. frostbite, trenchfoot and hypothermia. Indirectly, cold environments may exert a stress on human health. Cold weather in winter is a challenge and a significant risk factor, especially in the elderly, causing an excess mortality from cardiovascular diseases.

A short review of cold injuries and their treatment is presented in a recent paper [22]. Their occurrence in winter sports is fairly uncommon. The physicians of the Finnish elite skiing team and the mass skiing events report that during the last 5 years no cold injuries have been diagnosed (Dr P. Mäkelä, team physician, personal communication). An annual incidence of cold injuries in Finland is presently 2.5 cases per 100 000 inhabitants and they are mostly mild. The annual incidence of mild cold injuries varies from 2.3 to 22.4% of the population exposed to winter conditions by their recreational or professional activities [23]. The incidence of frostbite requiring hospitalization is far lower: 0.001–0.0016% [23]. On the other hand, fatal casualties have at all times occurred in conjunction with polar and high-altitude expeditions, and also in subjects using alcohol or drugs affecting the central nervous system in winter conditions.

Direct cold injuries

Frostbite and trenchfoot
Skin begins to freeze at temperatures between 0 and −2 °C. Vascular endothelium is damaged by ice crystals. Edema, inflammation and blisters develop. At lower temperatures larger skin areas freeze and become marble-white and hard. Symptoms are numbness, pain and cold, and pale or bluish skin. In mild cold exposures a small white area on skin (frostnip) develops, which disappears rapidly when warmed. For clinical reasons frostbite is divided into superficial and deep injuries; the former is limited to skin only but the latter extends to subcutis and muscles.

Trenchfoot or immersion foot develops usually when the feet are exposed for several hours (> 12 h) to wetness and temperatures between 1 and 10 °C (but not below zero). Trenchfoot is a vascular injury leading to edema. The foot is swollen, numb and often bluish. After some time there is a hyperemic phase with pain and ulcerations.

Treatment of frostbite and immersion foot
Local pain, frostnip and numbness in cold environment are warning signs of the development of frostbite. When frostbite has occurred, the following measures should be taken:
1 Prevent further heat loss, e.g. with warm clothing, drinks and shelter.
2 Immobilize the frostbite area and transfer the patient to first aid, or deep injuries to hospital.
3 If frostbite is deep, thawing during transport should be avoided if it is not absolutely certain that refreezing can be prevented.
The following measures are strictly forbidden: thawing and refreezing, rubbing with snow or hand, ointments, alcohol, local warming by fire.

First aid of superficial frostbite consists of thawing in a warm water bath, analgesic drugs, sterile bandages, immobilization and elevation of the frostbitten area.

Table 2.3.1 Symptoms and signs at different levels of hypothermia (after [51]).

Core temperature (°C)	Symptoms
36	Increased metabolic rate
35	Maximal shivering, hyperreflexia, speech disorders, delayed cerebration
34	Responsive and compatible with exercise, blood pressure normal
33–31	Amnesia, consciousness clouded, pupils dilated, blood pressure low
30–28	Slow pulse and breathing, cardiac arrhythmia, muscular rigidity
27–25	Unconscious, reflexes lost, 'cold and dead', ventricular fibrillation
24–20	Pulmonary edema, mortality high, cardiac arrest
17	Isoelectric ECG
9	Surgical hypothermia

Blisters should not be punctured. Deep injuries should always be treated in hospital. Recent information on the occurrence and modern treatment of frostbite is described by Paton [24].

Hypothermia (Table 2.3.1)
Whole-body cooling may occur during winter sports activities due to fatigue or accidents. In such situations of decreased heat production the clothing is no longer sufficient to maintain heat balance; this may also occur if the insulation effect of the clothing has become reduced due to soaking with sweat. Hypothermia may also occur after accidents in water. In this case the cooling is very rapid, and the victim may lose consciousness within 15–20 min.

The thermal conductivity and the specific heat capacity of water are, respectively, 25 and 1000 times that of air. This means that the heat loss to the environment is much greater in water than in air at the same temperature. Furthermore, the skin temperature becomes almost equal to the water temperature. The heat loss to the water is determined by the heat transport from the core to the skin surface, that is the 'conductance of the peripheral tissues', which depends on the skin circulation and also on the amount of the insulating fat tissue

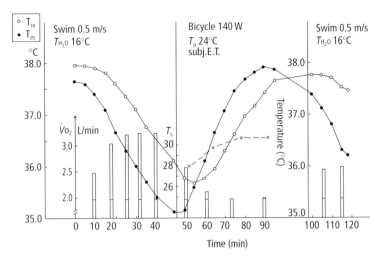

Fig. 2.3.8 Core temperature and oxygen uptake during swimming in water at 16 °C followed by cycling in 24 °C. Oxygen uptakes, $\dot{V}O_2$, are shown as bars, the shaded areas being the $\dot{V}O_2$ in thermoneutral condition, the light areas the extra $\dot{V}O_2$ due to shivering. One subject (from B. Nielsen. *Acta Physiol Scand* 1976; **97**: 129–38).

in the skin. The range of the prescriptive zone in water is very narrow compared to air, only 3–5 °C. A resting lean subject in water cannot maintain thermal balance at water temperatures below 32–33 °C. At water temperatures of 12–15 °C the core temperature will fall about 3–4 °C in 15 min in a swimmer despite swimming activity and maximal shivering (Fig. 2.3.8). The fall in core temperature causes a reduction in muscle force and contraction velocity, a fall in $\dot{V}O_{2\,max}$ and early fatigue [25]. Hypothermia is defined as a condition where deep body temperature is below 35 °C and actions have to be taken to restore the normal body temperature.

In hostile mountain conditions four states of hypothermia have been recognized: (i) below 36 °C full consciousness but shivering; (ii) impaired consciousness but no shivering; (iii) below 30 °C unconsciousness; and (iv) below 28 °C cardiac and respiratory arrest.

Treatment of hypothermia
When respiratory movements and heart function stop death will occur within minutes to half an hour, depending on the cooling rate. Even in this state patients can be revived. The proper procedure is under discussion, and depends on whether it takes place under field conditions, or in a hospital ward. If the deep temperature is below 35 °C, the physician/hospital should always be consulted. Outside the hospital ward further heat loss should be prevented, e.g. by warm blankets

and the patient must be handled cautiously (e.g. no unclothing). The general principle is that rewarming should take place from the interior to avoid the 'after-drop', the extra fall in core temperature, which takes place if the cold blood from the periphery is redistributed back into the core of the body. This may cause a sudden heart stop.

Indirect cold injuries
Cold climates also have indirect harmful effects on human health. Raynaud's syndrome or white finger disease is mostly an idiopathic phenomenon, in which cold or even emotional exposure leads to cold, pale and numb fingers. Long-lasting vasospasms may lead to ulceration. Raynaud's syndrome may also relate to smoking, previous frostbite, vascular diseases, abnormal plasma proteins or compression of thoracic nerves. The syndrome can be treated by vasodilating agents or by protecting hands from cold. Desensitization treatment (putting hands in cold water) is also often a good measure.

Cold urticaria is a skin allergy caused by local or general cold. Usually a large wheal appears on skin exposed to cold. The wheal disappears after 1–2 h in a warm environment.

In rare cases cold exposure causes angioedema (swelling of veins and tissues, which may be life-threatening and calls for immediate treatment in hospital if the throat and respiratory pathways are affected). The main treatment includes avoiding exposure to cold (water, air) and use of antihistamine drugs. Daily cold showers may also help, but the possible development of angioedema should be taken into account.

Cold-induced increases in blood pressure and hemoconcentration and increased sympathetic activity are well-known risk factors for heart diseases and may explain the high mortality from cardiovascular diseases in winter mentioned above.

Physiologic responses to hot (and humid) environments

Physiologic mechanisms activated by heat

Increased heat loss:
- Vasodilatation, increased skin blood flow
- Sweat secretion (evaporation)

Decreased heat production:
- Inertia
- Decreased food intake

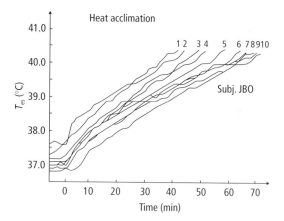

Fig. 2.3.9 Esophageal temperature during exercise in 40 °C dry heat till exhaustion for 10 consecutive days (one subject). The endurance time increased from 40 to 72 min with acclimatization (from [28]).

hyperthermia. Performance is markedly hampered under these adverse conditions, as athletes are forced to lower their exercise intensity (to reduce heat production) or they will attain critically high body temperatures of 40–41 °C, which *per se* will cause fatigue [27,28] (see Fig. 2.3.9).

Cardiovascular changes in hot conditions

The circulatory capacity also affects the ability to sustain exercise in the heat, and hence determines the upper critical temperature. The amount of blood needed for the transport of heat to the skin, H_{skin}, is expressed by the equation:

$$H_{skin} = Q_{skin} \cdot c \cdot (T_{ar} - T_v)$$

where Q_{skin} is blood flow to the skin in L/min, c the heat capacity of blood (approx. 4 kJ/kg) and $T_{ar} - T_v$ is the temperature of arterial and venous blood, respectively, reaching and leaving the skin. If we substitute T_{ar} with T_{re}, rectal or esophageal temperature, and T_v with T_{sk}, and rearrange the equation, we obtain:

$$Q_{sk} = H_{skin} / c(T_{re} - T_{sk}).$$

In warm conditions the difference $(T_{re} - T_{sk})$ becomes smaller, thus the skin blood flow necessary to carry the heat to the skin increases. At rest and during mild to moderate exercise this extra skin blood flow is adequately supplied by an increase in cardiac output and a

Sweating

The physiologic capacity for heat dissipation is closely linked to the ability to sweat. This depends on the size of the individual, on the physical fitness, and on the state of heat acclimatization. Maximal sweating rates may vary between 600 and 700 mL/h for a sedentary person, to about 4 L/h in very well trained and heat-acclimatized individuals exercising in dry heat. The evaporation of 1 L sweat removes approximately 2500 kJ (2430 kJ). However, in humid conditions the amount of sweat which can evaporate may be restricted (evaporation depends on the difference in water vapor pressure between skin and air). If the water vapor pressure difference is too small not all the sweat produced can evaporate; only the evaporated sweat removes heat, the rest drops off and is wasted [26]. Due to the physical limits for evaporation, heat loss is drastically impaired in hot humid environments, and exercise is often associated with advancing degrees of redistribution of blood flow (diminished renal and splanchnic flow). However, during more intense exercise or when hyperthermia is combined with dehydration, cardiac output is limited and skin tissue and active muscles must compete for the available blood flow. A limit is reached for the ability of the heart to supply blood both to the exercising muscles and to cover the thermoregulatory demand for skin blood flow. Under this condition, the core temperature increases, and the skin blood flow may be reduced (see equation). This is when the upper critical temperature is surpassed.

Hot environments represent an additional load on the circulatory system. The temperature-induced vasodilatation and increased skin circulation result in redistribution of blood volume to the periphery, and a fall in central blood volume and reduced filling of the heart. This becomes even worse in the case of dehydration (see below) where plasma volume is reduced. The stroke volume decreases and heart rate is increased to maintain blood pressure. Depending on the severity of the exercise, a compensatory increase in cardiac output may take place. The competition for blood flow between the thermoregulatory need for skin circulation, and the metabolic demand for blood flow to the exercising muscles results firstly in a reduction in skin circulation, and in increased heat storage as mentioned above. But ultimately, with advancing dehydration, blood pressure and cardiac output become reduced, and the blood flow to the exercising muscles also falls (Fig. 2.3.10). The performance/endurance for continued exercise declines, resulting in exhaustion, which is caused primarily not by metabolic alterations but by hyperthermia [27,29,30].

Dehydration

If no fluid is ingested during prolonged physical activity, sweating leads to dehydration, loss of water from the body water compartments. This is a problem, especially in warm environments. Sweat also contains electrolytes, but in lower concentration than the body fluids. So after sweating the body becomes *hypohydrated* and *hyperosmotic*. Both hypohydration and hyperosmolality impair performance by effects on cardiovascular function and sweating [27,31]. Thus, each 1% loss of body weight by dehydration increases heart rate by 6–8 beats/min, and core temperature by

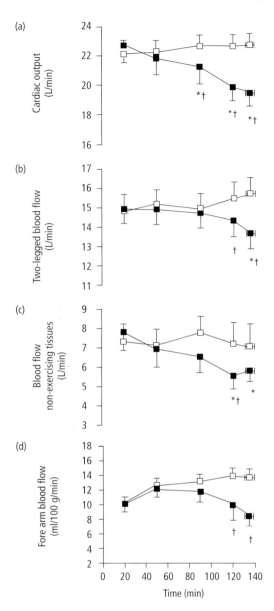

Fig. 2.3.10 Cardiac output and blood flows during dehydration and control trials (from [29]).

0.3 °C during exercise. Also the loss of sodium in the sweat (1–2 g NaCl per L sweat) can be a problem in prolonged exercise. This has to be taken into consideration together with the rehydration and food intake after exercise ('miner's cramp', see Chapters 2.4 and 2.8). With increasing dehydration performance is increasingly reduced, as a result of the reductions in the volume of circulating blood, and the rising core temperature. Severe dehydration during continued exercise leads to earlier fatigue due to hyperthermia; it may cause heat exhaustion or in extreme situations heat stroke (see below).

Heat injury

When the body core temperature increases above the normal level, due to internal or environmental heat stress, clinical symptoms of heat illness may develop. These symptoms range from mild discomfort, swelling of the legs, dizziness or ortostatic syncope in the upright position, heat cramps and heat exhaustion, to the severest form of heat illness, heat stroke, which may be lethal.

Heat exhaustion is usually the result of fluid loss from the vascular system with accompanying cardio-vascular disturbances, such as reductions in skin and splanchnic blood flow and a tendency for a fall in blood pressure. Of note is the fact that the environmental temperature is not necessarily very high in conditions where an endurance athlete performing at high metabolic rates becomes heat exhausted. The upper critical temperature for a good marathon runner may be as low as 20 °C (see Fig. 2.3.4). The treatment for heat exhaustion is to put the patient in a supine position, cool him or her, and supply ample water to drink. The heat exhaustion may develop into *heat stroke*, a potentially fatal syndrome, involving high core temperature, often but not always ceased sweating, unconsciousness, neurologic disorders, metabolic disturbances, cardiovascular failure with low blood pressure and weak pulse. This condition calls for immediate hospitalization and treatment with intravenous infusion and control of acid–base balance.

Causes for the development of the heat stroke syndrome are not fully understood (Fig. 2.3.11). It appears that endotoxins (lipopolysaccharides, LPS) from Gram-negative bacteria in the gastrointestinal tract are liberated, because the intestines become permeable to LPS due to the heat-induced reduction in splanchnic blood flow. This may add a fever to the already high core temperature. Furthermore, a multitude of cellular dysfunctions/damages due to high temperature may be involved in the clinical picture. Several factors such as age, state of training, exercise level, state of

> ## Case story 2.3.2 Copenhagen Marathon, heat exhaustion in temperate climate conditions
>
> A young student of physical education had prepared himself for the marathon; he had trained for several months and was well aware of the importance of keeping well hydrated. He had therefore planned to drink two cups of diluted 'Isostar' (200 mL) each 5 km, and arranged for his wife to follow him on bicycle to supply it. The air temperature was about 22–23 °C on a sunny day. All went well and as planned. After 15 km he overtook a friend, who he started to compete with. This resulted in him spilling half the fluid he was handed the following 4–5 times, but he felt all right until he stopped after 41.5 km to get his ration. He drank, and started off again after his friend, but began to stagger. A physician who happened to be nearby had a look at him, but decided that he would be able to run the final 700 m at a slower pace to complete his run. He ran on, but immediately fell to the ground and blacked out—and came to in the emergency ward, having 1.5 L isotonic fluid administered to him in drop infusion. His temperature was then still elevated.

hydration, heat acclimatization and effect of drugs play a role in the tolerance to heat stress [32] (see Case story 2.3.2).

Prevention and treatment of heat injuries

Procedures which improve conditions for heat loss and cardiovascular stability in warm conditions will be protective against heat injury. Since dehydration is a key factor in the development of heat illness, it is important to prevent dehydration by appropriate fluid intake. Water or isotonic fluid sufficient to replace the sweat loss should be drunk during ongoing exercise (see also Chapter 2.4). Two problems arise: firstly, the

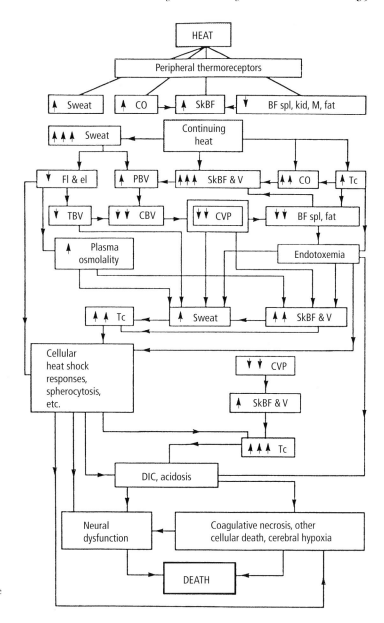

Fig. 2.3.11 Scheme of interacting sequences of events occurring from the beginning of exposure to hot environments to death from heat stroke. Arrows indicate (↑) increase or (↓) decrease in the parameter. BF = blood flow (spl, kid, M, respectively, Splanchnic, kidney and muscle). CBV = central blood volume. CO = cardiac output. CVP = central venous pressure. DIC = disseminated intravascular coagulation. F1 & el = fluid and electrolytes. PBV = peripheral blood volume. SkBF = skin blood flow. Tc = core temperature. V = volume. (From [32].)

sense of thirst is not a good indicator of water deficit. Persons offered fluid to replace a sweat loss stop drinking before the deficit has been compensated for. This 'voluntary dehydration' must be overcome by encouraging persons exercising in warm conditions to drink more than they feel is enough. The other problem is the limitation in the rate of gastric emptying. Fluid is transferred from the stomach to the gut, where absorption takes place at a maximum rate of approximately 1–1.2 L/h, while sweat rates during exercise in hot conditions may exceed 3 L/h. This means that even with optimal fluid intake dehydration cannot be totally prevented during prolonged exercise such as marathon running or military activity in warm

Table 2.3.2 Changes in physical parameters with altitude above sea level (s.l.).

Altitude (m)	Air pressure			Air density		Temperature and water content of air		
								Water content (at 100% saturation)
	Atmospheric (mmHg)	P_{O_2} (mmHg)	% of s.l. value	kg/m^3	% of s.l. value	°C	g/L	% of s.l. value
0	760	159	100	1.12	100	30	33.3	100
2000	600	125	79	1.01	90	17	15.4	46
3400	500	105	66	0.87	78	+7	8.1	24
5500	360	75	50	0.70	60	−7	3.0	9
8800	250	52	33	0.50	45	−29	0.5	2

climates [33]. Sports organizations, coaches and physicians responsible for events in hot and especially humid climates should agree on rules for the cancellation of competitions if temperature and humidity exceed certain limits, e.g. 35 °C, 60% relative humidity, to prevent heat illness [1].

Acclimatization

Acclimatization to heat is another important means of protection against heat stress. Stressful environments induce physiologic adaptive changes, which improve tolerance to the stress. When humans are exposed acutely to exercise in hot environments, their heart rate and core temperature increase more than under cool conditions, and their performance and endurance for prolonged exercise is reduced (Fig. 2.3.9). A prolonged stay in a hot climate, or repeated daily exposures in climatic chambers over a period of several days to weeks will induce physiologic changes, which include an increase in sweating rate, a lowering of resting core temperature and increased blood volume. These adaptations are beneficial for performance, since they lead to an increased evaporative heat loss, resulting in a lowering of the core and skin temperatures during work in hot environments [26,28]. Furthermore, the improved filling of the cardiovascular system results in a lower heart rate and improved endurance for exercise. However, in hot humid environments the improved sweating capacity does not help if the physical limits for evaporation of the produced sweat are exceeded.

High altitude

Introduction

Physical changes and their implications

Exposure to high altitude is associated with a reduction in barometric pressure, by one-third at an altitude of 3400 m, by half at an altitude of 5500 m, and by about two-thirds at the altitude of Mount Everest (8848 m). There is an almost parallel decline in partial pressure of oxygen and air density. Furthermore, temperature declines approximately by 1 degree per 150 m of altitude. As a consequence of the decrease in temperature, the water content of fully saturated air decreases dramatically because of falling water vapor pressure (see Table 2.3.2). In addition, the thinner overlying atmosphere absorbs less and snowfields reflect more radiation. Therefore solar radiation, especially of short wavelength near the ultraviolet spectrum, is increased at high altitude and calls for special protection of skin and eyes.

Table 2.3.2 also shows that there are already considerable physical changes in the environment at the highest altitudes at which athletes compete or perform classic high-altitude training (2000–2800 m). In brief, altitude can have the following principal effects on exercise performance.

1 As long as maximum voluntary power output is not affected, it will enhance performance in short anaerobic events involving high speed because of decreased air resistance.

2 It will decrease performance in events which depend predominantly on aerobic capacity because of a decreased ambient Po_2. Running over distances longer than about 1500 m will be affected as demonstrated by the results of the Olympic Games held in Mexico City (2200 m) in 1968.

3 The lower water content and lower temperature of ambient air may affect performance by exacerbating exercise-induced asthma in athletes with bronchial hyperreactivity or asthma.

4 At altitudes that are relevant for mountaineers (3000–4000 m and higher) the danger of acute altitude illnesses (see p. 243) and cold injuries (see p. 234) will increase.

This section will discuss in more detail acute adjustments and acclimatization to hypoxia, the effects of acute and chronic altitude exposure on aerobic performance, and the modalities and efficacy of high-altitude training. In addition, an overview of acute high-altitude illness is given. As cold injuries are not strictly related to hypoxia, they are discussed in a separate section.

Immediate adjustments and acclimatization to hypoxia

The energy requirement and thus the O_2 demand for performing a given task does not change with altitude. Because of the reduced partial pressure of oxygen, O_2 loading of the blood is incomplete at high altitude. The reduced O_2 content per volume unit of blood is compensated for at several levels.

Ventilation. Ventilation increases immediately and continues to rise further over the first 10–14 days at a given altitude. This further rise is called ventilatory acclimatization. As a consequence of this arterial Po_2 rises considerably during this time. On the other hand, more CO_2 will be blown off by the enhanced ventilation causing a relative increase of bicarbonate, i.e. a respiratory alkalosis. This is partially compensated for by increased renal bicarbonate excretion. This leads to a reduction in the blood buffer capacity [34].

Circulation. Cardiac output and heart rate are increased for a given submaximum workload. With acclimatization this increase declines but heart rate still remains elevated compared to sea level.

Blood. Oxygen-carrying capacity is increased per volume unit of blood, acutely by decreasing plasma volume and in the long range by increases in the number of circulating red cells, i.e. by increasing erythropoiesis through release of erythropoietin from the kidney. Furthermore, 2,3-diphosphoglycerate (2,3-DPG) increases in red cells and favors unloading of oxygen in the tissue. This effect may, depending on the altitude, be offset or even overridden by the respiratory alkalosis which favors loading of oxygen in the lung [35].

Muscle. There are no immediate adjustments in the muscle cell components for hypoxia. Training studies in hypobaric chambers suggest that acclimatization to altitudes below 4000 m may increase capillary density, mitochondrial density, aerobic enzymes and enzyme activities [36]. Furthermore, increase of myoglobin and other proteins accounts for the augmented buffer capacity of muscle tissue. At altitudes above 4000 m (Himalayan mountaineers) muscle mass, muscle fiber and oxidative capacity of muscle decrease [37], a surprising finding, for which the low level of exercise intensity and insufficient nutrition may account.

Aerobic performance

Maximum aerobic capacity

$\dot{V}o_{2\,max}$ decreases with acute exposure to high altitude by approximately 1% per 100 m above an altitude of 1500 m. In highly trained athletes hypoxia-induced reduction of $\dot{V}o_{2\,max}$ may be considerably greater (Fig. 2.3.12) and it can be detected at altitudes as low as 1000 m [36,38]. Thus, at elevations of 2000–2500 m at which altitude training is performed, athletes may have a considerably greater reduction of their aerobic capacity than the expected 5–10%. This forces them to reduce the training intensity. This reduction shows, however, considerable interindividual variability [39].

Despite improved oxygen delivery and utilization with acclimatization the depressed $\dot{V}o_{2\,max}$ increases little, if at all, with chronic exposure to hypoxia. This lack of improvement can in part be attributed to a reduction in maximal heart rate [40]. A young healthy mountaineer climbing at 8800 m without supplemental oxygen is left with less than one-third of his sea-level aerobic capacity. Expressed in O_2 uptake he is at

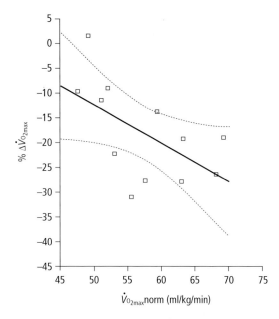

Fig. 2.3.12 Individuals with a higher $\dot{V}_{O_2 \max}$ show a greater loss of aerobic performance ($\Delta \dot{V}_{O_2 \max}$) when exercising at a simulated altitude of 3000 m in a hypobaric chamber. From [21].

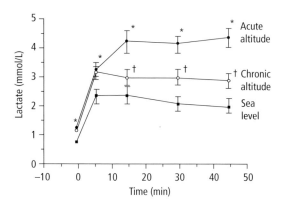

Fig. 2.3.13 Arterial plasma lactate significantly increases at high altitude when exercising at the same absolute workload at an intensity that elicited 50% of sea-level $\dot{V}_{O_2 \max}$ on day 1 and day 21 at an altitude of 4300 m. With acclimatization lactate levels fall significantly but remain elevated compared to sea-level values. From [43].

the level observed in patients with severe heart failure (15 mL/kg/min) and his rate of climbing is accordingly slow. The maximum power output of this individual is reduced to about 1.5 W/kg with maximal values of ventilation of 184 L/min, with a heart rate of 120/min and with lactate of 3.5 mmol/L [41]. Despite an arterial oxygen saturation of only 50%, the ECG is normal. The reduction in maximum heart rate, presumably due to a down-regulation of α-receptors, may protect his heart from ischemia by reducing the maximum workload on the heart.

Submaximum aerobic performance

At high altitude the same absolute submaximum workload elicits a higher ventilation, a greater cardiac output and thus a higher heart rate as well as a greater increase in plasma lactate than at low altitude. Acclimatization to high altitude improves submaximum performance as demonstrated by increased endurance time as well as a reduction of heart rate and plasma lactate (Fig. 2.3.13) for a given workload [42,43]. The fact that lactate is higher at a given submaximum exercise level while several studies found maximum lactate to

be reduced compared with exercise at sea level (see data from Mount Everest mentioned above) has been termed the 'lactate paradox'. This phenomenon, for which there is no clear explanation, has been questioned by recent findings of unchanged maximum lactate levels during the Chacaltaya expedition.

In summary, acclimatization to high altitude does not improve the reduced $\dot{V}_{O_2 \max}$ but it enhances performance at submaximum levels. This may help to explain why athletes competing at altitude must train and thereby acclimatize at this altitude prior to the competition. Furthermore, because of changes in the relationship between heart rate and workloads at altitude, it is necessary to adjust heart rate-based recommendations for training intensities.

Training at high altitude for sea-level competition

The hypothesis that high-altitude training improves sea-level performance is based on the assumption of beneficial effects by acclimatizing to high altitude and/or hypoxia being an additional training stimulus. Accordingly, three concepts have emerged:
• Live high—train high (classic high-altitude training).
• Live high—train low (high-altitude houses or hypoxic tents).

- Live low—train high (training in hypobaric chambers or in normobaric hypoxia).

The most important *beneficial effect of altitude acclimatization* for sea-level performance is the increase in erythropoiesis. Improvements of aerobic capacity after high-altitude training correlate with the increase in red cell mass (RCM). It appears that a significant increase in RCM only occurs when more than 3 weeks are spent at an altitude equivalent to 2300 m. Interestingly, an exposure of 8–10 h at night at an FIO_2 of 15.6% (equivalent to 3000 m) for 23 consecutive nights while living and training in normoxia for the rest of the day did not increase RCM [44]. There are preliminary reports of an increase in RCM by about 5–7% after living 12–16 h per day at normobaric hypoxia equivalent to an altitude of 2500 m for 25 days suggesting that this time and altitude may be sufficient for stimulation of erythropoiesis. Specific ventilation does not change after altitude training indicating that ventilatory acclimatization has no advantage for sea-level performance. The effects of acclimatization on the hemoglobin–O_2 affinity and on the plasma volume are rapidly reversible and most likely offer no benefit for sea-level performance. Increases of myoglobin and possibly another muscle protein (karosin) enhance the local buffer capacity of muscle tissue and overcome the potential disadvantage of reduced blood buffer capacity which is due to renal compensation of respiratory alkalosis. It has already been mentioned above that mountaineers living and exercising above altitudes of 4000–5000 m have a loss of muscle mass and a reduction in oxidative capacity. This is mostly a consequence of catabolism due to reduced food intake because of lack of appetite. Regularly exercising on a bicycle ergometer during a chamber study (Operation Everest II, described in reference [41]) could not prevent muscle loss.

Training at high altitude may have several negative aspects like reduction in absolute workload, lack of adequate facilities or locations, unfavorable climate and sleep disturbance. These may offset the benefits of altitude acclimatization. Therefore, the concept of living high and training low has become popular although the evidence in favor of this approach for the elite athlete is at best circumstantial. One well-controlled study, published in German only, demonstrated a greater improvement of performance after classic high-altitude training [46] and one equally well con-

trolled study found the same after living high and training low [45] compared to sea-level training. These studies were performed in moderately well trained athletes ($\dot{V}O_{2\,max}$ 55–65 mL/kg/min). There are no controlled data obtained in elite athletes that unequivocally demonstrate a benefit of either training modality. A recent investigation suggests that there is an individual response to training at high altitude that depends on how much erythropoiesis is increased and on the training intensity that can be maintained at high altitude [39].

Living in normoxia and *training in a hypoxic chamber* at simulated altitudes up to 5000 m leads to increases in myoglobin content, oxidative enzymes, capillaries and muscle fiber volume when training is performed at the same absolute workload as in normoxia. Thus, the beneficial effect can be attributed to more intense work rather than to hypoxia itself. Training at the same relative workload in hypoxia vs. normoxia also has no additional effects on endurance performance [47].

Acute high-altitude illnesses

Unacclimatized healthy individuals who ascend too fast to high altitudes are at risk of developing acute high-altitude illnesses. The faster they climb and the higher they go the greater the chances of developing a serious, possibly life-threatening illness. We distinguish between acute mountain sickness (AMS), an illness dominated by cerebral symptoms which can progress to overt cerebral edema (high-altitude cerebral edema, HACE) and high-altitude pulmonary edema (HAPE). AMS often also precedes the pulmonary form of high-altitude illnesses. There are distinct differences between these entities with regard to aspects of pathophysiology as well as prophylaxis and treatment with drugs (Table 2.3.3).

Acute mountain sickness (AMS) frequently occurs within 8–12 h after rapid ascent to altitudes above 2000–2500 m [48]. It is characterized by headache, nausea or loss of appetite, fatigue, dizziness and insomnia. AMS usually resolves spontaneously over the next 2 days when no further gain in altitude occurs. It may also progress to ataxia and clouded consciousness which are early signs of potentially lethal HACE [49]. The pathophysiology of this illness is poorly understood. While imaging techniques show cerebral edema when HACE is present, the cerebral changes accompa-

Table 2.3.3

	Acute mountain sickness	High-altitude pulmonary edema
Occurrence	Altitude > 2000–2500 m	Altitude > 3000 m
Latency	6–12 h	1–4 days
Leading symptoms	Cerebral symptoms: • Headache • Nausea, vomiting • Neurological abnormalities	Pulmonary symptoms: • Cough • Dyspnea and decreased exercise performance • Rales
Pathophysiology	Low hypoxic ventilatory response Sodium retention	Exaggerated hypoxic pulmonary vasoconstriction
	Increased cerebral blood flow and permeability of blood brain barrier?	Exaggerated hypoxic pulmonary vasoconstriction
Prophylaxis	Pre-acclimatization and slow ascent to altitudes > 2500 m (average daily ascent rate: 300–500 m above 2000 m)	Nifedipine: in case of known susceptibility and rapid ascent
	Acetazolamide: in case of known susceptibility and rapid ascent	Nifedipine: in case of known susceptibility and rapid ascent
Therapy		Descent by at least 1000 m of height, supplemental oxygen
	In addition: glucocorticoids	In addition: Nifedipine
Prognosis	• AMS: spontaneous resolution within 1–2 days • HACE: lethal without treatment, prolonged recovery of severe cases at low altitude	• 50% mortality without therapy • Clinical recovery at low altitude within 1–2 days

nying AMS are subtle and hardly detectable by conventional imaging techniques.

There is a large interindividual variability regarding susceptibility to AMS. While usually less than 10% have AMS (defined as headache and one additional symptom) at an altitude of 2500 m, about 40–50% have AMS after rapid ascent to 4500 m. For prevention it is important that the rate of ascent matches the degree of acclimatization and the individual tolerance. When symptoms occur, a day of rest should be taken. If this is not followed by improvement, one must descend. In severe and often rapidly progressive cases application of supplemental oxygen or treatment in a portable hyperbaric chamber and the administration of dexamethasone (4–8 mg every 6 h) should be given until descent is possible. Acetazolamide (2×250 mg) can be taken for prophylaxis when slow ascent in susceptible individuals is not possible.

High-altitude pulmonary edema (HAPE) presents after rapid ascent from low altitude within 2–5 days [50]. It is rarely observed below altitudes of 3000 m and after 1 week of acclimatization at a particular altitude. In most cases, it is preceded by symptoms of AMS. Early symptoms of HAPE include exertional dyspnea, cough and reduced exercise performance. As edema progresses, cough worsens, and breathlessness at rest and orthopnea occur. Gurgling in the chest and pink frothy sputum indicate advanced cases. There is large interindividual variability in susceptibility to HAPE. Individuals with a proven history of HAPE have a 60% chance of developing this illness again when the exposure is similar compared to the last episode [50].

The clinical examination reveals cyanosis, tachypnea, tachycardia, and elevated body temperature, which generally does not exceed 38.5 °C. Rales are discrete at the beginning, typically located over the middle lung fields. Often, there is a discrepancy between the minor finding at auscultation compared with the widespread disease on the chest radiograph. In advanced cases, signs of concomitant cerebral edema,

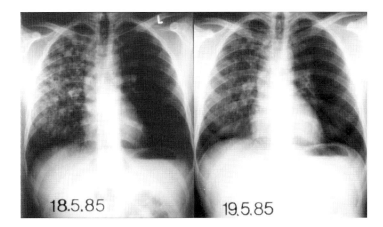

Fig. 2.3.14 Chest radiograph with patchy alveolar pulmonary edema of a 23-year-old mountaineer with HAPE on admittance to hospital (600 m) after evacuation by helicopter from an altitude of 4559 m (left side). Reduction of edema over 24 h with bed rest and supplemental oxygen (right side).

such as ataxia and decreased levels of consciousness, are frequent findings.

There are no characteristic findings in common laboratory examinations. Abnormal results may be due to accompanying dehydration, stress and preceding exercise. Arterial blood gas measurements of four cases of advanced HAPE at 4559 m showed a mean Po_2 of 23 mmHg and a mean arterial oxygen saturation of 48%. These findings demonstrate the severity of this illness. In early cases, values around 30 mmHg for Po_2 and 70% for S_aO_2 were observed at this altitude. Chest radiographs and CT scans of early HAPE cases show a patchy, peripheral distribution of edema (Fig. 2.3.14).

Cardiac catheterization of untreated cases of HAPE at high altitude revealed normal wedge pressure and pulmonary artery hypertension (systolic pressure in the order of 60 mmHg compared to 40 mmHg in controls at 4559 m). This increased pressure precedes edema formation. Lowering pulmonary artery pressure by nifedipine is effective for treatment and prevention of HAPE. The prevailing hypothesis to explain increased capillary filtration pressure is inhomogeneous hypoxic vasoconstriction accounting for increased capillary pressure in areas of overperfusion. Recent investigations by bronchoalveolar lavage suggest that early HAPE is caused by a pressure-induced leak without increased permeability due to an inflammatory reaction.

With the exception of the recommended drugs, the prevention and treatment of HAPE resemble those of AMS and are summarized in Table 2.3.4. The fol-

Table 2.3.4 How to avoid and treat high-altitude pulmonary edema.

Prevention
1 Slow ascent for susceptible individuals (average increase in sleeping altitude of 300–350 m/day above 2000 m).
2 No ascent to higher altitude with symptoms of acute mountain sickness (AMS).
3 Descent when symptoms of AMS do not improve after a day of rest.
4 Under circumstances of high risk avoid vigorous exercise when not acclimatized.
5 Nifedipine: 20 mg slow release formulation every 8 h (or 30–60 mg sustained release formulation once daily) for susceptible individuals when slow ascent is impossible.

Treatment
1 Descent by at least 1000 m of altitude (primary choice in mountaineering).
2 Supplemental oxygen: 2–4 L/min (primary choice in areas with medical facilities).
3 When **1** and/or **2** not possible:
20 mg nifedipine slow release formulation every 6 h.
Portable hyperbaric chamber.
Descent as soon as possible.

lowing case history demonstrates that HAPE can be a life-threatening illness from which one recovers rapidly at low altitude. It also demonstrates that a susceptible individual may continue mountaineering even as a mountain guide because HAPE can be avoided with adequate preventive measures (see Case story 2.3.3).

Case story 2.3.3

In the summer of 1984 a party of 12 people led by two mountain guides ascended by cable car from low altitude to 3887 m to climb for several days at altitudes between 3600 and 4500 m. On the third day one of the mountain guides, who was 25 years old, noticed unusual shortness of breath while climbing to 4075 m, which improved when descending to a hut at 3611 m. There his appetite was reduced, he had headache, felt weak and slept poorly. He did not want to leave a group of 12 people with only one guide and accompanied the party on the next day to the Margherita Hut (4559 m). On this ascent, he could not keep up with the group above 4000 m altitude because of severe shortness of breath. He also noticed a dry cough. After he had fought his way up to the hut, he did not recover, was cyanotic and had considerable dyspnea at rest. There were rales over both lungs. He showed truncal ataxia but his consciousness was not clouded. Arterial blood gas analysis, measured by a research team working in the hut, demonstrated severe hypoxemia with a P_{O_2} of 23.4 mmHg, a P_{CO_2} of 26.3 mmHg and a measured arterial oxygen saturation of 43%. He was immediately flown out by helicopter to a hospital at 600 m where the diagnosis of HAPE was confirmed by chest radiography (see Fig. 2.3.4). At low altitude, the patient felt immediately better; blood examinations including sedimentation rate and a differential white cell count were normal. He was on supplemental oxygen overnight. When he left the hospital the next morning arterial blood gases without supplemental oxygen showed increased ventilation in order to achieve normoxemia: P_{O_2} 73.8 mmHg, P_{CO_2} 33.4 mmHg (oxygen saturation 95%).

He continued to work as a mountain guide and had a similar episode of HAPE at the same location on day 3 after ascending from low altitude with only one night spent at 3611 m. Since then he pays attention to slow ascent (average rate of ascent 300–400 m per day above 2500 m) when staying for lengthy periods at altitudes above 4000 m. When slow ascent is not possible, he takes nifedipine, 20 mg every 8 h, during ascent until reaching the final altitude. With these measures, he is able to work normally as a mountain guide. He also accompanies groups in the Himalayas and in South America where he reached, without any problems, the top of Aconcagua (6990 m) after preacclimatizing by climbing the volcanoes in Ecuador (altitude between 2800 and 6300 m). Since 1986 he has had one further episode of threatened HAPE, at an altitude of about 6000 m, which he recognized so early that he was able to descend by himself.

Multiple choice questions

1 *The core temperature during exercise:*

a reaches a new level after 10 min exercise

b is increased during exercise in proportion to work intensity

c rises in proportion to the relative workload of the individual

d rises due to an insufficient heat loss

e is higher in trained than in untrained athletes at the same work intensity.

2 *The 'prescriptive zone' is:*

a a temperature range where body temperature is independent of environmental temperatures

b independent of the activity level

c affected by the sweating capacity

d the same as 'comfortable' temperature conditions

e the interval in which shivering responses occur

f reduced in water.

3 *In hot conditions:*

a maximal sweating rate is not so important for endurance performance

b competition between muscle and skin blood flows causes an increase in core temperature

c fatter individuals tolerate the heat better

d the process of heat acclimatization leads to increased blood volume *e* the air humidity has no effect on performance

f sweat loss impairs exercise performance.

4 *Heat illness is prevented by:*

a warming up before physical performance

b fluid intake during activity

c fluid intake after prolonged activity

d training without water for 1 week

e acclimatization to hot conditions.

5 *Cold exposure in humans leads to:*

a immediate shivering

b increase in serum norepinephrine

c loss of appetite

d extravasation

e increased serum FFAs.

6 *With regard to heat production:*

a it occurs mainly in the muscle

b uncoupling proteins are proton channels

c adult humans have no uncoupling proteins

d specific dynamic action is associated with exercise

e drugs increasing cAMP produce heat.

7 *With regard to heat loss and clothing:*

a radiation is the main avenue for heat loss in winter sports

b IREQ index relates to temperature and wind

c in winter sports the insulation of clothing is usually 5–6 clo units

d frostbite begins to develop when WCI is over 1600 W/m^2

e cold sensations acclimatize sooner than shivering.

8 *With regard to cold injuries:*

a ice crystals cause cold injuries

b local ointments protect from frostbite

c frostbite can be treated by fire

d comatose and cold patients should be warmed by active moving.

9 *Immediate adaptive responses to high altitude are:*

a increase of red blood cell mass

b decrease of plasma volume

c increase of ventilation

d increase of heart rate for a given workload

e increase of muscle oxidative capacity.

10 *The following statements about the effects of high altitude on aerobic performance are correct:*

a $\dot{V}o_{2\,max}$ decreases.

b $\dot{V}o_{2\,max}$ significantly increases with acclimatization.

c Maximal heart rate increases with acclimatization.

d Heart rate for a given workload decreases with acclimatization.

e An untrained individual has a greater decrease in aerobic performance than a well-trained individual.

11 *The following statements are correct regarding high-altitude training:*

a Training at high altitude improves performance at high altitude more than training at low altitude.

b Training in a hypobaric chamber is more effective than training in normobaric hypoxia.

c Increase in red cell mass is the principal factor for improvement of sea-level performance.

d The changes of hemoglobin affinity for oxygen are important for improvement of endurance performance at low altitude.

e Training at high altitude improves buffer capacity of muscle tissue.

12 *Acute mountain sickness (AMS): which statements are correct?*

a The most frequent symptom is vomiting.

b When symptoms of AMS occur, a mountaineer must always descend.

c Ataxia and decreased consciousness indicate progression to high-altitude cerebral edema (HACE).

d Slow ascent is the major preventive measure.

e The treatment of choice for HACE is descent, supplemental oxygen and glucocorticosteroids.

13 *High-altitude pulmonary edema (HAPE): which statements are correct?*

a An inadequate drop in performance accompanied by dyspnea and cough is an early sign of HAPE.

b Lowering pulmonary artery pressure is the principle of treatment.

c Acetazolamide has been shown to prevent HAPE.

d Clinical recovery at low altitude occurs within 1 or 2 days.

e An individual with a history of HAPE has a high probability of developing HAPE again under similar circumstances.

References

1 Nielsen B. Olympics in Atlanta: a fight against physics. *Med Sci Sports Exerc* 1996; **28**: 665–8.

2 Saltin B, Hermannsen L. Esophageal, rectal and muscle temperature during exercise. *Med Sci Sports Exerc* 1966; **21**: 1757–62.

3 Lind AR. A physiological criterion for setting thermal limits for everyday work. *J Appl Physiol* 1963; **18**: 51–6.

4 Nielsen M. Die Regulation der Körpertemperatur bei Muskelarbeit. *Skand Arch Physiol* 1938; **79**: 193–230.

5 Bittel JHM, Nonotte-Varly C, Livecchi-Gonnot GH, Savourey MJ, Hanniquit AM. Physical fitness and thermoregulatory reactions in a cold environment in men. *J Appl Physiol* 1988; **65**: 1984–9.

6 Wilber RL, Rundell KW, Szmedra L, Jenkinson DM, Im J, Drake SD. Incidence of exercise-induced bronchospasm in olympic winter sport athletes. *Med Sci Sports Exerc* 2000; **32**: 732–7.

7 Ricquier D, Fleury C, Larose M *et al.* Contribution of studies on uncoupling proteins to research on metabolic diseases. *J Intern Med* 1999; **245**: 637–42.

8 Danielsson U. Windchill and the risk of freezing. *J Appl Physiol* 1996; **81**: 2666–73.

9 ISO9920. Ergonomics of thermal environment—cold environments. 1995, Geneva: International Standard Organisation.

10 Thompson RL, Hayward JS. Wet-cold exposure and hypothermia: thermal and metabolic responses to prolonged exercise in rain. *J Appl Physiol* 1996; **81**: 1128–37.

11 ISO/TR-11079. Evaluation of cold environments—Determination of required clothing insulation (IREQ). 1993, Geneva: International Standard Organisation.

12 Bruck K, Baum E, Schwennike HP. Cold-adaptive modifications in man induced by repeated short-term cold exposures during a 10-day and -night cold exposure. *Pflügers Arch* 1976; **363**: 125–33.

13 Leppäluoto J, Korhonen J, Hassi J. Habituation of thermal sensations, skin temperature and norepinephrine in men exposed to cold. *J Appl Physiol* 2001; **90**: 1211–18.

14 Mager M, Robinson SM. Substrate mobilization and utilization in fasting men during cold exposure. *Bull New Jersey Acad Sci* 1969 (symposium issue); 6–30.

15 Keatinge WR. The effect of repeated daily exposures to cold and of improved physical fitness on the metabolic and vascular responses to cold air. *J Physiol* 1961; **177**: 207–20.

16 Scholander PF, Hammel TH, Lange Andersen K, Logning Y. Metabolic acclimation to cold in man. *J Appl Physiol* 1958; **12**: 1–8.

17 Park YS, Rennie DW, Lee IS *et al.* Time course of deacclimation to cold water immersion in Korean women divers. *J Appl Physiol* 1983; **54**: 1708–16.

18 Young AJ, Myza SR, Sawka MN, Gonzalez RR, Pandolf KB. Human thermoregulatory responses to cold air are altered by repeated cold water immersions. *J Appl Physiol* 1986; **60**: 1542–8.

19 O'Brien C, Young AJ, Lee DT, Shitzer A, Sawka MN, Pandolf KB. Role of core temperature as a stimulus for cold acclimation during repeated immersion in 20 °C water. *J Appl Physiol* 2000; **89**: 242–50.

20 Vuori I. Sudden death and exercise: effects of age and type of activity. *Sport Sci Rev* 1995; **4**: 46–84.

21 Galloway SD, Maughan RJ. Effects of ambient temperature on capacity to perform prolonged cycle exercise in man. *Med Sci Sports Exerc* 1997; **29**: 1240–9.

22 Sallis R, Chassay CM. Recognizing and treating common cold-induced injury in outdoor sports. *Med Sci Sports Exerc* 1999; **31**: 1367–73.

23 Hassi J, Mäkinen T. Frostbite: occurrence, risk factors and consequences. *Int J Circumpolar Health* 2000; **59**: 92–8.

24 Paton B. A history of frostbite treatment. *Int J Circumpolar Health* 2000; **59**: 99–107.

25 Berg U. Human power at subnormal body temperatures. *Acta Physiol Scand* 1980; **478**: 1–39.

26 Nielsen B, Strange S, Christensen NJ, Warberg J, Saltin B. Acute and adaptive responses in humans to exercise in a warm, humid environment. *Pflügers Arch* 1997; **434**: 49–56.

27 González-Alonso J, Teller C, Andersen SL, Jensen FB, Hylding T, Nielsen B. High body temperature causes fatigue during exercise in humans. *J Appl Physiol* 1999; **86**: 1032–9.

28 Nielsen B, Hales JRS, Strange S, Christensen JN, Warberg J, Saltin B. Human circulatory and thermoregulatory adaptations with heat acclimation and exercise. *J Physiol (Lond)* 1993; **460**: 467–85.

29 González-Alonso J, Calbert JA, Nielsen B. Metabolic and thermodynamic alterations with dehydration-induced reductions in muscle blood flow in exercising humans. *J Physiol (Lond)* 1999; **520**: 577–89.

30 González-Alonso J, Calbert JA, Nielsen B. Muscle blood flow is reduced with dehydration during prolonged exercise in humans. *J Physiol (Lond)* 1998; **513**: 895–905.

31 Sawka MN. Physiological consequences of hypohydration: exercise performance and thermoregulation. *Med Sci Sports Exerc* 1992; **24**: 657–70.

32 Hales JRS, Hubbard RW, Gaffin SL. Limitation of heat tolerance. In: Fregly MJ, Blatteis CM, eds. *Handbook of Physiology*, Section 4, Environmental Physiology. Bethesda MD: American Physiological Society, 1996: 285–355.

33 Nielsen B, Krog P. Optimal fluid replacement during long lasting exercise in 18 °C and 32 °C ambient temperature. *Scand J Med Sci Sports* 1994; **4**: 173–80.

34 Bender PR, McCullough RE, McCullough RG *et al.* Increased exercise S_aO_2 independent of ventilatory acclimatization at 4300 m. *J Appl Physiol* 1989; **66**: 2733–8.

35 Mairbäurl H, Schobersberger W, Oelz O, Bärtsch P, Eckardt KU, Bauer C. Unchanged in vivo P-50 at high altitude despite decreased erythrocyte age and elevated 2,3-diphosphoglycerate. *J Appl Physiol* 1990; **68**: 1186–94.

36 Terrados N. Altitude training and muscular metabolism. *Int J Sports Med* 1992; **13**: S206–S209.

37 Hoppeler H, Ceretelli P. Morphologic and metabolic response to chronic hypoxia: the muscle system. In: Fregly MJ, Blatteis CM, eds. *Handbook of Physiology*, Section 4, Environmental Physiology 2. Oxford: Oxford University Press, 1996: 1155–81.

38 Koistinen P, Takala T, Martikkala V, Leppäluoto J. Aerobic fitness influences the response of maximal oxygen uptake and lactate threshold in acute hypobaric hypoxia. *Int J Sports Med* 1995; **16**: 78–81.

39 Chapman RF, Stray-Gundersen J, Levine BD. Individual

variation in response to altitude training. *J Appl Physiol* 1998; **85**(4): 1448–56.

40 Gonzalez NC, Clancy RL, Moue Y, Richalet J-P. Increasing maximal heart rate increases maximal O_2 uptake in rats acclimatized to simulated altitude. *J Appl Physiol* 1998; **84**(1): 164–8.

41 Sutton JR, Reeves JT, Wagner PD *et al.* Operation Everest II: oxygen transport during exercise at extreme simulated altitude. *J Appl Physiol* 1988; **64**: 1309–21.

42 Maher JT, Jones LG, Hartley LH. Effects of high-altitude exposure on submaximal endurance capacity of men. *J Appl Physiol* 1974; **37**: 895–8.

43 Mazzeo RS, Bender PR, Brooks GA *et al.* Arterial catecholamine responses during exercise with acute and chronic high-altitude exposure. *Am J Physiol* 1991; **261**: E419–E424.

44 Ashenden MJ, Gore CJ, Dobson GP, Hahn AG. 'Live high, train low' does not change the total haemoglobin mass of male endurance athletes sleeping at a simulated altitude of 3000 m for 23 nights. *Eur J Appl Physiol* 1999; **80**: 479–84.

45 Levine BD, Stray-Gundersen J. 'Living high–training low'. effect of moderate-altitude acclimatization with low-altitude training on performance. *J Appl Physiol* 1997; **83**(1): 102–12.

46 Mellerowicz H, Meller W, Woweries J *et al.* Vergleichende Untersuchungen über Wirkungen von Höhentraining auf die Dauerleistung in Meereshöhe. *Sportarzt Sportmed* 1970; **21**: 207–40.

47 Desplanches D, Hoppeler H, Linossier MT *et al.* Effects of training in normoxia and normobaric hypoxia on human muscle ultrastructure. *Eur J Physiol* 1993; **425**: 263–7.

48 Johnson TS, Rock PB. Acute mountain sickness. *N Engl J Med* 1988; **319**: 841–5.

49 Houston CS, Dickinson J. Cerebral form of high-altitude illness. *Lancet* 1975; **II** (18 October): 758–61.

50 Bärtsch P. High altitude pulmonary edema. *Med Sci Sports Exerc* 1999; **31**(1): S23–S27.

51 Loyd EL. *Hypothermia and Cold Stress*. London: Croom-Helm, 1986.

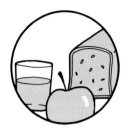

Chapter 2.4
Nutrition and Fluid Intake with Training

LEIF HAMBRÆUS,

STEFAN BRANTH &

ANNE RABEN

Classical reference

Ivy JL, Katz AL, Cutler CL, Sherman WM, Coyle
EF. Muscle glycogen synthesis after exercise: effect
of time of carbohydrate ingestion. *J Appl Physiol*
1988; **64**: 1480–1485.

The effect of the time of ingestion of a carbohydrate
supplement on muscle glycogen post exercise was examined. The authors investigated 12 male cyclists who
exercised continuously on a cycle ergometer at 68%
$\dot{V}_{O_{2\,max}}$ interrupted by six 2-min intervals of 88%
$\dot{V}_{O_{2\,max}}$ on two separate occasions. A 25% carbohydrate solution was ingested either immediately post
exercise or 2 hours post exercise.

Interestingly, the glycogen synthesis rate after exercise was markedly higher for the group who received
carbohydrate immediately after exercise compared
with the group that received it 2 hours after exercise.
The slower rate of glycogen storage in the group
receiving carbohydrate at a later time point occurred
despite the fact that the response in plasma glucose
and insulin to carbohydrate loading was similar in the
two groups.

The study was the first to show in humans that ingestion of a carbohydrate supplement immediately
post exercise will result in the most optimal recovery of
muscle glycogen storage.

Optimal nutrition for physical training and competition — a challenge for nutritional science

In order to perform optimally during daily training as
well as during competition, it is essential that an athlete's habitual diet contains enough of both required
nutrients and fluid. An optimal nutrient and fluid status is also important to avoid injuries and to optimize
the immune system. Not only nutrient composition,
but also timing and frequency of food and fluid intake
are critical for optimal performance.

One of the reasons for the common idea that athletes
need special diets might be based on the misconception
that an increased energy turnover *per se* leads to
increased needs for other nutrients. However, this is
not necessarily the case. Increased physical exercise is
essentially a question of increased energy turnover,
while the turnover of essential nutrients is usually not
related to energy turnover to such an extent that there
is a need for increased intakes. Most studies of food
habits have indicated that the nutrient density, i.e.
nutrients per energy unit, is the same in low-energy
consumers as in high-energy consumers. Thus the increased food intake in physically active individuals will
automatically have an increased intake of essential nutrients. To what extent the intake of essential nutrients
is a valid problem is consequently mainly due to two
factors: (i) are the athletes in energy balance? and (ii)
are they eating an optimal, nutritionally balanced diet
according to recommendations? For recreational athletes this also means that there is no need for specific
supplements or diets to cover their energy needs, as illustrated in Case story 2.4.1 below. This may also be
the case in elite athletes. However their often intensive
training programmes in combination with short times
for recovery between competitions may call for extra
nutritional support.

250

Case story 2.4.1 Energy in long distance biking might be obtained by sport drinks and carbohydrate loading.

62-year-old, non-athlete male: body weight 82 kg, height 187 cm, BMI 23.4 kg/m^2, body fat 22%, calculated BMR 6673 kJ, $\dot{V}O_{2\,max}$ 3.42 L/min or 41.7 mL/kg/min.

He participates in one of the classic Swedish sporting events (Vättern-rundan), a non-competitive endurance biking race with no exact completion times or publication of results. The 300-km Vätternrundan is a physically taxing event, as it will take the ordinary participant 15–20 h of cycling to complete. Most cyclists start in the evening and thus cycle a large part of the race throughout the night in the dark. The race comprises seven legs and nine stops where refreshments are available. At most stops blueberry soup, coffee, buns, and banana are available, but hot meals are offered after 109 km (milk, sausage and mashed potatoes, banana) and after 188 km (lasagne, milk). His mean speed was 27 km per hour, total energy cost during the race was 38 774 kJ (based on heart rate recording) and total energy intake from food and sport drinks during the race was 36 607 kJ.

His energy balance (in kJ) throughout the race is illustrated in this table. Note the essential energy (and fluid) supplement that is obtained from the sport drinks!

	Energy turnover (kJ)	Energy intake (kJ)	Energy balance (kJ)
Leg1/43 km	5507	4754+650*	−103
Leg2/36 km	4667	3153+650*	−864
Leg3/30 km	3757	4148+650*	+1041
Leg4/31 km	3991	3647+650*	+306
Leg5/38 km	5273	2247+650*	−2376
Leg6/32 km	4212	8333+650*	+4771
Leg7/22 km	2917	1753+650*	−514
Leg8/30 km	3484	2072+650*	−762
Legs 9 & 10/20 km + 18 km	4966	650*+650*	−3366
Total 300 km	38 774	30 757+5850*	−1867

* From half bottle of sports drink consumed during each leg.

The observed energy deficit (1867 kJ) corresponds to about 110 g glycogen which very well might be available, especially if the subject has performed carbohydrate loading before the race. The case illustrates that it is possible even during energy-demanding endurance performances to cover energy needs by combining carbohydrate loading with optimal food intake during a race.

Are requirement and recommended daily allowances equivalent to optimal nutrition?

For each nutrient there is a range of intakes from minimal requirement to prevent nutrient deficiency diseases to toxic levels. Somewhere in between is what is defined as *optimal intake*. According to the original definition, requirement refers to the minimal nutrient intake needed in order to prevent nutritional deficiency diseases. The recommended dietary allowance is defined as the mean of the requirement for a special population group + 2 standard deviations, thereby covering 97.5% of the need of a normal population. In order to compare the requirement vs. an adequate intake some concepts are introduced, as illustrated in Fig. 2.4.1.

A better distinction between the concepts 'requirement' and 'optimal intake' of nutrients is urgently needed. The mere fact that a more optimal restitution post exercise is reached at a higher nutrient intake does

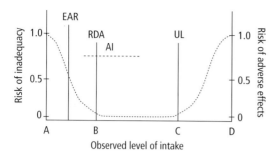

Fig. 2.4.1 Schematic illustration of various concepts used to express requirement and optimal intakes of nutrients. AI, adequate intake; EAR, estimated average requirement; RDA, recommended dietary allowances; UL, tolerable upper limit. (Source: Dietary reference intakes, National Academic Press, Washington, 1999).

not necessarily mean that there is an increased requirement in athletes as such in order to counteract any potential nutrient deficiency. This further accentuates the need to differentiate between various activity periods, whenever discussing the concept of nutritional perspectives on nutrient turnover in athletes. The daily nutritional requirements of nutrients have very little in common with specific nutritional needs pre-exercise and during exercise for optimal performance, which might also on the other hand be quite different from the nutritional needs post exercise for optimal recovery. Thus an optimal restitution of protein balance in the muscle due to heavy physical exercise might call for increased protein availability in the postexercise period although there is still no risk of protein malnutrition on a normal diet.

Energy requirement vs. nutrient requirement

Under normal conditions the body gives priority to covering its energy needs. In situations where its energy needs are not met, it will use all available energy-yielding substances in the food and body stores to cover energy requirements. This also means that the energy need essentially involves *quantitative* aspects of the dietary intake. The requirement for essential nutrients, i.e. protein, essential fatty acids, minerals and vitamins, is essentially related to fat-free mass and to a small degree to the extent of physical exercise. Thus nutrient requirement is related to age, sex

and body size and refers to a specific need for certain nutrients, involving *qualitative* aspects of the dietary intake.

When the energy intake via the diet, i.e. *exogenous energy*, does not meet energy requirements, *endogenous energy* is released from the mobilization of energy stores in the body (glycogen in liver and muscle; fat from subcutaneous and adipose tissue; gluconeogenesis from muscle catabolism).

Protein plays a two-fold role. There is (i) a *specific nutritional role* as source of essential amino acids for protein synthesis, i.e. building up, repairing and maintaining tissues; as well as (ii) a *non-specific role* as an energy-yielding nutrient. If energy needs are not met, protein will be used as an energy source, no matter whether protein needs are increased and not being met. It is consequently not possible to discuss energy and protein requirements separately. This is of special relevance when discussing nutritional problems in athletes.

Energy density vs. nutrient density

The energy density of a diet refers to the amount of energy per weight or volume, while the nutrient density refers to the amount of nutrient in relation to energy, i.e. g/10 MJ. Foods rich in fat and sugar have a high energy density, while their nutrient density is low. Persons with a high energy turnover, i.e. endurance athletes, may however cover their nutrient needs even on a diet with low nutrient density if they are in energy balance, while a low nutrient density may be detrimental in low-energy consumers. There are few examples, if any, where athletes consuming a normal diet in amounts relevant to cover their energy needs develop any objective signs of nutrient deficiency.

How to measure energy turnover

Figure 2.4.2 illustrates the various methods that can be used for studies of the various compartments in energy turnover in humans.

Energy turnover in the body comprises a conversion of energy between various forms:

mechanical energy as represented by physical exercise or muscular work;

heat production, which is also called thermogenesis. Sooner or later energy conversions result in heat production, i.e. dietary-induced thermogenesis

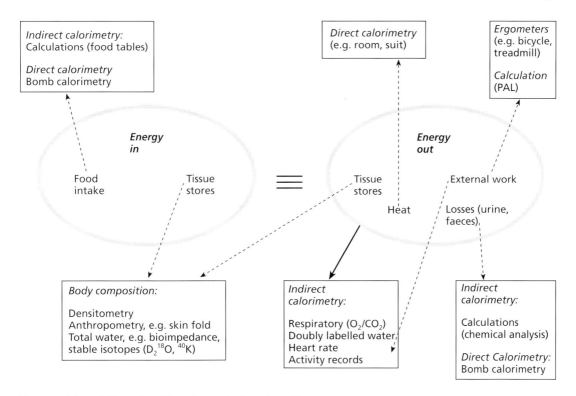

Fig. 2.4.2 Schematic illustration of the various methods used in studies on energy turnover.

(DIT), work-induced thermogenesis. The efficiency of the body in converting chemical energy to mechanical energy, i.e. physical work, is the same in normal and well-trained individuals, being about 25%, the remaining 75% being heat;

chemically bound energy, as in food and body stores of glycogen and fat, but also protein. Table 2.4.1 lists the types of energy stores and their role in exercise as a source for conversion into mechanical energy, as well as differences between trained and untrained individuals.

Energy turnover includes oxidation of biological substances, i.e. carbohydrate, fat, protein and alcohol, which yields heat. Energy turnover can thus be measured by analysing the heat produced as a result of the oxidation. This is usually called *direct calorimetry* and calls for advanced and sophisticated analytical methods, which are of little practical importance in field studies. Energy turnover is consequently usually estimated by means of *indirect calorimetry* based on

measuring consumption of oxygen or production of carbon dioxide as a result of oxidation of energy-yielding substrates. As oxidation is related to blood circulation and indirectly heart rate, a common method of indirect calorimetry measurement, especially in athlete physiology, is based on heart beat registration. The individual relationship between heart beat frequency and oxygen consumption, which is related to physical capacity, can be estimated in the laboratory. It is then possible to estimate the total energy turnover during physical performances using portable heart frequency recorders.

Calculation of energy turnover based on basal metabolic rate (BMR) and physical activity level (PAL)

The total energy turnover comprises basal metabolic rate (BMR) as well as the energy needed for daily life, i.e. characteristics of lifestyle including physical activity. Based on large population studies, equations have

Table 2.4.1 Energy stores, physical activity and training state.

Energy stores	Role in exercise	Difference in trained vs non-trained individuals
Muscle glycogen	Important energy source, influences endurance at moderate-intensity exercise This energy source is used to a large extent in: (i) high exercise intensity (ii) short-term exercise (iii) untrained subjects (iv) high intake of carbohydrate in the diet	Training increases the content by approximately 100%
Liver glycogen	Maintenance of blood glucose. To a certain extent, circulating blood glucose is taken up and catabolized in the working muscle	Training increases the content by approximately 100%
Triglycerides in adipose tissue and muscle tissue	Free fatty acids are produced during breakdown of triglycerides Free fatty acids as an energy source are to a large extent used in: (i) low intensity exercise (ii) long-term exercise (iii) trained subjects (iv) high fat intake in the diet	Exercise increases muscle triglyceride content to twice as much, but the percentage of body fat (and absolute fat mass) in the body drops
Muscle protein	Energy deficit leads to increased muscle catabolism due to increased gluconeogenesis. NB Muscle represents >20% of body energy stores in athletes	Energy deficit leads to more pronounced muscle catabolism in well-trained athletes with low body fat % than in-non-trained individuals with higher body fat %

Exercise: Calculate your own BMR

Table 2.4.2 Calculation of basal metabolic rate based on age, sex and body weight (W). From [1].

Age	Men		Women	
	MJ/24 h	kcal/24 h	MJ/24 h	kcal/24 h
0–3	0.255 W−0.226	60.9 W+54	0.255 W−0.214	61.0 W−51
3–10	0.0949 W+2.07	22.7 W+495	0.0941 W+2.09	22.5 W+499
10–18	0.0732 W+2.72	17.5 W+651	0.0541 W+3.12	12.2 W+746
19–30	0.0640 W+2.84	15.3 W+679	0.0615 W+2.08	14.7 W+496
31–60	0.0485 W+3.67	11.6 W+879	0.0364 W+3.47	8.7 W+829
>60	0.0565 W+2.04	13.5 W+487	0.0439 W+2.49	10.5 W+596

been established in order to calculate BMR with reasonable accuracy based on anthropometric data (weight, length, age and sex) [1].

It has been postulated that for survival, 24-h energy turnover represents about 1.27 times BMR, and for a sedentary lifestyle total energy turnover represents about 1.55 times BMR (Fig. 2.4.3).

Various activities in daily life as well as during

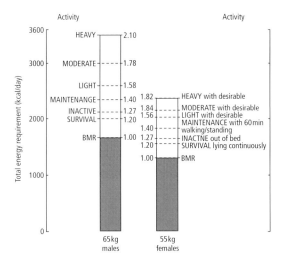

Fig. 2.4.3 Energy turnover expressed as multiples of BMR [1].

Table 2.4.3 Examples of MET values for various athletic activities. From [3].

Athletic activity	MET value
Badminton, competitive	7.0
Ballet dancing	6.0
Basketball, game	8.0
Bicycle ergometer 100 W	5.5
Biking > 32 km/h	16.0
Circuit training	8.0
Fencing	6.0
Golf, general	4.5
Horseback riding, general	4.0
Ice hockey	8.0
Jogging, general	7.0
Orienteering	9.0
Running, cross-country	9.0
Running 17 km/h	18.0
Sailing (Laser)	3.0
Scuba diving	12.0
Skiing, cross-country	7.0
Skiing, competition	16.5
Soccer, match	10.0
Squash	12.0
Skating, competition	15.0
Swimming, crawl	11.0
Table tennis	4.0
Volleyball, beach	8.0
Weight-lifting, training	6.0
Wrestling, one match	6.0

various forms of physical activities are expressed as multiples of BMR, often characterized as BMR factors [1,2] or metabolic energy turnover (MET) values (Table 2.4.3) [3,4]. The total energy turnover (ET) per 24 h can then be calculated based on BMR with the addition of energy for various physical activities based on intensity and duration throughout the day.

The relationship between the total energy turnover (ET) and BMR *per 24 h* is an indicator of the physical activity level (PAL) of the individual, thus expressing the lifestyle.

Is there a special nutritional problem in training athletes?

Elite athletes represent a group of individuals with usually high energy turnover, who experience intensive physical stress. The high energy turnover results in emptying their glycogen depots and in increased fat and protein turnover over shorter or longer intervals. Thus their training and competition schedule dominate their daily life and call for specific energy and nutrient demands and meal patterns. The principle behind any dietary advice to athletes is that priority should be given to covering the energy needs in addition to compensating for fluid losses. It is furthermore essential that all essential nutrients, i.e. vitamins, minerals, essential amino acids and fatty acids, are

Exercise: Calculate your own PAL

1 Calculate your BMR (as above).
2 Keep a record of your physical activity throughout 24 h:

Occupation	hours	factor BMR	Energy (kJ)
e.g. Sleeping	8	1.0	BMR/24 × 1.0
Sitting	6	1.5	BMR/24 × 1.5

etc.
3 Estimate total energy turnover per 24 h (ET).
4 Your PAL is calculated by dividing ET with BMR.

consumed not only in adequate amounts, which is usually a minor problem, but also in balanced amounts; the latter might be jeopardized when using food supplements. The meal pattern should always be adjusted to training and competition schedules.

However, the effect of physical exercise is not only related to energy turnover as such. Physical exercise also has an impact on substrate utilization and may help the individual to balance his/her body composition, metabolic regulation and homeostasis.

The protein debate

In athletic physiology the question as to whether there is a special need for protein in athletes is an ongoing matter of controversy. Critical analyses of the background data, however, show that there are a lot of conflicting opinions. When discussing protein needs, we must be certain that the studies performed have not been influenced by problems with energy deficiency, i.e. that the energy needs are not met [5]. This is of special concern in athletes with a high energy turnover as the body gives priority to covering its energy needs even when protein turnover is increased. Although it has essentially been the strength athletes that have been engaged in the discussions regarding increased protein needs of athletes, it seems, rather, that protein requirement is in fact a problem of endurance athletes.

An increased demand may be due to essentially three reasons. First, it is obvious that training leads to increased muscle mass, which may increase the protein requirement. Secondly, hard physical activity, especially endurance training, may lead to increased breakdown and muscle protein turnover. Thirdly, if energy needs are not met there is an increased gluconeogenesis from muscle protein, leading to muscle protein catabolism and negative nitrogen balance. Recent studies using stable isotope techniques [6,7] indicate that there seems to exist a compensatory reduction in leucine oxidation in the recovery phase after physical activity. This effect is most pronounced post exercise during fasting and might indicate a homeostatic response in order to preserve body protein. Furthermore, the effect of physical exercise on leucine oxidation seems to be reduced during feeding. This might indicate that increased leucine oxidation in the muscle might be compensated for by increased utilization of dietary protein. Interestingly earlier results from short-term studies (3–4 h) on protein turnover during physical exercise have not registered any compensatory reduction in leucine oxidation, as they have not continued their measurements long enough after the end of the physical exercise.

Both Wolfe and Rennie and their collaborators in a series of papers over the last few decades have also shown that protein turnover is increased during exercise. Nevertheless this does not necessarily mean that protein need is increased. Butterfield and Calloway [8] showed that physical activity improved protein utilization and in a recent review Rennie and Tipton [9] even suggested that protein metabolism may become more efficient as a result of training.

What do we know regarding gender differences?

Certain oscillations in the blood content of sex hormones are necessary in order for women to have a regular menstrual cycle. This also applies to female athletes, though they often have lower levels of these sex hormones than non-trained women [10,11]. This results in the absence of menstruation—amenorrhea—with the frequency related to exercise volume and intensity. Exercise-induced amenorrhea occurs in nearly 50% of female endurance athletes [12] and in athletes for whom esthetics and low body weight are important (gymnastics, sports with weight categories, dancing). Increase in running volume from 24 to 100 km/week for more than 1 year has resulted in amenorrhea in almost all women. The state of amenorrhea is, however, reversible and there are no indications of reduced fertility in former female elite athletes. Amenorrhea can be counteracted by a simple reduction in exercise volume.

There are several indications that an insufficient energy intake influences the development of bleeding disorders. In ballet dancers it is a well-known fact that reduced food intake is associated with amenorrhea. Furthermore, cross-sectional studies have shown that long-distance runners who do not increase their food intake to balance their energy output have a higher prevalence of amenorrhea. Surprisingly, these women do not lose weight in spite of a low energy intake. This may indicate that reduced energy intake is neutralized by a reduction in resting metabolic rate compared with non-trained women and trained women with normal menstruation patterns. Measurements of hormones in the blood support these theories, and the absence of bleeding could be an energy-sparing mechanism in women. Underreporting of food intake may also explain why the energy intake is unusually low.

The practical importance of the amenorrheal state with reduced plasma levels of sex hormones is a reduction in bone mineral content. In extremely well-trained female endurance athletes, a low bone mineral content close to the limit of fracture is often seen. In men also, intense exercise is known to cause a moderate reduction in sex hormones in the blood [13], but it has not yet been clarified whether this has any practical relevance in connection to performance [14a] and fertility or whether it relates to a reduced dietary intake.

Tarnopolsky has discussed in a series of papers the potential gender differences in substrate utilization during endurance exercise [15–17]. During moderate-intensity long-duration exercise he reported that female athletes showed greater lipid utilization and less carbohydrate and protein metabolism than equally trained males. In studies on substrate utilization and energy turnover in elite cyclists during a 7-h race we have not been able to show any gender differences in substrate utilization (Branth, Hambraeus *et al.* in press).

How to identify nutritional problems in athletes

Assessment of nutritional status

The nutritional status of an individual can be evaluated by various methods, i.e. anything from recording of dietary intake or analysis of physiologic parameters (i.e. body composition, physical capacity, immune defence system) to biochemical indicators (i.e. plasma levels of nutrients or endocrine response). Each of them will illustrate various stages in the nutritional status. While analysis of dietary intake will indicate potential risks of developing nutrient and energy deficiencies, changes in plasma levels of various nutrients or metabolites can be a result of physiologic adaptation to a changed nutrient balance as well as a serious indicator of nutrient imbalance. Likewise changes in body composition may represent an adaptive mechanism in the homeostatic regulation of metabolism, but also in-

dicate a developing nutrient deficiency state. Physiologic parameters such as decreased muscle strength, prolonged nerve reaction time and reduced immune response, however, may indicate more serious disturbances as a result of deterioration of the nutritional state of an individual.

Increased physical exercise is essentially a question of increased energy turnover, while the turnover of essential nutrients is usually not affected to such an extent that there is a need for an increased intake *per se*, provided the energy needs are covered. The debate as to whether the intake of nutrients in athletes is adequate is usually based on assessments of the dietary intake by various methods. Interestingly numerous food intake studies in elite athletes have been published based on dietary assessments where the energy intake is remarkably low and the discrepancy is obvious if the data are compared to calculated energy turnover from their training log. Thus the first step in analysing any possible nutrient deficiencies in athletes must be based on validation of reported dietary intakes. It is not scientifically relevant to draw any conclusions regarding the possible need for food supplements or increased requirement for specific nutrients in athletes as long as the energy needs are not being met by dietary intake.

Dietary recalls and/or records

There are several methods used for studies on dietary intake, both retrospective and prospective, based on anything from personal interviews, records and use of food frequency questionnaires to the double portion technique. Each of them has its pros and cons as illustrated in Table 2.4.4.

There is no single golden method for estimation of the dietary intake without error, and the goal of the study is of utmost importance when selecting the optimal method for dietary assessment. Furthermore, different types of errors have different effects in analysis and interpretation. Consequently, data collected by means of one dietary assessment in order to study the intake of one nutrient may not necessarily be as valid in evaluation of the intake of another nutrient.

The *retrospective methods* comprise dietary interviews in order to describe dietary habits from a longer-term perspective. This calls for a skilled interviewer and is time consuming. They can also be based on

Table 2.4.4 Summary of various methods for dietary assessments.

Method	Coverage	Advantage	Disadvantage
Dietary history	All food items or selected items	Long-term perspectives of dietary habits Individual data	Time consuming Skilled interviewer needed Memory demanding Quantitative data difficult to obtain Variations in dietary habits lost
24-h recall	All foods	Relatively rapid and simple Can be repeated Individual data	Selection of interview day critical Quantitative data difficult to obtain Skilled interviewer needed
Food frequency questionnaire (FFQ)	Only listed food items	Rapid and simple Easy to computerize Large groups covered by mail	Restricted number of food items Memory demanding No direct contact with interviewer
Food records	All foods	Individual data Intake during various days Quantitative data	Selection of day critical Dietary intake may be affected Needs resources Time consuming Collaboration necessary
Double portions	All foods	Exact data on nutrient content possible (not dependent on accuracy of food tables)	Dietary intake may be affected Resource demanding Collaboration necessary

repeated 24-h recalls. In this case it is essential to select various weekdays and training situations and also to be aware of seasonal variations throughout the year. The advantage of retrospective methods is that they do not usually interfere with the subjects' eating habits, as he/she does not know beforehand that their dietary habits will be analysed. However, the results obtained depend on the skill of the interviewer and on the subject being able to recall his/her dietary intake.

In order to cover larger number of individuals, *food frequency questionnaires* can be used. Such forms can be coded in order to simplify computer analysis. However, the selection of food items is limited, and furthermore there is little personal contact with the subject that would allow the reliability of the data recorded to be assessed.

Prospective methods comprise the use of food records, based on weighing all food items consumed or estimated from menu records or by observation. This can be performed over one or several days, usually 3–7 days. In the latter case it is essential that the records are performed continuously. A 7-day food record kept over 7 consecutive days is far more informative and

reliable than seven isolated 24-h records made over shorter or longer intervals. All prospective methods may have a more or less pronounced indirect impact on the dietary habits, as the subject is aware that they are being studied.

Validation of dietary assessments

Dietary assessment methods will almost without exception result in an underestimation of energy intake. Energy turnover should consequently be evaluated on the basis of studies of energy expenditure based on calculated BMR with the addition of a relevant PAL factor, which is based on the lifestyle including physical activity, and only in exceptional circumstances on determinations of energy intake. The energy equation fulfils the first law of thermodynamics: energy cannot be created nor destroyed, it can only be transferred from one form to the other. Available energy from energy intake and tissue breakdown must balance energy turnover if body weight is stable and body composition unchanged over a certain length of time. Thus an objective and reliable reference against which to validate data obtained on dietary intake can be based on a comparison between the observed or registered energy intake (EI) and the theoretical calculations of energy turnover based on calculated BMR with addition of a relevant PAL factor. In Case story 2.4.2 the flow chart for the estimation of energy turnover is illustrated.

Four different situations of nutritional significance in athletes

The *mean* intake of nutrients in athletes is of less importance and/or interest; rather nutritional problems should be divided into the following subheadings with regard to energy and nutrient intake:
1 *daily intake and food habits* (e.g. energy balance, nutrient density);
2 intake *pre-exercise* (loading phase) for optimal training effect or performance;
3 intake *during exercise* (nutrient and energy maintenance) for optimal performance;
4 intake *post exercise* (recovery phase) for optimal restoration of the energy and nutrient stores.

Nutritional problems *pre-exercise* are dominated by the carbohydrate loading as discussed below and in Chapter 1.2. *During exercise* the dominant problems are compensation for water and electrolyte losses and, if possible, energy turnover. *Post-exercise* nutrition should be directed towards the most rapid and efficient restoration of body stores and compensation for tissue damages.

Daily intake and food habits in athletes

Interestingly numerous published food intake studies in elite athletes are based on dietary assessments where the energy intakes are remarkably low. If the data from their training logs are compared to calculated energy turnover from anthropometric data, the discrepancy is obvious and the use of various forms of compensation for energy adjustments have been proposed. Whether athletes have a tendency to reduce their BMR values as a compensation for insufficient energy intake is still an open question. An increased BMR would in fact have been expected, as both the lower fat content of an athlete's body compared to that of an untrained individual and the excessive postexercise oxygen consumption (EPOC) should lead to an increased BMR.

Data on energy intake from any dietary assessment in athletes who maintain a constant body weight, which does not exceed the minimal energy require-

ment based on BMR and a suitable PAL factor, cannot be considered accurate for analysis of the relationship between dietary intake and health (Case story 2.4.3). In case the data should be considered as representative in a long-term perspective, energy balance must have been obtained. It is thus recommended that a validation based on calculated EI/BMR ratios should be included in dietary surveys [18]. The data must then account for at least the minimal energy needed for sedentary life (BMR × 1.55), with the appropriate addition for physical exercise, otherwise they represent an underestimation. It is then necessary to find out whether the missing energy units are supplied by qualitatively identical dietary components or whether other sources of energy have been consumed and not recorded. Furthermore, to what extent can we assume that the underestimation of dietary intake is the same for all nutrients?

An intake of about 8 g carbohydrate/kg/day is generally recommended for athletes today (Table 2.4.5). This corresponds to a total carbohydrate intake of 560 g per day in a 70-kg person or to 60% of total energy (60E%) if daily energy intake is 15 MJ/day (1 g carbohydrate-17 kJ). This is a considerable amount—both compared to the recommendations for the average population (55–60 E% = 324–353 g at 10 MJ/day) and compared to the average intake of the adult Danish population (256 g/day) [19].

The energy need of an athlete will normally be greater than the energy need of a sedentary person. However, carbohydrates give a higher degree of satiety and feeling of fullness per kJ than fat [20]. Furthermore, 1 g carbohydrate contains approximately half as many kJ as 1 g fat (17 kJ/g vs. 37 kJ/g). It is therefore necessary to consume twice as much carbohydrate than

Table 2.4.5 Nutrient recommendations.

	Average population * E%	Athletes E%	g/kg/day
Carbohydrate	55–60	60–65**	c. 8
Fat	max. 30	20–25	Not defined
Protein	10–15	10–15	1.2–1.7

E%, percentage of total energy.
* From [90].

Case story 2.4.2 How to validate dietary assessment by comparing energy intake (EI) and energy turnover (ET) based on BMR and PAL including one practical example

Step	Procedure			Example
1	Collect anthropometric data (age and sex, body weight, height)			Male, 25 years, weight 75 kg, height 180 cm
2	Verify that body weight has not changed = energy balance			Stable body weight
3	Calculate energy intake (EI) from dietary assessment			13 600 kJ
4	Calculate BMR according to FAO/WHO/UNU 1985 equation			7640 kJ/24 h or 318 kJ/h
5	Analyse physical activity from training report and lifestyle (hours of sleep, sitting, walking, etc.)			

Occupation	h	BMR factor	Energy (kJ)
Sleep	8	1	2544
Cross-country skiing, training	2	14	8904
Sitting, reading, TV	8	1.5	3814
Walking	1	2.5	795
Miscellaneous	3	2.5	2385

Step	Procedure	Example
6	Calculate total energy turnover (ET):	
	(a) using BMR factors from physical activity record (see Step 5)	ET = 18 442 kJ
	(b) using BMR factor for sedentary life (1.55)	ET = 11 842 kJ
7	Calculate PAL factor based on: ET (Step 6a)/BMR(Step 4)	ET/BMR = 2.4
8	Compare estimated EI from dietary assessment (13 600 kJ) with:	
	(a) estimated BMR (7640 kJ)	EI/BMR = 1.78
	(b) estimated ET from theoretical calculations of BMR and PAL	EI/(BMR×PAL) = 0.73

Comments

The EI/BMR ratio is 1.78, i.e. the energy intake only covers sedentary life. This is quite different from his PAL according to the lifestyle and training record (2.4). The difference between ET for sedentary life (11 842 kJ) and that according to the dietary record (13 600 kJ) is 1758 kJ which is energy available for training. Training intensity (MET = 14) corresponds to $14 \times 318 = 4457$ kJ/h. If this dietary assessment is correct it means that he would only be able to train for 1758/4457 = 0.39 h or 24 min, if it is assumed that he is in energy balance. If on the other hand he is training for the 2 h recorded in the physical activity diary his daily ET would be 18442, i.e. the recorded EI (13 600) would represent only 78% of ET. These values do not fit if he is maintaining his body weight and body composition. If he had been asleep in bed when not training, his ET would have been 11 453 kJ. This would mean that his EI should represent a BMR factor of 1.18, which is considered below survival needs. Another solution might be that he must reduce his BMR in order to maintain his body composition and energy balance and not develop a catabolic state. In this case he must reduce his BMR from 318 to 219 kJ/h, or 32% if the BMR factor of 1.55 is valid for his sedentary life when not training.

The most probable reason for the discrepancy between ET and EI is an underevaluation of his dietary intake!

Case story 2.4.3 Energy balance in a 20-year-old tennis-playing female (weight 61 kg, height 165 cm)

1 Her BMR calculated from anthropometric data was 5832 kJ/24 h or 243 kJ/h.

2 Her energy intake (EI) based on dietary records was 5016 kJ.

3 Her physical activity according to training report and lifestyle was as follows:

Occupation	h	BMR factor	Energy (kJ)
Sleep	8	1	1944
Tennis training	4	7	6804
Sitting, reading, TV	8	1.5	2916
Walking	1	2.5	608
Miscellaneous	3	2.5	1823
Total energy turnover (ET) using BMR factors			14095 kJ

4 Her PAL factor was:

based on ET/BMR	2.4
based on EI/BMR	0.86

5 EI in relation to ET from physical activity records 0.36

Comments

The EI/BMR ratio is 0.86, i.e. the energy intake does not even cover her BMR. This is quite different from her PAL according to lifestyle and training record (2.4). A dietician (who obviously had no experience or knowledge of athletic physiology) had recommended a low-fat diet, using skimmed milk, low-fat margarine and low-fat yoghurt, and this female started to develop anorexia.

Unfortunately this is an authentic case and not an unusual example of misinformation due to lack of knowledge that dietary counselling for athletes should be different from that intended for the general public. Low fat diets with low energy density usually lead to difficulties for athletes with high energy turnover in covering their energy needs with reasonable amounts of food. Furthermore the risk factor for cardiovascular disease secondary to fat intake has little relevance for athletes with high energy turnover as long as they are in energy balance.

---

fat in order to obtain the same energy intake. Finally, the so-called nutritious and recommended carbohydrates, which also contribute vitamins, minerals and dietary fiber (starch-rich carbohydrates and fruit), are characterized by a large volume and water content. This type of carbohydrate is therefore much less energy dense than fat, which means that a larger volume of food intake is needed in order to obtain the same energy intake on a carbohydrate-rich diet than on a fat-rich diet. An athlete may therefore find that satiety occurs before the meal is finished and consequently that their intake of energy and carbohydrate is not adequate. Evidence of this also comes from the numerous studies showing a spontaneous decrease in total energy and a reduction in body weight when a carbohydrate-rich diet is consumed *ad libitum* for weeks or months [14b,21,22].

From Table 2.4.5 it can be calculated that you have to eat 1.1 kg bread (23 slices of rye bread or 28 slices of wholemeal bread), 2.2 kg boiled rice or 4.3 kg apples, or drink 5–6 L of juice every day in order to obtain 560 g carbohydrates per day.

The volume problem of a very carbohydrate-rich diet can be managed partly through more frequent meals (six to eight per day), and partly by consuming some of the carbohydrates as concentrated carbohydrates or fluids such as dried fruits, sugar-rich sweets, juice, energy drinks, glucose or maltodextrin (glucose polymer) solution. In order to obtain essential vitamins and minerals, it is, however, necessary to ensure a daily intake of the nutritious carbohydrates as well. This recommendation is particularly important for subjects with a low fat intake (often women).

Since a very high intake of carbohydrates is recommended, the diets of athletes will mostly be based on vegetable food and hence the diet is likely to be semi- or totally vegetarian. It is difficult to design a vegetarian diet, especially a vegan diet (100% vegetable), which is sufficient in essential amino acids, vitamins and minerals. The latter applies especially to iron, zinc, calcium and vitamins D and B_{12}. In a lacto-ovovegetarian diet it is relatively easy to obtain essential amino acids, vitamin B_{12} and calcium, but iron intake is still a problem. This is primarily due to the fact that non-heme iron which is found in vegetables is more difficult to absorb than heme iron which is found in meat [23]. A vegetarian diet may reduce concentrations of sex hormones even when ideally balanced [13,14a], but the long-term effects on performance of a vegetarian diet have not been shown [14a,24].

Nutrient and fluid intake *before* training/exercise (loading phase)

Carbohydrate

The focus with regard to athletes' diets has been on carbohydrate intake in particular, since the body's glycogen stores are very limited. Although glycogen content is increased about two-fold in a well-trained athlete compared with a sedentary person (Table 2.4.6), the glycogen stores are still a limiting factor for exercise endurance and intensity (see Chapter 1.2). Compared with the fat stores, glycogen stores can supply energy for a few hours of medium-intensity work, whereas fat stores can supply energy for several days. It is also essential to remember that muscle protein also represents a substantial and potential endogenous energy source, constituting about 20% of the body's total energy store in a normal individual, probably more in a well-trained athlete.

Studies during the past century have also shown quite convincingly, that glycogen stores can be varied according to the dietary composition (Table 2.4.4) [25]. This is of great importance when heavy training takes place once or twice every day. In this case, the stores can be completely replenished if the diet is rich in carbohydrates. Therefore, the goal in dietary advice to athletes has first and foremost been to increase carbohydrate intake. However, it should always be remembered that a diet rich in carbohydrates which still does not meet energy needs is of little use.

An increase in muscle and liver glycogen content and an improvement in performance have been seen after the intake of a relatively large carbohydrate meal (approximately 200 g carbohydrate) 3–4 h before training compared with no intake [26–28]. Previous opinion was that high concentrations of insulin in the blood at the beginning of physical activity (as after intake of carbohydrate 30–60 min before training) were a disadvantage because blood glucose during training of medium severity might drop as a consequence of increased glucose absorption in the working muscula-

Table 2.4.6 Size of glycogen stores on different diets. From [25].

Stores	Total weight	Size of the glycogen stores		
		Mixed diet*	CHO-rich diet†	Fat-rich diet‡
Liver	1.2 kg	40–50 g	70–90 g	0–20 g
Muscle	32 kg	350 g	600 g	300 g

CHO, carbohydrate.
* 30 E% fat, 45–50 E% carbohydrate.
† 70 E% carbohydrate, 10 E% fat.
‡ 20 E% carbohydrate, 50 E% fat.

ture [29]. This risk is lower during intense muscular exercise of short duration (e.g. 7–10 min of rowing). Here the release of blood glucose-elevating hormones (counter-regulatory hormones), such as epinephrine, cortisol and growth hormone, is very powerful and can therefore match the extra glucose absorption in the muscle [30]. Several more recent studies have shown, however, that intake of glucose 30–60 min before training (cycling or running) does not result in reduced endurance capacity, sometimes even the contrary (for a review see [31]).

The glycemic index

More recently, not only the amount but also the types of carbohydrate have been included in the dietary guidelines to athletes. The concept of glycemic index (GI) was introduced in 1981 in order to be able to classify carbohydrates according to the postprandial increase in blood glucose [32]:

$$GI = [\text{blood glucose area of test food}]/$$
$$[\text{blood glucose area of white bread}] \times 100$$

According to the GI method, carbohydrates can be divided into high, medium and low GI foods. In general, GI is low for foods high in fructose, which have a high amylose/amylopectin ratio, contain large starch particles, are minimally processed or are ingested with fat and protein. However, there is no general rule that complex carbohydrates have a low glycemic index. Thus potatoes may have a high glycemic index while some pasta products have a very low glycemic index [33]. The GI for some selected foods is shown in Table 2.4.7. For a more extensive table, see Foster-Powell and Brand-Miller [34].

Some studies have suggested that low GI or slow carbohydrates should be preferred to high GI carbohydrate before exercise [35]. However, it seems that carbohydrate intake during exercise eliminates any difference in blood glucose, insulin, substrate oxidation and performance induced by pre-exercise carbohydrate intake [36].

Fluid

Fluid stores must be filled before exercise in order to prevent premature dehydration. About 500 mL of fluid about 2 h before exercise would promote ade-

Table 2.4.7 Carbohydrate content and glycemic index (GI)* (where known). From [91–93].

	g/100 g	GI
Glucose	100	138
Sucrose	100	89
Fructose	100	31
Candy	98	–
Cornflakes, unspecified	83	115
Muesli, unspecified	71	96
Liquorice	78	–
Liquorice allsorts	83	
Biscuits, digestive	66	82
Raisins	78	93
Chocolate, milk	59	–
White bread	51	100
Rye bread, dark	48	89
Wholemeal bread	49	99
Rye bread, wholegrain	49	58
Wine gums	79	–
Soya beans†	34	20
Boiled rice, brown†	25	96
Boiled pasta†	25	45–66
Corn	23	80–87
Banana	21	79–84
Fresh-boiled potatoes†	18	80
Orange juice	10	67
Apple/pear	13	53/47
Soft drink and syrup	10	–
Skimmed milk	5	46
Tomato/cucumber	6	–

* Compared to white bread = 100.
† GI varies according to method of preparation and temperature during intake.

quate hydration and allow time for excretion of excess ingested water. Of special interest in this context is the fact that glycogen binds 2.7 g water per gram of glycogen. Thus during carbohydrate loading it is also essential to have an accurate fluid intake.

Nutrient and fluid intake *during* training/exercise (maintenance phase)

See Case story 2.4.4.

Energy substrates

The metabolic fuels used during exercise depend on the training duration and intensity, the training state of the athlete, the fuel availability and reserves in the

Case story 2.4.4 Emergy balance not protein deficiency is the problem in athletes

21-year-old girl, elite athlete, active mountain biker: body weight 57.3 kg, height 171 cm, BMI 19.6, body fat 20.8%, BMR calculated 1369 kJ, $\dot{V}_{O_{2\,max}}$ 3489 mL/min (61 mL/kg/min).

She participates in a test training program involving cycling 200 km at a mean speed of 30 km/h. Duration of race 416 min. Breakfast before race contained juice, cereals, yoghurt, bread and butter, coffee. Intake during race: sports drinks, chocolate bars and bananas. The nutritional balance at the end of the race could be summarized as follows:

	Energy (kJ)	Protein (g)	Fluid (L)
Intake before race	979	31	0.72
Intake during race	1029	8	1.93
Losses during race	5404	20	1.78
Balance	−3396	+19	+0.83

Please note the pronounced negative energy balance! The protein balance does not represent a problem and it seems that she managed to maintain her fluid balance. (Fluid losses are calculated based on weight differences and measurements of body water using bioimpedance.)

---

body, the previous diet and possible intake during exercise. In general, the use of carbohydrate as substrate increases with increasing exercise intensity and falls with increasing exercise duration (due to depletion of the glycogen stores). Conversely, fat utilization is higher at low exercise intensities ($< 50\%$ $\dot{V}_{O_{2\,max}}$) and increases with longer exercise duration ($> 2–12$ h) [37].

The recommended carbohydrate intake is 1 g carbohydrate/min, since this is the maximal rate of carbohydrate oxidation during exercise [38]. A 10-g/100 mL glucose drink at a rate of about 600 mL/h would be a compromise between fluid intake recommendations and intake rates typically achieved by athletes in competitive situations [39]. There seem to be no important differences between different moderate to high GI carbohydrate sources ingested during prolonged, moderate-intensity exercise (except for fructose which is very slowly metabolized) [38]. Furthermore, the food form (fluid vs. solid) seems to be of no importance either.

Carbohydrate supplements have not been considered very relevant in exercise bouts lasting less than 1 h. However, recent studies have shown that in intermittent or high-intensity exercise of < 1 h, carbohydrate intake may also improve performance [40].

Protein

Physical exercise leads to an increased protein oxidation in the muscle in absolute terms. However, the contribution of protein to energy turnover is remarkably reduced in relation to carbohydrate and fat. Food intake seems to reduce leucine oxidation during exercise [41]. The changes in substrate oxidation during exercise at 24-h energy balance during fasting and feeding is illustrated in Fig. 2.4.4.

A high protein diet seems to have a carbohydrate-sparing effect as the surplus of protein is converted through gluconeogenesis and contributes to endogenous carbohydrate which is then oxidized. Interestingly a high protein diet also seems to stimulate fat oxidation [41]. Both these effects might be due to increased glucagon levels in the blood on a high protein diet.

Fat

The contribution of fat oxidation increases with improved training state [42]. But even for the well-trained athlete, the optimal situation during exercise is to maintain carbohydrate supply to the muscles, but slow the depletion of the glycogen stores by increasing the reliance on fatty acids and on glucose supplied from intake of carbohydrate.

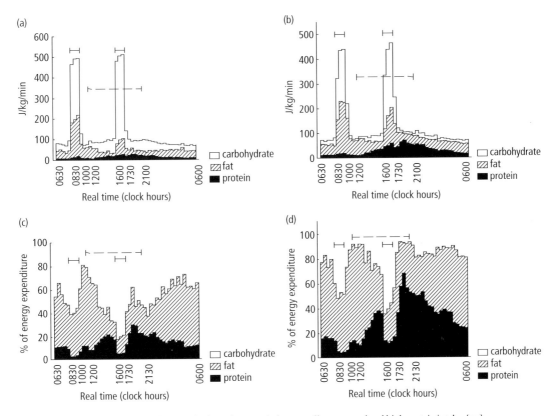

Fig. 2.4.4 Substrate utilization during exercise in 24-h energy balance studies at normal and high protein intakes [41].

In order to reduce carbohydrate oxidation and spare glycogen stores during exercise, it has been suggested that fat also could be ingested before and/or during work. Medium-chain triglycerides (MCTs) have been investigated in particular, since they are rapidly absorbed and enter the circulation directly through the portal vein. MCTs are rapidly oxidized both at rest and during exercise, especially when ingested with carbohydrate [43,44]. Conflicting results have, however, been produced, showing either a negative effect, no effect or a glycogen-sparing and performance-enhancing effect of MCTs. Ingestion of 30 g MCTs was found to contribute 5–8% of energy expenditure, but to have no effect on muscle glycogen breakdown or carbohydrate utilization [45]. Conversely, a large dose of 86 g MCTs was found to elevate plasma free fatty acid (FFA), decrease glycogen breakdown and increase performance in a time trial [46]. However, in another study a negative effect on performance was observed

after intake of 85 g MCTs alone even though FFA levels were increased. Also the subjects reported gastrointestinal discomfort, which may have been the reason for the decreased performance [47]. A more recent study showed no effect of carbohydrate + MCT ingestion on time trials after 2 h of constant-load exercise [48]. At present, data are therefore too conflicting to conclude whether MCTs should be used or not to enhance performance.

Optimal fluid intake

During physical activity fluid is lost at a rate dependent on the degree of work intensity, temperature and humidity of the surroundings. Often athletes have a water loss due to sweating of 1–2 L/h. For elite runners this may amount to 3.5–4 L in warm surroundings.

Studies have shown a tendency to drink too little (involuntary dehydration) since increased thirst during physical activity does not appear until the subjects dehydrate about 1% of their body weight. This should be viewed in light of the fact that even a dehydration of 1–2% of body weight reduces performance because of compromised temperature and adjustment of cardiovascular regulation [49]. It is therefore very important that athletes drink at least as much fluid as they lose. A good rule today is to drink at least every 20 min during a race. However, how much and what kind of fluid that can be consumed during exercise will vary for each individual and must therefore be decided individually during the actual exercise bout. It is consequently recommended that various kinds of fluids are tested during training in order to find the optimal solution and to try to estimate the water losses by recording body weight changes during the race. To what extent the glycogen-bound water is released and available for the homeostasis of water balance during endurance performance has to be further elucidated.

The rate of gastric emptying for fluids depends on the volume and concentration. It is possible to empty *c.* 1000 mL/h, but the amount is reduced during intense muscle activity ($>80\%\ \dot{V}_{O_2\,max}$) and with high osmolality in the consumed fluid. The latter is especially important in exercise of longer duration (>2–3 h). As long as the carbohydrate solution is 5–6% it does not, however, affect gastric emptying rate. Newer carbohydrate types (e.g. the glucose polymer maltodextrin) permit an intake of 10% solutions. This is due to the fact that the osmolality is too low to affect the gastric emptying rate.

During prolonged exercise (1–3 h) the fluid should contain carbohydrates and a small amount of electrolytes, primarily in order to increase intestinal absorption of carbohydrate. Even though sodium is lost in sweat, there is no sodium depletion until several hours of work have been performed.

Nutrient and fluid intake *after* training/exercise (recovery phase)

How soon post exercise?
Muscle glycogen repletion occurs most rapidly just after exercise. This is due partly to increased glycogen synthase activity and high permeability to glucose, and partly to increased insulin action in the exercised muscle [50,51]. Hence, the rate of glycogen storage was

Table 2.4.8 Examples of 'pick-me-up' food items for restoration of glycogen depot (all containing 100 g carbohydrate).

1.5 L sport drink (7% carbohydrate)	(0 g protein)
0.9 L blueberry soup	(3 g protein)
2 bananas (peeled)	(4 g protein)
1.5 dL raisins	(4 g protein)
1 L orange juice	(10 g protein)
4 dL cereal mix (muesli)	(15 g protein)
10 bread slices (wheat)	(17 g protein)
4 dL oats	(20 g protein)
0.7 L fruit yoghurt (0.5% fat)	(25 g protein)
2 L low-fat milk (0.5% fat)	(70 g protein)

found to be four times higher in the first hour after exercise than just 2 h after end of exercise, when carbohydrate was consumed 0 or 2 h post exercise, respectively [52]. Carbohydrate should therefore be consumed as soon as possible after exercise. Protein consumed in combination with carbohydrate may increase postexercise glycogen synthesis more than carbohydrate alone, due to increased insulin concentrations [53,54] (Table 2.4.8). Recent studies indicate that protein post exercise in the form of protein hydrolysates and amino acid–carbohydrate mixtures [55] will also optimize muscle protein recovery or even stimulate protein anabolism and increased muscle mass but this still has to be verified.

Fluid intake in connection with exercise must at least compensate for the fluid lost during exercise. Weighing (without any clothes) before and after exercise will show the approximate fluid loss during exercise. The color of an athlete's urine can also reveal whether overall fluid intake is sufficient.

Is there a need for a special diet post exercise?
After moderate-intensity exercise with glycogen depletion, muscle glycogen content (like liver glycogen) is regenerated to a normal level in 2–3 days on a mixed diet and in approximately 24 h on a carbohydrate-rich diet. Provided that the emptying of the muscle glycogen has been extensive and the following intake of carbohydrate is large, muscle glycogen will be regenerated to higher levels than before exercise (supercompensation).

The type of carbohydrate probably plays its most

important role in the postexercise diet. Thus, one study showed that the glycogen storage rate after glycogen-depleting exercise (1.5–2 h at 75% of $Vo_{2\,max}$) was higher 6 h after intake of high GI carbohydrates compared to low GI carbohydrates [56]. Faster glycogen resynthesis with glucose compared to fructose has also been found during the hours after exercise. After 20 h, however, no difference between the glycogen resynthesis was found after high or low GI carbohydrates. However, another study showed that after 24 h a high GI diet increased muscle glycogen stores 50% more than a low GI diet [57]. If exercise takes place once or twice daily, it is therefore advisable to choose high GI carbohydrates after training. With exercise only once a day or less and a recovery period of more than 24 h, the type of carbohydrate does not seem to be important for the training outcome, but this has not yet been completely clarified.

A problem often encountered by athletes is a decreased appetite for up to 2–3 h after heavy exercise [58]. To overcome this problem, a carbohydrate-containing drink is advisable. In this way both fluid balance and muscle glycogen can be rapidly restored. It has not yet been clarified, though, if additional protein intake—resulting in a positive nitrogen balance—can be advantageous with respect to muscle building and performance.

For most athletes, a sufficient protein intake will not be a problem. This implies, however, that the athletes are in energy balance and consume varied meals containing all the essential amino acids. In types of sport with frequent periods of energy deficiency during training (running, gymnastics, athletics, ballet) as well as for vegetarians (especially vegans), the diet may be low in proteins and insufficient with respect to essential amino acids [59]. Examples of complete protein combinations are: beans + rice, peas + corn, pulses + bread, cereals + milk or eggs, and potatoes + eggs or milk. One should also bear in mind that the bioavailability of vegetable protein from a fiber-rich diet is estimated to be 10% lower than the bioavailability of animal protein.

Studies on the dietary intake of Kenyan runners by Christensen and collaborators [60] were able to show, however, that the high carbohydrate and low fat intake, which was similar to that reported in endurance runners from other low-income countries, was suffi-

cient to cover energy as well as protein intake, including the need of essential amino acids, despite the diet being based on a small range of mainly vegetable food items.

The role of dietary supplements

Is there a need for food supplements?

Subnormal levels of one or more nutrients in body fluids cannot be taken as an indicator that there is a nutrient deficiency which calls for food supplements, unless the energy needs are covered. Several studies indicate that subnormal levels of nutrients can be restored by means of a well-balanced diet consumed in adequate amounts to cover energy requirements.

The motivation for athletes to use supplements can be divided into various categories:

1 use of supplements for optimal training effect, e.g. use of certain amino acids stimulating the release of growth hormone;
2 supplements to be used during competition, e.g. use of bicarbonate to counteract acidosis;
3 use of preparations for optimal restoration, e.g. creatinine for training effect at repetitive strength training;
4 use of supplements to increase psychological capacity, e.g. B vitamins against agony, branched chain amino acid supplements to counteract central tiredness, antioxidants against muscle tissue damage.

In all these circumstances there is a gray area between physiologic demands and doping effects, an issue which is still not resolved.

There are also various forms and types of supplements. *Complete supplements* represent an alternative to conventional food which are often used in clinical dietetics for tube feeding of patients with gastrointestinal problems. These products may be used as 'convenience foods' for athletes who have problems fitting their meal pattern around their training schedule. Food supplements comprising *vitamins and minerals* are often used. It is, however, essential that they are balanced in a defined mixture, usually as a multiple of the recommended intakes. Otherwise there is a risk that imbalanced intakes will cause problems. *Energy supplements*, often drinks or cakes with high energy density, usually based on carbohydrate, are often used to cover high energy turnover. However, there is a potential risk of high energy density products leading to nutrient imbalance as a result of low nutrient density of the diet. Finally there are the *ergogenic supplements* which usually include megadoses of vitamins, minerals, stimulators (e.g. caffeine), and others (e.g. creatinine, Q10, ginseng), in order to increase physical and mental capacity. In these cases we are also in the gray area between physiologic demands and doping effects.

Excessive dietary intake of certain minerals and trace elements may impair the balance of other minerals due to interactions affecting intestinal absorption; e.g. zinc intake above 50 mg per day impairs copper and iron metabolism and high iron supplementation impairs the uptake of other minerals, e.g. zinc. A high protein intake has also been reported to be deleterious for calcium, phosphorus, zinc and copper requirements.

Fat

More recently, a renewed interest in fat-rich diets as an ergogenic aid has emerged. Thus, several studies have investigated whether fat oxidation can be increased and thereby glycogen breakdown prolonged during exercise if the athlete is habituated to a more fat-rich diet instead of the recommended carbohydrate-rich diet [61–63]. The overall message from these studies seems to be, however, that a fat-rich diet consumed for at least 7 weeks does not improve performance or increase glycogen stores. On the contrary, a carbohydrate-rich diet still seems to be superior to a fat-rich diet.

A daily intake of at least 15 E% fat should be consumed in order to obtain enough essential fatty acids and fat-soluble vitamins in the diet. However, up to 25–30 E% fat would still ensure enough calories for carbohydrate and protein in the diet.

Protein

Protein is also metabolized during exercise, although to a lesser degree than carbohydrate and fat as long as the athlete is in energy balance. Furthermore, sufficient carbohydrate stores and carbohydrate administration during exercise have a sparing effect on protein utilization. It is recommended that an endurance athlete should consume 1.2–1.5 g protein/kg body weight/day, while strength-training athletes should consume 1.2–1.7 g protein/kg body weight/day [64] although the scientific evidence for a raised protein requirement in the diet is questioned by others. At a total energy intake of 15 MJ/day, where the protein intake corresponds to 15 E%, this means an intake of 134 g protein or 1.9 g protein/kg body weight in a 70-kg man, i.e. well above these recommendations. Most athletes even in their normal diet have >15 E% protein and a higher energy intake than 15 MJ. Thus there is no need for extra protein supplements in their diet in order to cover a protein requirement of 1.5–1.7 g/kg body weight/day. Of greater interest is, however, to what extent a more optimal muscle protein restoration could be obtained if protein is given post exercise. This, however, still has to be further elucidated.

Minerals

Minerals and trace elements constitute about 4% of the body. The dominant part is calcium phosphate in the skeleton, representing almost 2–3% of body mass, while the trace elements constitute less than 0.02%. As the latter play an essential role in the metabolic function of the body, trace elements represent essential nutrients which must be consumed regularly, albeit in small amounts. Today 21 minerals and trace elements have been identified as essential, but recommended daily allowances (RDA) have only been established for seven of these: calcium, iodine, iron, magnesium, phosphorus, selenium and zinc.

Intense physical exercise has been shown to increase the losses of minerals and trace elements in urine, sweat and feces to varying degrees. The magnitude of the losses is dependent not only on the type and intensity of exercise and individual homeostatic control, but also on the nutritional situation (nutrient intake and nutrient status of the individual). It is still an open question as to how to measure mineral status in an individual, as plasma levels are usually not appropriate indicators and may even be misleading due to the homeostatic regulation in the body.

It is generally agreed that moderate physical activity does not adversely affect mineral status when recommended amounts of minerals and trace elements are consumed in a mixed diet with a normal nutrient density [65]. Diets with high energy density and low nutrient density (often called empty calories), i.e. high carbohydrate and/or high fat diets, may potentially lead to deficiencies of essential nutrients for some athletes with high physical activity. Other risk groups are those engaged in sports which favor low body weights, leading to restricted dietary intakes (e.g. gymnasts, endurance runners). Nevertheless, very few studies have so far indicated reduced physical performance due to trace element deficiencies, with the exception of iron-deficiency anemia.

Calcium

Calcium is the most abundant mineral in the body, which contains about 0.8–1.2 kg. Approximately 99% of the body calcium is located in the skeleton, which serves as an important calcium depot, while the remaining 1% occurs as calcium ions of relevance for neuromuscular function. Severe hypocalcemia can cause serious muscle cramps and heart arrhythmias. However, there are no reliable data available concerning the potential effect of calcium supplementation in the treatment of muscle cramps in athletes. The homeostasis of calcium is tightly regulated by a complicated hormonal system in which vitamin D plays an important role.

Peak bone mass is achieved by the age of 25–30 years. An inadequate calcium intake before this age, which is common in many young females, may lead to consequences later in life with osteoporosis and fractures. Weight-bearing exercises such as running and weight-lifting have been shown to increase peak bone mass, especially before puberty, but are probably not as important as calcium intake. A physically active lifestyle throughout life does however have a positive effect on bone mass and a lifelong adequate calcium intake of over 800 mg/day reduces the risk for later osteoporosis [66]. A positive interaction between exercise and calcium has also been shown in young subjects but it seems likely that the calcium intake has to exceed 1000 mg, which many athletes do not achieve [67].

Athletes with stress fractures have been found to have low bone density associated with low calcium intake [68]. In contrast calcium supplements (500 mg/day) given to military recruits did not prevent stress fractures [69]. In osteoporosis, prophylactic studies indicate that an effect is obtained only when more than 1000 mg are given in supplements. There

are no studies or other evidence that calcium supplementation could give athletes any physical performance benefits. On the contrary, excess calcium intake may inhibit iron absorption.

Iron

The total content of iron in the body is 3–5 g. Iron is stored in the body bound to a protein, ferritin, and serum ferritin is considered to reflect total body iron stores. Transferrin is a transport protein in plasma and is usually only saturated with iron to 30%. The saturation decreases during iron depletion, but total transferrin content, often referred to as total iron binding capacity, is also increased during chronic infections and pregnancy, leading to a lower saturation. Serum iron is influenced by many factors including physical exercise and it is not considered as a suitable indicator of iron status of the individual.

Iron occurs in two forms in the diet: in an inorganic form in vegetable sources, non-heme iron, as well as in an organic form, heme iron, from animal products, i.e. meat and blood products. The absorption of non-heme iron is relatively low and inhibited by, for example, bran, cellulose, pectin and phytic acid, while protein such as meat and ascorbic acid enhance absorption. Heme iron has a higher bioavailability and this is not influenced by antinutrients to the same extent. Iron supplements are widely used by athletes but gastrointestinal side-effects are common, which decrease compliance and make the treatment complicated. Low dose iron supplementation seems to be a good practice (approximately 40 mg elemental Fe/day) [70].

The daily loss of iron is small (*c.* 1 mg/day for men and 2 mg/day for women—menses) because of an effective recycling system. In addition iron absorption increases when iron stores are depleted as occurs during growth and menstrual bleeding (up to 5 mg/day). Hence, recommendations have been fixed at 12 mg/day for men and 15 mg/day for women, respectively.

An increased incidence of reduced serum ferritin has been shown in many studies among athletes, where runners are most affected, especially females, but most types of training can affect serum ferritin concentration. However, most studies have shown that a low serum ferritin level without manifest anemia does not seem to affect performance capacity. Furthermore, low serum ferritin concentrations may only reflect a shift of iron from stores to functional compartments, e.g. myoglobin in muscle. Moreover, the widespread low or subnormal hemoglobin and hematocrit, often reported especially among endurance athletes, has been called 'sports anemia'. However, in most cases this is probably caused by physiologic adaptation with expanding baseline plasma volume (dilution pseudoanemia) due to the repetitive acute loss of plasma volume during intense physical exercise [71]. In addition, intensive prolonged or muscle-damaging exercise evokes an acute phase response which, among other reactions, causes a fall in serum iron and rise in ferritin levels. This makes the interpretation of iron status in athletes difficult.

Several suggestions have been proposed to explain how iron status can be affected by physical exercise, including increased gastrointestinal blood losses by hemorrhage erosions or ischemic colitis and/or reduced absorption. Hematuria occurs but is uncommon, and iron losses in the urine are small. Hemolysis due to erythrocyte rupture during strenuous training, especially running, where erythrocytes may be crushed within the foot, is also suggested as an explanation. There is also a possibility of increased red cell turnover and there might be increased red cell mass by training. Iron losses through sweat have been estimated to be 6–11% of absorbed iron per day during 1 h exercise and thus might be a problem for those with low iron intake and marginal stores [72].

The incidence of iron-deficiency anemia has not been shown to be high in athletes. Most studies have so far also shown that non-anemic iron depletion as well as iron supplementation does not seem to increase physical performance. However, some limited data suggest that female athletes with low ferritin values could benefit from iron supplementation [73,74] but this still has to be clarified. Increased iron intake by diet should always be the first choice.

Three groups have, however, been identified to be at greater risk for developing iron deficiency: female athletes, distance runners and vegetarian athletes. Attention has, however, to be focused on the fact that excess iron appears to lead to oxidative stress and may therefore aggravate exercise-induced oxidative stress. It could also be deleterious for those with the genetic disease hemochromatosis [75]. Furthermore, excess iron intake may reduce uptake of other trace elements, in particular zinc, and cause nutritional imbalances. Consequently iron supplementation to athletes should only involve small doses and should only be used when iron-deficiency anemia is properly documented by laboratory assessments [70].

Zinc

Zinc is a component of more than 200 enzymes involved in carbohydrate, fat and protein turnover. They are necessary for the immune system as well as for the endocrine response and protection against free radicals. Zinc is of vital importance for metabolic turnover during physical exercise. About 95% of the zinc is intracellular; only 0.1% of the total body content of zinc occurs in plasma while 60% is located in muscles. Thus the measurement of plasma zinc levels as an indicator of zinc status can be questioned.

Zinc needs for athletes are still not clarified although exercise may result in increased zinc losses in sweat and urine [76]. There is, however, so far no evidence that zinc supplementation may enhance physical performance in humans. It has however, been suggested that zinc depletion could increase exercise-induced stress, e.g. decreased immune defence and muscle damage secondary to changes in membrane stability [77]. Zinc supplementation is common among athletes. However, zinc overdose (>30 mg) may impair immune function as well as iron and copper status [78].

Magnesium

Magnesium is involved in more than 300 metabolic reactions of relevance for substrate turnover and utilization. It is also involved in neuromuscular, cardiovascular, immune and endocrine function, and has an antioxidant role.

Magnesium deficiency has been shown to occur in a wide variety of clinical conditions associated with oxidative stress, e.g. cardiovascular disorders and diabetes, where magnesium supplementation may be beneficial [79].

In athletes it has been suggested that magnesium deficiency is a contributing factor to exercise-induced muscle cramps, but this is still not proven. Serum magnesium is a poor indicator of magnesium status and there are still no reliable methods available for evaluating magnesium status. Although magnesium is excreted in the sweat, even during profuse sweating the magnesium losses are relatively small, probably due to an effective redistribution of magnesium within the body, especially thanks to the homeostatic control of the kidney. There might, however, be increased magnesium turnover and urinary losses during long and intensive training periods and stress [80]. So far there are, however, no studies that show that magnesium supplementation is beneficial for athletes despite the fact that magnesium has an essential function in energy turnover in the body.

Chromium

Although chromium is considered as an essential nutrient, its biologic role is still not fully understood. Strenuous exercise has been shown to increase urinary excretion of chromium markedly [81], but whether this leads to a risk of developing chromium deficiency is not known.

Selenium

Selenium functions as an antioxidant alone in the detoxification of heavy metals in the body and as a cofactor of the antioxidant enzyme glutathione peroxidase. Dietary selenium deficiency increases tissue oxidative damage and it seems that selenium has a sparing effect on tissue levels of vitamin E. However in experimental studies selenium deficiency does not impair endurance capacity in rats and supplementation in humans has no effect on physical performance [82]. Selenium has also been shown to be important for the immune system. This is of special concern in the Scandinavian countries, which have selenium-poor soils, and has led to specific programs to add selenium to fertilizers in Finland in order to increase the dietary intake of selenium. In this context it is of interest that it has been shown that selenium status in Swedish athletes is subnormal and lower than in Finnish athletes [83].

Sodium

As sodium plays an essential role in the regulation of fluid balance, prolonged strenuous exercise, especially in a hot environment, may result in acute sodium losses which lead to heat exhaustion or even heat cramps [84]. The daily intake of sodium is usually quite accurate and sodium replacement is seldom necessary during exercise. There is also an adaptation process in the body during heat environment leading to less sodium losses in sweat and urine, but if the athlete is not acclimatized, losses of sodium and minerals in a hot environment may be considerable.

Vitamins

Vitamins are essential nutrients which must be supplied on a regular basis. They are involved in many metabolic pathways, which often are stressed during intensive exercise, and include coenzymes essential in the metabolic system as well as antioxidants. Consequently it has been shown that a low vitamin status can reduce physical performance [85] although, to date, no controlled studies have shown that vitamin supplementation increases performance. Exercise appears to increase the turnover and losses of some B vitamins. Some studies indicate that nutritional status is impaired in some active individuals with insufficient energy intake and/or poor nutrient density in their diet such that it is deficient in certain B vitamins, i.e. thiamine, riboflavin and vitamin B_6.

Oxidative stress and antioxidants

Oxygen is essential for human life and necessary for energy production, but in some forms it can be damaging to the body as reactive oxygen species (ROS): free radicals. The majority of ROS are produced in the mitochondrial electron transport chain during energy production. Physical exercise augments the production of free radicals and other forms of reactive oxygen species. End-products of oxidative damage are observed in the blood and tissues after acute intensive exercise as well as signs of decreased levels of antioxidants in some studies. Strenuous exercise may manifest an imbalance between the production of ROS and antioxidant defences, resulting in an oxidative stress situation in the body [86]. In fact there is some evidence which implicates ROS as an underlying cause of exercise-induced muscle fatigue and damage. During an acute bout of strenuous exercise the immune system is activated and produces a substantial amount of ROS, which may cause an inflammatory process. The immune system produces ROS to kill bacteria and viruses. During β-oxidation of large amounts of fat, as occurs during starvation, there is a substantial production of ROS; this also occurs during oxidation of amino acids through degradation of xanthine to uric acid. In addition there is a ROS production during the autooxidation of catecholamines [87]. The body has created an extensive protective system against these potentially damaging species, the antioxidant system. If the production of free radicals is large enough to overcome the antioxidant defence system, oxidative stress will ensue. Training seems to induce an adaptation with elevation of antioxidant protection through increased levels of the key antioxidant enzymes: the zinc-containing superoxide dismutase, iron-containing catalase and selenium-containing glutathione peroxidase. Training also seems to reduce signs of oxidative stress.

Important dietary sources of antioxidants include vitamins C and E, carotenoids, zinc and selenium, whereas uric acid, bilirubin, ubiquinone (Q10) and the thiol glutathione are important endogenous antioxidants. It is not yet fully known whether the body's natural antioxidant defence system is sufficient to counteract the increase of free radical production during intense exercise. There is, however, evidence that antioxidant consumption increases during excessive prolonged exercise, but not to what extent.

Some studies have reported that supplementation with antioxidants, such as vitamins C and E and thiol compounds (e.g. *N*-acetyl-cysteine and α-lipoic acid) might have some protective properties against tissue damage induced by oxidative stress [82]. Antioxidant supplements have, however, not been shown to increase performance. The balance between ROS production and availability of antioxidants plays a very important role in maintaining an intact immune system. Antioxidant deficiencies have been shown to impair immune function and supplementation has been shown to improve protection against infections in some studies. However, megadoses and unbalanced supplementation with antioxidants may be deleterious as they may cause autoxidation and increased tissue damage and suppress immune functions [88]. Thus recommendations for athletes should give priority to increasing the dietary intake of food items containing naturally occurring antioxidants, such as vegetables and fruits.

Ergogenic substances

A number of diet-related supplements have been credited with the ability to improve performance. Today

some of these are included in the list of doping drugs, such as caffeine (max $12\,\mu g/mL$ is allowed in urine) and alcohol. Among the (still) legal and most often used diet supplements are creatine, Q10, antioxidants and ginseng.

The daily need of creatine is approximately $2\,g/day$ and it is covered through both the diet and the body's own production (through the amino acids arginine and methionine). In the diet, creatine is found especially in meat ($c.\,5\,g/kg$), fish and to a smaller extent in milk ($80–100\,mg/L$). If the intake of creatine is increased, the muscle tissue will reach a saturation limit after approximately 4 days whereafter the surplus is excreted in the urine. An increased intake of creatine may have a positive effect, especially after short-term explosive exercise [89]. Athletes who consume a well-balanced diet do not, however, need a creatine supplement.

Q10 (ubiquinone or vitamin Q) works as an electro-transporter in the respiratory chain of the mitochondria where it is involved in the energy-producing processes. Furthermore, studies have shown that Q10 has antioxidative qualities. During physical activity, the content of Q10 in plasma lipoproteins is reduced. This may be due to an increased incorporation of Q10 into the heart and skeletal muscle, or because Q10 is used or excreted in the intestine. Q10 supplementation is known to have a positive effect on the heart muscle of patients with particular heart diseases, but no studies have yet shown that athletes who consume a varied diet need additional Q10.

Ginseng (Russian root) has been shown to have an ability to prevent tiredness and increase work capacity. However, there are also studies which have not been able to show this positive effect.

In general, the effects of the diet supplements mentioned above have not been fully investigated for either possible positive qualities or toxicity, side-effects and long-term effects. Furthermore, the type of sport may influence the possible effects.

Practical dietary advice

In training camps and abroad

• In a training camp or at competitions it is not always possible to obtain the diet you are used to. It is therefore essential that you are prepared and plan in advance in order to keep to your normal dietary habits and meal order as far as possible. It is often possible to discuss the matter with your coach and to contact the hotel staff in advance to discuss your needs.

• Bring your own food (raisins, bread, biscuits) and some nutritionally well-balanced convenient food items in suitable portions if you know in advance that the food may be of poor quality. If you do not get enough food, it may be necessary to eat food of poor nutritional value, such as chocolate, crisps and sweets.

• Make sure that you consume plenty of bread together with the hot meal. It is always possible to get bread. Otherwise: insist on having bread! Pasta is another alternative that you can bring with you in order to get enough carbohydrate.

• Make sure that there is plenty of food and ask for more if you do not feel full.

• Make sure that it is possible to have a snack between meals, such as fresh fruit.

Important guidelines while abroad

• Buy bottled water if the tap water is not drinkable, but be sure that the bottle has been carefully sealed by the factory. Boil the tap water whenever you are uncertain of its quality.

• Never have ice in your drinks as it comes from tap water and may have been stored under less than hygienic conditions.

• Do not eat dishes containing mayonnaise or egg.

• Avoid eating fresh vegetables and raw fruits. Do not eat salad and cold mixed dishes. In a lot of countries, e.g. in Asia, the water is so polluted that bacteria in fresh vegetables may cause illness. Furthermore, avoid dishes which have been heated for a while and left to cool down.

• Eat only fruits which have a 'natural wrapping', such as bananas and oranges, and peel them yourself. Otherwise peel the fruit (e.g. apples, pears) yourself carefully. Do not eat 'ready-made' fruit salad.

• Do not eat ice-cream, or cakes with cream or filling, no matter how nice they look.

• Be sure that meat, fish, egg and chicken dishes are thoroughly boiled or fried. Do not eat raw meat.

Summary

Elite athletes represent a group of individuals with an unusually high energy turnover who experience intensive physical stress, and who regularly increase their fat and protein turnover and empty their glycogen depots. Training and competition schedules dominate their daily life and call for specific energy and nutrient requirements as well as meal patterns. Many athletes, especially in endurance sports, have problems satisfying their energy needs through a conventional diet according to recommendations.

The principle behind any dietary advice to athletes is that energy needs should be covered and fluid losses compensated for. All nutrients, i.e. vitamins, minerals and fatty acids, should be consumed in adequate and *balanced* amounts. The meal pattern should also be adjusted to the training/competition schedule. Furthermore, based on all available scientifically sound data the diet should take into account the specific demands that occur as a result of various physical and psychological stresses during training and competition. Special attention should also be given to the characteristics of each phase of training and competition within each specific type of athletic performance, i.e. strength as well as endurance sports.

This may call for dietary counselling regarding diet composition, meal order and meal frequency as well as energy-rich food supplements. A high energy intake is no guarantee *per se* that the need for essential nutrients is being satisfied. Increased use of energy-dense food items (empty calories) leads to a diet with low nutrient density.

The role of dietary intake for optimal performance can be divided into the following categories: (i) dietary habits in general (energy balance, nutrition density); (ii) intake of nutrients before competition (loading phase); (iii) intake of nutrients during performance (maintenance phase); and (iv) intake of nutrients after performance (recovery phase).

Dietary recommendations for the general population may not be valid for elite athletes as a high intake of carbohydrate and dietary fiber leads to bulkiness. A low fat intake leads to problems in supplying energy needs. A high intake of PUFA and iron may lead to increased formation of free radicals and increased need for antioxidants.

There are also various levels of motivation for the use of supplements: (i) for optimal training effect, e.g. amino acids stimulating growth hormone; (ii) use during competition, e.g. bicarbonate against acidosis; (iii) for optimal restoration, e.g. creatine for training effect at repetition; and (iv) to increase psychological capacity, e.g. B vitamins against agony, branched chain amino acids against central tiredness.

Subnormal levels of one or more nutrients in body fluids cannot be taken as an indicator that there is a nutrient deficiency unless it is known that the energy needs are being adequately fulfilled. Subnormal levels of nutrients can usually be restored by means of a well balanced diet consumed in adequate amounts.

Multiple choice questions

1 *Resynthesis of muscle glycogen after prolonged endurance exercise depends on:*
a only complex carbohydrate being taken
b intake of carbohydrate in a liquid form
c immediate intake of carbohydrate after exercise
d ensuring a high carbohydrate content in the food intake for the following 24 h.

2 *With regard to an athlete's diet it is important to:*
a have a high fat content in the diet
b have a minimum intake of 2 g protein/kg body weight/day
c ensure obligatory administration of antioxidants
d ensure that over 60% of the daily energy intake is from carbohydrate.

3 *With regard to energy intake during exercise it is correct that:*
a a solution with around 20% carbohydrate will provide the best source of carbohydrate during exercise
b carbohydrate intake during exercise helps prolong endurance by emptying the glycogen stores at a lower rate
c energy intake only plays a role during exercise if it lasts for more than 3 h
d fat intake will help improve fat combustion and therefore improve endurance.

4 *With regard to supplementation in regularly training individuals it is correct that:*
a all training female athletes will need iron implementation in order not to become anemic
b magnesium deficiency can easily be detected by blood sample
c extra administration of vitamin B will increase performance
d vitamins C and E might have some protective properties against tissue damage from oxidative stress.

References

1 FAO/WHO/UNU. *Energy and Protein Requirements.* WHO Technical Report Series No. 724. Geneva: WHO, 1985.

2 James WPT, Schofield EC. *Human Energy Requirements. A Manual for Planners and Nutritionists.* Oxford: Oxford Medical Publishers, 1990.

3 Ainsworth BE, Haskell WL, Leon AS, Jacobs DR Jr, Montoye HJ, Sallis JF, Paffenbarger RS Jr. Compendium of physical activities: classification of energy costs of human physical activities. *Med Sci Sports Exerc* 1993; **25**: 71–80.

4 Ainsworth BE, Haskell WI, Whitt MC, Irwin ML, Schwarz AM, Strath SJ, O'Brien WL, Bassett, DR Jr, Schmitz KH, Emplaincourt PO, Jacobs DR Jr, Leo AS. Compendium of physical activities: an update of activity codes and MET intensities. *Med Sci Sports Exerc* 2000; **32**: S498–504.

5 Butterfield GE. Whole-body protein utilization in humans. *Med Sci Sports Exerc* 1987; **19** (Suppl.): S157–65.

6 El-Khoury AE, Forslund A, Olsson ER, Branth S, Sjödin A, Andersson A, Atkinson A, Selvaraj A, Hambraeus L, Young VR. Moderate exercise at neutral energy balance does not affect total 24 h leucine oxidation or nitrogen excretion in healthy men. *Am J Physiol* 1997; **273** *(Endocrin Metab **36**)*: E394–407.

7 Forslund A, Hambræus L, Olsson R, El-Khoury AE, Yu Y-M, Young VR. The 24-h status of whole body leucine and urea kinetics at 'normal' and 'high' protein intakes, with exercise, in healthy adults. *Am J Physiol* 1998; **275** *(Endocrin Metab **38**)*: E310–20.

8 Butterfield GE, Calloway DH. Physical activity improves protein utilization in young men. *Br J Nutr* 1984; **51**: 171–84.

9 Rennie MJ, Tipton KD. Protein and amino acid metabolism during and after exercise and the effects of nutrition. *Annu Rev Nutr* 2000; **20**: 457–83.

10 Boyden TW, Pamenter RW, Stanforth T, Rotkis T, Wilmore JH. Sex steroids and endurance running in woman. *Fertil Steril* 1983; **39**: 629–32.

11 Bonen A, Ling WY, Macintyre KP, Neil R, McGrail JC, Belcastro AN. Effects of exercise on the serum concentrations of FSH, LH, progesterone and estradiol. *Eur J Appl Physiol Ocup Physiol* 1979; **42**: 15–9.

12 McArthur JW, Bullen BA, Beitins IZ, Pegano M, Badger TM, Klibanski A. Hypothalamic amenorrhea in runners of normal body composition. *Endocr Res Comm* 1980; **7**: 13–25.

13 Hackney AC, Sinning WE, Brout BC. Reproductive hormonal profiles of endurance-trained and untrained males. *Med Sci Sports Exerc* 1988; **20**: 60–5.

14a Raben A, Kiens B, Richter EA, Rasmussen LB, Svenstrup B, Micic S, Bennett P. Serum sex hormones and endurance performance after a lacto-ovovegetarian and a mixed diet. *Med Sci Sports Exerc* 1992; **24**: 1290–7.

14b Raben A, Jensen ND, Marckmann P, Sandström B, Astrup

A. Spontaneous weight loss during 11 weeks' ad libitum intake of a low fat/high fiber diet in young, normal weight subjects. *Int J Obes* 1995; **19**: 916–23.

15   Tarnopolsky LJ, MacDougall JD, Atkinson SA, Tarnopolsky MA, Sutton JR. Gender differences in substrate for endurance exercise. *J Appl Physiol* 1990; **68**: 302–8.

16   Tarnopolsky MA, Bosman M, MacDonald JR, Vandeputte D, Martin J, Roy BD. Postexercise protein–carbohydrate and carbohydrate supplements increase muscle glycogen in men and women. *J Appl Physiol* 1997; **83**: 1877–83.

17   Tarnopolsky MA. Gender differences in substrate metabolism during endurance exercise. *Can J Appl Physiol* 2000; **25**: 312–27.

18   Hambræus L. Dietary assessment: How to validate primary data before conclusions can be drawn. *Scand J Nutr* 1998; **42**: 66–8.

19   Andersen NL, Fagt S, Groth MV, Hartkopp HB, Møller A, Ovesen L, Warming DL. Danskernes kostvaner 1995. Copenhagen: Levnedsmiddelstyrelsen, 1996.

20   Astrup A, Raben A. Glucostatic control of intake and obesity. *Proc Nutr Soc* 1996; **55**: 485–95.

21   Raben A, Macdonald I, Astrup A. Replacement of dietary fat by sucrose or starch. Effects on 14 day ad libitum energy intake, energy expenditure and body weight in formerly obese and never-obese subjects. *Int J Obes* 1997; **21**: 846–59.

22   Siggard R, Raben A, Astrup A. Weight loss during 12 weeks' ad libitum carbohydrate-rich diet in overweight and normal-weight subjects at a Danish work site. *Obes Res* 1996; **4**(4): 347–56.

23   Monsen ER, Hallberg L, Layrisse M, Hegsted DM, Cook JD, Mertz W, Finch CA. Estimation of available dietary iron. *Am J Clin Nutr* 1978; **31**: 134–41.

24   Nieman DC. Physical fitness and vegetarian diets: is there a relation? *Am J Clin Nutr* 1999; **70** (Suppl.): 570S–575S.

25   Saltin B, Gollnick PD. Fuel for muscular exercise: role of carbohydrate. In: Horton ES, Terjung RL, eds. *Exercise, Nutrition and Energy Metabolism.* 1988: 47.

26   Chryssanthopoulos C, Hennessy LCM, Williams C. The influence of pre-exercise glucose ingestion on endurance running capacity. *Br J Sports Med* 1994; **28**: 105–9.

27   Decombaz J, Sartori D, Arnaud MJ, Thelin AL, Schurch P, Howald H. Oxidation and metabolic effects of fructose or glucose ingested before exercise. *Int J Sports Med* 1985; **6**: 282–6.

28   Sherman WM, Brodowicz G, Wright DA, Allen WK, Simonsen J, Dernbach A. Effects of 4 h preexercise carbohydrate feedings on cycling performance. *Med Sci Sports Exerc* 1989; **21**: 598–604.

29   Foster C, Costill DL, Fink WJ. Effects of pre-exercise feedings on endurance performance. *Med Sci Sports* 1979; **11**: 1–5.

30   Kjær M, Bangsbo J, Lortie G, Galbo H. Hormonal responses to exercise in humans: influence of hypoxia and physical training. *Am J Physiol* 1988; **254**: R197–R203.

31   Hawley JA, Burke LM. Effect of meal frequency and timing on physical performance. *Br J Nutr* 1997; **77** (Suppl.): S91–S103.

32   Jenkins DJA, Wolever TMS, Taylor RH, Barker H *et al.* Glycemic index of foods: a physiological basis for carbohydrate exchange. *Am J Clin Nutr* 1981; **34**: 362–6.

33   Björk I, Liljeberg H, Östman E. Low glucaemic-index foods. *Br J Nutr* 2000; **83** (Suppl.): S149–S155.

34   Foster-Powell K, Brand Miller J. International tables of glycemic index. *Am J Clin Nutr* 1995; **62**: S871–S893.

35   Thomas DE, Brotherhood JR, Brand JC. Carbohydrate feeding before exercise: effect of glycemic index. *Int J Sports Med* 1991; **12**: 180–6.

36   Burke LM, Claassen A, Hawley JA, Noakes TD. Carbohydrate intake during prolonged cycling minimizes effect of glycemic index of preexercise meal. *J Appl Physiol* 1998; **85**(6): 2220–6.

37   Romijn JA, Coyle EF, Sidossis LS, Gastaldelli A, Horowitz JF, Endert E, Wolfe RR. Regulation of endogenous fat and carbohydrate metabolism in relation to exercise intensity and duration. *Am J Physiol* 1993; **265**: E380–E391.

38   Hawley JA, Dennis SC, Noakes TD. Oxidation of carbohydrate ingested during prolonged exercise. *Sports Med* 1992; **14**: 27–42.

39   Noakes TD. Fluid replacement during exercise. *Exerc Sport Sci Rev* 1993; **21**: 297–330.

40   Jeukendrup A, Brouns F, Wagenmakers AJM, Saris WHM. Carbohydrate-electrolyte feedings improve 1 h time trial cycling performance. *Int J Sports Med* 1997; **18**: 125–9.

41   Forslund AH, El-Khoury AE, Olsson RM, Sjödin AM, Hambraeus L, Young VR. Effect of protein intake and physical activity on 24-h pattern and rate of macronutrient utilization. *Am J Physiol* 1999; **276** (*Endocrin Metab* **39**): E964–E976.

42   Hurley BF, Nemeth PM, Martain WH, Hagberg JM, Dalsky GP, Holloszy JO. Muscle triglyceride utilization during exercise: effect of training. *J Appl Physiol* 1986; **60**: 562–7.

43   Massicotte D, Peronnet F, Brison GR, Hillaire-Marcel C. Oxidation of exogenous medium-chain free fatty acids during prolonged exercise—comparison with glucose. *J Appl Physiol* 1992; **73**: 1334–9.

44   Jeukendrup AE, Saris WHM, Schrauwen P, Brouns F, Wagenmakers AJM. Metabolic availability of medium chain triglycerides co-ingested with carbohydrates during prolonged exercise. *J Appl Physiol* 1995; **79**: 756–62.

45   Jeukendrup AE, Saris WHM, Brouns F, Halliday D, Wagenmakers AJM. Carbohydrate (CHO) metabolism after ingestion of CHO and medium-chain triglycerides (MCT) during prolonged exercise. *Metabolism* 1996; **45**: 915–21.

46   Van Zeyl CG, Lambert EV, Hawley JA, Noakes TD, Dennis SC. Effects of medium-chain triglyceride inges-

tion on fuel metabolism and cycling performance. *J Appl Physiol* 1996; **80**(6): 2217–25.

47   Jeukendrup AE, Thielen JJHC, Wagenmakers AJM, Brouns F, Saris WHM. Effect of MCT and carbohydrate ingestion during exercise on substrate utilization and subsequent cycling performance. *Am J Clin Nutr* 1998; **67**(3): 397–404.

48   Goedecke JH, Elmer-English R, Dennis SC, Schloss I, Noakes TD, Lambert EV. Effects of medium-chain triacylglycerol ingested with carbohydrate on metabolism and exercise performance. *Int J Sports Nutr* 1999; **9**: 35–47.

49   Maughan RJ. Fluid and electrolyte loss and replacement in exercise. *J Sports Sci* 1991; **8**: 117–42.

50   Garetto LP, Richter EA, Goodman MN, Ruderman NB. Enhanced muscle glucose metabolism after exercise in the rat: the two phases. *Am J Physiol* 1984; **246**: E471–E475.

51   Price TB, Rothman DL, Taylor R, Avison MJ, Shulman GI, Shulman RG. Human muscle glycogen resynthesis after exercise: insulin-dependent and -independent phases. *J Appl Physiol* 1994; **76**: 104–11.

52   Ivy JL, Katz AL, Cutler CL, Sherman WM, Coyle EF. Muscle glycogen synthesis after exercise: effect of time of carbohydrate ingestion. *J Appl Physiol* 1988; **64**: 1480–5.

53   Zawadzki K, Yaspelkis B III, Ivy J. Carbohydrate–protein complex increases the rate of muscle glycogen storage after exercise. *J Appl Physiol* 1992; **72**: 1854–9.

54   Van Loon LJC, Saris WHM, Kruijshoop M, Wagenmakers AJM. Maximizing postexercise muscle glycogen synthesis: carbohydrate supplementation and the application of amino acid or protein hydrolysate mixtures. *Am J Clin Nutr* 2000; **72**: 106–11.

55   Van Loon LJC, Kruijshoop M, Verhagen H, Saris WHM, Wagenmakers AJM. Ingestion of protein hydrolysate and amino acid–carbohydrate mixtures increases postexercise plasma insulin responses in man. *J Nutr* 2000; **130**: 2508–13.

56   Kiens B, Raben AB, Valeur AK, Richter EA. Benefit of dietary simple carbohydrates on the early postexercise muscle glycogen repletion in male athletes. *Med Sci Sports Exerc* 1990; **22**: 588.

57   Burke LM, Collier GR, Hargreaves M. Muscle glycogen storage after prolonged exercise: effect of glycemic index of carbohydrate feedings. *J Appl Physiol* 1993; **75**: 1019–23.

58   King NA, Burley VJ, Blundell JE. Exercise-induced suppression of appetite: effects on food intake and implications for energy balance. *Eur J Clin Nutr* 1994; **48**: 715–24.

59   Acosta PB. Availability of essential amino acids and nitrogen in vegan diets. *Am J Clin Nutr* 1988; **48**: 868–74.

60   Christensen DL, van Hall G, Hambræus L. Food intakes in Kalenjin runners in Kenya: a field study. In: *Sport Science in a Changing World of Sports, 2nd Annual Congress of the European College of Sport Science.* Copenhagen, Denmark, 20–23 August 1997: 1076–7.

61   Lambert EV, Speechly DP, Dennis SC, Noakes TD. Enhanced endurance in trained cyclists during moderate

intensity exercise following 2 weeks adaptation to a high fat diet. *Eur J Appl Physiol* 1994; **69**: 287–93.

62   Pruett EDR. Glucose and insulin during prolonged work stress in men living on different diets. *J Appl Physiol* 1970; **2**: 199–208.

63   Helge JW, Richter EA, Kiens B. Interaction of training and diet on metabolism and endurance during exercise in man. *J Physiol* 1996; **292**: 293–306.

64   Lemon PWR. Effect of exercise on protein requirements. *J Sports Sci* 1991; **9**: 53–70.

65   Armstrong LE, Maresh CM. Vitamin and mineral supplements as nutritional aids to exercise performance and health. *Nutr Rev* 1996; **54**: 149–58.

66   Weaver CM. Calcium requirements of physically active people *Am J Clin Nutr* 2000; **72** (Suppl.): S579–S584.

67   Specker BL. Evidence for an interaction between calcium intake and physical activity on change in bone mineral density. *J Bone Min Res* 1996; **11**: 1539–44.

68   Myburgh KH, Hutchins J, Fataar AB, Hough SF, Noakes TD. Low bone density is an etiological factor for stress fractures in athletes. *Ann Intern Med* 1990; **113**: 754–9.

69   Schwellnus MP, Jordan G. Does calcium supplementation prevent bone stress injuries? A clinical trial. *Int J Sports Nutr* 1992; **2**: 165–8.

70   Beard J, Tobin B. Iron status and exercise. *Am J Clin Nutr* 2000; **72** (Suppl.): 594S–597S.

71   Weight LM. Sport anemia: does it exist? *Sports Med* 1993; **16**: 1–4.

72   Clarkson PM. Micronutrients and exercise. Antioxidants and minerals. *J Sports Sci* 1995; **13**: 11–24.

73   Rowland TW, Deisroth MB, Green GM, Kelleher JF. The effect of iron therapy on exercise capacity of non-anemic iron deficient adolescent runners. *Am J Dis Child* 1988; **142**: 165–9.

74   Yoshida T, Ido M, Chida M, Ichioka M, Makiguchi K. Dietary iron supplement during physical training in competitive distance runners. *Med Rehab* 1990; **1**: 279–85.

75   Jenkins RR, Krause K, Schoufield LS. Influence of exercise on clearance of oxidant stress products and loosely bound iron. *Med Sci Sports Exerc* 1993; **25**: 213–7.

76   Van Rij AM, Hall MT, Dohm G, Bray J, Porioes WJ. Change in zinc metabolism following exercise in human subjects. *Biol Trace Element Res* 1986; **10**: 99–106.

77   König D, Weinstock C, Keul J, Northhoff H, Berg A. Zinc, iron and magnesium status in athletes. Influence on regulation of exercise induced stress and immune function. *Exerc Immun Rev* 1998; **4**: 2–21.

78   Fosmire G. Zinc toxicity. *Am J Clin Nutr* 1990; **51**: 225–7.

79   Begona MK, Moorkens G, Vertommen J, Noe M, Nève J, De Leeuw I. Magnesium status and parameters of magnesium. *J Am Coll Nutr* 2000; **19**: 374–82.

80   Seelig MS. Consequences of magnesium deficiency on the enhancement of stress reactions: preventive and therapeutic implications. *J Am Coll Nutr* 1994; **13**: 429–46.

81   Anderson RA, Bryden NA, Polansky MM, Deutster PA. Exercise effects on chromium excretion of trained and untrained men consuming a constant diet. *J Appl Phys* 1988; **64**: 249–52.

82   Sen KC, Packer L. Thiol homeostasis and supplements in physical exercise. *Am J Clin Nutr* 2000; **72** (Suppl.): 653S–669S.

83   Wang W-C, Heinonen O, Mäkelä A-L, Mäkelä P, Näntö V, Branth S. Serum selenium, zinc and copper in Swedish and Finnish orienteers. A comparative study. *Analyst* 1995; **120**: 837–40.

84   Armstrong LE, Maresh CM. The exertional heat illness: a risk of athletic participation. *Med Exerc Nutr Health* 1993; **2**: 125–34.

85   Manroe MM. Effects of physical activity on thiamine, riboflavin, and vitamin B6 requirements. *Am J Clin Nutr* 2000; **72** (Suppl.): 598S–606S.

86   Li Li J. Antioxidants and oxidative stress in exercise. *Proc Soc Exp Biol Med* 1999; **222**: 283–92.

87   Clarkson PM, Thompson SH. Antioxidants. what role do they play in physical activity and health? *Am J Clin Nutr* 2000; **72** (Suppl.): 637S–646S.

88   Niess AM, Dickhuth HH, Northoff H, Fehrenbach E. Free radicals and oxidative stress in exercise — immunological aspects. *Exerc Immun Rev* 1999; **5**: 22–56.

89   Greenhaft PL, Casey A, Short AH, Søderlund K, Hultman E. Influence of oral creatine supplementation of muscle torque during repeated bouts of maximal voluntary exercise in man. *Clin Sci* 1993; **84**: 565–71.

90   Sandström B, Aro A, Becker W, Lyhne N, Pedersen JI, Pórsdóttir I. Nordic Nutrition Recommendations. Nordiska Ministerrådet, Köpenhamn. Nord Livsmedel: 28.

91   Møller A. *The Composition of Foods*, 4th edn. Copenhagen: Levnedsmiddelstyrelsen, 1996.

92   Jenkins DJA, Wolever TMS, Jenkins AL, Josse RG, Wong GS. The glycemic response to carbohydrate foods. *Lancet* 1984; **2**: 388–91.

93   Jenkins DJA, Wolever TMS, Jenkins AL. Starchy foods and glycemic index. *Diabetic Care* 1988; **11**: 149–59.

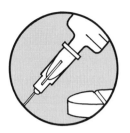

Chapter 2.5
Ergogenic Aids (Doping) and
Pharmacologic Injury Treatment

ULRICH FREDBERG, TIMO SÄPPÄLÄ,

RASMUS DAMSGAARD & MICHAEL KJÆR

Classical reference

Ekblom B, Berglund B. Effect of erythropoietin
administration on maximal aerobic power. *Scand J
Med Sci Sports* 1991; **1**: 88–93.
The effect of subcutaneous injections of recombinant
human erythropoietin (rhEPO) on the circulatory
response to submaximal and maximal exercise was
studied in healthy males. The study was the first to
describe the ergogenic effect in well-trained humans
of exogenous rhEPO. Seven weeks of rhEPO resulted
in increased [Hb] from 152 g/L to 169 g/L and in parallel maximal $\dot{V}O_2$ increased from 4.52 to 4.88 L/min
(Fig. 2.5.1). The improvement in $\dot{V}O_{2\,max}$ by rhEPO
administration was similar to that obtained by acute elevation of [Hb] with red blood cell reinfusion. After
stopping rhEPO administration $\dot{V}O_{2\,max}$ gradually returned to the initial value over 2–4 weeks. Interestingly, systolic blood pressure at 200 W increased after
rhEPO treatment.

Doping and ergogenic drugs

Introduction

The use of prohibited ergogenic aids to enhance sporting performance is referred to as doping (Table 2.5.1).
The word 'dope' arises from the Dutch word 'doop'
which means sauce or cream. In South Africa the word
referred to a drink that was used as a stimulant in reli-
gious ceremonies and during intensive hard work. In
1889 the word appeared for the first time in an English
dictionary, referring to a mixture of opium and narcotics used in horses. In 1933 the term 'doping' was

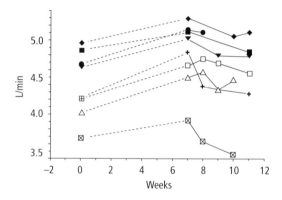

Fig. 2.5.1 Maximal oxygen uptake before and after rhEPO
administration in eight healthy young individuals.

found in an English sports lexicon, and included both
the medical use and the moral implications. Gradually
the term adopted a wider usage and in reference to
sport, it became known as 'doping'. In today's sporting
context, doping refers to the use by athletes of banned
substances or methods that may enhance performance.

Ancient and modern drug use

In the third century BC Greek athletes prepared different mushrooms in the belief that it would enhance
their performance. Similarly the Roman gladiators
used stimulants for faster recovery after injury and
chariot racers fed their horses 'potent' mixtures.
Members of the Inca people chewed coca leaves before
engaging in particularly intensive physical activities
and Vikings have been said to eat fly agaric when
fighting battles. Various stories about the use of different drugs by athletes emerge from the nineteenth

Table 2.5.1 Overall effect of ergogenic agents and procedures. Substances above the full line represent abandoned doping substances, whereas procedures and substances below the line represent legal or limited-legal approaches (caffeine below the allowed limit).

Substance	Mechanism and effect
Blood doping	Hgb and $\dot{V}_{O_2\,max}$ (10–15%)
Erythropoietin	Hgb and $\dot{V}_{O_2\,max}$ (10–15%)
Anabolic steroids	Protein synthesis and strength (10–30%)
GH/IGF-I	Protein synthesis and strength (?)
Beta-adrenergics	Protein synthesis and strength (5%)
Beta-blockers	Central (5–10%)
Amphetamine	Central (3–5%)
Altitude	Hgb and $\dot{V}_{O_2\,max}$ (3–6%)
Caffeine	Metabolism (5–15%), contraction (2–4%)
Creatine	Metabolism (3–5%), strength (10–20%)
Bicarbonate	Neutralize acidosis (3–4%)

GH, growth hormone; Hgb, hemoglobin; IGF-I, insulin-like growth factor 1.

century when sport became more organized and sophisticated, reflecting the industrialization and urbanization of society; drugs included strychnine, nitroglycerine, opium, alcohol, coca leaves and caffeine. The majority of stories were related to cycling and other endurance sports. The events leading to a banning of drugs in sports are listed in Table 2.5.2.

The Olympic Movement Anti-Doping Code

The use of drugs to improve athletic performance is strictly prohibited in sports, mainly on the grounds of fair play and health. From an ethical and moral standpoint doping contravenes the fundamental principles of Olympism, sports as well as medical ethics and is thus forbidden. Furthermore, recommending, proposing, authorizing, condoning or facilitating the use of any substance or method covered by the definition of doping or trafficking therein is also forbidden.

The International Olympic Committee (IOC) has considered the philosophy of control and the types of drugs to be classified as doping agents, and has established suitable methods for testing. These are included in the Olympic Movement Anti-Doping Code and may be changed by the IOC Executive Board. Legally

licensed athletes are bound by the regulations of their international federations. The regulations of the different federations vary in the details of their sanctions and restricted drugs. The IOC list of banned substances and methods consists of stimulants, narcotics, anabolic agents, diuretics and peptide hormones, masking agents, blood doping and manipulations (Table 2.5.4).

Doping agents and their function

Substances used to increase performance can be classified according to the parameters they will influence, i.e. (i) increasing endurance and aerobic capacity, (ii) increasing muscle mass and strength, (iii) decreasing feelings of fatigue and nervousness and (iv) improving recovery processes (Table 2.5.3).

Stimulants (amphetamine, ephedrine, cocaine and caffeine)

Substances belonging to this group range from the potent amphetamines to the weaker caffeine and ephedrine. The substances are called sympathomimetics and imitate the effects of the stress hormones epinephrine and norepinephrine. Amphetamines were synthesized first in 1887 and were initially commercially available as a nasal decongestant. They cause the release of excitatory neurotransmitters, such as dopamine, to stimulate the central nervous system (CNS). The main effects on the CNS include wakefulness, alertness and a decreased sense of fatigue, mood elevation, increased self-confidence and a decreased appetite. The physical effects include increased heart rate, redirection of blood flow from the gastrointestinal tract to the muscles, and an increased fat metabolism. Amphetamine carries a high potential of tolerance, i.e. dosage has to be increased after prolonged use to induce the same effect. Although several CNS-acting stimulants are suspected to be performance enhancing, amphetamine is among the few that has been evaluated scientifically and has been shown to improve performance by 3–5% [1]. Ephedrine's effect on the CNS is weaker than that of amphetamine and controlled studies on its effect are few. Evidently ephedrine has an energy expenditure enhancing effect which has been used in treatment of obesity, and thus could potentially—although this is unsubstantiated—lead to fat loss in athletes. Cocaine has not

Table 2.5.2 Chain of events finally leading to the banning of drugs in sport and the establishment of the independent World Anti-Doping Agency (WADA).

1896
The first recorded death was in 1896 when a cyclist, Arthur Linton, collapsed and died after finishing the first ever Paris Roubaix apparently after an overdose of strychnine

1904
The first near death in modern Olympics where a marathon runner, Thomas Hicks, was using a mixture of brandy and strychnine
No specific date
Most drugs involved alcohol and strychnine. Heroin, caffeine and cocaine were also widely used until heroin and cocaine became available only on prescription

1930s
Amphetamines were produced and quickly became the choice over strychnine. A wide use of amphetamine among soldiers was seen during the Second World War

1950s
The production and use of synthetic testosterone explains the extreme improvements in weight-lifters from the Soviet team at the World Championship in 1954. Accordingly the potent effect of testosterone and synthetic derivatives such as dianabol became common knowledge

1952
One of the first noticeable doping cases involving amphetamines, which occurred at the Winter Olympics. Several speed skaters became ill and needed medical attention

1960
At the Olympics in Rome, Danish cyclist, Kurt Jensen, collapsed and died from an amphetamine overdose

1963
The Council of Europe set up a Committee on drugs but couldn't decide on a definition of doping. The first ever antidoping law was approved in France and 2 years later in Belgium

1966
The first doping controls were carried out by FIFA during the World Championship in soccer in England

1967
The IOC took action after the death of Tommy Simpson (due to the illegal taking of amphetamines) in the Tour de France

1968
The IOC decided on a definition of doping and developed a banned list of substances. Testing began at the Olympic games

1988
At the Seoul Olympics, Ben Johnson tested positive for a banned anabolic steroid, was stripped of his gold medal and was suspended for 2 years

1999
The World Conference on Doping in Sport held in Lausanne on 2–4 February 1999 produced the *Lausanne Declaration on Doping in Sport*. This document provided for the creation of an independent international antidoping agency to be fully operational for the Games of the XXVII Olympiad in Sydney. Pursuant to the terms of the Lausanne Declaration, the World Anti-Doping Agency was established on 10 November 1999 to promote and coordinate the fight against doping in sport internationally

been found to have any performance-enhancing effect in athletes. Although this drug could contribute to a subjective feeling of 'doing well', the effects on peripheral reflexes of cocaine could in fact impair performance.

The effect on the CNS of amphetamine may lead to a distortion of the user's perception of reality and impairment of judgement, which may cause an athlete to continue participation while injured or exhausted leading to worse injuries or collapse. Other acute side-effects are headaches, insomnia, convulsions, halluci-

nations and paranoia and ultimately death due to ruptured blood vessels in the brain, heart attacks, heart rhythm abnormalities and heat stroke. Chronic side-effects consist of dyskinesia, compulsive and repetitive behaviors, schizophrenia and death from ruptured blood vessels throughout the body.

Caffeine, even in moderate doses (5–6 mg/kg body weight) that do not exceed the accepted amount of caffeine in the urine, will result in improved performance. Earlier results indicated that the primary effect of caffeine was to stimulate an increase in circulating

Table 2.5.3 Performance-enhancing drugs.

Performance aim	Ergogenic agent or method	Effect
Endurance	Erythropoietin Blood doping Hemopure/oxyglobin Caffeine	5–15%
Strength (Body composition)	Anabolic steroids Growth hormone Insulin-like growth factor 1 Beta-adrenergic	10–30%
Central fatigue Restitution (Nervousness) (Pain)	Amphetamine Ephedrine/cocaine Beta-blockers ACTH/cortisol Local anesthetics Glucose/insulin Alcohol	3–5%
Anti-test	Diuretics Probenecid/epitestosterone Human choriogonadotrophin Saline infusion	

Table 2.5.4 The IOC list of prohibited classes of substances and methods.

I Prohibited classes of substances
A Stimulants
B Narcotics
C Anabolic agents
D Diuretics
E Peptide hormones, mimetics and analogs

II Prohibited methods
A Blood doping
B Pharmacologic, chemical and physical manipulation

III Classes of substances prohibited in certain circumstances
A Alcohol
B Cannabinoids
C Local anesthetics
D Corticosteroids
E Beta-blockers

catecholamines which in turn mobilized free fatty acids (FFA) from adipocytes and improved muscular fat metabolism, sparing glycogen stores and improving endurance performance . However, more recently it has been shown that other mechanisms are also active, in that an enhanced performance effect of caffeine can be demonstrated in the absence of changes in catecholamines, and is found even in sports lasting only 5–30 min where fat metabolism does not play any major role. The effect has also been demonstrated *in vivo* in spinal cord injured individuals who underwent electrical stimulation of paralyzed muscle indicating that effects were local on the muscle rather than related to the brain, epinephrine or fatty acid mobilization [2].

Beta-2 agonists

These drugs are used for treatment of asthma (see Chapter 4.5) and do not improve aerobic performance in lung-healthy individuals. However, it has been documented that β-agonists administered orally have an anabolic effect. Clenbuterol increases muscle hypertrophy and decreases fat deposition in animals, and several studies on β₂-agonists in humans have shown increased strength gains [3].

Beta-blockers

By reducing sympathetic activity β-blockers cause a marked reduction in the maximal heart rate and thus reduce $\dot{V}_{O_{2\,max}}$ by 25–30% which is clearly unfavorable in the case of any components of a sport that demand circulatory loading. On the other hand, β-blockers have been shown to cause an improvement in pistol shooting, ski jumping and musical performance of 5–10% [4].

Anabolic androgen steroids

These substances, especially the hormone testosterone, are the doping substances most widely used for improving muscle mass and strength in association with regular training. Initially evidence for its effect was minor, due to the use of very small doses, but later studies have confirmed a significant effect. Body composition changes, with increased fat-free mass and reduced body fat. Some of this effect can be seen even without training, but is relatively more pronounced when added to resistance training [5–7]. Doses used

Table 2.5.5 Overview of anabolic steroids.

Drug	Administration	Side-effects	Comments
Testosterone esters	i.m. (in water) Subling/derm (oil)	Some risk of hepatotoxic and lipid effects Androgenic effects	Very potent, cleared rapidly
Stanozolol	Oral	Low hepatotoxic risk Very little fluid retention	Cleared slowly
Oxandrolone	Oral	Low androgen risk Very little fluid retention	Regarded as potent with few side-effects
Nandrolone	i.m. (in oil)	Low androgen risk	Regarded as potent with few side-effects

are variable depending upon the drug type, but it is not uncommon to use 50–100 mg/day for men and 25–50 mg/day for women. A study of female body builders who all had trained for 6 years showed that those who took anabolic steroids intermittently for around 4 years had markedly more muscle mass than the control group. Furthermore, reports on former German Democratic Republic athletes who took anabolic substances for several years estimated that improvements in already well trained athletes were up to 10–20% with regard to throwing events in track and field [8]. Interestingly, women performing running distances of 400, 800 and 1500 m also gained up to 8–10% improvement. Finally, in a well-controlled study, 10 weeks of 600 mg/week testosterone enanthate administered to healthy young males resulted in markedly enhanced muscle growth in the group that received the drug [7].

Drug users often use a mixture of steroids, or have preference for specific types of steroids, e.g. testosterone enanthate, nandrolone decanoate, stanozolol, oxymetholone or oxandrolone. This is due to differences in the profile of the various drugs with regard to effect vs. side-effects, especially anabolic vs. androgenic effects. Whereas some substances have a low androgen side-effect and are thus preferred by women users, other drugs are cleared more rapidly from the body, lowering the risk of being caught in a doping test (Table 2.5.5).

In general the side-effects associated with androgen abuse are three-fold: (a) hepatotoxic effects; (b) androgenic and reproductive side-effects; and (c) other effects on lipid and carbohydrate metabolism as well as

Table 2.5.6 Side-effects associated with intake of anabolic steroids in well-trained athletes (180 mg testosterone daily over 3 months). Data from Alen *et al. Int J Sports Med* 1984; **5**: 189–195.

	Before	3 months
ASAT (U/L)	30±3	46±7*
Testicular volume	19±2	13±1*
LH (IU/L)	5.0±2.4	2.5±2.1*
Sperm count (millions/mL)	55±15	2*
HDL cholesterol (mmol/L)	1.5±0.2	0.6±0.1*
LDL cholesterol (mmol/L)	3.1±0.5	4.1±0.9*
Hct (%)	45±2	48±2*

ASAT, aspartate aminotransferase; LH, luteinizing hormone; HDL, high-density lipoproteins; LDL, low-density lipoproteins; Hct, hematocrit.

psychologic effects. As substances are metabolized in the liver and are often used in high doses, it is clear that toxic parenchymal effects on the liver can occur, and elevation of aminotransferases is one of the first signs of anabolic substance abuse (Table 2.5.6) [6]. In addition, liver pathology such as cholestasis, blood cysts and primary liver tumors are observed. Suppression of sex hormones as well as testicular atrophy and infertility can be observed after only 3 months of abuse, and although these effects are thought to be reversible after drug use ceases, good long-term studies of chronic abusers are lacking. Male athletes often take human chorionic gonadotrophin (hCG) in order to maintain endogenous synthesis of substances needed for spermatogenesis. Administration of large amounts of testosterone can in males result in formation of estrogen and thus development of gynecomastia, and many male abusers take estrogen antagonists to counteract this. In women androgenous side-effects lead to virilization including a deepened voice, increased facial hair and clitoral hypertrophy [9]. Hair loss including balding has been observed in both female and male athletes. Likewise skin problems with acne appear in a dose-dependent manner in both sexes. Changes in blood lipid profile are seen rapidly after androgen intake commences, and interestingly the cholesterol profile after 3 months of use seems more unfavorable than in untrained healthy individuals [6]. Likewise a dramatic change in insulin sensitivity has been seen, providing the basis for development of glucose intolerance. Good studies are, however, lacking with regard to reversibility, as well as to any later development of cardiovascular disease and/or type II diabetes. Psychologic side-effects have been difficult to assess, but studies have suggested an increase in psychologic pathologies such as anxiety, psychosis, irritability, aggression and violent behavior [10]. The exact mechanisms are not obvious but could be related to changes in neurotransmitter systems or hypogonadism.

Diuretics

These substances are used in sports where body weight is important such as wrestling, boxing, light-weight rowing and horse riding, and weight loss of several percent has been observed overnight, resulting in unfavorable dehydration and subsequent reduced performance (see Chapter 2.3). Previously, diuretics were also used for diluting the urine in order to pass doping tests, but today the determination of the urine mass weight has stopped this.

Human growth hormone (hGH) and insulin-like growth factor (IGF-I)

Intake of growth hormone (GH) has been used for years in the belief that it has an anabolic effect on skeletal muscle. It has been demonstrated that GH administration in GH-deficient individuals can improve fat-free body mass and thus muscle, and animal studies have documented a GH-mediated stimulation of muscle hypertrophy. In spite of this, there have been no studies robustly documenting any muscle mass-increasing effect of GH in addition to strength training

in either untrained or well-trained individuals [11]. What has been shown is an enhancing effect of GH on lipid oxidation and thus on body composition. Growth hormone administration results in several side-effects, in both the short and long term. Immediate side-effects are fluid accumulation in the legs and carpal tunnel syndrome, whereas impaired glucose metabolism (glucose intolerance), hyperlipidemia and cardiomegaly can develop with long-term misuse. IGF-I has become used as a doping substance but no good experiments have documented any major effect of its administration in relation to muscle growth and performance.

Erythropoietin (rhEPO)

The development of erythropoietin in recombinant form to use in patients with anemia has led to it totally replacing blood doping as the doping choice in endurance athletes. It has been demonstrated in both untrained and well-trained athletes with normal hematocrit and hemoglobin values that rhEPO can increase hemoglobin concentration, endurance performance, maximal aerobic power and arterial pressure during exercise [12–14]. Improvements by rhEPO administration are similar to those seen previously with blood transfusion, and it is thus likely that improvements in real sports performance are equally as good as those achieved by blood transfusion (see also Classical reference). It has been documented that performance in cross-country skiing and 10-km running has been shown to be increased by 3–5% up to 5–10 days after blood transfusion. More recently it has been shown in monkeys that genetic engineering was able to produce erythropoietin in muscle and that hematocrit rose. Unfortunately, the increase in hemoglobin production led to a rise to unacceptably high levels. However, the finding points to the fact that genetic doping could very well be used in the future for other categories of doping substances. Another area of interest for doping attempts is the production of stable hemoglobin without erythrocytes from bovine blood (hemopure, oxyglobin) which is being developed for emergency cases involving blood loss. Use of this formulation is expected to provide higher oxygen uptake and delivery capacity in athletes, and is likely to become a used substance within the next few years.

Legal substances or procedures

In addition to the doping substances described above, it is clear that legal approaches can also result in performance enhancement. With regard to endurance, it has been documented that altitude training, especially if training is carried out at a moderate altitude (~ 1000 m) and the rest of the time is spent at a somewhat higher altitude (~ 2500 m), can result in some marginal improvement. Furthermore, the use of artificial low-oxygen 'altitude' houses has been shown to increase Hb concentration and hematocrit, if sufficient time is spent in hypoxia (> 8–10 h). The improvement is, however, not as large as that seen with rhEPO.

The intake of bicarbonate has been shown to result in a small improvement in performance of events such as the 800-m run where both aerobic and anaerobic systems are heavily taxed.

One of the most debated substances lately has been creatine (Cr), and its performance-enhancing effects. Research indicates that Cr supplementation (initially 20 g/day followed by 3–4 g/day) can increase muscle PCr content in some individuals. Exercise performance involving short periods of extremely powerful activity can be enhanced, especially during repeated bouts of activity [15], whereas performance in aerobic exercise is not influenced. Furthermore, it has been demonstrated that Cr results in increased improvement of muscle strength with strength training but the mechanism behind this has not been discovered [16]. So far there are no documented gastrointestinal, renal or muscle side-effects associated with Cr intake.

Doping analyses

Doping analyses have been used for doping control in a variety of sports for some 30 years now [17]. National and international sports associations and their anti-doping authorities are responsible for the selection of the athletes to be tested, for maintaining the testing organization and for handing down judgements. Athletes are tested at competitions and during training (out-of-competition tests). To ensure the quality and reliability of testing, the protocol of sample collection is clearly specified and standardized. At present in most sports, only urine is collected from an athlete as a doping sample. The sample is divided between two glass bottles, each of which bears a distinguishable code. To guarantee the security of processing and storage of the test samples, the bottles are sealed and transported to the laboratory in special containers. The analysis itself has to rely on an adequate sample collection. In some countries certified quality systems for doping control based on ISO-9000 series standards and International Anti-Doping Arrangement (IADA) standards for doping control have been established already and in several other countries quality certification is in progress.

Analysis in all official doping control tests is carried out exclusively in doping control laboratories accredited by the IOC, at present 25 in the world. The laboratories follow the guidelines and procedures set by the IOC. The accreditation must be reapplied for each year. In the near future, WADA, founded by the IOC and nations throughout the world in 1999, will take the leadership in organizing and harmonization of worldwide doping control.

Methods of detection

The requirements of the IOC for the accreditation of doping laboratories include sophisticated instrumentation. Most of the methods are based on gas chromatography and sensitive and selective detectors.

Development of analytic techniques and instrumentation has been fast in recent years allowing ever better resolution, identification and detection of smaller and smaller amounts of analytes with sufficient certainty. High-resolution and tandem mass spectrometry, liquid chromatography combined with mass spectography (HPLC/MS) with various configurations and even gas chromatography/combustion/carbon isotope ratio mass spectrometry (GC/C/CIRMS) are coming into routine use [18–20].

The IOC list of banned substances consists of numerous compounds with a wide range of chemical structures. The actual laboratory analysis consists of two steps: screening and confirmation analysis. From seven to nine separate analytic procedures are needed to cover all banned substances. After screening, all suspected samples are reanalyzed by gas chromatography/mass spectrometry (GC/MS) to provide fully reliable results.

Some peptide hormones with large molecules such as human chorionic gonadotrophin (hCG) are still detected by immunoassays since sufficiently sensitive mass spectrometry methods are not yet available.

However, if appropriately standardized and validated methods are used, investigators should be able to detect self-administration of hCG in men as reliably as anabolic steroids and testosterone are now being detected by mass spectrometry methods [21].

Reliability of the doping result is of crucial importance. The consequence of a false finding of doping in an innocent athlete is personal disaster. Therefore, the ratio of true-positive to false-positive doping results must be extremely high. The personal opinion of the author is that 99.9% of the cases decided as 'doping' should be true positive. Because approximately 100 000 doping tests performed annually in the whole world yield more than 1000 positive findings the application of the 99.9% principle would lead to false positive tests of one or two non-users throughout the world each year.

All tests used for doping control purposes should be well validated. The positive predictive value (PPV) of the test can be estimated by routine measures using Bayesian rule [22] provided that the sensitivity and specificity of the test have been studied. The accurate value is, however, hardly ever obtained since the relative number of drug users has a marked effect on PPV.

IOC requirements for doping laboratories guarantee that the reliability of the doping tests is high in general. This in no way precludes the existence of various uncertainties in the test results (or in judgements).

Testing of some doping agents of interest

Non-physiologic agents

Misuses of central nervous system stimulants, narcotic analgesics and β-blocking agents are all controlled at competitions only, and are easily controlled by the present analytic techniques, e.g. [17]. Sensitivities of the assays are nearly 100% for these agents, and analyses are reliable and specific. The ion mass spectrum indicative of the parent drug or its metabolite detected from the sample can be considered as a fingerprint of the banned substance in the body.

Since stimulants, narcotics and β-blocking agents are allowed to be used during the training period for therapeutic purposes there is a risk for careless athletes of stopping the treatment too late before the competition to give sufficient time for elimination of the drug from the body. Such cases do not lead to sanctions and

Table 2.5.7 Summary of urinary concentrations above which IOC-accredited laboratories must report findings for specific substances.

Caffeine	>12 µg/mL
Carboxy-THC	>15 ng/mL
Cathine	>5 µg/mL
Ephedrine	>5 µg/mL
Epitestosterone	>200 ng/mL
Methylephedrine	>5 µg/mL
Morphine	>1 µg/mL
19-Norandrosterone	>2 ng/mL in males
19-Norandrosterone	>5 ng/mL in females
Phenylpropanolamine	>10 µg/mL
Pseudoephedrine	>10 µg/mL
Testosterone/epitestosterone ratio	>6

in order to decrease this risk the IOC has set limits for urinary concentrations of e.g. ephedrine and ephedrine derivatives for which the laboratories declare the results as negative (Table 2.5.7). Similar to this, morphine positive samples are reported to doping authorities only when the urinary morphine concentration exceeds a certain limit. The rationale for this is that several unbanned antidiarrheals and narcotics, e.g. codeine, are metabolized in part into morphine. Ingestion of poppy seeds may also be the reason for the existence of small amounts of morphine in urine.

Caffeine which is daily consumed in many beverages and foods belongs to the list of prohibited substances. The definition of a positive result depends on the concentration of caffeine in urine. This concentration may not exceed 12 mg/L. The restricted level is only occasionally exceeded by common habitual intake [23]. In any case, excretion of caffeine into urine shows large interindividual variation due to several factors including differences in genetically determined enzyme profile [24,25]. Before doping sanctions based on urinary caffeine concentrations can be considered reliable much more research is needed.

Anabolic steroid agents are used during the training period and therefore out-of-competition tests are of utmost importance to reveal the users. Conventional urine testing for anabolic steroids reliably identifies either the banned drug, its metabolites or both by GC/MS [26,27]. Increased knowledge of their metabolism has made it possible to select metabolites with long elimination half-lives and different from naturally occurring steroids for monitoring. On the other hand, the recent development of high-resolution equipment has lowered the detection limit for these agents. Accordingly, the number of anabolic steroid-positive findings has clearly increased over the last few years. Moreover, very small amounts of nandrolone metabolites, which may be physiologic in certain conditions (e.g. pregnancy) can be detected nowadays and the IOC has set the maximum allowable urine concentrations for these substances. It is well known that use of anabolic androgenic steroids has a long-term influence on the production and excretion of various endogenous steroids. In looking at methods of broadening the time window of detection of anabolic androgen use, the influence of these steroids on the hormone to hormone ratios derived from the measurement of several endogenous steroid hormones and metabolites ('urinary steroid profile') has been considered (see [28]). It has been shown that when appropriately calibrated the chemometric evaluation of urinary steroid profiles makes a distinction between control and user groups and may delineate androgenic steroid users directly from the routine screening procedure [28]. Validation of the procedure and confirmation of the results may be laborious. Further, the procedure is extremely vulnerable to exogenous manipulation.

Therefore, steroid profile and chemometric methods are not in official use.

Physiologic agents

There are two possible strategies for revealing doping with an agent which naturally occurs or may occur in some physiologic conditions in the human body. The more laborious way to find the solution is to make quantitative determinations of the agent itself, e.g. growth hormone (GH), and of a number of potential 'markers' of its effects. In the case of GH such markers could be e.g. insulin-like growth factor (IGF-I) and IGF binding proteins. Measurements should be made in the blood and urine. Samples should be taken in rest and exercise situations from healthy subjects with varying demography and athletes representing different sports. The results should be submitted to extensive statistic modelling and analysis to obtain reference values or indexes with sufficient reliability to reveal the exogenous use of the agent. The second way is more challenging: attempt to set up a method which allows discrimination between the endogenous and exogenous molecule.

The current assay methods for testosterone do not distinguish synthetic (exogenous) testosterone from physiologic (endogenous) testosterone. Detection of doping with testosterone is based on measuring the testosterone to epitestosterone ratio (T/E) in urine by GC/MS [26]. The T/E ratio in healthy males who have not used testosterone is usually lower than or around 1.0. Athletes who have a urinary T/E ratio >6 are suspected of testosterone doping. The difficult aspect of the T/E test is that a small number of males have been found with T/E ratios in the range 6–10 in the absence of testosterone administration [20] and a strict application of the T/E >6 criterion would falsely classify these subjects as testosterone users. Attempts to distinguish testosterone users from non-users in this population have included measuring the urinary ratio of testosterone to luteinizing hormone, measuring serum testosterone/17-hydroxyprogesterone ratio, carrying out the ketoconazole test, measuring different ratios of testosterone and epitestosterone sulfate and glucuronide conjugates as well as measuring several ratios based on testosterone precursors and metabolites. At present, sports authorities do not act on the basis of a single result T/E >6, instead additional tests are carried out on the suspected athlete to follow the changes in the T/E ratio which has been to found to be relatively stable in healthy drug-free males. Not only may the current methodology applied to reveal testosterone doping lead to erroneous reporting of cases in which the T/E ratio >6 might be natural due to a physiologic or pathologic condition, it may also miss the cases with urinary T/E <6 in which exogenous testosterone, alone or together with epitestosterone and/or hCG, might have been used. Therefore assays for exogenous testosterone would be more reliable if identification of injectable testosterone esters, occurring in the body only after the use of testosterone preparations, were possible. Recently, a promising method utilizing HPLC/MS analysis of serum testosterone esters has been published [29]. With further development a method might be adopted in sports doping control provided that blood samples will be allowed to be collected.

The most promising approach for confirming the abuse of exogenous testosterone is based on gas chromatography/combustion/carbon isotope ratio mass spectrometry (GC/C/CIRMS) in which the changes in carbon isotope ratios ($^{13}C/^{12}C$) of urinary testosterone, its precursors and metabolites are detected [20]. Synthetic testosterone is derived from chemical sources whilst physiologic testosterone is of natural origin with a much higher carbon isotope ratio. Accordingly, decreased isotope ratio is indicative to a great extent of the use of exogenous testosterone. High costs may restrict the adoption of this method into routine use, as well as the lack of knowledge of the effects of dietary habits, variability of different pharmaceutical batches, etc. on the results [30].

The pregnancy hormone human chorionic gonadotrophin (hCG) has so far been measured by commercial immunoassays. According to the IOC recommendations hCG should be determined by two different immunoassays. Since hCG-like immunoreactivity occurs at low concentration in the plasma and urine of normal healthy males the analyses are quantitative in nature. Some uncertainties are included in the different immunoassays because hCG occurs in various molecular forms including the intact hCG heterodimer, its free a and b subunits, proteolytically cleaved forms and fragments, and these different forms cross-react to various degrees in immunoassays. Therefore, in each laboratory the assay procedure for urinary hCG has to be validated carefully in control and athletic populations before running the tests routinely. After the appropriate validation the self-administration of hCG can be reliably detected [21] provided that pregnancy or diseases associated with endogenous hCG production are excluded.

Although human growth hormone (hGH) is easily measured by simple immunoassays the fact is that there are currently no valid methods of detecting its abuse. Based on quantitative determination of urinary hGH by immunoassays detection of hGH doping would be feasible provided that urine samples could be obtained in the basal states without exogenous intake [31]. The problem is that renal clearance of the hGH increases drastically during strenuous effort preventing relevant interpretation of the results. GH-2000 is a European multinational research project, the aim of which is to produce an indirect method of revealing hGH doping by measuring hGH, growth factors, IGF binding protein and connective tissue metabolites as potential markers [32]. As for testosterone, the $^{13}C/$$^{12}C$ isotope ratios have been measured for natural hGH and commercial recombinant rhGH products in an attempt to differentiate endogenous and exogenous origins of the hGH by high-performance liquid chromatography/isotope ratio mass spectrometry (HPLC/IRMS) [30]. However, only one preparation studied differed markedly from natural hormone in its carbon isotope ratio. Further, the low renal clearance of GH reduces the applicability of this concept. The assay might work better with serum GH. So far, there are no reliable methods available to reveal the abuse of hGH.

Erythropoietin (EPO) is a physiologic glycoprotein hormone involved in the regulation of erythropoiesis. The pharmacokinetics and pharmacodynamics of recombinant human EPO (rhEPO) are well clarified [33]. The produced rhEPO is homogenous with respect to the peptide sequence of natural EPO, but rhEPO contains heterogeneous carbohydrate moiety and this difference in carbohydrate structure is an important factor for identifying the administration of exogenous rhEPO [34] as is the consequent difference in electric charges of natural EPO and rhEPO detectable by electrophoresis [35,36]. At the Sydney Olympic Games a combination of an indirect method utilizing blood samples [14] and a direct method utilizing urine samples [36] was used for the first time in a preliminary manner to reveal the use of rhEPO. Validation of methods reliable for doping control purposes is in progress.

Pharmacologic treatment of sports injuries

The objective for medical treatment of sports injuries is primarily to shorten the rest period by reducing inflammation and pain so active rehabilitation can start as soon as possible before the deconditioning rest period has seriously reduced the physical properties of the soft tissues. Medical treatment is therefore only an adjuvant therapy in the overall management of sports injuries. The main treatment is 'active' rest and gradual rehabilitation within the limits of pain. If you are not familiar with the principles of rehabilitation, do not use medicine in the treatment of sports injuries.

The indications for using medicine in sports medicine are (i) pain control: simple analgesics (e.g. paracetamol), non-steroid anti-inflammatory drugs (NSAIDs) and weak opioids (e.g. tramadol) and (ii) inflammation control: NSAIDs and corticosteroids.

Simple analgesics and weak opioids

Indications
Analgesics can be used to a limited extent to reduce the pain in minor injuries when there is no risk of aggravating the injury by continuing the sports activity, for example hematomas under nails and excoriations. Of course analgesics can be used to reduce all forms of pain if the sports activity is stopped. Because of its few side-effects paracetamol is recommended.

Pharmacodynamics
Paracetamol has an analgesic and antipyretic effect. Mode of operation is partly unknown but it seems probable that it has both a peripheral and central component.

Pharmacokinetics
Ninety per cent is absorbed and maximal plasma concentration of paracetamol is reached after 0.5–1 h after oral administration. The duration of effect is 4–6 h. Only 60% of paracetamol is absorbed by rectal administration.

Adverse events
In contrast to weak opioids and acetylsalicylate derivatives paracetamol at the recommended dose has virtually no side-effects [36a].

Contraindications
Analgesics should never be used to allow an athlete to continue a sports activity when there is a risk of aggravating the injury. Paracetamol and other analgesics with antipyretic effects must never be used to reduce the body temperature before sports activity. Several viral infections can invade heart muscle and produce myocarditis. This risk of myocarditis is increased in strenuous physical activity during the acute phase of viral infection, and there are reports of spontaneous death and serious complications occurring in previously fit young adults who undertake vigorous exercise

when in the acute phase of a viral illness [37,38]. Fever indicates an infection and sports activity must be stopped and temperature normalized before resuming sports activity.

Administration
Paracetamol 1–2 g 3–4 times daily by oral administration. Rectal administration gives a slower but longer effect.

Conclusion
Because of the very few side-effects of paracetamol it is recommended as the drug of choice in treatment of pain without inflammation.

NSAIDs
NSAIDs are widely used in sports medicine (i) to control pain, (ii) as anti-inflammatory agents that presumably allow early activity that speeds the healing process, and (iii) to decrease inflammation presumably to speed healing directly.

Indications
Tendon injuries. Several randomized, placebo-controlled short-term studies of NSAID treatment in acute tendon injuries have been done. Healing was slightly more rapid and inflammation slightly decreased in treated patients compared with placebo-treated patients in most studies [39–43], while no effect was found in other studies [44,45], and some studies showed increased instability and reduced range of motion [43].

Acute muscular injuries (strains and contusions). Only a few animal studies [46,47], and a single double-blind, placebo-controlled human study [48] are available. Increased contractile force was found in the NSAID-treated muscles early following the injury, but the treatment was associated with a delayed degradation of damaged tissue later on and a delayed muscle regeneration. Similarly, muscle regeneration appeared to be slowed by the NSAID treatment. The human study showed no beneficial effect.

Myositis ossificans. One study showed that ossifications after non-cemented total hip arthroplasty appeared significantly less frequently in patients postoperatively treated with anti-inflammatory drugs [49]. No studies concerning athletes exist.

Chronic muscle and tendon injuries. There is no convincing scientific support in literature for using NSAID treatment in chronic muscle and tendon injuries [50,51].

Pharmacodynamics
NSAIDs have analgesic, antipyretic and anti-inflammatory effects. NSAIDs act by inhibiting the synthesis of prostaglandins, which are capable of mediating the inflammatory response following injury by the enzyme cyclooxygenase (COX). Two isoforms are now recognized. COX-1, which is constitutively expressed, sustains the routine physiologic function of prostaglandins, including gastric mucosal protection. COX-2 is induced chiefly in response to pathologic processes, including pain and inflammation. Prostaglandins synthesized by the inducible COX-2 isoform mediate acute inflammatory responses in animal models. NSAIDs are non-isoform specific, inhibiting both the COX-1 and COX-2 isoforms. Since prostaglandins are involved in the maintenance of gastrointestinal (GI) mucosal integrity and since only the COX-1 isoform is present in the normal GI mucosa, the GI toxicity of NSAIDs has been proposed to result largely from inhibition of COX-1 activity. The therapeutic effects of NSAIDs may be primarily attributable to COX-2 inhibition. By selective inhibition of the COX-2 enzyme it is possible to reduce inflammation almost entirely without serious GI side-effects.

A recent animal study [52] indicates that a new isoform of the enzyme cyclooxygenase (COX-3) has anti-inflammatory activity equivalent to or greater than that seen with steroids [53] and can be an important part of the regeneration process.

Pharmacokinetics
All NSAIDs are almost completely absorbed after oral administration and the half-life in the body ($t_{1/2}$) is from a few hours to more than 1 day.

Adverse events
Adverse GI effects are frequently seen in patients who are given NSAIDs and include dyspepsia, nausea and ulcer. The new selective COX-2 inhibitors are largely free of serious GI side-effects. Serious adverse events are rare, but anaphylactic shock, nephritis and aplastic anemia are described. Only very few side-effects are associated with the use of topical NSAIDs (allergy).

Contraindications
In healthy athletes only allergy is a contraindication. Be careful with ulcer disease, hypertension and insufficiency of the kidney, heart and liver.

Administration
Oral administration is recommended. A few placebo-controlled studies [54–56] all suggest that topical NSAIDs may indeed be significantly better than placebo in treating acute injuries although the blood concentration after topical administration will reach less than 10% of levels after oral or intramuscular administration [57]. There is no scientific support in literature for using intramuscular administration. No scientifically based conclusion as to the ideal time to start and the ideal duration of NSAID treatment can be drawn.

Discussion
It remains controversial whether inhibiting the acute inflammatory response is of uniform advantage. Pain and disability following the injury are at least in part due to the inflammatory response. Decreasing the inflammation decreases the symptoms and may allow earlier rehabilitation. On the other hand, inflammatory cells are responsible for clearing away cell debris and necrotic muscle fibers. Without this phagocytic function healing, in particular regeneration, may not be able to begin. Studies involving anabolic steroids (which are not allowed in sport) and muscle injuries have found increased numbers of progenitor cells [57a] and more rapid healing and restoration of force [58]. Interestingly, both studies found this was associated with an initial increase in inflammatory cells. This suggests that the initial inflammatory response is indeed a crucial part of the healing response. The future will show whether the new isoform of the enzyme cyclooxygenase (COX-3) can be an important part of this regeneration process. Inhibiting the enzyme cyclooxygenase can theoretically result in a reduced spontaneous regeneration after an injury.

Conclusions

Although several clinical trials indicate that treatment with NSAIDs has some effect in sports injuries it is not clear that the difference between NSAIDs and placebo is clinically significant and clear-cut indications cannot be given. The indication for suppressing the acute inflammatory response is questionable. Theoretically it could reduce regeneration of the injured tissue. Adverse events after oral NSAIDs are common, but rarely serious. With this background it does not seem reasonable to recommend the use of NSAIDs routinely in acute muscle and tendon injuries. If treatment with NSAIDs is indicated, topical administration is recommended whenever possible. When systemic treatment is indicated it seems rational to use a COX-2 inhibitor because of the fewer side-effects although there is no documentation of the effect in athletes. If treatment with NSAIDs is misused as a 'pain killer' in order to send athletes back to full sport activity without rehabilitation and correction of training failures the medical treatment can indirectly result in a chronic injury.

Other pharmaceutical agents

Systemic injected heparin has been used in the treatment of peritendinitis crepitans. At the moment there is little scientific basis for this treatment [59] and the adverse events are so serious that the treatment cannot be recommended [60]. Local injections of polysulfated glycosaminoglycan [61], one of the constituents of the base substance, and the protease inhibitor aprotinin [62], have been used in the management of peri- and intratendinous pathologies. For these experimental treatments also there is currently little scientific basis.

Corticosteroids

No legal treatment in sport has been so controversial as local injected corticosteroids. Intratendinous injection of corticosteroid has resulted in some animal studies in a directly deleterious effect on the tendon [63–65], and should be unanimously condemned. Obviously not all studies agree [66–68]. No proof of any deleterious effect of peritendinous injections exists in the literature [69–71]. Generally the literature concerning injection of local corticosteroids is very sparse and too many conclusions are based on poor scientific evidence.

Injection of corticosteroids is used in sports medicine: (i) to decrease acute inflammation in bursitis, tendovaginitis and peritendinitis; and (ii) to reduce the deleterious effect of chronic inflammation in chronic overuse symptoms.

Indications

Arthritis. Intra-articular injected corticosteroid is one of the most widespread treatments in rheumatology. Placebo-controlled studies have proved the effectiveness of the treatment in arthritis [72,73].

Chronic tendinopathy. There are only very few randomized, placebo-controlled studies concerning the effect of local corticosteroids and chronic tendon injuries, but some effect has been recognized in the treatment of tennis elbow [74,75], rotator cuff tendinitis [76] and plantar fasciitis [72]. Often the effect has been of short duration. Newer randomized, double-blind, placebo-controlled studies [76a,76b] have shown a significant effect of ultrasound-guided peritendinous injection of long-acting corticosteroids in athletes with the most severe ultrasonography-verified jumper's knee or Achilles tendinopathy. Despite having had symptoms for an average of $1\frac{1}{2}$ years 50% of the athletes were free of symptoms after 3 months but only 20% were free of symptoms after 6 months. The increased tendon diameter and the edema evaluated by ultrasonography were highly significantly reduced every week for the first 4 weeks following an injection despite the fact that the tendons were never totally normalized after the maximum of three peritendinous corticosteroid injections. The high frequency of relapse of symptoms in the study can be explained by the very aggressive training involving starting running a few days after injection. Another explanation could be the degenerative changes in the tendon. Although there is only sparse documentation of inflammatory cells in biopsies from chronically affected tendons the significant reduction in edema and thickness of the treated tendons is most likely due to a reduction in the inflammatory process. The corticosteroid seems to reduce the inflammation and edema of the tendon, but steroid cannot, however, repair the degenerative changes. When maximal training intensity is resumed the degenerative changes will cause relapse of the inflammation. A third explanation of the relapse of symptoms could be the limited duration of the steroid effect.

Peritendinitis. A retrospective study reported significant reduction in pain after corticosteroid injection for peritendinitis [71]. No controlled studies exist.

Myositis ossificans. One article has reported seven cases demonstrating the beneficial effect of local corticosteroid injection in myositis ossificans [77]. No controlled studies exist.

Bursitis. The effect of injected corticosteroid in bursitis is safe but sparsely documented [78].

Muscle strain. To date, there are no reported human or animal studies where corticosteroids have been injected locally into strained muscle.

Pharmacodynamics

The mechanism of the anti-inflammatory action of corticosteroid is not completely understood, but corticosteroids inhibit both the early vascular phase of inflammation and the late inflammatory and regenerative phase. Corticosteroids seem to modulate the inflammation not only through an effect on prostaglandin production but also by modulating the cytokine activity in both the parenchymal tissue and the cellular components.

Pharmacokinetics

Most preparations are microcrystallic suspensions of glucocorticoid esters. The less soluble the preparation the longer the duration of effect and the higher the risk of systemic effect. The long-acting corticosteroid triamcinolone has effects lasting for 6 weeks.

Adverse events

Introduction of infection is a possible adverse effect when using local steroid injection therapy. However, this risk can be almost completely eliminated by using a meticulous aseptic, no-touch technique, and by avoiding injections in areas with suspected infection. Atrophy of the overlying skin with telangiectasia and increased hyperesthesia or hypoesthesia and transparency or subcutaneous fat necrosis is often seen when subcutaneous structures are injected. In the above mentioned study [76a,76b] where Achilles and patellar tendons were injected, nearly 50% had atrophy, which disappeared in most cases after 6 months and in no cases caused embarrassing symptoms. Generally this atrophy seems to do little harm and recedes with time.

Systemic effects from the corticosteroid are only a theoretical risk. Although locally injected corticosteroids are designed to be most effective where they are injected, a proportion of the substance penetrates to the bloodstream, and flushing, menstrual disturbances and fluctuations in blood glucose have been reported. Anaphylactic shock is a theoretical complication which doctors must be prepared to treat since cortisone allergy is a rare but possible form of allergy.

Unintended injection in total or partial ruptured Achilles tendons is not unheard of [82,83] as the diagnosis can be difficult without ultrasonography and it is impossible to feel the erroneous intratendinous injection in degenerated tendons (see Figs 2.5.2–2.5.4). Unintentional damage to other structures is minimized when ultrasound-guided injections are used.

The doping supervisors must be informed if the athlete is chosen for doping control during the 8 weeks following an injection.

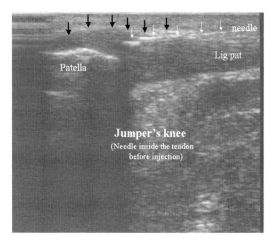

Fig. 2.5.2 Athlete with jumper's knee before injection. The erroneous placement of the needle inside the thick inflamed tendon is seen. The black arrows show the superficial border of the inflamed patellar ligament. The white arrows show the needle.

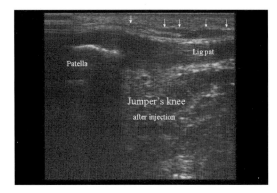

Fig. 2.5.3 The same athlete as in Fig. 2.5.2 before injection. After correction the correct peritendinous placement of the needle is seen. The white arrows show the needle.

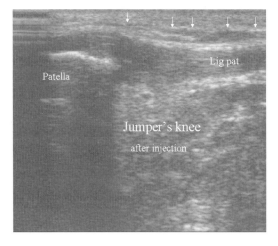

Fig. 2.5.4 The same athlete as in Fig. 2.5.2 after injection. The injection fluid is seen peritendinous. The white arrows show the peritendinous corticosteroid and local anesthesia.

Contraindications

Avoid injection in areas with suspected infection. Active tuberculosis is an absolute contraindication. There is not enough practical or scientific experience with local injection with corticosteroids in children. Injecting children for sports injuries is almost never indicated.

Administration

Dilute the corticosteroid with local anesthetic before the injection. The diluted solution decreases the risk of adverse effects, and the anesthetic-induced disappearance of pain helps to confirm the diagnosis. The literature on the comparative efficacy of different preparations, doses and number of injections is scanty [74,79]. Price *et al.* [74] concluded in a double-blind study that more rapid relief of symptoms of tennis elbow was achieved with 10 mg triamcinolone than with 25 mg hydrocortisone and there was less need to repeat injections in the former group, and Vogel [79] showed an increase in the tensile strength of tendons after corticosteroid injections, but repetition of injections progressively weakened the tendons, suggesting a relationship between cumulative dose and the adverse effect.

Systemic treatment with corticosteroids is not allowed in sports and no studies in the literature find any beneficial effects of this treatment.

Corticosteroids may also be delivered with phonophoresis or iontophoresis [80,81]. The literature is also unclear concerning the efficacy and potential side-effects when corticosteroids are used in this manner. These are common physical therapy modalities used especially to treat some of the most chronic problems in athletes, such as tendinopathy or bursitis.

Discussion

Peritendinous injection of corticosteroids can be used as an adjuvant therapy of severe chronic tendon injuries. The main treatment is of course 'active' rest and gradual rehabilitation for several months within the limits of pain. Only when the injured structure is trained to withstand the maximal stress, should full sports activity be allowed. If the athlete does not follow the rules for graduated rehabilitation over several months after a chronic injury and returns to full sports activity before the weakened tissue is strong enough, there is of course a risk of rupturing the tissue. Incorrect rehabilitation is obviously the greatest risk in treating athletes with local corticosteroid injections. It is necessary to verify the diagnoses by ultrasonography (or MRI) and make the injection under ultrasonographic guidance especially when the big tendons are being treated (Achilles and patellar tendons and the plantar fascia). If there is no effect from one ultrasound-guided steroid injection there is no indication for a second (or third) injection. If there is a partial effect it might be reasonable to repeat the injection once or twice at 4–6-week intervals.

Conclusions

Local injection of corticosteroids seems to be an effective treatment in acute bursitis, tenosynovitis, peritendinitis, plantar fasciitis and (traumatic) arthritis even though the documentation is sparse.

Performed where indicated, on the basis of an ultrasonography-verified diagnosis, ultrasound-guided peritendinous injection with a long-acting corticosteroid is safe and can be a powerful supplement to the basic rehabilitation of severe chronic tendon injuries when normal conservative rehabilitation has failed. If the treatment is misused to send athletes back to full sport after a few weeks the medical treatment can indirectly result in chronic injuries.

Summary

Medical treatment is only an adjuvant therapy in the overall management of sports injuries. On the basis of a correct diagnosis and indication medical treatment can reduce the deconditioning rest period so that active rehabilitation can start as soon as possible before the physical properties of the soft tissues are seriously impaired. Before full participation in sports activities a period with gradual increased rehabilitation with respect for pain is necessary to reduce the risk of relapse of symptoms. Without this period of active rehabilitation medical treatment can be misused and increase the risk for chronic injuries.

The use of ergogenic aids is subject to doping regulations, and urine analysis provides the basis for detection of several doping agents. In endurance sports use of erythropoietin (5–10% improvement) and in power sports anabolic steroids (10–30% improvement) is documented to improve performance but simultaneously to cause major side-effects.

Multiple choice questions

1 *Corticosteroids can be administered in sport as a:*
a tablet
b suppository
c intramuscular injection
d intra-articular injection
e peritendinous injection.

2 *In chronic tendinopathy in the groin unalleviated by rest and graduated training it seems reasonable to try the following medical treatment:*
a paracetamol
b weak opioids
c heparin
d NSAIDs
e local injected steroid.

3 *Why should ultrasound be used when local steroid injection is planned?*
a For correct diagnosis.
b To decrease the risk of unintended puncture of vessel and nerves.
c To decrease the risk of erroneous intratendinous injection.
d To decrease the risk of skin atrophy.
e To allow evaluation of the effect of treatment.

4 *What are the documented risks after a peritendinous injection of corticosteroid?*
a Skin atrophy.
b Tendon rupture.
c Adrenal suppression.
d Fat necrosis.
e Unintended injection in other structures.

5 *What are possible facts concerning acute inflammation after injury?*
a It is necessary for clearing away cell debris and necrotic muscle fibers.
b It is necessary for regeneration and healing.
c It causes pain.
d Treatment with anti-inflammatory drugs reduces the risk for myositis ossificans (after hip arthroplasty).
e When left unchecked it can lead to a chronic situation and destruction of tendons and surrounding tissue resulting in ruptures of tendons, scar tissue and adherence.

References

1 Clarkson PM, Thomson HS. Limits to research on drugs and sport. In: Reilly T, Orme M, eds. *The Clinical Pharmacology of Sport and Exercise*. Amsterdam: Excerpta Medica, 1997: 25–35.
2 Graham T. The possible actions of methylxantines on various tissues. In: Reilly T, Orme M, eds. *The Clinical Pharmacology of Sport and Exercise*. Amsterdam: Excerpta Medica, 1997: 257–71.

3   Choo JJ, Horan MA, Little RA, Rothwell NJ. Anabolic effects of clenbuterol on skeletal muscle are mediated by beta2-adrenoreceptor activation. *Am J Physiol* 1992; **263**: E50–E56.

4   Kruse P, Ladefoged J, Nielsen U, Pavlev P, Sørensen JP. The effect of beta blockers on shooting performance. *J Appl Physiol* 1986; **61**: 417–23.

5   Hervey GR, Knibbs AV, Burkinshaw L, Jones PRM, Norgan NG, Levell MJ. Anabolic effects of methadienone in men undergoing athletic training. *Lancet* 1976; **2**: 702–5.

6   Alen M, Hakkinen K, Komi PV. Changes in neuromuscular performance and muscle fiber characteristics of elite power athletes self-administering androgenic and anabolic steroids. *Acta Physiol Scand* 1984; **122**: 535–44.

7   Bhasin S, Storer TW, Berman N, Callegari C, Casaburi R. The effects of supraphysiological doses of testosterone on muscle size and strength in normal men. *N Engl J Med* 1996; **335**: 1–7.

8   Franke WW, Berendonk B. Hormonal doping and androgenization of athletes: a secret program of the GDR government. *Clin Chem* 1997; **43**: 1262–79.

9   Strauss RH, Liggett M, Lanese RR. Anabolic steroid use and percieved effects in ten weight-trained women athletes. *J Am Med Assoc* 1985; **253**: 2871–3.

10   Pope HG, Katz DL. Psychiatric and medical effects of anabolic-androgenic steroid use. *Arch Gen Psych* 1998; **51**: 375–82.

11   Yarasheski K, Zachwieja JJ, Bier DM. Short-term growth hormone treatment does not increase muscle protein synthesis in experienced weight lifters. *J Appl Physiol* 1993; **74**: 3073–6.

12   Ekblom B, Berglund B. Effect of erythropoietin administration on maximal aerobic power. *Scand J Med Sci Sports* 1991; **1**: 88–93.

13   Birkeland KI, Stray-Gundersen J, Hemmersbach P, Hallen J, Haug E, Bahr R. Effect of rhEPO administration on serum levels of sTfR and cycling performance. *Med Sci Sports Exerc* 2000; **32**: 1238–43.

14   Parisotto R, Gore JC, Emslie KR, Ashenden MJ, Brugnara C, Howe C, Martin DT, Trout GJ, Hahn AG. A novel method utilizing markers of altered erythropoiesis for the detection of recombinant human erythropoietin abuse in athletes. *Haematologica* 2000; **85**: 564–72.

15   Söderlund K, Balsom PD, Ekblom B. Creatine supplementation and high-intensity exercise: influence on performance and muscle metabolism. *Clin Sci* 1994; **87**: 120–1.

16   Vandenberghe K, Goris M, Van Hecke M, Van Leemputte L, Van Gerven L, Hespel P. Long term creatine intake is beneficial to muscle performance during resistance training. *J Appl Physiol* 1997; **83**: 2055–63.

17   Hemmersbach P, de la Torre R. Stimulants, narcotics and β-blockers: 25 years of development in analytical techniques for doping control. *J Chromatogr B (Biomed Appl)* 1996; **687**: 221–38.

18   Mueller RK, Grosse J, Lang R, Thieme D. Chromatographic techniques—the basis of doping control. *J Chromatogr B (Biomed Appl)* 1995; **674**: 1–11.

20   Aguilera R, Becchi M, Casabianca H, Hatton CK, Catlin DH, Starcevic B, Pope HG Jr. Improved method of detection of testosterone abuse by gas chromatography/ combustion/isotope ratio mass spectrometry analysis of urinary steroids. *J Mass Spectrometr* 1996; **31**: 169–76.

21   Stenman U-H, Unkila-Kallio L, Korhonen J, Alfthan H. Immunoprocedures for detecting human chorionic gonadotropin. clinical aspects and doping control. *Clin Chem* 1997; **43**: 1293–8.

22   Pauker SG, Kassirer JP. Decision analysis. *N Engl J Med* 1987; **316**: 250–8.

23   Tarnopolsky MA. Caffeine and endurance performance. *Sports Med* 1994; **18**: 109–25.

24   Ullrich D, Compagnone D, Münch B, Brandes A, Hille H, Bircher J. Urinary caffeine metabolites in man. Age-dependent changes and pattern in various clinical situations. *Eur J Pharmacol* 1992; **43**: 167–72.

25   Vistisen K, Poulsen E, Loft S. Foreign compound metabolism capacity in man measured from metabolites of dietary caffeine. *Carcinogenesis* 1992; **13**: 1561–8.

26   Catlin DH, Cowan DA, de la Torre R, Donike M, Fraisse D, Oftebro H, Hatton CK, Starcevic B, Becchi M, de la Torre X, Norli H, Geyer H, Walker CJ. Urinary testosterone (T) to epitestosterone (E) ratios by GC/MS. 1. Initial comparison of uncorrected T/E in six international laboratories. *J Mass Spectrometr* 1996; **31**: 397–402.

27   Schänzer W. Metabolism of androgenic steroids. *Clin Chem* 1996; **42**: 1001–20.

28   Norli HR, Esbensen K, Westad F, Birkeland KI, Hemmersbach P. Chemometric evaluation of urinary steroid profiles in doping control. *J Steroid Biochem Molec Biol* 1995; **54**: 83–8.

29   Schackleton CHL, Chuang H, Kim J, de la Torre X, Segura J. Electrospray mass spectrometry of testosterone esters: potential for use in doping control. *Steroids* 1997; **62**: 523–9.

30   Abramson FP, Osborn BL, Teffera Y. Isotopic differences in human growth hormone preparations. *Anal Chem* 1996; **68**: 1971–2.

31   Saugy M, Cardis C, Schweizer C, Veuthey J-L, Rivier L. Detection of human growth hormone doping in urine: out of competition tests are necessary. *J Chromatogr B (Biomed Appl)* 1996; **687**: 201–11.

32   Kickman AT, Miell JP, Teale JD, Powrie J, Wood PJ, Laidler P, Milligan PJ, Cowan DA. Serum IGF-I and IGF binding proteins 2 and 3 as potential markers of doping with human GH. *Clin Endocrinol* 1997; **47**: 43–50.

33   Soullaird A, Audran M, Bressolle F, Gareau R, Duvallet A, Chanal J-L. Pharmacokinetics and pharmacodynamics of recombinant human erythropoietin in athletes. Blood sampling and doping control. *Br J Clin Pharmacol* 1996; **42**: 355–64.

34   Choi D, Kim M, Park J. Erythropoietin. physico- and

biochemical analysis. *J Chromatogr B (Biomed Appl)* 1996; **687**: 189–99.

35 Wide L, Bengtsson C, Berglund B, Ekblom B. Detection in blood and urine recombinant erythropoietin administered to healthy men. *Med Sci Sports* 1995; **27**: 1569–76.

36 Lasne F, de Ceaurriz J. Recombinant erythropoietin in urine. *Nature (Brief Comm)* 2000; **8**: 405 (6787): 635–6.

36a Garcia Rodriguez LA, Hernandez-Diaz S. Relative risk of upper gastrointestinal complications among users of acetaminophen and non-steroidal anti-inflammatory drugs. *Epidemiology* 2001; **12**: 570–6.

37 Roberts JA. Viral illnesses and sports performance. *Sports Med* 1986; **3**: 298–303.

38 Friman G, Ilbäck NG. Acute infection. metabolic responses, effects on performance, interaction with exercise, and myocarditis. *Int J Sports Med* 1998; **19**: 172–82.

39 Blazina ME. Oxyphenbutazone as an adjunct to the conventional treatment of athletic injuries. *Clin Med* 1969: 76.

40 van Marion WF. Indomathacin in the treatment of soft-tissue lesions: a double-blind trial against placebo. *J Int Med Res* 1973; **1**: 151–8.

41 Hutson MA. A double-blind study comparing ibuprofen 1800 mg or 2400 mg daily and placebo in sports injuries. *J Int Med Res* 1986; **14**: 142–7.

42 Bahamonde SLA, Saavedra CH. Comparison of the analgesic and anti-inflammatory effects of diclofenac potassium versus piroxicam versus placebo in ankle sprain patients. *J Int Med Res* 1990; **18**: 104–11.

43 Slatyer MA, Hensley MJ, Lopert R. A randomized controlled trial of pirioxicam in the management of acute ankle sprain in Australian regular army recruits. *Am J Sports Med* 1997; **25**: 544–53.

44 Huskisson EC, Berry H, Strect FG. Indomethacin for soft-tissue injuries: a double-blind study in football players. *Rheumatol Rehabil* 1973; **12**: 159–60.

45 Fredberg U, Hansen PA, Skinhej A. Ibuprofen in the treatment of acute ankle joint injuries: a double-blind study. *Am J Sports Med* 1989; **17**: 564–6.

46 Obremsky WT, Seaber AV, Ribbeck BM. Biomechanical and histologic assessment of a controlled strain injury treated with piroxicam. *Am J Sports Med* 1994; **22**: 558–61.

47 Almekinders LC, Gilbert JA. Healing of experimental muscle strains and the effect of non-steroidal anti-inflammatory medication. *Am J Sports Med* 1986; **14**: 303–8.

48 Reynolds JF, Noakes TD, Schwellnus MP. Non-steroidal anti-inflammatory drugs fail to enhance healing of acute hamstring injuries with physiotherapy. *S Afr Med J* 1995; **85**: 517–22.

49 Kjaersgaard Andersen P, Sletgaard J, Gjerleff C, Lund F. Location of ectopic bone and the influence of postoperative antiinflammatory treatment. *Clin Orth* 1990; **252**: 156–62.

50 Adebajo AOP, Nash P, Hazleman BL. A prospective double blind dummy placebo controlled study comparing tri-

amcinolone hexacetonide injection with oral diclofenac 50 mg tds in patients with rotator cuff tendinitis. *J Rheumatol* 1990; **17**: 1207–10.

51 Astrom M, Westlin N. No effect of piroxicam on achilles tendinopathy: a randomized study of 70 patients. *Acta Orthop Scand* 1992; **63**: 631–4.

52 Willoughby DA, Moore AR, Colville-Nash PR. COX-1, COX-2, and COX-3 and the future treatment of chronic inflammatory disease. *Lancet* 2000; **355**: 646–8.

53 Willis D, Moore AR, Frederick R, Willoughby DA. Heme oxygenase: a novel target for the modulation of the inflammatory response. *Nat Med* 1996; **2**: 87–90.

54 Russel AL. Pirioxicam 0.5% topical gel compared to placebo in the treatment of acute soft tissue injuries: a double-blind study comparing efficacy and safety. *Clin Invest Med* 1991; **14**: 35–43.

55 Thorting J, Linden B, Berg R. A double-blind comparison of naproxen gel and placebo in the tretment of soft tissue injuries. *Curr Med Res Opin* 1990; **12**: 242–8.

56 Ginsberg F, Famaey JP. Double-blind, randomized cross-over study of the percutaneous efficacy and tolerability of a topical indomethacin spray versus placebo in the treatment of tendinitis. *J Int Med Res* 1991; **19**: 131–6.

57 Dominkus M, Nicolakis M, Kotz R. Comparison of tissue and plasma levels of ibuprofen after oral and topical administration. *Arzneimihelforschung* 1996; **46**: 1138–43.

57a Beiner JM, Jokl P, Cholewicki J. The effects of anabolic steroids and corticosteroids on healing of a muscle contusion injury. *Am J Sports Med* 1999; **27**: 2–9.

58 Sloper JC, Pegmm GD. Regeneration of crushed mammalian skeletal muscle and the effect of steroids. *J Pathol Bacteriol* 1967; **93**: 47–63.

59 Larsen AI, Egfjord M, Jelsdorff HM. Low-dose heparin in the treatment of calcaneal peritendinitis. *Scand J Rheumatol* 1987; **16**: 47–51.

60 Rydholm U, Rööser B, Lidgren L. Risk for severe hemorrhagic complication in heparin treatmeat of peritendinitis. *Lähartidningen* 1985; **82**: 4008–9.

61 Sundqvist H, Forsskahl B, Kvist M. A promising novel therapy for achilles peritendinitis. double-blind comparison of glycosaminoglycan polysulfate and high-dose indomethacin. *Int J Sports Med* 1987; **8**: 298–303.

62 Capasso G, Testa V, Maffulli N. Aprotinin, corticosteroids and normosaline in the management of patellar tendinopathy in athletes: a prospective randomized study. *Sports Exerc Injury* 1997; **3**: 111–5 19–22.

63 Noyes FR, Nussbaum NS. Biomechanical and ultrastructural changes in ligaments and tendons after local corticosteroid injections. *J Bone Joint Surg* 1975; **57A**: 876–7.

64 Kennedy JC, Baxter R. The effects of local steroid injections on tendon: a biomechanical and microscopic correlative study. *Am J Sports Med* 1976; **4**: 11–21.

65 Kapetanos G. The effect of the local corticosteroids on the healing and biomechanical properties of the partially injured tendon. *Clin Orth* 1982; **163**: 170–9.

66 Phelps D, Sonstegard DA, Mathews LS. Corticosteroid injection effects on the biomechanical properties of rabbit patellar tendons. *Clin Orth* 1974; **100**: 345–8.

67 Mackie JW, Goldin B, Foss ML, Cockrell JL. Mechanical properties of rabbit tendons after repeated anti-inflammatory steroid injections. *Med Sci Sports* 1974; **6**: 198–202.

68 Matthews LS, Sonstegard DA, Phelps DB. A biomechanical study of rabbit patellar tendon: Effects of steroid injection. *J Sports Med* 1974; **2**: 349–57.

69 McWhorter W, Francis RS, Heckmann RA. Influence of local steroid injections on traumatized tendon properties: a biomechanical and histological study. *Am J Sports Med* 1991; **19**: 435–9.

70 Fredberg U. Local corticosteroid injection in sport. Review of literature and guidelines for treatment. *Scand J Med Sci Sports* 1997; **7**: 131–9.

71 Read MTF. Safe relief of rest pain that eases with activity in achillodynia by intrabursal or peritendinous steroid injection: the rupture rate was not increased by the steroid injections. *Br J Sports Med* 1999; **33**: 134–5.

72 Gudeman SD, Eisele SA, Heidt RSJ, Colosimo AJ, Stroupe AL. Treatment of plantar fasciitis by iontophoresis of 0.4% dexamethasone. A randomized, double-blind, placebo-controlled study. *Am J Sports Med* 1997; **25**: 312–6.

73 Luukkainen R, Nissilä M, Asikainen E, Sanila M, Lehtinen K, Alanaatu A. Periarticular corticosteroid treatment of the sacroiliac joint in patients with seronegative spondylarthropathy. *Clin Exp Rheumatol* 1999; **17**: 88–90.

74 Price R, Sinclair H, Heinrich T, Gibson T. Local injection treatment of tennis elbow—hydrocortisone, triamcinolone and lignocaine compared. *Br J Rheumatol* 1991; **30**: 39–44.

75 Day BH, Govindasamy N, Patnaik R. Corticosteroid injec-

tions in the treatment of tennis elbow. *Pract Med* 1978; **220**: 459–62.

76 Petri M, Dobrow R, Neiman R. Randomized, double-blind, placebo-controlled study of the treatment of the painful shoulder. *Arthritis Rheum* 1987; **30**: 1040–5.

76a Pfeiffer-Jensen M, Fredberg U, Clemmensen D, Bolvig L, Jacobsen BW, Stengaard-Pedersen K. Pain assessment in inflamed tendons before and after placebo and local glucocorticoid treatment. *Scand J Rheumatol* 1998; **108S**: 146.

76b Fredberg U, Pfeiffer-Jensen M, Bolvig L, Clemmensen D, Jacobsen BW, Stengaard-Pedersen K. Ultrasonographic visualisation and pain assessment of inflamed tendons before and after local glucocorticoid treatment. *Arthritis Rheum* 1998; **41**: 166.

77 Molloy JC, McGuirk RA. Treatment of traumatic myositis ossificans circumscripta: use of aspiration and steroids. *J Trauma* 1976; **16**: 851–7.

78 Smith DL, McAfee JH. Treatment of non-septic olecranon bursitis. A controlled, blinded prospective trial. *Arch Intern Med* 1989; **149**: 2527–30.

79 Vogel HG. Correlation between tensile strength and collagen content in the rat skin; effect of age and cortisol treatment. *Connective Tissue Res* 1974; **2**: 177–82.

80 Byl NN, McKenzie A, Halliday B, Wong TO, Connell J. The effects of phonophoresis with corticosteroids: a controlled pilot study. *J Orth Sports Phys Ther* 1993; **18**: 590–600.

81 Martin DF, Carlson CS, Berry J, Reboussin BA, Gordon ES, Smith BP. Effect of injected versus iontophoretic corticosteroid on the rabbit tendon. *South Med J* 1999; **92**: 600–8.

82 Ljungqvist R. Subcutaneous partial rupture of the Achilles tendon. *Acta Orthop Scand Suppl* 1968: 113.

83 Shields CL. The Cybex II evaluation on surgical repaired Achilles tendon ruptures. *Am J Sports Med* 1978; **7**: 15–17.

Part 3
Physical Activity: Health Achievements vs. Sports Injury

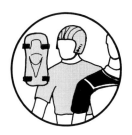

Chapter 3.1
Epidemiology and Prevention
of Sports Injuries

ROALD BAHR, PEKKA KANNUS &
WILLEM VAN MECHELEN

Classical reference

Ekstrand J, Gillquist J, Liljedahl SO. Prevention of
    soccer injuries. Supervision by doctor and
    physiotherapist. *Am J Sports Med* 1983; **11**:
    116–120.

This study is recognized as the first randomized
controlled trial (RCT) examining the effects of an injury prevention program in sports. Ekstrand and his
coworkers used the classic four-sequence injury
prevention approach in a series of studies. Firstly, they
described the magnitude of the problem of soccer
injuries in terms of their incidence and severity,
demonstrating an incidence of 7.6 injuries per 1000
practice-hours and 16.9 per 1000 game-hours. Secondly, they described risk factors and injury mechanisms in their cohort. Among several factors identified
in their first studies, the content of the warm-up the
teams used appeared to be inadequate, previous injury
and persistent instability was a significant risk factor
for reinjury to the ankle and knee, and traumatic lower
leg injuries occurred in players with inadequate or no
shin guards. The two final steps in the injury prevention sequence, introducing measures that are likely to
reduce the risk of injuries and evaluating the effect of
these measures, were completed in the RCT described
in this 'Focus on Research'. Twelve teams (180 players)
in a male senior soccer division were followed for the
first 6 months of the 1980 and 1981 seasons. Between
these two observation periods, the teams were al-
located at random to two groups of six teams, one being
given a prophylactic program and the other serving as
control. The program was based on previous studies of

injury mechanisms. It comprised: (i) correction of
training; (ii) provision of optimum equipment; (iii)
prophylactic ankle taping; (iv) controlled rehabilitation; (v) exclusion of players with grave knee
instability; (vi) information about the importance of
disciplined play and the increased risk of injury at
training camps; and (vii) correction and supervision
by doctor(s) and physiotherapist(s). The six control
teams had a mean of 2.6 injuries per month during
the first 6 months of 1981, an incidence equal to the
mean for all 12 teams in the division during the same
period in 1980. After the introduction of the prophylactic program, the six test teams reduced the
incidence to 0.6 injuries per month in 1981, which was
75% less than in the control group (P<0.001). The
most common types of soccer injuries, sprains and
strains to ankles and knees, were all significantly re-

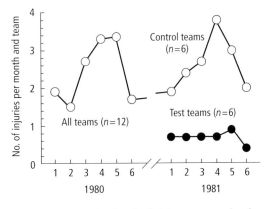

Fig. 3.1.1 In this landmark study, the injury rate was reduced
by 75% through simple preventive measures.

duced. Ekstrand and coworkers concluded that the prevention program, including close supervision and correction by doctors and physiotherapists, significantly reduces soccer injuries. This landmark study has served as a model in this research area, and most of the elements in their prevention program have been incorporated into the training program of Scandinavian soccer clubs.

Introduction

A physically active lifestyle and active participation in sports and physical activity is important for all age groups. Reasons to participate in sports and physical activity are many, such as pleasure and relaxation, competition, socialization, and maintenance and improvement of fitness and health. However, sports participation also entails a risk for overuse injuries as well as acute injuries, which may even lead to death or permanent disability.

In the following chapters the health benefits of exercise across the lifespan for both healthy and disabled persons are discussed. This chapter describes some current concepts regarding sports injury epidemiology, as well as the general principles for injury prevention research. The chapter will focus mainly on Scandinavian team sports and use examples from research performed in the region to describe the range of injuries that may be expected in this area. Also, these examples will illustrate some of the limitations that apply when interpreting research in this area. Finally, since potential injury prevention strategies may differ considerably between sports, it is not possible to describe practical preventive strategies for specific sports within the confines of the present chapter. However, some models will be presented and examples will be given from randomized controlled trials (RCTs) to illustrate the principles involved when trying to prevent injuries. These models may, in turn, be applied to the specific sport in question by the clinician.

First, a different question will be addressed: do the health benefits of regular exercise outweigh the risk of injury and long-term disability, especially in high-performance athletes? Sarna *et al.* have studied the incidence of chronic disease and life expectancy of Finnish male world-class athletes[1]. Finnish team members in the Olympic games, World or European championships or intercountry competitions from 1920 to 1965 in track and field athletics, cross-country skiing, soccer, ice hockey, basketball, boxing, wrestling, weight-lifting and shooting were compared with a reference cohort of men selected from the Finnish Defence Forces conscription register, all classified as completely healthy at the time of induction to military service. The mean life expectancy adjusted for occupational group, marital status and the age at entry to the cohort was 75.6 years in endurance sports (long-distance running and cross-country skiing), 73.9 years in team games (soccer, ice hockey, basketball) and jumpers and short-distance runners from track and field, 71.5 years in power sports (boxing, wrestling, weight lifting, and throwers from field athletics), and 69.9 years in the reference group. The increased mean life expectancies were mainly explained by decreased cardiovascular mortality.

These results are corroborated by a second study from the same group by Kujala *et al.* [2] where they investigated the postcareer use of hospital care from all causes in the same groups based on national hospital discharge registry data. Compared with controls, the rate ratios for all-cause hospital care were lower in athletes from endurance sports, mixed sports (including endurance and weight training) and power sports compared with the reference group. The lower rate of hospitalization among athletes was largely explained by lower rates of hospital care for heart disease, respiratory disease and cancer. However, the rate of hospitalization for musculoskeletal disorders was higher in all groups of athletes than the control group. This may be partly explained by the increased risk of osteoarthritis in former elite athletes [3].

In other words, former elite athletes, particularly those in aerobic sports, live longer, and while they need less overall hospital care, they suffer more from frequent musculoskeletal problems. These health benefits cannot be attributed to their athletic career alone, but may in part be explained by the fact that elite athletes are healthier than the controls already at baseline (selection bias), and are likely to maintain a physically active lifestyle in later life. Also, it is important to keep in mind that the intensity of training and competition in sports has increased several-fold over the last two decades. This means that acute injuries as well as long-term musculoskeletal problems are likely be more prevalent and more severe today than >35 years ago.

However, the benefits in terms of increased longevity and reduced morbidity due to reduced risk of cardiovascular disease in athletes may be even greater today, when contrasted to the gradually more sedentary lifestyle observed in the general population.

Undoubtedly, there is an increased risk of short- and long-term musculoskeletal problems associated with physical activity, particularly in competitive sports. As sports medicine professionals and promoters of sports and physical activity from a health perspective, we have an obligation to make sports participation as safe as possible. In order to reduce the risk of injury associated with sports, it is necessary to use advances in the epidemiology of sports injuries as a basis for sports policy. In order to set out effective prevention programs, epidemiologic studies need to be done on incidence, severity and etiology of sports injuries. Also, the effect of preventive measures needs to be evaluated as they are introduced.

The sequence of prevention

Measures to prevent sports injuries do not exist in isolation. They form part of what might be called a sequence of prevention [4] (Fig. 3.1.2).

First, the magnitude of the problem must be identified and described in terms of incidence and severity of sports injuries. Second, the risk factors and injury mechanisms that play a part in the occurrence of sports injuries must be identified. The third step is to introduce measures that are likely to reduce the future risk and/or severity of sports injuries. Such measures should be based on information about the etiologic factors and the injury mechanisms as identified in the second step. Finally, the effect of the measures must

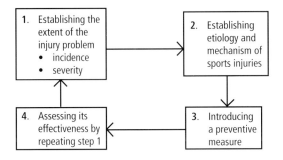

Fig. 3.1.2 The sequence for prevention of sports injuries [18].

be evaluated by repeating the first step, which will lead to so-called time-trend analysis of injury patterns. However, from an epidemiologic standpoint it is preferable to evaluate the effect of preventive measures by means of an RCT. Unfortunately, relatively few RCTs have been conducted in sports injury prevention studies [5–13].

The magnitude of the problem

One way of getting an impression of the magnitude of the sports injury problem is by counting the absolute number of injuries. When these absolute numbers are compared with, for instance, the number of traffic accidents or the number of work-related injuries the relative extent of the sports injury problem can be revealed.

Table 3.1.1 shows data from selected community-based studies from Scandinavia that describe the proportion of sports injuries as a percentage of the total number of acute injuries, as well as the distribution of injuries by sport. In these studies, between 6.3% and 18.1% of all acute injuries seen in an emergency room, casualty department or outpatient clinic setting are sports induced.

A consistent finding across these studies is that in the total population, soccer is the number one sport in terms of the absolute number of injuries (Table 3.1.1). After soccer, other team games such as European team handball, volleyball, basketball and ice hockey also cause a significant proportion of the absolute number of injuries. Note that the proportions vary considerably between countries. A good example is ice hockey and skating injuries, which are common in Sweden and Finland, but rare in Norway. It is important to note that this injury pattern is a result of not only the risk involved when playing each of these sports, but also differences in participation rate for each sport. Soccer is a very popular sport in all of the Nordic countries, and ice hockey is very popular in Sweden and Finland, but not in Norway. This is reflected in concomitant differences in the number of injuries seen between these countries (Table 3.1.1). Consequently, these studies provide information about the magnitude of the sports injury problem and in particular which sports are responsible for the largest absolute number of injuries. They are therefore important from a public health perspective, but do not give estimates of injury risk.

Table 3.1.1 Total population distribution of sports-related injuries by sport. Selected studies conducted in an emergency room setting in Scandinavia have been included.

	Lindqvist *et al.* [38]	Mæhlum & Daljord [39]	Ytterstad [40]	Sandelin *et al.* [41]	de Loës [37]
	Motala, Sweden (pop. 40 000), 1983–84	Oslo, Norway (pop. 650 000), 1981–82	Harstad, Norway (pop. 22 600), 1985–93	Helsinki, Finland (pop. 800 000), 1978	Falköping, Sweden (pop. 31 260), 1984
Soccer	39	25	45	24	42
Handball		7	11		5
Volleyball			7		
Basketball		2	4		
Ball games (unspecified)	11			23	5
Ice hockey/bandy/skating	12	3		19	6
Alpine skiing	4	7	11		5
Cross-country skiing	2	7			
Skiing (unspecified)				7	
Horse riding	6				6
Gymnastics	2			4	4
Martial arts		2		5	2
Cycling	1	6			
Orienteering	4				
Athletics	1			2	2
Racket sports	3			5	2
Motor sports	3				3
Jogging and recreational walking	1	2		7	5
Other	10		20	4	11
No. of injuries (% of total injuries)	993 (18.9%)	3434 (6.3%)	2234 (17.2%)	2493 (10%)	571 (18.1%)

The only Scandinavian population-based study which takes time at risk into account and which therefore provides risk estimates is the one by de Loës and Goldies [14]. This study shows that the incidence rate is highest in ice hockey, horseback riding, team handball and soccer among men, and team handball and soccer among women.

Similarly, Table 3.1.2 provides similar data on absolute numbers of acute injuries among children and adolescents. Not surprisingly, since participation in sports is more prevalent among children than adults, it appears that sports participation causes a larger proportion of injuries in the younger population, between 18% and 35% in the Scandinavian studies. Similar to adults, soccer is the sport causing the most injuries among boys, except in Finland, where ice hockey dominates. Among girls a significant proportion of injuries is caused by team handball, horse riding and gymnastics. Again, this is a reflection of participation rates and not of the risk associated with each sport. In Scandinavia, team handball, horse riding and gymnastics are generally more popular among girls than boys. For true risk estimates it is necessary to collect information on exposure, and to compute incidence rates.

Sports injury incidence

The most appropriate indication of the spread of disease in the population or in a section of the population is incidence. If one substitutes 'sports injury or sports accident' for 'disease', incidence can be defined as 'the number of new sports injuries or accidents sustained during a particular period, in a particular population at risk (i.e. the number of newly sustained sports injuries per year divided by the population at risk)'. Incidence

Table 3.1.2 Injury distribution by sport in children and adolescents. Selected prospective studies conducted in an emergency room setting in Scandinavia have been included.

	Sahlin [42]		Sørensen et al. [43]		Kvist et al. [44]	
	Trondheim, Norway, 1985–86, age 5–14		Esbjerg, Denmark, 1988–92, age 6–17		Turku, Finland, 1980–82, age 6–15	
	Boys (%)	Girls (%)	Boys (%)	Girls (%)	Boys (%)	Girls (%)
Soccer	33	13	39	11	20	7
Handball	5	30	7	19		
Basketball			5	6	3	4
Volleyball					1	3
Volleyball/basketball	2	3				
Ball games (unspecified)	4	7			1	
Ice hockey/skating	5	6	12	2	42	21
Alpine skiing	15	7			3	4
Cross-country skiing	11	6			4	6
Ski jumping	3					
Horse riding	1	6	1	18		18
Gymnastics	5	6	7	15	3	14
Martial arts	2	1				
Swimming	2	2			5	3
Running					4	6
Athletics		1			3	3
Roller skating			3	5		
Skateboard			10	2		
Baseball					2	3
Other	14	12	24	23	9	8
No. of sports-related injuries	359	399	3322	2774	772	352
(% of total injuries)	27%		35%		18%	

thus defined also gives an estimate of risk. If one multiplies the obtained figure by 100, one gets the incidence percentage rate [15]. Expressed in this way, sports injury incidence figures give insight into the extent of the sports injury problem in a particular population at risk. It is clear from this definition of incidence that incidence can only be assessed properly if clear definitions of both sports injury and of the population at risk are present.

In many studies the incidence rate of sports injuries is usually defined as the number of new sports injuries during a particular period (e.g. 1 year) divided by the total number of sports persons at the start of that period (population at risk). When interpreting and comparing incidence rates found in different studies it is important to know what definition of sports injury was used. Information on the comparability of the populations at risk is also needed. It is clear that the methods used to count injuries and to count the population at risk will also influence sports injury incidence figures. Finally the length of the observation period has to be taken into account, since different lengths of observation periods will have a distinct influence on the incidences calculated.

In terms of risk assessment another problem lies in the way incidence rates are expressed. In most cases, the number of injuries in a particular category of sports persons per season or per year is taken, or the number of injuries per player per match. In both examples no allowance is made for any differences in the actual exposure to injury risk (i.e. the number of hours of active play during which the sports person actually runs the risk of being injured). This is peculiar because this factor certainly has great influence on the risk of sustaining a sports injury. Incidence figures that take no account of exposure are therefore not a good indication of the 'true' risk one runs, nor can such incidence rates be used for a comparison of risk between different sports or between age and sex groups participating in the same sport. It would therefore be better to calculate the incidence of sports injuries in relation to exposure time (for example, per 1000 game-hours).

This is commonly done in cohort studies, where a particular athlete population, e.g. one or several teams in a league, is followed prospectively. In this type of study it is often possible to collect detailed participation records for training as well as games to calculate exposure. Incidence is normally expressed as the number of injuries per 1000 player-hours. The equation of Chambers [16], adapted by De Loës and Goldie [14], can be used to calculate injury incidence taking exposure into account:

$$\text{injury incidence} = \frac{[(\text{no. of sports injuries}/\text{year}) \times 10^4]}{[(\text{no. of participants})}$$
$$\times (\text{hours of sports participation}/\text{week})$$
$$\times (\text{weeks of season}/\text{year})].$$

Expressing incidence this way, as the number of injuries per 1000 athlete-hours, yields convenient numbers (usually between 1 and 100) and allows comparison between various sports, settings and populations. This method may have to be adjusted to particular research settings. When studying alpine skiing injuries it may be more valid to express incidence per 1000 days on ski (since exposure registration is often linked to lift pass sales) or, even better, to skiing distance. To this end, Rønning *et al.* have developed the distance-correlated injury index (DCI), expressing incidence as the number of injuries per 100 000 km on skis [17]. This obviously requires the ability to record exposure through the actual use of ski lift passes and not only lift pass sales.

Table 3.1.3 shows the incidence rates for some team sports commonly played in Scandinavia. Although there is a limitation to the number of studies available in some sports, the trend seems relatively clear. Ice hockey is the game with the highest rate of injuries by far, in most studies 50–80 injuries per 1000 player-

hours during games. Ice hockey is followed by soccer with a match injury incidence of 18–35 per 1000 player-hours. There is only one study available from European team handball, showing an incidence slightly lower than soccer, and volleyball appears to have the lowest injury rate of the most popular Scandinavian team sports. There is no prospective study available from Scandinavian basketball, but other studies have shown rates just slightly higher than volleyball [18–21].

Table 3.1.3 also shows other interesting trends. It appears that within a certain sport, competing at a high level increases sports injury risk and more injuries are sustained during matches than during training. This is primarily due to the higher intensity during matches, and most likely also due to the fact that athletes do not take the same risks when training with their teammates as they do in games. The high difference in injury rates between games and training seen in Swedish and Finnish elite ice hockey can be explained by the fact that the teams have an intense match schedule and mainly use their training sessions during the season for recovery and basic skill training purposes.

Methodologic issues

When conducting (and also when interpreting the outcomes of) epidemiologic sports injury studies one is confronted with a number of methodologic issues. The first issue of importance here is the definition of sports injury. In general, sports injury is a collective name for all types of damage that can occur in relation to sporting activities. Various studies of incidence define the term 'sports injury' in different ways. In some studies a sports injury is defined as any injury sustained during sporting activities for which an insurance claim is submitted; in other studies the definition is confined to injuries treated at a hospital casualty or other medical department [4].

As shown in Table 3.1.3, different injury definitions have been used in the Scandinavian studies. These definitions can be grouped into three categories: (i) time loss injuries, where the definition is usually that the player is unable to participate in the next match or training session because of injury; (ii) game interruption injuries, where the player has to interrupt the game or training session because of an injury; or

Table 31.3 Injury incidence in soccer, ice hockey, volleyball and handball. *Time loss: Player unable to participate in next match or training session because of injury; Interruption: Player has to interrupt game or training session because of injury; Medical attention: Player seeking medical attention for evaluation and/or treatment.

Reference	Country and period	Population	Sample size	Injury definition*	Injury rate (per 1000 player-hours)		
					Total	Game	Training
Soccer							
Arnason et al. [45]	Iceland, May–Sept 1991	5 of 10 div. I teams	84 players	Acute & overuse; Time loss	12.4±1.4	34.8±5.7	5.9±1.1
Drogset & Midthjell [46]	Norway, late 80s, 17 months	Three div. VI teams	~75 players	Acute & overuse; Time loss or Interruption	13	27	3
Ekstrand [47]	Finland, Jan–Oct 1993	12 div. IV teams	180 players	Acute; Time loss		16.9	7.6
Lüthje et al. [48]		All 12 div. I teams	263 players	Acute & overuse; Interruption or Medical attention		11.3	1.8
Nielsen & Yde [49]	Denmark, Jan–Nov 1986	One club, div. II & lower div.	34 div. II & 59 lower div. players	Acute; Time loss	Div. II: 18.5 Lower div. 11.9	Div. II: 2.3 Lower div. 5.6	
Poulsen et al. [50]	Denmark, 1996, one year	Three teams, div. I & lower div.	34 div. I & 59 lower div. players	Acute & overuse; Time loss	Div. I: 19.8 Lower div. 20.7	Div. I: 4.1 Lower div. 5.7	
Ice hockey							
Lorentzon, Wedren & Pietilä [51]	Sweden, 1982–84, two seasons	One div. I team	24–25 players	Acute & overuse; Time loss		28.8	1.5
Lorentzon et al. [52]	Sweden, 1984–85, 40 games	Swedish national team	22–25 players	Acute; Time loss		79.2	
Lorentzon, Wedren & Pietilä [53]	Sweden, 1982–85, three seasons	One div. I team	24–25 players	Acute & overuse; Time loss		78.4	1.4
Mölsa et al. [54]	Finland, 1988–89, one season	4 div. I teams & 3 div. II teams	21 players per team	Acute; Time loss		Div. I: 66 Div. II: 36	
Mölsa et al. [55]	Finland, 1976–79 & 1988–89 & 1992–93	3–7 div. I teams	17–22 players per team	Acute; Treatment		1970s:54 1980s:55 1990s:83	1.5
Petterson & Lorentzon [56]	Sweden, 1986–90	One div. I team	22–25 players	Acute & overuse; Time loss		74.1	2.6
Tegner & Lorentzon [57]	Sweden, 1986–90, one season	12 div. I teams	?	Acute & overuse; Time loss		53.0	
Volleyball (indoor)							
Aagaard, Scavenius & Jørgensen [58]	Denmark, 1993–94, one season	36 teams, div. I–IV	286 players	Acute & overuse; Treatment	4.2	4.8	4.1
Bahr & Bahr [29]	Norway, 1992–93, one season	26 teams, div. I–II	273 players	Acute; Time loss	1.7	3.5	1.5
Yde & Buhl Nielsen [59]	Denmark, September 1985–April 1986	One club, div. II & lower div.	136 players	Acute & overuse; Time loss	2.8	5.7	2.1
Handball							
Nielsen & Yde [60]	Denmark, Sep.1985— May 1986	One club, div. I & lower div.	127 players	Acute; Time loss		Males: 13.3 Females: 13.8	Males: 2.4 Females: 0.7

(iii) medical attention injuries, where the player has to seek medical attention for evaluation and/or treatment because of an injury.

Differences in the injury definition used may partly explain the differing injury rates observed, but the study setting also plays a role. Apparently, all of the studies cited in Table 3.1.3 have been performed in the same setting, by collecting injury and exposure information for the team through the coach, medical personnel or players directly. However, one should bear in mind that if a study is conducted in a setting where courtside medical support is readily available, using a 'medical attention' injury definition is likely to result in a higher injury incidence rate than a 'time loss' definition; in such a situation players are likely to seek medical attention for minor injuries not involving time loss. This may be the case in ice hockey, where medical staff is required to be present at all times during training and matches. Conversely, if a study is done in volleyball, where professional medical support is not as readily available, a 'time loss' definition is likely to result in a higher injury rate than a 'medical attention' definition. Players do not always seek medical attention for injuries, not even for time loss injuries.

The results of various sports injury incidence surveys are not necessarily comparable, if the study setting differs. If sports injuries are recorded through medical channels (for instance through hospital emergency rooms or insurance records), a fairly large percentage of serious, predominantly acute injuries will be observed and less serious and/or overuse injuries will not be recorded. If such a 'limited' definition is used, only part of the total sports injury problem is revealed. This 'tip-of-the-iceberg' phenomenon is commonly described in epidemiologic research [15]. This problem is to a large extent found in sport injury epidemiology in the young where many overuse injuries are thought to be found, as well as 'minor' acute injuries.

To make sports injury surveys comparable and to avoid the 'tip-of-the-iceberg' phenomenon as far as possible, an unambiguous, universally applicable definition of sports injury is the first prerequisite. This definition should be based on a concept of health different than that customary in standard medicine, and should for instance, take incapacitation for sports or school into account.

Research design

The extent to which sports injury incidence and sports injury risk can be assessed depends not only on the definition of sports injury or the study setting, but also on the methods used to count injuries, to establish the population at risk and to verify that the sample is representative. Here proper research design comes into play. Injuries as well as time at risk can be assessed retrospectively or prospectively, using questionnaires or person-to-person interviews. However, prospective studies can, by closely monitoring exposure time and injury outcome, more accurately estimate the risk and incidence of sports injury according to the level of sports participation and type of exposure of an athlete. They are therefore superior to retrospective studies. One of the main problems of retrospective studies is the inherent recall bias of the subjects participating in such a study.

A word should be said here about case studies. In sports medical journals clinical case series are commonly described. Conclusions are drawn from these case series regarding the incidence and the risk of sustaining sports injuries. However, case studies have the drawback that no information on the population at risk is available. Consequently, no valid conclusions can be drawn from case studies; neither with respect to sports injury incidence, nor with respect to injury risks [15].

Depending on the methods used the researcher will be confronted to a greater or lesser extent with phenomena such as recall bias, overestimation of the hours of sport participation [22], incomplete responses, non-response, dropout, invalid injury description and problems related to the duration and cost of research. These factors will clearly affect the internal validity of a study.

Special attention has to be paid to the method of assessing the population at risk and to ascertaining that the sample is representative. If the population at risk is not clearly identified it is not possible to calculate reliable incidence data. With regard to representative samples, consideration has to be taken of the fact that the performance of athletes in sports, and therefore the incidence of sports injuries, is highly determined by selection. Bol *et al.* [23] recognized four different kinds of selection: (i) self-selection (personal preferences) and/or selection by social environment (parents, friends, school, etc.); (ii) selection by the sports environment (trainer, coach, etc.); (iii) selection by sports organizations (organization of competition by age and gender, the setting of participation standards, etc.); and (iv) selection by social, medical and biologic factors (socioeconomic background, mortality, age, aging, gender, etc.). All these issues should be taken into account in the study design or, if this is not possible, limitations must be readily acknowledged when interpreting the results.

The severity of sports injuries

A description of the severity of sports injuries is important in making a decision about whether or not preventive measures are needed, since the need to prevent serious injuries in a particular sport does not need to coincide with a high overall incidence of injuries in that sport. According to the literature the severity of sports injuries can be described on the basis of six criteria [24]. These criteria are briefly described below.

Nature of sports injuries

The nature of sports injuries can be described in terms of medical diagnosis, e.g. sprain (of joint capsule and ligaments), strain (of muscle or tendon), contusion (bruising), dislocation or subluxation, fracture (of bone). It is the nature of the sports injury that determines whether assistance (medical or otherwise) is sought. The Abbreviated Injury Scale (AIS) has been developed as a direct measure of the severity of an injury based on patient status upon presentation in the emergency room, originally developed for motor vehicle accidents [25]. Recording of the nature of sports injuries enables those sports with relatively serious injuries to be identified. Information on which body part is injured can also give important information.

As an example, studies from European team handball show that there is a high incidence of anterior cruciate ligament (ACL) injuries, especially among female players. Myklebust *et al.* [26] and Strand *et al.* [27] have found an incidence of 0.91 and 0.82 per 1000 player-hours for women during competition in Norwegian team handball, compared with 0.10 injuries per 1000 player-hours in soccer [28]. This means that the rate of ACL injuries in handball almost equals the rate of ankle sprains in volleyball [29,30]. Since one can

predict a high frequency of future disability and functional impairment after an ACL rupture, an ACL injury is a much greater source of concern than an ankle sprain.

Duration and nature of treatment

Data on the duration and nature of treatment can be used to determine the severity of an injury more precisely, especially if it is a question of what medical bodies are involved in the treatment and what therapies are used.

Sports time lost

It is important for a sports person to be able to take up his or her sport again as soon as possible after an injury. Sport and exercise play an essential part in people's free time and thus influence their mental well-being. The loss of sporting time is an important psychosocial factor. Also, for the professional athlete or the elite level team loss of sporting time is directly related to salary (or the opportunity to earn prize money or appearance fees) or to the relative success of the individual or his team. Thus, the length of sporting time lost gives the most precise indication of the consequences of an injury to a sports person.

Working or school time lost

Like the cost of medical treatment, the length of working or school time lost gives an indication of the consequences of sports injuries at a societal level. Data on working or school time lost is used to compare the cost to society of sports injuries with that of other situations involving risks, such as traffic accidents.

Permanent disability

The vast majority of sports injuries heal without permanent disability. Serious injuries such as fractures, ligament, tendon and intra-articular injuries, concussions, spinal injuries and eye injuries can leave permanent damage (residual symptoms). Excessive delay between the occurrence of an injury and medical assistance can aggravate the injury. If the residual symptoms are slight, they may cause the individual to modify his or her level of sporting activity. In some cases, however, the sports person may have to choose another sport or give up sport altogether. Serious physical damage can cause permanent disability, thus reducing or eliminating the individual's capacity for work or school, or even death. When taking precautions, then, priority should be given to measures in sports where such serious injuries are common, even though the particular sport itself may be characterized by a low incidence of sports injuries and/or a low absolute number of participants.

As an example, we have already mentioned the high incidence of ACL injuries in female team handball, which causes concern even if the total injury incidence in the sport is thought to be moderate. Ice hockey, in turn, represents a sport where the total incidence is high, and where even a high frequency of concussions and spinal cord injuries is seen [31,32].

Costs of sports injuries

The calculation of the costs of sports injuries essentially involves the expression of the above-mentioned five categories of seriousness of sports injuries in economic terms. The economic costs can be divided into: (i) direct costs, i.e. the cost of medical treatment (diagnostic expenses such as X-rays, doctors' fees and costs of medicines, hospital admission and rehabilitation); and (ii) indirect costs, i.e. expenditure incurred in connection with the loss of productivity due to increased morbidity and mortality levels (loss of school or working time and loss of expertise due to death or disability).

Conceptual models for the etiology of sports injuries

Risk indicators for sports injuries can be divided into two main categories: internal personal risk indicators and external, environmental risk indicators [4]. This division is based on partly proven and partly supposed causal relationships between risk factors and sports injuries. However, merely to establish the risk factors for sports injuries, i.e. the internal and external factors, is not enough; the mechanisms by which they occur must also be identified.

As can be seen in Fig. 3.1.3 sports injuries result from a complex interaction of multiple risk factors of which only a fraction have been identified. Despite this multicausality many epidemiologic studies have concentrated on identifying single internal or external risk indicators from a medical, monocausal point of view, rather than from a multicausal point of view. However,

studies on the etiology of sports injuries require a dynamic model that accounts for this multifactorial nature of sports injuries, and that also takes the sequence of events eventually leading to an injury into account. One such dynamic model is described by Meeuwisse [33]. This model describes how multiple factors interact to produce injury (Fig. 3.1.4).

In studies on the etiology of sports injuries this model can be used to explore the interrelationships between risk factors and their contribution to the occurrence of injury. Meeuwisse classifies the intrinsic or athlete-related factors as predisposing factors that are necessary, but seldom sufficient, to produce injury. In his theoretical model extrinsic risk factors act on the predisposed athlete from without and are classified as enabling factors in that they facilitate the manifestation of injury. It is the presence of both intrinsic and extrinsic risk factors that render the athlete susceptible to injury, but the mere presence of these risk factors is usually not sufficient to produce injury. It is the sum of these risk factors and the interaction between them that 'prepare' the athlete for an injury to occur at a given place, in a given sports situation. Meeuwisse describes an inciting event to be the final link in the chain of causation to sports injury and states that such an inciting event is usually directly associated with the onset of injury. Such events are regarded as necessary causes. The term injury mechanism is often used to describe the inciting event in biomechanical terms. Studies on the etiology of sports injuries tend to focus on factors proximal to the injury event (i.e. the inciting events) and tend to neglect factors more distant from the injury event (i.e. the intrinsic and extrinsic risk factors), thereby revealing only a small fraction of the factors and events that lead to sports injury. Although understandable, focusing on inciting events may lead to overweighing the importance of such events in the etiology and prevention of sports injuries. If in etiologic studies distant factors are studied it usually concerns intrinsic, person-related risk factors. These factors are relatively easier to measure than extrinsic risk factors. A multifactorial model like the model of Meeuwisse should be used to study the etiology of sports injuries.

Although there are a fair number of studies available documenting the incidence, severity and injury profile of most major sports, we have very little information available on risk factors and injury mechanisms. As

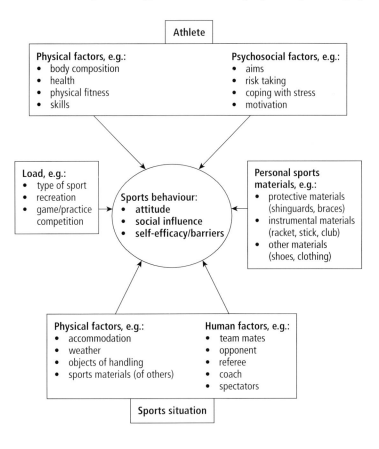

Fig. 3.1.3 Risk indicators for sports injuries and determinants of sports and preventive behavior [18].

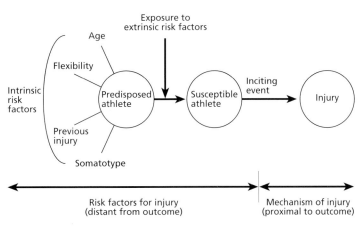

Fig. 3.1.4 A dynamic, multifactorial model of sports injury etiology [37]. (Reprinted with permission from *Clinical Journal of Sports Medicine*, Lippincott, Williams and Wilkins) [33].)

already mentioned, most studies have focused on single risk factors. And although the inciting event may be the most obvious causative factor in the chain of events leading to an injury, this has been neglected or at best described in broad terms in most studies. For instance, describing an ACL injury as a non-contact or contact injury does provide meaningful information, but leaves us far from having a complete understanding of the injury mechanism. Also, in most studies information on injury mechanisms has been collected using questionnaires given to the injured athlete, often weeks after the injury occurred. Recall bias is an obvious problem using this approach, but another important limitation is that injuries often happen in a split second, and the athlete is not always aware of what really happened. When completing a questionnaire, the information collected probably reflects the sum of what the athlete perceived and remembered, plus what he has been told by the coach, team mates or spectators. In future studies, more detailed information on injury mechanisms can probably be obtained by systematic examination of video recordings of injuries. Also, such systematic evaluation should not be limited to some biomechanical description of, e.g. knee motion, but should also describe the events leading up to the injury. This is especially important in team sports like soccer or team handball, where application of sport science methods may provide a better understanding of the chain of events preceding an injury.

Sports behavior

When trying to prevent sports injuries one should realize that participation in sports is a form of behavior. Usually the introduction of preventive measures implies a change or modification of behavior of the athlete. It may very well be that the desired preventive behavior conflicts with the actual sport behavior, for instance because it is believed by the athlete that the preventive behavior will affect sports performance negatively. When introducing preventive measures and when evaluating the effect of such measures it is therefore necessary to have knowledge of the determinants of both sports and preventive behavior. Many models are used to explain preventive behavior. In general these models include three sets of determinants: (i) knowledge and attitude; (ii) social influence; and (iii) barriers and self-efficacy [34] (see Fig. 3.1.3). These determinants can be described as follows:

'Attitude' refers to the knowledge and beliefs of a person concerning the specific consequences of a certain form of behavior. An attitude is the weighing of all consequences of the performance of the behavior, as seen by the individual. Health is only seen as one of the considerations, and is often an unimportant one.

When health is part of attitude one may suppose that healthy motivation is a combination of the perceived severity of the health risk, the perceived susceptibility to the health risk, and the effectiveness of the preventive behavior. 'Social influence' is the influence by others; directly by what others expect, indirectly by what others do (modelling). 'Social influence is often underestimated as a determinant of behavior. It can lead to behavior that conflicts with previous attitudes. Most sports situations are social situations. 'Self-efficacy-cum-barriers' stands for the determinant whether one is able to perform the (desired) behavior. It involves an estimation of ability, taking into account possible internal (e.g. insufficient skill, knowledge, endurance) or external barriers (e.g. resistance from others, time and money not available, etc.). Self-efficacy is people's perception of their ability to perform the behavior, and barriers are the real problems they face in actually performing the behavior. These determinants should be accounted for when trying to prevent sports injuries.

A model for sports injury prevention

Given the limited information available on risk factors and injury mechanisms, it comes as no surprise that very few studies are available on injury prevention. Only 10 RCTs on sports injury prevention can be found in the literature [5–13,35]. However, strategies for injury control have been developed from other energy exchange areas, particularly from research on motor vehicle accidents. One such model, the so-called Haddon matrix [25], is actually a family of matrices varied to suit the area it is applied to, in this case sports injuries (Table 3.1.4).

As shown in Table 3.1.4, the matrix has two dimensions. The first dimension is based on the fact that processes that naturally divide into three stages precede the end results of damaging interactions with environmental hazards. These three stages can be labeled the 'precrash', 'crash' and 'postcrash' phases. For the sports injury application the second dimension of the matrix can be divided into at least three factors, 'athlete', 'equipment' and 'environment'. A considerable host of literature illustrates the practical application of such matrices to the study of motor vehicle crashes and their results [25]. Table 3.1.4 lists a num-

Table 3.1.4 Haddon's matrix applied to sports injury prevention.

	Precrash	Crash	Postcrash
Athlete	Skills Neuromuscular control	Training status Falling technique	Rehabilitation
Environment	Floor friction Game rules	Safety net	Medical coverage
Equipment	Shoe friction	Tape/brace Ski bindings Shin guards	First aid equipment Ambulance

ber of injury control measures that may be effective in sports.

Precrash measures

The precrash phase includes measures designed to prevent a potentially dangerous situation to occur at all. An example from the motor vehicle accident area would be four-lane highways built to avoid head-on collisions.

In sports, examples of athlete-related precrash measures include increasing the skill level of an alpine skier to prevent falls or improving neuromuscular control around the knee or ankle to prevent the athlete from landing without proper alignment. Examples of precrash environmental measures include modifying the friction of the playing surface (too high may lead to twisting injuries to the lower extremity, too low may lead to slipping and falling injuries) or rule changes to avoid dangerous plays (e.g. checking from behind in ice hockey to avoid injuries to the spine, or a red card for tackling from behind in soccer). Equipment-related precrash measures include modifying shoe friction or cleat length to the playing surface and weather conditions.

Several RCTs have applied precrash measures or actions to examine the efficacy of the intervention on occurrence of sports injuries. One of the very first was the study of Ekstrand *et al.* (for a detailed description, see 'Focus on Research' above): the study showed that by a multifactorial prevention program the injury rate in soccer could be reduced by 75% [36]. Since the program was multifactorial, it remains unclear which parts of the program were effective and which were

not. Jakobsen *et al.* investigated whether a multipart preventive program would decrease the number of injuries among long-distance runners [6]. The program consisted of a health examination, instructions on proper warm-up and stretching, selection of well-fitting running shoes, individually tailored running programs, and easy access to medical treatment. As a result, the risk of injury decreased 50% in competition, while no change was seen in training-induced injuries. Again, the effectiveness (or ineffectiveness) of any single action in the program remains unclear. Van Mechelen *et al.* examined, in turn, the effect of warm-up, cool-down and stretching on injuries of recreational long-distance runners, but could not find any effect [12]. This conclusion was recently supported by Pope *et al.* who studied the effect of pre-exercise stretching on risk of lower-limb injury in male army recruits [7].

Wedderkopp *et al.* investigated whether a program consisting of balance-board training and careful warming-up activities could reduce the high risk of lower-limb injuries in European team handball among girls [13]. The program was effective, since the risk of injury was reduced by more than 70% in the intervention group. This was the case for injuries occurring during games as well as practice. Recently, Heidt *et al.* examined the effect of a preseason conditioning program on the rate and severity of injuries in adolescent female soccer players aged 14–18 years [35]. The 7-week program combined sports-specific cardiovascular conditioning, plyometric work, sport cord drills, strength training and flexibility exercises to improve speed and agility. After the playing season, 14% of the players randomized to the training program had sustained injuries, compared to 34% of those in the control group.

Crash measures

The crash phase includes measures designed to protect the athlete from being injured, even when there is an accident. Examples of crash measures from the area of traffic accidents include seat belts and air bags to protect passengers from being injured in collisions, and use of safety helmets in cyclists.

Athlete-related crash measures mainly focus on the physical preparation of athletes to allow them to withstand the forces involved when a collision or a fall occurs. Athlete-related crash measures could involve, for example, a general strength training program or falling techniques. Environmental crash measures include safety nets to avoid falling alpine skiers from flying into the crowd or soft mats protecting gymnasts who fail a dismount or fall down from apparatus. There are many examples of equipment-related crash measures in sports, possibly because they are the most obvious to consider, or because there is a potential sales profit involved. Equipment-related measures include release bindings for alpine skiing, helmets for various sports, taping and braces for ankles and other joints, shin guards for soccer players, eye guards for squash and racquetball, and visors for ice hockey.

Examples of crash measures in sports traumatology (as tested in RCTs) include knee and ankle injuries. Sitler *et al.* (1990) showed that it was possible to reduce the risk of medial collateral ligament injuries of the knee in defensive American football players by the use of a prophylactic knee brace [8]. For ankle injuries, similar results have been obtained by balance-board training [11] and semirigid ankle stabilizers [9,10]. The risk of ankle sprains in particular in players with previous injuries could be reduced by these measures.

Postcrash measures

Postcrash measures are designed to minimize the damage resulting from an injury and the risk of reinjury (which is a strong risk factor for sports injuries), and mainly relates to the chain of medical treatment provided after an injury. Postcrash measures in sports may include the training of athletes and coaches to provide adequate on-field first aid, providing adequate

medical services during sports events (personnel and equipment), including quick evacuation procedures to a hospital in the case of severe injuries, and adequate rehabilitation programs for injured athletes before they return to competition. Unfortunately, in sports medicine there are no examples known of effective postcrash measures that have been tested in RCTs.

Practical application of the Haddon matrix

The Haddon matrix may be applied to any sport, thereby providing a means for identifying and considering, cell by cell: (i) prior and possible future resource allocations and activities, as well as the efficacies of each; (ii) the relevant research and other knowledge — both that already available and that needed for the future; and (iii) the priorities for injury countermeasures, judged in terms of their costs and their effects on undesirable injury results.

Summary

The outcome of research on the extent of the sports injury problem is highly dependent on the definitions of 'sports injury', 'sports injury incidence' and 'sports participation'. The outcome of sports epidemiologic research also depends on the research design and methodology, the representativeness of the sample, and on whether or not exposure time was considered when calculating incidence. The severity of sports injuries can be expressed by taking six indices into consideration. The etiology of sports injuries is highly multicausal. This fact, as well as the sequence of events leading to a sports injury, should be accounted for when studying the etiology of sports injuries and when trying to prevent them. Finally, one should take determinants of sports and preventive behavior into account in attempts to solve the sports injury problem.

Multiple choice questions

1 *Is the risk of post-career musculoskeletal problems increased in former elite athletes?*
a Yes.
b No.
2 *Which of the following factors are important to take into account if you want to compare the magnitude of sports injuries between different sports?*
a The total number of injuries.
b The training level of the athletes.

c The number of athletes involved in the sport.

d The severity of injuries sustained.

e All of the above.

3 *Which of the following team sports has the highest incidence of injuries during games?*

a Soccer.

b Team handball.

c Volleyball.

d Ice hockey.

e Basketball.

4 *Which of the following team sports causes the highest number of injuries in Scandinavia?*

a Soccer.

b Team handball.

c Volleyball.

d Ice hockey.

e Basketball.

5 *Ankle tape and braces are commonly used to prevent ankle sprains in sport, and their preventive effect has been investigated in some clinical studies. What is the result from these studies?*

a Using ankle braces prevents ankle sprains.

b Using ankle braces prevents ankle sprains, but their effect is most pronounced in players with former ankle injuries.

c There is no protective effect of using ankle braces.

References

1 Sarna S, Sahi T, Koskenvuo M, Kaprio J. Increased life expectancy of world class athletes. *Med Sci Sports Exerc* 2000; **25**: 237–44.

2 Kujala UM, Sarna S, Kaprio J, Koskenvuo M. Hospital care in later life among former world-class Finnish athletes. *J Am Med Assoc* 1996; **276**: 216–20.

3 Roos H, Lindberg H, Gardsell P, Lohmander LS, Wingstrand H. The prevalence of gonarthrosis and its relation to meniscectomy in former soccer players. *Am J Sports Med* 1994; **22**: 219–22.

4 van Mechelen W, Hlobil H, Kemper HC. Incidence, severity, aetiology and prevention of sports injuries. A review of concepts. *Sports Med* 1992; **14**: 82–99.

5 Ekstrand J, Gillquist J, Liljedahl SO. Prevention of soccer injuries. Supervision by doctor and physiotherapist. *Am J Sports Med* 1983; **11**: 116–20.

6 Jakobsen BW, Kroner K, Schmidt SA, Kjeldsen A. Prevention of injuries in long-distance runners. *Knee Surg Sports Traumatol Arthrosc* 1994; **2**: 245–9.

7 Pope RP, Herbert RD, Kirwan JD, Graham BJ. A randomized trial of preexercise stretching for prevention of lower-limb injury. *Med Sci Sports Exerc* 2000; **32**: 271–7.

8 Sitler M, Ryan J, Hopkinson W *et al.* The efficacy of a prophylactic knee brace to reduce knee injuries in football. A prospective, randomized study at West Point. *Am J Sports Med* 1990; **18**: 310–5.

9 Sitler M, Ryan J, Wheeler B *et al.* The efficacy of a semirigid ankle stabilizer to reduce acute ankle injuries in basketball. A randomized clinical study at west point. *Am J Sports Med* 1994; **22**: 454–61.

10 Surve I, Schwellnus MP, Noakes T, Lombard C. A fivefold reduction in the incidence of recurrent ankle sprains in soccer players using the Sport-Stirrup orthosis. *Am J Sports Med* 1994; **22**: 601–6.

11 Tropp H, Askling C, Gillquist J. Prevention of ankle sprains. *Am J Sports Med* 1985; **13**: 259–62.

12 van Mechelen W, Hlobil H, Kemper HCG, Voorn WJ, Jongh DHR. Prevention of running injuries by warm-up, cool-down, and stretching exercises. *Am J Sports Med* 1993; **21**: 711–9.

13 Wedderkopp N, Kaltoft M, Lundgaard B, Rosendahl M, Froberg K. Prevention of injuries in young female players in European team handball. A prospective intervention study. *Scand J Med Sci Sports* 1999; **9**: 41–7.

14 de Loes M, Goldie I. Incidence rate of injuries during sport activity and physical exercise in a rural Swedish municipality: incidence rates in 17 sports. *Int J Sports Med* 1988; **9**: 461–7.

15 Walter SD, Sutton JR, McIntosh JM, Connolly C. The aetiology of sport injuries. A review of methodologies. *Sports Med* 1985; **2**: 47–58.

16 Chambers RB. Orthopaedic injuries in athletes (ages 6–17). Comparison of injuries occurring in six sports. *Am J Sports Med* 1979; **7**: 195–7.

17 Ronning R, Gerner T, Engebretsen L. Risk of injury during alpine and telemark skiing and snowboarding. The equipment-specific distance-correlated injury index. *Am J Sports Med* 2000; **28**: 506–8.

18 Arendt E, Dick R. Knee injury patterns among men and women in collegiate basketball and soccer. NCAA data and review of literature. *Am J Sports Med* 1995; **23**: 694–701.

19 Colliander E, Eriksson E, Herkel M, Skold P. Injuries in Swedish elite basketball. *Orthopedics* 1986; **9**: 225–7.

20 Yde J, Nielsen AB. Sports injuries in adolescents' ball games: soccer, handball and basketball. *Br J Sports Med* 1990; **24**: 51–4.

21 Zelisko JA, Noble HB, Porter M. A comparison of men's and women's professional basketball injuries. *Am J Sports Med* 1982; **10**: 297–9.

22 Klesges RC, Eck LH, Mellon MW, Fulliton W, Somes GW, Hanson CL. The accuracy of self-reports of physical activity. *Med Sci Sports Exerc* 1990; **22**: 690–7.

23 Bol E, Schmickli SL, Backx FJG, van Mechelen W. *Sportblessures onder de knie*. Papendal. Amsterdam, Holland: NISGZ publication 38, 1991.

24 van Mechelen W. The severity of sports injuries. *Sports Med* 1997; **24**: 176–80.

25 Haddon W. Advances in the epidemiology of injuries as a basis for public policy. *Pub Health Rep* 1980; **95**: 411–21.

26 Myklebust G, Maehlum S, Holm I, Bahr R. A prospective cohort study of anterior cruciate ligament injuries in elite Norwegian team handball. *Scand J Med Sci Sports* 1998; **8**: 149–53.

27 Strand T, Tvedte R, Engebretsen L, Tegnander A. [Anterior cruciate ligament injuries in handball playing. Mechanisms and incidence of injuries]. *Tidsskrift for Den Norske Laegeforening* 1990; **110**: 2222–5.

28 Bjordal JM, Arnly F, Hannestad B, Strand T. Epidemiology of anterior cruciate ligament injuries in soccer. *Am J Sports Med* 1997; **25**: 341–5.

29 Bahr R, Bahr IA. Incidence of acute volleyball injuries: a prospective cohort study of injury mechanisms and risk factors. *Scand J Med Sci Sports* 1997; **7**: 166–71.

30 Bahr R, Lian Ø, Karlsen R, Øvrebø RV. Incidence and mechanisms of acute ankle inversion injuries in volleyball—a retrospective cohort study. *Am J Sports Med* 1994; **22**: 601–4.

31 Molsa JJ, Tegner Y, Alaranta H, Myllynen P, Kujala UM. Spinal cord injuries in ice hockey in Finland and Sweden from 1980 to 1996. *Int J Sports Med* 1999; **20**: 64–7.

32 Tegner Y, Lorentzon R. Concussion among Swedish elite ice hockey players. *Br J Sports Med* 1996; **30**: 251–5.

33 Meeuwisse WH. Assessing causation in sport injury: a multifactorial model. *Clin J Sport Med* 1994; **4**: 166–70.

34 Kok G, Bouter LM. On the importance of planned health education. Prevention of ski injury as an example. *Am J Sports Med* 1990; **18**: 600–5.

35 Heidt R, Sjr Sweeterman LM, Carlonas RL, Traub LA, Tejkulve FX. Avoidance of soccer injuries with preseason conditioning. *Am J Sports Med* 2000; **28**: 659–62.

36 Ekstrand J. *Soccer injuries and their prevention*. Thesis, Linköping University, 1982.

37 de Loes M. Medical treatment and costs of sports-related injuries in a total population. *Int J Sports Med* 1990; **11**: 66–72.

38 Lindqvist KS, Timpka T, Bjurulf P. Injuries during leisure physical activity in a Swedish municipality. *Scand J Social Med* 1996; **24**: 282–92.

39 Maehlum S, Daljord OA. Acute sports injuries in Oslo: a one-year study. *Br J Sports Med* 1984; **18**: 181–5.

40 Ytterstad B. The Harstad injury prevention study. the epidemiology of sports injuries. An 8 year study. *Br J Sports Med* 1996; **30**: 64–8.

41 Sandelin J, Kiviluoto O, Santavirta S, Honkanen R. Outcome of sports injuries treated in a casualty department. *Br J Sports Med* 1985; **19**: 103–6.

42 Sahlin Y. Sport accidents in childhood. *Br J Sports Med* 1990; **24**: 40–4.

43 Sorensen L, Larsen SE, Rock ND. The epidemiology of sports injuries in school-aged children. *Scand J Med Sci Sports* 1996; **6**: 281–6.

44 Kvist M, Kujala UM, Heinonen OJ *et al.* Sports-related injuries in children. *Int J Sports Med* 1989; **10**: 81–6.

45 Arnason A, Gudmundsson A, Dahl HA, Johannsson E. Soccer injuries in Iceland. *Scand J Med Sci Sports* 1996; **6**: 40–5.

46 Drogset JO, Midthjell K. [Injuries among soccer players in lower division clubs]. *Tidsskrift for Den Norske Laegeforening* 1990; **110**: 385–9.

47 Ekstrand J, Gillquist J. Soccer injuries and their mechanisms: a prospective study. *Med Sci Sports Exerc* 1983; **15**: 267–70.

48 Luthje P, Nurmi I, Kataja M *et al.* Epidemiology and traumatology of injuries in elite soccer: a prospective study in Finland. *Scand J Med Sci Sports* 1996; **6**: 180–5.

49 Nielsen AB, Yde J. Epidemiology and traumatology of injuries in soccer. *Am J Sports Med* 1989; **17**: 803–7.

50 Poulsen TD, Freund KG, Madsen F, Sandvej K. Injuries in high-skilled and low-skilled soccer: a prospective study. *Br J Sports Med* 1991; **25**: 151–3.

51 Lorentzon R, Wedren H, Pietila T. [The occurrence of injuries in first class ice hockey]. *Läkartidningen* 1986; **83**(3432–3): 3435.

52 Lorentzon R, Wedren H, Pietila T, Gustavsson B. Injuries in international ice hockey. A prospective, comparative study of injury incidence and injury types in international and Swedish elite ice hockey. *Am J Sports Med* 1988; **16**: 389–91.

53 Lorentzon R, Wedrén H, Pietelä T. Incidence, nature and causes of ice hockey injuries. *Am J Sports Med* 1988; **16**: 392–6.

54 Molsa J, Airaksinen O, Nasman O, Torstila I. Ice hockey injuries in Finland. A prospective epidemiologic study. *Am J Sports Med* 1997; **25**: 495–9.

55 Molsa J, Kujala U, Nasman O, Lehtipuu TP, Airaksinen O. Injury profile in ice hockey from the 1970s through the 1990s in Finland. *Am J Sports Med* 2000; **28**: 322–7.

56 Pettersson M, Lorentzon R. Ice hockey injuries. a 4-year prospective study of a Swedish elite ice hockey team. *Br J Sports Med* 1993; **27**: 251–4.

57 Tegner Y, Lorentzon R. Ice hockey injuries. incidence, nature and causes. *Br J Sports Med* 1991; **25**: 87–9.

58 Aagaard H, Scavenius M, Jorgensen U. An epidemiological analysis of the injury pattern in indoor and in beach volleyball. *Int J Sports Med* 1997; **18**: 217–21.

59 Yde J, Nielsen AB. [Epidemiologic and traumatologic analysis of injuries in a Danish volleyball club] Epidemiologisk og traumatologisk analyse af skader i en dansk volleyball-klub. *Ugeskr Læger* 1988; **150**: 1022–3.

60 Nielsen AB, Yde J. An epidemiological and traumatologic study of injuries in handball. *Int J Sports Med* 1988; **9**: 341–4.

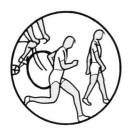

Chapter 3.2
Exercise as Disease Prevention

ILKKA VUORI & LARS-BO ANDERSEN

Classical reference

Nilsson BE, Westlin NE. Bone density in athletes.
    Clin Orth Rel Res 1971; **77**: 179–182.
Commensurate with the fact that osteoporosis may be caused by inactivity, physical exercise is used clinically for its prevention and cure. There is, however, no convincing evidence that exercise will actually increase the bone mass in pathologic cases nor that physical exercise should in any way influence the bone mass in man. Some circumstantial evidence may be extracted from the positive relationships between body weight and bone mass in women and between weight bearing and bone density in rats. The objective of the present study was to evaluate the influence of physical activity on bone mass in healthy young men.

The bone density was evaluated in 64 male athletes and compared to 29 healthy age-matched non-athletes (Fig. 3.2.1). The athletes had significantly denser bone in the distal end of the femur than the non-athletes. Within the group of athletes there was evidence that sports activities including heavy loads on the lower limbs were associated with higher bone density. Also in the athletes, the dominant leg had a denser femur. Among the controls, those who regularly exercised had a higher bone density than those who did not.

Introduction

Exercise has been claimed to be healthy since ancient times. However, scientific evidence for specific health benefits of exercise began to accumulate only about 50 years ago. Since then the amount and quality of information on the potential for exercise in disease prevention has increased greatly. The latest comprehensive review covering this topic at large is the Report of the Surgeon General [1], but a large number of nar-

rative reviews, meta-analyses and critical systematic Cochrane reviews on more limited topics have been published since then.

This chapter presents a short overview of the evidence of the potential value of physical activity in prevention or slowing down of the development of non-communicable diseases. Table 3.2.1 gives an evidence-rated list of these conditions. This review is limited to those conditions that are prevalent in the population and in which there is strong or at least moderate evidence of preventative effectiveness of physical activity supported by evidence that offers plausible biologic mechanism(s) related to the etiopathogenesis of the diseases.

Cardiovascular disease

Over the last five decades cardiovascular disease (CVD) has been the most common cause of death in the Western world. Inside the EU, 44% of all deaths are attributed to CVD and this is almost twice as many as all cancers put together [2]. CVD rates have decreased during the last few decades in Western countries especially in men below the age of 75 years [3,4]. This development is in contrast to the Eastern European countries, where CVD rates have increased. The positive trend in the Northern European countries parallels a positive change in CVD risk factor levels [5,6].

The most common cardiovascular diseases are ischemic or coronary heart disease (CHD) and stroke. CHD and thrombotic stroke are characterized by a gradual development of atherosclerosis that obstructs the vessels supplying the heart and brain, respectively, with blood. Atherosclerosis development is influenced by many factors. Although there is genetic predisposition, most risk factors are modifiable. The probability of developing CHD can to a large extent be predicted

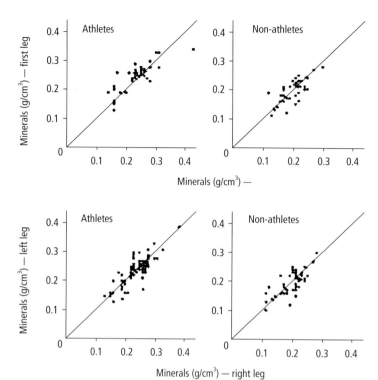

Fig. 3.2.1 Left–right and preference–non-preference side relationships of bone density.

from the risk factor levels. The three traditional risk factors are smoking, high blood pressure and abnormal blood lipid levels. Other risk factors also predict risk of CHD. Currently there is evidence to conclude that physical inactivity is about as strong but even more prevalent a risk factor for CHD as the other major risk factors. Furthermore, physical activity modifies most of the other risk factors in a positive direction, i.e. type 2 diabetes, hypertension, hypercholesterolemia, fibrinogen and obesity, and protects against a number of other diseases including osteoporosis and some cancers [1].

Epidemiologic studies of CVD

The first good study showing that physical inactivity was associated with CVD was published in 1953 [7]. In the early studies, subjects were classified according to their physical activity at work. At that time this made sense, because most of the physical activity people were engaged in was job related, but this has changed since. In 1962 another large population study was initi-

ated [8]. This study was based on detailed information of self-reported physical activity. Paffenbarger and Hyde found that age-adjusted CHD rates were 84% higher among sedentary compared to physically active alumni from Harvard. Many different physical activity variables were assessed, i.e. walking, stair climbing, recreational sports, vigorous sports and total energy expenditure. All physical activity variables predicted future CHD, and higher rates were found among the less physically active.

More than a hundred studies have been published, and the methods of assessing different types and intensities of physical activities have been refined in the later studies. Morris *et al.* [9] analysed the importance of the frequency of participation in vigorous aerobic activities [9]. Those who most frequently participated in vigorous aerobic activities only experienced one-third of the myocardial infarctions of the sedentary group (RR=0.35; 95% confidence interval (CI) 0.21–0.57). Further, a dose–response relationship was found between the four groups analysed. Morris *et al.* did not

Table 3.2.1 The health benefits of regular physical activity (adapted from [121]). The table is based on a total physical fitness program that includes physical activity designed to improve both aerobic and musculoskeletal fitness.

Physical activity benefit	Surety rating	Physical activity benefit	Surety rating
Fitness of body		Cancer	
Improved heart and lung fitness	****	Prevention of colon cancer	****
Improved muscular strength/size	****	Prevention of breast cancer	**
Osteoporosis		Prevention of uterine cancer	**
Helps build up bone density	****	Prevention of prostate cancer	**
Prevention of osteoporosis	***	Infection and immunity	
Treatment of osteoporosis	**	Prevention of the common cold	**
Osteoporotic fractures		Improvement in overall immunity	**
Prevention of fractures	**	Improvement in life quality with HIV infection	***
Arthritis		Psychological well-being	
Prevention of arthritis	*	Elevation in mood	****
Treatment of arthritis	**	Buffering of effects of mental stress	***
Improvement in life quality/fitness	****	Alleviation/prevention of depression	****
Low back pain		Anxiety reduction	****
Prevention of low back pain	**	Improvement in self-esteem	****
Treatment of low back pain	**	Nutrition and diet quality	
Blood cholesterol/lipoproteins		Improvement in diet quality	**
Lower blood total cholesterol	*	Increase in total energy intake	***
Lower LDL-cholesterol	*	Cigarette smoking	
Lower triglycerides	***	Improvement in success in quitting	**
Raised HDL-cholesterol	***	Sleep	
High blood pressure		Improvement in sleep quality	***
Prevention of high blood pressure	****	Children and youth	
Treatment of high blood pressure	****	Prevention of obesity	***
Diabetes		Control of disease risk factors	***
Prevention of NIDDM	****	Reduction of unhealthy habits	**
Treatment of NIDDM	***	Improved odds of adult activity	**
Treatment of IDDM	*	Special issues for women	
Improvement in diabetic life quality	***	Improved total body fitness	****
Weight management		Improved fitness while pregnant	****
Prevention of weight gain	****	Improved birthing experience	**
Treatment of obesity	**	Improved health of fetus	**
Maintenance of weight loss	***	Improved health during menopause	***
Cardiovascular disease		Elderly and the aging process	
Coronary heart disease prevention	****	Improvement in physical fitness	****
Regression of atherosclerosis	**	Countering of loss of heart/lung fitness	**
Treatment of heart disease	***	Countering of loss of muscle	***
Prevention of stroke	***	Countering of gain in fat	***
Asthma		Improvement in life expectancy	****
Improvement in life quality	***	Improvement in life quality	****
Digestive diseases			
Prevention of gallstone disease	**		

**** Strong consensus, with little or no conflicting data.
*** Most data are supportive, but more research is needed for clarification.
** Some data are supportive, but much more research is needed.
* Little or no data support.

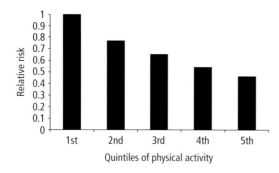

Fig. 3.2.2 Age-adjusted rates of cardiovascular disease (CVD) events in quintiles of physical activity index among 72 488 female nurses (from [10]).

find the same protective effect against CHD with physical activity at moderate intensities, but this has convincingly been shown in other studies. Most studies only include men, but a few recent studies have included large cohorts of women [10,11]. Manson *et al.* [10] analysed CHD rates in 107 000 female nurses in relation to different types of physical activity. A dose–response relationship was found over all quintiles (Fig. 3.2.2). After multivariate adjustment for all the measured risk factors the estimate was still 0.66. Just as convincing, and graded, a relationship was found between quintiles of kilometres walked per week (RR = 0.46; 95% CI 0.33–0.63). In an analysis of walking speed, those with a walking speed above 3 miles/h experienced 0.41 the CHD rate of the slow walkers after exclusion of women who participated in vigorous sport.

In a recent study from Copenhagen, Andersen *et al.* found half the mortality rate in the physically active compared to the sedentary [11]. The study included more than 30 000 subjects and half of them were women. The same relative risk was found in both genders and all age groups. Those who participated in sports had only half the mortality rate of the moderately active, and those who did not cycle to work had a 40% higher mortality rate even after adjustment for other types of physical activity and other CHD risk factors.

A number of studies have analysed the effect of changes in physical activity habits. These studies are important because they exclude the possibility that the

lower CHD rate among the physically active is caused by a selection bias at baseline. Healthier people may be more likely to participate in physical activity. Further, it is important to elucidate whether it can be too late to start to exercise to obtain health benefits and lower the risk of CVD. At least five studies have analysed the effect of changes in physical activity or aerobic fitness against either all-cause mortality or CVD [12–16]. Paffenbarger *et al.* found a graded, dose–response relationship between changes in physical activity in 10 000 men in relation to all-cause mortality, adjusted for baseline physical activity level. Subjects who increased their energy expenditure by more than 1250 kcal/week experienced less than half the mortality rate of subjects who decreased their level similarly. The studies from Copenhagen included more than 17 000 men and women, and a similar dose–response relationship was found in those who decreased physical activity most, having a CHD rate of three to four times the rate of those who increased most [17a].

Blair *et al.* [14] studied the effect of changes in fitness. Genetics play a role in a subject's fitness level and in fitness-related fat and carbohydrate metabolism that in turn are related to risk of developing atherosclerosis. Those who belonged to the lowest quintile of fitness had an age-adjusted mortality rate that was five times the rate of the most fit [17]. This difference could theoretically be caused by a link between genes for fitness and genes for health parameters even if the most plausible explanation is a difference in physical activity levels, and the current fitness level most likely reflects the past few months' physical activity. However, an increase in physical fitness level can only be caused by an increase in aerobic physical activity or a decrease in body weight, which can be adjusted for. It is therefore interesting that Blair *et al.* found that those who were unfit at the first measurement and fit at a second measurement 5 years later had only half the mortality rate of those who were unfit both times [14].

There is consensus that there is a large preventive potential in increasing physical activity in the population. This is caused by a large decrease in incidence rates in people adopting a more active lifestyle, but also by the fact that the prevalence of physical inactivity is very high in the population. In a recent study, Haapanen-Niemi *et al.* [18] collected data from

Table 3.2.2 Prevalence, adjusted relative risks and population attributable risks for coronary heat disease deaths among Finnish men aged 30-63 years according to the different risk factors. From [18].

Risk factor	Prevalence	Lowest values		Highest values	
		RR	PAR (%)	RR	PAR (%)
Physical inactivity (3 h/w)	71%	1.4	22.1	1.9	39.0
Smoking	43%	1.3	9.5	2.4	32.9
Elevated cholesterol (> 6.5 mmol/L)	26%	1.4	9.4	2.0	20.6
Hypertension (SBP > 160 mmHg)	15%	1.4	5.7	2.2	15.3
Obesity (BMI > 30 kg/m^2)	15%	1.2	2.9	1.4	5.7
(BMI > 27 kg/m^2)	37%	1.2	6.9	1.4	12.9

BMI, body mass index; PAR, population attributable risk; RR, relative risk; SBP, systolic blood pressure.

different published studies on Finnish men and calculated the population-attributable risk (PAR) of CHD for different risk factors (Table 3.2.2). The cut-off points for risk may be arbitrary and can be discussed, but the relative risk between groups are calculated from the same cut-off points, and if cut-off points are changed the RR changes too, leaving the calculated PAR at almost the same level. Highest and lowest values are calculated on data from different studies.

Even if these kinds of calculations include several inaccuracies and uncertainties and do not take into account the fact that it is not realistic to change risk levels in all subjects at risk, it is obvious that there is a great preventive potential in behavioral change in physical activity habits.

Stroke

There are two types of stroke, hemorrhagic and thrombotic, which only partly have the same etiology. A thrombotic stroke is caused by clot formation (atherosclerosis) and is therefore caused by the same risk factors as CHD. A hemorrhagic stroke is a bleeding event and one of the main risk factors for this is high blood pressure. Only few epidemiologic studies separate these two conditions even if risk factors partly differ and physical activity may act differently on these two types of stroke. Systolic blood pressure can increase during maximal isometric contractions to more than 300 mmHg and this type of physical activity may therefore be a risk factor for hemorrhagic stroke.

However, intensive isometric contractions increase lipoprotein lipase activity [19] which is favorable in terms of protecting against atherosclerosis. During dynamic exercise almost no change is found in transmural blood pressure in cerebral arteries and this type of exercise may therefore have a different effect on the risk of stroke. These differences may explain varying outcomes from the published studies.

In the Surgeon General's Report [1], 14 studies of physical activity and stroke were reviewed. Most studies included less than 200 endpoints, and in eight of them an inverse association was found between physical activity and stroke. The report concluded that there was not yet consensus about the effect of physical activity on risk of stroke.

Since 1995, a number of good studies have been published [20–23]. Gillum *et al.* [20] followed 8000 subjects who experienced more than 600 strokes. They found a dose–response relationship between physical activity and low incidence of stroke with a relative risk of two in the sedentary. Lee and Paffenbarger [21] analysed the association between physical activity and stroke in 11 130 former Harvard alumni who had 378 strokes. The relationship was somewhat U-shaped, with subjects expending between 2000 and 3000 kcal/week having only half the risk of the sedentary. This activity level equals the international recommendations of 30 min accumulated physical activity a day. The most active did not exceed the sedentary in risk. Only a few studies include women, but in the Copenhagen City Heart Study 7060 women experienced 265 strokes [23]. The physically inactive had 45% higher risk of stroke compared to the physically active.

In conclusion, the evidence of physical activity as protection against stroke is less than for CHD, but it is likely that moderate physical activity has a protective effect. However, it is much more doubtful if high-intensity physical activity has a positive effect and isometric contraction may even increase the risk of hemorrhagic stroke.

Osteoporosis and related fractures

Osteoporosis is characterized by low bone mass and microarchitectural deterioration of bone tissue. These changes lead to enhanced bone fragility and increased risk of fractures. Osteoporosis as such without fracture is usually symptomless and the diagnostic criterion is bone mass. The most commonly used indicator of bone mass is areal bone mineral density (BMD, g/m^2), which can be measured accurately by dual-energy X-ray absorptiometry (DXA). Bone density accounts for 75–85% of the variance in ultimate bone strength. The diagnostic criterion for osteoporosis is BMD at least 2.5 standard deviations (SD) and for osteopenia (low bone mass) 1–2.5 SD below the mean of young adult women [24]. One SD is usually around 12–14% of a given BMD value.

Osteoporosis is most commonly related to aging. The rate of bone loss varies largely between individuals and by site. At the femoral neck BMD is decreased on average by 1 SD at the age of 60 and by 2.5 SD at the age of 90 (Fig. 3.2.3). By the age of 75, an estimated 94% of white women are osteopenic and 38% are osteoporotic [25]. Fracture risk increases 1.5- to 3-fold for each SD fall in BMD. Nearly 20% of women 50 years of age and older suffer from hip fracture during their later years, and for vertebral fracture the corresponding figure is 10–25%.

Prevention of osteoporosis can be defined as preventing BMD from dropping lower than 2.5 SD below the mean for young adult women. Two factors determine the amount of bone later in life: the bone mass accumulated during youth (peak bone mass) and the subsequent rate of bone loss. Peak bone mass and the rate of bone loss are thought to be equally important in determining bone mass at the age of 70. Although genetic factors are the most powerful determinants of

bone mass, at least 20% of it is determined by modifiable factors, physical activity being one of them.

Physical activity and bone mass

Physical activity can influence bone mass by causing compressive or bending loads on bone. If these are sufficiently strong, they can cause a temporary deformation, strain, in bone. As a result, primary and secondary responses occur that stimulate bone formation. The purpose of the increased bone formation can be thought to act as part of a homeostatic mechanism that aims to keep deformation of bone due to mechanical loading within narrow limits in order to avoid damage of the bone structure. Low loading leads to decreased bone formation and increased resorption (Fig. 3.2.4).

Physical activity can substantially increase peak bone mass in youth and it can deter significantly bone loss with aging. Cross-sectional studies in athletes suggest that intensive sports training for many years can increase bone mass at the loaded sites by 20–30% [26], even over 50% [27]. These findings are not due to selection bias (individuals with strong bones or with bones that respond unusually well to physical loading would become superior athletes), as shown by studies comparing the bones of the right and left extremities of athletes practising unilateral sports such as tennis [28]. However, these very high bone mass values are seen

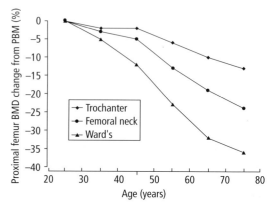

Fig. 3.2.3 Average bone mineral density (BMD) change from peak bone mass (PBM) at different areas of the proximal femur, trochanter, neck, and Ward's triangle in women. (From [119], with permission.)

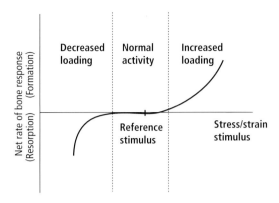

Fig. 3.2.4 Hypothetical relationship between the applied stress or strain stimulus and the net rate of bone resorption or formation. (From [120], with permission.)

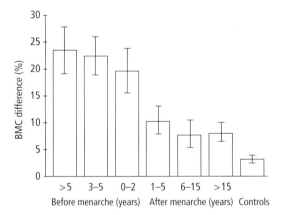

Fig. 3.2.5 Benefit of mechanical loading with respect to bone mineral content (BMC) in growing girls. The BMC of the playing arm (humeral shaft) of the subjects was about two times greater if the girls started playing at or before, rather than after, menarche. The bars represent the 95% confidence intervals. (From [29], with permission.)

only in athletes who have begun systematic training before puberty. It has been shown that bone responds maximally to physical loading during prepuberty and puberty and much less before and after those few years (Fig. 3.2.5) [29,30]. Studies on non-elite athletes and physically active young subjects show bone mass values 5–15% greater than those in their sedentary counterparts. Training studies on young subjects have

resulted in bone mass increases of a few per cent. The high bone mass that has been attained by athletic training or other physical activity cannot be maintained without continuous activity. It seems, however, that less activity is required to maintain the high bone mass or at least a substantial part of it than the amount needed to gain it [31–34]. However, it seems that much or most of the high peak bone mass attained by athletic training is lost before reaching old age [35–37].

In adulthood a substantial increase of bone mass by exercise has not been observed, but in premenopausal women physical activity can maintain the bone mass and in postmenopausal women regular exercise can substantially decrease loss of bone. In quantitative analyses of published studies this effect was on average about 1% per year in favor of the exercising subjects [38,39] and it is mainly due to decreased rate of loss of bone in the exercisers. Importantly, in randomized controlled trials the size of the effects was only about half of that observed in non-randomized studies [38]. The beneficial effect of exercise has been observed in both pre- and postmenopausal women and in both the proximal femur and the lumbar spine. On the basis of the size of the effect of exercise on bone mass it can be estimated that regular physical activity can prevent the development of osteoporosis until even very old age in women who have average or somewhat low bone mass in middle age. However, currently available methods for applying physical loading are not sufficiently effective to compensate for low bone mass.

In addition to prevention of age-related osteoporosis, physical activity is important also in prevention of bone loss in conjunction with injuries and surgical operations. Permanent osteopenia or even osteoporosis may develop if immobilization is long and complete or if the functional results remain poor and loading of the affected body part remains insufficient [28,40].

The effectiveness of physical activity as an osteogenic stimulus is determined by its characteristics in relation to causing strain in bone. These strain-related characteristics are weight-bearing, magnitude of force, rate of application of force, number of cycles of force (repetitions), and pattern of distribution of force in the bone (variability of movements). Table 3.2.3 shows a descriptive assessment of these characteristics in a number of sports. In sports with beneficial loading characteristics such as tennis and squash bone

Table 3.2.3 Assessment of the loading characteristics of the different sports in which bone measurements of female athletes have been made [26].

Sport	Loading characteristics				
	Weight-bearing	High-magnitude	High-impact	Repetitive	Varied
Strength sports					
Body-building	xxx	xxx	x	x	x
Power-lifting	xxx	xxx	x	x	x
Weight-lifting	xxx	xxx	xx	x	xx
Endurance sports					
Running	xx	x	xx	xxx	xx
Orienteering	xx	x	xx	xxx	xx
Speed skating	xx	x	xx	xxx	xx
Cross-country skiing	xx	x	x	xxx	x
Rowing	x	x	x	xxx	x
Cycling	x	x	x	xxx	x
Swimming	0	x	x	xxx	x
Speed and power					
Aerobic dancing	xxx	xx	xxx	xxx	xxx
Ballet dancing	xxx	xx	xxx	xx	xxx
Gymnastics	xxx	xx	xxx	xx	xxx
Figure skating	xxx	xx	xxx	xx	xxx
Basketball	xxx	xx	xxx	xx(x)	xxx
Soccer	xxx	xx	xxx	xx(x)	xxx
Volleyball	xxx	xx	xxx	xx	xxx
Squash	xxx	xx	xxx	xx	xxx
Tennis	xxx	xx	xxx	xx	xxx

Assumption: duration of exposure is sufficient.
xxx, high, broad; xx, medium; x, low, limited; 0, none.

mass at the loaded sites has been found to be high as compared with sports with weak loading characteristics and with referents (Fig. 3.2.6) [26]. Quantitative analyses of results of clinical trials agree well with these cross-sectional observations and strongly support the notion that only high-intensity activity significantly influences bone mass except possibly in osteoporotic subjects. Both endurance or aerobic and dynamic strength or progressive resistance training as well as impact and non-impact exercises have been found effective and thus far no definite differences in the effectiveness between the types of training have been found in quantitative analyses, possibly due to small number of studies in some categories. Static exercises and slow movements do not influence bone

mass in normal subjects. Also movements that are repeated in a similar fashion even in large amounts, e.g. walking, are weak or insufficient loading stimuli for healthy young and middle-aged subjects. However, smaller loading can be osteotrophic for weakened bones. Thus, walking has been found effective in osteoporotic subjects [41]. Data are not sufficient to reach firm conclusions as to the required number of loadings in one session, but on the basis of animal experiments it is likely to be only a few regarding stimulation of a small bone site. However, in order to stimulate sufficiently large bone sites, the total number of loadings from different directions has to be quite large. The optimal frequency of training sessions is likely to be a few times a week. The duration of training that is toler-

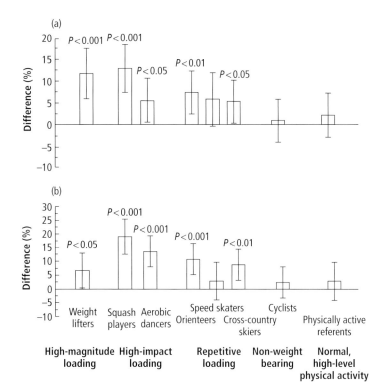

Fig. 3.2.6 Relative difference in weight-adjusted bone mineral density (BMD) at the most loaded lower limb sites of different female athlete groups ($n = 18–30$) and a physically active reference group ($n = 25$) compared with that of the sedentary reference group ($n = 25$). (a) Proximal tibia BMD and (b) calcaneus BMD. The grouping of the athletes was based on the specific bone-loading characteristics of the respective sports. The bars indicate the 95% confidence intervals. (From [120], with permission.)

able to ordinary subjects should be more than half a year in order to begin to see its effects. During the post-menopausal years physical activity in combination with estrogen replacement therapy is more effective in maintaining bone mass than estrogen alone, but without the influence of estrogen physical activity is hardly effective [31].

The effects of physical activity on bone geometry, internal architecture and material properties have not yet been thoroughly studied. The few published observations suggest that physical loading can lead to increased diameter and strength of bone [42,43]. These kinds of changes may substantially influence the breaking strength of bone without marked changes in bone mass or areal density.

Physical activity can also be detrimental to bone. Large amounts of intensive training for prolonged periods such as seen in military training and in competitive athletes can lead to stress fractures and osteopenia. The mediating mechanisms of development of os-

teopenia are complicated and not completely understood, but one mechanism is disruption of normal ovarian function that leads to inhibition of the production of gonadotrophin-releasing hormone by the hypothalamus and to decreased estrogen content in blood. These athletes have oligo- or amenorrhea and gradually bone mass decreases or in young athletes peak bone mass remains low. As a consequence, the risk of stress fractures increases but it is not definitively known whether the risk of osteoporosis is also increased [44,45]. In addition to hormonal disturbances low body mass and, frequently, eating disorders can contribute to athletes' osteopenia.

Physical activity and prevention of osteoporotic fractures

The lifetime risk of having at least one osteoporotic fracture is greater than 50% for women. This includes a lifetime risk of approximately 32% for vertebral fractures, 16% for hip fractures, 15% for wrist fractures and 8% for humerus fractures [46]. Most verte-bral fractures occur without trauma, solely as a result of osteoporosis. Most wrist and hip fractures are caused by a combination of mild or moderate trauma, usually a fall from a standing level, and osteoporosis. Thus, prevention of falls or decreasing their severity is an important part of prevention of osteoporotic fractures.

Falls are common among elderly people. Each year, approximately 30% of community-dwelling older people fall at least once and 10–20% fall twice or more. Although less than 5% of falls among older adults lead to bone fracture, multiple falling in particular is clearly an indicator of increased risk of fracture. Established risk factors for falls include older age, impaired balance and orthostatic hypotension, lower-extremity muscle weakness, decreased reaction time, impaired vision and cognition, decreased lean body mass and overall impaired mobility. Also several factors related to use of medications and alcohol, environment and the acute situation influence the risk of fall and its seriousness [47].

Physical activity may influence the risk of fall and its consequences through several mechanisms. The most likely effects are mediated through musculoskeletal and neuromuscular systems and can be measured by performance in strength, balance, coordination, postural stability, gait and mobility. Review of the currently published studies [47] revealed that randomized controlled exercise trials aiming at decreasing the risk of falls have produced inconclusive results. No exercise modalities have shown to be consistently effective in reducing risk for falls, but balance and strength training exercise programs have shown promising results in recent studies. Most case-control studies of physical activity and hip fracture have shown a 20–60% reduction in odds of fracture among women engaging in moderate physical activity vs. control. Most prospective studies on the topic have found 30–50% smaller risk in physically active as compared with sedentary subjects. The consistency, magnitude of effect and diversity of populations across these studies strongly suggest that a physically active lifestyle can help reduce the incidence of hip fractures in the population. It is unclear whether physical activity is associated with risk of osteoporotic fractures at sites other than the hip. It is important to notice that es-pecially in subjects with impaired movement abilities physical activity may also increase the risk of falls and consequently osteoporotic fractures. On the basis of the current evidence a pertinent message to older people would be to recommend a physically active lifestyle including a variety of customary tasks performed in a safe environment and requiring moderate amounts of muscle strength, balance, coordination and mobility. More studies are needed before evidence-based recommendations for specific exercise regimens tailored for various population groups can be given. It seems obvious, however, that physical activities that maintain and improve both muscle strength and abilities for a wide variety of physical tasks are favorable in terms of both bone strength and risk of falls.

Physical activity and low back pain

Low back pain is pain, muscle tension or stiffness localized below the costal margin and above the inferior gluteal folds, with or without leg pain (sciatica). About 85% of low back pain cases are non-specific, not attributable to recognizable pathology. The poorly defined pathophysiology and mechanism of pain explain to a large degree the difficulties of prevention and treatment of low back pain.

Low back pain is a common disorder, the lifetime incidence being around 60–80%. Most cases are resolved within 2–4 weeks and 90% recover by 12 weeks [48]. However, in a follow-up study nearly one-third of cases had not recovered completely in 1 year [49,50], and recurrence of low back pain is very frequent with rates of up to 50% in the year following the initial episode.

The origin and mechanisms of low back pain are not exactly known, but it seems that the symptoms originate from tissue injury or inflammation and from the resulting irritation, nociception [51]. This in turn causes increased muscular tension in order to decrease movements that cause pain. Thus, trunk muscles are an important element related to low back pain syndrome, and these muscles have a decisive role in protecting back structures from excessive mechanical loading.

Physical activity might relate to the development of low back pain as a provoking or preventing factor. Heavy physical work, frequent bending, twisting, lifting, pulling and pushing, repetitive work and static postures as well as reduced muscle strength in back, abdominal and thigh muscles, reduced endurance in back muscles, hypermobility in the lumbar column and hypomobility of hip joints are commonly listed, activity-related risk factors for low back pain [52]. The theoretical rationale for the role of physical activity (PA) in the causation or prevention of low back pain includes the following ideas: (i) PA can induce acute and repetitive subclinical or more severe injuries in the back structures; (ii) higher strength of the muscles of the back and trunk could protect the back from injury or minimize the effects of injurious events; (iii) higher endurance of the trunk muscles helps to maintain motor control due to less fatigue in various tasks thus decreasing the risk of high loading of spine structures or occurrence of malfunctions and consequently development of injury; (iv) better flexibility may decrease the risk of injury especially during lifting and bending activities; (v) good motor skills decrease the risk of injury in various tasks; and (vi) good general or aerobic endurance helps to counteract fatigue and development of injury [53]. Additional suggested mechanisms include improved circulation to the back structures and improved mood that would influence favorably sensitivity to pain [51]. In addition, PA may influence the development or the course of low back pain episodes in indirect, unspecific ways, e.g. through influences on body mass, mood, perceptions and motivation, and by decreasing or abolishing the effects of physiologic deconditioning due to inactivity or hypoactivity.

Current scientific evidence on the role of physical activity in provoking or preventing low back pain can be summarized as follows. Prolonged, repetitive, heavy physical activity at work or in sports can cause low back pain in susceptible individuals, but the ultimate contributory role of injury is not known. The most commonly practised leisure-time physical activities have not been found to increase the risk of low back pain. Strong evidence indicates that physical activity can have a preventive effect on low back pain and is currently the only effective tested modality for this purpose [51,54]. However, all studies do not show physical activity to be effective for prevention of low back pain. Further, the characteristics of an effective exercise program have not been defined. It is worth noting, however, that trunk muscle endurance in some

cross-sectional studies and endurance training of these muscles in controlled trials has been associated with positive preventative findings [55].

Overweight and obesity

The most commonly used measure to define overweight and obesity is body mass index (BMI, in kg/m^2). Currently the most widely accepted cut-off point for overweight is BMI ≥ 25.0 and for obesity BMI ≥ 30. BMIs in the range of 25.0–29.9 indicate only overweight, but not obesity. BMIs ≥ 30.0 assume that persons categorized at this level are obese, i.e. overweight because of excess adiposity.

Overweight and obesity constitute an important health problem because of two reasons. First, the risk of a number of somatic disorders as well as psychological and social consequences increases sharply with increasing overweight and obesity [56–58]. However, part of the increased morbidity and mortality associated with increased BMI may not be due to excess fat *per se* but to physical inactivity and low fitness associated with and probably causally related to overweight and obesity [59,60]. Secondly, overweight and obesity are very common and increasingly prevalent conditions in European as well as in other populations, nearly one in three EU citizens being overweight and one in 10 being obese [56].

Regulations of body fat mass and body weight are extremely complicated phenomena, but in essence they are functions of energy intake by eating and energy expenditure by resting metabolism and various forms of physical activity (Fig. 3.2.7). Overweight and obesity are due to excess energy intake in relation to energy expenditure for a lengthy time period. The factors related to and mechanisms involved in both of these basic processes and in their interactions are very complex and not completely understood. Data from several national surveys indicate that over the past few decades, there has been either a slight increase or very modest decline in total energy and fat intake. At the same time work-related physical activity and the energy expenditure required for daily living have substantially decreased. Participation in leisure-time physical activity is rather low in most populations, and it has showed only modest changes. Cross-sectional and population studies consistently show a negative relationship between level of physical activity and indices

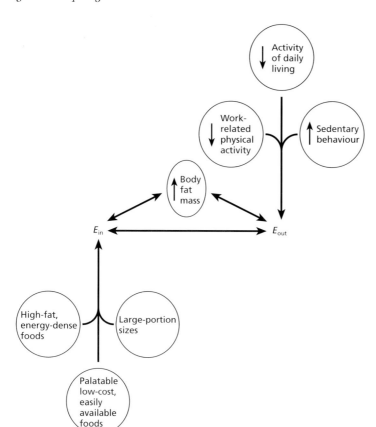

Fig. 3.2.7 The effect of environmental factors on energy balance. When energy intake (E_{in}) equals energy expenditure (E_{out}), the system is in energy balance and body fat mass stable. In the current environment, factors (in circles) on the left are driving E_{in} up, whereas factors on the right are driving E_{out} down, creating a state of positive energy balance, leading to an increase in the body fat mass. (From [61], with permission.)

of obesity. The few published cohort studies show that high levels of physical activity are protective against obesity. Thus, although there are no definitive prospective studies to show that a low level of physical activity is a risk for obesity development and that a high level of physical activity is protective against obesity, an overwhelming amount of indirect evidence suggests that this is the case. The major factor explaining the current obesity epidemic is most likely the continued decline in daily energy expenditure that has not been matched by equivalent reduction in energy intake. For most people it is difficult to restrict intake to meet energy requirements, and thus an increase in physical activity is necessary to curtail the increasing prevalence of obesity [61,62].

Although the biologic basis is sound and evidence from ecologic and observational studies strongly sup-

port the value of physical activity in the prevention of overweight and obesity, data from prospective studies and clinical trials are less consistent. Systematic review of studies on physical activity and weight gain shows that results from the studies using baseline physical activity data were variable. When physical activity data at follow-up were used, four studies out of five found that a large volume of physical activity at follow-up was associated with less weight gain. If physical activity increased during the follow-up, less weight gain was observed in most studies [63]. Observational studies and clinical trials on the effect of physical activity on weight change after intentional weight reduction in previously obese subjects show that the effects of prescribed exercise training in preventing weight regain is on average only very modest, about 600 g/year.

The discrepancy between observational studies suggesting a substantial potential for physical activity in preventing weight gain and clinical trials indicating this effect to be very modest only can be explained by several factors. The two most important reasons are the great amount of physical activity needed to influence body weight significantly and the commonly poor adherence to prescribed exercise training. These same reasons largely explain also the good results in short-term but poor results in long-term weight reduction programs based on exercise training [63,64]. In observational studies the comparison is made between those who have chosen to be highly active for a long time and those who have been sedentary, but in clinical trials even the prescribed activity is often modest and only part of that has actually been realized due to poor compliance. The amount of physical activity that is necessary to prevent weight gain is not yet definitively known, but a summary of the evidence suggests that approximately 6900–8400 kJ/week (1500–2000 kcal/week) in addition to energy consumed in daily living improves weight maintenance, but some studies suggest smaller and some studies larger amount of energy expenditure in physical activity for this purpose [63].

Overweight and obesity are health problems as such but largely also because of the great number of serious comorbidities. Even though the physiologic potential of physical activity for weight maintenance and particularly for weight reduction is hard to realize in practice, physical activity has significant independent beneficial effects on several comorbidities of obesity, and it appears to attenuate morbidity and mortality risk in overweight and obese individuals [65] even to the extent that active obese individuals have lower morbidity and mortality than normal-weight individuals who are sedentary (Fig. 3.2.8) [22,66]. These effects of physical activity have been observed even when changes in weight have been modest or negligible. Thus, physical activity should be an important part of the effort to decrease the health consequences of obesity regardless of its effectiveness to influence body weight and fat mass.

Type 2 diabetes

In early studies it was shown that the prevalence of

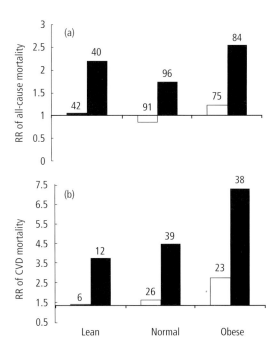

Fig. 3.2.8 Body fatness and relative risks (RRs) of (a) all-cause and (b) cardiovascular disease (CVD) mortality by cardiorespiratory fitness categories in men: □, fit; ■, unfit. Fit, lean men comprised the reference category, represented by the heavy line at 1.0. Unfit men were the lowest quartile of oxygen uptake (mL/kg/FFM/min) in each age group, and fit refers to all other men. RRs were adjusted for age (single year), examination year, smoking habit, alcohol intake and parental history of ischemic heart disease. Body fatness categories were, in percentage body fat, lean (<16.7%), normal (16.7% to 25.0%) and obese (≥25.0%). Numbers above or below the bars represent the number of deaths. From [22], with permission.)

type 2 diabetes increased in societies where a rapid change from a traditional physically active lifestyle to a more technologic sedentary lifestyle had occurred [67]. Also, in cross-sectional studies low glucose and insulin levels are associated with higher physical activity levels [68]. In training studies, insulin sensitivity increases after a period of aerobic training in both diabetics and healthy subjects [69], and this increase is a local response in the trained muscle [69a]. Possible mechanisms for the improved glucose transport are an increase in GLUT-4-mediated transport [70], increased number of insulin receptors, and an increased density of capillaries. Further, glucose is transported into the muscle cell independently of insulin by Ca^{2+} channels in the membrane, and Ca^{2+} is released when the muscle contracts, so glucose transport is enhanced by the physical activity itself. It seems that the insulin sensitivity is closely related to capillary density [71], which again is highly associated with aerobic fitness [72].

In a prospective study, Heinrich *et al.* [73] found an inverse relationship between physical activity and risk of type 2 diabetes, and physical activity was more important in men with a high body mass index, elevated blood pressure or a genetic disposition for diabetes. Every extra energy expenditure of 500 kcal/week, equivalent to 1 h walking, decreased the risk of developing diabetes by 6%. Sports participation was more protective than walking. Similarly, Manson *et al.* [74] found that women participating at least once a week in vigorous physical activity had a 16% lower risk of developing diabetes.

Hypertension

Current classification [75] defines blood pressure <120/<80 mmHg as optimal, <130/<85 as normal, 130–139/85–89 as high normal, 140–159/90–99 as mild (grade 1) hypertension (140–149/90–94 as borderline), 160–179/100–109 as moderate (grade 2) hypertension and ≥180/≥110 as severe (grade 3) hypertension.

The risk of cardiovascular events is related to the level of blood pressure, e.g. a prolonged 5 mmHg higher level of usual diastolic pressure is associated with a 35–40% higher risk of stroke. Most studies have found a continuous increase of risk of cardiovascular events with increasing blood pressure [76], but a recent analysis of the Framingham data found a sharp stepwise increase of mortality at high blood pressure level [77]. Lowering of elevated blood pressure leads to decreased cardiovascular events, e.g. each reduction of 10–14 mmHg in systolic and 5–6 mmHg in diastolic pressure confers a benefit of about two-fifths less stroke and one-sixth less coronary heart disease. In patients with grade 1 hypertension, monotherapy usually produces reductions in blood pressure of about 10/5 mmHg.

The most reliable data of the prevalence of various categories of blood pressure in Europe are from the MONICA Project. They show a very wide distribution of, for example, systolic blood pressure over 160 mmHg: 2% in Toulouse, France and 21% in North Karelia, Finland in 35–64-year-old men [78].

The ultimate cause of blood pressure elevation is not known. Risk factors for hypertension include genetic factors, high intake of salt, fat and alcohol, insulin resistance and hyperinsulinemia, overweight and obesity, psychic stress and physical inactivity. Increased sympathetic activity seems to be an important factor in the genesis of hypertension and it may also be involved in the genesis or worsening of several pressure-independent risk factors of cardiovascular diseases [79].

Role of physical activity

Only a few studies have been published on the association between level of blood pressure and its development and physical activity. The observational studies before mid-1998 reviewed by Hagard [80] and some others [81,82] show quite consistently that higher levels of physical activity or fitness are associated with a lower blood pressure level and 30–70% lower incidence of hypertension.

The effects of exercise training on blood pressure show wide variation in different studies. A recent meta-analysis of 44 randomized controlled trials found that aerobic or endurance exercise on normotensive and hypertensive men and women resulted on average 3.4/2.4 mmHg net decrease in systolic and diastolic blood pressure, respectively, adjusted for control observations and for the number of trained participants [83]. The effect depends on the initial blood pressure being greater in hypertensive subjects. Another meta-analysis of 10 randomized controlled trials on the effect of aerobic exercise on blood pressure of normotensive and hypertensive women revealed a 2/1 mmHg decrease in systolic and diastolic blood pressure, respectively [84]. A comparable meta-analysis on the effect of progressive resistance exercise including 11 studies found an average 3/3 mmHg blood pressure decrease [85]. Hagberg *et al.* [86] reported in their updated review of all studies on the effect of exercise training on hypertensive subjects an average blood pressure reduction of 11/8 mmHg and exercise was effective in approximately 75% of individuals with hypertension. The decreased systolic blood pressure was on average 142 mmHg and thus remained inside the hypertension range. The corresponding decreased diastolic blood pressure was on average 89 mmHg. The greater reduction of blood pressure found in this review as compared with the results of the three meta-analyses is likely to be mainly due to the fact that Hagberg and coworkers included studies on hypertensive subjects only and they included both randomized and non-randomized trials. The reviews largely agree on some important aspects. The effect of exercise on resting blood pressure seems to be independent of change of body weight, moderate and vigorous exercise is equally effective and the effects are seen in both men and women and across a wide range of age. In an additional analysis of randomized controlled trials focusing on dose–response relationships Fagard [87] found that the changes in blood pressure were not significantly related to training frequency (1–7 sessions per week, but in two-thirds of the studies the frequency was 3 sessions per week) or to time per session (15–70 min). Thus, on the basis of current evidence exercise regimens that vary greatly in their content can be effective in reducing blood pressure.

The mechanisms that are responsible for the blood pressure lowering effect of exercise training are not definitively known, but the possible mechanisms include attenuation of adrenergic sympathetic activity, increased cellular insulin sensitivity and decreased level of circulating insulin, decreased peripheral resistance, increased baroreflex sensitivity, changes in the renin–angiotensin aldosterone system and reduction in body fat. Improved relaxation and decreased tension and anxiety are examples of indirect mechanisms.

The risk of cardiovascular events associated with hypertension depends not only on the blood pressure level but to a large extent also on the presence of other risk factors. This is demonstrated by wide differences in the risk of cardiovascular mortality at the same absolute level of blood pressure in different populations [76]. Therefore, it is important that exercise training improves, for example, the blood lipid profile and insulin sensitivity of hypertensive subjects to the same degree as in normotensive individuals. Some evidence also suggests that exercise training in hypertensive patients may result in regression of pathologic left ventricular hypertrophy and attenuate exaggerated

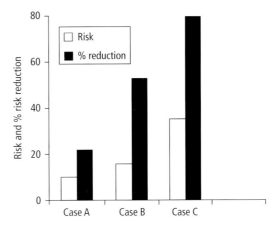

Fig. 3.2.9 Risk of developing cardiovascular (CV) disease for hypertensive individuals with different combinations of CV disease risk factors and the reductions in risk expected with exercise training. Case A: Average 10-year risk for a 50-year-old man and woman with systolic/diastolic blood pressure (BP) of 153/97 mmHg, cholesterol of 206 mg/dL, high density lipoprotein cholesterol (HDL-C) of 42 mg/dL, non-smoking and not having diabetes mellitus or left ventricular hypertrophy (LVH). Percentage risk reduction in these individuals is that resulting from usual CV disease risk factor changes with exercise training in patients with hypertension (ΔBP=-11/ -8 mmHg, ΔHDL-C=$+3$ mg/dL). Case B: Same man and woman as in case A except that both have type 2 diabetes mellitus (non-insulin-dependent diabetes mellitus, NIDDM). The type 2 diabetes mellitus is eliminated with exercise training in both the man and woman, and as in case A all other expected changes occur with exercise training. Case C: Same man and woman as in case A except that both have type 2 diabetes mellitus and LVH. Type 2 diabetes mellitus and LVH are eliminated with exercise training in both the man and the woman, and as in case A all other expected changes occur with exercise training. All risks are calculated using the equations of Anderson *et al.* based on the Framingham Study. (From [86], with permission.)

blood pressure response during physical exertion [86,88]. The recent finding that exercise training also decreases blood pressure response to mental stress in hypertensive subjects may be important in terms of the risk of developing end-organ damage [89]. Taken together, the effects of exercise training may decrease the risk of acute cardiovascular complications and development of cardiovascular diseases (Fig. 3.2.9), reduce antihypertensive and other medication requirements and improve the quality of life of hypertensive patients.

Cancer

Studies have investigated the relationship between physical activity and a number of different cancers. Among these are colon, rectal, lung, prostate, pancreatic and breast cancer. In the prospective studies, the number of cases is the limiting factor, and we have the best knowledge about the relationship in the most common cancers.

Many studies have investigated colon cancer. Colditz *et al.* [90] reviewed 41 studies and found that even though many had not controlled thoroughly for confounders, the results were very consistent. They concluded that colon cancer rates were lower with higher physical activity levels both at work and during leisure time. There is a dose–response relationship between total amount of physical activity and colon cancer risk, but little is known about the effect of different types and intensities of physical activity. Different hypotheses exist concerning the mechanisms behind the protective effect. The most plausible explanation seems to be that the transit time in the intestine is lower in the physically active. This decreases the time carcinogenic material spends in contact with the mucosa [91]. The reason for this may be that the peristaltic movements in the intestine are controlled by vagal nerve, and the vagal activity is higher in more fit individuals. Another hypothesis is that insulin is a strong growth factor for colon mucosal cells and the insulin level increases with physical inactivity [92]. Other mechanisms may be possible.

Hormone-dependent cancers

The relationship between physical activity and breast, ovarian or uterine cancers has been investigated in more than 20 studies. Most of the cohort studies suffer from methodologic problems involving the assessment of physical activity, lack of statistical power and a very long follow-up period. The latter increases misclassification because of true changes in behavior since the baseline measurement. A recent Norwegian study included 25 624 women with 351 cases of breast cancer [93]. After adjustment for age, BMI, number of children and socioeconomic background, the physically active at work had only half the rate of the physically inactive and in the analysis of physical activity in leisure time, the active had a 0.63 lower rate. However,

more good studies are needed before sound conclusions can be drawn about the relationship between physical activity and these types of cancers.

In men, the association between physical activity/fitness and risk of prostate and testicular cancers has been studied. Oliveria *et al.* [94] found in a study including 13 000 men that the most fit men had a relative risk of prostate cancer of 0.26 (95% CI 0.10–0.63) compared to the unfit after adjustment for age, BMI and smoking. This conclusion is supported by other studies of the general population, but in some studies where the incidence is compared between athletes and non-athletes, the athletes have had a higher rate [95]. Only a few studies have been published on physical activity and testicular cancer. Therefore, it is too early to conclude that there is an association between physical activity and these cancers.

Immune system

During both moderate and vigorous physical activity leukocytes in the blood increase, which is a strengthening of the defence system. However, after prolonged intensive exercise with a duration of more than an hour at above 75% of aerobic capacity, a weakening of the immune system is found hours to days afterwards. Experimental research in animals support this hypothesis [96], but in humans the risk of infections has been studied in epidemiologic studies. About 10 studies have reported on upper respiratory tract infections within the week after a marathon [97]. Compared to control groups, marathon runners report increased number of infections. In the largest study, 12.9% of 2311 participants in the Los Angeles Marathon in 1987 reported infections during the following week vs. only 2.2% in the control group. In three studies, self-reported symptoms have been investigated in relation to more moderate exercise. In all these studies a lower frequency of illness was found [97].

Mental health

Epidemiologic studies have shown associations between physical activity and symptoms of depression [98–101], clinical depression [102] and general well-being. Most studies have used self-report questions for the assessment of both physical activity and mental health. These questions are useful to identify persons with perceived mental stress, but there is a poor relationship between questionnaire variables and clinical diagnoses of stress and depression [103].

Subjects with mood disturbances have benefited by participating in physical activity programs [104,105]. Improvements in symptoms of anxiety [106] and depression [107], and in patients with non-psychotic depression have been reported [108]. Most interventions have used aerobic exercise.

Some prospective cohort studies have been published. Farmer *et al.* [100] found among 1900 adults an association between lack of exercise and depressive symptoms at the baseline investigation. After 8 years' follow-up, lack of recreational physical activity predicted an increase in depressive symptoms in women, who at baseline had few symptoms. In men with many symptoms at baseline, lack of exercise predicted continuing symptoms. The Harvard Alumni Study collected questionnaire data on physician-diagnosed depression in 1988 and information on suicide from death certificates [109]. These data were analysed in relation to their detailed information of the subjects' former physical activity levels collected from 1962–66. Suicide was not related to baseline physical activity level, but the relative risk of depression was 27% less in subjects who had participated in sports at least 3 hours a week compared to the sedentary. When the risk of depression was analysed in relation to energy expenditure in physical activity, a dose–response relationship was found.

The evidence of the effect of physical activity on mental health in well-functioning individuals are less clear. Some studies have shown positive effects on mood, perceived stress and anxiety [110,111], while others have failed to show this. This is not surprising because well-functioning persons have 'less room' for improvement. The psychological measures used are 'state' and 'trait' anxiety, where state anxiety is a 'here and now feeling' of anxiety and trait anxiety is a more permanent personal characteristic. The most common effect of physical activity is a transient reduction in anxiety [112,113].

The biologic mechanisms are unknown, but researchers have suggested that physical activity induces changes in the neurotransmitters norepinephrine, dopamine, serotonin and endorphins [114,115]. The elevated temperature may have an impact on muscle tension [113], but this effect could be mediated through hormonal or nervous changes. It is well known that training induces changes in circulating epinephrine and norepinephrine [116]. A less described, but important factor for mental health, is the social factor in sports participation. Much physical activity is performed in some social setting, which is rarely included in cohort studies, but of course has an effect on mental health [117,118].

Multiple choice questions

1 *The population-attributable risk of coronary heart disease is given in a table. This measure is:*

a the decrease in risk a subject will get if he/she changed the level of a risk factor to the level recommended in the table

b the number of deaths that would be prevented if a successful campaign were carried out

c the number of deaths that theoretically could be prevented if all subjects had the most favorable behavior

d the percentage that would survive if the risk factor levels were above the level recommended in the table.

2 *Why do most published prospective studies on the risk of physical inactivity only include men?*

a Because most scientists are men and they are mainly interested in research they can benefit from themselves.

b Women are less physically active and it is difficult to assess their activity level.

c Rates of many diseases are higher in men than women and it is cheaper to conduct the investigation.

d The follow-up time would be too long in women before a sufficient number had experienced disease, and during that time many would have changed their behavior.

3 *Physical inactivity has been accepted as a strong risk factor for many diseases much later than many other risk factors, and authorities have not until recently taken steps to organize prevention through increased physical activity. Why has it taken so long?*

a The evidence has been less convincing compared to smoking and alcohol because no randomized controlled trials have been conducted with physical activity in relation to disease.

b The mechanisms behind the preventive effect of physical activity are not fully known, which they are for other important risk factors.

c It is easier to get people to stop smoking or abusing alcohol than to make them physically active.

d There is much more to gain by giving hypertensives or hypercholesterolemia pills to patients to decrease the risk factor levels.

e There are no economic interests in prevention through physical activity.

4 *Why is our knowledge limited about the association between physical activity and ovarian, breast and uterine cancers?*

a Only few scientists are interested in preventing diseases in women.

b These diseases are rare and studies are expensive to conduct.

c There is no association and it is difficult to get negative results published.

References

1 US Department of Health and Human Services, Centers for Disease Control and Prevention, National Center for Chronic Disease Prevention and Health Promotion. *Physical Activity and Health. A Report of the Surgeon General.* Atlanta, GA, 1996.

2 European Commission. *The State of Health in the European Community: Report from the Commission.* Luxembourg: European Commission, 1999.

3 Juel K, Sjøl A. Decline in mortality from heart disease in Denmark: some methodological problems. *J Clin Epidemiol* 1995; **48**: 467–72.

4 Sans S, Kesteloot H, Kromhout D. The burden of cardiovascular diseases mortality in Europe. Task force of the European society of cardiology on cardiovascular mortality and morbidity statistics in Europe. *Eur Heart J* 1997; **18**: 1231–48.

5 Sjøl A, Grunnet K, Schroll M. Secular trends in serum cholesterol, high density lipoproteins and triglycerides 1964–87. *Int J Epidemiol* 1991; **20**: 105–13.

6 Sjøl A, Thomsen KK, Schroll M. Secular trends in blood pressure levels in Denmark 1964–91. *Int J Epidemiol* 1998; **27**: 614–22.

7 Morris JN, Heady JA, Raffle PAB, Roberts CG, Parks JW. Coronary heart-disease and physical activity of work. *Lancet* 1953; **1**: 1053–7.

8 Paffenbarger RS, Hyde RT, Wing AL, Hsieh C. Physical activity and longevity of college alumni. *N Engl J Med* 1986; **315**: 399–401.

9 Morris JN, Clayton DG, Everitt MG, Semmence AM, Burgess EH. Exercise in leisure time: coronary attack and death rates. *Br Heart J* 1990; **63**: 325–34.

10 Manson JE, Hu FB, Rich-Edwards JW, Colditz GA, Stampfer MJ, Willett WC, Speizer FE, Hennekens CH. A prospective study of walking as compared with vigorous exercise in the prevention of coronary heart disease in women. *N Engl J Med* 1999; **341**: 650–8.

11 Andersen LB, Schnohr P, Schroll M, Hein HO. All-cause mortality associated with physical activity during leisure time, work, sports, and cycling to work. *Arch Intern Med* 2000; **160**: 1621–8.

12 Paffenbarger RS, Hyde RT, Wing AL, Lee I-M, Dexter L, Kampert JB. The association of changes in physical-activity level and other lifestyle characteristics with mortality among men. *N Engl J Med* 1993; **328**: 538–45.

13 Paffenbarger RS. Influence of adopting a physically active lifestyle on mortality rates of middle-aged and elderly men. *ICHPER* 1994; **30**: 5–10.

14 Blair SN, Kohl HW, Barlow CE, Paffenbarger RS, Gibbons LW, Macera CA. Changes in physical fitness and all-cause mortality. *J Am Med Assoc* 1995; **273**: 1093–8.

15 Lissner L, Bengtsson C, Björkelund C, Wedel H. Physical activity levels and changes in relation to longevity. A prospective study of Swedish women. *Am J Epidemiol* 1996; **143**: 54–62.

16 Wannamethee G, Shaper AG, Walker M. Changes in physical activity, mortality, and incidence of coronary heart disease in older men. *Lancet* 1998; **351**: 1603–8.

17 Blair SN, Kohl HW, Paffenbarger RS, Clark DG, Cooper KH, Gibbons LW. Physical fitness and all-cause mortality. A prospective study of healthy men and women. *J Am Med Assoc* 1989; **262**: 2392–401.

17a Andersen LB, Schroll M, Saunamäki K, Kanstrup I-L, Hansen JF, Nielsen JR, Videbæk J. Redegørelse om fysisk aktivitet i fritiden. Copenhagen, Hjerteforeningen, 1999: 1–24.

18 Haapanen-Niemi N, Vuori I, Pasanen M. Public health burden of coronary heart disease risk factors among middle-aged and elderly men. *Prev Med* 1999; **28**: 343–8.

19 Booth FW, Gordon SE, Carlson CJ, Hamilton MT. Waging war on modern chronic diseases: primary prevention through exercise biology. *J Appl Physiol* 2000; **88**: 774–87.

20 Gillum RF, Mussolino ME, Ingram DD. Physical activity and stroke incidence in women and men. The NHANES 1 epidemiologic follow-up study. *Am J Epidemiol* 1996; **143**: 860–9.

21 Lee I-M, Paffenbarger RS. Physical activity and stroke incidence. The Harvard Alumni Study. *Stroke* 1998; **29**: 2049–54.

22 Lee CD, Blair SN, Jackson AS. Cardiorespiratory fitness, body composition, and all-cause and cardiovascular disease mortality in men. *Am J Clin Nutr* 1999; **69**: 373–80.

23 Lindenstrøm E, Boysen G, Nyboe J. Lifestyle factors and risk of cerebrovascular disease in women. The Copenhagen city heart study. *Stroke* 1993; **24**: 1468–72.

24 World Health Organization. Assessment of fracture risk and its application to screening for postmenopausal osteoporosis. *WHO Technical Report Series* No. 843. Geneva: WHO, 1994.

25 National Osteoporosis Foundation. Osteoporosis: review of the evidence for prevention, diagnosis, and treatment and cost-effectiveness analysis. Status report. *Osteoporos Int* 1998; 8: S1–S88.

26 Vuori I, Heinonen A. Sport and Bone. In: Drinkwater BL, ed. *Women in Sport*. Oxford: Blackwell Science, 2000: 280–300.

27 Dickerman RD, Pertusi R, Smith GH. The upper range of lumbar spine bone mineral density? An examination of the current world record holder in the squat lift. *Int J Sports Med* 2000; 21: 469–70.

28 Kannus P, Järvinen M, Sievänen H, Järvinen TAH, Oja P, Vuori I. Reduced bone mineral density in men with a previous femur fracture. *J Bone Min Res* 1994; 9: 1729–36.

29 Kannus P, Haapasalo H, Sankelo M, Sievänen H, Pasanen M, Heinonen A, Oja P, Vuori I. The effect of the starting age of physical activity on bone mass in the dominant arm of tennis and squash players. *Ann Intern Med* 1995; 123: 27–31.

30 Haapasalo H, Kannus P, Sievänen H, Pasanen M, Uusi-Rasi K, Heinonen A, Oja P, Vuori I. Effect of long-term unilateral activity on bone mineral density of female junior tennis players. *J Bone Min Res* 1998; 13: 310–9.

31 Bass S, Pearce G, Bradney M *et al.* Exercise before puberty may confer residual benefits in bone density in adulthood: studies in active prepubertal and retired female gymnasts. *J Bone Min Res* 1998; 13: 500–7.

32 Heinonen A, Kannus P, Sievänen H, Pasanen M, Oja P, Vuori I. Good maintenance of high-impact activity-induced bone gain by voluntary, unsupervised exercises: an 8-month follow-up of a randomized controlled trial. *J Bone Min Res* 1999; 14: 125–8.

33 Kontulainen S, Kannus P, Haapasalo H *et al.* Changes in bone mineral content with decreased training in competitive young adult tennis players and controls: a prospective 4-yr follow-up. *Med Sci Sports Exerc* 1999; 31: 646–52.

34 Kontulainen S, Kannus P, Haapasalo H, Sievänen H, Pasanen M, Heinonen A, Oja P, Vuori I. Good maintenance of exercise-induced bone gain with decreased training of female tennis and squash players: a prospective 5-year follow-up study of young and old starters and controls. *J Bone Min Res* 2001; 16: 195–201.

35 Karlsson MK, Johnell O, Obrant KJ. Is bone mineral density advantage maintained long-term in previous weight lifters? *Calcified Tissue Int* 1995; 57: 325–8.

36 Karlsson MK, Hasserius R, Obrant KJ. Bone mineral density in athletes during and after career: a comparison between loaded and unloaded skeletal regions. *Calcified Tissue Int* 1996; 59: 245–8.

37 Karlsson MK, Linden C, Karlsson C, Johnell O, Obrant K, Seeman E. Exercise during growth and bone mineral density and fractures in old age. *Lancet* 2000; 355: 469–70.

38 Wolff I, Van Croonenborg J, Kemper HCG, Kostense PJ, Twisk JWR. The effect of exercise training programs on bone mass: a meta-analysis of published controlled trials in pre- and postmenopausal women. *Osteoporos Int* 1999; 9: 1–12.

39 Wallace BA, Cumming RG. Systematic review of randomized trials of the effect of exercise on bone mass in pre- and postmenopausal women. *Calcified Tissue Int* 2000; 67: 10–8.

40 Leppälä J, Kannus P, Niemi S, Sievänen H, Vuori I, Järvinen M. An early-life femoral shaft fracture and bone mineral density at adulthood. *Osteoporos Int* 1999; 10: 337–42.

41 Iwamoto J, Takeda T, Otani T, Yabe Y. Effect of increased physical activity on bone mineral density in postmenopausal osteoporotic women. *Kei J Med* 1998; 47(3): 157–61.

42 Uusi-Rasi K, Sievänen H, Vuori I, Pasanen M, Heinonen A, Oja P. Associations of physical activity and calcium intake with bone mass and size in healthy women at different ages. *J Bone Min Res* 1998; 13: 133–42.

43 Haapasalo H, Kontulainen S, Sievänen H, Kannus P, Järvinen M, Vuori I. Exercise-induced bone gain is due to enlargement in bone size without a change in volumetric bone density: a peripheral quantitative computed topography study of the upper arms of male tennis players. *Bone* 2000; 27: 351–7.

44 Bennell KL, Malcolm SA, Wark JD, Brukner BD. Skeletal effects of menstrual disturbances in athletes. *Scand J Med Sci Sports* 1997; 7: 261–73.

45 Gibson JH, Harries M, Mitchell A, Godfrey A, Lunt M, Reeve J. Determinants of bone density and prevalence of osteopenia among female runners in their second to seventh decades of age. *Bone* 2000; 26: 591–8.

46 Ross PD, Santora A, Yates AJ. Epidemiology and consequences of osteoporotic fractures. In: Rosen CJ, Glowacki J, Bilezikian JP, eds. *The Aging Skeleton*. San Diego: Academic Press, 1999: 339–57.

47 Gregg EW, Pereira MA, Caspersen CJ. Physical activity, falls, and fractures among older adults: a review of the epidemiological evidence. *J Am Geriatr Soc* 2000; 48: 883–93.

48 Andersson GBJ. Epidemiology of low back pain. *Acta Orthop Scand* 1998; 69 (Suppl. 281): 28–31.

49 Von Korff M, Saunders K. The course of back pain in primary care. *Spine* 1996; 21: 2833–7.

50 Von Korff M, Dey RA, Cherkin GD, Barlow W. Back pain in primary care: outcomes at one year. *Spine* 1993; 18: 855–62.

51 Ont i ryggen, ont i nacken. En evidensbaserad kunskapssammanställning, Vol. 1–2. Stockholm: Statens Beredning För Medicinsk Utvärdering, 2000: 806.

52 Hilde G, BØK. Effect of exercise in the treatment of chronic low back pain. a systematic review, emphasising type and dose of exercise. *Phys Ther Rev* 1998; 3: 107–17.

53 Suni J. *Health-related fitness test battery for middle-aged adults with emphasis on musculoskeletal and motor tests.* Doctoral dissertation, University of Jyväskylä, Jyväskylä, Finland, 2000.

54 Van Tulder MW, Malmivaara A, Esmail R, Koes BW. Exercise therapy for low back pain. *Cochrane Database Syst Rev* 2000: 2: CD000335.

55 Vuori I. Dose–response of physical activity and low back pain, osteoarthritis and osteoporosis. *Med Sci Sports Exerc* 2001; 33: S551–S586.

56 Must A, Spadano J, Coakley EH, Field AE, Colditz G, Dietz WH. The disease burden associated with overweight and obesity. *J Am Med Assoc* 1999; 282: 1523–9.

57 Seidell JC, Visscher TLS, Hoogeveen RT. Overweight and obesity in the mortality rate data: current evidence and research issues. *Med Sci Sports Exerc* 1999; 31 (11 Suppl.): S597–S601.

58 Pi-Sunyer FX. Comorbidities of overweight and obesity: current evidence and research issues. *Med Sci Sports Exerc* 1999; 31 (11 Suppl.): S602–S608.

59 Wei M, Kampert JB, Barlow CE *et al.* Relationship between low cardiorespiratory fitness and mortality in normal-weight, overweight, and obese men. *J Am Med Assoc* 1999; 282: 1547–53.

60 Haapanen-Niemi N, Miilunpalo S, Pasanen M, Vuori I, Oja P, Malmberg J. Body mass index, physical inactivity and low level of physical fitness as determinants of all-cause and cardiovascular disease mortality — 16 year follow-up of middle-aged and elderly men and women. *Int J Obes* 2000; 24: 1465–74.

61 Hill JO, Melanson EL. Overview of the determinants of overweight and obesity: current evidence and research issues. *Med Sci Sports Exerc* 1999; 31 (11 Suppl.): S515–S521.

62 Jebb SA, Moore MS. Contribution of a sedentary lifestyle and inactivity to the etiology of overweight and obesity: current evidence and research issues. *Med Sci Sports Exerc* 1999; 31 (11 Suppl.): S534–S541.

63 Fogelholm M, Kukkonen-Harjula K. Does physical activity prevent weight gain — a systematic review. *Obesity Rev* 2000; 1: 95–111.

64 Ross R, Freeman JA, Janssen I. Exercise alone is an effective strategy for reducing obesity and related comorbidities. *Exerc Sport Sci Rev* 2000; 28(4): 165–70.

65 Grundy SM, Blackburn G, Higgins M, Lauer R, Perri MG, Ryan D. Physical activity in the prevention and treatment of obesity and its comorbidities: evidence report of independent panel to assess the role of physical activity in the treatment of obesity and its comorbidities. *Med Sci Sports Exerc* 1999; 31 (11 Suppl.): 1393–500.

66 Blair SN, Brodney S. Effects of physical inactivity and obesity on morbidity and mortality: current evidence and research issues. *Med Sci Sports Exerc* 1999; 31 (11 Suppl.): S646–S662.

67 West KM. *Epidemiology of Diabetes and its Vascular Lesions.* New York: Elsevier, 1978.

68 Wang JT, Ho LT, Tang KT, Wang LM, Chen Y-DI, Reaven GM. Effect of habitual physical activity on age-related glucose intolerance. *J Am Geriatr Soc* 1989; 37: 203–9.

69 Dela F, Larsen JJ, Mikines KJ, Plough T, Petersen LN, Galbo H. Insulin-stimulated muscle glucose clearance in patients with NIDDM. *Diabetes* 1995; 44: 1010–20.

69a Dela F. On the influence of physical training on glucose homeostasis: 1–41. The Copenhagen Muscle Research Center, Rigshospitalet, Copenhagen, 1996.

70 Dela F, Plough T, Handberg A, Petersen LN, Larsen JJ, Mikines KJ, Galbo H. Physical training increases muscle GLUT4 protein and mRNA in patients with NIDDM. *Diabetes* 1994; 43: 862–5.

71 Saltin B, Helge JW. Skeletmuskulaturens metaboliske kapacitet og sundhed. *Ugeskr Læger* 2000; 162: 2159–64.

72 Klausen K, Andersen LB, Pelle I. Adaptive changes in work capacity, skeletal muscle capillarization and enzyme levels during training and detraining. *Acta Physiol Scand* 1981; 113: 9–16.

73 Heinrich CH, Going SB, Pamenter RW, Perry CD, Boyden TW, Lohman TG. Bone mineral content of cyclically menstruating female resistance and endurance trained athletes. *Med Sci Sports Exerc* 1990; 22: 558–63.

74 Manson JE, Rimm EB, Stampfer MJ, Colditz GA, Willett WC, Krolewski AS *et al.* Physical activity and incidence of non-insulin-dependent diabetes mellitus in women. *Lancet* 1991; 338: 774–8.

75 World Health Organization — International Society of Hypertension Guidelines for the management of hypertension. *J Hypertension* 1999; 17: 151–83.

76 Van den Hoogen PCW, Feskens EJM, Nagelkerke NJD, Menotti Al Nissinen A, Kromhout D. The relation between blood pressure and mortality due to coronary heart disease among men in different parts of the world. *N Engl J Med* 2000; 342: 1–8.

77 Port S, Demer L, Jennrich R, Walter D, Garfinkel A. Systolic blood pressure and mortality. *Lancet* 2000; 355: 175–80.

78 Rayner M, Petersen S. *European Cardiovascular Disease Statistics 2000 Edition.* Oxford: British Heart Foundation, 2000.

79 Julius S, Majahalme S. The changing face of sympathetic overactivity in hypertension. *Ann Med* 2000; 32: 365–70.

80 Hagard RH. Physical activity in the prevention and treatment of hypertension in the obese. *Med Sci Sports Exerc* 1999; 31 (11 Suppl.): S624–S630.

81 Haapanen N, Miilunpalo S, Vuori I, Oja P, Pasanen M. Association of leisure time physical activity with the risk of coronary heart disease, hypertension and diabetes in middle-aged men and women. *Int J Epidemiol* 1997; 26: 739–47.

82 Wareham NJ, Wong M-Y, Hennings S, Mitchell J, Rennie K, Cruickshank K, Day NE. Quantifying the association between habitual energy expenditure and blood pressure. *Int J Epidemiol* 2000; **29**: 655–60.

83 Fagard RH. Physical activity in the prevention and treatment of hypertension in the obese. *Med Sci Sports Exerc* 1999; **31**: S624–S630.

84 Kelley GA. Aerobic exercise and resting blood pressure among women; a beta-analysis. *Prev Med* 1999; **28**: 264–85.

85 Kelley GA, Kelley KS. Progressive resistance exercise and resting blood pressure: a meta-analysis of randomized controlled trials. *Hypertension* 2000; **35**: 838–43.

86 Hagberg JM, Park J-J, Brown MD. The role of exercise training in the treatment of hypertension. An update. *Sports Med* 2000; **30**(3): 193–206.

87 Fagard RH. The influence of exercise intensity on the blood pressure response to dynamic physical training. *Med Sci Sports Exerc* 2001; **33**: S484–S492.

88 Kokkinos PF, Papademetriou V. Exercise and hypertension. *Coronary Artery Dis* 2000; **11**: 99–102.

89 Georgiades A, Sherwookd A, Gullette ECD, Babyak MA, Hinderliter A, Waugh R, Tweedy D, Craighead L, Bloomer R, Blumenthal JA. Effects of exercise and weight loss on mental stress-induced cardiovascular responses in individuals with high blood pressure. *Hypertension* 2000; **36**: 171–6.

90 Colditz GA, Cannuscio CC, Frazier AL. Physical activity and reduced risk of colon cancer: implications for prevention. *Cancer Causes Control* 1997; **8**: 649–67.

91 Burkitt DP. Epidemiology of cancer of the colon and rectum. *Cancer* 1971; **28**: 3–13.

92 Tran T, Medline A, Bruce W. Insulin promotion of colon tumors in rats. *Cancer Epidemiol Biomark Prev* 1996; **5**: 1013–5.

93 Thune I, Brenn T, Lund E, Gaard M. Physical activity and the risk of breast cancer. *N Engl J Med* 1997; **336**: 1269–75.

94 Oliveria SA, Kohl HW, Trichopoulos D, Blair SN. The association between cardiorespiratory fitness and prostate cancer. *Med Sci Sports Exerc* 1996; **28**: 97–104.

95 Polednak AP. College athletes, body size, and cancer mortality. *Cancer* 1976; **38**: 382–7.

96 Woods JA, Davis JM, Smith JA, Nieman DC. Exercise and cellular immune function. *Med Sci Sports Exerc* 1999; **31**: 57–66.

97 Mackinnon LT. Chronic exercise training effects on immune function. *Med Sci Sports Exerc* 2000; **32**: S369–S376.

98 Ross CE, Hayes D. Exercise and physiologic well-being in the community. *Am J Epidemiol* 1988; **127**: 762–71.

99 Stephens T. Physical activity and mental health in the United States and Canada: evidence from four population surveys. *Prev Med* 1988; **17**: 35–47.

100 Farmer ME, Locke BZ, Moscicki EK, Dannenberg AL, Larson DB, Radloff LS. Physical activity and depressive symptoms: the NHANES I epidemiologic follow-up study. *Am J Epidemiol* 1988; **128**: 1340–51.

101 Camacho TC, Roberts RE, Lazarus NB, Kaplan GA, Cohen RD. Physical activity and depression: evidence from the Alameda County Study. *Am J Epidemiol* 1991; **134**: 220–3.

102 Weyerer S. Physical inactivity and depression in the community: evidence from the Upper Bavarian Field Study. *Int J Sports Med* 1992; **13**: 492–6.

103 Fechner-Bates S, Coyne JC, Schwenk TL. The relationship of self-reported distress to depressive disorders and other psychopathology. *J Consult Clin Psyc* 1994; **62**: 550–9.

104 Simons CW, Birkimer JC. An exploration of factors predicting the effects of aerobic conditioning on mood state. *J Psychosom Res* 1988; **32**: 63–75.

105 Wilfley D, Kunce J. Differential physical effects of exercise. *J Couns Psych* 1986; **33**: 337–42.

106 Steptoe A, Edwards S, Moses J, Mathews A. The effects of exercise training on mood and perceived coping ability in anxious adults from the general population. *J Psychosom Res* 1989; **33**: 537–47.

107 Morgan WP, Roberts JA, Brand FR, Feinerman AD. Psychological effect of chronic physical activity. *Med Sci Sports* 1970; **2**: 213–7.

108 Martinsen EW, Medhus A, Sandvik L. Effects of aerobic exercise on depression: a controlled study. *Br Med J* 1985; **291**: 109.

109 Paffenbarger RS, Lee I-M, Leung RW. Physical activity and personal characteristics associated with depression and suicide in American college men. *Acta Psychiatr Scand Suppl* 1994; **377**: 16–22.

110 Cramer SR, Nieman DC, Lee JW. The effects of moderate exercise training on psychological well-being and mood state in women. *J Psychosom Res* 1991; **35**: 437–49.

111 King AC, Taylor CB, Haskell WL. Effects of differing intensities and formats of 12 months of exercise training on psychological outcomes in older adults. *Health Psychol* 1993; **12**: 292–300.

112 Morgan WP. Anxiety reduction following acute physical activity. *Psychiatr Ann* 1979; **9**: 36–45.

113 deVries HA. The tranquilizer effect of exercise: a critical review. *Physician Sportsmed* 1981; **9**: 47–55.

114 Ransford CP. A role for amines in the antidepressant effect of exercise: a review. *Med Sci Sports Exerc* 1982; **14**: 1–10.

115 Moore M. Endorphins and exercise: a puzzling relationship. *Physician Sportsmed* 1982; **10**: 111–4.

116 Kjær M. Epinephrine and some other hormonal responses to exercise in man. *Int J Sports Medicine* 1988; **9**: 1–48.

117 Hughes JR, Casal DC, Leon AS. Psychological effects of exercise: a randomized cross-over trial. *J Psychosom Res* 1986; **30**: 355–60.

118 Simons AD, McGowan CR, Epstein LH, Kupfer DJ, Robertson RJ. Exercise as a treatment for depression: an update. *Clin Psyc Rev* 1985; **5**: 553–68.

119 Mautalen CA, Oliveri B. Densitometric manifestations in age-related bone loss. In: Rosen CJ, Glowacki J, Bilezikian JP, eds. *The Aging Skeleton*. San Diego: Academic Press, 1999: 263–76.

120 Heinonen A. *Exercise as an osteogenic stimulus*. Academic dissertation, University of Jyväskylä, Jyväskylä, 1997.

121 Haskell WL. The benefits of regular exercise. In: Nieman DC, ed. *The Exercise Health Connection*. Champaign, IL: Human Kinetics, 1998: 301–9.

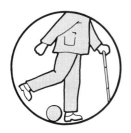

Chapter 3.3
Physical Activity in the Elderly

STEPHEN HARRIDGE & HARRI SUOMINEN

Classical reference

Fiatarone, M *et al.* Exercise training and nutritional supplementation for physical frailty in very elderly people. *N Engl J Med* 1994; **330**: 1169–1175.

This study was one of the first to focus on the adaptability to muscle strengthening exercise in the 'oldest old', the group of individuals where the largest relative population increases are to be seen in future years. Yet it is these individuals who are among society's most vulnerable. These have a high risk of falling and sustaining life-threatening fractures or at best a loss of independence as progressive declines in muscle strength and power mean that simple physical tasks become increasingly difficult and eventually impossible to perform.

In this study [1], Fiatarone and coworkers examined 100 nursing home residents in the USA who ranged in age from 72 to 98 years of age. They conducted a randomized, placebo-controlled trial which focused on the effects of 10 weeks of progressive resistance exercise (strength training), combined with a caloric boosting nutritional supplement. Subjects were randomly assigned to either strength training, strength training and nutritional supplementation, nutritional supplementation only, or control groups. Those that underwent strength training exercised the hip and knee extensors 3 days per week, at 80% of the amount of weight that could be lifted once (1 RM). Muscle strength was tested weekly and the training load adjusted accordingly. The nutritional supplement was a mixture of carbohydrate, fat and protein and was designed to increase caloric intake by 20%.

The results of the study showed that muscle strength as determined by the 1 RM increased by on average 113% in those that undertook the strength training exercise ($P < 0.001$), a value similar to that which is achieved by young subjects undergoing similar training (Fig. 3.3.1). The nutritional supplement was without significant effect.

The authors concluded that even in very frail individuals high-resistance training is a feasible and effective means of counteracting muscle weakness in older people. In practical functional terms, gait velocity and stair climbing power also improved in the exercisers compared with the non-exercisers. In general agreement with these researchers an earlier, non-controlled, study on 10 90-year-old men and women [2], where strength training increased thigh cross-sectional area by on average 9%, quadriceps size as determined

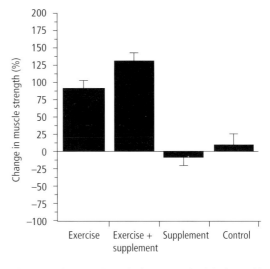

Fig. 3.3.1 The mean change in the amount of weight that could be lifted once (1-RM) by the hip and knee extensor muscles following 10 weeks of strength training in frail elderly people aged 72–98 years of age. (From [1].)

337

by CT scanning also showed a tendency (2.7%) to increase.

This article and subsequent studies have shown the importance of resistance-type exercise training for improving muscle mass and function in the very oldest of individuals. It is recommended that exercise that involves the use of relatively large muscle forces, which may in absolute terms be very light, be encouraged as part of any exercise program developed for older people.

Introduction

Demographic evidence suggests that the developed world is faced with an increasingly aged population. In particular, it is in the 'oldest old' where the greatest increase will be seen. For example, in the countries of Western Europe the percentage of the total population over the age of 80 years is predicted to rise from between 2.6 and 4.9% in 1997 to 4.2–8.1% in 2025 [3]. This increased life expectancy relates, in part, to improvements in medicine and nutrition, but there is no guarantee that the quality of these extra years will be high, in other words free from illness and disease. It is now becoming clear that higher levels of physical activity may help to improve the quality of later life through improved levels of fitness and general health. It is the aim of this chapter to outline briefly the effects the aging process has on the major systems of the body relating to physical activity, how the older person may respond to a bout of exercise and how elderly people may adapt to exercise training and benefit from increased levels of physical activity.

What is aging?

It is clear that the functioning of many of the systems of the body declines as we get older and this is evident not only in athletic and sports performance, but also in the ability to perform simple physical tasks needed for everyday living. Whilst it is beyond the scope of this chapter to enter in to a full discussion into the many theories of aging [4], it is important to briefly discuss what we actually mean by the term 'aging' when interpreting the age-related studies on human physical performance.

The term 'aging' may imply development, because in the strictest sense of the word from the day we are conceived we are all in fact 'aging'. Senescence on the other hand implies deteriorative changes which occur during the adult period of life and underlie an increasing vulnerability to challenges, a vulnerability which ultimately impairs the ability of an organism to survive. Indeed, Holliday [4] defined aging as the 'eventual breakdown of tissue maintenance'. Rowe and Kahn [5] proposed a concept of 'successful aging'. This is characterized by a low risk of disease and disease-related disability, high mental and physical function and active engagement with life. The challenge for those interested in the study of aging is therefore to be able to differentiate between the changes in physiologic function which may be due simply to getting older and those which may be as a result of illness or disease. The study of healthy older individuals, excluding those with underlying disease etc., is one way in which the effects of the aging process have been studied in humans. However, a major limitation with this approach is that completely healthy older people do not reflect society at large, as such people, free from age-associated diseases, are actually an elite minority and not the norm.

A further complication is that some 'diseases' might be considered to be an integral part of the aging process. In other words the boundary between that which constitutes a pathophysiologic condition and that which is part of the aging process is often arbitrarily set. The loss of bone mineral density and osteoporosis is one example of this.

In this chapter an objective examination of the effects of aging in relation to physical activity will draw upon both cross-sectional and longitudinal studies. Neither of these provide completely perfect models when considering the question of aging. In cross-sectional studies, where comparisons are made between people of different ages at a given point in time, any differences observed may not necessarily reflect the effects of aging on a particular physiologic characteristic. For example, some of the problems of making comparisons between a group of 80-year-old men and a group of 20-year-old men include the fact that the 80-year-old men were born and grew up in conditions where the health care systems were less well developed, their nutritional status generally poorer and the socioeconomic environment very different. In other words, the present-day younger men may not be an accurate reflection of how present-day 80-year-old men were 60 years ago. Furthermore, with cross-sectional studies the question of selective mortality must be considered. Those individuals who have survived to later life, although possibly very frail, may well actually represent the elite of their generation and thus are probably not going to be equally represented in a random group of young individuals.

Longitudinal studies, where the same group of individuals are followed throughout a prolonged period of time, overcome some of the problems of cross-sectional studies. However, these studies are more difficult to perform in terms of time and resources needed and are also not without problems of interpretation. Changes in the lifestyle of the individuals under study may occur within the study period, whilst changes in research personnel and equipment during a 20-year study may also serve to influence data collection and interpretation.

Physical activity, exercise and sport

There are important distinctions between the terms 'physical activity' and 'exercise'. Physical activity may be considered as any body movement produced by skeletal muscle that results in energy expenditure, and as such includes dressing, walking to the shops and gardening as well as participating in sport or attending an aerobics class. Exercise on the other hand might be considered one subset of physical activity defined as planned, structured and repetitive movement aimed at improving or maintaining one or more components of fitness. Participation in exercise involving a competitive element might be considered as sporting activity and as such is a further subdivision of physical activity [6]. The terminology has particular relevance for older people, many of whom may benefit from increasing their overall levels of physical activity even though this may not necessarily be considered preplanned exercise or participation in sport (Table 3.3.1).

Epidemiology of exercise, health and aging

A wide perspective to exercise, health and aging is provided by studies investigating the relationships between physical activity, longevity and morbidity. One of the first well-controlled studies in the area was published by Paffenbarger *et al.*[7]. The authors examined physical activity levels and other lifestyle characteristics of about 17 000 Harvard alumni, aged 35–74 years, over a 12–16-year period. Exercise, reported as walking, stair climbing and participation in sport, was

inversely related to total mortality and to death due to cardiovascular and respiratory causes. Death rates were one-quarter to one-third lower among those expending 2000 or more kcal during exercise per week than among less active men. Mortality rates of the physically active were significantly lower even after controlling for the effects of smoking, body weight, hypertension and early parental death. Depending on the age and activity perspective, the number of additional years attributable to exercise was 1–3 years.

In another well-controlled study, Sarna *et al.* [8] examined the life expectancy of the athletes representing Finland in international competitions during 1920–65. The athletes were compared with a reference cohort of healthy men matched on age and area of residence. The mean life expectancy of long-distance runners and cross-country skiers was more than 5 years longer than that of the referents (Fig. 3.3.2). The increased life expectancy of the endurance athletes was mainly explained by decreased cardiovascular mortality (odds ratio 0.49 compared to referents). No differences between the groups were observed for maximum lifespan. The authors concluded that the active and healthy lifestyle adopted by the athletes prevented the premature deaths rather than extended the possibly genetically determined maximum lifespan.

Furthermore, a 10-year longitudinal study carried out in Finland [9] showed that the survival functions of

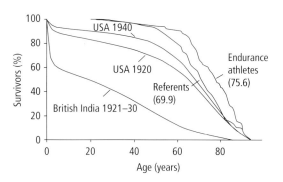

Fig. 3.3.2 Survival curves with mean life expectancies in endurance athletes and referents adjusted by occupational group. The figure also shows examples of population survival curves becoming more rectangular in the developed world. (Data from [8,70,71].)

Table 3.3.1 Recommended quantity and quality of exercise for older adults. Adapted from [72,73].

Variable	Cardiovascular system	Skeletal muscle	Bone	Connective tissue
Frequency of training	3–5 days/week	2–3 days a week		
Duration of training	20–60 min of continuous or intermittent (minimum of 10-min bouts accumulated throughout the day)	<60 min		
Intensity of training	40–50% of maximum $\dot{V}O_2$ or heart rate reserve or 55–65% of maximum heart rate. Higher intensities are possible for healthy elderly persons, but medically supervised exercise testing and individual tailoring is imperative	One set of 8–10 exercises with 10–15 repetitions for the major muscle groups		
Mode of activity	Large muscle rhythmic aerobic forms of exercise such as walking, running, swimming, cycling, and dancing added into individual's habitual lifestyle	Resistance training with equipment, calisthenics and other types of resistive activities	Resistance training as above to maintain or increase bone strength and dynamic balance and to prevent osteoporotic fractures	Aerobic and resistance training as above to strengthen the tendons, ligaments, and other connective tissue structures; static and/or dynamic stretching of major muscle groups included in the exercise programs to increase and maintain range of motion
Overall aim	To counteract the changes with aging in the cardiovascular system and related disease risk factors and to benefit the quantity and quality of life	To improve and maintain muscle strength and power and to increase functional capacity		

men and women, aged 60–70 years at baseline, were significantly better among those who reported walking more than 10 km per week than among their more sedentary counterparts. The effect of exercise remained significant after controlling for self-rated health.

In a way, these examples further point out the importance of the increased population survival which has been obvious in the developed world (Fig. 3.3.2) and which was briefly described above. It might be suggested that athletes and other physically active people are forerunners, where increased longevity is manifested as an increased number of healthy and active extra years rather than of increasing disability.

Sports performance with increasing age

Elite veteran athletes are, by definition, not representative of the aged population, but nevertheless provide a valuable insight into the potential of the human body to cope with the aging process and give an indication of the limits to which an aging population might aspire. These performers have often maintained high levels of physical training throughout their lives, but importantly still show marked declines in performance over time with increasing age. This simple observation tells us that the decline in physical performance is not simply due to a disuse phenomenon. Figure 3.3.3 shows the world records for three track athletic events: the 100-m sprint, the 800 m and the 10 000 m. In all three events in both men and women, the decline in performance occurs in an almost linear manner until around 70–75 years, whereupon the decline in performance begins to accelerate. The extent to which this reflects a population effect is unclear, as participation in masters or veterans sports is on the increase. As more competitors continue to take part in veterans athletics it is likely that the records shown in Fig. 3.3.3, particularly in the older age groups, will show considerable improvements.

Indeed, it has been argued that even frail elderly people are in some ways like athletes, in that both groups of people must often perform at the limits of their physical capability, the athlete to win medals and break records, the frail older person to rise from a chair or walk home from the shops carrying heavy bags [10].

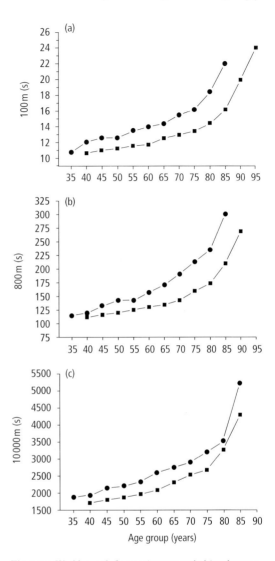

Fig. 3.3.3 World records for men (square symbols) and women (round symbols) for the 100 m (a), 800 m (b) and 10 000 m (c) track events as at 1st September 1999. Data from the World Veterans Athletic Association.

The effects of aging on the body

Body composition

Aging is associated with alterations in body composition such that there is an increase in fat mass and a decrease in muscle mass. This results in whole-body mass remaining relatively unchanged. Tzankoff and Norris [11] demonstrated using creatinine excretion as a marker of total body protein content that, in men, fat-free body mass declines progressively from 40 to 80 years of age at a rate equating to ~5% per decade. In a 5-year longitudinal study in Finland, the change in lean body mass (estimated by bioimpedance) between 75 and 80 years of age was 2.4% in men and 3.1% in women, and between 80 and 85 only 0.5% in men but 2.8% in women [12].

Aging results in a decrease in resting energy expenditure primarily as a consequence of this decline in muscle mass. Fat distribution also alters with aging, such that truncal and intra-abdominal fat content increase. In addition, the reference criteria of stature changes with age. Because of increasing kyphosis, compression of intervertebral discs and even vertebral collapse, stature has usually decreased 1–2 cm by the age of 60 years, with an accelerating decrease thereafter. These important factors need to be considered when physiologic data such as muscle strength or maximal oxygen consumption are normalized to anatomic measures such as body mass.

Skeletal muscle

Strength and power loss

Skeletal muscle is the largest organ in the body and has numerous functions most of which are impaired as a result of the aging process. Its prime role is to produce force and generate movement. It generates power during movement and also acts to brake movement. The force-generating ability of a muscle is primarily determined by its physiologic cross-sectional area. Measures of muscle strength made under isometric (static) conditions have shown that in both large and small muscles, in both men and women, there is a reduction in strength with increasing age which begins to become evident in the sixth decade [13]. Cross-sectional data on the knee extensor muscles of healthy older people aged 65–85 years imply that this decline occurs at a rate of about 1–2% per year (of a 77-year-old's value) [14]. These data are generally confirmed by the results of recent longitudinal studies. The decline in muscle strength is most closely associated with a reduction in muscle cross-sectional area. However, it is clear that not only does a loss of muscle mass contribute to the decline in strength, there is also a further loss of strength such that there is a reduction in force per unit

area. This can be attributed, in part, to the fact that with increasing age skeletal muscle is encroached by fat and connective tissue. This leads to an overestimate of the actual contractile material within a given anatomic area of muscle.

Recently, evidence from studies on the adductor pollicis muscle suggests that a sudden loss of specific force occurs in women at the time of the onset of the menopause [15]. In this cross-sectional study, this phenomenon was not observed in women taking estrogen and progesterone supplements (hormone replacement therapy, HRT). The mechanisms by which this should occur are not clear. However, the general findings of this study are supported by a longitudinal study on postmenopausal women, in which 6 months of HRT increased adductor pollicis specific force by 12% [16].

A reduction in voluntary strength with increasing age could also be due to an inability of older people to recruit and optimally fire motor units during a maximal voluntary contraction. It remains unclear as to whether or not such a limitation is responsible for a decline in specific force, at least in healthy older people and whether there may be differences depending upon the muscle group tested.

The ability to generate explosive power is a characteristic of muscle which has been closely related to the ability to perform simple functional tasks [17]. Muscle power, the product of force of contraction and speed of movement, has been shown to decline at a greater rate than the decline in isometric force muscle under some testing situations. One explanation for this phenomenon is that when faced with a given resistance or inertia, such as body mass during a vertical jump, the forces required to overcome this load represent a greater proportion of a weaker elderly person's maximum force-generating capacity. Because of the nature of the force–velocity relation of skeletal muscle, the weaker older muscle has to contract more slowly to produce these forces. This results in a less optimum speed for power generation.

A further contributory factor in the decline in muscle power with increasing age could be a change in muscle composition. Muscle fibers are characterized by three types of molecular motor allowing them to be classified into MHC-I, MHC-IIa and MHC-IIx isoform-expressing fibers. Using traditional ATPase histochemistry, these equate to type I, type IIa and type IIb fibers. Recent technical developments have allowed experiments to be performed on chemically skinned single muscle fibers obtained from a needle biopsy sample of muscle. Bottinelli *et al.* [18] confirmed the results of studies on animal muscle by showing that human fibers which expressed the MHC-I isoform were slower to shorten, generated slightly less force per unit area and generated approximately one-third of the power of the MHC-IIa fibers and one-fifth of that generated by the MHC-IIx fibers. At the whole-muscle level, Harridge *et al.* [19] reported an association between the amount of fast myosin MHC-II in the soleus and gastrocnemius muscles and the ability to generate electrically evoked plantar flexor torque at high speeds in older men. It is thus clear that a change in muscle fiber myosin composition could potentially have a dramatic effect on whole-muscle power output in older people. In a study in which whole sections of the vastus lateralis obtained from cadavers were examined, Lexell *et al.* [20] reported no effect of age on the relative distribution of type I and type II fibers, although in agreement with other needle biopsy studies an atrophy of type II fibers in later life was observed. Type II fiber atrophy would itself, however, lead to less of a whole muscle being occupied by fast myosin molecules. Recently though, more sensitive electrophoretic techniques have shown that muscles from older people have relatively more fibers which express more than one MHC isoform [21]. The increased number of these 'hybrid' fibers is perhaps indicative of an ongoing transformation process which might be suggested by the results of neurophysiologic studies which suggest that the larger fast-twitch motor units are preferentially lost in old age.

In recent studies of single muscle human fibers obtained from young and older individuals Larsson *et al.* [22] reported both a lower specific force and maximum shortening velocity in fibers expressing the MHC-I isoform if they originated from an older muscle. This suggests a fundamental age-related alteration in the way molecular motors, the cross-bridges which drive muscle contraction, behave in old age.

The functional consequences for older people of losing muscle strength and power are important. Physical tasks ultimately require the generation of certain muscle forces and power outputs [17]. With

diminishing strength and power, the relative percentage of an older person's maximum capability which has to be used to perform these tasks increases. With a progressive decline in muscle function the margin for safety becomes eroded until tasks become more difficult and eventually impossible to perform [10]. This may be exacerbated in thin elderly people in poorly heated accommodation where a cold muscle will further reduce power-generating potential. This in turn increases the already elevated risk of falling. The cascade of detrimental effects that a loss of muscle mass has for an older person is summarized in Fig. 3.3.4.

Why is muscle mass lost in old age?

In addition to its mechanical function muscle plays other roles, including that of a dynamic metabolic store, a generator of heat [23] and a source of protective padding. These other roles are also impaired as a result of the aging process and these changes relate principally, although not exclusively, to the loss of muscle mass, a process recently termed 'sarcopenia'. The loss of muscle mass is associated with a reduced rate of muscle protein synthesis [24]. At the anatomic level however, it appears that the main reason for the loss of muscle mass is a loss of motor units (the muscle fibers and the motoneurons which innervate them) [20]. The remaining motor units appear to be larger in older muscle as many, but not all, of the abandoned fibers from dying units are taken up by those remaining motor units through a process of collateral sprouting. The mechanism for such a loss of motor units remains unknown and remains one of the critical issues to be resolved in the study of aging muscle. It is possible that such changes are of both neuro- and myogenic origin.

Muscle damage

Anecdotal evidence has long suggested that as they approach the end of their careers sportsmen and women acquire injuries more easily, and once sustained, injuries take longer to heal. Although difficult to study in humans, there is evidence from animal experiments which suggest that aging may be associated with a slower repair process following muscle injury. Brooks and Faulkner [25] developed a method for evoking controlled eccentric muscle lengthening contractions of anesthetized rats. Eccentric exercise causes damage

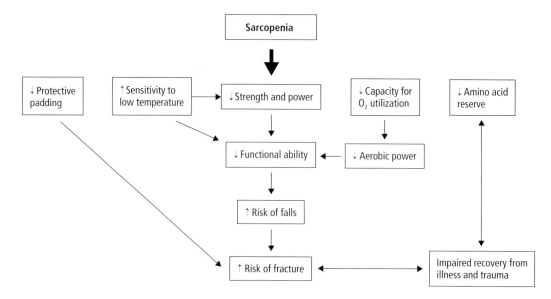

Fig. 3.3.4 This flow diagram illustrates a cascade of effects that a loss of muscle mass (sarcopenia) may have for an older person.

to muscles. In young animals they reported that following this procedure it took 18 days for isometric force to recover to the pre-exercise level. When a similar protocol was performed on aged animals, force failed to recover to the pre-exercise level. In a second important study, Carlson and Faulkner [26] reported that if a muscle from an old animal was transplanted into a young animal then that muscle would take on the properties of the muscles of the young host. However, if a muscle from a young animal was transplanted into an old host then the implanted muscle failed to regain its young characteristics. These two experiments provide important evidence for an impairment in the repair process of aged muscle and that there might well be both local and systemic factors that could contribute to this phenomenon. The role of locally produced growth factors such as insulin-like growth factor I (IGF-I) and their interaction with the satellite cells of the muscle fiber are likely to be important factors involved in the repair process.

Cardiovascular and respiratory systems

The delivery of O_2 to and the removal of the end product of metabolism (CO_2) from the working muscles are prime functions of the pulmonary and cardiovascular systems. Maximal oxygen uptake ($\dot{V}O_{2\,max}$) or maximal

aerobic power is the recognized measure of aerobic fitness and represents the maximum ability of the body to utilize O_2. Both cross-sectional and longitudinal studies have demonstrated a decline in $\dot{V}O_{2\,max}$ with increasing age. When data are expressed in absolute terms (i.e. L/min), this decline corresponds to a rate of about 10% per decade from the late twenties [27]. A significant decline in aerobic power is also observed when $\dot{V}O_{2\,max}$ is normalized to body mass (mL/kg/min). The contributions of different mechanisms to this phenomenon are not completely clear.

There are a number of changes in both the cardiovascular and pulmonary systems which could contribute. In terms of the respiratory system, the vital capacity of the lungs, lung power, forced expiratory volume in 1 s (FEV_1) and maximal voluntary ventilation are all reduced with age. These changes relate to changes in lung and chest wall function resulting from decreased lung elastic recoil, increased chest wall stiffness and decreased respiratory muscle strength. Due to the high prevalence of heart disease in the elderly population it has been somewhat difficult to determine the effects of aging on the cardiovascular system. At rest, overall cardiac function in most older people free from heart disease is adequate to meet the body's circulatory requirements. During submaximal exercise the

O_2 cost is similar between young and old subjects. During exercise at exhaustion, however, $\dot{V}O_{2\,max}$ is directly related to maximum cardiac output and with increasing age maximum cardiac output declines. This phenomenon is due almost entirely to a reduction in maximum heart rate, which is apparently brought about by a decreased responsiveness to β-adrenergic stimulation. Stroke volume does not show a dramatic decline with age in either men or women. Indeed during submaximal exercise cardiac output may be maintained in older people through an increased reliance on the Frank–Starling mechanism, namely the increased contractility conferred by a greater stretching of the ventricles prior to systole.

It has been suggested that the 50% decline in $\dot{V}O_{2\,max}$ between the ages of 20 and 80 years is approximately 30% attributable to a decline in cardiac output and 20% to a decreased O_2 utilization, directly relating to the decreased muscle. For when $\dot{V}O_{2\,max}$ is normalized to muscle mass and not to whole-body mass the age-related decline is significantly diminished [28].

The functional implications of a reduction in $\dot{V}O_{2\,max}$ are, in some senses, similar to that which occur in terms of strength and power. Namely, that to perform a given physical task will require a certain O_2 cost. In older people a given O_2 consumption represents a greater proportion of $\dot{V}O_{2\,max}$ (their maximum ability) and therefore represents a higher relative intensity. Furthermore, this situation may be exacerbated as the absolute cost of some activities may increase with age, for example the increased energy cost of walking may be explained by the shortening of stride length as age increases.

Bone

The usual aging pattern of the skeleton involves the gain of peak bone mass during growth, a plateau in adulthood, and bone loss during aging (Fig. 3.3.5). Bone tissue is renewed throughout life by organized bone cell activities such as osteoclastic bone resorption and osteoblastic bone formation. Bone modeling, which is particularly active during growth, improves bone strength by adding mass and changing the shape and geometry of bone. Remodeling, on the other hand, provides a mechanism for maintaining bone mass and structure in the adult skeleton by replacing the damaged and degraded tissue with new bone tissue. With aging and osteoporosis, however, the remodeling tends to remain uncoupled, in that packets of bone removed during resorption are not completely replaced during formation resulting in a net loss of bone.

Bone mass and structural integrity start to decline

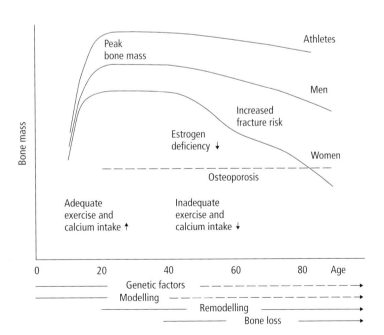

Fig. 3.3.5 Schematic presentation of age-related changes in bone mass and associated factors.

after the age of 35–40 years, the changes becoming more obvious around 50 years of age, particularly in trabecular bone during the female menopause [29]. Higher bone loss in women compared with men also occurs in the older age groups [30], which makes older women more likely to have osteoporotic bone mineral density (BMD) values. It has been estimated that women lose on average about 50% of their trabecular and 30% of their cortical bone mass during their lives, the corresponding figures for men being 30% and 20% [29]. Bone loss in early menopause results in an increased risk of fractures of the vertebrae and distal radius, while osteoporosis in older persons, which also involves cortical structures, is manifested mainly by hip and vertebral fractures. As such, the association between BMD and fracture risk is similar in men and women [30], but due to the greater number of older women and their lower bone mass, osteoporosis appears as a major public health problem for women.

Although genetic factors largely determine the development of bone mass, several external factors such as disuse or, conversely, increased physical activity, calcium nutrition and hormonal factors may significantly modify the bone modeling and remodeling processes. There is evidence from both animal and human studies that bone mass and mechanical competence is achieved and maintained by homeostatic mechanisms which adjust bone architecture to control the strains produced by mechanical load and functional activity and perceived by osteocytes and bone-lining cells. A widespread failure of these mechanisms occurs with postmenopausal osteoporosis which is characterized by an increased bone resorption and a decline in bone strength associated with the absence of estrogen. According to recent findings, estrogen may alter the mechanosensory set point for skeletal adaptation [31] and play a key role in bone loss in elderly men as well [32].

Connective tissue

In addition to the loss of the ability to develop force, musculoskeletal aging is characterized by an increase in the stiffness of movements. Most of the stiffness affecting the movements resides in the soft connective tissues of muscles, tendons and joint capsules. Connective tissue is instantly involved with both active and passive functions of force transmission in muscles and tendons, thus providing a potentially unique environment for studying the accommodation of the extracellular matrix to alterations such as muscle atrophy during aging and hypertrophy after resistance training.

The major macromolecule of soft connective tissues is collagen which represents about one-third of all protein in tissues and over 80% of the dry weight in tissues such as tendon. Although the concentration of collagen in skeletal muscle is much lower (less than 10%), the collagenous matrix plays an important role in the alignment of muscle fibers, providing structural support and strength, storing elastic energy during stretching, and participating in muscle remodeling during growth and regeneration. Of the 19 distinct collagen types found so far, types I, III, IV and V are the most abundant in skeletal muscle [33].

In the human body, the total amount of collagen increases from about 0.5 kg at the age of 1 year to 3–4 kg in adulthood and middle age. Collagen accumulation is accompanied by decreased collagen turnover, particularly during the growth period. With maturation, the area and diameter of collagen fibrils and the content of pyridinoline and sugar-derived pentosidine cross-links are increased while the number of fibroblasts is decreased in tendons [34,35]. There is also an increase in muscle collagen content and a decrease in the activity of the enzymes of collagen biosynthesis with age [36]. Animal experiments have shown that the relative proportion of collagen and pyridinoline cross-links increases up into old age, particularly in slow postural muscles such as the soleus, where the concentration of all major collagen types is generally higher than in muscles containing mainly fast-twitch fibers [36,37]. The ratio of type I to type III collagen may also increase with aging [36]. Increased accumulation of collagen and fibrosis of skeletal muscle with age is not the result of increased collagen gene expression, but is most likely due to an impaired degradation [38].

The mechanical performance of tissues such as muscles, tendons, ligaments and skin is clearly improved by strengthening of the collagen fibers during growth. In older age, however, the stiffening of collagen matrix, wasting of other proteins, and finally the deterioration of collagen fibers as well, make the tissues more brittle and vulnerable to mechanical stress. Whilst the age-related increase in muscle stiffness and decrease in the viscous and plastic properties is not, as such, detrimental to the transfer of muscular force, increased passive resistance of the connective tissue structures, particularly when occurring in the antagonistic muscles, may act against rapid elongation and therefore also against rotation of joints in old age. The experiments in old rats suggest that increased flexor muscle stiffness during extension is not due to a reflex response, but depends chiefly on overgrowth of non-elastic connective tissue replacing degenerated active muscle fibers [39].

Endocrine system

Aging is associated with many changes in endocrine function and a number of these changes are important with regard to physical activity. During growth and development an important role is played by growth hormone (GH) which is secreted by the anterior pituitary gland. The secretion of this hormone falls with increasing age. The fall in growth hormone secretion is particularly marked around 40 years and occurs at approximately 14% per decade [40]. The decrement in growth hormone secretion has been linked to decreases in protein synthesis and increases in adiposity. The major mediator of its muscle-building actions is through the synthesis of insulin-like growth factor I (IGF-I). GH stimulates the synthesis of IGF-I in the liver. Circulating IGF-I levels are also decreased in older people. Administration of recombinant GH to chronically GH-deficient young adults has been shown to have some benefits for muscle mass and function. This led to the suggestion that frail older people may benefit from it as an anabolic agent, in addition to its use as an anticatabolic agent in patients undergoing surgery. The results regarding its efficacy remain inconclusive. However, in one study in healthy older men, no additional benefit in muscle strength was observed when treatment with recombinant growth hormone was added to strength training [41].

With aging there are changes in both the male and female sex hormones which may alter muscle function. In men, serum testosterone levels fall with increasing age and in one study this has been correlated with the decline in muscle strength [42]. The administration of testosterone can increase circulating levels to values

comparable with those found in young men and this may have an effect of increasing muscle protein synthesis and muscle strength [43]. In women, as mentioned earlier, changes in estrogen and progesterone levels which occur at the time of the menopause appear to be associated with a loss in specific strength [15,16].

Another important change in endocrine function that occurs in aging and which has relevance for physical activity is the decreased ability of a high proportion of men and women over 65 years to maintain glucose homeostasis. This is through both alterations in insulin action and defects in carbohydrate metabolism. Type II, or adult onset, diabetes is characterized by a decrease in insulin resistance, resulting in increased circulating levels of glucose in spite of elevated insulin levels. The increased glucose concentrations are detrimental to number of organs and to the central nervous system. There is now good evidence to suggest that exercise can play an important role in the prevention of diabetes, by enhancing the transport of glucose into muscle cells during contraction.

Adaptability of older people to exercise

Cross-sectional perspective

In Fig. 3.3.3 the decline in sports performance that occurs with increasing age was described in terms of changes in world record performances. These athletes represent a highly elite population of individuals, some of whom have continued in competition since adulthood, whilst others are those who have come into a sport as a master or veteran competitor. Physiologic analysis in the laboratory of these athletes reveals that as a general rule, and as with their performance or competition data, there is a decline in a number of laboratory-based physiologic parameters. Nevertheless, it must be remembered that, although in decline, in absolute terms these individuals are considerably superior when compared with their non-active age-matched counterparts.

Strength and power

In an important study, Klitgaard *et al.* [44] investigated muscle function and composition in four groups of men aged 69 years, who had undertaken different types of physical training (swimming, endurance running, weight-lifting) over the previous 6 years and compared them with non-active men of a similar age and a group of young men who were also non-trained. They reported that among the older subjects the size and strength of the knee extensor muscles was greatest in those older men who had been strength training and that their strength values were actually similar to those of the non-trained young men (Fig. 3.3.6). In a similar study Sipilä *et al.* [45] studied 82 Finnish master athletes and confirmed that this (as well as other major muscle groups) group was stronger in weight lifters when compared with non-trained and endurance-trained individuals. In addition, Harridge *et al.* [46] reported that although having a high level of aerobic power (35.6–46.8 mL/kg/min in those aged 70–76 years), lifelong orienteering athletes of up to 95 years of age were no stronger than those of non-active individuals. These data suggest that for the maintenance of muscle strength, exercise which involves high muscle forces is of critical importance.

The explanation for the superior muscle function described for strength and power athletes appears to lie in a larger muscle mass, relatively greater type II muscle fiber area [44] and an apparent maintenance of sarcoplasmic reticulum function [47].

Aerobic power

As with muscle strength and power, it is clear that master athletes have $\dot{V}_{O_2\,max}$ values considerably higher than those of non-active individuals. Saltin [48] reported that inactive and still active elite orienteers differed in their $\dot{V}_{O_2\,max}$ values, but not the rates of decline (about 10% per decade). Endurance training however, does not appear to affect the decline in maximum heart rate. Cardiac output is better maintained in these individuals through increased stroke volume and they appear to retain a greater peripheral vasodilatory response. At the level of skeletal muscle it is unclear as to whether there is an age-related effect on the ability of muscle to utilize O_2. This uncertainty arises because in old as well as young subjects muscle capillary density and oxidative enzyme levels are highly sensitive to activity levels. Indeed, in a study by Coggan *et al.* [49], which compared master athletes

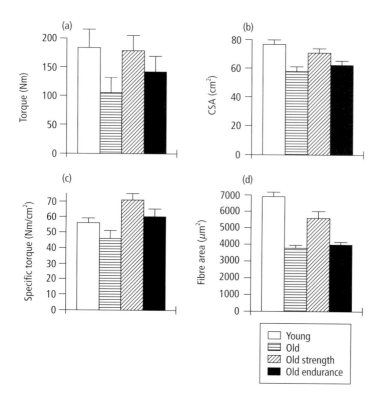

Fig. 3.3.6 Muscle strength (a), size (b), torque per unit area (c) and the size of type II muscle fibers (d) in different populations of older men aged 70 years (strength trained, running endurance trained, non-active) and a group of non-active young men. (Data from [47].) These cross-sectional data highlight the likely effects of different training regimens on muscle size and strength and emphasize the need for resistance-type exercise for maintaining muscle mass and strength. For clarity endurance swimmers are not shown.

with young runners matched for amount and absolute training intensity, the muscle biopsies from the older athletes were found to have higher oxidative enzyme activities and capillary/fiber ratios than their younger counterparts.

Bone

It is well known that if bones are not subjected to mechanical load, as happens with extreme forms of physical inactivity, reduced mass and strength are readily observed. Prolonged bed rest and limb immobilization may result in an average bone loss of 1–2% per week in trabecular bone sites such as the calcaneus [50]. Reversal of the bone loss is poor, though substantial individual differences may be observed.

The evidence in human studies supporting an association between increased physical exercise and bone mass first came from studies of athletes. The top curve outlined in Fig. 3.3.5 is warranted by the results of numerous cross-sectional and some longitudinal observational studies which show that athletes from various sports, especially from strength and power events, achieve and preserve superior bone mass compared to their non-athletic counterparts. In elderly males, the differences in BMD in the loaded bone sites and in the dominant/non-dominant bone comparisons in unilateral sports have been in the order of 10–20% [51]. Studies in elderly female athletes have, however, been fewer and shown less pronounced differences, probably because of their less intensive exercise habits and the greater role of body weight and fat mass as determinants of BMD.

Connective tissue

As with bones, immobilization deteriorates the soft connective tissue structures thus precipitating the reduction of their mechanical competence with aging. In skeletal muscle, immobilization in a shortened position results in a loss of serial sarcomeres and an increase in the proportion of collagen, less extensible collagen fibers, and an increased stiffness [52]. Such an immobilization is also accompanied by decreased collagen biosynthesis in muscle and tendon [33].

One of the first cross-sectional studies to suggest a responsiveness of human muscle collagen to physical training was reported by Suominen and Heikkinen [53] who found an increased prolyl 4-hydroxylase ac-

tivity (PH) in the vastus lateralis in middle-aged and elderly male endurance-trained athletes when compared to sedentary controls. The trained and untrained men also showed differences in 'non-loaded' connective tissue, the athletes having higher values in skin thickness, stiffness and elastic efficiency [54]. In subsequent studies, older endurance and power athletes were suggested to have maintained better muscle architecture with firmer fasciae and connective tissue septa and wider Achilles tendons than men in a population sample when assessed by ultrasonography [55,56].

Longitudinal perspective

It is clear that the performance by master athletes in both competitive sporting events and in physiologic tests in the laboratory is significantly better than that of older people who do not take regular exercise. This suggests that many inactive older people would benefit from taking regular exercise. The following section deals with the question as to whether elderly and very elderly individuals, who are not active, are able to adapt positively to increased levels of physical activity.

Strength and power

In the last decade a number of trials have been undertaken in which traditional strength training programs have been undertaken by older people. The findings of these studies suggest that the muscles of older people are able to adapt to progressive resistance exercise training and that this is true for both men and women. The adaptations to strength training can be considered at a number of different levels. For example the gains in the amount of weight that can be lifted once (1 RM) may increase some 174% in even very frail elderly people [2], similar relative gains to those achieved in young adults (see also 'Classical reference'). With strength training it is clear that the gains in isometric strength are lower than that of the 1 RM. However, in older people the gains in isometric strength are also similar in percentage terms to young people. Skelton *et al.* [57], for example, reported a 23% increase in isometric knee extensor strength in older women aged 75–80 years of age following 12 weeks of training, with the resistance provided by elastic tubing. These increases in muscle strength have been shown to be accompanied by increases in anatomic cross-sectional area. For example, even in very elderly frail men and women aged over 85 years, quadriceps muscle cross-sectional area increased by on average 10% after 12 weeks of heavy strength training of the knee extensor muscles [58] (Fig. 3.3.7). In those studies in which muscle biopsy samples have been obtained, both type I and type II fibers have been shown to hypertrophy. For instance, after 12 weeks of training the knee extensor muscles in 66-year-old men, Frontera *et al.* [59] reported a mean increase of 14% increase in type I fiber area and a 30% increase in type II fiber area.

Aerobic power

As with increases in muscle strength, it is now becoming clear that provided the exercise intensity is of suffi-

cient magnitude (and this for older people requires more individual tailoring), then even in very late life, individuals are able to increase their aerobic power through training. For example Seals *et al.* [60] reported that 12 months of aerobic training in 60–70-year-old subjects resulted in a mean increase of 30% in $\dot{V}o_{2\,max}$. In 70–79-year-old men and women 26 weeks of endurance training resulted in an increase in $\dot{V}o_{2\,max}$ of 22% [27]. Two recent studies on the oldest old suggest that, as with positive adaptations to strength training, even very elderly people may adapt to aerobic-based physical training. Maltbut–Shannan *et al.* [61] reported a 15% increase in $\dot{V}o_{2\,max}$ in women aged 80–93 years of age following 24 weeks of progressive aerobic training; however, no change was observed in the older men. In a second recent study on the oldest old, Puggaard *et al.* [62] reported a similar increase in $\dot{V}o_{2\,max}$ of 18% in women, also over the age of 80 years, following 8 months of general training.

Bone

The experimental evidence on the possibility of increasing bone strength by exercise in older adults is still weak compared to the 'training effects' indirectly obtained in the athlete studies. Several exercise interventions have shown positive changes in BMD, but the magnitude of these changes (on average 1–2% per year vs. controls) [63], at least in the short term, remains low in terms of bone strength and fracture prevention. The question remains as to whether more strength-demanding, fast and unusual loading patterns which have been suggested to be osteogenic in premenopausal women and early postmenopausal women with hormone replacement therapy are at all feasible for most older people, or whether outcomes other than BMD (e.g. moment of inertia and mass distribution, see [30], or collagen structure and metabolism) would be more relevant and sensitive to the effects of exercise.

However, even moderate exercise may be beneficial in the long run and improve and maintain muscle mass and strength, balance and coordination which, in addition to bone properties, are all independent risk factors for fracture. There is growing evidence that participation in exercise programs may improve postural stability and reduce the number of falls and severity of fall injuries. A meta-analysis of randomized trials [64] suggested that assignment to an exercise group with a

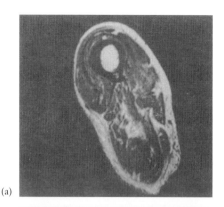
(a)

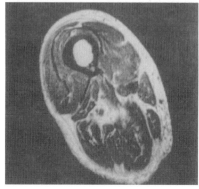
(b)

Fig. 3.3.7 MRI images on the same scale taken from a 90-year-old male subject (a) before and (b) after 12 weeks of resistance training of the knee extensors and flexors. This individual showed a 44% increase in muscle cross-sectional area of the quadriceps muscle. Data from [58].

wide range of treatments was associated with a decrease in the risk of falling even in the frail elderly. Although direct experimental evidence on the specific effects of physical activity on fracture risk is still missing, exercise may be the best single means of simultaneously modifying the key risk factors for osteoporotic fractures, and when prescribed appropriately, be a potential therapy to also improve the quality of life in osteoporotic patients.

Connective tissue

Hardly any longitudinal experimental studies have been conducted to investigate the effects of exercise on connective tissues in older adults. Suominen *et al.* [65] observed an increased PH activity in the vastus lateralis muscle after 2 months of training in 69-year-old women. Modern techniques allowing *in vivo* determination of tissue concentrations and release rates of substances such as those involved in collagen synthesis have, together with other methods, suggested that connective tissue, e.g. in the human peritendinous region, may be extremely adaptive to muscular activity [66]. In addition, there is quite a lot of evidence from animal studies to support a dynamic adaptation potential of connective tissues up into old age. For example, Simonsen *et al.* [67] showed that the tensile strength of the Achilles tendon, which was decreased with aging, was influenced by endurance training, but not by strength training in rats. Higher PH and galactosyl-hydroxylysyl glycosyltransferase (GGT) activities together with higher collagen concentration and mechanical strength of the soleus muscle were observed in rats trained on a treadmill for 2 years when compared to untrained rats of similar age [36]. The increase in hydroxypyridinium cross-linking normally seen with aging in the soleus was attenuated in both middle-aged and trained animals in the study by Zimmermann *et al.* [67], which fits in with the possibly increased turnover of muscle collagen, but shows some discrepancy with increased mechanical stiffness. Long-term training may also have systemic effects on connective tissues in a 'younger' direction. Supporting the aforementioned observations on non-loaded connective tissue, a recent series of studies [69] has shown that continuous training on a treadmill delays the age-related changes in the thermal stability and biomechanical properties of rat tail tendon.

Summary

The economic and social implications of an increasingly aged population are considerable. With this realization has come an increased focus upon the possible benefits of increased physical activity and the dangers of inactivity for older people. The aging process is associated with many changes in the functioning of the body. These changes appear to affect all systems needed for undertaking exercise, namely muscle, tendon, bone, heart, lungs, etc. In youth there is a generous safety margin for undertaking physical tasks; in other words, the difference between a maximum ability, whether it be $\dot{V}O_2$ or muscle strength, is considerably greater than the amount required to perform a task. With the decline in physiologic function this difference becomes eroded, until even in health, a point is reached where physical tasks become impossible to perform. Older people, do however, represent a heterogeneous mix of physical abilities and health statuses. Some older people can be considered to be physically fit, free from disease and independent, whilst others may be physically unfit with chronic and debilitating diseases and require full-time care. However, it is clear that even in the latter group of individuals, who often reside in nursing and care homes, significant improvements in physical function can be improved by exercise. Furthermore, not only are there physical benefits, but there is considerable evidence of improvements in the quality of sleep, improvements in mood and well-being and reduced anxiety and depression which combined with improved physical function lead to improvements in the quality of life.

Master or veteran athletes have shown that it is possible to perform extraordinary physical feats even very late in life. That is not to say that performance does not decline in these individuals: it does. However, relative to their non-active counterparts, they may be in some senses years younger.

Multiple choice questions

1 *The loss in muscle mass with aging is characterized by the following:*

a an unchanged muscle mass up to the age of 70

b a linear reduction in muscle mass from the age of 20

c a preferential loss of slow type I fibers with aging

d a curve-linear decrease in muscle mass with aging within approximate 1–2% loss in muscle mass per year.

2 *The maximal cardiovascular function during exercise is reduced with aging because:*

a there is a reduced stroke volume capacity but an unchanged maximal heart rate

b the oxygen uptake rate decreases with age solely due to an increase in body weight

c during submaximal work load, cardiac output can be maintained in the elderly due to a compensatory increase in stroke volume

d when maximal oxygen uptake is normalized to muscle mass and not to whole-body mass, the age-related decline is significantly enlarged.

3 *Endocrine responses in the elderly are characterized by:*

a a decrease in growth hormone secretion

b an increasing level of serum testosterone in males

c an increased insulin sensitivity

d unchanged levels of estrogen and progesterone in women.

4 *Training in the elderly and the effect on bone are characterized by the following:*

a Training has no effect on bone mineral density in elderly women.

b Several exercise interventions have demonstrated positive changes in bone mineral density of 5–10% per year.

c Several exercise interventions have demonstrated positive changes in bone mineral density of 1–2% per year.

d Effects on bone with training in postmenopausal women can only be obtained if simultaneous treatment with hormones is given.

References

1 Fiatarone MA, O'Neill EF, Ryan ND *et al.* Exercise training and nutritional supplementation for physical frailty in very elderly people. *N Engl J Med* 1994; **330**: 1769–75.

2 Fiatarone MA, Marks EC, Ryan ND, Meredith CN, Lipsitz LA, Evans WJ. High-intensity strength training in nonagenarians. *J Am Med Assoc* 1990; **263**: 3029–34.

3 United States Bureau of the Census. *International Data Base.* Washington, DC: International Programmes Center, US Bureau of the Census, 1998.

4 Holliday R. *Understanding Ageing.* Cambridge: Cambridge University Press, 1995.

5 Rowe JW, Kahn RL. *Successful Ageing.* New York: Pantheon, 1988.

6 Casperson CJ. Physical activity, exercise and physical fitness. Definitions and distinctions for health-related research. *Pub Health Rep* 1985; **100**: 126–30.

7 Paffenbarger RS Jr, Hyde RT, Wing AL, Hsieh CC. Physical activity, all-cause mortality, and longevity of college alumni. *N Engl J Med* 1986; **314**: 605–13.

8 Sarna S, Sahi T, Koskenvuo M, Kaprio J. Increased life expectancy of world class male athletes. *Med Sci Sports Exerc* 1993; **25**: 237–44.

9 Heikkinen E, Era P, Jokela J, Jylhä M, Lyyra AL, Pohjolainen P. Socioeconomic and life-style factors as modulators of health and functional capacity with age. In: Schroots JJF, ed. *Aging, Health and Competence.* Elsevier Science Publishers, 1993: 65–86.

10 Young A. Exercise physiology in geriatric practice. *Acta Med Scand Suppl* 1986; **711**: 227–32.

11 Tzankoff SP, Norris AH. Effect of muscle mass decrease on age-related BMR changes. *J Appl Physiol* 1977; **43**: 1001–6.

12 Suominen H. Changes in physical characteristics and body composition during 5-year follow-up in 75 and 80-year-old women. *Scand J Soc Med Suppl* 1997; **53**: 19–24.

13 Vandervoort AA, McComas AJ. Contractile changes in opposing muscles of the human ankle joint with aging. *J Appl Physiol* 1986; **61**: 361–7.

14 Skelton DA, Greig CA, Davies JM, Young A. Strength, power and related functional ability of healthy people aged 65–89 years. *Age Ageing* 1994; **23**: 371–7.

15 Phillips SK, Rook KM, Siddle NC, Bruce SA, Woledge RC. Muscle weakness in women occurs at an earlier age than in men, but strength is preserved by hormone replacement therapy. *Clin Sci* 1993; **84**: 95–8.

16 Skelton DA, Phillips SK, Bruce SA, Naylor CH, Woledge RC. Hormone replacement therapy increases isometric muscle strength of adductor pollicis in post-menopausal women. *Clin Sci* 1999; **96**: 357–64.

17 Bassey EJ, Fiatarone MA, O'Neill EF, Kelly WJ, Evans WJ, Lipsitz LA. Leg extensor power and functional performance in very old men and women. *Clin Sci* 1992; **82**: 322–7.

18 Bottinelli R, Canepari M, Pellegrino MA, Reggianai C. Force-velocity properties of human skeletal muscle fibres: myosin heavy chain isoform and temperature dependence. *J Physiol* 1996; **495**: 573–86.

19 Harridge SDR, White MJ, Carrington CA, Goodman M, Cummings P. Electrically evoked torque-velocity characteristics and isomyosin composition of the triceps surae in young and elderly men. *Acta Physiol Scand* 1995; **154**: 469–77.

20 Lexell J, Taylor CC, Sjöström M. What is the cause of the ageing atrophy? Total number, size and proportion of different fiber types studied in whole vastus lateralis muscle from 15- to 83-year-old men. *J Neurol Sci* 1988; **84**: 275–94.

21 Andersen JL, Terzis G, Kryger A. Increase in the degree of coexpression of myosin heavy chain isoforms in skeletal muscle fibers of the very old. *Muscle Nerve* 1999; **22**: 449–54.

22 Larsson L, Li X, Frontera WR. Effects of ageing on shortening velocity and myosin isoform composition in single human skeletal muscle cells. *Am J Physiol* 1997; **272**: C638–49.

23 Griffiths RD, Newsholme EA, Young A. Muscle as a dynamic metabolic store. In: Evans JG, Williams TF, Beattie BL, Michel JP, Wilcock CK, eds. *Oxford Textbook of Geriatric Medicine*, 2nd edn, Section on 'Muscle' (Young A, section ed.). Oxford: Oxford University Press, 1993; 972–9.

24 Welle S, Thornton C, Jozefowicz R, Statt M. Myofibrillar protein synthesis in young and old men. *Am J Physiol* 1993; **264**: E693–8.

25 Brooks SV, Faulkner JA. Contraction-induced injury: recovery of skeletal muscles in young and old mice. *Am J Physiol* 1990; **258**: C436–42.

26 Carlson BM, Faulkner JA. Muscle transplantation between young and old rats: age of host determines recovery. *Am J Physiol* 1989; **256**: C1262–6.

27 Hagberg JM. Effect of training on $\dot{V}O_{2\,max}$ with ageing. *Fed Proc* 1987; **46**: 1830–3.

28 Fleg JL, Lakatta EG. Role of muscle loss in the age associated reduction in $\dot{V}O_{2\,max}$. *J Appl Physiol* 1988; **65**: 1147–51.

29 Riggs BL, Melton LJ III. The prevention and treatment of osteoporosis. *N Engl J Med* 1992; **327**: 620–7.

30 Cheng S, Suominen H, Sakari-Rantala R, Heikkinen E. Calcaneal bone mineral density predicts fracture occurrence —a 5-year follow-up study in elderly people. *J Bone Min Res* 1997; **12**: 1075–82.

31 Turner RT. Mechanical signaling in the development of post menopausal osteoporosis. *Lupus* 1999; 8: 388–92.

32 Riggs BL, Khosla S, Melton LJ III. Primary osteoporosis in men: role of sex steroid deficiency. *Mayo Clinic Proc* 2000; **75** (Suppl.): S46–50.

33 Takala TE, Virtanen P. Biochemical composition of muscle extracellular matrix: the effect of loading. *Scand J Med Sci Sports* 2000; **10**: 321–5.

34 Nagawa Y, Majima T, Nagashima K. Effect of ageing on ultrastructure of slow and fast skeletal muscle tendon in rabbit Achilles tendons. *Acta Physiol Scand* 1994; **152**: 307–13.

35 Naresh MD, Brodsky B. X-ray diffraction studies on human tendon show age-related changes in collagen packing. *Biochim Biophys Acta* 1992; **1122**: 161–6.

36 Kovanen V. Effects of ageing and physical training on rat skeletal muscle. An experimental study on the properties of collagen, laminin, and fibre types in muscles serving different functions. *Acta Physiol Scand* 1989; **135** (Suppl. 577): 1–56.

37 Palokangas H, Kovanen V, Duncan A, Robins SP. Age-related changes in the concentration of hydroxypyridinium crosslinks in functionally different skeletal muscles. *Matrix* 1992; **12**: 291–6.

38 Goldspink G, Fernandes K, Williams PE, Wells DJ. Age-related changes in collagen gene expression in the muscles of mdx dystrophic and normal mice. *Neuromusc Disord* 1994; **4**: 183–91.

39 Wolfarth S, Lorenc-Koci E, Schulze G, Ossowska K, Kaminska A, Coper H. Age-related muscle stiffness. predominance of non-reflex factors. *Neuroscience* 1997; **79**: 617–28.

40 Rudman DM, Kutner MH, Rogers CM, Lubin MF, Fleming GA, Bain RP. Impaired growth hormone secretion in the adult population: relation to age and adiposity. *J Clin Invest* 1981; **67**: 1361–9.

41 Yarasheski KE, Zachwieja JJ, Campbell JA, Bier DM. Effect of growth hormone and resistance exercise on muscle growth and strength in older men. *Am J Physiol* 1995; **268**: E268–E276.

42 Häkkinen K, Pakarinen A. Muscle strength and serum testosterone, cortisol and SHBG concentrations in middle-aged and elderly men and women. *Acta Physiol Scand* 1993; **148**: 199–207.

43 Urban RJ, Bodenburg YH, Gilkison C *et al*. Testosterone administration to elderly men increases muscle strength and protein synthesis. *Am J Physiol* 1995; **269**: E820–E826.

44 Klitgaard H, Mantoni M, Schiaffino S *et al*. Function, morphology and protein expression of ageing skeletal muscle: a cross-sectional study of elderly men with different training backgrounds. *Acta Physiol Scand* 1990; **140**: 41–54.

45 Sipilä S, Vitasalo J, Era P, Suominen H. Muscle strength in male athletes aged 70–81 years and a population sample. *Eur J Appl Physiol* 1991; **63**: 399–403.

46 Harridge SDR, Magnusson G, Saltin B. Life-long endurance trained elderly men have high aerobic power, but have similar muscled strength to non-active elderly men. *Aging Clin Exp Res* 1997; **9**: 80–7.

47 Klitgaard H, Ausoni S, Damiani E. Sarcoplasmic reticulum of human skeletal muscle, age-related changes and effect of training. *Acta Physiol Scand* 1989; **137**: 23–31.

48 Saltin B. The aging endurance athlete. In: Sutton JR, Brock RM, eds. *Sports Medicine for the Mature Athlete*. Indianapolis: Benchmark Press, 1986: 59–80.

49 Coggan AR, Spina King DS *et al*. Skeletal muscle adaptations to endurance training in 60–70 year old men and women. *J Appl Physiol* 1992; **72**: 1780–6.

50 LeBlanc A, Schneider W, Evans H, Engelbretson D, Krebs J. Bone mineral loss and recovery after 17 weeks of bed rest. *J Bone Min Res* 1990; **5**: 843–50.

51 Suominen H. Bone mineral density and long-term exercise: an overview of cross-sectional athlete studies. *Sports Med* 1993; **16**: 316–30.

52 Williams PE, Goldspink G. Connective tissue changes in immobilized muscle. *J Anat* 1984; **138**: 343–50.

53 Suominen H, Heikkinen E. Enzyme activities in muscle and connective tissue of M. vastus lateralis in habitually training and sedentary 33–70-year-old men. *Eur J Appl Physiol* 1975; **34**: 249–54.

54 Suominen H, Heikkinen E, Moisio H, Viljamaa K. Physical and chemical properties of skin in habitually trained and sedentary men. *Br J Dermatol* 1978; **99**: 147–54.

55 Kallinen M, Suominen H. Ultrasonographic measurements of the Achilles tendon in elderly athletes and sedentary men. *Acta Radiol* 1994; **35**: 560–3.

56 Sipilä S, Suominen H. Ultrasound imaging of the quadriceps muscle in elderly athletes and untrained men. *Muscle Nerve* 1991; **14**: 527–33.

57 Skelton DA, Young A, Greig CA, Malbut KE. Effects of re-

sistance training in strength, power, and selected functional abilities of women aged 75 and older. *J Am Geriatr Soc* 1995; **43**: 1081–7.

58 Harridge SDR, Kryger A, Stensgaard A. Knee extensor strength, activation and size in very elderly people following 12 weeks strength training. *Muscle Nerve* 1999; **22**: 831–9.

59 Frontera WR, Meredith CN, O'Reilly KP, Knuttgen HG, Evans WJ. Strength conditioning in older men. Skeletal muscle hypertrophy and improved function. *J Appl Physiol* 1998; **64**: 1038–44.

60 Seals DR, Hagberg JM, Hurley BF, Eshani AA, Holloszy JO. Endurance training in older men and women. I. Cardiovascular responses to exercise. *J Appl Physiol* 1984; **57**: 1024–9.

61 Malbut-Shennan K, Dinan S, Young A. Aerobic training can increase maximal oxygen uptake in women over 80. *Med Sci Sports Exerc* 1998; **5** (Suppl.): S138.

62 Puggaard L, Larsen JB, Stovring H, Jeune B. Maximal oxygen uptake, muscle strength and walking speed in 85-year-old women: effects of increased physical activity. *Aging* 2000; **12**: 180–9.

63 Wolff I, van Croonenborg JJ, Kemper HC, Kostense PJ, Twisk JW. The effect of exercise training programs on bone mass: a meta-analysis of published controlled trials in pre- and postmenopausal women. *Osteoporos Int* 1999; **9**: 1–12.

64 Province MA, Hadley EC, Hornbrook MC *et al.* The effects of exercise on falls in elderly patients: a preplanned meta-analysis of the FICSIT Trials — Frailty and Injuries. Cooperative Studies on Intervention Techniques. *J Am Med Assoc* 1995; **273**: 1341–7.

65 Suominen H, Heikkinen E, Parkatti T. Effect of eight weeks' physical training on muscle and connective tissue of the m. vastus lateralis in 69-year-old men and women. *J Gerontol* 1977; **32**: 33–7.

66 Kjaer M, Langberg H, Skovgaard D *et al.* In vivo studies of peritendinous tissue in exercise. *Scand J Med Sci Sports* 2000; **10**: 326–31.

67 Simonsen EB, Klitgaard H, Bojsen-Moller F. The influence of strength training, swim training and ageing on the Achilles tendon and m. soleus of the rat. *J Sports Sci* 1995; **13**: 291–5.

68 Zimmerman SD, McCormick RJ, Vadlamudi RK, Thomas P. Age and training alter collagen characteristics in fast- and slow-twitch rat limb muscle. *J Appl Physiol* 1993; **75**: 1670–4.

69 Viidik A, Nielsen HM, Skalicky M. Influence of physical exercise on aging rats. II. Life-long exercise delays aging of tail tendon collagen. *Mech Age Dev* 1988; **17**: 139–48.

70 Comfort A. *The Biology of Senescence*. Edinburgh: Churchill Livingstone, 1964.

71 Fries JF, Crapo LM. *Vitality and Aging*. New York: Freeman, 1981.

72 American College of Sports Medicine. Position stand. The recommended quantity and quality of exercise for developing and maintaining cardiorespiratory and muscular fitness, and flexibility in healthy adults. *Med Sci Sports Exerc* 1998; **30**: 975–91.

73 American College of Sports Medicine. Position stand. Exercise and physical activity for older adults. *Med Sci Sports Exerc* 1998; **30**: 992–1008.

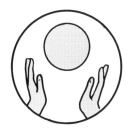

Chapter 3.4
Exercise in Healthy and Chronically Diseased Children

HELGE HEBESTREIT, ODED BAR-OR
& JØRN MÜLLER

Classical reference

Åstrand PO. *Experimental Studies of Physical Working Capacity in Relation to Sex and Age.* Copenhagen: Munksgaard, 1952.
These studies were some of the first to systematically evaluate maximal oxygen uptake in relation to age and development in both boys and girls. It is shown that in the teenage period a larger increase in maximal oxygen uptake is found in boys. Furthermore, the studies also established a linear relationship in children between running speed and oxygen uptake. For a given speed, the oxygen uptake per kg body weight decreases with increasing age from the age of around 6 to the age of 17 (Fig. 3.4.1).

Introduction

Physical activity is an integral part of every child's life. While in former years, children used to participate in a large variety of non-organized games, they nowadays either live a sedentary life or engage in one or two competitive sports. Consequently, physicians have to deal with the effects of low physical activity in a major section of the pediatric population. For young competitive athletes, regular medical guidance is required to avoid the adverse effects of intense sports participation. In this chapter, we will first address some developmental aspects of exercise physiology, since the understanding of basic principles will facilitate the decision process in daily medical practice. This will be followed by discussion of the benefits and risks of exercise at different levels in healthy children and in those with a chronic disease.

Developmental aspects of exercise science

Performance in various tasks such as running, swimming, jumping, throwing, etc. improves during childhood and adolescence. For most variables, girls reach their peak performance at about the age of 14 years. Thereafter, performance either remains constant or declines. The performance of boys usually improves up to the age of 16 years.

Several dimensional and functional changes occur during childhood and adolescence which may influence performance during exercise. Some of these changes are listed below.

Changes in body size

Performance in many tasks depends on body size. Especially during laboratory-based tasks, in which maximal power or peak oxygen uptake are determined, a close relationship between performance and size-related variables such as body weight has been observed. Therefore, during childhood and adolescence, a person's power or oxygen uptake measured in the laboratory is usually corrected for the influence of body size. The reason behind this procedure is that two people's performance can then be better compared and that one person's performance can be compared to normative data.

Traditionally, this correction is made by dividing the performance variable, e.g. oxygen uptake or power, by body mass. In cardiology, a ratio with body surface area in the denominator is commonly used. However, these ratio standards have an important limitation: the performance variable is usually not related to body

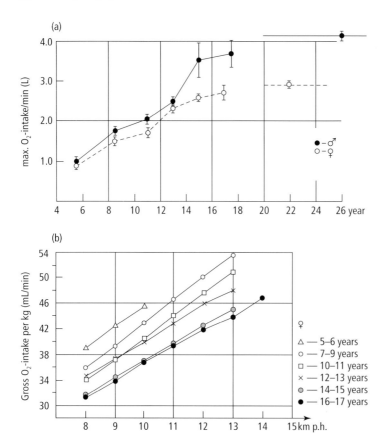

Fig. 3.4.1 (a) $\dot{V}_{O_2 max}$ in girls and boys.
(b) O_2 cost of locomotion in girls.

mass or surface area such that the intercept of a linear regression line would be zero. Therefore, after correcting for differences in body size using ratio standards, small subjects may appear more powerful than bigger subjects. To avoid this phenomenon, different ways of correcting for differences in body size (scaling) have been suggested. The limited space in this chapter does not allow discussion of the approaches in detail. The reader is referred to recent reviews on this topic [1,2].

Changes in body proportions

From birth to adulthood, the size of the head, trunk and extremities increases by different percentages of the initial size. In general, young children have relatively larger heads and shorter extremities compared to older individuals. Furthermore, there are considerable differences in growth rates and peak growth velocities

among body parts. The lower extremities reach their peak growth velocity earlier than the trunk or the arms. And even within an extremity, the growth is not synchronized. The proximal parts of the arms and legs reach their respective adult dimensions later than the more distal parts. Consequently, the proportions of one body segment relative to the others change continuously during growth. These changes affect biomechanics and power generation during different tasks. Furthermore, motor coordination has continuously to adapt to the changed body proportions.

Changes in muscle mass

Muscle mass relative to total body weight increases during childhood and adolescence in boys from about 42% to 53% [3]. In girls, relative muscle mass remains more or less constant at around 40–46% between the ages of 5 years and 29 years [3].

Changes in muscle fiber type

For ethical reasons, muscle biopsy data are scarce in children. While older reviews did conclude that there is no difference in muscle fiber distribution between children at the age of 5–6 years and adults [4], more recent studies found a relatively larger proportion of slow oxidative type I fibers and fewer type II fibers in younger individuals [5,6].

Development of neuromotor control

There is a large base of evidence that there is a considerable improvement of coordination during childhood. The development of neural control of locomotion during childhood is only partly understood. Increasing ramification of neurons with higher density of interneuron contacts, which is stimulated by motor learning, plays an important role. Increased myelinization of peripheral neurons allows for faster transmission of information. Improvements in neuromotor control may explain, for example, the increase in running economy with age during childhood and adolescence [7,8], and the faster reaction time in adolescents compared with children.

Physical activity in children and adolescents

Physical activity (PA) is a complex variable which is difficult to assess. A subject's PA is commonly described in various dimensions [9]: (i) duration of any given activity; (ii) intensity; (iii) frequency of activity sessions; and (iv) mode or type of the activity. For some research questions, overall PA is expressed as energy expenditure.

Various methods have been employed to determine the level of PA in children, but none of them is optimal for each possible question about activity in this age group. In other words, each method has its strengths and limitations, and the choice has to be made related to the research or clinical question being asked. Often, more than one method has to be used to collect relevant data.

In spite of their low validity and fair reliability, questionnaires and proxy reports of parents and teachers are the main methods available for clinicians and for population-based studies. An increase in validity and reliability can be achieved by conducting a face-to-face interview with the child and/or parent. Direct observation is very labor-intensive and is therefore only used for studies with a small sample size over a short period of time. Heart rate monitoring combined with an individual oxygen uptake over heart rate calibration curve can yield estimates of PA which are reasonably reliable and valid. There are, however, some limitations of the method, since, in addition to PA, heart rate is affected by emotions, ambient temperature, state of hydration, posture and the muscle groups involved. Motion sensors, like heart rate monitoring, have an acceptable reliability and validity. However, activities such as cycling are not detected well. Furthermore, there is a problem with non-random missing data in some subjects since the sensors are often removed during water-based activities and not put back on again afterwards. The gold standard for the measurement of overall energy expenditure over several days to weeks is the doubly labeled water technique. This method is very costly and does not allow detection of patterns of physical activities.

It is generally agreed that children are physically more active than adolescents or adults. However, the answer to the question whether they are active enough to stay healthy and to 'build health' remains unknown. A study of English children [10] has shown that only 4% of 92 boys and 1% of 138 girls aged 11 to 16 years experienced at least one sustained 20-min period per day with a heart rate above 139 beats/min. The respective values for heart rate above 159 beats/min were 2% and 0%. These thresholds were considered optimal exercise intensities for the promotion of cardiopulmonary fitness in children and adolescents. However, when using a different criterion, the conclusions can change considerably. Energy expenditure of 12.6 kJ/kg/day or more has been shown to be associated with health in adults [11]. When this criterion for an 'active' lifestyle was used for 10–18-year-old children and adolescents, 94% of 1307 boys and 88% of 843 girls were classified as active [12].

Potential health gains from physical activity and sports during childhood and adolescence

Although epidemologic studies show a relationship between PA and health in adults, there is not much proof for such a relationship in children and adolescents.

Prevention of cardiovascular disease

The Bogalusa heart study has shown that atherosclerosis begins early in life [13]. The following risk factors were identified as predictors of fatty streaks and fibrous plaques in the coronary arteries and aorta of young individuals [13]: body mass index, systolic and diastolic blood pressure, serum concentrations of total cholesterol, triglycerides, low-density lipoprotein cholesterol and smoking habits.

A large number of studies has been performed to assess the effects of increased PA on the above risk factors. This chapter will focus on some findings from intervention studies. Since an in-depth description of all studies on PA and cardiovascular health is beyond the limited space available for this chapter, the reader is referred to some recent reviews for more details [14,15].

Adiposity

Common sense would suggest that active children should be less obese than inactive children since the former expend more energy compared with the latter. It may thus seem surprising that several studies have failed to document an effect of enhanced PA on body fatness of non-obese children. In the SPARK project, fourth- to fifth-grade USA students were taught physical education by either physical education specialists or trained classroom teachers over 2 years [16]. These groups were compared with children attending ordinary physical education classes. Although the intervention groups spent significantly more time per week being physically active (40 min and 33 min) compared with the control group (18 min), there was no difference among groups in calf or triceps skinfolds at the end of the 2-year intervention [16]. Likewise, no effect of 3 hours of additional physical education per week was observed on triceps skinfold and body mass index in the Odense schoolchild study [17]. In contrast to these findings, an Australian school intervention program did show effects of increased physical education on skinfold thickness: a group of 10-year-old children receiving 75 min of endurance exercises during physical education classes per day over 14 weeks showed a decrease in skinfold thickness, while two control groups, one receiving ordinary physical education and one engaging in skill-oriented physical education

75 min per day, experienced no change in skinfold thickness [18]. The different findings in these studies might reflect the differences in training volume and intensity among the studies.

Blood pressure

Endurance training was shown to lower systolic and diastolic blood pressure in hypertensive adolescents [19,20]. In the Odense schoolchild study, a blood pressure lowering effect of 3 hours of additional physical education was also shown for hypertensive and non-hypertensive children after 8 months of intervention, but not after 3 months [17]. However, no effects of 14 weeks of additional PA on systolic and diastolic blood pressure was observed in the Australian school intervention program [18].

Serum lipid concentrations

In the Australian school intervention program, blood was analysed for plasma total cholesterol, high-density lipoprotein (HDL)-cholesterol, and triglycerides in a subsample of the children. Following 14 weeks of intervention, no change in blood lipid levels was observed in either the endurance or the control group [18].

Smoking habits

Several cross-sectional studies have suggested a negative relationship between self-reported tobacco use and self-reported PA or participation in organized sports [21]. After controlling for the effects of age, gender and/or race, the relationship disappeared in some of the studies.

In summary, proof for the effect of enhanced PA on cardiovascular risk factors during childhood and adolescence is equivocal. This might be attributed to several reasons.

1 Cardiovascular risk factors might not be influenced by PA during childhood at all. This assumption is very unlikely, since a positive effect of training has been observed under certain conditions.

2 A very high level of PA over an extended period of time might be required to elicit any change in a given risk factor in young individuals. This hypothesis could explain the different results among the studies cited above.

3 The baseline PA of subjects was relatively high compared to the small increment in PA imposed by the study design.

4 Children and adolescents participating in the above studies might have experienced a low risk profile to begin with, so that the intervention could show no additional effects.

5 Cardiovascular risk factors are influenced not only by PA but also by other factors such as nutrition, growth and development, and genetics. If the relative importance of PA is small, it might be difficult to discern any effect.

Most likely, more than one of the above hypotheses is correct.

Prevention of osteoporosis and fractures later in life

PA, and especially exercise which poses high strain on the bones, is associated with an elevation in bone mass and bone mineral density during childhood and adolescence [22,23]. It has been estimated that a level of PA achievable by a large proportion of children and adolescents may increase peak bone mass by approximately 7–8% [24].

If the activity-related increase of bone mineral density during adolescence is maintained through adulthood, this increase might be sufficient to prevent premature osteoporosis in old age.

Prevention of accidents

It is well documented that injuries during childhood and adolescence occur during play and sports. Very little is known, however, as to whether enhanced PA might help to reduce the number of accidents and injuries. In a study conducted in Germany [25], children of 94 kindergartens were divided into two groups. One group (16 kindergartens) received 15 min of supervised physical education per day in addition to the usual time scheduled for play and sports, while the other group (78 kindergartens) served as control. The number of accidents reported to the accident insurance companies declined in the children participating in the activity group considerably. At the same time, the frequency of accidents increased marginally in the control group. Possible reasons for the observed effect of a physical education program in kindergartens

might be either improved coordination, better concentration, or a reduction in risky behavior (less hyperactivity).

Improved psychological profile

Various psychological benefits from regular PA have been reported [21]. In children with a chronic disease, these benefits may be the primary goal for a rehabilitative program which includes physical exercise. The benefits which may be derived from regular PA include improvements in self concept, self-esteem, body image, self-efficacy, perceived competence, academic functioning and social skills. PA may also reduce depressive symptoms and stress.

Lifetime increase in physical activity

In adults, a sedentary lifestyle has been linked to a higher morbidity and mortality from cardiovascular disease, a higher risk for certain types of cancer, compromised mental health, and a higher incidence of non-insulin-dependent diabetes mellitus, obesity and osteoporosis [26]. One key question when assessing the benefits from PA during childhood is therefore whether the level of PA during childhood might affect the level of PA during adulthood. Unfortunately, there are only relatively few studies that have addressed this question. Data from the Amsterdam growth study show no significant tracking of total weekly PA from the teens (age 13–16 years) to age 27 years in females and males [27]. However, a long-term follow-up of the Trois-Rivières experiment demonstrates that an intense involvement in physical education during primary school may enhance PA in females in their thirties, but not in males [28].

Prevention of future back pain

Back pain is one of the leading causes for morbidity and absenteeism from work during adulthood. To our knowledge, there is only one study investigating the effects of a high level of PA during childhood on the prevalence of back pain in adulthood [28]. The follow-up of former participants of the Trois-Rivières study showed a significantly lower frequency of back pain in the females who had received 5 hours of physical education per week during grades 1–6 compared with the females who received only 1 hour. There was no effect of additional physical education on future back pain in the males.

Potential health gains from physical activity and sports specific to children and adolescents with a chronic disease

Children and adolescents suffering from a chronic disease may experience the same benefits from PA as do their healthy peers. In some variables, such as self-confidence, the positive effects of sport may even be more pronounced in children with a chronic disease [29]. Furthermore, for some children with a chronic health condition, the ability to be physically active is a more important criterion for feeling healthy than the absence of symptoms related to the disease or the ability to live without medications [30].

Asthma

There are some studies showing a reduction in asthma symptoms and severity with a structured exercise program [31]. Whether regular exercise may also reduce exercise-induced bronchoconstriction is not clear.

Cystic fibrosis

Some evidence shows a slowing of lung destruction in patients with cystic fibrosis by regular physical training [32,33]. Although experimental proof is lacking, it may also be speculated that long-term sport involvement may also reduce the incidence or severity of cystic fibrosis-related diabetes mellitus and osteoporosis.

Cerebral palsy

A general exercise program may improve walking proficiency in patients with cerebral palsy [34].

Hypertension

As discussed above, regular exercise may lower blood pressure in healthy children and those with hypertension. This effect may be used therapeutically in adolescents with moderate hypertension [19,20]. Interestingly, resistance training following an aerobic training program was effective in maintaining the reduction in blood pressure [19]. However, blood pressure increased back to pretraining levels once the program was concluded.

Insulin-dependent diabetes mellitus (IDDM)

Several intervention studies have shown that regular PA does not improve the long-term control of blood glucose in most subjects with IDDM. However, in patients with insulin resistance, exercise may increase insulin sensitivity and may, thereby, improve control. Regular sports involvement can possibly help to reduce or delay long-term complications resulting from diabetes mellitus such as angiopathy or neuropathy [35].

Obesity

While regular exercise has little or no effect on adiposity in normal-weight children, it is commonly recommended as part of the treatment and rehabilitation in patients with obesity. The reason for this approach is not that exercise in itself will induce a fast and considerable loss of body fat. However, if exercise is combined with diet, two benefits of exercise may be perceived. (i) When weight loss is achieved by a low calorie diet only, muscle tissue mass is decreased in addition to the loss of fat tissue. An exercise program in addition to the diet may prevent the loss of muscle mass. (ii) When caloric intake is reduced, basal metabolic rate decreases. By adding an exercise program to diet, the decrease in metabolic rate may be abolished.

Rheumatoid arthritis

With chronic joint inflammation the strength of ligaments and tendons stabilizing the joint to withstand tear forces is reduced. On the other hand, the joint capsule and the surrounding ligaments shrink so that flexibility of the inflamed joint is lost. Furthermore, a local decrease of bone mineralization leading to a circumscript osteoporosis may occur in proximity to the joint. Consequently, the joints are prone to injuries including distortion and fractures. Physiotherapy and exercise programs are recommended to prevent these complications [36].

Potential risks from physical activity and sports in childhood and adolescence

Adverse effects on growth and puberty

Linear growth and pubertal development are important elements of normal childhood and adolescence.

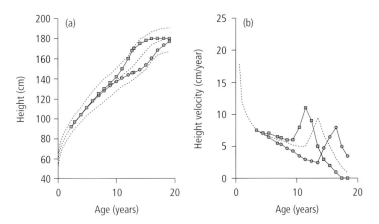

Fig. 3.4.2 (a) Normal growth curve in an early- and a late-maturing boy. Note the difference in height before and particularly during puberty. (b) Growth velocity curve in an early- and a late-maturing boy. Note that peak height velocity decreases with increasing age at the start of the pubertal growth spurt. Peak height velocity in girls occurs on average 2 years earlier than in boys. Danish reference data.

The tempo of growth and puberty as well as adult stature are primarily genetically determined. However, environmental factors such as e.g. nutrition, psychological stress and chronic medication may be important modulators of the normal maturation processes. It is also possible that intense physical activity may influence linear growth and the time of onset of puberty. The pubertal period is by far the most sensitive phase of the growth process, and females seem to be more sensitive to adverse influences than males. Thus, in analysing the possible adverse effects of physical activity on growth it is important to include information on parental stature and puberty, and to distinguish between prepubertal and pubertal growth.

The normal growth curve is shown in Fig. 3.4.2. In girls, puberty starts between 8 and 13 years, in boys between 9 and 14 years. The average age at menarche differs between countries, but in most places it occurs between 12 and 13 years of age.

Linear growth

Only few studies have dealt exclusively with linear growth before puberty in children taking part in sport at a competitive level. In a study of 184 children participating in swimming, team handball, tennis and gymnastics, it was found that height at the age of 9–11 years was significantly lower in children participating in gymnastics compared with the other sports [37]. These children, however, were also short at the age of 2–4 years, many years before starting their sports activities, indicating that selection rather than an influence

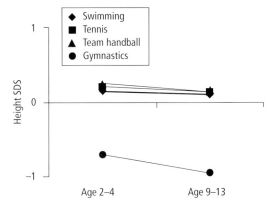

Fig. 3.4.3 Median height SDS (standard deviation score) in females participating in swimming, tennis, team handball and gymnastics at ages 2–4 and 9–13 years, respectively. No significant change in height SDS during this period was found in any of the sports. On both occasions, girls in gymnastics were significantly shorter than the participants in the three other sports. Boys in the same investigation displayed similar changes. Adapted from [37].

of the physical activity had taken place (Fig. 3.4.3) [37,38]. The number of training hours was not associated with actual stature. These data support a previous investigation of Polish athletes [39], although this study did not include children participating in gymnastics.

Several studies have indicated that linear growth in female gymnasts is compromised [40–42]. The Swiss study of pubertal growth in female swimmers and gymnasts showing reduced pubertal growth in the latter group has raised particular concern. However, the data should be interpreted with caution since height and height velocity were related to skeletal age rather than chronologic age. In an earlier study, it was suggested that the height of the gymnasts at start of puberty corresponded to the genetic potential [43]. In a longitudinal study of children participating in gymnastics, soccer, swimming and tennis no training effect on stature could be demonstrated [42]. However, the authors could not exclude the possibility that a training effect had occurred prior to the investigation. Thus, it has not yet been convincingly shown whether short stature in female gymnasts is due to constitutional factors, nutritional factors or the impact of the physical training.

On the other hand, available data have indicated that girls participating in swimming, track, rowing, tennis and volleyball had normal stature or were taller than average [44–47]. Similarly, no effect of sport participation has been demonstrated in boys [37,39,41,42,48]. Height differences between boys participating in different sports do occur; however, the variation may simply reflect differences in skeletal maturation, and it is most likely a result of selection rather than a training effect.

In conclusion, prepubertal and pubertal growth has not unambiguously been shown to be affected by participation in sport.

Age at onset of puberty

It is only possible to assess the age at onset of puberty in longitudinal studies, and data are scarce. Several cross-sectional studies have described differences in attained pubertal stage or age at peak height velocity among children participating in different sports. Skeletal maturation has also been used as a surrogate for pubertal maturation in several studies. In boys, only gymnasts seem to exhibit a small delay of 1–2 years compared with the reference population. In contrast, advanced body maturation has been reported in soccer players [39,49], and in other sports as well [50]. Again, these differences are most likely a result of selection. In a recent study of 88 boys 11–13 years of age participating in swimming, tennis, team handball and gymnastics, no difference in testicular volume was found when age was controlled for [38].

Female gymnasts have consistently been reported to have delayed pubertal development [40,46,47,51]. One

Table 3.4.1 Age at menarche in female athletes.

Sport	N	Mean age
Control subjects in US	63	12.8
Gymnastics	201	15.6
Figure skating	30	15.0
Ballet	75	14.5
Running	17	13.8
Rowing	59	13.7
Swimming	52	13.1
Volleyball	63	13.1
Handball	98	13.0

N, number of subjects. Adapted from [81] and [82], with permission.

study, however, could not confirm these observations [52]. Girls participating in other sports do not seem to differ from the reference population with regard to pubertal development [53].

Age at menarche

Age at menarche is a milestone in female puberty and is easier to assess than other aspects of maturation. In accordance with the above-mentioned findings, most studies agree that female gymnasts have delayed menarche [44,54–56]. The same phenomenon has been observed in girls participating in diving, figure skating, distance running and ballet (Table 3.4.1). Interestingly, some studies indicate a correlation between age at menarche in athletes and their mothers [44,47], again indicating that constitutional factors rather than the participation in sports may play a role.

Female reproductive function, nutritional disorders and bone mineral content

If menarche is delayed beyond the age of 16, the condition is referred to as primary amenorrhea. Secondary amenorrhea is defined as a period of more than 6-months without menstruation, in a girl who has experienced her menarche. These conditions may be a consequence of poor nutrition and low body weight or, rather, low body fat. This is known for a fact from disorders of malabsorption. It is also known that the psychiatric disorder anorexia nervosa is accompanied by delayed puberty and primary or secondary amenorrhea, probably due to a combination of neuroendocrine disturbances and low body fat. It is much less

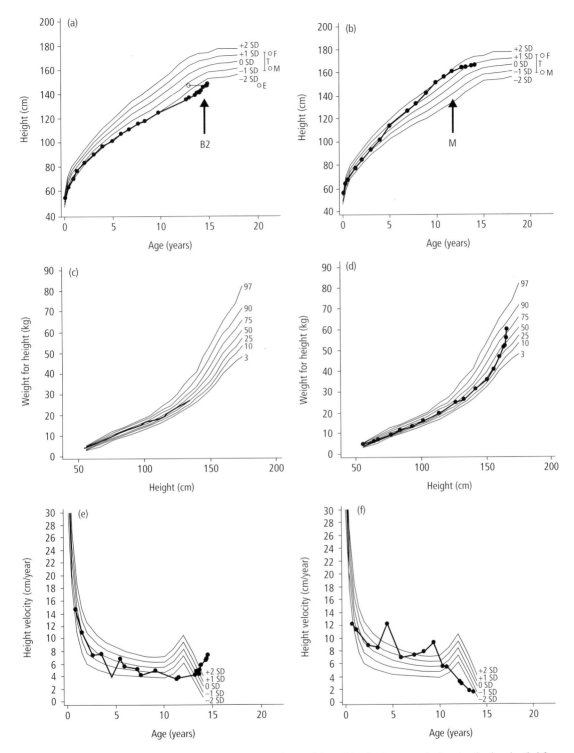

Fig. 3.4.4 Linear growth, growth velocity and weight for height in two girls participating in gymnastics (a,c,e) and swimming (b,d,f), respectively. Note that the growth patterns are representative for an early- and a late-maturing girl, and that the difference in growth pattern of the girls started long before participation in sport. Both girls will reach their target height.

Case history

Julie is a 15-year-old girl, who has participated in gymnastics at a national competitive level since the age of 8 years. Currently, she is active in sport 6 hours a week. Julie is healthy and takes no medication. There is no indication of anorexia. Julie's birth weight and length were 3.0 kg and 49 cm. Her mother experienced late puberty with menarche at age 15 years. At the age of 15, Julie is in breast stage 2 and pubic hair stage 1 with sign of early pubertal growth spurt (Fig. 3.4.4). Note that weight for height is well within the normal limits, between the 25th and the 50th percentile.

Marie is also 15 years old and she has been active in swimming at a competitive level since the age of 8 years. She is swimming 9 hours a week. She is healthy, takes no medication, and has normal eating habits. She is in breast and pubic hair stage 5, and Marie had menarche at the age of 11.4 years. Marie's birth weight and length were 3.4 kg and 52 cm. Her mother had menarche at the age of 12 years. She has a growth pattern in keeping with her early maturation (Fig. 3.4.4) with age at peak height velocity at 9.5 years. Note that her weight for height is similar to Julie's up to a height of approximately 150 cm.

Comment. These two girls represent the extremes of growth and maturation among girls participating in sport. Their growth patterns are in accordance with the literature; however, it should be noted that both girls have followed their initial growth pattern, and the gymnast has a genetic disposition for late puberty in contrast to the swimmer whose mother had first menstruation at the age of 12 years. Both girls had normal birth weights and lengths, and both girls had similar body mass indices up to a height of 150 cm.

Table 3.4.2 Prevalence of eating disorders in female athletes.

Activity	N	Eating disorder (%)
Non-athletes	101	6
Activities emphasizing leanness		
Dancing	55	33
Gymnastics	19	74
Track	40	35
Combined activities	35	20
Activities without emphasis on leanness		
Tennis	25	24
Volleyball	14	21
Combined activities	32	0

Adapted from [81] and [82], with permission.

clear, however, whether excess of exercise *per se* results in disturbances of female reproductive function. In a study of 22 female gymnasts and 22 healthy girls, a significantly reduced energy intake compared to nutritional recommendations was found in both groups, but more so in the group of gymnasts who also had the highest energy expenditure [57].

The sports associated with primary and secondary amenorrhea (gymnastics, figure skating, running and ballet) are also sports in which a slender physique is valued. Thus, a low body weight is prevalent in women participating in these sports. A high prevalence of eating disorders including anorexia nervosa and bulimia is also associated with these sports (Table 3.4.2). A comparison of body composition in female distance runners, gymnasts and anorexia nervosa patients showed no difference, indicating that the specific phenotype may be achieved by different mechanisms [58]. Measurements of serum leptin showing comparable low levels in elite gymnasts and patients with anorexia nervosa have also indicated similarities between the two conditions [59].

The above mentioned menstrual disturbances are associated with low serum levels of estrogens and progesterone. Both steroids are of paramount importance for accretion of calcium into the skeleton during adolescence. Therefore, athletes with primary or secondary amenorrhea or even anovulatory cycles are at high risk of reduced bone mineral content and subsequent osteoporosis and spontaneous fractures. The research field of bone mineral content is associated with methodologic difficulties; however, available data suggest that female athletes have bone deficits of 0.9–20% (for review, see [60]). The pathogenesis of the reduced bone mineralization is most likely decreased sex steroid production possibly combined with insufficient calcium intake, since physical activity is known to promote bone accretion.

In summary, certain female sports are associated with eating disorders, both anorexia and bulimia, and the consequences of an excess energy expenditure compared to energy intake may lead to delayed menarche and secondary amenorrhea, which in its turn may cause decreased bone mineral content. There is no evidence that physical activity *per se* results in disturbances of gonadal function and bone mineralization.

Sudden death

Sudden death within one hour after performing sport is fortunately rare. The prevalence of sudden cardiac death among adolescent athletes has been estimated to range between 1 in 100 000 and 1 in 300 000 [61]. In most cases a congenital cardiovascular defect (aortic valve stenosis, anomalies of the coronary arteries) or a connective tissue disorder such as Marfan's syndrome was present, leading to acute aortic dissection [62]. Hypertrophic cardiomyopathy is another cause of sudden death in athletes (for review, see [63]). Systematic screening of young athletes for cardiac disease has been attempted [64]; however, the benefit seems doubtful since only 0.07% of 33 735 athletes had signs of hypertrophic cardiomyopathy, and none of these died during a follow-up period of 8.2 ± 5 years. A detailed medical history including the family history and a thorough clinical examination plus a 12-lead ECG recording may, however, help to detect subjects at risk of Marfan's syndrome (ectopia lentis, hyperflexible joints, scoliosis), aortic stenosis (systolic murmur), and hypertrophic cardiomyopathy (family history, signs of left ventricular hypertrophy in ECG). Children with anomalies of the coronary arteries may present with chest pain during exercise. However, many of these children will not have any symptoms at all. If one of the above diseases is suspected, an echocardiogram should be performed to verify or exclude the diagnosis. A chest X-ray is less helpful in the evaluation of suspected heart disease.

Doping

The prevalence of doping in children is difficult to assess. Figures are obtained most often by self-reporting, a method that carries an inherited bias. In a meta-analysis of 16 studies of children and adolescents between 6 and 19 years of age, frequencies between 0.6% and 15% were found [65]. Misuse of anabolic steroids was most often reported. However, both human growth hormone and stimulants were also mentioned. Males in the highest age group had the highest prevalence of doping in accordance with a previous study [66]. It was difficult to assess which sports had the biggest problem. Abuse of steroids and growth hormone may cause serious adverse effects (impaired gonadal function, aggressive and risky behavior, liver carcinoma, adverse lipid profile and development of acromegalic features). The pubertal and adolescent periods are particularly vulnerable. Therefore, every effort should be made to minimize doping in this age group.

Acute and overuse injuries

Both acute and overuse sport injuries are common in children and adolescents and account for a significant proportion of visits to the primary care physician. Minor injuries that do not lead to medical attention are even more frequent and may only be recognized if they cause loss of participation in practice or competition. In a recent Dutch study of children 4–13 years of age, the incidence of school sport injuries was lower in the younger children than in the older (0.5/1000 in the 4–5-year olds compared with 4.8/1000 in the 12–13-year olds) [67]. The risk of injury in adolescents is even higher.

The pattern of injuries in children is similar to that of adults with a few exceptions. The fact that the child is growing with open epiphyses implies a risk of damage to the growth plate. In practice, however, growth plate injuries from sport are relatively rare. Problems located in the foot and ankle are the most common complaints and may be due to both acute and overuse injuries [68]; however, knee injuries are also frequent, particularly in sports such as downhill skiing, gymnastics, team handball and soccer [69]. Injuries of the hip are less common, and it is difficult to assess how much sport contributes to the numerous complaints of back pain. Overuse and acute injuries to the upper limb include glenohumoral instability, shoulder dislocation, elbow pain, and strains, sprains and fractures of the wrist.

Boys participating in soccer, basketball and football seem to be at greatest risk for acute injuries. Sprains (injury to ligaments) or strains (injuries to muscles or tendons) are common, whereas fractures are less frequent. First aid in acute injuries includes immobilization, cooling and, if required, pain relief. The subsequent treatment depends on the type, severity and location of the injury. The approach to acute injuries in children is similar to that in adults unless the growth plate is injured. The reader is therefore referred to the chapters on injuries in this textbook. Children with growth plate injuries should be seen by an experienced pediatric orthopedic surgeon.

With increasing training load in children and adolescents over the last decades, overuse injuries have become more and more frequent in this age group. These injuries usually present initially with pain during exercise, but may, if not treated appropriately, lead to continuous pain, loss of function and disability. During physical examination, overuse injuries present with pain which is elicited by pressure or stress applied to the body part under examination. Most injuries involve the muscle–tendon unit (e.g. tennis elbow, little league elbow, shin splints). However, other structures may also be affected. Repetitive stress to the apophyses may induce a disruption of the apophyseal structure (Osgood–Schlatter disease). Likewise, repetitive stress to bones during training may lead to stress fractures, especially in long-distance runners and gymnasts. Various bones in the foot, the tibia and lumbar vertebra (spondylolysis) are especially prone to overuse fractures. The fractures are often difficult if not impossible to identify by standard radiologic procedures. Therefore, if a stress fracture is suspected, scintigraphy of the bones or, preferably, MRI may be required. In the treatment of overuse injuries, restriction of training, at least for the exercises putting stress on the injured body part, is extremely important. The short-term use of non-steroidal, anti-inflammatory drugs may also be helpful. Injections of steroids should only be considered in extremely selected cases. In children, restriction from physical activities is usually sufficient to allow a full recovery from stress injuries within 3–12 weeks.

It is an important responsibility of the physician to repeatedly remind the pediatric athlete, her or his parents and the coach that stress injuries can be prevented. Inappropriate biomechanics which may result from wrong techniques or equipment (for example old, worn sport shoes), and pain during exercise, increase the risk of overuse injuries. A sudden increase in training volume or running on a hard surface may also injure the musculoskeletal system.

Thermoregulation

During exercise in very hot or cold ambient conditions, children are less able than adults to maintain thermal homeostasis [70]. For example, while exercising in a very hot and dry environment, children's core temperature increases faster than in adults. Likewise, when swimming in cool water, children cannot maintain their core temperature as well as adults. Reasons for the relative heat intolerance of children are: (i) a lower sweating rate and, consequently, evaporative heat dissipation in children compared to adolescents and adults; (ii) a larger body surface area/body mass ratio in children, which allows for a higher radiative and convective heat exchange; and (iii) a higher metabolic heat production/kg body mass in children. Based on these considerations, children should be at increased risk of heat- or cold-related illnesses. Although epidemiologic data on this issue are lacking, special attention should be given to climate when organizing a training or competition involving children.

Potential risks from sports participation in children and adolescents with a chronic disease

Children and adolescents with a chronic disease who engage in physical activities face the same risks as do healthy individuals. They may, however, experience additional risks which are specific to the disease and which should be addressed by the caring physician. Due to the limited space only some important aspects can be highlighted in this chapter. The reader is referred to recent textbooks for further information [34,71–73]. Possible risks perceived by patients, parents and physicians should, however, not lead to cessation of all PA. Instead, the target for a medical counseling should always be to suggest activities with a low risk profile for the given condition and to teach appropriate behavior to avoid risks.

Congenital heart disease and arrhythmia

There are several different congenital heart defects and arrhythmias, most of which may be subdivided according to their severity. Furthermore, surgical corrections and individual factors may further influence hemodynamics at rest and during exercise.

In the 1960s and 1970s, a restriction in physical activities and sports participation was implemented in almost every child with a suspected or proven congenital heart disease or arrhythmia. The discussion and guidelines over the recent years, however, has reflected a more liberal approach towards exercise in several of the children in this group.

Currently, medical counseling regarding sports participation of patients with heart disease is based on detailed guidelines [74] which are modified according to individual factors. In many cases, exercise testing is necessary to determine the individual risk of specific physical activities.

Asthma

In most patients with bronchial asthma, exercise can trigger an asthma attack if the exercise is of sufficient intensity and duration. The risk for exercise-induced asthma further increases if the exercise is performed in a cold climate and/or the patient is especially vulnerable due to infections, allergen exposure or lack of medication. Attacks triggered by exercise usually resolve spontaneously within 60 min; however, in rare cases, the attack may lead to hospitalization and even death. A proper education and the use of sufficient medication will help to allow most children with asthma to engage in whatever type of sport she or he chooses. Specifically, consistent suppression of airway inflammation employing inhaled cromoglycate or steroids plus short-acting β_2-agonists 10–20 min before exercise combined with a proper warm-up should be recommended. Possibly, leukotriene antagonists such as montelukast may also have a role in the medical treatment of exercise-induced asthma. In cold climates, a face mask is helpful to prevent attacks. It is important to realize that national or international sports organizations need to be notified about athletes with asthma prior to large competitions so that their inhaled medication is not considered as doping. More detailed information on sport and asthma is provided elsewhere [31].

Insulin-dependent diabetes mellitus

In healthy children, insulin levels decrease with exercise so that glucose can be liberated from stores in the liver and blood levels are maintained despite an increase in glucose uptake into the exercising muscle. Children suffering from insulin-dependent (type 1) diabetes mellitus have to inject insulin into the subcutaneous fat tissue. In consequence, insulin is liberated at a constant rate from the subcutaneous injection site, irrespective of glucose demand. Since insulin sensitivity increases during and following exercise, these children are at a high risk of experiencing severe hypoglycemia with exercise, resulting in a loss of consciousness or epileptic seizures. Low blood glucose levels have been described for up to 24 h following exercise in patients with insulin-dependent diabetes. In a survey of parents whose children had suffered from severe hypoglycemia, many parents blamed preceding exercise as trigger. Children should therefore be advised to measure blood glucose before exercise and intermittently thereafter. They should avoid exercise when blood glucose is low and ingest additional carbohydrates before, during and after exercise. In preparation for prolonged activities, the insulin dose should be reduced. However, periodic drinking of a carbohydrate beverage provides more flexibility, as the amount can be modified as the activity progresses [75]. To teach a patient the individual effect of a specific exercise on blood glucose, a simulation of the activity under medical supervision may prove helpful.

Children with type 1 diabetes mellitus may, however, not only experience hypoglycemia with exercise. When insulin levels are insufficient, exercise may lead to ketoacidosis. Therefore, not only low but also high blood glucose levels may indicate possible risks of subsequent physical activities.

It is important to realize that a well-educated patient with diabetes may participate in nearly any sport. There are patients who have achieved world-class performance in various sports.

Cystic fibrosis

Patients with cystic fibrosis may suffer from oxygen desaturation during exercise. Therefore, exercise testing is recommended in all patients with moderate to advanced lung disease to check for this condition. Patients with exercise-induced hypoxemia should be

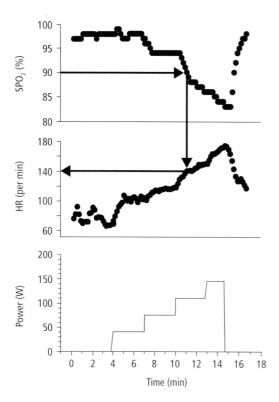

Fig. 3.4.5 Oxygen saturation and heart rate in a 16-year-old boy during an incremental cycle ergometry to volitional fatigue. Oxygen saturation was measured by pulse oximetry, heart rate by ECG. Based on the guideline that exercise with an oxygen saturation below 90% should be avoided, this boy was told not to exercise with a heart rate above 140 beats/min unless he is using additional oxygen.

advised to keep exercise intensity in a range which does not induce a fall in oxygen saturation below 90% [76]. Usually, this recommendation is accommodated by providing a heart rate margin (Fig. 3.4.5). Alternatively, patients may be offered oxygen supplementation with exercise.

Patients with cystic fibrosis often suffer from intolerance to hot climates. One possible cause is suppression of their thirst mechanism, which results in marked dehydration [77]. Addition of NaCl (e.g. 50 mmol/L) to a flavoured beverage will increase their voluntary drinking rate and reduce the likelihood of exercise-induced dehydration [78].

Some patients with cystic fibrosis suffer from liver cirrhosis, resulting in venous congestion in the esophagus (varicosis) and splenomegaly. Trauma may result in severe hemorrhage which can sometimes be fatal.

Therefore, contact sports and bungee jumping should not be recommended to patients with liver cirrhosis [79].

Further, less common risks of exercise in cystic fibrosis include pneumothorax, hemoptysis, and right heart failure. Scuba diving with pressurized air is especially dangerous in this respect.

Epilepsy, hemophilia, cancer and juvenile rheumatoid arthritis

In these four diseases, the risk of sports participation and exercise tolerance depends mainly on the severity of the disease itself, on the positive or negative effects of therapy, and on possible sequelae of the disease or therapy. By contrast, the age of the patient does not usually have a major impact on the ability to engage in physical activities or sports. Due to limited space, we refer to recent reviews and books for a more detailed description of diseases and exercise recommendations [71,80].

Conclusion

Physical activity in early life is an important element in a child's development, well-being and social interactions. It may also yield dividends regarding health in adult years. Health practitioners should encourage children and their families to adopt an active lifestyle. It is important though to recognize potential risks which may accompany enhanced physical activity of healthy children and those with a chronic disease. Such recognition is a prerequisite for the prevention of such risks.

Summary

Children differ from adults in many aspects. During childhood and adolescence, body size and body proportions change markedly. Furthermore, body composition, muscle fiber type and neuromuscular control develop during the first 12–18 years of life. All these changes have an impact on performance during exercise. The relative weakness of epiphyseal and apophyseal growth plates puts children at risk for epiphyseal fractures and apophyseal diseases such as Osgood–Schlatter disease. Due to a lower sweating rate and a larger surface area per body mass in children, compared with adults, the former are less able to maintain thermal homeostasis in very hot conditions.

Although children are usually more active than

adults, their physical activity may not be high enough to improve current and future health. Methodologic problems with the assessment of physical activity may explain some differences between studies looking at the effects of physical activity on health in children. Furthermore, there might be only small effects of childhood physical activity on risk factors for future cardiovascular disease such as adiposity, blood pressure and blood lipid profile in healthy children. However, an active lifestyle may also have direct positive effects in children such as a reduction in accidents and psychological benefits. Children with a chronic disease may further experience a direct improvement in the disease itself or in the symptoms of the disease. For example, patients with asthma may have less attacks when they exercise regularly. In cystic fibrosis, regular physical training may slow the process of lung destruction, and in diabetes mellitus an active lifestyle may slow or postpone the development of long-term complications.

Engagement in physical activity and sport, however, is not risk free in children and adolescents. The risk of growth plate injuries and hyperthermia has been mentioned above. Sudden death during exercise is rare in children and mostly related to cardiac disease. Further risks of sports participation include nutritional disorders, abnormalities of the menstrual cycle and doping. Like adults, children may also suffer from acute and overuse injuries. A negative effect of an intense athletic engagement on growth has not been observed for most sports; the evidence in gymnastics is equivocal. Children with a chronic health condition have additional risks from physical activity and sports, which depend on their disease and the disease severity.

Physicians caring for healthy children and those with a chronic health condition should be familiar with possible benefits and risks of physical activity and sport in this population. This knowledge is a prerequisite for adequate counseling and the prevention of damage.

Multiple choice questions

1 *Tom, a 12-year-old prepubertal boy, weighs 52 kg and has a maximal oxygen uptake of 37 mL/kg/min. His best friend Mike is also 12 years old and prepubertal, weighs 34 kg and has a maximal oxygen uptake of 50 mL/kg/min. The two boys would like to know who is aerobically more fit. Which statement is correct?*

a Mike is more fit because he has the higher maximal oxygen uptake per kg body weight.

b Tom is more fit because he has the higher maximal oxygen uptake in absolute terms (1924 mL/min vs. 1700 mL/min).

c Neither of the above two answers is optimal because neither ratio standards nor absolute values should be used to compare performance in subjects with different body sizes (or age, or gender).

2 *Which of the following sentences is correct?*

a Asking a child whether she or he is active will provide a valid measure of physical activity.

b The pattern of physical activity can be measured by the doubly labeled water technique.

c Heart rate monitoring cannot be used to determine physical activity since heart rate is influenced by ambient temperature and emotions.

d Motion sensors are valid instruments for monitoring all types of activities.

3 *Routine preparticipation examination in children should include:*

a past medical history

b family history

c sports history

d physical examination

e chest X-ray.

4 *Which statements reflect true child–adult differences.*

a Children cannot suffer from overuse injuries.

b Children are more prone than adults to experience heat intolerance in hot, dry climates.

c The level of physical activity is generally higher in children than in adults.

d Children do not benefit from physical activity.

5 *Which of the following statements is/are correct:*

a Children with a congenital heart disease should generally not be allowed to engage in competitive sports.

b Children with insulin-dependent diabetes mellitus might need to reduce their insulin dose prior to a bicycle tour.

c Children with asthma cannot participate in international competitions since their inhaled medication is considered as doping.

d Children with cystic fibrosis should be encouraged to engage in any type of physical activity.

References

1 Nevill AM. The appropriate use of scaling techniques in exercise physiology. *Pediatr Exerc Sci* 1997; **9**: 295–8.

2 Welsman JR. Interpreting young people's exercise performance: sizing up the problem. In: Armstrong N, Kirby BJ, Welsman JR, eds. *Children and Exercise XIX. Promoting Health and Well-Being.* London: E & FN Spon, 1997: 191–203.

3 Malina RM. Quantification of fat, muscle and bone in man. *Clin Orthopaed* 1969; **65**: 9–38.

4 Malina RM, Bouchard C. *Growth, Maturation, and Physical activity.* Champaign, IL: Human Kinetics, 1991: 115–32.

5 Elder GCB, Kakulas BA. Histochemical and contractile property changes during human muscle development. *Muscle Nerve* 1993; **16**: 1246–53.

6 Lexell J, Sjöström M, Nordlund AS, Taylor CC. Growth and development of human muscle: a quantitative morphological study of whole vastus lateralis from childhood to adult age. *Muscle Nerve* 1992; **15**: 404–9.

7 Allor KM, Pivarnik JM, Sam LJ, Perkins CD. Treadmill economy in girls and women matched for height and weight. *J Appl Physiol* 2000; **89**: 512–6.

8 Frost G, Dowling J, Bar-Or O. Cocontraction in three age groups of children during treadmill locomotion. *J Electromyogr Kinesiol* 1997; **7**: 179–86.

9 Harro M, Riddoch C. Physical activity. In: Armstrong N, van Mechelen W, eds. *Paediatric Exercise Science and Medicine.* Oxford: Oxford University Press, 2000: 77–84.

10 Armstrong N, Williams J, Balding J, Gentle P, Kirby B. Cardiopulmonary fitness, physical activity patterns, and selected coronary risk factor variables in 11- to 16-year-olds. *Pediatr Exerc Sci* 1991; **3**: 219–28.

11 Blair SN, Clark DG, Cureton KJ, Powell KE. Exercise and fitness in childhood: implications for a lifetime of health. In: Gisolfi CV, Lamb DR, eds. *Youth, Exercise, and Sport.* Carmel, IN: Benchmark Press, 1989: 401–30.

12 Ross JG, Dotson CO, Gilbert GG. Are kids getting appropriate activity? The national children and youth fitness study. *J Phys Educ Recreat Dance* 1985; **82**: 40–3.

13 Berenson GS, Srinivasan SR, Bao W, Newman WP III, Tracy RE, Wattigney WA. Association between multiple cardiovascular risk factors and atherosclerosis in children and young adults. *New Engl J Med* 1998; **338**: 1650–6.

14 Cheung LWY, Richmond JB. *Child Health, Nutrition, and Physical Activity.* Champaign, IL: Human Kinetics, 1995.

15 Twisk JWR. Physical activity, physical fitness and cardiovascular health. In: Armstrong N, van Mechelen W, eds. *Paediatric Exercise Science and Medicine.* Oxford: Oxford University Press, 2000: 253–63.

16 Sallis JF, McKenzie TL, Alcaraz JE, Kolody B, Faucette N, Hovell MF. The effects of a 2-year physical education program (SPARK) on physical activity and fitness in elementary school studies. *Am J Public Health* 1997; **87**: 1328–34.

17 Hansen HS, Froberg K, Hylderbrandt N, Nielsen JR. A controlled study of eight months of physical training and reduction of blood pressure in children: the Odense schoolchild study. *Br Med J* 1991; **303**: 682–5.

18 Dwyer T, Coonan WE, Leitch DR, Hetzel BS, Baghurst RA. An inestigation of the effects of daily physical activity on the health of primary school students in South Australia. *Int J Epidemiol* 1983; **12**: 308–13.

19 Hagberg JM, Ehsani AA, Goldring D, Hernandez A, Sinacore DR, Holloszy JO. Effect of weight training on blood pressure and hemodynamics in hypertensive adolescents. *J Pediatr* 1984; **104**: 147–51.

20 Hagberg JM, Goldring D, Ehsani AA, Heath GW, Hernandez A, Schechtman K, Holloszy JO. Effect of exercise training on the blood pressure and hemodynamic features of hypertensive adolescents. *Am J Cardiol* 1983; **52**: 763–8.

21 Tortolero SR, Taylor WC, Murray NG. Physical activity, physical fitness and social, psychological and emotional health. In: Armstrong N, van Mechelen W, eds. *Paediatric Exercise Science and Medicine.* Oxford: Oxford University Press, 2000: 273–93.

22 Bradney M, Pearce G, Naughton G, Sullivan C, Bass S, Beck T, Carlson J, Seeman E. Moderate exercise during growth in prepubertal boys: change in bone mass, size, volumetric density and bone strength: a controlled prospective study. *J Bone Min Res* 1998; **13**: 1814–21.

23 Welten DC, Kemper HCG, Post GB, van Mechelen W, Twist J, Lips P, Teule GJ. Weight bearing activity during youth is a more important factor for peak bone mass than calcium intake. *J Bone Min Res* 1994; **9**: 1029–96.

24 Vuori I. Peak bone mass and physical activity: a short review. *Nutr Rev* 1996; **54**: S11–S14.

25 Kunz T. *Weniger Unfälle Durch Bewegung.* Schorndorf: Verlag Karl Hofmann, 1993.

26 US Department of Health and Human Services. *Physical activity and health: a report of the Surgeon General*, 1996.

27 Van Mechelen W, Kemper HCG. Habitual physical activity in longitudinal perspective. In: Kemper HCG, ed. *The Amsterdam Growth Study. A Longitudinal Analysis of Health, Fitness, and Lifestyle.* Champaign, IL: Human Kinetics, 1995: 135–58.

28 Trudeau F, Laurencelle L, Tremblay J, Rajic M, Shephard RJ. A long-term follow-up of participants in the Trois-Rivières semi-longitudinal study of growth and development. *Pediatr Exerc Sci* 1998; **10**: 366–77.

29 Gruber JJ. Physical activity and self-esteem development in children: a meta-analysis. In: Stull GA, Eckert HM, eds. *Effects of Physical Activity on Children.* Champaign, IL: Human Kinetics, 1986: 30–48.

30 Kieckhefer GM. The meaning of health to 9-, 10-, and 11-year-old children with chronic asthma. *J Asthma* 1988; **25**: 325–33.

31 Hebestreit H. Exercise and physical activity in the child with asthma. In: Armstrong N, van Mechelen W, eds. *Paediatric Exercise Science and Medicine.* Oxford: Oxford University Press, 2000: 323–30.

32 Nixon PA, Orenstein DM, Kelsey SF, Doershuk CF. The prognostic value of exercise testing in patients with cystic fibrosis. *N Engl J Med* 1992; **327**: 1785–8.

33 Schneiderman-Walker J, Pollock SL, Corey M, Wilkes DD, Canny GJ, Pedder L, Reisman JJ. A randomized controlled

trial of a three year home exercise program in cystic fibrosis. *J Pediatr* 2000; **136**: 304–10.

34 Bar-Or O. *Pediatric Sports Medicine for the Practitioner. From Physiological Principles to Clinical Applications.* Berlin: Springer-Verlag, 1983.

35 LaPorte RE, Dorman JS, Tajima N, Cruickshanks KJ, Orchard TJ, Cavender DE, Becker DJ, Drash AL. Pittsburgh insulin-dependent diabetes mellitus morbidity and mortality study. Physical activity and diabetic complications. *Pediatrics* 1986; **78**: 1027–33.

36 Joffe I, Epstein S. Osteoporosis associated with rheumatoid arthritis: pathogenesis and management. *Semin Arthritis Rheum* 1991; **20**: 256–72.

37 Damsgaard R, Bencke J, Matthiesen G, Petersen JH, Müller J. Is prepubertal growth adversely affected by sport? *Med Sci Sports* 2000; **31**: 1698–1703.

38 Damsgaard R, Bencke J, Matthiesen G, Petersen JH, Müller J. Body proportions, body composition and pubertal development of children in competitive sports. *Scand J Med Sci Sports*; 2001; **11**: 54–60.

39 Malina RM, Woynarowska B, Bielicki T, Beunen G, Eweld D, Geithner CA, Huang YC, Rogers DM. Prospective and retrospective longitudinal studies of the growth, maturation, and fitness of Polish youth active in sport. *Int J Sports Med* 1997; **18**: S179–S185.

40 Theintz GE, Howald H, Weiss U, Sizonenko PC. Evidence for a reduction of growth potential in adolescent female gymnasts. *J Pediatr* 1993; **122**: 306–13.

41 Malina RM. Physical activity and training: effects on stature and the adolescent growth spurt. *Med Sci Sports Exerc* 1994; **26**: 759–66.

42 Baxter-Jones AD, Helms P, Maffulli N, Baines-Preece PJ, Preece M. Growth and development of male gymnasts, swimmers, soccer and tennis players: a longitudinal study. *Ann Hum Biol* 1995; **22**: 381–94.

43 Theintz GE, Howald H, Allemann Y, Sizonenko PC. Growth and pubertal development of young female gymnasts and swimmers: a correlation with parental data. *Int J Sports Med* 1989; **10**: 87–91.

44 Baxter-Jones ADG, Helms PJ. Effects of training at a young age: a review of the training of young athletes (TOYA) study. *Pediatr Exerc Sci* 1996; **8**: 310–27.

45 Malina RM. Attained size and growth rate of female volleyball players between 9 and 13 years of age. *Pediatr Exerc Sci* 1994; **6**: 257–66.

46 Peltenburg AL, Erich WB, Zonderland ML, Bernink MJ, VanDenBrande JL, Huisveld IA. A retrospective growth study of female gymnasts and girl swimmers. *Int J Sports Med* 1984; **5**: 262–7.

47 Peltenburg AL, Erich WB, Bernink MJ, Zonderland ML, Huisveld IA. Biological maturation, body composition, and growth of female gymnasts and control groups of schoolgirls and girl swimmers, aged 8–14 years: a cross-sectional survey of 1064 girls. *Int J Sports Med* 1984; **5**: 36–42.

48 Beunen GP, Malina RM, Renson R, Simons J, Ostyn M, Lefevre J. Physical activity and growth, maturation and

performance: a longitudinal study. *Med Sci Sports Exerc* 1992; **24**: 576–85.

49 Hansen L, Klausen K, Bangsbo J, Muller J. Short longitudinal study of boys playing soccer: parental height, birth weight and length, anthropotry and pubertal maturation in elite and non-elite players. *Pediatr Exerc Sci* 1999; **11**: 199–207.

50 Malina RM, Bielicki T. Retrospective longitudinal growth study of boys and girls active in sport. *Acta Paediatr* 1996; **85**: 570–6.

51 Bass S, Bradney M, Pearce G, Hendrich E, Inge K, Stuckey S, Lo SK, Seeman E. Short stature and delayed puberty in gymnasts: influence of selection bias on leg length and the duration of training on trunk length. *J Pediatr* 2000; **136**: 149–55.

52 Caldarone G, Leglise M, Giampietro M, Berlutti G. Anthropometric measurements, body composition, biological maturation and growth predictions in young male gymnasts of high agonistic level. *J Sports Med Phys Fitness* 1986; **26**: 406–15.

53 Malina RM, Katzmarzyk PT, Bonci CM, Ryan RC, Wellens RE. Family size and age at menarche in athletes. *Med Sci Sports Exerc* 1997; **29**: 99–106.

54 Claessens AL, Malina RM, Lefevre J, Beunen G, Stijnen V, Maes H, Veer FM. Growth and menarcheal status of elite female gymnasts. *Med Sci Sports Exerc* 1992; **24**: 755–63.

55 Lindholm C, Hagenfeldt K, Ringertz BM. Pubertal development in elite juvenile gymnasts. Effects of physical training. *Acta Obstet Gynecol Scand* 1994; **73**: 269–73.

56 Pigeon P, Oliver I, Charlet JP, Rochiccioli P. Intensive dance practice. Repercussions on growth and puberty. *Am J Sports Med* 1997; **25**: 243–7.

57 Lindholm C, Hagenfeldt K, Hagman U. A nutrition study in juvenile elite gymnasts. *Acta Paediatr* 1995; **84**: 273–7.

58 Bale P, Doust J, Dawson D. Gymnasts, distance runners, anorexics body composition and menstrual status. *J Sports Med Phys Fitness* 1996; **36**: 49–53.

59 Matejek N, Weimann E, Witzel C, Molenkamp G, Schwidergall S, Bohles H. Hypoleptinaemia in patients with anorexia nervosa and in elite gymnasts with anorexia athletica. *Int J Sports Med* 1999; **20**: 451–6.

60 Bennell KL, Malcolm SA, Wark JD, Brukner PD. Skeletal effects of menstrual disturbances in athletes. *Scand J Med Sci Sports* 1997; **7**: 261–73.

61 Maron BJ, Shirani J, Poliac LC, Mathenge R, Roberts WC. Sudden death in young competitive athletes. Clinical, demographic, and pathological profiles. *J Am Med Assoc* 1996; **276**: 199–204.

62 Fikar CR, Koch S. Etiologic factors of acute aortic dissection in children and young adults. *Clin Pediatr* 2000; **39**: 71–80.

63 Futterman LG, Myerburg R. Sudden death in athletes. *Sports Med* 1998; **26**: 335–50.

64 Corrado D, Basso C, Schiavon M, Thiene G. Screening for hypertrophic cardiomyopathy in young athletes. *N Engl J Med* 1998; **339**: 364–9.

65 Laure P. Epidemiologic approach of doping in sport. *J Sports Med Phys Fitness* 1997; **37**: 218–24.

66 DuRant RH, Rickert VI, Ashworth CS, Newman C, Slavens G. Use of multiple drugs among adolescents who use anabolic steroids. *N Engl J Med* 1993; **328**: 922–6.

67 Kingman J, Ten Duis HJ. Injuries due to school sports accidents in 4–13-year-old children. *Percept Mot Skills* 2000; **90**: 319–25.

68 Omey ML, Micheli LJ. Foot and ankle problems in the young athlete. *Med Sci Sports Exerc* 1999; **31** (Suppl.): S470–S486.

69 DeLoes M, Dahlstedt LJ, Thomee R. A 7-year study on risks and costs of knee injuries in male and female youth participants in 12 sports. *Scand J Med Sci Sports* 2000; **10**: 90–7.

70 Bar-Or O. Temperature regulation during exercise in children and adolescents. In: Gisolfi CV, Lamb DR, eds. *Perspectives in Exercise Science and Sports Medicine*, Vol. 2. Indianapolis: Benchmark Press, 1989: 335–67.

71 Armstrong N, van Mechelen W. *Paediatric Exercise Science and Medicine*. Oxford: Oxford University Press, 2000.

72 Bar-Or O. *The Child and Adolescent Athlete. The Encyclopaedia of Sports Medicine VI.* Oxford: Blackwell Science, 1996.

73 Goldberg B. *Sports and Exercise for Children with Chronic Health Conditions*. Champaign, IL: Human Kinetics, 1995.

74 Sklansky MS, Bricker JT. Guidelines for exercise and sports participation in children and adolescents with congenital heart disease. *Prog Pediatr Cardiol* 1993; **2**: 55–66.

75 Riddell MC, Bar Or O, Ayub BV, Calvert RE, Heigenhauser GJ. Glucose ingestion matched with total carbohydrate utilization attenuates hypoglycemia during exercise in adolescents with IDDM. *Int J Sport Nutr* 1999; **9**: 24–34.

76 Boas SR. Exercise recommendations for individuals with cystic fibrosis. *Sports Med* 1997; **24**: 17–37.

77 Bar-Or O, Blimkie JCR, Hay JT, Macdougall JD, Ward DS, Wilson WM. Voluntary dehydration and heat intolerance in cystic fibrosis. *Lancet* 1992; **339**: 696–9.

78 Kriemler S, Wilk B, Schurer W, Wilson WM, Bar-Or O. Preventing dehydration in children with cystic fibrosis who exercise in the heat. *Med Sci Sports Exerc* 1999; **31**: 774–9.

79 Hebestreit H, Hebestreit A, Kriemler S. Körperliche Aktivität und Training bei Mukoviszidose. *Dt Zeitschr SportMed* 2000; **51**: 85–93.

80 Hebestreit H, Bar-Or O. Chronic conditions. In: Sullivan JA, Anderson SJ, eds. *Care of the Young Athlete*. American Academy of Orthopaedic Surgeons and American Academy of Pediatrics, 2000: 219–26.

81 Constantini NW, Warren MP. Special problems of the female athlete. *Baillière's Clin Rheumatol* 1994; **8**: 199–219.

82 Warren MP, Stiehl AL. Exercise and female adolescents. effects on the reproductive and skeletal systems. *J Am Med Women's Assoc* 1999; **54**: 115–20.

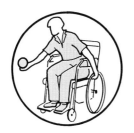

Chapter 3.5
Disabled Individuals
and Exercise

FIN BIERING-SØRENSEN & NILS HJELTNES

Classical reference

Kralj A, Bajd T, Turk R. Electric stimulation
    providing functional use of paraplegic patient
    muscles. *Med Progr Technol* 1980; **7**:3–9.
Much of the fundamental research on electrical stimulation to obtain function of paralyzed muscles had
its origin in Ljubljana, Yugoslavia, at the Faculty of
Electrical Engineering, Edvard Kardelj University, in
cooperation with the Rehabilitation Institute:

The research work reported in this paper is
directed toward the exploration of methods for
applying functional electrical stimulation (FES) to
the paraplegic patients enabling them to regain
different locomotor functions, which are activated
by their own muscles being stimulated
electrically . . . the FES method for paraplegic
patients has numerous advantages which have to be
explored, and proven in the near future. Among
problems of interest are also spasticity reduction
and contracture prevention, improvement of
different physiological functions, etc. This report
should be considered an attempt to gain knowledge
and to prove some expectations on the following
topics: condition of paraplegic patient muscles,
their reinforcement by the use of electrical
stimulation and training procedures, the
performance of reinforced muscles regarding
exerted force, fatigue and functional usefulness for
standing and primitive walking.

The study included two paraplegic patients with
complete upper motor neuron lesions at the thoracic
level, 5 and 10 months after a car accident, respectively.
Surface electrodes were used with stimulation pulses
of 0.3 ms pulse duration, and a stimulation frequency

of 20–40 Hz was applied. The program was 4 s stimulation and 8 s pause. Muscle strengthening was the first
step, and the paraplegic muscles were stimulated to
obtain a good tetanic muscle contraction. Because of
stimulated muscle fatigue at the beginning the program lasted only for half an hour per day. Each week
another half-hour was added so that by the end the
program lasted for 6 hours. The muscle force evoked
by the titanic contraction caused by electrical stimulation was measured with the aid of special joint torque
measuring braces. The joint torque was measured at
different stimulation voltage amplitudes. The measurements were taken approximately every 2 weeks
during the muscle strengthening program.

Figure 3.5.1 gives joint torque plots of the quadriceps muscle, measured as a function of the stimulation
amplitude at different dates of the program. After 6
weeks of exercising the increase of muscle torque has
reached a saturation level.

The study also showed that the lowest frequency of
stimulation produced the lowest muscle fatigue. Further, the lowest torque drop occurred at 20 Hz stimulation. It was also found that the normally innervated
muscles had the same fatigue properties.

FES was used to facilitate standing by stimulation of
both the quadriceps and hip abductors, as well as other
muscles. The swing phase in a primitive gait pattern
was generated by the flexor reflex mechanisms (afferent stimulation), which gives knee and hip joint flexion
and ankle dorsiflexion.

The authors believe that FES of spinal cord injured
patients is a promising application, where vital
functions of severely handicapped patients can be
restored. The work reported in this paper shows
that by means of electrical stimulation it is possible

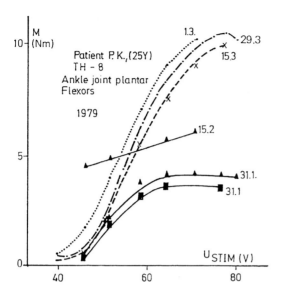

Fig. 3.5.1 Knee joint torque measured versus the stimulation amplitude at different dates during the muscle strengthening program.

to retrain and to exercise the paraplegic patients' weakened muscles. In addition we have demonstrated that the fatiguing of stimulated muscles can be overcome and that the paralyzed muscles can be used to perform functional movements.

Introduction

The beneficial health-promoting effects of physical exercise and sports in the general population are widely accepted and thoroughly documented. These effects are even more needed when persons are potentially more inactive due to a physical disability.

At all times members of the medical profession concerned with the treatment of deformities and other forms of disability have included physical exercise in their treatment; and gymnastics has through the centuries become a household word for remedial exercise[1].

Sir Ludwig Guttmann introduced sport as part of the physically disabled patient's hospital program in 1944 [1]. For some years the development continued within rehabilitation medicine, but since then the participation of physically disabled people has devel-

oped to be included in recreation, health, fitness and competition.

The level of physical activity among individuals with locomotor disabilities is low, but it seems likely that early exposure to physically active pursuits may be an important factor in determining activity level later in life in a locomotor-disabled population [2].

Sports participation is often associated with younger age, less severe disability, disability sustained at an earlier stage, and otherwise good health [2,3]. In a study of spinal cord injured people no significant differences were found on any of the used psychometric measures of depression and trait anxiety between those participating or not participating in sports activities [3]. On the other hand a recent study has demonstrated that sports activity can improve the psychological status, and the psychological benefits are emphasized by sports at high frequency. In addition no difference was found between the more severely disabled tetraplegics in comparison with the less disabled paraplegics [4].

Hutzler and Felis [5] made a literature search for the period 1983–97 related to disability and exercise and sport. They found 253 published records of which 70% were original papers and 30% review articles; 41% were categorized as physiological, 28% psychological and 20% biomechanical. The disability involved was wheelchair users in 55%, and 10% of the papers were focused on children and youngsters.

In this chapter we will give an overview of the exercise physiology in selected locomotor disability groups with the emphasis on spinal cord injured (SCI) individuals, due to the fact that the majority of the research has been carried out in this disability group. In addition the chapter will give an introduction to sport for the disabled.

Exercise physiology in selected groups of physically disabled people

Spinal cord injuries

The establishment of specialized SCI units using the concept of comprehensive treatment and rehabilitation for SCI patients has revolutionized their prognosis [6]. Today SCI individuals survive long enough to grow old with their injuries [7,8]. In parallel with a longer total lifetime, the causes of illness and death in the SCI population approach the causes in the non-disabled population [7,8]. In fact long-term survival studies demonstrate that cardiovascular mortality rates have continued to increase relatively more than in the general population, to become one of the most frequent causes of illness and death also in the SCI population [9].

Physiological and metabolic consequences of physical inactivity

Chronic SCI changes the body composition. Reduced lean body mass (bone mass, muscle mass and essential fat), and increased body fat (storage fat) has been documented in longstanding para- and tetraplegia [10]. Fat accumulation was documented even though the SCI individuals were not overweight and had a normal body mass index. The fat seems to 'replace' lost muscular tissue, and also accumulates in increasing amounts intracellularly in the decentralized muscles [11]. However, whole-body ^{40}K recordings [10] and muscle mass calculations based on basal energy expenditure [12] as well as the more than 40% reduction in muscle fiber cross-sectional area that was observed [13], provide estimates of even lower lean body mass. The primary reason for altered body composition in chronic SCI persons is physical inactivity, owing to paralysis and bed rest in the acute phase of the injury, and continued paralysis and reduced physical activity in the chronic phase [14]. Due to physical inactivity, a daily caloric requirement for a tetraplegic person is only 50% of that for able-bodied people [15]. Accordingly, the caloric intake, especially in tetraplegic subjects, can easily become too great with an unrestricted diet. Thus, physical inactivity and a relatively high caloric intake contribute to a vicious circle leading to metabolic disturbances that result in altered body composition (increased fat mass and decreased lean body mass). The changes in body composition may subsequently lead to an imbalance in glucose homeostasis, which may cause chronic metabolic disorders.

When a muscle is inactivated for an extended period of time, it ends up with predominantly type IIb fibers, or fibers containing only MHC-IIb [16]. Longstanding decentralized skeletal muscles in SCI subjects are also dominated by type IIb fibers [17]. Other fiber distribution patterns have been reported in such muscles,

only when the muscles were extremely spastic [18], or when biopsies were analysed a short time after injury [19]. On the basis of myofibrillar ATPase staining, type IIb fibers were found to be predominant ($66 \pm 6\%$) in tetraplegic vastus lateralis muscle, compared with control subjects ($29 \pm 2\%$) [13]. A pronounced muscle fiber atrophy was demonstrated among all the fiber types in the same tetraplegic group, and the number of capillaries per mm^2 was doubled compared with the controls while the number of capillaries per muscle fiber was significantly reduced. More general staining of connective tissue was observed intramuscularly in the tetraplegic subjects than in the controls [13].

Despite reduced whole-body glucose uptake, glucose transport activity in isolated skeletal muscle was similar in tetraplegic and control subjects. Similarly, the muscular crude membrane content of the glucose transporter protein (GLUT-4), and the glycogen stores were comparable in tetraplegic and able-bodied subjects [13]. Thus the reduced insulin-mediated whole-body glucose uptake in chronic tetraplegic subjects may be explained solely from their reduced muscle mass. Although altered microcirculation cannot be excluded in the tetraplegic subjects, recorded hormone levels were found to be within the reference interval compared to healthy individuals [20].

Arm exercise

Physical exercise and sports in the SCI population have three dimensions. The first is to promote good health and well-being. The second is to make daily life activities easier to perform. And the third is to achieve better results in sports and competition. The common denominator to reach success at all levels is physical training.

SCI subjects need increased muscle strength to lift themselves to and from their bed, wheelchair, toilet chair, car, etc. They need endurance and technique to drive their wheelchair, and they need endurance, strength and technique to walk with crutches and long leg bracelets. Muscle strength training and lifting technique were therefore integrated into rehabilitation treatment from the early days [6]. Lung function training was also adapted early in the tetraplegic group to compensate for their loss of expiratory muscle strength. Endurance training, on the other hand, was not appreciated until the last three decades. As late as 1972, medical authorities spoke against endurance activities for tetra- and high paraplegic individuals due to their inability to control body temperature and blood pressure. A close negative correlation between peak $\dot{V}o_2$ during arm exercise and ascending injury level was observed in recently spinal cord injured patients [21]. Corresponding observations have been reported for SCI subjects with longstanding injury [22]. The results in the recently injured SCI patients were not biased by training, and therefore more convincingly reflect the influence of decreasing volatile muscle mass on peak $\dot{V}o_2$.

Today it has been documented that although there are great individual differences, SCI subjects with low neurologic level injuries can reach an endurance capacity (peak $\dot{V}o_2$) that is close to peak $\dot{V}o_2$ during arm exercise in well-trained able-bodied individuals, while the endurance capacity in tetraplegic subjects is only one-third of this [22]. Therefore paraplegic subjects are considered to have the potential to maintain or improve their cardiovascular capacity, while tetraplegic individuals and some subjects with high neurologic level paraplegia probably continue to lose cardiovascular capacity during the chronic phase [23]. On the other hand, endurance capacity expressed as endurance time and peak oxygen uptake, has been found to increase following a 10-week strictly scheduled arm-cycle program even in chronic tetraplegic subjects [24]. In addition tetraplegic wheelchair marathoners achieve surprisingly elevated fitness levels (Fig. 3.5.2) [25]. Thus, physical training in tetraplegic subjects should consider not only their functional abilities, but also their physical endurance capacity or their peak $\dot{V}o_2$, which is so closely related to health risk factors in the able-bodied population. In a clinical rehabilitation context one must find the optimal balance between time spent on physical endurance training to improve metabolic functions (peak $\dot{V}o_2$), and time spent on functional improvements in daily life. So far, there is no documentation that rehabilitation in recently injured tetraplegic patients improves their aerobic capacity to an optimal level [26].

In SCI subjects muscles above injury level that still function normally are used relatively more than in able-bodied persons. Overuse injuries in shoulders are therefore common. In adaptation to increased de-

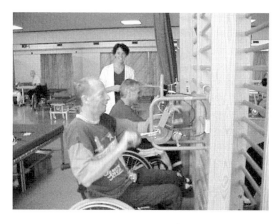

Fig. 3.5.2 The arm ergometer is recommended for endurance training and testing especially during the early rehabilitation period for the spinal cord injured when wheelchair driving technique has not yet been acquired.

mands, intact arm and shoulder muscles are altered both metabolically and morphologically compared to corresponding muscles in untrained and trained able-bodied individuals [27].

Tetraplegic individuals demonstrate a reduced stress response emanating from the sympathetic system, and this probably contributes to the low endurance capacity which was observed both during orthostatic maneuvers [28] and following arm exercise [29]. Low and synchronized activity in postganglionic sympathetic nerves to skin and muscles has also been observed in tetraplegic persons during resting conditions and during afferent stimulation below injury level [30]. A detailed study of catecholamine and blood pressure response during arm exercise using continuous intra-arterial blood pressure recordings and frequent measurements of arterial catecholamine concentrations demonstrated low blood pressure levels and low, but variable, concentrations of catecholamines. A scattered profile of moderate peaks of catecholamines in the blood, as well as a characteristic increase in blood pressure during inspiration compared to expiration, were also noted in the same study. The latter observations may be interpreted as signs of spinal sympathetic reflex activation. Spinal sympathetic reflex activation has also been observed in tetraplegic subjects during inspiration in resting conditions, during bladder activity and cutaneous stimulation [31], and during postural changes [28]. These reflexes are likely to play a key role during the 'boosting' maneuvers (see below), which lead to increased blood pressure and improved performance in tetraplegic athletes [32]. Whether the blood pressure during daily life activities or during ordinary arm exercise is influenced by the low but variable catecholamine concentrations is still an open question. Conversely, spinal sympathetic reflexes contribute to the pathologic condition autonomic dysreflexia, which is characterized by the pathologic elevation of the blood pressure. Results provide evidence to suggest that spinal sympathetic reflexes may be of importance in avoiding a greater drop in blood pressure during ordinary arm exercise in the sitting position, and may therefore lead to less extensive reduction in endurance capacity [33].

Electrically stimulated leg cycle (ESLC) training in SCI individuals

A large increase in ESLC peak $\dot{V}O_2$ in tetraplegic persons following ESLC training is demonstrated in many studies (Fig. 3.5.3) [34]. Since ESLC peak $\dot{V}O_2$ after the training has been found to be significantly

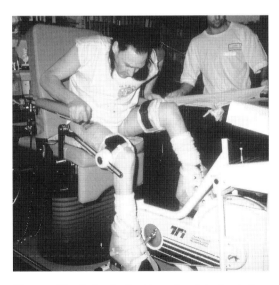

Fig. 3.5.3 Electrically stimulated leg cycle training in spinal cord injured individuals can increase peak $\dot{V}O_2$, muscle volume in the stimulated muscles, muscle glucose transport, the transformation from muscle fiber IIb to IIa, and bone mineral density in the proximal part of the tibial bone.

greater than peak $\dot{V}O_2$ during arm exercise, ESLC is likely to increase the volume load of the heart more than arm exercise. Thus, ESLC may be an effective means of improving myocardial function. ESLC has been shown to reverse left ventricular atrophy in tetraplegic persons [23]. Consequently, if ESLC is supplemented with arm exercise (hybrid exercise), an even greater load on the cardiovascular system will be achieved [35]. Some studies report low mechanical efficiency and high blood lactate levels with various training protocols for tetraplegic persons during ESLC [20]. Thus, ESLC activates the musculature in an 'unphysiologic' manner. In contrast to voluntary activation, electrical stimulation is likely to activate different types of motor units in a synchronized manner. The antagonistic muscles may also be activated and stimulation of afferent nerve fibers may provoke spinal reflexes. A previous study provided evidence for a relatively high increase in body temperature during ESLC [36]. Resent data do not provide evidence for such a marked increase in body temperature with ESLC [20].

ESLC activates larger muscle groups than arm exercise, without any serious side-effects. Thus, ESLC is highly recommended as supplementary endurance training for SCI persons. Better compliance is achieved in patients who have been physically active before the injury, and who are realistic as to the effects of ESLC. Evidence that ESLC training leads to altered body composition in SCI has been provided [20]. Previously magnetic resonance imaging (MRI) scans taken from electrically stimulated thigh muscles have implied that muscle hypertrophy occurs in association with training [34].

It has also been shown that cellular glucose transport capacity was markedly increased per unit muscle mass after ESLC training in SCI persons, and reached values significantly above those of able-bodied persons. The four-fold increase in GLUT-4 protein expression demonstrated at the same time is likely to account for the observed increased muscle glucose transport, since the basal glucose transport was also increased in the skeletal muscle from the same SCI persons [33]. The first demonstration of a direct connection between overexpression of GLUT-4, hexokinase (HKII) and glycogen synthase (GS) through exercise (ESLC) and enhanced glucose transport and metabolism in human skeletal muscle was provided from a study in tetraplegic subjects [33]. The results of this study provide a molecular mechanism by which chronic muscle contraction leads to enhanced glucose uptake and metabolism through increased protein expression and activity of GLUT-4, HKII and GS in skeletal muscle.

Mohr and coworkers [34] assessed muscle fiber type composition in para- and tetraplegic subjects following ESLC training (30 min, three times a week for 12 months) and noted large-scale transformations from type IIb to type IIa, with no transformation to type I fibers. Spasticity has been shown to influence muscle fiber type transformation [18]. Electrical stimulation may activate the muscles through efferent as well as afferent stimulation and the sum of stimulation most likely decides the degree of muscle fiber transformation [37]. Myosin heavy chain assessment indicated gradual transformation from IIb fibers to IIa through intermediate fibers with both types of heavy chain myosin [38]. Muscle fiber transformation from type II to type I was observed in tibialis anticus muscles in high-level SCI subjects exposed to electrical stimulation without external muscular resistance for more than 2 hours daily for 24 weeks [39]. Extreme muscle fiber atrophy was not reversed after ESLC. Therefore, it seems necessary both to increase the stimulation time and to exert additional external load to normalize the decentralized muscle fiber type pattern.

A longitudinal study of bone mineral content in the lower extremities after SCI has shown a decrease of around 50% in the proximal part of the tibial bone within the first couple of years after injury, with the greatest decrease in the first few months [40]. ESLC has been able to increase the bone mineral density by 10% years after the SCI [41].

Efforts should be taken for more extensive treatment involving early activation and mobilization of the paralyzed part of the body after SCI in order to avoid the profound alterations in metabolism and body composition which result from the injury during the first few months after injury. To accomplish this, new and more 'user friendly' electrical stimulation training equipment may be a possibility. More extensive metabolic research in chronic SCI may also highlight the metabolic consequences of physical inactivity for able-bodied persons in general. Future investigations of the relative importance of different cardiovascular risk factors in SCI individuals are needed. On the molecular level, future investigations of different electrical stimulation exercise programs should address both the stimulation qualities and the thermoregulatory parameters which are altered, since electrically stimulated exercise is mechanically different compared to voluntary exercise by physical training.

Neuromuscular disorders

The neuromuscular disorders include a variety of myopathies, i.e. muscular dystrophy and other disorders originating in the nervous system, e.g. motoneuron diseases. Due to the difficulty in recruiting participants, only few larger studies exist on the effect of endurance and strength training in these individuals.

Muscular dystrophies are today incurable inherited disorders characterized by progressive muscle degeneration. There is a great variability in the severity of symptoms and the rate of progression among the different disorders under this heading. Probably due to the diminished muscle mass and strength there is a restricted aerobic exercise capacity and lower power outputs in individuals with Duchenne dystrophy, the most severe type of muscular dystrophy.

In a study of six myopathy patients in a 12-week cycle ergometer training program improvements were found in their maximal oxygen uptake from approximately 13% to 47%, and a reduction in their heart rate at submaximal exercise. These changes were comparable to those in matched control subjects. Although these results are encouraging, two of the participants, one with limb-girdle and one with congenital dystrophy had 30% increases in plasma creatinine kinase and myoglobulin, which may indicate muscle damage induced by the training [42]. In a recent study of six myotonic dystrophy ambulatory persons, who completed a 12-week progressive high-resistance training program for their knee extensor muscles, the muscle strength improved without any observed negative side-effects [43]. In a larger randomized clinical trial on the effects of strength training including 33 participants with myotonic dystrophy neither positive nor negative effects of the training protocol were shown [44]. High-resistance weight training in 16 individuals with gradually progressive neuromuscular disorders increased the muscle performance significantly if the initial muscle strength was greater than 15% of normal [45].

The above-mentioned randomized clinical trial did also include 29 participants with hereditary motor and sensory neuropathy, and after the 24 weeks of training three times a week with weights adapted to their force, a moderate increase in strength and leg-related functional performance was found [44].

In another study 16 postpolio syndrome patients were trained three times a week for 16 weeks on a cycle ergometer at 70% of the maximal heart rate. This resulted in reductions in resting heart rate, systolic and diastolic pressures of up to 7%, and increases in maximal oxygen uptake and peak power output of 15% and 18%, respectively. None of the participants had signs or symptoms of muscle damage, and those with pre-existing atrophy actually increased their maximal oxygen uptake by almost twice the group average [46]. Muscle biopsies of the anterior tibial muscle of individuals with prior poliomyelitis with paresis and excessive and low use of the residual muscle during walking have been investigated. Antibodies directed against cytoskeletal proteins, spectrin and desmin, and against a myoblast and satellite cell-related antigen were applied. Increased staining for these three substances in atrophic fibers could indicate an ongoing denervation process which has been suggested as an important factor for the development of postpolio muscular atrophy. In the polio individuals the number of residual motoneurons is low and the amount of fibers reinnervated by collateral sprouting high. This ongoing denervation–reinnervation process might lead to an exhaustion of the sprouting capacity resulting in muscle weakness [47].

For the metabolic myopathies there is skeletal muscle dysfunction due to disorders of muscle energy production. There may be a coexistence of cardiac and systemic metabolic function, and the symptoms are often intermittent and provoked by exercise or changes in supply of lipid and carbohydrate. Evaluation of these myopathies may actually often require provocation exercise testing. These tests may include ischemic forearm exercise, aerobic cycle exercise and ^{31}P magnetic resonance spectroscopy with exercise [48]. Several metabolic myopathies are known, but the best studied in relation to exercise performance

is McArdle's disease, a phosphofructokinase deficiency. It is characteristic for both syndromes that the muscle strength is adequate at rest and light exercise can be performed, but heavy exertion causes pain, muscle contractures and evidence of muscle damage.

In the presented studies large variations were found, primarily due to the large variability in the participants included in the investigations. The general impression is that training of progressive disorders with low muscle strength may not be useful, and may be potentially harmful, while some of the less severe neuromuscular disorders seem to benefit from endurance as well as strength training. The evidence is still very sparse and further studies are needed.

Cerebral palsy

According to a recent study cardiorespiratory endurance does not differ significantly between people with cerebral palsy (CP) and the able-bodied, and it is independent of their locomotion ability. But the highest physical working capacity performed by the CP participants was significantly lower than in the controls [49].

In CP children of 5–7 years the lung function was reduced in comparison with normative data for children of the same age. But with a 6-month training program including swimming sessions twice weekly and physical activity in a gym once a week, each session lasting 30 min, it was possible to improve the baseline vital capacity by 65%, while a control group only improved by 23% [50].

Strength training for CP has been controversial, as it has been postulated that this training will increase the spasticity, but so far this has not been proven scientifically, and coaches involved with CP athletes claim not to have this experience (Fig. 3.5.4). Furthermore in mildly involved adolescents with CP and ambulatory children with spastic diplegia muscle training programs of 6–8 weeks have been able to improve muscle strength significantly to make them similar in magnitude to values obtained in able-bodied individuals [51,52]. A 10-week muscle strengthening and physical conditioning program in chronic stroke survivors likewise resulted in increased muscle strength *without* concomitant increase in spasticity [53].

Spasticity can be affected by many factors, includ-

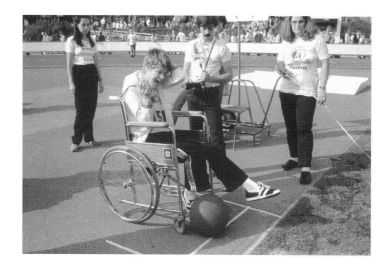

Fig. 3.5.4 'Medicine ball' kick for severely disabled cerebral palsy athletes.

ing fatigue, and therefore the spasticity can fluctuate, which may imply large fluctuations in the economy of motion. This may have a major impact on performance in endurance sports such as distance running and swimming. For years this particular issue has been debated in sport for the disabled when different disability groups compete together. At the present time it is difficult to substantiate the problem and find solutions acceptable to all involved.

Similar to the situation for the neuromuscular disorders, large-scale research related to exercise and CP is scarce. Many of the existing beliefs are based on case stories and anecdotal observations and are not evidence based.

Sports for disabled people

The aims of sport embody the same principles for the disabled as they do for the able-bodied. In addition, sport may be of therapeutic value and play a role in the physical, psychological and social rehabilitation of the disabled.

History

Sports organizations for the deaf were set up many years before the First World War. They really are the forerunners of the modern sports organizations for the disabled and, with greatly improved educational and other social services, for the deaf. As early as 1924 the first world sports organization for the hearing disabled was created (Table 3.5.1).

Table 3.5.1 The history of international organizations in sports for the disabled.

Year formed	International organizations for sports for various disability groups
1924	Comité International des Sports Silencieux (CISS)
1952	International Stoke Mandeville Games Federation (ISMGF) — changed to:
1990	International Stoke Mandeville Wheelchair Sports Federation (ISMWSF)
1964	International Sports Organization for the Disabled (ISOD)
1978	Cerebral Palsy — International Sports and Recreation Association (CP-ISRA)
1981	International Blind Sports Association (IBSA)
1982	International Sports Federation for Persons with a Mental Handicap (INAS-FMH)
1984	International Coordinating Committee of World Sports Organizations for the Disabled (ICC) — changed to:
1989	International Paralympics Committee (IPC)

On 28 July 1948 the Stoke Mandeville Games for the Paralysed were founded as the first officially organized competition for physically disabled athletes. It took place on the same day the Olympic Games were opened in London, and demonstrated to the public that competitive sport is not the prerogative of the able-bodied, but that the severely disabled, even those with a disablement of such magnitude as spinal paraplegia, can become sportsmen and women in their own

right. In 1952 the Games became international, and led to the creation of the International Stoke Mandeville Games Federation (ISMGF). In Rome in 1960 a tradition was started to have international competitions for the disabled following the Olympics for the able-bodied. These games were attended by 400 paralyzed sportsmen and women representing 23 countries, and were held at the Olympic Stadium [1]. In 1990 ISMGF changed its name to the International Stoke Mandeville Wheelchair Sports Federation (ISMWSF).

When the International Sports Organization for the Disabled (ISOD) was founded it was intended primarily to be a coordinating body for disabled athletes, including amputees, the blind and those with cerebral palsy or spinal cord afflictions, as well as other disabilities. Subsequently the first international competition for amputees was held in Brussels in Belgium in 1968, and in 1976 amputees took part in both the Winter and Summer Olympics for the Disabled in Sweden and Canada, respectively.

In 1978 the Cerebral Palsy—International Sports and Recreation Association (CP-ISRA) was formed. CP-ISRA includes all athletes with cerebral upper motoneuron lesions, both congenital and acquired.

Visually impaired athletes also had their own international organization created in 1981, the International Blind Sports Association (IBSA).

At this time all larger physically disabled groups were organized internationally, each with their special diagnosis-related classification system, i.e. spinal cord injured, cerebral palsy and amputee athletes [54], as well as the deaf and the blind. At the same time there was an increasing awareness that a large and very varied group of physically disabled people did not fit into the mentioned categories. Therefore a new classification system was developed to accommodate 'the others', also known as 'Les Autres'. Les Autres includes athletes with polio, muscular dystrophy, arthrogryposis, dwarfism and other conditions, as well as injuries to the musculoskeletal or nervous systems. This group of athletes was first challenged internationally in Oslo, Norway 1981 [55], and took part in the Olympics for the Disabled in 1984. Due to the development of international organizations described, ISOD now only oversaw sport for amputees and Les Autres [56,57].

An international organization, the International Sports Federation for Persons with a Mental Handicap (INAS-FMH) was set up for mentally retarded or athletes with learning difficulties in 1982. But in the USA Special Olympics for this disability group had already started in 1968 on the initiative of the Kennedy family.

Due to these many sports organizations for the disabled there was a need for a new coordinating body for the various international multidisability games, not least the Olympics for the Disabled. Therefore the International Coordinating Committee of World Sports Organizations for the Disabled (ICC) was created. The work by the ICC was continued in the International Paralympics Committee (IPC) (Table 3.5.1), but by 1985 the ICC agreed to the name Paralympic Games instead of the Olympics for the Disabled because this term was not acceptable to the IOC. Paralympics means 'parallel' to the Olympics.

At the 1984 Olympics two demonstration wheelchair track races were staged: a men's 1500-m and a women's 800-m event were an illustration of how far the concept of competitive sport for the disabled had advanced.

In the year 2000 Paralympics in Sydney 4000 disabled people participated, including athletes with visual impairment, learning difficulties, spinal cord paralysis, cerebral palsy, amputation and Les Autres, from 125 nations. It is the world's second largest sports event, only surpassed by the Olympics. It is noteworthy that the number of countries attending the Paralympics in Sydney equaled the number participating in the Olympics in Munich in 1972.

Some sports have created their own international organizations, e.g. the International Wheelchair Basketball Federation (IWBF). This development will probably continue in the coming years, to make sport for the disabled more and more like the able-bodied sports organizations.

Winter sports for people with disabilities began in Switzerland as early as 1935. Attempts were made to use underarm crutches with skis. In 1942 Franz Wendel of Germany, who was a leg amputee, was the first person with a disability to enter ski competition using crutches attached to short skis. By the late 1950s Austria had a ski school for amputees, and by the early 1960s the United States had several ski schools for

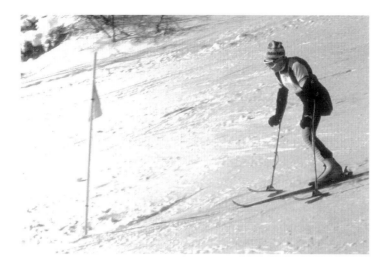

Fig. 3.5.5 One-leg skier using three-track skiing, one ski and two outriggers—forearm crutches attached to short skis.

amputees that used three-track skiing (Fig. 3.5.5), one ski and two outriggers—forearm crutches attached to short skis [58,59]. With the rapidly evolving technology, including ice sledge, sit-ski, mono-ski and downhill sledge a variety of winter sports became available for people with many different forms of impairment. Ski competitions in North America began in the early 1970s. In Ornfeldvik, Sweden the Winter Olympics for the Disabled were arranged by ISOD for the first time in 1976. Demonstrations of disabled skiers had already occurred in 1984 at the Winter Olympics. At the Winter Paralympics in 1998 at Nagano, Japan, 571 disabled athletes from 32 countries participated.

Classification systems

When taking part in competitions, classifications of the disabled athletes may be necessary for the competition to be fair. This is comparable to weight classes in various able-bodied sports. You don't match flyweight with heavy weight. Likewise you don't match slightly disabled with severely disabled in one-to-one competitions. Still one has to remember that we all are more or less different in character and physical possibilities, disabled or not. Therefore no one can expect any classification system to be perfect, in the sense that it can equalize the competitors completely. Like the non-disabled, disabled athletes have to choose their sports in accordance with their personal capacity.

Hearing impaired

To take part in CISS (Comité International des Sports Silencieux) sports competitions for the hearing impaired the only requirement is to fulfil the minimum disability of a hearing deficit of minimum 55 dB on the better ear.

Visually impaired (Fig. 3.5.6)

The minimum disability for the visually impaired to be allowed to compete under the international organization IBSA is a maximal visual power of 6/60 on the better eye with optimal correction or a visual field of maximum 20°.

The visually impaired are for many competitions divided into three groups.

Class B1   From complete inability to perceive light to inability to recognize the form of a hand at any distance or in any direction.

Class B2   From ability to recognize the form of a hand up to visual power of 2/60 or visual field up to 5°.

Class B3   From a visual power over 2/60–6/60 or a visual field over 5° and up to 20°.

Intellectually impaired

The INAS-FMH has established evaluation criteria in relation to intellectual function and social adaptability for participation in competitions. This means to be eligible the person must be or have been in receipt of

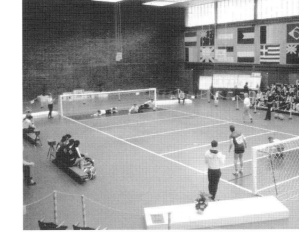

Fig. 3.5.6 Goal-ball for visually impaired athletes. There are three on each team defending their goal and attacking the opposite goal. The ball has a bell in it. The ball is thrown by one team towards the opposite goal, and the other team by listening to the sound from the bell in the ball try to prevent it from passing into their goal. To allow not completely blind visually impaired athletes into the game all players on the field wear eyeshades.

education or social services training opportunities for those who have mental handicap/intellectual disability, as defined by WHO, i.e. falling below the IQ level of 70. Persons can be identified as those who are eligible to receive education, accommodation, employment, guardianship, counselling, financial support or special schooling because they have a mental handicap/intellectual disability. In addition the athlete's learning difficulties must have been recognized before the age of 18.

Locomotor disabled

For many years specific *diagnosis-related classifications* have been available for spinal cord injured (eight classes), cerebral palsy (eight classes), amputee (nine classes) and Les Autres (six classes—depending on the sport) athletes. Due to the difficulty in carrying out competitions with so many classes, classifications are today more sports specific and functional. For example, amputees in the early days had 27 classes, but these were later reduced to nine, not least because competitions became difficult due to insufficient numbers of athletes in most of the classes.

At multidisability games the number of different classes for the 100-m freestyle, despite the reduction in the amputee classes, could reach 31. This is of course due to the large differences among the many locomotor disabled, including athletes with tetra- and paraplegia,

poliomyelitis sequelae, various degrees of cerebral palsy, hemiplegia, brain injury, muscular dystrophy, amputations, congenital dysmelia, anchylosis, severe scoliosis, burns sequelae, etc.

Some competitions are still arranged for only one diagnosis group of locomotor disabled, and during these competitions these classifications are sometimes used, although more and more competitions even in these situations are carried out using the sports-specific classifications.

From the early 1980s the development was from diagnosis-oriented to the more *sports-specific and functional classifications* [55]. This development has been natural in the sense that the sport itself became more essential, while the rehabilitation aspects were very prominent in the early years. At the same time, the previous very large medical involvement has been changed to a much more sports technical approach.

Table 3.5.2 shows an example of a sports-specific functional classification as it appears in an abbreviated form for two of the 10 classes in swimming—S-classes are for the butterfly, backstroke and freestyle strokes. Because the functional profile is different for breast-stroke, this stroke has a somewhat different classification. Class S1 is for the most disabled and S10 for the least disabled.

In team sports it is possible to have athletes with dif-

Table 3.5.2 Examples from the swimming classification — not the complete classification for the particular class! The classification is used for all locomotor disabled, i.e. spinal cord lesioned including poliomyelitis sequelae, cerebral palsy including head injured, amputees including dysmelia, and all other locomotor disabled including muscular dystrophy, multiple sclerosis, dwarfs, arthrogryposis, etc. The functional classification in swimming measures coordination (dysfunction), muscle strength, joint mobility, amputation and body height. In addition to the medical test a functional water test is part of the classification. This functional classification system undergoes continual study and fine tuning. In the S-classes for butterfly, backstroke and freestyle the total number of points a non-disabled person can have is 300 (arms 130, legs 100, trunk 50, start 10 and turns 10 points, respectively). For minimum disability a minus of 15 points must be met (*IPC Swimming Classification Manual*, IPC Swimming, December 1998, www.paralympic.org).

CLASS S1 (THE MOST DISABLED CLASS): 40–65 POINTS *Practical profile*		CLASS S10 (THE LEAST DISABLED CLASS): 266–285 POINTS *Practical profile*	
Hands	Unable to catch the water due to inability of hand or wrist functional control.	Hands	Able to catch the water gaining full propulsion from; OR control of catch phase and propulsion is gained. Minimal involvement of spasticity/ataxia; OR able to catch the water gaining full propulsion from one hand only with some propulsion being gained with the other.
Arms	Has no or severely affected biceps or triceps; OR may have involuntary or minimal movements. Has a restriction in the full range of movement and no coordination.		
Trunk	Has no control, therefore very unstable in the water. May have involuntary movements.	Arms	Full controlled arm cycle gaining full propulsion; OR able to maintain a full controlled arm cycle.
Legs	No leg mobility and normally a severe leg drag. Legs in a flexed position and lack muscle control. May have involuntary movements.	Trunk	Full trunk control.
		Legs	Propulsive kick is possible; OR propulsive kick with minimal involvement in the feet; OR propulsive kick is possible with one leg with minimal propulsion possible of the other leg, which is used for stability; OR full propulsive kick is possible with one leg with satisfactory propulsion with the other leg; OR full propulsive kick.
Others	Swimmers of this class would normally only perform the double arm backstroke. Would normally not be possible for them to perform freestyle as they are unable to control the head, or lack muscle groups to perform this movement.		
Disability profile		*Disability profile*	
1	Tetraplegia, complete below C4/5 or comparable polio.	1	Polio and cauda equina syndrome S1/2 minimal affected lower limbs.
2	Very severe quadriplegia with poor head and trunk control and very limited movements of all limbs for propulsion.	2	Clear evidence of slight spasticity and/or ataxia in specific tests.
		3	(a) Paresis on one leg. (b) Severe restriction of one joint.
		4	(a) Single below-knee amputation. (b) Double foot amputation. (c) Hand amputation, loss of half of the hand.

ferent degrees of disability on the court at the same time, due to a point system as exemplified for basketball. This functional classification system ensures that players with limited or absent lower limb or trunk movement will have an opportunity to play and that the strategies and skills of competing teams, not the amount of physical movement of their players, would be the factors determining success in competition (International Wheelchair Basketball Federation, IWBF). This classification has been modified since its first introduction in 1984. Players are divided into classes 1, 2, 3, 4 and 4.5 according to key functional abilities. When a player does not fit clearly into the descriptions of either one class or the next class, they are assigned a half-point, creating classifications of 1.5, 2.5 and 3.5. In IWBF international competitions, the maximum number of allowable points for the five players on the floor is 14.0. Examples of typical functions evaluated in the classification are given in Table 3.5.3.

Table 3.5.3 Example of functions used in the evaluation of wheelchair basketball players according to the International Wheelchair Basketball Federation (www.iwbf.org).

Function	Class 1	Class 2	Class 3	Class 4	Class 4.5
Shooting	Loses trunk stability during minimal contact	Able to rotate the trunk towards the basket while shooting with both hands	The trunk moves toward the basket with shooting movement, without loss of stability	Is able to move the trunk forcefully in the direction of the follow-through after shooting	Is able to move the trunk forcefully in all directions during shooting
Passing	A forceful one-handed pass requires grasping with the off hand to maintain stability	Fair stability when catching passes in an upright position	Can exert force in passing by trunk extension before initiating trunk flexion movement	Able to lean laterally to at least one side while executing a two-handed pass in the same lateral direction	Able to move the trunk in all directions with good stability while passing
Rebounding	Almost always reaches with one hand while holding the wheelchair to stabilize the trunk with opposite hand	Usually rebounds with one hand, with minimal to moderate loss of stability	Can rebound forcefully with two hands from overhead by moving the trunk forward while reaching for the ball	Can lean forward and to at least one side to grasp an over-the-head rebound with both hands	Can lean forward or to either side with arms overhead to grasp the ball
Pushing the wheelchair	In an upright position the player leans into the back of the wheelchair with head movement forward and back with each push	Able to push the wheelchair without total support of the back of the wheelchair	Able to push the wheelchair forcefully with no loss of anterior or posterior stability	Able to push and stop the wheelchair with rapid acceleration and maximal forward movement of the trunk	Same as Class 4
Dribbling	Usually performed at the side of the wheelchair with trunk instability and slow acceleration	Usually dribbles the ball beside the front castors, particularly when starting this action it is often accompanied by loss of stability	Can dribble the ball in front of the castors with one hand while simultaneously accelerating at a rapid rate by pushing forcefully with the other hand	Can dribble the ball in front of the front castors while pushing with the other hand	Same as Class 4
Typical disability	T1–T7 paraplegia	T8–L1 paraplegia	L2–L4 paraplegia. Hip disarticulation or above-knee amputees with very short residual limbs	L5–S1 paraplegia Hemipelvectomy. Most double above-knee amputees	Single below-knee amputees

Exercise and sports possibilities

It is important to realize that exercise and sport is not only for those who want to take part in competitions. Today sports clubs for the disabled organize all those who are interested in doing exercise and sport together with fellow men and women. In many clubs only 10% or less of the members take part in competitive sports, while the others only take part in the training and exercise activities. On the other hand, several high-level competition athletes are coached in clubs for the able-bodied, e.g. in swimming, athletics and table tennis. Today the standard of elite disabled sports performance demands the very best of coaching, sports science and sports medicine support.

Depending on the disability, including how severe it is, it will always be possible to find some exercise and even competition activities which it will be possible to carry out.

The Paralympics includes many sports, such as archery, shooting, fencing, judo, power-lifting, wheelchair rugby, soccer, swimming, table tennis, wheelchair tennis, riding, cycling, track and field events, wheelchair basketball, volleyball (Fig. 3.5.7), goal-ball for the visually impaired and yachting in summer competitions, and both Nordic and alpine skiing and skating and sledge events in winter competitions.

One major issue to be aware of is the development inherent with integration with the Olympics. This level of performance may be achievable and attractive to the less impaired athletes. The more severely impaired athletes, despite great excellence of performance, may present a less exciting performance to the general spectator and are at risk of being eliminated from elite-level competitions.

Another issue is the possibility of the able-bodied participating in wheelchair sports. The wheelchair could be considered as a piece of sports equipment like a cycle, a kayak or a canoe. But what would happen to the credibility of the sport for the disabled, if this practice became widespread, e.g. in the situation where the winner of a wheelchair marathon race stood up from the chair after the race and received his honour without being physically impaired?

Technical developments

During the last few decades technical developments have been central in relation to many sports and disability groups.

Wheelchairs for road-racing, track and field events, wheelchair basketball (Fig. 3.5.8) and wheelchair rugby are all different and made for their particular purpose. Through years of trials and modifications racing wheelchairs have evolved with the use of basic vehicle mechanics and technical innovations implemented in wheelchair designs. Ergonomics have led to improved fitting of the individual wheelchair (Fig. 3.5.9). Today further developments include advanced engineering and materials, computer simulations and wind tunnel testing [60]. Differences in push rim and wheel diameter, etc. are of importance for the propul-

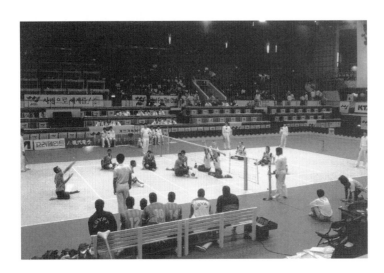

Fig. 3.5.7 Sitting volleyball is very popular, in particular for amputee athletes.

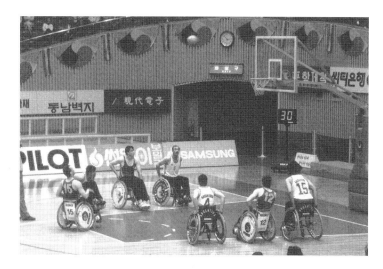

Fig. 3.5.8 Wheelchair basketball. Notice the oblique position of the wheels, which prevent the athletes' fingers being trapped when the chairs come close to each other.

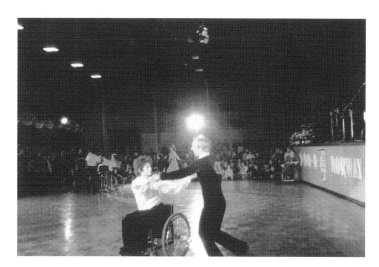

Fig. 3.5.9 Wheelchair dance, with one wheelchair athlete and one ambulant athlete. It is currently being negotiated for this discipline to be on the Paralympic Winter sports program.

sion kinematics. These changes in, for example, road-racing wheelchairs are also a part for the explanation of the development in performance in the wheelchair marathon. The first appearance of wheelchair athletes in the 1977 Boston Marathon was with a finishing time of 2 h 45 min, but since then wheeling marathon racers have been repeatedly below 1 h 30 min.

Prostheses for amputee athletes have likewise developed considerably over the years. An investigation was even able to conclude that prosthetic limb kinematics in transtibial amputee athletes were similar to those for the sound limb, and individuals achieved an 'up-on-the-toes' gait typical of able-bodied sprinting

[61]. Indeed, currently the 100-m able-bodied world record is 9.83 s, but the same distance has been run in 11.31 s by a below-knee amputee and, for further comparison, in 10.72 s by an athlete with a shoulder disarticulation.

Buoyant artificial limbs are also available to allow people who have an amputation to take part in water sport. An artificial limb that is buoyant, however, can interfere with the function of a life jacket and prevent a person who is floating face down in water from turning over [62].

Among other sports equipment which has developed considerably over the years special skis and sledges should be mentioned; these include water-ski seating systems and much more.

Injuries

Ferrara *et al.* [63] carried out a retrospective cross-disability survey in 426 disabled athletes who participated in national competitions in the USA in 1989. Of these 32% reported at least one injury occurring during a practice, training or competition session, which had caused the athlete to stop, limit or modify participation for 1 day or more over the past 6 months. A total of 178 acute injuries were reported by 95 (22.3%) athletes, and 61 athletes (14.3%) reported 210 chronic injuries. The injuries were distributed with 44.3% to the upper and 42.8% to the lower extremities, while 8.2% were located to the neck or spine and 3.6% to the trunk, and 1.1% to the head and face. Among the athletes grouped for spinal cord injury sports 57% of all injuries were to the shoulder and arm/elbow, corresponding to the excess of wheelchair athletes. Among the visually impaired 53% of the injuries involved the lower extremities. For the cerebral palsy athletes knee

injuries accounted for 21%, shoulder for 16%, forearm/wrist for 16%, and leg/ankle for 15% of all the injuries. Relatively this group had the lowest frequency of injuries.

In a study on soft tissue injuries to USA paralympians at the 1996 Summer Games there was found a decreased incidence of shoulder injury among wheelchair athletes suggesting that the injury prevention advice provided by previous studies is being implemented among athletes at this competitive level [64] (Fig. 3.5.10).

The relative risk of injury among disabled athletes is approximately the same as that reported by able-bodied athletes. The most frequent injuries are soft tissue injuries, blisters, other overuse injuries, and abrasions [58,65]. Similarly it has been concluded that skiers with a disability incur approximately the same proportion of injuries as skiers without a disability [66].

The athletes with sports-related injuries took their primary medical advice from a physician in 45.5%, an athletic trainer in 18.8% and a physiotherapist in

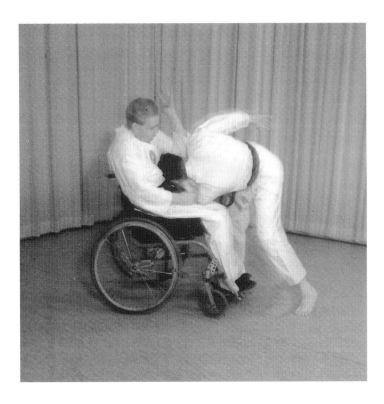

Fig. 3.5.10 Even sports like Daito-ryu Aiki Jujutsu Roppokai can be performed in a wheelchair.

6.8% of cases. Less than one-fifth of the injuries were not medically evaluated [63].

Wilson and Washington [65] investigated a pediatric population with a mean age of 12.9 years at the 1990 Junior National Wheelchair Games in the USA. Of the 83 athletes who responded 77% had a spinal cord lesion, in particular caused by spina bifida. Of those participating in track events 97% reported injuries; the corresponding numbers were 22% for field and 91% for swimming participants. Apart from blisters in track and field, wheelburns and bruises in track, foot scrapes in swimming, abrasions, soft tissue injuries and a few fractures, it was noteworthy that 49% of those with injuries in track reported hyperthermia or over-heating, 22% bladder infection and 14% pressure sores. In swimming hypothermia was reported by 9%.

Special precautions for certain disabled groups

Locomotor disabled
Blisters, wheelburns, abrasions and bruises can be re-duced with proper protective equipment and padding. Individuals involved in wheelchair track events can protect hands from blistering with proper gloves. Wheelburns on the arms and chest can be decreased by utilization of protective garments like arm guards. Bruises may be prevented by padding restraining straps, padding bony prominences, and protecting vul-nerable areas during transfers, including placing mats at poolsides to allow safer transfers [65].

For individuals with *spinal cord lesions* without sen-sation in areas below the level of the lesion there must be maximum awareness of the risk of developing fric-tion blisters and pressure ulcers. This means, for ex-ample, that these individuals should not participate in sitting volleyball and similar activities. Generally ex-tended periods of sitting should be avoided, and the athletes should use proper cushions and regular weight shifts. In wheelchair races the popular seating position distributes the body weight over a small surface area, thus predisposing the athlete to pressure sores [65].

SCI individuals are also susceptible to urinary tract infections. In particular residual urine in the bladder should be avoided, as this is the single most frequent cause for the infections. Sufficient hydration and the possibility for regular bladder emptying are important.

Wheelchair athletes or athletes using crutches may be prone to carpal tunnel syndrome.

Precautions have to be taken, such as for example body restraining straps, in people with spinal cord lesions prone to spasms, to prevent them from being thrown out of the wheelchair.

Horseback riding may not be recommended for SCI tetraplegics [58].

Thermoregulation is impaired in SCI individuals, due to the loss of autonomic nervous system control of skin blood flow and sweating below the level of the spinal cord lesion. Therefore the core temperature rises more during exercise in the athlete with a spinal cord lesion than in an able-bodied athlete, and the temperature rises more the higher the spinal cord le-sion is localized [36,67]. To avoid heat cramps, heat ex-haustion or even heat stroke during exercise or sport in high temperatures, in particular when associated with high humidity, it is important to have shaded facilities near by, ready access to drinking water, and water for wetting exposed body surface areas. Adequate hydra-tion is fundamental, and daily weighing may be a prac-tical way to keep track of hydration status if exercising or competing in very hot and humid environments [68].

Not all disabilities are static: some medical con-ditions such as *multiple sclerosis* may have a variable course and others such as *muscular dystrophy* are pro-gressive. The sporting activity that is possible at one stage may not be so in the future, and therefore re-assessments of the individual's capacity to participate in sport may be necessary [62]. As already mentioned, training of progressive muscular dystrophy with low muscle strength may be potentially harmful.

For persons with *osteogenesis imperfecta* contact sports like football (tackle), ice hockey, sledge hockey and soccer should be discouraged due to the risk of fractures. Similarly it is not recommended that indi-viduals with *hemophilia* take part in football (tackle) or ice hockey [58].

Persons with many other locomotor disabilities, in-cluding lower extremity amputations, cerebral palsy, neuromuscular disorders, arthrogryposis, juvenile rheumatoid arthritis and skeletal dysplasias, have to take their individual circumstances into account in re-lation to many individual as well as team sports [58].

In addition the presence of *pre-existing medical*

problems, like orthopaedic disability and limited range of motion should be acknowledged as areas of higher risk of injury due to unusual stress to joints, tendons and muscles. Orthotics and other such devices may sometimes be used to correct structural deformities and reduce unnecessary biomechanical stress. In *young athletes* possible damage to growth-specific areas, such as epiphyses, articular surfaces and tendon apophyses may result from repetitive stress [65].

Intellectually impaired

Mentally handicapped persons who suffer from genetic disorders may have associated, potentially dangerous physical abnormalities such as congenital heart disease [62].

In individuals with *Down's syndrome* the potential instability of the atlantoaxial joint is of particular concern. Hyperextension or severe flexion of the cervical spine may produce neurologic deficits or even death caused by compression of the lower brain stem and upper spinal cord. Opinions differ as to whether people with Down's syndrome should be allowed to take part in a contact sport. The American Academy of Paediatrics suggests that athletes with radiographic atlantoaxial instability participate only in non-contact sports limited to moderately strenuous or non-strenuous intensity. Acceptable sports include badminton, curling, table tennis, archery, golf and swimming, provided that the athletes do not dive or perform the butterfly or breaststroke [69]. Riding is not recommended for mentally handicapped people who have communication difficulties or behavioral disorders [62].

Epilepsy

Epileptic people who have occasional and unpredictable fits, particularly if there is no aura, require attention. These individuals should not be allowed to participate in subaqua diving. Activities such as canoeing or water skiing are not encouraged. The wearing of life jackets is an important addition to safety when sailing or rowing. The normal function of a life jacket is to turn the wearer on his or her back; a person who has suffered a seizure and is wearing a life jacket has a small risk of airway obstruction by the tongue falling back. An epileptic person should therefore be paired with a capable person who is familiar with the condition and knows what action to take if a seizure occurs. Sports that are solitary such as hang gliding should not be encouraged. People with epilepsy should be advised to take part in sporting activities where they do not endanger themselves or others and should be accompanied by someone who is familiar with their needs [62].

Doping and boosting

People with a disability may be taking medications for control of a disease process or specific symptoms, or both. Advising doctors should be aware of drugs that, if used, may be on the International Olympic Committee (IOC) list of doping substances, and in particular of certain products sold over the counter as remedies for the common cold, cough, pain, indigestion, etc., which may contain banned substances.

During the Barcelona Paralympic Games in 1992, 217 tests were performed and three were positive. One wheelchair basketball player had used dextropropoxifen, while two had taken anabolic steroids, athletes in judo and field events, respectively. For comparison 1817 tests were carried out during the Olympics the same year, and three were positive.

In the Atlanta Paralympics in 1996 approximately 480 doping tests were taken in about 460 competitors. No positive tests were found, except for six competitors, who were registered in advance on the Medications Advisory Panel.

Boosting

Boosting is the intentional induction of autonomic dysreflexia to enhance performance. This condition is unique to SCI individuals with a neurologic level at or above T6. Therefore in individuals with high-level paraplegia or tetraplegia a nociceptive stimulus below the level of the lesion may result in increased sympathetic outflow with exaggerated norepinephrine response. Hypertension, bradycardia and piloerection occur. Above the level of the lesion the individual may experience flushing, vascular headache and nasal congestion. This condition can be induced by noxious stimuli below the level of the neurological lesion such as clamping of a urinary catheter to produce bladder distension, excessive tightening of the leg straps, twisting or sitting on the scrotum, or similar 'pain'-producing situations. The potential danger is uncontrolled hypertension, which may lead to cerebral hemorrhage and death. Burnham *et al.* [32] found that in eight athletes who could introduce autonomic dysreflexia by this procedure, they were able to improve race performance time by 9.7%. It was also demonstrated that the reported ability to control the response was fallacious.

Boosting was deemed a banned method by the IPC in 1994, but there is a real practical problem with enforcement. The concern is for the safety of the athletes, but 'unless you catch the athlete in the act, how do you detect it?' [70]. The way forward in preventing a potential disaster is education of athletes and a dialogue with athletes. For the sports physician working with athletes with this disability it is important to be aware of this condition. The immediate management is to remove the nociceptive stimulus where possible and to administer sublingual nifedipine (10 mg) to reduce the blood pressure.

Summary

An overview is given of exercise physiology in spinal cord injured (SCI) individuals with regard to physiologic and metabolic consequences of physical inactivity, arm exercise and the use of electrically stimulated leg cycle training. Efforts should be taken for more extensive treatment involving early activation and mobilization of the paralyzed part of the body after spinal cord injury in order to diminish the reduction in lean body mass, the increase in body fat, the muscle atrophy, the reduction in glucose uptake, the loss in bone mineral density, etc. For persons with neuromuscular disorders and cerebral palsy the corresponding knowledge is summarized although it is much more sparse.

Organized sport for the physically disabled dates back to the 1940s, but during the last half-century it has grown stronger, even leading to participation in the Olympic Games. To make competition fair classification of the participants for the various disciplines is necessary. For many years diagnosis-related classifications were used, but today the sports-specific and functional approach is utilized. Still, competition is only for the few while participation in exercise and sport in general can be enjoyed by virtually everyone regardless of the disability. Many possibilities exist for the disabled to focus on their abilities more than the opposite in performing exercise and sport. This is also accomplished by technical developments of various

kinds, e.g. wheelchairs and prostheses. When competing, disabled athletes have a relative risk of injury similar to that of the able-bodied. Special precautions have to be taken for certain disability groups in relation to the exercise and sport performed. Doping does also exist in sport for disabled. Boosting, which is the induction of autonomic dysreflexia in SCI individuals with lesions above T6, is potentially dangerous.

Multiple choice questions

1 *Glucose homeostasis in chronic high-level spinal cord injuries is disturbed by:*

a altered hormonal balance
b reduced transport of glucose into each muscle cell
c reduced whole-body lean body mass
d low levels of circulating catecholamines
e increased fat mass.

2 *Arm endurance exercise in tetraplegic persons is limited by:*

a cardiac output
b ventilatory capacity
c exercise-induced hypotension
d local muscular fatigue in the exercising muscles
d blood volume.

3 *In what year did the first officially organized competition for the physically disabled take place:*

a 1940
b 1948
c 1956
d 1964
e 1972.

4 *In what time will an international wheelchair marathon race often be won?:*

a between 1 h 15 min and 1 h 30 min
b between 1 h 30 min and 1 h 45 min
c between 1 h 45 min and 2 h
d between 2 h and 2 h 15 min
e between 2 h 15 min and 2 h 30 min.

5 *What is boosting?*

a The use of amphetamines to enhance athletic performance.
b The use of anabolic steroids to increase muscle strength.
c The induction of autonomic dysreflexia in spinal cord injured athletes.
d The use of growth hormone to increase muscle strength.

e The use of pain killers to induce higher performance.

References

1 Guttmann L. *Textbook of Sport for the Disabled*. Aylesbury, Bucks, UK: HM&M Publishers Ltd, 1976.

2 Washburn R, Hedrick BN. Descriptive epidemiology of physical activity in university graduates with locomotor disabilities. *Int J Rehabil Res* 1997; **20**: 275–87.

3 Foreman PE, Cull J, Kirkby RJ. Sports participation in individuals with spinal cord injury: demographic and psychological correlates. *Int J Rehabil Res* 1997; **20**: 159–68.

4 Muraki S, Tsunawake N, Hiramatsu S, Yamasaki M. The effect of frequency and mode of sports activity on the psychological status in tetraplegics and paraplegics. *Spinal Cord* 2000; **38**: 309–14.

5 Hutzler Y, Felis O. Computerized search of scientific literature on sport for disabled persons. *Percept Mot Skills* 1999; **88**: 1189–92.

6 Guttmann L. New hope for spinal cord sufferers. *New York Med Times* 1945; **73**: 318–27.

7 Hartkopp A, Brønnum-Hansen H, Seidenschnur AM, Biering-Sørensen F. Survival and cause of death after traumatic spinal cord injury. A long-term epidemiologic survey from Denmark. *Spinal Cord* 1997; **35**: 76–85. [Corrigendum: *Spinal Cord* 1997; **35**: 862–4.]

8 Whiteneck GG, Charlifue SW, Frankel HL, Fraser MH, Gardner BP, Gerhart KA, Krishnan KR, Menter RR, Nuseibeh I, Short DJ, Silver JR. Mortality, morbidity, and psychosocial outcomes of persons spinal cord injured more than 20 years ago. *Paraplegia* 1992; **30**: 617–30.

9 Krause JS, Sternberg M, Lottes S, Maides J. Mortality after spinal cord injury: An 11-year prospective study. *Arch Phys Med Rehab* 1997; **78**: 815–21.

10 Spungen AM, Bauman WA, Wang J, Pierson RN Jr. Measurement of body fat in individuals with tetraplegia: a comparison of eight clinical methods. *Paraplegia* 1995; **33**: 402–8.

11 Scelsi R, Marchetti C, Poggi P, Lotta S, Lommi G. Muscle fiber type morphology and distribution in paraplegic patients with traumatic cord lesion. *Acta Neuropathol (Berlin)* 1982; **57**: 243–8.

12 Aksnes A-K, Brundin T, Hjeltnes N, Wahren J. Metabolic, thermal and circulatory effects of intravenous infusion of amino acids in tetraplegic patients. *Clin Physiol* 1995; **5**: 377–96.

13 Aksnes A-K, Hjeltnes N, Wahlström EÖ, Katz A, Zierath J, Wallberg-Henriksson H. Intact glucose transport in morphologically altered denervated skeletal muscle from quadriplegic patients. *Am J Physiol* 1996; **271** *(Endocrin Metab* **34**): E593–600.

14 Dallmeijer AJ, Hopman MT, van As HH, van der Woude LH. Physical capacity and physical strain in persons with tetraplegia; the role of sport activity. *Spinal Cord* 1996; **34**: 729–35.

15 Mollinger LA, Spurr GB, El Ghatit AZ, Barboriak JJ, Rooney CB, Davidoff DD, Bongard RD. Daily energy expenditure and basal metabolic rates of patients with spinal cord injury. *Arch Phys Med Rehab* 1985; **66**: 420–6.

16 Pette D, Vrbova D. Adaptation of mammalian skeletal muscle fibers to chronic electrical stimulation. *Rev Physiol Biochem Pharmacol* 1992; **120**: 115–202.

17 Grimby G, Broberg C, Krotkiewska I, Krotkiewski M. Muscle fiber composition in patients with traumatic cord lesion. *Scand J Rehab Med* 1976; **8**: 37–42.

18 Scelsi R, Poggi P, Padovani R, Lotta S, Cairoli S, Saitta A. Skeletal muscle changes following myelotomia in paraplegic patients. *Paraplegia* 1986; **24**: 250–9.

19 Rochester L, Barron MJ, Chandler CS, Sutton RA, Miller S, Johnson MA. Influence of electrical stimulation of the tibialis anterior muscle in paraplegic subjects. 2. Morphological and histochemical properties. *Paraplegia* 1995; **33**: 514–22.

20 Hjeltnes N, Aksnes AK, Birkeland KI, Johansen J, Lannem A, Wallberg-Henriksson H. Improved body composition after 8 weeks of electrically stimulated leg cycling in tetraplegic patients. *Am J Physiol* 1997; **273** *(Regulat Integr Comp Physiol* **42**): R1072–9.

21 Hjeltnes N. Cardiorespiratory capacity in tetra- and paraplegia shortly after injury. *Scand J Rehab Med* 1986; **18**: 65–70.

22 Wicks JR, Oldridge NB, Cameron JB, Jones NL. Arm cranking and wheelchair ergometry in elite spinal cord-injured athletes. *Med Sci Sports Exerc* 1983; **15**: 224–31.

23 Nash MS, Bilsker M, Marcillo AE, Isaac SM, Botelho LA, Klose KJ, Green BA, Rountree MT, Shea JD. Reversal of adaptive left ventricular atrophy following electrically-stimulated exercise training in human tetraplegics. *Paraplegia* 1991; **29**: 590–9.

24 McLean KP, Skinner JS. Effect of body training position on outcomes of an aerobic training study on individuals with quadriplegia. *Arch Phys Med Rehab* 1995; **76**: 139–50.

25 Eriksson P, Lofstrom L, Ekblom B. Aerobic power during maximal exercise in untrained and well-trained persons with quadriplegia and paraplegia. *Scand J Rehab Med* 1988; **20**: 141–7.

26 Hjeltnes N, Wallberg-Henriksson H. Improved physical work capacity but unchanged peak oxygen uptake during primary rehabilitation in tetraplegic patients. *Spinal Cord* 1998; **36**: 691–8.

27 Schantz PG, Sjöberg B, Widebeck A-M, Ekblom B. Skeletal muscle of trained and untrained paraplegics and tetraplegics. *Acta Physiol Scand* 1997; **161**: 31–9.

28 Corbett JL, Frankel HL, Harris PJ. Cardiovascular responses to tilting in tetraplegic man. *J Physiol* 1971; **215**: 411–31.

29 Bloomfield SA, Jackson RD, Mysiw WJ. Catecholamine response to exercise and training in individuals with spinal cord injury. *Med Sci Sports Exerc* 1994; **26**: 1213–9.

30 Stjernberg L, Wallin GB. Sympathetic neural outflow in spinal man. A preliminary report. *J Autonom Nerv Syst* 1983; **7**: 313–8.

31 Corbett JL, Frankel HL, Harris PJ. Cardiovascular reflex

responses to cutaneous and visceral stimuli in spinal man. *J Physiol* 1971; **215**: 395–409.

32 Burnham R, Wheeler G, Bhambhani Y, Belanger M, Eriksson P, Steadward R. Intentional induction of autonomic dysreflexia among quadriplegic athletes for performance enhancement: efficacy, safety and mechanism of action. *Clin J Sport Med* 1994; **4**: 1–10.

33 Hjeltnes N, Björnholm M, Aksnes AK, Lannem A, Galuska D, Zierath J, Wallberg-Henriksson H. Exercise induced over-expression of key regulatory proteins involved in glucose uptake and metabolism in tetraplegic persons: molecular mechanism for improved glucose homeostasis. *FASEB J* 1998; **12**: 1701–12.

34 Mohr T, Andersen JL, Biering-Sørensen F, Galbo H, Bangsbo J, Wagner Å, Kjær M. Long term adaptation to electrically induced cycle training in severe spinal cord injured individuals. *Spinal Cord* 1997; **35**: 1–16.

35 Mutton DL, Scremin AME, Barstow TJ, Scott MD, Kunkel CF, Caggle TG. Physiologic responses during functional electrical stimulation leg cycling and hybrid exercise in spinal cord injured subjects. *Arch Phys Med Rehab* 1997; **78**: 712–8.

36 Petrofsky JS. Thermoregulatory stress during rest and exercise in heat in patients with a spinal cord injury. *Eur J Appl Physiol* 1992; **64**: 503–7.

37 Stein RB, Gordon T, Jefferson J, Scharfenberger A, Yang JF, Totosy de Zepetnek J, Belanger M. Optimal stimulation of paralyzed muscle after human spinal cord injury. *J Appl Physiol* 1992; **72**: 1393–400.

38 Andersen JL, Mohr T, Biering-Sørensen F, Galbo H, Kjær M. Myosin heavy chain isoform transformation in single fibres from m. vastus lateralis in spinal cord injured individuals: Effects of long-term functional electrical stimulation (FES). *Pflügers Arch – Eur J Physiol* 1996; **431**: 513–8.

39 Martin TP, Stein RB, Hoeppner PH, Reid DC. Influence of electrical stimulation on the morphological and metabolic properties of paralyzed muscle. *J Appl Physiol* 1992; **72**: 1401–6.

40 Biering-Sørensen F, Bohr HH, Schaadt OP. Longitudinal study of bone mineral content in the lumbar spine, the forearm and the lower extremities after spinal cord injury. *Eur J Clin Invest* 1990; **20**: 330–5.

41 Mohr T, Pødenphant J, Biering-Sørensen F, Galbo H, Thamsborg G, Kjær M. Increased bone mineral density after prolonged electrically induced cycle training of paralyzed limbs in spinal cord injured man. *Calcified Tissue Int* 1997; **61**: 22–5.

42 Florence JM, Hagberg JM. Effect of training on the exercise responses of neuromuscular disease patients. *Med Sci Sports Exerc* 1984; **16**: 460–5.

43 Tollbäck A, Eriksson S, Wredenberg A, Jenner G, Vargas R, Borg K, Ansved T. Effects of high resistance training in patients with myotonic dystrophy. *Scand J Rehab Med* 1999; **31**: 9–16.

44 Lindeman E, Leffers P, Spaans F, Drukker J, Reulen J, Kerckhoffs M, Köke A. Strength training in patients with myotonic dystrophy and hereditary motor and sensory neu-

ropathy: a randomized clinical trial. *Arch Phys Med Rehab* 1995; **76**: 612–20.

45 Milner-Brown HS, Miller RG. Muscle strengthening through high-resistance weight training in patients with neuromuscular disorders. *Arch Phys Med Rehab* 1988; **69**: 14–9.

46 Jones DR, Speier J, Canine K, Owen R, Stull A. Cardiorespiratory responses to aerobic training by patients with post-poliomyelitis sequelae. *J Am Med Assoc* 1989; **261**: 3255–8.

47 Borg K, Edström L. Prior poliomyelitis: an immunohistochemical study of cytoskeletal proteins and a marker for muscle fibre regeneration in relation to usage of remaining motor units. *Acta Neurol Scand* 1993; **87**: 128–32.

48 Martin A, Haller RG, Barohn R. Metabolic myopathies. *Curr Opin Rheumatol* 1994; **6**: 552–8.

49 Tobimatsu Y, Nakamura R, Kusano S, Iwasaki Y. Cardiorespiratory endurance in people with cerebral palsy measured using an arm ergometer. *Arch Phys Med Rehab* 1998; **79**: 991–3.

50 Hutzler Y, Chacham A, Bergman U, Szeinberg A. Effects of a movement and swimming program on vital capacity and water orientation skills of children with cerebral palsy. *Dev Med Child Neurol* 1998; **40**: 176–81.

51 Damiano DL, Vaughan CL, Abel MF. Muscle response to heavy resistance exercise in children with spastic cerebral palsy. *Dev Med Child Neurol* 1995; **37**: 731–9.

52 MacPhail HE, Kramer JF. Effect of isokinetic strength-training on functional ability and walking efficiency in adolescents with cerebral palsy. *Dev Med Child Neurol* 1995; **37**: 763–75.

53 Teixeira-Salmela LF, Olney SJ, Nadeau S, Brouwer B. Muscle strengthening and physical conditioning to reduce impairment and disability in chronic stroke survivors. *Arch Phys Med Rehab* 1999; **80**: 1211–8.

54 Biering-Sørensen F. Classification of paralysed and amputed sportsmen. In: Natvig H, ed. *The First International Medical Congress on Sports for the Disabled*. Royal Ministry of Church and Education State Office for Youth and Sports, Oslo, 1980: 44–53.

55 Natvig H, Biering-Sørensen F, Jørgensen P. Proposal for classification of athletes with 'other locomotor disabilities'. In: Natvig H, ed. *The First International Medical Congress on Sports for the Disabled*. Royal Ministry of Church and Education State Office for Youth and Sports, Oslo, 1980: 76–84.

56 Biering-Sørensen F. The classification system of ISOD (International Sports Organisation for the Disabled). In: Hoeberigs JH, Vorsteveld H, eds. *Proceedings of the Workshop on Disabled and Sports*. Ebu, Maastricht, 1983: 97–105.

57 Biering-Sørensen F. Problems of the ISOD classification system. In: Heoberigs JH, Vorsteveld H, eds. *Proceedings of the Workshop on Disabled and Sports*. Ebu, Maastricht, 1983: 106–10.

58 Clark MW. The physically challenged athlete. *Adolescent Med* 1998; **9**: 491–9.

59 Laskowski ER. Snow skiing for the physically disabled. *Mayo Clinic Proc* 1991; **66**: 160–72.

60 MacLeish MS, Cooper RA, Harralson J, Ster JF III Design of a composite monocoque frame racing wheelchair. *J Rehabil Res Dev* 1993; **30**: 233–49.

61 Buckley JG. Sprint kinematics of athletes with lower-limb amputations. *Arch Phys Med Rehab* 1999; **80**: 501–8.

62 Chawla JC. Sport for people with disability. *Br Med J* 1994; **308**: 1500–4.

63 Ferrara MS, Buckley WE, McCann BC, Limbird TJ, Powell JW, Robl R. The injury experience of the competitive athlete with a disability: prevention implications. *Med Sci Sports Exerc* 1992; **24**: 184–8.

64 Nyland J, Snouse SL, Anderson M, Kelly T, Sterling JC. Soft tissue injuries to USA paralympians at the 1996 summer games. *Arch Phys Med Rehab* 2000; **81**: 368–73.

65 Wilson PE, Washington RL. Paediatric wheelchair athletes. sports injuries and prevention. *Paraplegia* 1993; **31**: 330–7.

66 Ferrara MS, Buchley WE, Messner DG, Benedict J. The injury experience and training history of the competitive skier with a disability. *Am J Sports Med* 1992; **20**: 55–60.

67 Price MJ, Campbell IG. Thermoregulatory responses of spinal cord injured and able-bodied athletes to prolonged upper body exercise and recovery. *Spinal Cord* 1999; **37**: 772–9.

68 McCann BC. Thermoregulation in spinal cord injury: the challenge of the Atlanta Paralympics. *Spinal Cord* 1996; **34**: 433–6.

69 Smith J, Wilder RP. Musculoskeletal rehabilitation and sports medicine. 4. Miscellaneous sports medicine topics. *Arch Phys Med Rehab* 1999; **80**: S68–89.

70 Webborn ADJ. 'Boosting' performance in disability sport. *Br J Sports Med* 1999; **33**: 74–5.

Part 4
Exercise in Acute and Chronic Medical Diseases

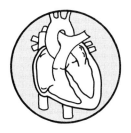

Chapter 4.1
Cardiovascular and Peripheral Vessel Diseases

MATS JENSEN-URSTAD &
KERSTIN JENSEN-URSTAD

Classical reference

Excerpt translated from Henschen SE. Om skidlöpning och skidtäfling ur medicinsk synpunkt [about skiing and skiing competition from a medical viewpoint]. Upsala Universitets Årstidskrift 1897 Medicin II: 49–50.

This demonstrates:

(1) that skiing induces enlargement of the heart; and

(2) that this enlarged heart can perform more work than the normal heart; and also

(3) that athletic activity thus induces a physiologic enlargement—an athlete's heart.

We thus meet the same relationship as in the

5 kilometer race—the large hearts win.

If I was generally surprised that so many of the competitors had large hearts, this was especially the case when such hearts were found in the three Lapps [16]. The heart in all three—in addition frequent prize winners—was, especially in relation to their small bodies and their weights, nearly a *cor bovinum*. The cardiac thrust was in two significantly, and in one insignificantly, beside the midmamillary line. It was furthermore markedly lifting and broad; and as this was the case in all three, one cannot avoid relating the hypertrophy to their lifestyle. The form and volume of the pulse also showed a hypertrophied heart. The heart sounds were normal in one; in two the first sound was a little blurred.

Considering that two of them came in at nos 1 and 3 and that the third was an old prize winner, who got behindhand however, probably due to his years (37 years) and his relatively severe bronchitis, one may dare to state that these large hearts could perform, and due to their way of living did perform, a very large work.

Rimpi was an example of the fact that such a heart does not have to *degenerate* rapidly. His pulse was regular, large and forceful, both before and after the race.

Maybe these *large hearts*, together with their *light bodies*, are one of the reasons for their success in competition.

Athlete's heart

It is now over 100 years since Henschen described the physiologic adaptation of the heart to physical training and distinguished this from cardiac enlargement due to heart disease[1]. However there still exist confusion and misconcepts regarding so-called athlete's heart. The term 'athlete's heart' is commonly used for the increased left ventricular dimensions seen in trained athletes. The adaptation to intense physical training, especially endurance training, also comprises, however, enlargement of other heart chambers and resting bradycardia.

Left ventricular and right ventricular cavity dimension and wall thickness

The advances in non-invasive techniques like ultrasound and magnetic resonance imaging have made studies of left ventricular (LV) dimensions in athletes easy and accurate and there are now numerous concordant studies. Most studies have used echocardiography. LV end-diastolic diameter is normally between 43 and 59 mm in adult men and 40–52 mm in women, depending mostly on body size. Wall thickness refers to the interventricular septum which is normally 8–12 mm or the LV posterior wall which is slightly thinner than the interventricular septum. Left ventricular systolic function at rest is similar in athletes and control subjects.

The heart muscle responds to physical training depending on the type of exercise performed. With pure endurance training LV cavity dimensions and LV wall dimensions increase similarly with a mainly unchanged ratio between wall thickness and LV end-diastolic dimension. In contrast athletes training in strength sports, such as weight-lifting and wrestling, have high values for wall thickness relative to cavity dimension. In combined dynamic and static sports (for example cycling and rowing) a combination of this is seen with both increased LV cavity dimensions and relatively more increased wall thickness.

In a study of 1309 Italian athletes (including 25% women) 14% had a LV cavity >60 mm, which was used as an arbitrary cut-off value for upper limit of normal LV size. The major determinants of a large cavity dimension were greater body surface area and participation in endurance sports. The few athletes with >60 mm LV cavities had normal left ventricular systolic function and no regional wall motion abnormalities [2].

Female athletes have, as male athletes do, larger LV cavity dimensions than controls although somewhat smaller dimensions than males of the same age and body size training in the same sport. In a study of 600 women athletes four women had left ventricular cavity diameter >60 mm [3].

The right ventricle is enlarged in athletes in endurance sports to the same degree as the left ventricle, i.e. larger than in controls, but usually within the upper normal limit.

Left ventricular mass is larger in athletes in strength-trained sports and endurance sports, and a combination of these, compared to controls. Those with larger muscle mass usually have larger LV cavity diameter. Athletes training in strength sports, such as weight-lifting, have high values for wall thickness relative to cavity dimension, but their absolute wall thickness usually remains within normal limits.

The upper limit to which the thickness of the left ventricular wall may be increased by athletic training appears to be 16 mm. Athletes with a wall thickness of more than 16 mm and a non-dilated left ventricular cavity are likely to have pathologic hypertrophy, such as hypertrophic cardiomyopathy [4]. It may be difficult to distinguish between physiologic hypertrophy and pathologic changes and in some cases cessation of training may be necessary to see if the hypertrophy is reversible, meaning that there was physiologic hypertrophy. A study of six Olympic rowers after the 1988 Seoul Olympic Games who voluntarily rested for 6–34 weeks after the games showed that the ventricular septal thickness decreased from a mean of 13.8 mm in the trained state to a mean of 10.5 mm in the deconditioned state (change 15–33%) [5]. Aging does not seem to influence the effect of detraining on left ventricular morphology. In a comparison of cyclists, detraining in a 50–60-year age group induced fairly similar left ventricular morphologic changes to those in a 20-year age group.

Athletes with a higher left ventricular mass do not show the slower diastolic filling of the LV seen in patients with pathologic left ventricular hypertrophy where left ventricular filling during diastole is abnormal and slow.

Conclusion

Although there are clearly different cardiac adaptations to the different types of exercise, with few exceptions athletes' LV dimensions are usually within the upper reference level of normal limits—the athlete's heart is a normal heart. LV wall thickness above normal (>12–13 mm) is found in only a few per cent of athletes (most likely cyclists or rowers) and is associated with an enlarged left ventricular cavity.

ECG findings in athletes

Resting bradycardia is common in athletes and heart rate values below 30 beats/min during the night are not uncommon [6,7]. Pauses (long R–R intervals) in sinus rhythm of 2–2.5 s are often seen and pauses over 3 s have been reported (Fig. 4.1.1). Pronounced sinus bradyarrhythmias during the night are due to a vagal influence on the heart and a normal finding.

Sporadic atrial and ventricular premature beats are common and do not require investigation or treatment.

The majority of athletes have normal ECGs or only minor alterations. Conduction abnormalities such as first- and second-degree (Mobitz type 1) atrioventricular block are common, and complete heart block has also been described, usually at night and resolving during exercise.

Grossly 10–20% of athletes have aberrancies in their ECGs, usually increased voltage (high QRS am-

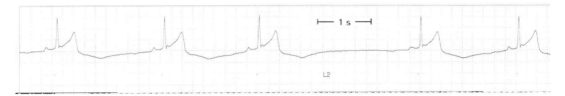

Fig. 4.1.1 Sinus bradycardia at night in a 1500-m runner, longest R–R interval in sinus rhythm 3.06 s. (Reproduced with permission from [6].)

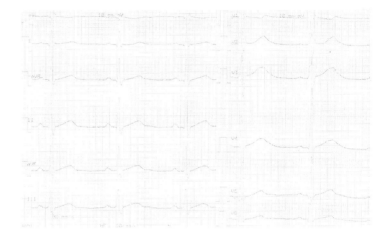

Fig. 4.1.2 Resting ECG from a long-distance runner. Heart rate 60 beats/min. Paper speed 50 mm/s.

plitudes) which may reflect the increased cardiac volume and muscle mass (and the leaner body of the athlete). Other features include ST elevation, high T waves, prominent U waves and intraventricular conduction abnormalities, usually affecting the right branch bundle. Figure 4.1.2 shows an ECG from a healthy long-distance runner.

In an athlete without evidence of cardiac disease the above-mentioned ECG changes should be considered a normal variant.

Among the total population of athletes there are a few, 2–5%, with highly abnormal ECGs but without clinical symptoms and without evidence of pathologic structural or morphologic changes on echocardiography. However, in athletes presenting with symptoms such as syncope, near-syncope, sudden dizziness, etc., as for other patients a thorough investigation must be made as arrhythmias can also be symptoms of underlying structural heart disease, such as hypertrophic cardiomyopathy, arrhythmogenic right ventricular

dysplasia, acquired heart block, sinus node disease or myocarditis.

If an ECG is taken for any other reason than the patient's symptoms and is highly abnormal, or abnormal in an unexpected way, an echocardiography could be performed to rule out hypertrophic cardiomyopathy, arrhythmogenic right ventricular dysplasia (ARVD), or other structural cardiac disease. Figure 4.1.3 shows an ECG from a patient with hypertrophic cardiomyopathy.

Veteran athletes

Some studies have shown an increased prevalence of supraventricular and ventricular ectopic beats and complex ventricular premature beats in older athletes compared to controls [8–10]; there are however, also studies that do not show any difference in incidence of arrhythmias between athletes and controls. These arrhythmias found in elderly athletes seldom require treatment and evidence from epidemiologic studies

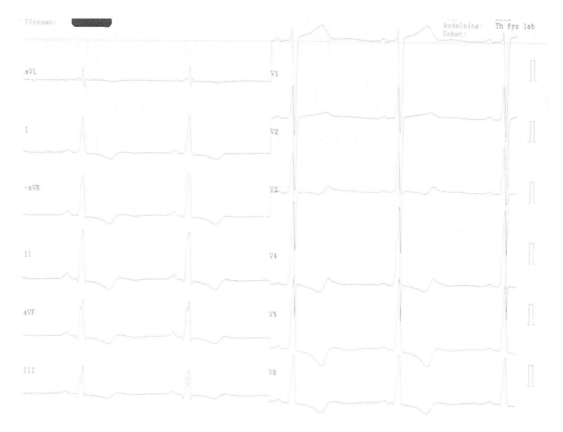

Fig. 4.1.3 Resting ECG from a patient with hypertrophic cardiomyopathy. Heart rate 55 beats/min. Paper speed 50 mm/s.

shows that a physically active lifestyle reduces risk of cardiac death [11].

Heart and vessel diseases and training

From the patient's point of view the main questions are:

If I have a cardiovascular disease and want to participate in aerobic exercise, is it safe?

Might the training have any positive effects?

Does regular exercise increase the exercise ability and make it possible to increase the ability to handle daily life?

Does regular exercise improve the prognosis?

The term exercise below generally refers to aerobic exercise, such as walking, swimming, jogging and running.

Exercise has been studied in terms of clinical outcomes (morbidity and mortality), exercise tolerance (effect on $\dot{V}_{O_2}$) and effects on risk factors like blood lipids, body weight, and blood pressure and on quality of life. There are other aspects of exercise such as health economy which will not be dealt with.

While total mortality among physically active people is less than among the inactive, there is an increased risk for sudden death or myocardial infarction during physical activity as compared to during rest. This is because the increased load on circulation and metabolism leads to long-term beneficial effects on the development of cardiovascular diseases, but in predisposed subjects the acute strain on the circulation might trigger myocardial infarction or a life-threatening arrhythmia. During exercise blood pressure and heart rate increase, resulting in increased myocardial oxygen demand. The autonomic tone is changed towards increased sympathetic activity. Depending on the exercise intensity and duration and climatic conditions metabolic changes such as lactic acidosis and/or electrolyte imbalances might occur. A vulnerable atherosclerotic plaque could then disrupt in response to the hemodynamic stress with subsequent platelet activation, aggregation and thrombus formation. Regional ischemia, blood pressure changes and increased sympathetic tone could trigger ventricular fibrillation in subjects with coronary abnormalities or stenosis, cardiomyopathies or myocarditis. It should, however, be emphasized that higher levels of physical fitness appear to delay all-cause mortality, with mortality rates found to be 3.4 and 4.6 times higher among the least fit men and women compared to the most fit men and women, respectively [12].

The different cardiovascular diseases have different pathophysiologic features which make the impact of the hemodynamics at rest and during exercise extremely variable in each of these conditions. The impact of training on the different cardiovascular diseases has been concluded from studies of groups of patients.

The largest group of patients with cardiovascular disease are patients with atherosclerosis-related diseases like angina pectoris or myocardial infarction. Atherosclerosis is a disease of the intimal layer of large and medium-sized arteries developing silently for decades before onset of clinical manifestations such as an acute myocardial infarction or a stroke. Risk factors for atherosclerosis include smoking, high blood lipids, hypertension and a sedentary lifestyle, and are discussed in Chapter 3.2.

Exercise after acute myocardial infarction

In the 18th century William Heberden and Caleb H. Parry recommended physical activity for patients with angina pectoris [13,14]. Other views soon became dominant and for almost 200 years rest was a major part in the treatment of angina pectoris and in myocardial infarction. In the 1950s the bed rest period after a myocardial infarction was shortened and it was reported that the patients having shorter bed rest after a myocardial infarction returned to normal activities sooner. It was shown that patients who were mobilized early had a lower mortality rate and lower morbidity up to a year after acute myocardial infarction (AMI).

Over the last few decades the length of hospital stay after an AMI has been reduced and exercise programs have been safely and increasingly used since the 1960s.

The overall idea of postinfarction rehabilitation programs is to reduce the physiologic effects of the cardiac illness, to increase psychological well-being and to reduce morbidity and mortality. Training is often used in the context of a rehabilitation program with multiple risk factor modification but it seems that training in itself also reduces morbidity [15].

Aerobic exercise improves functional capacity and the higher the exercise intensity the higher the improvement in $\dot{V}o_2$. Patients with the lowest $\dot{V}o_2$ improve most with training programs but patients that at baseline have a preserved exercise capacity also improve with exercise. Patients with reduced LV function also improve their $\dot{V}o_{2\,max}$ with exercise [16].

Rehabilitation programs including exercise have been shown to reduce ischemic symptoms, reduce the risk of new coronary events and reduce cardiac mortality [17], and may prevent the progression or reduce the severity of coronary atherosclerosis [18].

After AMI, a predischarge symptom–limited exercise test [19], or a test done 2–4 weeks after discharge can guide exercise prescription. Symptoms (chest pain or chest discomfort), ST depression, arrhythmias and a low blood pressure increase during exercise are predictors of adverse events following AMI and these patients should be further investigated and treated. A new exercise test should be done after treatment before patients are allowed to exercise. Previously patients with anterior MI (who usually have larger infarctions than patient with inferior infarctions) were restrained from early testing and training but newer studies have shown that patients recovering from anterior MI may exercise with moderate intensity.

The long-term beneficial effects of supervised conventional exercise programs post-MI have been questioned: 1 year after a completed post-MI training program there were only marginal improvements in physical performance [20]; other studies show that fitness level is maintained if the training is maintained.

Exercise recommendations. The patient is recommended at discharge to take daily walks at comfortable speed and increase the time, length and speed of the walk gradually to moderate dynamic exercise (to toler-

Case study 4.1.1

A 70-year-old man with a lifelong history of strenuous training underwent cardiovascular testing in a study of veteran male athletes. He had no symptoms. ECG showed signs of an old myocardial infarction. Echocardiography showed a dilated left ventricle with regional hypokinesia of the LV wall and reduced LV function. Nuclear angiography showed decreased left ventricular function both at rest and during exercise. Myocardial scintigraphy revealed a large perfusion abnormality. Despite these findings he cycled on an ergometer cycle with gradual increase of workload of 20 W/min to 180 W. Running on a treadmill his pulmonary oxygen uptake was 39 mL/kg/min which is higher than in healthy 70–75-year-old controls. This suggests that the endurance training compensated for the deteriorating effect of the myocardial infarction via both central and peripheral mechanisms.

ance). Training in groups supervised by a physiotherapist is an alternative (See Case Study 4.1.1).

Stable angina pectoris

This group of patients has been studied less extensively than post-MI patients. Studies show that training improves exercise tolerance and retards disease progression [21]. Measures of ischemia such as ST depression are reduced after a training program [22] and exercise may improve symptomatology.

The earlier used rehabilitation programs often excluded patients older than 65 whereas later studies have shown that patients ≥75 years of age with coronary artery disease show improvements in exercise capacity, lipid levels and quality of life parameters [23].

After bypass surgery

This group of patients have also been studied less than post-MI patients. It seems that exercise improves functional capacity but there is a lack of controlled

studies. Patients in a rehabilitation group lower their blood lipids compared to controls which probably improves prognosis.

Exercise in patients with stable heart failure

In congestive heart failure exercise tolerance is severely limited; the peak pulmonary oxygen uptake may be less than 10 mL O_2/kg/min. This is due to central factors like attenuated myocardial function (the cardiac ejection fraction is often less than 20%), decreased inotropic response and increased diastolic pressures, and peripheral factors such as reduced vasodilator response, increased activity of sympathetic afferents and impaired muscle function.

Exercise training programs, for example ergometer cycling three times a week at 60% of $\dot{V}_{O_2 max}$ improves exercise capacity and reduces symptoms.

In a prospective study of 80 patients with class II and III chronic heart failure physical training was safe and resulted in improvements in exercise time, anaerobic threshold and quality of life [24]. Exercise improves blood flow to exercising muscles [25] and work capacity of the trained peripheral muscle [26]. Exercise also results in an increase in peak heart rate and a partial reversal of chronotropic incompetence among patients with stable heart failure.

Exercise with small muscle groups, one at a time, may be an alternative to whole-body exercise in patients severely limited by low cardiac output. Light strength training is also possible to carry out due to its low loading on the cardiovascular system.

Exercise programs have been shown to increase heart rate variability (HRV) [27] which is a measure of autonomic function, both vagal control on the heart and sympathetic control on the peripheral vessels [28].

There are no data at present on the impact of exercise training on mortality and morbidity in heart failure patients.

Exercise recommendations: mild to moderate dynamic exercise (to tolerance) such as walking or easy bike riding.

Hypertension

In the middle-aged age groups 15–30% of the population in Western countries have hypertension (resting blood pressure $\geq 140/90$ mmHg). Regular aerobic exercise lowers blood pressure in patients with essential hypertension.

Exercise in the form of walking and jogging is predominantly used in studies, often showing reductions in systolic and diastolic blood pressure of 10 mmHg in around 75% of hypertensive patients. An exaggerated blood pressure response during physical exertion attenuates after regular training. The blood pressure response to mental stress has also been shown to be attenuated in borderline hypertensive persons after a training program.

The greatest effect of exercise training on hypertension is observed after around 10 weeks of regular training, whereas training more than three times per week or for more than 50 min at a time does not lower the blood pressure further.

In mildly hypertensive men, short-term physical activity decreases blood pressure for 8–12 h after exercise. Average blood pressure is lower on exercise than non-exercise days [29].

Mild to moderate intensity exercise (intensities of 40–70% $\dot{V}\mathrm{O_{2\,max}}$) appears to lower systolic blood pressure more and diastolic blood pressure to the same degree as higher intensity training and may be more effective in lowering blood pressure and attenuating an exaggerated blood pressure response to exercise than higher intensity exercises.

Exercise also seems to be safe and to lower blood pressure in patients with severe hypertension and left ventricular hypertrophy.

No gender differences in the antihypertensive effect of exercise is observed although most studies have been performed in men. Few studies have been performed in older patients; there does not, however, appear to be an age-dependent antihypertensive effect of exercise.

A swimming training program reduces arterial blood pressure at rest in individuals with hypertension. Swimming is an alternative for patients that prefer swimming and for those that cannot walk or jog because of, for example, obesity or orthopedic problems [23].

Exercise recommendations: mild to moderate exercise.

Valvular disease

Generally, mild valvular regurgitations, usually in the mitral and tricuspid valves, are a normal finding on echocardiography, and do not warrant further investigation or any restriction in activity.

Mitral valve prolapse is a common disorder that affects a few per cent of the adult population and may cause mitral regurgitation. Some patients with mitral prolapse have supraventricular and/or ventricular arrhythmias. The prognosis regarding arrhythmias in these patients is, however, good.

Patients with more than mild valvular regurgitations or patients with valvular stenoses should be followed for progress of valvular disease (for timing of valve repair or valve replacement) and should have an individualized exercise prescription from a cardiologist. In patients with significant aortic stenosis in particular, heavy exercise might be dangerous.

Cardiomyopathies

Hypertrophic cardiomyopathy

Hypertrophic cardiomyopathy (HCM) is one of the most common causes of sudden death in young athletes. Athletes with symptoms such as syncope, near-syncope or sudden dizziness, who have pathologic ECG findings with increased QRS amplitudes and ST–T changes or a family history of HCM should therefore be investigated. HCM is a cardiomyopathy with varying degrees of hypertrophy of the left ventricle, often with obstruction of the left ventricular outflow tract. The mechanism for sudden death is presumably malign ventricular arrhythmias although bradycardia also may occur.

Subjects with suspected HCM should not exercise and should be investigated; an echocardiographic examination is generally diagnostic while chest X-ray may show an enlarged heart or be normal. A risk assessment should be made, including an exercise stress test and electrophysiologic evaluation. If an athlete wants to continue training at a high level treatment with an implantable defibrillator may be warranted.

Figure 4.1.3 shows an ECG from a patient with hypertrophic cardiomyopathy and Fig. 4.1.4 shows LV cavity and wall dimensions measured at echocardiography in the same patient.

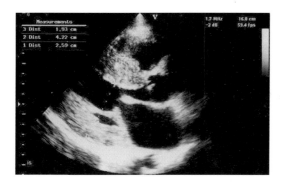

Fig. 4.1.4 Echocardiography frame showing left ventricular cavity and wall dimensions in a patient with hypertrophic cardiomyopathy (ECG Fig. 4.1.3), septum thickness 26 mm and posterior wall thickness 19 mm compared to normal 9–12 mm.

Arrhythmogenic right ventricular dysplasia

Arrhythmogenic right ventricular dysplasia (ARVD) or arrhythmogenic right ventricular cardiomyopathy (ARVC) is a disease in the myocardium of the right ventricle. Muscle tissue in the right ventricle is replaced with fibrous and fatty tissue. A familial occurrence has been documented but the etiology is largely unknown.

Symptoms are arrhythmias (ventricular) or syncope caused by arrhythmia. Typical ECG findings are inverted T waves in the right precordial leads (and this is *not a* normal finding among athletes), so-called epsilon waves and ventricular arrhythmias.

Echocardiography findings include right ventricular dilatation, changes in the right ventricular wall with focal wall thinning and focal aneurysms. The right ventricle is difficult to assess with echocardiography and in patients with any suspicion of ARVD magnetic resonance imaging and/or right ventricle angiography should be performed.

ARVD is a cause of sudden death in young athletes and it is of utmost importance to recognize and diagnose these patients early. These patients should be restricted from sports. Implantable defibrillator treatment may be warranted.

Myocarditis

A person with suspected acute myocarditis should not exercise. After the acute phase is over and the myocarditis is healed a maximal exercise stress test should

be done to reveal any tendency for malign arrhythmias. An echocardiographic examination should also be made. If all investigations are normal, exercise can be resumed. Sometimes an athlete will have obtained the diagnosis of myocarditis on weak or faulty grounds and the athlete is unnecessarily restrained from training. However, a diagnosis of myocarditis may also indicate other diseases such as cardiomyopathies and an investigation can be warranted to reveal this. This is particularly important if any symptoms are present. In this context one should also keep in mind that congenital coronary artery abnormalities are not an uncommon cause of sudden death among young athletes as well as early coronary artery disease.

Arrhythmias

Atrial fibrillation

Exercise increases vagal tone and may decrease the need for rate regulation by drugs. When heart rate is well controlled during exercise, the subject may exercise to tolerance. Patients with atrial fibrillation are, however, often treated with anticoagulants and should therefore avoid contact sports. Patients with chronic atrial fibrillation can improve functional capacity through an exercise rehabilitation program [30]. Subjects with atrial fibrillation may compete at high level even in endurance sports as demonstrated by one orienteer who, despite a history of atrial fibrillation since youth, competed at national level and at 75 years of age still had an exercise capacity of 240 W or 3.4 W/kg on the bicycle and an oxygen uptake of 36 mL O_2/kg (Jensen-Urstad *et al.*, unpublished data).

Atrial flutter

The same considerations as for atrial fibrillation may be applied for atrial flutter. Atrial flutter may, however, constitute a larger problem for the subject as rate control may be more difficult. Atrial flutter can in many cases be cured by a radiofrequency ablation procedure [31]. Electrophysiologic evaluation and possibly curative radiofrequency ablation should therefore be considered.

Supraventricular tachycardias

Subjects with paroxysmal supraventricular tachycardias, with a sudden onset and abrupt ending, usually have an AV nodal re-entry tachycardia or an atrioventricular re-entry tachycardia utilizing an accessory pathway with or without pre-excitation in the resting ECG. More rarely ectopic atrial tachycardias are found. The tachycardia often starts during exercise when catecholamine levels increase. Patients may feel shortness of breath, palpitations, dizziness and in some cases also syncope. These arrhythmias are generally considered relatively benign but depending on the situation the abrupt onset can make them dangerous, e.g. during diving, cycling, driving etc. In older subjects they may also give more serious symptoms. Individuals with a history of tachycardias with sudden onset especially with symptoms such as dizziness or syncope should be investigated for a diagnosis. Today the arrhythmia can in most cases be cured by radiofrequency ablation. Of note is that resting ECG in most cases is totally normal. Subjects with overt pre-excitation in their ECG can sometimes have an accessory pathway capable of conducting at very high frequencies making a paroxysmal atrial flutter or fibrillation dangerous. The accessory pathway may also facilitate development of atrial fibrillation. These individuals may not have a history of tachycardias, but can present with syncope or aborted sudden death as their first symptom (See Case Study 4.1.2). Electrophysiologic evaluation should be recommended until a curative radiofrequency ablation is done. After successful radiofrequency ablation the patient is not restricted from any sport.

Ventricular arrhythmias

Except for ventricular ectopic beats without symptoms, all ventricular arrhythmias should be thoroughly investigated. Subjects with a history of tachycardia and symptoms such as sudden dizziness, near-syncope or syncope should be restricted from physical activity until malignant arrhythmias are ruled out.

Cardiac transplantation

Preoperatively these patients are severely physically limited. The transplanted heart is denervated and reliant on circulating cathecholamines for increasing heart rate during exercise, although reinnervation may occur. There is a delayed heart rate response at the onset of exercise and with change of exercise level. Exercise intensity cannot therefore be guided by heart rate monitoring and perceived exertion can be used instead.

Exercise in these patients increases maximal oxygen uptake, reduces perceived exertion, heart rate and blood pressure during submaximal exercise, and results in a lower resting heart rate and blood pressure. No influence on rejection has been shown.

Peripheral vessel diseases

In patients with intermittent claudication, arterial insufficiency in the legs, the major goal is to improve the ability to walk. Exercise training programs have great impact on functional capacity. Pain-free walking time may increase almost 200% and maximal walking time may be more than doubled in patients participating in an exercise program, and walking speed may increase substantially with an exercise program.

A treadmill training program improves functional status during daily activities, 24 weeks of training being more effective than 12 weeks. Treadmill training (walking) alone is more effective in improving functional status in patients with intermittent claudication than strength training or combinations of the training modalities [32]. In one study comparing angioplasty to exercise training in the treatment of stable claudication the exercise training group had the greatest improvement in terms of improved walking performance

---

Case study 4.1.2

A 14-year-old boy with no previous history of arrhythmias or syncope suddenly loses consciousness during an ice hockey game. He is unconscious for about a minute. When he arrived in the emergency department he had a fast irregular pulse. Systolic blood pressure was 70 mmHg. ECG showed pre-excited atrial fibrillation with a ventricular rate of 220–250 beats/min (Fig. 4.1.5a). ECG in sinus rhythm showed pre-excitation (Fig. 4.1.5b). He was successfully treated with radiofrequency ablation and could resume full activity with no restrictions.

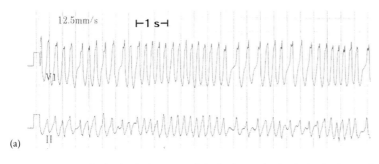

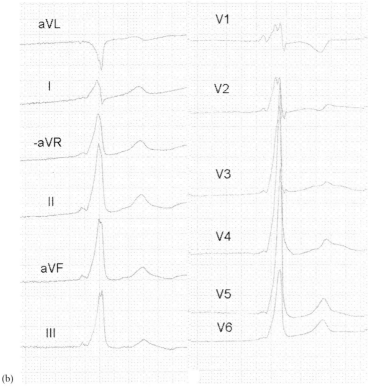

Fig. 4.1.5 (a) Atrial fibrillation with rapid conduction over an accessory pathway, heart rate around 240 beats/ min. (b) Pre-excitation in sinus rhythm.

and less pain [33]. The effects of exercise on atherosclerosis *per se* in peripheral arteries have been less studied than in coronary arteries but good cardiorespiratory fitness is associated with slower progression of early atherosclerosis, at least in the carotid arteries [34].

Exercise recommendations: walking to tolerance.
For further recommendations regarding eligibility

for competition in athletes with cardiovascular abnormalities, the 26th Bethesda Conference [35] provides panel consensus recommendations.

Summary

Over 100 years ago Henschen described the physiologic adaptation of the heart to physical training and distinguished this from cardiac enlargement due to heart disease. The term 'athlete's heart' is commonly

Table 4.1.1 Which patients should not exercise?

> Patients with:
>   uncontrolled hypertension
>   untreated congestive heart failure
>   severe stenotic or regurgitant valvular disease
>   hypertrophic cardiomyopathy
>   acute myocarditis
>   arrhythmogenic right ventricular dysplasia
>   unclear dysrhythmias

used for the increased left ventricular dimensions seen in trained athletes. The adaptation to intense physical training, especially endurance training, also comprises enlargement of other heart chambers and resting bradycardia.

Physical exercise has well-documented positive effects on the cardiovascular system in both healthy and diseased subjects. In healthy subjects regular exercise has large long-term benefits with very few direct risks. For the vast majority of individuals with known cardiovascular disease physical exercise has positive effects regarding quality of life, and may decrease morbidity and mortality. In patients with known cardiovascular disease exercise programs should, however, be individualized with respect to the underlying disease. There is a small number of subjects where exercise might be contraindicated at least until they have received proper treatment (Table 4.4.1).

Athletes with symptoms such as syncope, near-syncope and sudden dizziness or with highly abnormal ECGs should be investigated to rule out an underlying possibly life-threatening disease.

Multiple choice questions

1 *A 24-year-old middle-distance runner experiences a syncope during interval training; during a 400-m run at maximal speed he falls and is unconscious for a couple of minutes before he wakes up and feels quite OK apart from a hurting arm. Which (one or more) of the following statements is/are correct?*

a Syncope during exercise is normal and no further investigation is warranted.

b Syncope during exercise only needs investigation if it happens more than once.

c Syncope during exercise may be a sign of life-threatening disease and the patient should be promptly investigated.

2 *Which (one or more) of the following statements about ECG and echocardiography findings in endurance-trained athletes is/are normal findings:*

a first-degree atrioventricular block

b low resting heart rate, below 40 beats/min

c large QRS amplitudes and high T waves

d slightly enlarged left ventricle on echocardiography.

3 *A strength-training athlete is investigated because of fatigue over the last few months. Echocardiography shows a left ventricle diameter of 40 mm and a thickness of the posterior and septal wall of 18–19 mm. There is normal left ventricular function. Which (one or more) of the following statements is/are correct?*

a This is a normal finding.

b The left ventricular walls are thick but this is normal finding in a strength-trained athlete.

c The LV hypertrophy in this athlete is probably a pathologic finding and further investigation is warranted.

4 *An otherwise healthy patient with treated essential hypertension wants to start jogging. Which (one or more) of the following statements is/are correct?*

a Exercise in contraindicated as it may be harmful.

b Moderate aerobic training is recommended.

c Moderate aerobic training is recommended but only once a week.

d Exercise a few times a week may reduce resting systolic blood pressure by 10 mmHg.

5 *Which (one or more) of the following statements is/are correct about moderate aerobic exercise 6 weeks after uncomplicated acute myocardial infarction?*

a Not allowed because of risk of arrhythmias.

b Leads to increased exercise ability and $\dot{V}_{O_2}$.

c Improves the prognosis.

d Improves blood lipid status.

References

1   Henschen SE. *Om Skidlöpning och Skidtäfling ur Medicinsk Synpunkt.* Upsala Universitets Årstidskrift. Medicin II. 1897: 49–50.

2   Pelliccia A, Culasso F, Di Paolo FM, Maron BJ. Physiologic left ventricular cavity dilatation in elite athletes. *Ann Intern Med* 1999; **130**: 23–31.

3   Pelliccia A, Maron BJ, Culasso F, Spataro A, Caselli G.

Athlete's heart in women. Echocardiographic characterization of highly trained elite female athletes. *J Am Med Assoc* 1996; **276**: 211–15.

4   Pelliccia A, Maron BJ, Spataro A, Proschan MA, Spirito P. The upper limit of physiologic cardiac hypertrophy in highly trained elite athletes. *N Engl J Med* 2000; **31**: 295–301.

5   Maron BJ, Pelliccia A, Spataro A, Granata M. Reduction in left ventricular wall thickness after deconditioning in highly trained Olympic athletes. *Br Heart J* 1993; **69**: 125–8.

6   Jensen-Urstad K, Saltin B, Ericsson M, Storck N, Jensen-Urstad M. Pronounced resting bradycardia in male elite runners is associated with high heart rate variability. *Scand J Med Sci Sports* 1997; **7**: 274–8.

7   Rost R, Hollmann W. Athlete's heart—a review of its historical assessment and new aspects. *Int J Sports Med* 1983; **4**: 157–64.

8   Grimby G, Saltin B. Physiological analysis of physically well-trained middle-aged and old athletes. *Nord Med* 1966, 513–26.

9   Jensen-Urstad K, Saltin B, Jensen-Urstad M. High prevalence of arrhythmias in elderly male athletes with a lifelong history of regular strenuous exercise. *Heart* 1998; **79**: 161–4.

10 Northcote RJ, Canning GP, Ballantyne D. Electrocardiographic findings in male veteran endurance athletes. *Br Heart J* 1988; **61**: 155–60.

11 Leon AS, Connett J, Jacobs DR Jr, Rauramaa R. Leisure-time physical activity levels and risk of coronary heart disease and death. The Multiple Risk Factor Intervention Trial. *J Am Med Assoc* 1987; **258**: 2388–95.

12 Blair SN, Kohl HW III, Paffenberger RS Jr, Clark DG, Cooper KH, Gibbons LW. Physical fitness and all-cause mortality. A prospective study of healthy men and women. *J Am Med Assoc* 1989; **262**: 2395–401.

13 Heberden W. Some account of a disorder of the breast. *Med Trans Coll Physiol* 1772; **II**: 59–67.

14 Parry CH. *An Inquiry Into the Symptoms and Causes of Syncope Anginosa, Commonly Called Angina Pectoris; Illustrated by Dissections*. London: R Cutwell for Caldell and Davies, 1799.

15 Hambrecht R, Niebauer J, Marburger C et al. Various intensities of leisure time physical activity in patients with coronary heart disease: effects of cardiorespiratory fitness and progression of coronary atherosclerosis. *J Am Coll Cardiol* 1993; **22**: 468–77.

16 Balady GJ, Fletcher BJ, Froelicher EF et al. Statement on cardiac rehabilitation programmes. *Circulation* 1994; **90**: 1602–10.

17 Hedback B, Perk J, Wodlin P. Long term reduction of cardiac mortality after myocardial infarction: 10-year results of a comprehensive rehabilitation programme. *Eur Heart J* 1993; **14**: 831–5.

18 Haskell WL, Alderman EL, Fair JM et al. Effects of intensive multiple risk factor reduction on coronary atherosclerosis and clinical cardiac events in men and women with coronary artery disease. The Stanford Coronary Risk Intervent Project (SCRIP). *Circulation* 1994; **89**: 975–90.

19 Jensen-Urstad K, Samad B, Bouvier F et al. Improved prognostic value of symptom-limited vs low-level exercise stress test after thrombolytically treated myocardial infarction. *Heart* 1999; **82**: 199–203.

20 Holmback AM, Sawe U, Fagher B. Training after myocardial infarction: lack of long-term effects on physical capacity and psychological variables. *Arch Phys Med Rehabil* 1994; **75**: 551–4.

21 Niebauer J, Hambrecht R, Velich T et al. Attenuated progression of coronary artery disease after 6 years of multifactorial risk intervention: role of physical exercise. *Circulation* 1997; **96**: 2534–41.

22 Todd IC, Ballantyne D. Effects of exercise training on the total ischaemic burden: an assessment by 24 hour ambulatory electrcardiographic monitoring. *Br Heart J* 1992; **68**: 560–6.

23 Stahle A, Mattsson E, Ryden L, Unden A, Nordlander R. Improved physical fitness and quality of life following training of elderly patients after acute coronary events. A 1 year follow-up randomized controlled study. *Eur Heart J* 1999; **20**: 1475–84.

24 Wielenga RP, Huisveld IA, Bol E et al. Safety and effects of physical training in chronic heart failure. Results of the Chronic Heart Failure and Graded Exercise study. *Eur Heart J* 1999; **20**: 872–9.

25 Tanaka H, Bassett DRJ, Howley ET, Thompson DL, Ashraf M, Rawson FL. Swimming training lowers the resting blood pressure in individuals with hypertension. *J Hypertension* 1997; **15**: 151–5.

26 Magnusson G, Gordon A, Kaijser L et al. High intensity knee extensor training in patients with chronic heart failure. Major skeletal muscle improvement. *Eur Heart J* 1996; **17**: 1048–55.

27 Coats AJS, Adamopoulos S, Radaelli A et al. Controlled trial of physical training in chronic heart failure: exercise performance, hemodynamics, ventilation, and autonomic function. *Circulation* 1992; **85**: 2119–31.

28 Radaelli A, Coats AJ, Leuzzi S et al. Physical training enhances sympathetic and parasympathetic control of heart rate and peripheral vessels in chronic heart failure. *Clin Sci* 1996; **91**: 92–4.

29 Pescatello LS, Fargo AE, Leach CN, Scherzer HH. Short term effect of dynamic exercise on arterial blood pressure. *Circulation* 1991; **83**: 1557–61.

30 Mertens DJ, Kavanagh T. Exercise training for patients with chronic atrial fibrillation. *J Cardiopulm Rehabil* 1996; **16**: 193–6.

31 Waldo AL. Treatment of atrial flutter. *Heart* 2000; **84**: 227–32.

32 Regensteiner JG, Steiner JF, Hiatt WR. Exercise training improves functional status in patients with peripheral arterial disease. *J Vasc Surg* 1996; **23**: 104–15.

33 Perkins JM, Collin J, Creasy TS, Fletcher EW, Morris PJ. Exercise training versus angioplasty for stable claudication. Long and medium term results of a prospective, randomised trial. *Eur J Endovasc Surg* 1996; **11**: 409–13.

34 Lakka TA, Laukkanen JA, Rauramaa R *et al.* Cardiorespiratory fitness and the progression of carotid atherosclerosis in middle-aged men. *Ann Intern Med* 2001; **134**: 12–20.

35 Maron BJ, Isner JM, Mckenna WJ. 26th Bethesda Conference: recommendations for determining eligibility for competition in athletes with cardiovascular abnormalities. Task force 3: hypertrophic cardiomyopathy myocarditis and other myopericardial diseases and mitral valve prolapse. *J Am Coll Cardid* 1994; **24**: 880–5.

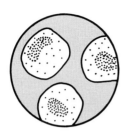

Chapter 4.2
Exercise and Infectious Diseases

BENTE KLARLUND PEDERSEN,
GÖRAN FRIMAN & LARS WESSLÉN

Classical reference

Peters EM, Bateman ED. Ultramarathon running and
upper respiratory tract infections and
epidemiological survey. *S Afr Med J* 1983; **64**:
582–4.
This was one of the first studies to demonstrate a
relationship between acute stress and susceptibility to
upper respiratory tract infections. A prospective study
of the incidence of symptoms of upper respiratory
tract infections in 150 randomly selected runners, who
took part in a 56-km run, was performed. Incidences
were compared with individually matched controls
who did not run.

Symptoms of upper respiratory tract infections
occurred in 33% of the runners compared with 15% of
controls and were most common in those who achieved
the faster race times. The incidence in slow runners
was no greater than in controls.

It is suggested that intense physical stress increases
the susceptibility to upper respiratory tract infections
(Fig. 4.2.1).

Introduction

Compared with a sedentary lifestyle, the practice of
moderate, regular physical training is generally considered to be associated with improved health including, for example, lower blood pressure and body
weight, as well as improved glucose tolerance. The issues raised in this chapter are: (i) to what extent exercise and training influence susceptibility to infections;
(ii) the potential risks of strenuous exercise during
infections; (iii) to what extent infections influence
performance; and (iv) suggestions as to practical
guidelines for exercise with symptoms of infectious
diseases.

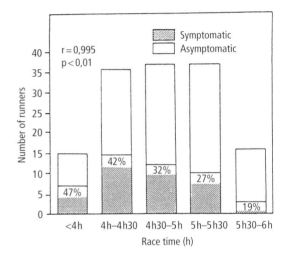

Fig. 4.2.1 Distribution of symptomatic and asymptomatic
runners according to time taken to complete the race ($n = 141$).

Exercise and the immune system

Research during the last decade has demonstrated that
an acute bout of physical activity induces pronounced
changes in the immune system (for a recent review see
[1]). Thus, the fact that leukocytes are mobilized to the
blood during moderate as well as intense exercise is
generally considered as an enhancement of the immune function. However, following intense exercise
($>75\%$ of $\dot{V}O_{2\,max}$) of long duration (>1 h) the immune
system is impaired for several hours or even days (Fig.
4.2.2). Thus, in the recovery period after exercise, the
lymphocyte concentration declines and the ability of
the lymphocytes to proliferate and mediate cytotoxici-
ty against virus-infected or malignant cells is impaired
[2]. The use of *in vivo* immunologic methods supports
these findings. Furthermore, salivary IgA levels
decline with intense exercise [3]. Also, animal experi-

ments tend to show that a given microorganism becomes more invasive and pathogenic if the animal performs intense physical activity during the incubation period or during the acute disease. This has been demonstrated for polio- and coxsackie virus B infection, as well as for influenza and others.

After intense long-term exercise, not only is the immune system characterized by impairment of the cellular immune system but, concomitantly, markedly enhanced levels of pro- and anti-inflammatory cytokines can be demonstrated. A fully developed cytokine cascade develops within the first few hours of strenuous exercise, having some similarities to the acute phase response to trauma and sepsis (Fig. 4.2.3) [4].

One indicator of chronic exercise as a lifestyle factor is to compare resting levels of any immune parameter in untrained controls and in conditioned athletes. Most studies show that trained subjects compared to untrained subjects have enhanced natural immunity [1]. Animal experiments support these findings; thus, trained animals have enhanced survival when they are infected at rest with *Salmonella typhimurium* [5] or influenza virus [6].

Thus, there is no doubt that exercise and training influence the concentration of immunocompetent cells in the circulating pool, as well as the function of these cells. An important question is, however, to what degree these cellular changes are of clinical significance

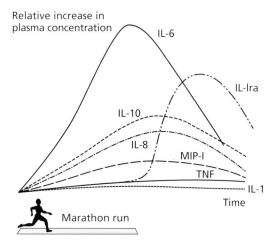

Fig. 4.2.3 Schematic changes in a number of cytokines in relation to strenuous exercise.

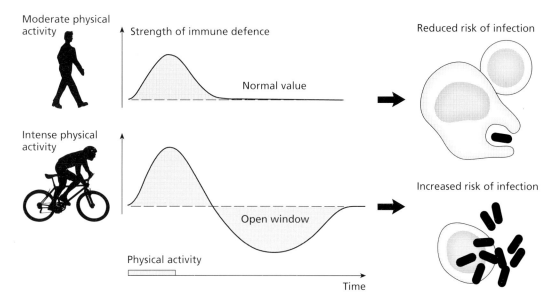

Fig. 4.2.2 During moderate to intense exercise the immune system is enhanced (as shown by mobilization of lymphocytes to the circulation), but intense exercise is followed by a period of immune impairment (decreased natural killer cell activity, lymphocyte proliferation and levels of salivary IgA) during which there is an 'open window' of opportunity for pathogens.

in humans, especially with respect to resistance to infectious diseases.

Exercise and infections

Myocarditis

One reason why clinicians advise against performing vigorous exercise during acute infections is the potential for supervening myocarditis [7,8]. Acute exercise during ongoing viral myocarditis causes increased viral replication, inflammation and necrosis in the myocardium. Thus, swimming during the initial phase of coxsackie virus B3 infection in immunologically immature (2-week-old suckling) mice increased mortality [9]. Many of the affected mice died of congestive heart failure while swimming, with massive cardiac dilatation and necrosis upon autopsy. In another study of coxsackie virus B3 infection in 8–14-week-old mice, exercise on a motor-driven treadmill to exhaustion at 48 h after the inoculation of virus did not influence lethality but the myocarditic lesions were aggravated by the exercise [10]. As compared to the situation in infected control mice who were allowed to rest, the exercise-associated increased myocardial inflammation and necrosis were related to a decreased number of cells expressing major histocompatibility complex class II, such as macrophages. Thus, the extent of tissue damage in these exercised mice may be related to decreased macrophage mobilization followed by increased destruction of the myocardium, possibly mediated by cytotoxic T cells.

Myocarditis may be an acute, subacute or chronic disease and most studies show acute myocarditis to be the most common of these manifestations (Fig. 4.2.4). Myocarditis may be either asymptomatic (subclinical) or cause chest symptoms of variable severity, ranging from vague oppression to sharp pain, as well as dyspnea and irregular heart rhythm. The observation that myocarditis can exist without any cardiac symptoms [11] is in line with the finding of active myocarditis in 1% of unselected autopsies performed during a 10-year period [12]. Commonly, symptoms from other organs precede the onset of cardiac symptoms, such as symptoms of upper respiratory tract infection [13]. Acute infectious myocarditis is usually a benign condition, which has a favorable long-term prognosis in the great majority of cases [14–16].

Sudden unexpected death (SUD) in the acute phase

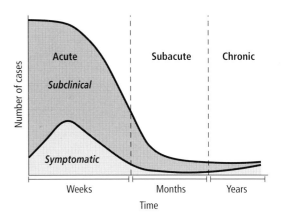

Fig. 4.2.4 Spectrum of infectious myocarditis/cardiomyopathy. Reproduced with permission from [47].

of symptomatic or asymptomatic myocarditis is a well-known but rare phenomenon. SUD from cardiac causes in the young (below 35 years of age) may be caused by several underlying conditions and is often precipitated by exercise [17,18]. Several studies have shown that an average of 10% of cases of SUD in young athletes have been caused by myocarditis [18] and in only a few studies has myocarditis been a more frequent cause of SUD [19,20]. Clustering of SUD is rare [21]. During 1979–92, however, an increased rate of SUD was reported among young Swedish orienteers; there were 15 men and one woman (Fig. 4.2.5) and myocarditis was the most frequent histopathologic feature [20,22]. The inflammatory process was subacute to chronic. All but two of the SUDs were associated with exercise. It has previously been found that loss of performance may be the only symptom of ongoing myocarditis [23] but all of these deceased people had performed at, or close to, their individual maximum shortly before they died. Five of them, however, had experienced heart-related symptoms prior to death, such as fainting during exercise, tachycardia or chest pain, but the majority had not reported any prior warning symptoms. Since late 1992 there have been no new cases of SUD among young (<35-year) Swedish orienteers. It seems plausible that the various measures taken at that time, including the introduction of a 6-month intermission in training and competition in early 1993, may have had a favorable effect in changing behavioral patterns; previously, the training habits among young elite orienteers had been extreme

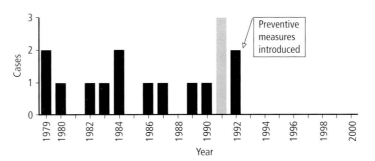

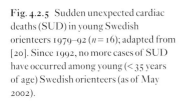

Fig. 4.2.5 Sudden unexpected cardiac deaths (SUD) in young Swedish orienteers 1979–92 (*n* = 16); adapted from [20]. Since 1992, no more cases of SUD have occurred among young (< 35 years of age) Swedish orienteers (as of May 2002).

[20,21]. Continued research has shown subacute *Bartonella* infection to be the suggested cause of the orienteers' heart disease [51,52]. For details see http://publications.uu.se/theses/fulltext/91-554-4986-7.pdf

Poliomyelitis

In the 1930s and 1940s, it was demonstrated that polio took a more serious course if patients had exercised during the early stages of the disease. The idea that physical exercise might influence the clinical outcome of poliomyelitis was based on case reports of strenuous physical exertion prior to the onset of severe paralysis. In total, 100 cases of poliomyelitis were reported and it was found that physical activity of any kind during the preparalytic stage increased the danger of severe paralysis. This observation was confirmed in epidemiologic studies and animal studies [24,25].

HIV infection

The primary immunologic defect in individuals infected with human immunodeficiency virus (HIV) is a depletion of the CD4+ T cell subset. However, conjoint effects have been reported on the function of other lymphocyte subpopulations, including the natural killer (NK) and lymphokine-activated killer (LAK) cells and cytokines.

In healthy subjects exercise-induced alterations in the immune system include changes in blood mononuclear cells, proliferative responses as well as NK and LAK cell functions. A study [26] on acute exercise was designed to determine to what extent HIV-infected individuals were able to mobilize immunocompetent cells to the blood in response to a physical exercise challenge. Interestingly, HIV-seropositive subjects were shown to possess an impaired ability to mobilize neutrophils, and cells mediating NK cell activity. Furthermore, only seronegative persons showed increased LAK cell activity in the blood in response to exercise, whereas HIV-seropositive subjects did not.

There are only few controlled studies on the effect of chronic exercise on the immune system in HIV-seropositive subjects. Despite significant increases in neuromuscular strength and cardiorespiratory fitness, there were no significant effects on the CD4 cell numbers or other lymphocyte subpopulations [27]. Similar observations have been found in a number of other studies (reviewed in [1]).

However, recent findings in HIV-positive homosexual men suggest that exercising 3–4 times a week is associated with a temporary slowing down of the progression toward AIDS, compared with the situation in a non-exercising control group [28]. Taken together, however, the available data do not allow any firm conclusions to be drawn regarding possible beneficial or detrimental effects of exercise training on the immune system in HIV-positive individuals.

Thus, although the case of 'Magic' Johnson highlights the fact that HIV infection is an issue also within elite sports and athletics, the current knowledge does not allow for any scientifically based guidelines regarding the advisability for an individual asymptomatic athlete to continue practising his sport at the elite level.

Upper respiratory tract infections

In contrast to the limited experimental evidence, there are several epidemiologic studies on exercise and upper respiratory tract infection (URTI). These studies are based on self-reported symptoms rather than clinical verification. In general, an increased number of URTI symptoms have been reported in the days following strenuous exercise (e.g. a marathon race) [29–32], whereas moderate training has been claimed to reduce the number of symptoms [33,34]. It has been suggested that a 'J'-shaped curve best describes the relationship between the intensity of physical activity, ranging from a sedentary lifestyle to the activity of the high-performance endurance athlete (along the *x*-axis) and the sensitivity to upper respiratory tract infections (Fig. 4.2.6). The finding of an increased frequency of infections following intense exercise may be causally linked to the postexercise impairment of immune function.

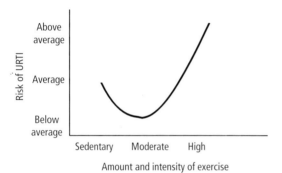

Fig. 4.2.6 A J-shaped curve describes the concept that the relative risk of acquiring upper respiratory tract infections (URTI) is decreased in individuals who practice moderate exercise, but increased in those who 'overtrain', compared to the risk in sedentary subjects.

Metabolic responses to infections and effects on performance

Acute infections in general evoke a multitude of host responses, some of which are directed toward the causative microorganism, including specific cellular and humoral immunity, whereas others have the purpose of adapting the metabolism of the host in order to increase its potential for survival. This non-specific, systemic 'acute phase reaction' includes the mobilization of nutrients from body tissues, predominantly from muscle tissue (Fig. 4.2.7). This is to satisfy the increased nutritional needs of the activated immune system and to provide substrates for the accelerated energy production during fever, which is generally associated with anorexia and decreased food intake. The elevated insulin levels during infection and fever generally hamper the mobilization of fatty acids from fat depots. The generalized catabolism of muscle protein progresses throughout the acute phase of the infection and includes skeletal muscles, as well as the heart muscle, regardless of whether or not there is a coexisting myocarditis. Several mild infections, however, such as an uncomplicated common cold, may not give rise to any significant muscle protein degradation (for review, see [7,21,48,49]).

When an acute infection is over, the decline in muscle strength and endurance from the individual's baseline conditions when healthy is correlated to the muscle protein loss caused by the infection. In studies of otherwise healthy young male adults, a week-long uncomplicated febrile infection of a severity that re-

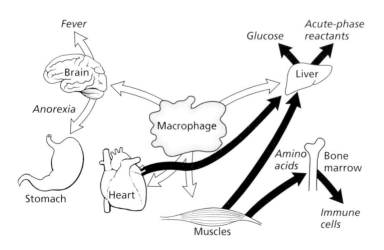

Fig. 4.2.7 Schematic description of cytokine effects in acute infectious diseases. Cytokines stimulate muscle protein degradation by mediating release of amino acids from muscles and increased uptake of amino acids in the liver and other organs. Similarly, cytokines are involved in the fever response and in the development of anorexia during infection and fever. Reproduced with permission from [21].

quired 'clinical bed rest' resulted in a decrease in the isometric strength of 5–15% [35], and in the isometric endurance of 13–18% [36] in various major muscle groups tested shortly after the disappearance of clinical symptoms of disease, as compared to subsequent repeated individual baseline results when the patients were healthy. Furthermore, in both young male and young female adults, such infections caused a decrease in the aerobic exercise capacity, as determined from the heart rate response during submaximal exercise, by approximately 25% [37].

The aerobic exercise capacity is dependent on central factors, such as the plasma volume, the total hemoglobin and the myocardial function, as well as on peripheral factors, i.e. the state of the skeletal muscles [38]. Potentially, all these factors may be negatively influenced by either the infection or the clinical bed rest that is part of the treatment, or both. In a group of healthy young adult males who served as controls in the studies described above [35,36,37], one week of bed rest, similar to the clinical bed rest of the patients in those studies, resulted in a decrease in the heart rate-related submaximal exercise capacity of 10–13% [37], whereas the maximal oxygen uptake decreased by only 6%, the plasma volume by 7% and the total hemoglobin by 6% [39]. (For obvious ethical reasons, maximal oxygen uptake studies could not be carried out in the patients, who were tested on day 1 after abatement of fever.) Thus, in the patients, the infection and the associated bed rest both contributed to the deterioration in aerobic exercise capacity. Conversely, neither the isometric muscle strength nor the isometric muscle endurance was influenced by the clinical bed rest in the healthy control subjects [35,36]. The recorded decreases in the isometric strength and endurance of up to 15 and 18%, respectively, in the patients on day 1 after abatement of fever were thus solely linked to the infection as a result of the catabolic effects on muscle tissue (Fig. 4.2.8).

During even the very early phase of ongoing infection and fever the muscle capacity, as well as the aerobic capacity, is already decreased, and these events are unrelated to the muscle catabolism, which is minimal at this early stage [41]. Furthermore, during ongoing infection and fever, muscle coordination and 'motor precision' required for carrying out 'synthetic work' are impaired [42]. This may potentially increase the risk of

ankle sprains, dislocations, etc. in many sports [21]. The underlying mechanisms explaining the deterioration in muscle function during early infection and fever are not fully understood; one study showing the safety margin of the neuromuscular transmission to be decreased during various ongoing febrile infections is suggestive of unspecific involvement of the nervous system, although that particular disturbance cannot account for any muscle weakness [43].

During infections that are severe enough to evoke a systemic acute phase reaction, the magnitude of the resulting muscle protein catabolism is the major determinant of the length of the convalescent period, provided there is no complicating myocarditis. For example, following a brief, flu-like illness with about 36 h of fever, as in sandfly fever, as long as 2 weeks is required for the accumulated muscle protein losses to be replenished. This period is longer after more long-lasting or severe infections [44]. Available evidence suggests that the time to full replenishment of the muscle protein and resumed performance can be shortened by physical training once the infection is over [7,21].

Guidelines

In general it may be said that physical activity in connection with infections is associated with certain medical risks, both for the infected individual and for fellow sportsmen, who may in turn become infected. The latter risk has relevance mainly in team sports, but is also possible in other sports where the participants are in close physical contact before, during or after the sporting event. Several previous publications include pertinent information on the handling of infections in athletes and on what to tell the patient [45–50].

Recently, the following considerations and suggestions for guidelines for management and counseling the athlete, primarily intended for the general practitioner, have been published [21].

The risk to the individual

The risks of deleterious effects of physical activity in an infected person vary considerably, depending both on the location, degree and cause of the infection and on the intensity and type of physical activity. Vigorous or prolonged physical activity as well as intensive mental stress can lower the defense against infection.

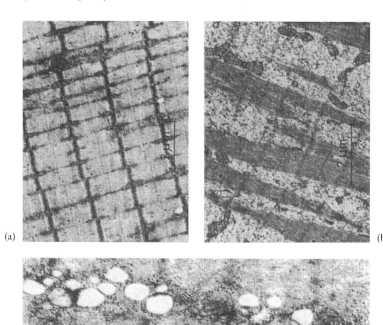

(a)

(b)

(c)

Fig. 4.2.8 Transmission electron micrographs of quadriceps muscle biopsies from: (a) a healthy subject after 1 week of 'clinical bed rest' showing normal ultrastructure (magnification × 10 000); (b) a patient who has suffered a week-long influenza type A infection showing degeneration of myofilaments; biopsy taken 3 days after abatement of fever (magnification × 12 000); and (c) a patient suffering from acute coxsackie virus type B2 infection with complicating myocarditis showing distended sarcoplasmic reticulum; biopsy taken after 1 week of symptoms (magnification × 28 000). Changes occurred regardless of symptoms of myalgia [40].

Furthermore, a subclinical complication of infection, e.g. myocarditis, can be aggravated by physical exertion. The risk level is generally higher in a competing sportsman than in the ordinary jogger, for example. The physician's advice to different patients therefore needs to be individualized.

The muscular and cardiac capacity is reduced in connection with most infections, especially if the infection is accompanied by fever. Continuing to train during the infection cannot generally prevent this temporary impairment of physical capacity. On the contrary, training during the course of an infection can lead to further reduction of the capacity, infection complications and other damage.

The nervous system is affected in general by infection and fever, with impairment of the coordination ability (the 'motor precision'). This can influence physical performance, especially in sports that demand high precision. In addition, the risk of damage to joints, ligaments and tendons is increased.

Physical exertion in the presence of fever means an increased hemodynamic load on the heart compared with such exertion in the healthy individual. This may lead to the manifestation, sometimes in the form of fatal dysrhythmia, of perhaps previously undiagnosed heart disease, e.g. coronary sclerosis or hypertrophic cardiomyopathy. Further, for example in respiratory tract infections, a heavy physical load may aggravate the infection, with more pronounced or prolonged symptoms, or development of complications, such as sinusitis and pneumonia. This applies even in the absence of fever. Myocarditis is the complication that has been discussed most in this connection. It should be pointed out, however, that in the majority of cases infectious myocarditis resolves, when properly attended to, without residual symptoms and that in myocarditis sudden death is rare.

A large number of different viruses and bacteria can infect the heart and give rise to myocarditis. Some microorganisms are more prone than others to attack the heart, while others do this very rarely. The former group includes enteroviruses (mainly coxsackie virus), and the latter group includes common cold viruses (rhinovirus and coronavirus). There is no quick test for demonstrating these viruses in an infected person. Moreover, many other microorganisms associated with a varying degree of risk of myocarditis often give rise to similar symptoms. There are certain rules of thumb (see below), but their precision varies. In clinical practice, therefore, conclusions drawn from the symptomatology and clinical picture regarding the microbial cause and hence the risk of myocarditis can be uncertain. As a general rule, the physician should adopt a more cautious attitude towards physical activity in infected sportsmen who are under 'pressure' to achieve their maximal performance than in infected joggers, for example, as mental stress can also lower the defense against infection. Special attention must be paid to elite athletes, where the environmental demands and expectations regarding participation and success, as well as their own demands, are particularly high. In certain sports the impairment of performance associated with the infection can be compensated by the sportsman's routine and skill, which may lead to increased risk-taking.

Mononucleosis can often be diagnosed by a rapid test. This disease can be associated with myocarditis. Further, mononucleosis is not infrequently accompanied by splenic enlargement, which has an impact on counseling, especially of persons practicing contact sports and weight-lifting.

Tonsillopharyngitis with β-streptococci can also be diagnosed by a quick test, and penicillin therapy should be given. There is some risk of myocarditis, despite treatment, during the first week.

Gastroenteritis is associated with fluid losses, which reduce performance as a result of a decreased plasma volume. Fluid losses through sweating in connection with physical exercise accentuate this effect and in-

crease the risk of collapse and of manifestation of undiagnosed heart diseases. Myocarditis can sometimes occur as a complication of gastroenteritis.

Skin infections of different kinds are common in sports, usually in the form of infected chafing sores, athlete's foot, infected eczema and plantar warts. Dermal borreliosis (erythema migrans in Lyme disease) is common among sportsmen who are exposed to ticks. Myocarditis is a rare but well-known complication of borreliosis. Sometimes even minor skin infections, on account of their location, can form a hindrance to sports activities and in occasional cases can constitute a port of entry for bacteria that give rise to septicemia. Small superficial skin infections are seldom contraindications to training and competitions. One exception is herpes infection in the skin, particularly in wrestlers. During wrestling viruses can easily be transmitted to other wrestlers via skin lesions.

Genital infections give rise to local and general symptoms of varying degrees of severity, or may be asymptomatic. It is uncommon for the microorganisms involved in such infections to lead to myocarditis.

There is currently no evidence that the course of the disease in asymptomatic HIV infection is influenced unfavorably by physical activity and sports. On the contrary, it has been documented that training and competitive activities have an important effect in improving the quality of life in many HIV patients.

Suggestions for guidelines for management and counseling

• In people with fever (38 °C or more), rest should always be recommended.

• People who know their normal temperature and pulse curves should rest if their resting temperature has increased by 0.5–1 °C or more and at the same time their resting pulse has risen by 10 b.p.m. or more, in combination with general symptoms (malaise, muscle pains, muscle tenderness, diffuse joint pains, headache).

• General malaise of acute onset, especially in combination with muscle pains, muscle tenderness, diffuse joint pains and headache, should give reason to recommend rest, even when the body temperature is normal.

• In all infections, caution should be observed during the first 1–3 days of symptoms, even with a normal body temperature, until the body defense against infection has had time to become mobilized and until the further development of the infection becomes clear. Serious infections often have prodromal symptoms, and in such cases it may take 1–3 days before the serious nature of the infection becomes evident.

• In people with nasal catarrh without a sore throat, cough or general symptoms, caution is recommended during the first 1–3 days, after which training can gradually be resumed, if the symptoms do not become intensified.

• If a cold is accompanied by further symptoms, e.g. sore throat, hoarseness or cough, the recommendation should be more restrictive, depending on the degree and development of the symptoms.

• In people with a sore throat without any other manifestations, caution is advised until this has begun to improve. In cases of β-streptococcal tonsillopharyngitis, which should be treated with penicillin for 10 days, rest is recommended until the symptoms have disappeared, and caution during the first week of treatment even in the absence of symptoms.

• In cases of mononucleosis, the general recommendation is rest until the symptoms have disappeared. Sometimes, however, fatigue can persist for several months after this disease, and in such cases a suitable time for resuming training has to be judged individually. Further, mononucleosis is often accompanied by splenic enlargement, and an enlarged spleen in mononucleosis is fragile and can rupture if it is subjected to a blow or increased pressure. Thus people engaged in contact sports such as football, wrestling and so on, and weight-lifting, should wait 1 month after they have become free from fever before taking up these sports again.

• In gastroenteritis, heavy physical exercise should be avoided.

• In skin infections, the recommendations need to be individualized. All athletes should observe caution in episodes of herpes accompanied by regional lymphadenitis or general symptoms. Individuals practicing contact sports should be screened for dermal herpes lesions and infected individuals should wait until the vesicles have dried before resuming these activities. Erythema migrans should be treated with penicillin or doxycycline for 10 days and caution should be recommended during the first week.

• In cystitis, which mainly affects women, strenuous physical exertion should be avoided until the symptoms have subsided.

• People with ongoing genital infections should avoid strenuous physical exertion. In asymptomatic genital chlamydial infection it seems reasonable to restrict the physical activity during the period of antibiotic therapy.

• Asymptomatic HIV infection constitutes no hindrance to exercise and sports (as far as the infected person is concerned—see below).

• In most cases of febrile infectious diseases, training can be resumed as soon as the fever has abated. It is important, however, that the training should be resumed gradually, and with attention paid to the 'body signals'. If unexpected symptoms referable to the heart should appear, for example pain, a sense of pressure or discomfort in the chest, irregular heart beats, abnormal breathlessness or fatigue or exertional syncope, the training should be discontinued and a physician consulted, because myocarditis can occur in connection with a number of different infections. It is important to point out that myocarditis can develop even without prior symptoms of infection. In persons who have reached middle age, the possibility of coronary disease or myocardial infarction should also be considered with symptoms of this type.

• In general, it may be said that in infections, as in other situations, it is important to 'listen to the body signals'.

Risks to the environment—epidemiologic aspects

Plantar warts are readily spread via shower floors and changing-rooms. These warts should therefore be treated quickly in athletes.

Respiratory tract infections can be readily transmitted both by droplet infection (sneezing/cough) and by contact (direct skin contact such as hand-shaking, or indirect contact via objects) among sportsmen who are in close proximity before, during or after a training or competitive event. Examples of this are countless. In addition, the fact that strenuous or prolonged physical exertion can reduce the defense against infection increases the susceptibility to respiratory tract infection.

Because prevention of exposure is the only prophylactic measure available in the vast majority of respiratory tract infections, the above aspects should be carefully considered by the individual athlete, as well as by trainers and sports leaders, before an infected individual allows himself or is allowed to meet his fellow participants prior to important training and competitive events. Annual immunization against influenza should be recommended for elite athletes.

Generally, athletes with HIV infection should be allowed to participate in sports just like any others. Physicians of HIV patients who are engaged in sports associated with a risk of exposure of blood, such as wrestling, boxing, football and so on, should inform the patients concerned of the theoretical risk that the infection can be transmitted further and strongly advise against their continuing to take part in sports of that kind. It is important to consider the anonymity aspects and to ensure that the infection status of the person concerned does not come to the knowledge of leaders or team-mates unless the individual has given his/her consent.

Summary

Exercise induces dramatic changes in the immune system. In essence, moderate exercise stimulates the immune system, whereas long-lasting intense exercise is followed by immune impairment, which may last from several hours to days. During this postexercise immune impairment, called 'the open window in the immune system', microorganisms may invade the host and establish an infection. Thus, it has been shown that several microorganisms become more invasive after strenuous exercise. A J-shaped curve describes the concept that the relative risk of acquiring upper respiratory tract infections is lower in individuals who practise moderate exercise, but higher in those who 'overtrain', compared to the risk in sedentary subjects. During infections the muscle capacity, as well as the aerobic capacity, is decreased and, in addition, muscle coordination and 'motor precision' are impaired, which may increase the risk of ankle sprains and dislocations in many sports. After abatement of fever, performance is impaired until the muscle protein loss, resulting from the infection, has been replenished. Although the physician's advice to different patients needs to be individualized, the general advice is to rest when ill. This advice can be modified when the symptoms have lasted for a couple of days and are strictly 'above the neck' (stuffy or running nose, sneezing, watery eyes, scratchy throat and no fever). However, when 'below the neck' symptoms exist (aching muscles, malaise, hacking cough, nausea, vomiting, diarrhea, fever), exercise training should always be avoided.

Multiple choice questions

1 *Exercise influences the following immune parameters:*
a lymphocytes
b neutrophils
c natural killer cells
d salivary IgA
e cytokines.

2 *When trained animals and humans are examined at rest, you will find:*
a enhanced natural immunity
b decreased natural immunity
c enhanced survival of infections
d decreased survival of infections
e no changes from untrained controls.

3 *Metabolic responses to infections and effects on performance.*
a Nutrients are mobilized, especially from muscle, during infection.
b The declines in muscle strength and endurance do not correlate with muscle protein loss caused by infection.
c Bed rest induces a decrease in exercise capacity.

4 *Guidelines for athletes are:*
a In persons with fever (38°C or more), rest should always be recommended.
b In persons with nasal catarrh without a sore throat, cough or general symptoms, caution is recommended during the first 1–3 days, after which training can gradually be resumed, if the symptoms do not become intensified.
c In gastroenteritis heavy physical exercise should be avoided.
d Asymptomatic HIV infection constitutes no hindrance to exercise and sports.

References

1 Pedersen BK, Hoffman-Goetz L. Exercise and the immune system: regulation, integration and adaptation. *Physiol Rev* 2000; **80**: 1055–81.

2 Hoffman-Goetz L, Pedersen BK. Exercise and the immune system. A model of the stress response? *Immunol Today* 1994; **15**: 345–92.

3 Gleeson M, McDonald WA, Pyne DB *et al.* Salivary IgA levels and infection risk in elite swimmers. *Med Sci Sports Exerc* 1999; **31**: 67–73.

4 Pedersen BK. Exercise and cytokines. *Immunol Cell Biol* 2000; **78**: 532–5.

5 Cannon JG, Kluger MJ. Exercise enhances survival rate in mice infected with *Salmonella typhimurium* (41830). *Proc Soc Exp Biol Med* 1984; **175**: 518–21.

6 Ilbäck NG, Friman G, Beisel WR, Johnson AJ, Berendt RF. Modifying effects of exercise on clinical course and biochemical response of the myocardium in influenza and tularemia in mice. *Infect Immun* 1984; **45**: 498–504.

7 Friman G, Ilbäck NG. Acute infection: metabolic responses, effects on performance, interaction with exercise, and myocarditis. *Int J Sports Med* 1998; **19**: S172–82.

8 Friman G, Ilbäck NG. Exercise and infection — interaction, risks and benefits. *Scand J Med Sci Sports* 1992; **2**: 177–89.

9 Gatmaitan BG, Hanson JL, Lerner AM. Agumentation of the virulence of murine coxackievirus B3 myocardiopathy by exercise. *J Exp Med* 1970; **131**: 1121–36.

10 Ilbäck NG, Fohlman J, Friman G. Exercise in coxsackie B3 myocarditis: effects on heart lymphocyte subpopulations and the inflammatory reaction. *Am Heart J* 1989; **117**: 1298–302.

11 Karjalainen J, Heikkilä J, Nieminen M *et al.* Etiology of mild acute infectious myocarditis. Relation to clinical features. *Acta Med Scand* 1983; **213**: 65–73.

12 Gravanis MG, Sternby NH. Incidence of myocarditis. *Arch Pathol Lab Med* 1991; **15**: 390–2.

13 Karjalainen J, Heikkilä J. Incidence of three presentations of acute myocarditis in young men in military service. *Eur Heart J* 1999; **20**: 1120–5.

14 Bergström K, Erikson U, Nordbring F *et al.* Acute non-rheumatic myopericarditis: a follow-up study. *Scand J Infect Dis* 1970; **2**: 7–16.

15 Giesecke J. The long-term prognosis in acute myocarditis. *Eur Heart J Suppl* 1987; **J**: 251–3.

16 Remes J, Helin M, Vaino P *et al.* Clinical outcome and left ventricular function 23 years after acute coxsackievirus myopericarditis. *Eur Heart J* 1990; **11**: 182–8.

17 Maron B, Shirani J, Poliac L, Mathenge R, Roberts W, Mueller F. Sudden death in young competitive athletes. *J Am Med Assoc* 1996; **276**: 199–204.

18 McCaffrey FM, Braconier DS, Strong WB. Sudden cardiac death in young athletes. *Am J Dis Child* 1991; **145**: 177–83.

19 Phillips M, Robinowitz M, Higgins JR, Boran KJ, Reed T, Virmani R. Sudden cardiac death in air force recruits. *J Am Med Assoc* 1986; **256**: 2696–9.

20 Wesslén L, Påhlson C, Lindquist O *et al.* An increase in sudden unexpected cardiac deaths among young Swedish orienteers during 1979–1992. *Eur Heart J* 1996; **17**: 902–10.

21 Friman G, Wesslén L. Infections and exercise in high-performance athletes. *Immunol Cell Biol* 2000; **78**: 510–22.

22 Larsson E, Wesslén L, Lindquist O *et al.* Sudden unexpected cardiac deaths among young Swedish orienteers — morphological changes in hearts and other organs. *APMIS* 1999; **107**: 325–36.

23 Roberts JA. Viral illnesses and sports performance. *Sports Med* 1986; **3**: 296–303.

24 Hargreaves ER. Poliomyelitis. Effect of exertion during the pre-paralytic stage. *Br Med J* 1948; **2**: 1021–2.

25 Horstmann DM. Acute poliomyelitis. Relation of physical activity at the time of onset to the course of the disease. *J Am Med Assoc* 1950; **142**: 236–41.

26 Ullum H, Palmo J, Halkjaer Kristensen J *et al.* The effect of acute exercise on lymphocyte subsets, natural killer cells, proliferative responses, and cytokines in HIV-seropositive persons. *J Acquir Immune Defic Syndr* 1994; **7**: 1122–33.

27 Rigsby LW, Dishman RK, Jackson AW, Maclean GS, Raven PB. Effects of exercise training on men seropositive for the human immunodeficiency virus-1. *Med Sports Exerc* 1992; **24**: 6–12.

28 Mustafa T, Sy FS, Macera CA *et al.* Association between exercise and HIV disease progression in a cohort of homosexual men. *Ann Epidemiol* 1999; **9**: 127–31.

29 Kendall A, Hoffman-Goetz L, Houston M, Macneil B, Arumugam Y. Exercise and blood lymphocyte subset responses: intensity, duration, and subject fitness effects. *J Appl Physiol* 1990; **69**: 251–60.

30 Nieman DC, Johanssen LM, Lee JW. Infectious episodes in runners before and after a roadrace. *J Sports Med Phys Fitness* 1989; **29**: 289–96.

31 Nieman DC, Johanssen LM, Lee JW, Arabatzis K. Infectious episodes in runners before and after the Los Angeles Marathon. *J Sports Med Phys Fitness* 1990; **30**: 316–28.

32 Peters EM, Bateman ED. Ultramarathon running and upper respiratory tract infections. An epidemiological survey. *S Afr Med J* 1983; **64**(15): 582–4.

33 Nieman DC, Henson DA, Gusewitch G *et al.* Physical activity and immune function in elderly women. *Med Sports Exerc* 1993; **25**: 823–31.

34 Nieman DC, Nehlsen Cannarella SL, Markoff PA *et al.* The effects of moderate exercise training on natural killer cells and acute upper respiratory tract infections. *Int J Sports Med* 1990; **11**: 467–73.

35 Friman G. Effect of acute infectious disease on isometric muscle strength. *Scand J Clin Lab Invest* 1977; **37**: 303–8.

36 Friman G. Effect of acute infectious disease on human isometric muscle endurance. *Upsala J Med Sci* 1978; **83**: 105–8.

37 Friman G. Effects of acute infectious disease on circulatory function. *Acta Med Scand Suppl* 1976; **592**: 1–62.

38 Åstrand P-O, Rodahl K. *Textbook of Work Physiology: Physiological Bases of Exercise*, 3rd edn. McGraw-Hill Co, 1986: 1–608.

39 Friman G. Effect of clinical bed rest for seven days on physical performance. *Acta Med Scand* 1979; **205**: 389–93.

40 Åström E, Friman G, Pilström L. Effects of viral and mycoplasma infections on ultrastructure and enzyme activities in human skeletal muscle. *Acta Pathol Microbiol Scand Sect* 1976; **84**: 113–22.

41 Friman G, Wright JE, Ilbäck N-G, Beisel WR, White JD, Sharp DS, Stephen EL, Daniels WL, Vogel JA. Does fever or myalgia indicate reduced physical performance capacity in viral infections? *Acta Med Scand* 1985; **217**: 353–61.

42 Alluisi EA, Beisel WR, Bartelloni PJ, Coates GD. Behavioral effects of tularemia and sand fly fever in man. *J Infect Dis* 1973; **128**: 710–7.

43 Friman G, Schiller HH, Schwartz MS. Disturbed neuromuscular transmission in viral infections. *Scand J Infect Dis* 1977; **9**: 99–103.

44 Beisel WR, Sawyer WD, Ryll ED, Crozier D. Metabolic effects of intracellular infections in man. *Ann Intern Med* 1967; **67**: 744–79.

45 Eichner ER. Infection, immunity, and exercise. *Phys Sports Med* 1993; **21**: 125–35.

46 Nieman DC. Exercise immunology: practical applications. *Int J Sports Med* 1997; **18** (Suppl. 1): 91–100.

47 Pedersen BK. Exercise and infection. In: Pedersen BK, ed. *Exercise Immunology*. New York: Springer, 1997: 133–47.

48 Shephard RJ. Exercise, immune function and HIV infection. *J Sports Med Phys Fitness* 1998; **38**: 101–10.

49 Simon HB. Exercise and infection. *Phys Sports Med* 1987; **15**: 135–41.

50 Brenner IKM, Shek PN, Shephard RJ. Infection in athletes. *Sports Med* 1994; **17**: 86–107.

51 Wesslén L, Ehrenbory C, Holmberg M. Subacute *Bartonella* infection in Swedish orienteers succumbing to sudden unexpected cardiac death or having malignant arrhythmias. *Scand Infect Dis* 2001; **33**: 429–38.

52 McGill S, Wesslén L, Hjelm E, Holmb M, Rolf C, Friman G. Serological and epidemiological analysis of the prevalence of Bartonella Spp: antibodies in Swedish elite orienteers 1992–93. *Scand Infect Dis* 2001; **33**: 423–8.

Chapter 4.3
Osteoarthritis

L. STEFAN LOHMANDER &
HARALD P. ROOS

Classical reference

Fairbanks TJ. Knee joint changes after meniscectomy. *J Bone Joint Surg* 1948; **30B**: 664–670.
This paper records an investigation of changes found in the knee joint at intervals ranging from 3 months to 14 years after meniscectomy.

Radiologic study. After excluding all cases with definite osteoarthritis, a comparison was made between the preoperative and postoperative X-ray films in 107 cases of meniscectomy. Owing to difficulty in securing identical views on separate occasions, the changes described were accepted as convincing only because they were seen repeatedly; occasionally a film of the normal knee provided better comparison. The changes noted, alone or in combination, were of three types: formation of an anteroposterior ridge projecting downwards from the margin of the femoral condyle over the old meniscus site; generalized flattening of the marginal half of the femoral articular surface—a reaction similar to but more diffuse than the ridge; and narrowing of the joint space on the side of the operation. The changes were within 5 months of operation on many occasions, but they tend to become more obvious with time. No correlation was found between clinical and radiologic findings, many knee joints with the most marked radiographic changes being functionally perfect. The frequency of such changes after medial meniscectomy in 80 cases was: no change 33%, ridge 43%, narrowing 32%, flattening 18%.

Investigations. It is submitted that these changes result chiefly from loss of the weight-bearing functions of the meniscus—a function which has not been accepted universally.

Discussion. Meniscectomy must therefore result in the relative overloading of the articular surfaces on that side of the joint, with increasing compression of the cartilage. But narrowing of the joint space after operation was seen in X-ray films of the recumbent patient, and if such changes are permanent, and radiographically demonstrable, it must be due either to structural changes in the articular cartilages which impair the power of recoil, or to actual loss of tissue.

Summary and conclusion. Changes in the knee joint after meniscectomy include ridge formation, narrowing of the joint space and flattening of the femoral condyle. Investigations suggest that these changes are due to loss of the weight-bearing function of the meniscus. Meniscectomy is not wholly innocuous; it interferes, at least temporarily, with the mechanics of the joint. It seems likely that narrowing of the joint space will predispose to early degenerative changes, but a connection between these appearances and later osteoarthritis is not yet established and is too indefinite to justify clinical deductions.

Background

The benefits of physical activity are well documented and positive effects on diabetes, asthma and body weight have been postulated (see Chapters 4.4, 4.5 and 4.7). Physical activity also seems to decrease the risk of cardiovascular disease and its associated mortality. The positive effects of physical activity on the musculoskeletal system are also well documented, even extending to being a recommended treatment of osteoarthritis. However, vigorous physical activity and associated injuries are associated with short- and long-term side-effects.

Osteoarthritis (OA) in the lower extremity as a consequence of sports activities is the focus of this chapter. OA is characterized by a general loss of articular cartilage accompanied by an attempted repair of the articular cartilage, with remodeling and sclerosis of the subchondral bone. In many instances there is formation of bone cysts and osteophytes [1,2]. These changes in articular cartilage could be induced either by the physical activity itself or by associated joint injuries. It is important to point out that OA as discussed here is based on radiographic criteria and that there is an inconsistent relationship between symptoms and radiographic findings in OA. However, the presence of radiographic signs of OA increases the risk of current or future OA symptoms.

The course of OA induced by exercise or trauma is not fully understood. There is no clear evidence that the progression of OA is faster in sports-related OA compared to primary (idiopathic) OA, but since the initiating events tend to occur at a young age, especially when trauma is concerned, both radiographic signs and symptoms of OA occur at a much younger age than in primary OA.

Since the probable onset of the disease process, defined as the time of trauma, can be identified in most cases, post-traumatic OA is an attractive model for studying the course of OA and homogenous cohorts can be defined for this purpose.

There are many risk factors for the development of OA, age being the most important [3–5]. Sex, race, obesity, biomechanical factors and inherited susceptibility together with use and abuse of joints and joint trauma influence the development of OA [3,6]. The hand, knee and hip are most frequently affected by OA and the risk factors associated with OA differ according to the joint involved [3,4]. Hand and knee OA have a stronger female preponderance and knee OA also has a more solid association with obesity than hip OA [3,4,7]. However, a recent report suggested an association between OA and overweight also for the hip [8]. Risk factors are probably additive and Doherty *et al.* [9] noted an increased risk for developing knee OA after meniscectomy in patients with interphalangeal OA in the hand, suggesting that systemic factors can influence the course of postmeniscectomy OA [9]. This is in agreement with progressive joint space narrowing being more common in patients with multiple joint involvement [10,11].

Joint injury is a known risk factor for OA (secondary or post-trauma OA). Joint subluxation, dysplasia or incongruity as a consequence of a fracture with joint involvement will cause an abnormal contact stress on the articular surface [12]. However, joint trauma without overt skeletal injury, such as soft tissue trauma and contusion injuries to the joint cartilage, also probably increase the risk for OA. However, an experimental model on the effects of contusion injuries to the knee in dogs did not show consistent OA development [13]. Many studies have shown early cartilage changes secondary to meniscus and ACL injuries in the knee [5,14–20].

Sports-induced osteoarthritis

Physical activity and osteoarthritis

The amount of loading appears to be an important factor for OA development. Moderate running (4 km/day) increased the indentation stiffness of the cartilage and the cartilage matrix content of proteoglycan in beagle dogs [21–23], while running exercise of 20 km/day for 15 weeks in the same type of dogs decreased the proteoglycan content [22,24,25]. Long-term (1 year) strenuous running exercise (40 km/day) resulted in a depletion of proteoglycans and a softening of the cartilage [26]. It is however, unknown whether these changes will cause OA, since the depletion of proteoglycans and softening of the cartilage might also represent a normal physiologic adaptation to enhanced mechanical stress induced by vigorous running [21] (see Chapter 1.7).

A relationship between OA of the hip and knee, and heavy work or sports activities has been postulated. Sports activities with intense high impact and torsional loading are associated with an increased prevalence of OA [27]. Examples of such sports are soccer, American football, rugby, team handball, basketball, competitive running and water skiing [28].

Physical activities associated with knee bending have been suggested to increase the risk of knee OA [29]. There is also a correlation between heavy physical work that involves squatting and kneeling, and knee OA [6,29–32]. A relation between occupational loading and hip OA has been demonstrated [32,33], exemplified by the increased prevalence of hip OA in farmers [34] and ballet dancers [35,36], and an increased prevalence of knee and hip OA in coal miners [37], shipyard laborers [31], fire-fighters, food-processing workers, physical education teachers (Sandmark) and construction workers [32].

Long-distance running is an example of a sports activity that mainly consists of repetitive loading without traumatic injuries, and could thus serve as a model in the attempts to study the relationship between exercise and OA. Most studies on runners have failed to find a correlation between running and OA [38,39]. In a 5-year follow-up of runners, with a mean age of 65 at follow-up, both runners and controls had a significant progression of radiographic features of OA, but running did not appear to accelerate the development of OA [39]. However, one study showed more radiographic hip joint changes in a group of former national team long-distance runners compared to bobsled competitors and a reference group [40]. In a study by Konradsen *et al.* [38], 2 out of 33 former long-distance runners had hip OA, compared to none of the 27 controls [38]. Thus, high-mileage running on a competitive level may increase the risk of hip OA, but the evidence is weak.

Soccer and osteoarthritis

Soccer is the most popular sport in the world and is believed to have some 40 million amateur participants [41]. During the last decade female soccer has become popular and now attracts a fair number of women, not least in North America. It has been estimated that at least half of the sports injuries in Europe are soccer related [42].

In a review on sports practice and OA the authors concluded that some sports, especially practiced on a high level, comprise an increased risk for OA in hip and/or knee joints [27]. Soccer is such an activity with a calculated relative risk of hip and knee OA compared to controls of 2.3–3.7 and 4.4–5.2, respectively. However, these risk estimates are only valid as far as elite players are concerned [43–46].

Soccer as a cause of hip OA was described by Klünder *et al.* [47] and an increased prevalence of knee OA in former elite soccer players was reported by Chantraine [48]. The latter study was handicapped by a lack of a control group and considerable drop-out. Subsequent studies of former Finnish elite athletes found a prevalence of tibiofemoral knee OA of 29% in soccer players, and patellofemoral OA in 31% of weight-lifters. No premature knee OA in runners or shooters was found in that study [43].

Swedish studies on hip and knee OA in former soccer players [44,45] found a prevalence of hip and knee OA of 14–15% in former top-level players with a mean age of 63 years, compared to 3–4% in an age-matched control group. However, there was no increased prevalence of either hip or knee OA among former non-elite players compared to age-matched controls.

The increased prevalence of knee OA in former soccer players might be expected in the light of the high incidence of knee injuries in soccer. However, even after excluding patients with known injuries, 11% of the former players had knee OA, compared to 4% among controls, suggesting that soccer even in the absence of known injuries constitutes a risk factor for knee OA [45].

Female soccer is a more recent sport and long-term follow-up studies are thus lacking. In a Swedish study 66 retired female soccer players with a mean age of 43 years were radiographically examined [49]. The exposure to soccer was on average 13 years. The prevalence of hip OA was comparable to age- and gender-matched controls. In contrast, knee OA was present in 17% of the female players, compared to 2% of the age-matched male soccer ex-players and 0% of the age-matched female controls. The females were recruited from all levels of competitive soccer and no differences according to level of soccer playing could be detected, which contrasts with the findings among male ex-players. Spector *et al.* [50] studied the risk of knee OA defined as the presence of osteophytes in female ex-athletes and similarly demonstrated an increased prevalence of knee OA, especially among tennis players and runners. Tennis players were more prone to have tibiofemoral knee OA while former runners showed patellofemoral involvement, especially on the lateral facet of the patella.

Knee injuries and osteoarthritis

Experimental models of joint degeneration show that mechanical instability created by transection of the anterior cruciate ligament (ACL) and meniscectomy often leads to progressive joint degeneration. Joint instability combined with loss of sensory innervation greatly increases the susceptibility of the articular cartilage to damage [28].

The association between primary knee OA and female gender is well known [3,4], but in OA induced by an injury no such association has yet been shown [5,14,18,51]. A prospective study of 1300 students examined the relation between trauma and hip and knee OA and found a relative risk of 5.17 for subsequent knee OA after a trauma at that site, and 3.50 for hip OA [52]. The reported rate of OA after knee injuries varies considerably between different studies (Fig. 4.3.1) [53]. Possible explanations for these considerable differences are: (a) the majority of the studies are cross-sectional and show a considerable drop-out rate; (b) the age at onset of symptoms, trauma and surgery differs within and between the studies and is sometimes not defined; (c) associated injuries are not often described or taken into account; (d) different radiographic classifications are used; and (e) appropriate controls are lacking.

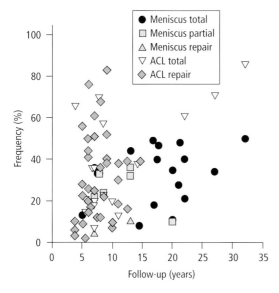

Fig. 4.3.1 Published outcomes for radiologic signs of osteoarthritis following knee ligament injury and intervention. Modified from [53]. Each symbol represents published results in the scientific literature for a specific patient group and intervention.

Anterior cruciate ligament injuries

ACL injuries may result in a faster development of joint cartilage changes than isolated meniscus tears, and radiographic evidence of OA will be seen in about 50% of the subjects 10–15 years after an ACL injury [53]. The possibly faster progression of OA after an ACL injury could be explained by the high forces involved in the initial trauma, with considerable injuries of associated structures in the joint, such as menisci, joint capsule and collateral ligaments. The bone bruises that can be visualized on MR images, often located in the lateral compartment of the joint, represent the effect of a contusion injury and may contribute to the initiation of the OA development [54,55]. Changes in gait pattern [56] and loss of proprioception are other factors that have been proposed as causative for the development of OA after an ACL injury [57,58].

The risk of post-traumatic OA increases with time so that an injury in the teenage period will cause visible radiographic changes of OA early in life. A recent nationwide study on female soccer players with ACL injury showed that one-third had radiographic OA 12 years after the injury and another 40% had other visible radiographic changes, but without reaching the criteria for OA. In this study, radiographic OA was defined as slight joint space narrowing (grade 1) combined with osteophytes or definite joint space narrowing (grade 2) according to the OARSI criteria [59]. This definition of radiologic OA corresponds to Kellgren and Lawrence grade II [60]. The mean age at time of trauma was 19 years and accordingly the age at follow-up 12 years later was 31 years of age. Postinjury treatment (ACL reconstruction or not) did not significantly alter the risk for developing OA. At the 12-year follow-up some 50% of these young females experienced problems such as pain and restricted ability to participate in physical activity. However, there was no association between the presence of radiographic OA and symptoms. This finding is in accordance with other studies [61].

Meniscus injuries

It is questionable whether a meniscus tear early in life represents the same disease as a tear in a 40-year-old patient. Tears in younger patients are usually caused by a trauma, whereas a tear later in life may be a part of a degenerative joint disease including the menisci. Following a meniscus tear the radiographic changes appear after a shorter time interval in those who suffered from the injury over 30 years of age as compared to younger people with a meniscus tear [5]. A follow-up of patients who underwent meniscectomy in adolescence showed three times more radiographic changes in the operated knee compared to the opposite knee after 30 years [62]. Seventy per cent were still satisfied with their knee, but the progression of changes paralleled a reduction in activity. In a Swedish study, mild radiographic changes were present in 75% of the patients 21 years after total meniscectomy. The mean age of the cohort at follow-up was 55 years, thus representing the 'average' age group of meniscectomy patients. More advanced changes, corresponding to Kellgren and Lawrence grade II [60], were present in 48% [18]. The corresponding figures for the occurrence of mild and more advanced radiographic changes in an age- and gender-matched control cohort were 17 and 7%, respectively. The risk ratios for radiographic changes of mild and more advanced OA compared to the age- and gender-paired controls were 9.8 and 14.0 for mild or advanced changes, respectively. However, as in the ACL study described above, the correlation between radiographic findings and experienced symptoms was limited. On the other hand, considerably more knee-related symptoms were seen in the meniscectomy group compared to the controls, suggesting that the loss of a meniscus causes symptoms independently of the presence of joint cartilage changes [18].

Treatment of knee injuries and development of osteoarthritis

No controlled studies on OA after ACL disruption comparing surgical vs. non-surgical treatment are available. The fact that an ACL reconstruction decreases the risk for a later meniscus injury appears to be an advantageous effect of surgical stabilization [63]. In a prospective uncontrolled outcome study Daniel *et al.* [64] concluded that patients who had undergone a reconstruction of the ACL had more radiographic OA than non-surgically treated patients, which is in accordance with the study on female soccer players cited above [59]. The suggested increased risk of OA in surgically treated patients could be caused by the fact that

they have a greater ability to return to knee-demanding activities after knee stabilization. On the other hand it could be that the patients with the most severe symptoms of their injury, and also the more severe associated injuries, are the ones recommended for surgery. The surgical procedure may also be harmful to the joint cartilage either by direct insult during the surgery or by the altered biomechanical situation in the knee after a ligament reconstruction [64].

Theoretically, a preservation of the meniscus by a repair or a very located resection should be advantageous. However, no data supporting this theory are available, although suggested by some authors [65–67]. The only randomized study comparing subtotal and partial meniscectomy could not verify a positive long-term effect of saving a part of the meniscus [68]. On the other hand, supporting the theory that the meniscus is of importance for the knee function, patients with a more extensive resection of the meniscus had more knee-related symptoms compared to those who had the meniscus partially resected [19]. However, a recent study on the outcome after meniscus resection comparing subtotal and partial resection, showed no differences between the groups. If the tears were divided into degenerative and traumatic tears, more complaints were found after a degenerative tear, confirming that these meniscus tears may represent different conditions [69]. Meniscus repair, a demanding intervention for the patient with an extensive rehabilitation program, has not yet with certainty been shown to prevent later OA. A reduced incidence of OA after meniscus repair compared to resection was shown by Sommerlath [20], but different types of tears were compared in this study. A difficulty in conducting a randomized study comparing equivalent meniscal tears is that reparable tears in stable knees are rare, and when they do occur they may be associated with degenerative changes in the meniscus substance [70]. Accordingly, a recent follow-up of meniscus repairs showed a prevalence of OA comparable to that after meniscus resection [67]. No controlled studies on meniscus transplantation are available yet [71].

In conclusion, as described in many publications, knee injuries increase the risk for OA considerably. ACL injuries seem to be more deleterious than an isolated meniscus tear. However, it must be kept in mind that the majority of ACL injuries are combined with meniscus tears. There is no scientific evidence that ACL reconstruction, meniscus repair or meniscus transplantation reduces the risk of OA developing as a consequence of the initial injury.

Treatment of osteoarthritis

For the 'common or garden' variety of patient with OA the disease is recognized as a slowly progressive condition that sometimes results in serious pain and functional impairment leading to a requirement for joint replacement. This disease stage for the hip and knee is frequently reached around the age of 70, an age where expectations of activity level have decreased.

For the joint-injured athlete the situation is often different, with onset of radiographic changes and symptoms of increasing severity at a considerably younger age [5,18,44,45,53,69,72,73]. These individuals at the time of onset of symptoms have a longer life expectancy and expectations of a higher level of physical activity, even after joint surgery. The remarkable success of arthroplasty as a treatment for older individuals with severe OA is replaced by a high rate of implant failure and revision surgery among those operated on at a younger age [74–76]. Osteoarthritis in the young, often resulting from joint injury during athletic activities, thus represents a continued and unresolved challenge for the sports medicine community.

The most important symptoms of OA are joint pain, stiffness and decreased range of motion. Pain is what brings the patient to the doctor and is the focus of most treatments for OA. There is no treatment that can change the course of joint destruction, but a range of modalities are effective in decreasing pain and retaining or improving function. Several recent reviews provide further information on OA and its management [3,77–81] but few are evidence based [82]. This chapter is based on these reviews, favoring those based on evidence.

Prevention

In view of our lack of effective means for dealing with OA in the young and our lack of treatments that could slow disease progression, much effort needs to be directed towards the prevention of joint injuries in young athletes.

A recent study of proprioceptional training indicates that it may be possible to reduce the incidence rate of ACL injuries in soccer [83], but the results of this single study has to be verified further. The prevention of ACL injuries in female players is particularly important, since females have a higher incidence of this injury, get injured earlier in life and, in addition, have a greater risk of knee OA even when injuries are excluded. The increased popularity of female soccer, not least at high-school level, shows a clear path towards a problematic situation some years ahead. Knee injuries occurring at 18 years of age, with radiographic OA in the early thirties and onset of symptoms perhaps a few years later or even before, may result in patients requiring OA surgery in their early forties. A study of injury risk factors in female soccer revealed that neither physical capacity, functional performance, nor muscle strength correlated to injuries [84]. In that study increased joint laxity was the only significant risk factor.

In those who are overweight, even a moderate decrease in body weight results in decreased symptoms and perhaps also a decreased risk for further development of knee and perhaps also hip OA [3]. Weight loss is thus an important advice for the overweight with OA.

As discussed above, there is little or no evidence that surgical reconstruction of a torn cruciate ligament or meniscus prevents the development of knee OA at a later time. The rationale for these interventions thus need to be sought elsewhere.

Non-surgical treatment of OA

Treatment of OA varies with patient, disease stage, local resources and traditions. As with any chronic condition, the informed and empowered patient is a most important factor. Decisions on treatment should be based on three dimensions: patient, joint and environment.

Information and education about the disease, and what will likely happen in the future is an important aspect of OA treatment. The message to give to the patient with early-stage OA is that the condition develops very slowly and that for many individuals exercise, training, simple aids and sometimes analgesics provide excellent relief. For a few, the disease will progress and require additional treatment.

Pain is what the patient initially seeks help for. Information and (perhaps also printed) advice about weight loss, shoes with shock-absorbing soles, maintenance of physical activity and training programs and 'over-the-counter' (OTC) analgesics are often effective. The interested and educated physical therapist has an important role in guiding the patient to the right kind of exercises and encouraging compliance. Some reports suggest that quadriceps weakness is a primary risk factor for knee pain, disability and progression of joint damage in persons with osteoarthritis of the knee [85]. Several other studies support the beneficial effects of exercise on OA symptoms [86–90].

Aids and adjustment of home or work environment can be very helpful. A knee brace can be used in unilateral knee OA. One randomized clinical trial showed significant benefits from valgus-producing knee braces, unloaders, in patients with medial compartment OA, compared with a neoprene sleeve [91].

Drugs

Drugs have a very dominant position in the treatment of OA, despite the fact that many patients report that the effect of analgesics on OA pain is limited. Clinical trials have in fact shown that for many patients information, training programs, etc. are as effective as drugs against OA pain [81]. Any choice of analgesics should be made in the light of the fact that OA is a chronic disease and that medication may be long term.

Paracetamol (acetaminophen) is recommended as a first choice for pain relief in OA, in doses of up to 4 g/24 h. The frequency of side-effects is low, compared to the alternatives, and those that occur are mainly associated with the combination of alcohol and paracetamol. Several randomized, controlled and blinded trials have shown a similar OA pain relief from paracetamol as from non-steroidal anti-inflammatory drugs (NSAIDs) [92].

NSAIDs. For those patients in whom paracetamol is insufficiently effective it is appropriate to try some form of NSAID. The effect on pain is similar to that of paracetamol, but some patients that do not respond to paracetamol respond to NSAIDs. There is no differ-

ence in effect on OA pain between the different members of this class of compounds or between those compounds that inhibit both cyclooxygenase-1 and -2, or are selective for cyclooxygenase-2 (COX-2) [81]. Several of the non-selective inhibitors have been in use for many years, such as diclofenac, ibuprofen and naproxen, and some are available OTC. The adverse effects of this class of compounds are significant and well known, affecting the gastrointestinal lining (dyspepsia, gastritis, gastrointestinal bleeding), kidney function, nervous system and thrombocyte function (clot inhibition). The risk of serious gastrointestinal bleeding, sometimes leading to death, varies significantly between different members of the class, and those mentioned above constitute a low-risk group within the class [93,94]. The risk of adverse effects increases with age. The patient should use the lowest effective dose for the shortest time needed.

The coxibs constitute a recently introduced subgroup of NSAIDs, and selectively inhibit COX-2. The pain relief is comparable to that for the non-selective COX inhibitors, but these compounds have the advantage of a lower risk of gastrointestinal bleeding and do not affect thrombocyte function. However, the adverse effects on e.g. the kidneys and cardiovascular system appear to be similar to those for the non-selective inhibitors. The absence of an effect on thrombocyte aggregation by the coxibs, which in some circumstances may be an advantage, means that an apparent protective effect of the traditional NSAIDs against thromboembolic disease is absent. This new class of compounds should be prescribed with the same care as non-selective COX inhibitors until our knowledge of their advantages and disadvantages has expanded [95].

Other analgesics, such as opioids (tramadol, codeine, etc.), may provide good relief for some patients with OA pain. However, side-effects and dependency limit their usefulness.

For those ageless athletes with OA pain that does not respond well to analgesics, the addition of an *antidepressant* may be tried.

Topical treatment of the knee or other joints with painful OA with gels containing NSAIDs has demonstrated effectiveness in some trials [96]. Gels containing capsaicin have also been effective in some trials and are available in some countries.

Intra-articular injections are frequently used in the treatment of OA of the knee and some other joints. This treatment should not be considered a first-line treatment, but may be considered for those patients that experience insufficient effect of the treatments discussed above. The placebo effect of any intra-articular intervention, including injections, is considerable.

Steroid injections are commonly used, but the treatment rests on a weak base of evidence. A few well-designed and controlled trials show a moderate and short-lived effect of a few weeks on OA pain.

Hyaluronan is an endogenous molecule that occurs naturally in connective tissues, cartilage and joint fluid. A review of the results of recent controlled clinical trials of intra-articular knee injections of hyaluronan in OA show a modest effect on pain over and above that of placebo injections [97]. Some individual patients may experience a more marked and extended pain relief. There is no support for a difference in efficacy or side-effects for the different preparations of hyaluronan now being marketed, irrespective of hyaluronan source or molecular size.

Adverse effects of knee injections are rare, but potentially severe in the form of septic arthritis. Steroids may mask an intra-articular infection.

Acupuncture, given as an adjunct to drugs and other treatments for OA, has been reported to provide significant pain relief in some patients.

Other treatments for OA than those described above are commonly used. Unless asked, the patient may not, however, reveal these to the treating doctor. In the USA more than half of OA patients use treatments other than those prescribed by their treating doctor. Examples of such treatments are glucosamine, chondroitin sulfate, vitamins and other 'nutraceuticals'. The scientific evidence for an effect of these treatments on OA symptoms (or disease progression) is still limited, and the mechanisms of action unknown. A recent review of glucosamine and/or chondroitin sulfate treatment suggested that the weight of evidence favored a modest symptomatic effect on OA pain, but

recommended additional trials to confirm this [98]. A common problem for many of the compounds of this group is uncertainty regarding quality control, purity and dosing.

Surgical treatment of OA

For the patient in whom the treatment modalities discussed above do not provide sufficient pain relief, surgical treatment has to be considered. While the treatment methods used are the same as for any patient with OA, the often younger age of the patient with postinjury OA provides an important confounding factor in the decision. As mentioned, these patients often have expectations of a continued high level of physical activity and usually have a longer life expectancy than the average patient with OA. Joint replacement in these young patients is associated with a much higher risk of implant wear, loosening and revision than the average OA patient around the age of 70 [74–76]. The risk for loosening and revision of a knee implant is more than three times higher in the patient operated on while younger than 65, than if older than 75 at surgery [74]. For this reason, surgical interventions other than joint replacement should be considered first if at all possible.

Cartilage or bone–cartilage transplantation in various forms are currently being developed to explore the benefits for the patient with symptomatic joint cartilage damage. However, although there are encouraging case reports [99], no results of randomized controlled trials have yet been published. This treatment should therefore be regarded as experimental and recommended for use only within the envelope of carefully monitored clinical studies [100]. No results are as yet available to show if these forms of treatment of cartilage damage can prevent the later development of OA in the injured joint [100]. It also needs to be emphasized that no results have yet been presented to prove the utility of this treatment for the OA joint. Altered biomechanics and dynamic forces in the unstable and osteoarthritic joint provide a challenge for the repair and regeneration of joint cartilage.

Joint lavage with physiologic salt solutions and/or arthroscopic debridement is frequently used. However, the evidence base for other than a temporary relief of pain is very weak and very few well-designed controlled studies exist that allow an analysis of the relative contributions to the effect of the debridement, the lavage or the placebo effect, which may be expected to be considerable [101].

Osteotomy, intended to correct unfavorable loading of the OA joint, is a treatment best suited for the patient younger than 60 years and with high activity expectations. The rehabilitation is, compared to joint replacement, more demanding and extended. The surgery can in the knee be performed as a 'closing wedge' high tibial osteotomy for moderately advanced medial compartment knee OA, or as 'callus distraction' osteotomy [102]. Osteotomy has so far provided the best results for the valgus knee with medial compartment OA. Done on the right patient and with the same care in planning and precision as joint replacement the 'survival' of this intervention is as good as for unicompartmental knee replacement and may delay the need for replacement for at least 10 years [103].

In young patients with knee OA after an ACL tear there is both pain and an instability problem. In such cases a combination of ACL reconstruction and an osteotomy may provide an acceptable solution [104,105]. It is usually recommended that the procedures are carried out separately, with an interval of 6–8 months between surgery. It is, however, possible to perform the procedures simultaneously, especially if the osteotomy is performed as a callus distraction. No clinical trial reports on the complication rate or outcome after such procedures are available yet. When required, a joint replacement can be done with good results in the postosteotomy knee [106,107].

Unicompartmental knee replacement is best suited for patients with stable knees and OA in one compartment only, usually the medial. Due to the previously discussed limitations of implant survival in younger patients [74,108], they should if possible be older than 60 at the time of surgery, with no upper age limit. A considerable advantage of unicompartmental knee replacement is the limited need for hospital stay and the short rehabilitation. Minimally invasive surgery is increasingly used. These developments may warrant a future re-evaluation of the current limitations for this intervention, although 'uni' knees still have a higher

revision rate than 'total' knees [108,109]. Unicompartmental replacements can be successfully revised to total knee replacements if required [110].

Bi- or tricompartmental knee joint replacement is best suited for those patients with severe OA in more than one knee joint compartment. For those patients where the patellar joint contributes significantly to the symptoms, this may be the preferred treatment. Similar to unicompartmental knee arthroplasty, young age at surgery and high physical activity levels contribute significantly to the risk for subsequent wear and loosening. It is therefore often recommended that the patient should be over the age of 60 at surgery. The surgical procedure is more extensive than for unicompartmental replacement. The results of both knee and hip joint replacements have continuously improved over the last few decades, with revision rates fairly similar for hip and knee OA, and more than 90% of the average patients having a well-functioning knee or hip at 10 years after surgery [75,108,111]. Deep infections are rare and below the 1% level, wear and loosening being responsible for the majority of problems.

The adverse effects of arthroplasty, except for those related to the implant as such, are similar to those with other forms of surgery. An increased risk of deep vein thrombosis and lung embolism has been reported.

Patients operated on with joint replacement need to recognize that they have been provided with a new joint, but not a normal joint. They should expect a stable and pain-free joint with a good range of motion that allows regular daily activities such as walking, cycling, swimming and other moderate physical activities or work. Patients wanting to engage in heavy physical activity or work should be informed that this will come at the price of a significantly higher risk of implant failure.

As noted above, OA in the young and physically active is a largely unresolved problem. While nonsurgical treatments often provide relief from pain and support a maintained function, there is little to offer those young individuals with progressive and severe OA except joint surgery. The current limited survival of implants in the young and physically active would make us suggest that joint replacement should be delayed 'until later and older'. However, the other view may well be that it is 'now' when young and active that the individual wants and needs the pain relief and improvement in function that can be provided by the replaced joint, even if the price is a higher risk of implant failure. It is in this context important to note that the relationship between the severity of radiologic change and symptoms in OA is only weak [3]. There is thus no reason to delay joint replacement, waiting for the severity of radiologic change to increase: young patients with symptomatic hip OA reach a higher score for patient-relevant outcome after joint replacement than do older patients (Nilsdotter, personal communication).

Summary

Some sports activities, just like some occupations, are associated with an increased risk of knee and hip OA. Soccer is clearly such an activity, even in the absence of reported injuries. The risk of OA after knee injuries is well documented and some 50% of the subjects who suffer a knee injury will develop radiographic knee OA after 15 years. Surgical treatment after a knee injury to repair or replace the injured structure has not yet been shown to influence the risk for postinjury OA. OA in the ageless athlete is treated like other OA with information, weight loss, exercise, aids, analgesics or surgery. However, the younger age at onset of symptoms compared to most other forms of OA influences the choice of surgical procedure for those with advanced disease.

Multiple choice questions

1 *An increased risk of development of osteoarthritis in the knee is seen among:*
a marathon runners
b female competitive soccer players
c patients who have undergone meniscectomy
d patients who have chronic patella tendinosis ('jumper's knee').
2 *Which of the following statements are correct?*
a Running will reverse manifest osteoarthritis in the knee and improve radiologic findings.
b Surgical reconstruction of a cruciate ligament or a meniscus will fully prevent the development of osteoarthritis.
c Osteoarthritis was observed in 50% of the middle-aged patients who had meniscus operation performed around 20 years earlier.
d The suggested radiographic classification of osteoarthritis (Osteoarthritis Research Society) includes separate grading (from 0 to 3) of joint space narrowing, osteophytes and sclerosis.

References

1 Buckwalther JA, Mankin HJ. Articular cartilage. Part I. Tissue design and chondrocyte–matrix interactions. *J Bone Joint Surg* 1997; **79A**: 600–11.
2 Buckwalther JA, Mankin HJ. Articular cartilage. Part II. Degeneration and osteoarthrosis, repair, regeneration and transplantation. *J Bone Joint Surg* 1997; **79A**: 612–32.
3 Felson DT, Lawrence RC, Dieppe PA *et al.* Osteoarthritis: New insights. Part 1: The disease and its risk factors. *Ann Intern Med* 2000; **133**: 635–46.
4 Dieppe P. Osteoarthritis. Clinical and research perspective. *Br J Rheum* 1991; **30** (Suppl. 1): 1–4.
5 Roos H, Adalberth T, Dahlberg L *et al.* Osteoarthrosis of the knee after injury to the anterior cruciate ligament or meniscus. The influence of time and age. *Osteoarthritis Cartilage* 1995; **3**: 261–7.
6 Kohatsu ND, Schurman DJ. Risk factors for the development of osteoarthrosis of the knee. *Clin Orth* 1990; **261**: 242–6.
7 Leach RE, Baumgard S, Broom J. Obesity: its relation to osteoarthritis of the knee. *Clin Orth* 1973; **93**: 271–3.
8 Karlson E, Mandle LA, Sangha O *et al.* Risk factors for severe hip osteoarthritis in a large female cohort study. *ACR* 2000; **64**: 946–52.
9 Doherty M, Watt I, Dieppe P. Influence of primary generalized osteoarthritis on development of secondary osteoarthritis. *Lancet* 1983; **8340**: 8–11.
10 Dougados M, Gueguen A, Nguyen M *et al.* Longitudinal radiologic evaluation of osteoarthritis of the knee. *J Rheumatol* 1992; **19**: 378–83.
11 Spector TD, Dacre JE, Harris PA *et al.* Radiological progression of osteoarthritis; an 11 year follow up study of the knee. *Ann Rheumatic Dis* 1992; **51**: 1107–10.
12 Brown TD, Anderson DD, Nepola JC *et al.* Contact stress aberrations following imprecise reduction of simple tibial plateau fractures *J Orth Res* 1988; **6**(851): 862.
13 Thompson RC, Oegema TR, Lewis JL, Wallace L. Osteoarthrotic changes after acute transarticular load. An animal model. *J Bone Joint Surg* 1991; **73A**: 990–1001.
14 Allen PR, Denham RA, Swan AV. Late degenerative changes after meniscectomy. Factors affecting the knee after operation. *J Bone Joint Surg (Brit)* 1984; **66**: 666–71.
15 Appel H. Late results after meniscectomy in the knee joint. A clinical and roentgenologic follow–up investigation. *Acta Orthop Scand Suppl* 1970; **133**: 1–111.
16 Johnson RJ, Kettelkamp DB, Clark W *et al.* Factors affect-

ing late results after meniscectomy. *J Bone Joint Surg* 1974; **56A**: 719–29.

17 Jørgensen U, Sonne-Holm S, Lauridsen F *et al*. Long-term follow-up of meniscectomy in athletes. A prospective longitudinal study. *J Bone Joint Surg* 1987; **69B**: 80–3.

18 Roos HP, Laurén M, Adalberth T *et al*. Knee osteoarthritis after meniscectomy. The prevalence of radiographic changes after 21 years, compared to matched controls. *Arthritis Rheum* 1998; **41**: 687–93.

19 Rockborn P, Gillquist J. Outcome of arthroscopic meniscectomy. *Acta Orthop Scand* 1995; **66**: 113–7.

20 Sommerlath KG. Results of meniscal repair and partial meniscectomy in stable knees. *Int Orthop* 1991; **15**: 347–50.

21 Helminen HJ, Kiviranta I, Säämänen A-M *et al*. Effect of motion and load on articular cartilage in animal models. In: Kuettner KE, Schleyerbach R, Peyron JG, Hascall VC, eds. *Articular Cartilage and Osteoarthritis*. New York: Raven Press, 1992: 501–10.

22 Jurvelin J, Kiviranta I, Säämänen A-M *et al*. Indentation stiffness of young canine knee articular cartilage — influence of strenuous joint loading. *J Biomech* 1990; **23**: 1239–46.

23 Säämänen A-M, Tammi M, Kiviranta I *et al*. Levels of chondroitin-6-sulfate and non-aggregating proteoglycans at articular contact sites in the knees of young dogs subjected to moderate running exercise. *Arthritis Rheum* 1989; **32**: 1282–92.

24 Kiviranta I, Tammi M, Jurvelin J *et al*. Articular cartilage thickness and glycosaminoglycan distribution in the canine knee joint after strenuous (20 km/day) running exercise. *Clin Orth* 1992; **283**: 302–8.

25 Säämänen AM, Kiviranta I, Jurvelin J *et al*. Proteoglycan and collagen alterations in canine knee articular cartilage following 20-km running exercise for 15 weeks. *Connective Tissue Res* 1994; **30**: 191.

26 Arokoski J, Kiviranta I, Jurvelin J *et al*. Long-distance running causes site-dependent decrease of cartilage glycosaminoglycan content in the knee joints of beagle dogs. *Arthritis Rheum* 1993; **36**: 1451–9.

27 Lequesne MG, Dang N, Lane NE. Sport practice and osteoarthritis of the limbs. *Osteoarthritis Cartilage* 1997; **5**: 75–86.

28 Buckwalther JA, Lane NE. Athletics and osteoarthritis. *Am J Sports Med* 1997; **25**: 873–81.

29 Felson DT, Hannan MT, Naimark A *et al*. Occupational physical demands, knee bending, and knee osteoarthritis: results from the Framingham study. *J Rheumatol* 1991; **18**: 1587–92.

30 Kirkeskov Jensen L, Eenberg W. Occupation as a risk factor for knee disorders. *Scand J Work Environ Health* 1996; **22**: 165–75.

31 Lindberg H, Montgomery F. Heavy labor and the occurrence of gonarthrosis. *Clin Orth* 1987; **214**: 235–6.

32 Vingård E, Alfredsson L, Goldie I *et al*. Occupation and osteoarthrosis of the hip and knee: a register-based cohort study. *Int J Epidemiol* 1991; **20**: 1025–31.

33 Lindberg H, Danielsson LG. The relation between labor and coxarthrosis. *Clin Orth* 1984; **191**: 159–61.

34 Axmacher B, Lindberg H. Coxarthrosis in farmers. *Clin Orth* 1993; **287**: 82–6.

35 Andersson S, Nilsson B, Hessel T *et al*. Degenerative joint disease in ballet dancers. *Clin Orth* 1989; **238**: 233–6.

36 Revel M, Thiesce A, Amour B. Danse professionnelle et coxarthrose. *Rev Rhum* 1989; **56**: 84–7.

37 Kellgren JH, Lawrence JS. Rheumatism in miners. X-ray study. *Br Med J* 1952; **9**: 197–207.

38 Konradsen L, Berg Hansen E-M, Söndergaard L. Long distance running and osteoarthrosis. *Am J Sports Med* 1990; **18**: 379–81.

39 Lane NE, Michel B, Bjorkengren A *et al*. The risk of osteoarthritis with running and aging: a five year longitudinal study. *J Rheumatol* 1993; **20**: 461–8.

40 Marti B, Knobloch M, Tschopp A, Jucker A, Howald H. Is excessive running predictive of degenerative hip disease? Controlled study in former elite athletes. *Br Med J* 1989; **299**: 91–3.

41 Janda DH, Bir C, Wild B *et al*. Goal post injuries in soccer. *Am J Sports Med* 1995; **23**: 340–4.

42 Maehlum S, Daljord OA. Football injuries in Oslo: a one year study. *Br J Sports Med* 1984; **18**: 186–90.

43 Kujala UM, Kettunen J, Paananen H *et al*. Knee osteoarthritis in former runners, soccer players, weight lifters, and shooters. *Arthritis Rheum* 1995; **38**: 539–46.

44 Lindberg H, Roos H, Gärdsell P. Prevalence of coxarthrosis in former soccer players: 286 players compared with matched controls. *Acta Orthop Scand* 1993; **64**: 165–7.

45 Roos H, Lindberg H, Gärdsell P *et al*. The prevalence of gonarthrosis in former soccer players and its relation to meniscectomy. *Am J Sports Med* 1994; **22**: 219–22.

46 Vingård E, Alfredsson L, Goldie I *et al*. Sports and osteoarthrosis of the hip. An epidemiologic study. *Am J Sports Med* 1993; **21**: 195–200.

47 Klünder K, Rud B, Hansen J. Osteoarthritis of the hip and knee joint in retired football players. *Acta Orthop Scand* 1980; **51**: 925–7.

48 Chantraine A. Knee joint in soccer players. osteoarthritis and axis deviation. *Med Sci Sports Exerc* 1985; **17**: 434–9.

49 Roos H, Lindberg H, Ornell M *et al*. Soccer as a cause of hip and knee osteoarthrosis. *Ann Rheum Dis* 1996; **55**: 690.

50 Spector TD, Harris PA, Hart DJ *et al*. Risk of osteoarthritis associated with long term weight-bearing sports — a radiologic survey of the hips and knees in female ex-athletes and population controls. *Arthritis Rheum* 1996; **39**: 988–95.

51 Kannus P, Järvinen M. Age, overweight, sex and knee instability: their relationship to the posttraumatic osteoarthrosis of the knee joint. *Injury* 1988; **19**: 105–8.

52 Gelber AC, Hochberg MC, Mead LA, Wang N-Y, Wigley FM, Klag MJ. Joint injury in young adults and risk for subsequent knee and hip osteoarthritis. *Ann Intern Med* 2000; **133**: 321–8.

53 Lohmander LS, Roos H. Knee ligament injury, surgery and osteoarthrosis. Truth or consequences? *Acta Orthop Scand* 1994; **65**: 605–9.

54 Engebretsen L, Arendt E, Fritts HM. Osteochondral lesions and cruciate ligament injuries. MRI in 18 knees. *Acta Orthop Scand* 1993; **64**: 434–6.

55 Adalberth T, Roos H, Laurén M et al. Magnetic resonance imaging, scintigraphy, and arthroscopic evaluation in traumatic hemarthrosis of the knee. *Am J Sport Med* 1997; **25**: 231–7.

56 Berchuck M, Andriacchi TP, Bach BR et al. Gait adaptations by patients who have an deficient anterior cruciate ligament. *J Bone Joint Surg* 1990; **72A**: 871–7.

57 Barrack RL, Skinner HB, Buckley SL. Proprioception in the anterior cruciate deficient knee. *Am J Sports Med* 1989; **17**: 1–6.

58 Corrigan JP, Cashman WF, Brady MP. Proprioception in the cruciate deficient knee. *J Bone Joint Surg* 1992; **74B**: 247–50.

59 Roos H, Östenberg A. A prospective study of female soccer players with anterior cruciate ligament tear. Radiographic findings and symptoms 12 years after injury. *ACR* 2000; **64**: 917–22.

60 Kellgren JH, Lawrence JS. Radiological assessment of osteo-arthrosis. *Ann Rheum Dis* 1957; **16**: 494–502.

61 Lethbridge-Cejku M, Scott WW, Reichle R et al. Association of radiographic features of osteoarthritis of the knee with knee pain: Data from the Baltimore longitudinal study of aging. *Arthritis Care Res* 1995; **8**: 182–9.

62 McNicholas MJ, Rowley DI, McGurty D, Adalberth T, Abdon P, Lindstrand A, Lohmander LS. Total meniscectomy in adolescence. A thirty-year follow-up. *J Bone Joint Surg* 2000; **82B**: 217–21.

63 Andersson C, Odensten M, Good L et al. Surgical or non-surgical treatment of acute rupture of the anterior cruciate ligament. A randomized study with long-term follow-up. *J Bone Joint Surg (Am)* 1989; **71A**: 965–974.

64 Daniel DM, Stone ML, Dobson BE et al. Fate of the ACL injured patient. A prospective outcome study. *Am J Sports Med* 1996; **22**: 632–44.

65 Bolano LE, Grana WA. Isolated arthroscopic partial meniscectomy. Functional radiographic evaluation at five years. *Am J Sports Med* 1993; **21**: 432–7.

66 McGinty JB, Geuss LF, Marvin RA. Partial or total meniscectomy. *J Bone Joint Surg* 1977; **59A**: 763–66.

67 Rockborn P, Messner K. Long term results of meniscus repair and meniscectomy; a 13 year functional and radiographic follow up study. *Knee Surg Sports Traum Arthrosc* 2000; **8**: 1–7.

68 Hede A, Larsen E, Sandberg H. Partial versus total meniscectomy. A prospective, randomized study with long-term follow-up. *J Bone Joint Surg* 1992; **74B**: 118–21.

69 Englund M, Roos EM, Roos HP, Lohmander LS. Patient-relevant outcomes fourteen years after meniscectomy. Influence of type of meniscal tear and size of resection. *Rheumatology* 2001; **40**: 631–9.

70 Gillquist J, Messner K. Long-term results of meniscal repair. *Sports Med Arthroscopy Rev* 1993; **1**: 159–63.

71 Gobble EM, Verdonk R, Kohn D. Arthroscopic and open techniques for meniscus replacement. *Scand J Med Sci Sports* 1999; **9**: 168–76.

72 Roos H, Ornell M, Gärdsell P et al. Anterior cruciate ligament injury and soccer — an incompatible combination? A national survey of incidence and risk factors and a 7-year follow-up. *Acta Orthop Scand* 1995; **66**: 107–12.

73 Roos E, Östenberg A, Roos H, Ekdahl C, Lohmander LS. Long-term results of meniscectomy symptoms, function, and performance tests in patients with or without radiographic osteoarthritis compared to matched controls. *Osteoarthritis Cartilage* 2001; **9**: 316–24.

74 Knutson K, Lewold S, Robertsson O, Lidgren L. The Swedish knee arthroplasty register. A nation-wide study of 30 003 knees 1976–1992. *Acta Orthop Scand* 1994; **65**: 375–86.

75 Robertsson O, Lewold S, Knutson K, Lidgren L. The Swedish Knee Arthroplasty Project. *Acta Orthop Scand* 2000; **71**: 7–18.

76 Malchau H, Herberts P, Ahnfeldt L. Prognosis of total hip replacement in Sweden. Follow-up of 92 675 operations performed 1978–1990. *Acta Orthop Scand* 1993; **64**: 497–506.

77 Brandt KD, Doherty M, Lohmander LS. *Osteoarthritis*. Oxford: Oxford University Press, 1998.

78 Dieppe P, Basler HD, Chard J et al. Knee replacement surgery for osteoarthritis: effectiveness, practice variations, indications and possible determinants of utilization. *Rheumatology* 1999; **38**: 73–83.

79 American College of Rheumatology Subcommittee on Osteoarthritis Guidelines. Recommendations for the medical management of osteoarthritis of the knee: 2000 update. *Arthritis Rheum* 2000; **43**: 1902–15.

80 Pendleton A, Arden N, Dougados M, Doherty M, Bannwarth B, Bijlsma J, Cluzeau F, Cooper C, Dieppe P, Häuselmann H, Herrero-Beaumont G, Kaklamanis P, Leeb B, Lequèsne M, Littlejohn P, Lohmander S, Mazières B, Martin-Mola E, Pavelka K, Serni U, Swoboda B, Verbruggen G, Weseloh G, Zimmermann-Gorska I. EULAR recommendations for the management of knee osteoarthritis. Report of a task force of the Standing Committee of clinical trials and epidemiological studies. *Ann Rheum Dis* 2000; **59**: 936–44.

81 Felson DT, Lawrence RC, Dieppe PA et al. Osteoarthritis: new insights. Part 2: Treatment approaches. *Ann Intern Med* 2000; **133**: 726–37.

82 Dieppe P, Chard J, Faulkner A, Lohmander S. Osteoarthritis. In: Godlee F, ed. *Clinical Evidence. A Compendium of the Best Evidence for Effective Health Care*. London: BMJ Publishing Group, 2001; **6**: 902–17.

83 Caraffa A, Cerulli G, Projetti M et al. Prevention of anterior cruciate ligament injuries in soccer. A prospective controlled study of proprioceptive training. *Knee Surg Sports Traum Arthrosc* 1996; **4**: 19–21.

84 Ostenberg A, Roos H. Injury risk factors in female soccer. A prospective study of 123 players during one season. *Scand J Med Sci Sports* 2000; **10**: 279–85.

85 Slemenda C, Brandt KD, Heilman DK *et al.* Quadriceps weakness and osteoarthritis of the knee. *Ann Intern Med* 1997; **127**: 97–104.

86 Allegrante JP, Kovar PA, MacKenzie CR, Peterson MG, Gutin B. A walking education program for patients with osteoarthritis of the knee: theory and intervention strategies. *Health Educ Q* 1993; **20**: 63–81.

87 Deyle GD, Henderson NE, Matekel RL, Ryder MG, Garber MB, Allison SC. Effectiveness of manual physical therapy and exercise in osteoarthritis of the knee. *Ann Intern Med* 2000; **132**: 173–81.

88 Ettinger WH Jr, Burns R, Messier SP *et al.* A randomized trial comparing aerobic exercise and resistance exercise with a health education program in older adults with knee osteoarthritis. The Fitness Arthritis and Seniors Trial (FAST) [see comments]. *J Am Med Assoc* 1997; **277**: 25–31.

89 Minor MA. Exercise in the treatment of osteoarthritis. *Rheum Dis Clin N Am* 1999; **25**: 397–415.

90 O'Reilly SC, Muir KR, Doherty M. Effectiveness of home exercise on pain and disability from osteoarthritis of the knee: a randomised controlled trial. *Ann Rheumatic Dis* 1999; **58**: 15–9.

91 Kirkely A, Webster-Bogaert S, Litchfield R, Amendola A, MacDonald S, McCalden R, Fowler P. The effect of bracing on varus gonarthrosis. *J Bone J Surg* 1999; **81A**: 539–48.

92 Bradley JD, Brandt KD, Katz BP, Jalasinski LA, Ryan SI. Comparison of an anti-inflammatory dose of ibuprofen, an analgesic dose of ibuprofen and acetaminophen in the treatment of patients with osteoarthritis of the knee. *N Engl J Med* 1991; **325**: 87–91.

93 Langman MJS, Well J, Wainwright P *et al.* Risks of bleeding peptic ulcer associated with individual non-steroidal anti-inflammatory drugs. *Lancet* 1994; **343**: 1075–8.

94 Garcia Rodriguez LA, Jick H. Risk of upper gastrointestinal bleeding and perforation associated with individual non-steroidal anti-inflammatory drugs. *Lancet* 1994; **343**: 769–72.

95 Goetsche PC. Non-steroidal anti-inflammatory drugs. *Br Med J* 2000; **320**: 1058–61.

96 Moore RA, Tramèr MR, Carroll D, Wiffen PJ, McQuay HJ. Quantitative systematic review of topically applied anti-inflammatory drugs. *Br Med J* 1998; **316**: 333–8.

97 Brandt KD, Smith GN, Simon LS. Intraarticular injection of hyaluronan as treatment for knee osteoarthritis: what is the evidence? *Arthritis Rheum* 2000; **43**: 1192–203.

98 McAlindon TE, La Valley MP, Gulin JP, Felson DT. Glucosamine and chondroitin for treatment of osteoarthritis. A systematic quality assessment and meta-analysis. *J Am Med Assoc* 2000; **283**: 1469–75.

99 Brittberg M, Lindahl A, Nilsson A, Ohlsson C, Isaksson O, Petterson L. Treatment of deep cartilage defects in the knee with autologous chondrocyte transplantation. *N Engl J Med* 1994; **331**: 889–95.

100 Lohmander LS. Cell-based cartilage repair — do we need it, can we do it, is it good, can we prove it? *Curr Opin Orthop* 1998; **9**: 38–42.

101 Buckwalter JA, Lohmander LS. Surgical approaches to preserving and restoring cartilage. In: Brandt KD, Doherty M, Lohmander LS, eds. *Osteoarthritis*. Oxford: Oxford University Press, 1998: 378–88.

102 Magyar G, Ahl TL, Vibe P, Toksvig-Larsen S, Lindstrand A. Open-wedge osteotomy by hemicallotasis or the closed wedge technique for osteoarthritis of the knee. *J Bone Joint Surg (Brit)* 1999; **81**: 449–51.

103 Odenbring S, Egund N, Knutson K, Lindstrand A, Toksvig Larsen S. Revision after osteotomy for gonarthrosis. A 10–19-year follow-up of 314 cases. *Acta Orthop Scand* 1990; **61**: 128–30.

104 Latterman C, Jacob RP. High tibial osteotomy alone or combined with ligament reconstruction in ligament deficient knees. *Knee Surg Sports Traum Arthroscopy* 1996; **4**: 32–8.

105 Noyes FR, Barber-Westin SD, Hewett TE. High tibial osteotomy and ligament reconstruction for varus angulated anterior cruciate ligament deficient knees. *Am J Sports Med* 2000; **28**: 282–6.

106 Meding JB, Keating EM, Ritter MA, Faris PM. Total knee arthroplasty after high tibial osteotomy. A comparison study in patients who had bilateral total knee replacement. *J Bone Joint Surg (Am)* 2000; **82**: 1252–9.

107 Meding JB, Keating EM, Ritter MA, Faris PM. Total knee arthroplasty after high tibial osteotomy. *Clin Orth* 2000; **375**: 175–84.

108 Robertsson O, Dunbar M, Pehrsson T, Knutson K, Lidgren L. Patient satisfaction after knee arthroplasty. A report on 27 372 knees operated on between 1981 and 1995 in Sweden. *Acta Orthop Scand* 2000; **71**: 262–7.

109 Robertsson O, Borgquist L, Knutson K, Lewold S, Lidgren L. Use of unicompartmental instead of tricompartmental prostheses for unicompartmental arthrosis in the knee is a cost-effective alternative. *Acta Orthop Scand* 1999; **70**: 170–5.

110 Lewold S, Robertsson O, Knutson K, Lidgren L. Revision of unicompartmental knee arthroplasty: outcome in 1135 cases from the Swedish Knee Arthroplasty Study. *Acta Orthop Scand* 1998; **68**: 469–74.

111 Herberts P, Malchau H. Longterm registration has improved the quality of hip replacement: a review of the Swedish THR register comparing 160 000 cases. *Acta Orthop Scand* 2000; **71**: 111–21.

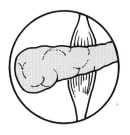

Chapter 4.4
Exercise in the Treatment of Type 2 and 1 Diabetes

HANNELE YKI-JÄRVINEN & FLEMMING DELA

Classical reference

Lawrence RD. The effect of exercise on insulin action in diabetes. *Br Med J* 1926; 1: 648–650.

In 1926, R. D. Lawrence, MD published in the *British Medical Journal* the first evidence on the additive effect of insulin and exercise on glucose uptake.

Based upon observations from his insulin-treated patients of incidences of hypoglycemic symptoms when exercise was taken, he conducted two experiments with one patient. On both occasions insulin was omitted for 20 h and uniform conditions of the diet were observed, which included breakfast and lunch taken as usual. An hour and a quarter after lunch the patient was given a dose of 10 units of insulin. On one day the patient then started a strenuous exercise bout for $2\frac{1}{2}$ hours, only interrupted by blood sampling, and on another day no exercise was taken.

With insulin alone blood glucose decreased as expected, but when exercise was added a clear hypoglycemic effect was observed and hypoglycemic symptoms were present during the last half-hour of exercise. R. D. Lawrence concluded: '. . . it seems clear that muscular activity greatly enhances the action of insulin.' Carbohydrates were given at the end of exercise and normoglycemia was restored, but after an additional 2 h the hypoglycemic symptoms recurred, and it was stated that: 'Even after exercise, when the carbohydrate stores have been partially depleted, it is usually advisable to reduce the next dose of insulin.' R. D. Lawrence recognized that people with diabetes should not be restricted to a sedentary life: 'It should be the object of all treatment to enable a diabetic to lead a normal and varied life . . .' and continued, 'Patients should and do easily learn to reduce their insulin before unaccustomed exercise or activity, or they must take vigorous exercise only at times when the effect of their injections has worn over.'

Physical inactivity and the epidemic of type 2 diabetes

Physical inactivity predicts type 2 diabetes

Data from several prospective epidemiologic studies have shown an inverse association between physical activity and the incidence of type 2 diabetes [1–3]. Recently, Wei *et al.* extended these findings, which were based on self-reporting of physical activity and type 2 diabetes, by examining the relationship of objectively measured cardiorespiratory fitness to the incidence of impaired fasting glucose and type 2 diabetes [4]. This analysis included 8633 mostly white men with non-insulin-treated type 2 diabetes, who were followed for 6 years after baseline assessment of cardiorespiratory fitness by a maximal exercise test on a treadmill. Men in the low fitness group (the least fit 20% of the cohort) had a 1.9-fold risk for impaired fasting glucose and a 3.7-fold risk for diabetes compared to those in the high fitness group (the most fit 40% of the cohort) after adjusting for age, smoking, alcohol consumption and parental diabetes. After additional adjustment for body mass index, high-density lipoprotein (HDL) cholesterol and triglycerides and hypertension, the low fitness group still had a significantly increased risk of impaired fasting glucose (1.7-fold increase compared to the high fitness group) and diabetes (2.6-fold increase) (Fig. 4.4.1). These data support the hypothesis

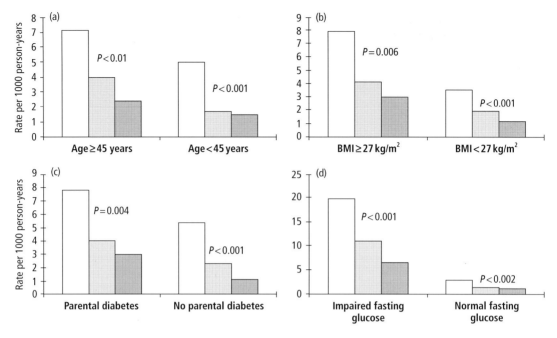

Fig. 4.4.1 Incidence of type 2 diabetes per 1000 person-years by cardiorespiratory fitness levels according to age group (a), body mass index (BMI, b), history of parental diabetes (c), and impaired fasting glucose (d). White bars represent the low fitness group, light tinted bars represent the moderate fitness group, and dark tinted bars represent the high fitness group. Reproduced with permission from [4].

that physical inactivity plays a significant role in the pathogenesis of type 2 diabetes. Similar data have also recently been reported for women participating in the Nurses' Health Study. This prospective study included self-reported data on physical activity in women surveyed in the United States in 1986 with updates in 1988 and 1992 [5]. During 8 years of follow-up, 1419 cases of diabetes were documented. After adjusting for age, smoking, alcohol use, history of diabetes and hypertension, menopausal status and high cholesterol, the relative risks of developing diabetes across quintiles of increasing physical activity decreased from 1.0 to 0.54 [5]. After further adjustment for body mass index, the relative risk reduction was still significant and fell from 1.0 to 0.74 (lowest vs. highest quintile of physical activity). Importantly, equivalent energy expenditures from walking and vigorous activity resulted in comparable magnitudes of risk reduction [5]. These data suggested that in women also, greater physical activity level is associated with a sub-stantial reduction in risk for type 2 diabetes and also suggested that physical activity of moderate intensity and duration is beneficial.

Physical inactivity and the burden of cardiovascular disease in type 2 diabetes

Patients with type 2 diabetes have a two- to four-fold increased mortality from cardiovascular disease [6]. The ultimate goal of all therapies in type 2 diabetes is to reduce this burden. In the Aerobic Center Longitudinal Study discussed above [7], the association between low cardiorespiratory fitness and physical inactivity and total mortality in 1263 men with type 2 diabetes was also studied. After adjustment for age, pre-existing and family history of cardiovascular disease, fasting glucose and cholesterol concentrations, overweight and hypertension, type 2 diabetic men in the low fitness group had a risk for all-cause mortality of 2.1. The majority of deaths were attributable to cardiovascular disease [7].

Physical training as a tool to prevent and treat type 2 diabetes

Prevention of type 2 diabetes

The convincing epidemiologic evidence linking physical inactivity to the development of type 2 diabetes is supported by a few intervention studies. In the 6-year Malmö feasibility study, 181 subjects with impaired glucose tolerance (IGT) and 41 type 2 diabetic patients participated in an intervention program which consisted of supervised training and dietary advice organized either as group sessions or individually for 1 year [8]. The subjects were then encouraged to continue exercise without supervision from the investigators for 5 years. At 6 years, body weight was reduced 2.3–3.7% amongst participants as compared to 0.5–1.7% in non-intervened subjects. Maximal oxygen uptake was increased by 10–14% vs. decreased by 5–9% in participants vs. control subjects. Glucose tolerance was normalized in 52% of the subjects with IGT and in 23% in those with type 2 diabetes in the intervention groups, as compared to 36% in an IGT control group [8]. These encouraging data may not, however, be generally applicable since the participants were not randomly assigned to intervention and control groups. This study also could not distinguish between physical activity vs. diet in the prevention of type 2 diabetes. These limitations do not apply to the Da-Qing study, where 577 subjects were randomized to either a control group or to one of three active treatment groups: diet only, exercise only or diet plus exercise [9]. The diet, exercise, and diet plus exercise interventions were associated with 31%, 46% and 42% reductions in developing diabetes over a 6-year period. All reductions were statistically significant. These data are novel in being the first to demonstrate in a randomized controlled trial that exercise alone can prevent type 2 diabetes. Recently, a lifestyle modification program, with the goals of at least a 7% weight loss and at least 150 min of physical activity per week, was shown in a large randomized trial in subjects with impaired glucose tolerance in the US to reduce the incidence of diabetes by 58% over a 2.8 year follow-up period [10]. Average weight loss was 5.6 kg in the lifestyle intervention and 0.1 kg in the placebo group. Similar data were reported in a Finnish study also in overweight subjects with IGT [11]. The contribution of weight loss as compared to increased physical activity to the observed reduction in the incidence of diabetes was not determined in these studies.

Treatment of type 2 diabetes

Effects of aerobic and resistive training on glycemic control

Data on effects of aerobic and resistance training on glycemic control in established type 2 diabetes are summarized in Tables 4.4.1 and 4.4.2. Many studies lacked an appropriate sedentary control group. This limitation is a concern as intensified patient–doctor interaction may itself improve glycemic control and other metabolic parameters. In many studies, the patients lost weight, which may or may not be a consequence of physical activity and confounds, as does small sample size, interpretation of effects of exercise as compared to weight loss *per se* on metabolic control. Overall effects of physical training on glycemic control have been modest and in roughly half of the studies non-significant. There are several potential explanations for the failure of exercise to be an effective antihyperglycemic therapy. First, physical training primarily improves insulin sensitivity in skeletal muscle (see below) rather than in the liver, which is the ultimate target of any antihyperglycemic drug[12]. Second, an increase in insulin sensitivity implies that the same amount of glucose can be utilized as before but less insulin is required. In the presence of endogenous insulin secretion, the expected effect of insulin sensitization is thus a decrease in the circulating insulin concentration and an unchanged or slightly lowered blood glucose concentration. However, even this effect has been poorly documented since insulin secretion remained unchanged in 7 out of 9 studies where it was measured (Table 4.4.1). Since muscle insulin sensitivity has improved when it has been quantified directly without reliance on endogenous insulin concentrations [13], it is possible that physical training improves both insulin secretion and sensitivity and that the net effect of these two changes is an unchanged insulin concentration. In this respect resistive training seems more effective since the insulin concentration has consistently been found to decrease

Table 4.4.1 Effects of aerobic exercise training on glycemic control and other parameters in patients with type 2 diabetes.

Year (ref)	Intervention/ Control (n[a])	Exercise program[b] times/ week, duration/session	Duration	Blood glucose	Serum insulin	HbA$_{1C}$	Lipids	BP	BW	Improvement in fitness significant[c]
Trials with a sedentary control group										
1985 [13]	33/13	3/week	3 months	↓	↔	–	↔	↔	↔	Yes
1991 [98]	30/56	1.7 aerobics sessions/week	37 weeks	→	–	–	–	–	↔→	No
1992 [99]	38/40	3–4/week, 30–60 min	1–2 months	→[e]	–	↓[e]	↑HDL-C ↓Tg ↓Chol	–	↔	No
1995 [100]	16/13	3–4/week, 30–90 min	3 months	↔	–	↔	↑HDL-C ↓Tg	→	↔	Yes
1997 [101]	25/26	3/week, 60 min	26 weeks	↔	↔	↔→	↓Tg	–	↔→↔	Yes
1997 [102]	11/12	3/week, 30–40 min	8 weeks	↔	–↑	↔→	–	–	↔	Yes
1997 [103]	10/11	2/week, 45 min	8 weeks	↔	←		–	–	↔	Yes
Trials without a sedentary control group										
1979 [104]	6	5/week, 30 min	6 weeks	↔	↔	–	↓Tg ↓Chol	–	↔	Yes
1984 [105]	6	7/week, 60 min	6 weeks	→→	↔	–→	–	–	↔	Yes
1984 [106]	5	3/week, 60 min	6 weeks	↔	↔	↔↔	–	–	↔↔	Yes
1988 [107]	7	3/week, 30 min	10–15 weeks	↔↔	↔	↔→↔	↔↔	↔→↔	↔↔↔	–
1990 [17]	13	4/week, 40–60 min	12–14 weeks	→→→	–	→↔→	↓Tg ↑HDL-C ↓Chol ↓LDL-C ↓Tg	→↔	→↔	–
1992 [108]	111	6/week, 30 min	3 months	→	–	–		–	↔	–
1993 [109]	10–12	Daily exercise[d]	1–2 months							
1994 [110]	652		3 weeks							
1994 [111]	9	3/week, 30 min	2 years	→	–	→	↔Chol	→	→	–
1996 [112]	20	3/week, 60 min	6 months	↔	↔↓[f]	↔	↔Chol ↑Chol	–	↔	Yes
2000 [113]	13	3/week, 40 min	3 months	↔	–	↔	↔↓Tg ↑HDL-C	→	↔	No

[a] Number of subjects.

[b] In most studies, exercise intensity was between 60 and 80% of $\dot{V}_{O_2\,max}$ and was performed using a bicycle or treadmill.

[c] Implies no data; 'No' implies $\dot{V}_{O_2\,max}$ or some other measure of fitness was measured but no significant change was observed.

[d] Primarily walking.

[e] Effect observed in women but not in men.

[f] Reduction in insulin dose.

BP, blood pressure; BW, body weight; Chol, serum total cholesterol; HbA$_{1C}$, glycosylated hemoglobin A$_{1C}$; HDL-C, serum high-density lipoprotein cholesterol; LDL-C, serum low-density lipoprotein cholesterol; Tg, serum triglycerides; $\dot{V}_{O_2\,max}$, maximum aerobic power; –, no data; ↔, no change; ↓, decrease; ↑, increase.

Table 4.4.2 Effects of resistive exercise training on glycemic control and other parameters in non-diabetic subjects and patients with type 2 diabetes.

Year (ref)	Intervention/ Control (n[a])	Exercise program	Duration	Blood glucose	Serum insulin	HbA$_{1c}$	Lipids	BP	BW	$\dot{V}_{O_2\,max}$ measured (change)[b]
Trials with a sedentary control group										
1998 [26]	11/10 Type 2 DM	CWT[d] 3/week	8 weeks	↔	↔	↔	–	↔	↔	↔
1998 [114]	9/8 Type 2 DM	CWT 5/week	4–6 weeks	↔	↓[e]	↔	–	Fat % ↔	↔ BW ↔	↔
Trials without a sedentary control group										
1988 [115]	11 NGT[c]	CWT 3–4/week	16 weeks	↔	↓	–	↑HDL-C ↓LDL-C	↓	Fat % ↔ BW ↔	↔
1989 [116]	15 NGT	CWT	12 weeks	↔	↓	–	–	–	BW ↔ Fat % ↓ FFM ↑	↔
1994 [117]	11 NGT	CWT	16 weeks	↔	↓	–	–	–	BW ↔ Fat % ↓ FFM ↑	↔
1997 [118]	18/20 Type 2 DM	Strength training 2/week	5 months	↔	↓	↔	↓Chol ↓Tg ↓LDL-C	↔	↔	↔
1998 [119]	8 Type 2 DM	CWT 2/week	3 months	↔	↓	↔	↔	↔	–	↔

[a] Number of subjects participating in the intervention vs. control group.

[b] Change in $\dot{V}_{O_2\,max}$ is denoted by arrows: ↔, no change; ↑ significant increase.

[c] NGT, normal glucose tolerance; Type 2 DM, type 2 diabetes.

[d] CWT, circuit weight training.

[e] Insulin sensitivity measured by the clamp technique improved 48%. Other abbreviations as in Table 4.4.1.

(Table 4.4.2). The mechanism underlying this change is, however, likely to be different from that of aerobic training.

Effects of aerobic and resistive training on insulin sensitivity and markers of cardiovascular risk

Data are limited regarding non-glycemic effects of physical training in type 2 diabetes. In many of the aerobic training studies, potentially beneficial effects in serum lipids (8 out of 14 studies, 57%) and blood pressure (5 out of 7 studies, 71%) were observed (Tables 4.4.1 & 4.4.2). Data are too sparse (no study with a control group) to allow conclusions to be made regarding the effects of resistive training on lipids and lipoproteins in type 2 diabetic patients. In non-diabetic power athletes, serum triglycerides, HDL and low-density lipoprotein (LDL) cholesterol are comparable to those of sedentary controls [14], and thus lack the changes characterizing aerobically trained athletes.

Hypertriglyceridemia, the hallmark of the dyslipidemia characterizing type 2 diabetic patients [15], is associated with abnormalities in fibrinolysis and coagulation such as increases in factor VII (FVII) and plasminogen-activator inhibitor 1 (PAI-1) concentrations [16]. In non-diabetic subjects, physical training has been consistently shown to enhance fibrinolysis by decreasing concentrations of PAI-1 but data on training effects on such parameters are very limited in type 2 diabetes. Three months of aerobic training, which increased $\dot{V}o_{2\,max}$ significantly by 12.5%, was associated with no changes in coagulation parameters, including plasminogen or α_2-antiplasmin, or in the measures of fibrinolysis but did cause a significant decrease in fibrinogen [17].

Oxidative stress is increased in patients with type 2 diabetes, at least when measured from the total antioxidant trapping capacity of plasma, which is inversely related to the HbA_{1c} concentration [18]. The concentration of superoxides and free radicals is also increased and can be reduced by antioxidants such as raloxifene [19], allopurinol [20] and tetrahydrobiopterin [21]. Numerous studies have demonstrated that free radical production (superoxides, hydrogen peroxide, hydroxyl radicals) is increased as oxygen production increases by stimuli such as aerobic exercise [22]. Free radical generation results in lipid peroxida-

tion, which is considered harmful. For example, intense, long-duration aerobic exercise has been shown, at least transiently, in two studies to increase LDL susceptibility to oxidation in non-diabetic subjects [23,24]. These data raise the possibility that type 2 diabetic patients may be even more susceptible to exercise-induced oxidative damage. On the other hand, aerobic training is also able to increase the activity of free radical scavenging enzyme systems in red blood cells and skeletal muscle [25]. Thus, training might either deplete or restore antioxidant defense mechanisms in type 2 diabetic patients but there are currently very limited data addressing this issue. F2-isoprostanes consist of a series of chemically stable prostaglandin F2 (PGF_2)-like compounds generated from the peroxidation of unsaturated fatty acids in membrane phospholipids independently of the cyclooxygenase enzyme. The urinary excretion rate of F2-isoprostanes is increased in patients with type 2 diabetes and is thought to reflect increased *in vivo* lipid peroxidation [19,26]. In the study of Mori *et al.* [26], urinary excretion of F2-isoprostanes was not altered by 8 weeks of aerobic training consisting of 30-min bicycle ergometer exercise 3 times a week. More data on this topic would, however, be of interest as the abovementioned antioxidants (allopurinol, raloxifene, tetrahydrobiopterin) not only reduce oxidative stress but also ameliorate endothelial dysfunction in patients with type 2 diabetes [19–21], a change which might serve to protect against future development of atherosclerotic vascular disease [27,28]. In this respect it is of interest that high-intensity aerobic training in normal subjects depletes antioxidants and has been associated with a decrease in endothelial function [29], although less intensive aerobic training regimens have improved endothelial function in healthy subjects [30], in patients with essential hypertension with [31] or without [32] dyslipidemia, in hypercholesterolemia [33], in chronic heart failure [34] and in patients with coronary artery disease [35]. There are no data on effects of aerobic or resistive training on endothelial function in patients with type 2 diabetes.

Mechanisms underlying improvements in insulin action by aerobic and resistive training

Insulin has multiple actions *in vivo* in normal subjects, all of which could be considered potentially antiatherogenic. These include the abilities of insulin to acutely: (i) decrease circulating glucose levels via inhibition of glucose production and stimulation of glucose uptake in skeletal muscle; (ii) decrease serum triglyceride concentrations via inhibition of hepatic VLDL production [36]; (iii) diminish large artery stiffness [37]; (iv) inhibit platelet aggregation [38]; and (v) regulate the autonomic nervous system [39]. All these actions are defective in insulin-resistant conditions [37,39–41] and are likely to contribute to hypertriglyceridemia [42], increased artery stiffness [43], abnormalities in platelet function [40] and inflexibility of the autonomic nervous system [39]. Data on effects of physical training in type 2 diabetic patients are, however, largely confined to insulin stimulation of skeletal muscle glucose uptake.

Insulin-stimulated glucose uptake across skeletal muscle can be calculated by multiplying glucose extraction and delivery [44]. During exercise, glucose uptake increases in the face of a marked increase in blood flow (glucose delivery) and a fall in glucose extraction [45,46]. This implies that blood flow is an important determinant of glucose uptake during exercise. In response to aerobic training, blood flow increases and this occurs similarly in normal subjects and patients with type 2 diabetes [45] (Fig. 4.4.2). The ability of high insulin concentrations to stimulate blood flow after training is better than before training in both normal subjects [47] and patients with type 2 diabetes [45]. Despite a normal blood flow response, the ability of skeletal muscle to extract glucose from the circulation in response to insulin remains lower than in non-

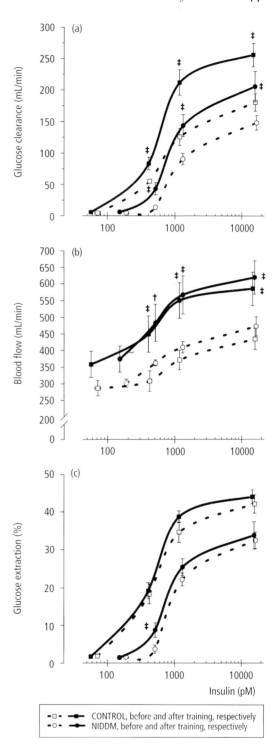

Fig. 4.4.2 Effect of a 10-week one-legged training program on glucose clearance (a), leg blood flow (b) and glucose extraction (c) in eight non-diabetic (squares) and seven type 2 diabetic patients (circles). The measurements were made before and during three sequential intravenous insulin infusions. Euglycemia was maintained using a variable rate glucose infusion. The type 2 diabetic patients had normal leg blood flows both basally and during the three insulin infusions compared to the non-diabetic subjects. Leg blood flow increased significantly and similarly in the trained leg in both groups. Glucose extraction was lower both before (open circles) and after (closed circles) training in the type 2 diabetic patients compared to normal subjects. A significant improvement was observed in the type 2 diabetic patients in response to physical training at all insulin infusion rates employed. Reproduced with permission from [45].

diabetic subjects in patients with type 2 diabetes [45]. A normal response of flow to insulin but a defect in insulin stimulation of glucose extraction has also been found in most [48–50], although not all [51] studies in patients with type 2 diabetes in the untrained state. These data are similar to those recently documented using positron emission tomography-based techniques in insulin-sensitive and insulin-resistant normal subjects [46]. In both sensitive and resistant subjects, acute exercise increased blood flow markedly but similarly in both groups and glucose extraction decreased significantly. However, in the resistant subjects glucose extraction and glucose uptake remained lower than in the sensitive subjects. These data demonstrate that while exercise stimulates glucose uptake by enhancing glucose delivery, differences in this response appear intact in non-diabetic and diabetic insulin-resistant subjects. In insulin-resistant patients such as those with type 2 diabetes, glucose uptake is determined under both resting and exercising conditions by the ability of skeletal muscle to extract glucose.

Regarding the cellular mechanisms contributing to glucose extraction, it is now clear that insulin and exercise stimulate this process by independent mechanisms. In normal subjects, physiologic hyperinsulinemia stimulates glucose uptake in skeletal muscle via the classic insulin signaling pathway, i.e. by stimulating insulin receptor and insulin receptor substrate 1 (IRS-1) tyrosine phosphorylation, association of the p85 regulatory subunit of phosphatidylinositol (PI) 3-kinase with IRS-1 and glycogen synthase fractional velocity [52]. In contrast, exercise has no effect on IRS-1 tyrosine phosphorylation and even decreases tyrosine phosphorylation of the insulin receptor [52]. After one-legged acute exercise in normal men, insulin-stimulated glucose uptake is higher in the exercised than the rested leg but this is accompanied by no change in insulin receptor or IRS-1 tyrosine phosphorylation [53,54], and by a decrease in IRS-1-associated PI 3-kinase activity [54]. In mice which lack insulin receptors selectively in skeletal muscle, insulin has no effect on muscle glucose uptake while the ability of exercise to stimulate glucose uptake is intact [55]. As in humans, acute exercise has no effect on insulin receptor tyrosine phosphorylation or PI3-kinase activity. Regarding the mechanism of contraction-stimulated glucose uptake, 5′-AMP-activated protein kinase (AMPK) is one candidate [56] (Fig. 4.4.3). AMPK, especially its α2 isoform, is activated by muscle contractions in human skeletal muscle. Activation of AMPK results in GLUT-4 translocation and an increase in glucose transport [57]. In animal studies, contractions but not insulin have been shown to increase AMPK activity [56]. The PI 3-kinase inhibitor wortmannin completely blocks insulin-stimulated glucose transport but has no effect on stimulation of glucose transport by contractions or an adenosine analog that stimulates AMPK [56]. On the other hand, in glycogen-loaded slow-twitch muscle, glucose transport increases sixfold by contractions despite an unchanged AMPK activity [58]. These data suggest that mechanisms other than AMPK may contribute to contraction-induced

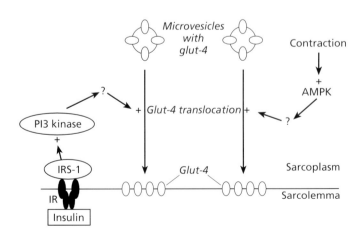

Fig. 4.4.3 Exercise and insulin stimulate glucose uptake in skeletal muscle by distinct mechanisms. The classic insulin signaling molecules such as the insulin receptor (IR), the insulin receptor substrate 1 (IRS-1) and phosphatidylinositol 3-kinase (PI3-kinase) are necessary for insulin- but not contraction-stimulated glucose uptake. Contractions have been suggested to trigger glucose uptake by increasing the activity of an adenosine 5′-monophosphate-activated kinase (AMPK). Both insulin- and exercise-stimulated pathways result in recruitment of glucose transporters (GLUT-4) to the cell surface, which leads to glucose transport. Reproduced with permission from [97].

glucose transport under conditions where AMPK has been deactivated by increasing muscle glycogen content.

In insulin-resistant patients with type 2 diabetes, the ability of insulin to stimulate tyrosine phosphorylation of the insulin receptor and of IRS-1, and to stimulate IRS-1-associated PI3-kinase activity is blunted. Furthermore, the ability of insulin to translocate GLUT-4 [59], the insulin-sensitive glucose transporter, is subnormal [60]. Few data are available regarding the ability of acute exercise or physical training to reverse defects in insulin signaling. In the study of Cusi *et al.* [61], type 2 diabetic patients had higher basal levels of tyrosine phosphorylation of the insulin receptor and IRS-1 and blunted phosphorylation responses to insulin. After acute exercise, the increased basal levels decreased, the insulin-stimulated levels remained unchanged but the fold-response to insulin increased. These changes were not accompanied by any change in insulin-stimulated glucose uptake [61]. On the other hand, aerobic training in patients with type 2 diabetes, as in normal subjects, has been shown to significantly increase the content of GLUT-4 in skeletal muscle [62] (Fig. 4.4.4) and also to significantly increase the expression and activity of glycogen synthase [45] and the ability of insulin to increase PI3-kinase activity [63]. There are currently few data available regarding the integrity of the insulin-

independent exercise-stimulated glucose transport pathway in patients with type 2 diabetes. A single bout of acute exercise, in contrast to insulin, seems to induce normal translocation of GLUT-4 from an intracellular pool to the sarcolemma in patients with type 2 diabetes [64]. Taken together these data are encouraging as they suggest that signaling defects, which are important for insulin action, may be enhanced by aerobic training. The data also suggest that the signaling pathways via which exercise stimulates glucose uptake in patients with type 2 diabetes may be intact. This has the practical implication that the glycemic response to exercise is unlikely to be blunted by insulin resistance.

In contrast to aerobic training, resistive training does not increase capillary density [65] or activity of oxidative enzymes [66–68]. Absence of these changes may explain why glucose uptake per muscle mass is similar in untrained subjects and weight lifters [69,70]. In studies comparing weight lifters or non-steroid-using body builders to sedentary subjects, a critical question is how the sedentary group is matched with the resistive-trained athletes. If muscular subjects are compared to equally heavy adipose subjects, insulin concentrations after an oral glucose load are lower in the muscular subjects [14,71]. This result could be explained by obesity-associated insulin resistance rather than enhanced sensitivity in muscular subjects. How-

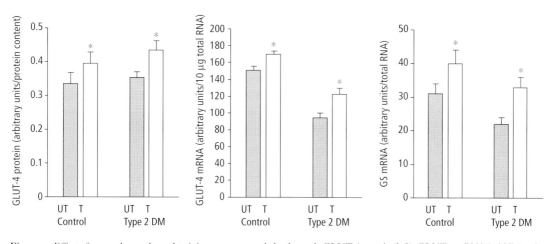

Fig. 4.4.4 Effect of 10-weeks one-legged training program on skeletal muscle GLUT-4 protein (left), GLUT-4 mRNA (middle) and glycogen synthase (GS) mRNA (right) content in eight non-diabetic (control) and seven patients with type 2 diabetes mellitus (Type 2 DM). *Increased in trained (T) compared with untrained (UT) leg ($P < 0.05$). Reproduced with permission from Dela *et al.* [62].

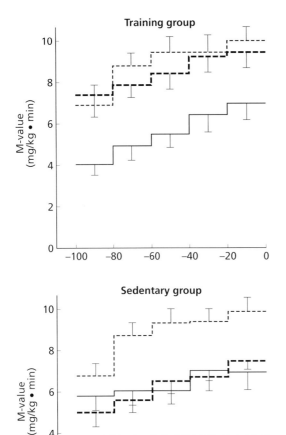

Fig. 4.4.5 Insulin sensitivity of glucose uptake in patients with type 1 diabetes before and after 6 weeks of bicycle exercise training (4 times/week 4 × 15 min at an intensity corresponding to 70% $\dot{V}O_{2\,max}$ with a 5-min rest period between exercise periods). Two control groups were studied: a group of sedentary type 1 diabetic patients who had similar and good glycemic control during treatment with continuous subcutaneous insulin infusion therapy as did the exercise group; and a group of normal subjects. The sedentary control group with type 1 diabetes was studied at 0 and 6 weeks. Body weight and HbA$_{1c}$ remained unchanged in both type 1 diabetic groups. In the training group, $\dot{V}O_{2\,max}$ increased significantly by 8%. This was sufficient to normalize insulin sensitivity. Reproduced with permission from [77].

ever, even when muscular subjects are compared to normal-weight men with similar $\dot{V}O_{2\,max}$, both glucose and insulin concentrations are still significantly lower in muscular than the normal-weight subjects [14]. In both comparisons, the muscular subjects have relatively less fat, which could itself enhance insulin sensitivity, e.g. via free fatty acids, but this remains speculative. If insulin sensitivity is quantified in muscular and normal-weight sedentary subjects, who are matched with respect to $\dot{V}O_{2\,max}$, insulin-stimulated rates of glucose uptake expressed per unit muscle weight are identical [69,70] (Fig. 4.4.5, Plates 2 and 3 facing p. 192). These data could mean that the lower glucose insulin responses during an oral glucose tolerance test (OGTT) [14] can be attributed to a larger muscle mass rather than to enhanced insulin sensitivity if defined as increased glucose uptake per unit muscle mass. Thus, both aerobic and resistive training enhance insulin sensitivity but via fundamentally different mechanisms.

Physical training in the treatment of type 1 diabetes

The role of physical activity has been emphasized in improving well-being and self-esteem in type 1 diabetic patients also. Although data specifically addressing type 1 diabetic patients are not available, exercise should have the same cardiovascular benefits in type 1 diabetic as in type 2 diabetic patients, provided the insulin treatment regimen and diet can be accurately adjusted to maintain normal glucose homeostasis during exercise.

Effect of physical training on glucose control and insulin requirements

Most studies have found no difference in glycemic control between type 1 diabetic patients who are physically active compared to those who are inactive [64,72,73], and no improvement in glycemic control by physical training [74–77]. On the other hand, physical training does improve and even normalize insulin sensitivity in type 1 diabetic patients [77] (Fig. 4.4.5), and this is associated with slight (5%) decreases in insulin requirements [75,77].

Effect of physical training on vascular function and cardiovascular risk markers in type 1 diabetic patients

Endothelial dysfunction, defined as an inability of the endothelium to release normal amounts of nitric oxide, characterizes some [78–81] but perhaps not all [82–86] patients with type 1 diabetes. The impact of physical activity on endothelial dysfunction has been sparsely studied. In one cross-sectional analysis, endothelial function, measured from perfusion changes in the skin microcirculation during iontophoresis with acetylcholine, was similar between physically active and inactive patients with type 1 diabetes [64]. Exercise does seem to have favorable effects on serum lipids and lipoproteins also in type 1 diabetic patients. In controlled studies, physical training has also been shown to lower total [76] and LDL [74] cholesterol and triglyceride [74] concentrations and to increase HDL cholesterol [74], HDL cholesterol/total cholesterol [74,76,77] and apoA-I [76] concentrations. In all of the controlled studies, these changes occurred independent of glycemic control and body weight and composition [74,76,77]. In uncontrolled or cross-sectional analyses, physical activity is associated with increases in HDL_2 cholesterol and decreases in serum triglycerides and LDL cholesterol [87,88].

Poorly controlled patients with type 1 diabetes are characterized by changes in markers indicative of increased oxidative stress such as increased levels of plasma thiobarbituric acid reactive substance (TBARS), reduced total radical trapping capacity [89], increased levels of oxidized LDL [89] and antibodies against oxidative LDL [90]. During acute exercise (40 min at 60% $\dot{V}_{O_{2\,max}}$), markers of oxidative stress such as TBARS and blood oxidized glutathione concentrations increase by 50% [91]. The significance of this with regards to long-term effects of training on cardiovascular function is unknown.

Little information is available on effects of different types of training on markers of metabolic control or cardiovascular risk. Aerobic circuit exercise training has been suggested to induce similar changes in body composition and lipids in type 1 diabetic patients as in normal subjects and type 2 diabetic patients but this study was uncontrolled [92] (Table 4.4.2).

Diet and insulin treatment during exercise

In normal subjects, the serum insulin concentration decreases during prolonged exercise in response to a slight decrease in glucose concentrations and protects against hypoglycemia [73]. In patients with type 1 diabetes, the serum free insulin concentration is determined by the amount of insulin injected, its rate of absorption, insulin antibodies and insulin clearance. During exercise, the serum free insulin concentration is frequently higher than in normal subjects. This can be due to overinsulinization or injection of insulin before exercise, inability of glucose to regulate insulin concentrations or acceleration of insulin absorption by exercise, if insulin has been injected in a region which is actively exercising [93]. Overinsulinization increases the risk of hypoglycemia. On the other hand, if the insulin concentration is subnormal, this will allow the exercise-induced increase in counterregulatory hormones to stimulate hepatic glucose production excessively, which leads to hyperglycemia. Excessive counterregulatory responses in poorly controlled patients may further exaggerate hyperglycemia [94].

In a well-controlled type 1 diabetic patient, it is usually recommended to increase carbohydrate intake by 20–40 g/h before or during exercise to prevent hypoglycemia. If hypoglycemia occurs despite this, the insulin dose should be reduced. To avoid changes in insulin absorption by exercise, insulin should be injected in a region which is inactive, and it is not recommended to exercise immediately after injection of regular insulin or a rapid-acting insulin analog [95]. Use of short-acting analogs has been shown to increase the risk of hypoglycemia if exercise is performed shortly (40 min) after a meal but reduce it by approximately 50% if exercise is performed 3 h after a meal [95].

In addition to the precautions necessary to minimize the occurrence of exercise-induced hypo- or hyperglycemia, the presence of complications should also be considered. This applies to type 1 [73] as well as type 2 [96] diabetic patients. Patients with proliferative retinopathy, poorly controlled hypertension or evidence of cardiovascular disease should avoid strenuous activities such as heavy weight-lifting and sprints. Individuals with autonomic neuropathy may experience postural hypotension after exercise. Heart rate responses may also be abnormal, which is why ratings of perceived exhaustion rather than heart rate should guide intensity of exercise. Non-weight-bearing activities should be preferred by patients with foot problems and peripheral neuropathy to avoid injuries and additional damage to feet [73,96].

Summary

The observational and trial evidence supporting the hypothesis that both type 2 diabetes and its cardiovascular complications can be prevented by being physically moderately active is rapidly emerging. The question of how beneficial exercise is in the treatment of type 2 diabetes is more difficult to answer. If one neglects the potentially important effects of physical activity on subjective well-being and self-esteem, and considers the metabolic effects of physical activity, glycemic control has been slightly improved in approximately half of the studies and in some independent of changes in body weight and composition. Data are sparse on cardiovascular risk markers or factors but physical activity appears to have beneficial effects on blood pressure, lipids and insulin sensitivity. In type 1 patients physical activity has consistently not been found to improve glycemic control but has been shown to improve insulin sensitivity and induce potentially antiatherogenic changes in lipids and lipoproteins. According to the American College of Sports Medicine position stand, exercise is a major therapeutic modality in type 2 diabetes and regular physical activity is imperative to sustain any glucose-lowering effects. It was also recommended that patients with type 2 diabetes should strive to expend at least 1000 kcal/week in physical activities. Both aerobic and resistance training were recommended [96]. In patients with type 1 diabetes, special precautions are necessary to avoid exercise-induced hypo- and hyperglycemia. In both types of diabetes, metabolic and physical screening should be performed in all patients with micro- or macrovascular complications and in those who are poorly controlled with respect to cardiovascular risk factors or who have longstanding disease.

Questions

For the following statements, please answer true (a) or false (b).

1 *Physical activity can prevent type 2 diabetes and reduce the burden of cardiovascular disease.*
2 *Resistive training increases capillary density in skeletal muscle.*
3 *An intact insulin signaling cascade is necessary for exercise to stimulate glucose uptake in type 2 diabetes.*
4 *Physical training improves glycemic control in type 1 diabetes.*
5 *Physical training improves insulin sensitivity and induces potentially antiatherogenic changes in lipids and lipoproteins in type 1 diabetes.*

References

1 Helmrich SP, Ragland DR, Leung RW, Paffenbarger RS. Physical activity and reduced occurrence of non-insulin-dependent diabetes mellitus. *N Engl J Med* 1991; **325**: 147–52.
2 Manson J, Rimm EB, Stampfer MJ *et al.* Physical activity and incidence of non-insulin-dependent diabetes mellitus in women. *Lancet* 1991; **338**: 774–8.
3 Manson JE, Nathan DM, Krolewski AS, Stapfer MJ, Willett WC, Hennekens CH. A prospective study of exercise and incidence of diabetes among US male physicians. *J Am Med Assoc* 1992; **268**: 63–7.
4 Wei M, Gibbons LW, Mitchell TL, Kampert JB, Lee CD, Blair SN. The association between cardiorespiratory fitness and impaired fasting glucose and type 2 diabetes mellitus in men [published erratum appears in *Ann Intern Med* 1999; **131**(5): 394]. *Ann Intern Med* 1999; **130**: 89–96.
5 Hu FB, Sigal RJ, Rich-Edwards JW *et al.* Walking compared with vigorous physical activity and risk of type 2 diabetes in women: a prospective study. *J Am Med Assoc* 1999; **282**: 1433–9.
6 Haffner SM, Lehto S, Rönnemaa T, Pyörälä K, Laakso M. Mortality from coronary heart disease in subjects with type 2 diabetes and in nondiabetic subjects with and without prior myocardial infarction. *N Engl J Med* 1998; **339**: 229–34.
7 Wei M, Gibbons LW, Kampert JB, Nichaman MZ, Blair SN. Low cardiorespiratory fitness and physical inactivity as predictors of mortality in men with type 2 diabetes [see comments]. *Ann Intern Med* 2000; **132**: 605–11.
8 Eriksson K-F, Lindgärde F. Prevention of type 2 (non-insulin-dependent) diabetes mellitus by diet and physical exercise. *Diabetol* 1991; **34**: 891–8.
9 Pan XR, Li GW, Hu YH *et al.* Effects of diet and exercise in preventing NIDDM in people with impaired glucose tolerance. The Da Qing IGT Diabetes Study. *Diabetes Care* 1997; **20**: 537–44.
10 Diabetes Prevention Progranm Research Group. Reduction in the incidence of type 2 diabetes with lifestyle intervention or metformin. *N Engl J Med* 2002; **346**: 393–403.
11 Tuomiletho J, Lindström J, Eriksson J *et al.* Prevention of

type 2 diabetes mellitus by changes in life-style among subjects with impaired glucose tolerance. *N Engl J Med* 2001; **344**: 1343–50.

12 Consoli A. Role of liver in pathophysiology of NIDDM. *Diabetes Care* 1992; **15**: 430–41.

13 Krotkiewski M, Lonnroth P, Mandroukas K *et al*. The effects of physical training on insulin secretion and effectiveness and on glucose metabolism in obesity and type 2 (non-insulin-dependent) diabetes mellitus. *Diabetol* 1985; **28**: 881–90.

14 Yki-Järvinen H, Koivisto VA, Taskinen M-R, Nikkilä E. Glucose tolerance, plasma lipoproteins and tissue lipoprotein lipase activities in body builders. *Eur J Appl Physiol* 1984; **53**: 253–9.

15 Syvanne M, Taskinen MR. Lipids and lipoproteins as coronary risk factors in non-insulin-dependent diabetes mellitus. *Lancet* 1997; **350** (Suppl. 1): S120–S123.

16 Juhan-Vague I, Alessi MC, Vague P. Thrombogenic and fibrinolytic factors and cardiovascular risk in non-insulin-dependent diabetes mellitus. *Ann Med* 1996; **28**: 371–80.

17 Hornsby WG, Boggess KA, Lyons TJ, Barnwell WH, Lazarchick J, Colwell JA. Hemostatic alterations with exercise conditioning in NIDDM. *Diabetes Care* 1990; **13**: 87–92.

18 Mäkimattila S, Liu M-L, Vakkilainen J, Schlenzka A, Lahdenperä S, Syvänne M, Mäntysaari M, Summanen P, Bergholm R, Taskinen M-R, Yki-Järvinen H. Impaired endothelium-dependent vasodilatation in NIDDM: relation to LDL size, oxidized LDL and antioxidants. *Diabetes Care* 1999; **22**: 973–81.

19 Chowienczyk PJ, Brett SE, Gopaul NK *et al*. Oral treatment with an antioxidant (raxofelast) reduces oxidative stress and improves endothelial function in men with type II diabetes. *Diabetol* 2000; **43**: 974–7.

20 Butler R, Morris AD, Belch JJ, Hill A, Struthers AD. Allopurinol normalizes endothelial dysfunction in type 2 diabetics with mild hypertension. *Hypertension* 2000; **35**: 746–51.

21 Heitzer T, Krohn K, Albers S, Meinerz T. Tetrahydrobiopterin improves endothelium-dependent vasodilatation by increasing nitric oxide activity in patients with type II diabetes mellitus. *Diabetol* 2000; **43**: 1435–8.

22 Sen CK. Oxidants and antioxidants in exercise. *J Appl Physiol* 1995; **79**: 675–86.

23 Liu ML, Bergholm R, Makimattila S *et al*. A marathon run increases the susceptibility of LDL to oxidation in vitro and modifies plasma antioxidants. *Am J Physiol* 1999; **276**: E1083–E1091.

24 Sanchez-Quesada JL, Homs-Serradesanferm R, Serrat-Serrat J, Serra-Grima JR, Gonzalez-Sastre F, Ordonez-Llanos J. Increase of LDL susceptibility to oxidation occurring after intense, long duration aerobic exercise. *Atherosclerosis* 1995; **118**: 297–305.

25 Clarkson PM. Antioxidants and physical performance. *Crit Rev Food Sci Nutr* 1995; **35**: 131–41.

26 Mori TA, Dunstan DW, Burke V *et al*. Effect of dietary fish and exercise training on urinary F2-isoprostane excretion in non-insulin-dependent diabetic patients. *Metabolism* 1999; **48**: 1402–8.

27 Schachinger V, Britten MB, Zeiher AM. Prognostic impact of coronary vasodilator dysfunction on adverse long-term outcome of coronary heart disease. *Circulation* 2000; **101**: 1899–906.

28 Suwaidi JA, Hamasaki S, Higano ST, Nishimura RA, Holmes DRJ, Lerman A. Long-term follow-up of patients with mild coronary artery disease and endothelial dysfunction. *Circulation* 2000; **101**: 948–54.

29 Bergholm R, Makimattila S, Valkonen M *et al*. Intense physical training decreases circulating antioxidants and endothelium-dependent vasodilatation in vivo. *Atherosclerosis* 1999; **145**: 341–9.

30 DeSouza CA, Shapiro LF, Clevenger CM *et al*. Regular aerobic exercise prevents and restores age-related declines in endothelium-dependent vasodilation in healthy men. *Circulation* 2000; **102**: 1351–7.

31 Lavrencic A, Salobir BG, Keber I. Physical training improves flow-mediated dilation in patients with the polymetabolic syndrome. *Arterioscler Thromb Vasc Biol* 2000; **20**: 551–5.

32 Higashi Y, Sasaki S, Kurisu S *et al*. Regular aerobic exercise augments endothelium-dependent vascular relaxation in normotensive as well as hypertensive subjects: role of endothelium-derived nitric oxide. *Circulation* 1999; **100**: 1194–202.

33 Lewis TV, Dart AM, Chin-Dusting JP, Kingwell BA. Exercise training increases basal nitric oxide production from the forearm in hypercholesterolemic patients. *Arterioscler Thromb Vasc Biol* 1999; **19**: 2782–7.

34 Hornig B, Maier V, Drexler H. Physical training improves endothelial function in patients with chronic heart failure [see comments]. *Circulation* 1996; **93**: 210–4.

35 Hambrecht R, Wolf A, Gielen S *et al*. Effect of exercise on coronary endothelial function in patients with coronary artery disease [see comments]. *N Engl J Med* 2000; **342**: 454–60.

36 Malmström R, Packard CJ, Watson TDG *et al*. Metabolic basis of hypotriglyceridemic effects of insulin in normal men. *Arterioscler Thromb Vasc Biol* 1997; **17**: 1454–64.

37 Westerbacka J, Wilkinson I, Cockcroft J, Utriainen T, Vehkavaara S, Yki-Järvinen H. Diminished wave reflection in the aorta: a novel physiological action of insulin on large blood vessels. *Hypertension* 1999; **33**: 1118–22.

38 Trovati M, Anfossi G, Massucco P *et al*. Insulin stimulates nitric oxide synthesis in human platelets and, through nitric oxide, increases platelet concentrations of both guanosine-3′, 5′-cyclic monophosphate and adenosine-3′, 5′-cyclic monophosphate. *Diabetes* 1997; **46**: 742–9.

39 Bergholm R, Westerbacka J, Vehkavaara S, Seppälä-Lindroos A, Goto T, Yki-Järvinen H. Insulin sensitivity regulates autonomic control of heart rate variation independent of body weight in normal subjects. *J Clin Endocrinol Metab* 2001; **86**: 1403–9.

40 Anfossi G, Mularoni EM, Burzacca S *et al.* Platelet resistance to nitrates in obesity and obese NIDDM, and normal platelet sensitivity to both insulin and nitrates in lean NIDDM. *Diabetes Care* 1998; **21**: 121–6.

41 Yki-Järvinen H. Pathogenesis of non-insulin-dependent diabetes mellitus. *Lancet* 1994; **343**: 91–5.

42 Malmstrom R, Packard CJ, Caslake M *et al.* Defective regulation of triglyceride metabolism by insulin in the liver in NIDDM. *Diabetol* 1997; **40**: 454–62.

43 Salomaa V, Riley W, Kark JD, Nardo C, Folsom AR. Non-insulin-dependent diabetes mellitus and fasting glucose and insulin concentrations are associated with arterial stiffness indexes. The ARIC Study. *Circulation* 1995; **91**: 1432–43.

44 Zierler KL. Theory of the use of arteriovenous concentration differences for measuring metabolism in steady-state and non-steady-states. *J Clin Invest* 1961; **40**: 2111–25.

45 Dela F, Larsen JJ, Mikines KJ, Ploug T, Petersen LN, Galbo H. Insulin-stimulated muscle glucose clearance in patients with NIDDM. Effects of one-legged physical training. *Diabetes* 1995; **44**: 1010–20.

46 Nuutila P, Peltoniemi PO, Ikonen V *et al.* Enhanced stimulation of glucose uptake by insulin increases exercise-stimulated glucose uptake in skeletal muscle in humans: studies using $[15O]O_2$, $[15O]H_2O$, $[18F]$fluoro-deoxy-glucose, and positron emission tomography. *Diabetes* 2000; **49**: 1084–91.

47 Hardin DS, Azzarelli B, Edwards J *et al.* Mechanisms of enhanced insulin sensitivity in endurance-trained athletes: effects on blood flow and differential expression of GLUT 4 in skeletal muscles. *J Clin Endocrinol Metab* 1995; **80**: 2437–46.

48 Dela F, Larsen JJ, Mikines KJ, Galbo H. Normal effect of insulin to stimulate leg blood flow in NIDDM. *Diabetes* 1995; **44**: 221–6.

49 Utriainen T, Nuutila P, Takala T *et al.* Intact insulin stimulation of skeletal muscle blood flow, its heterogeneity and redistribution but not of glucose uptake in non-insulin-dependent diabetes mellitus. *J Clin Invest* 1997; **100**: 777–85.

50 Yki-Järvinen H, Utriainen T. Insulin-induced vasodilatation: physiology or pharmacology? *Diabetol* 1998; **41**: 369–79.

51 Baron AD, Laakso M, Brechtel G, Edelman SV. Reduced capacity and affinity of skeletal muscle for insulin-mediated glucose uptake in non-insulin-dependent diabetes mellitus. *J Clin Invest* 1991; **87**: 1186–94.

52 Koval JA, Maezono K, Patti ME, Pendergrass M, DeFronzo RA, Mandarino LJ. Effects of exercise and insulin on insulin signaling proteins in human skeletal muscle. *Med Sci Sports Exerc* 1999; **31**: 998–1004.

53 Wojtaszewski JF, Hansen BF, Gade X *et al.* Insulin signaling and insulin sensitivity after exercise in human skeletal muscle. *Diabetes* 2000; **49**: 325–31.

54 Wojtaszewski JF, Hansen BF, Kiens B, Richter EA. Insulin signaling in human skeletal muscle: time course and effect of exercise. *Diabetes* 1997; **46**: 1775–81.

55 Wojtaszewski JF, Higaki Y, Hirshman MF *et al.* Exercise modulates postreceptor insulin signaling and glucose transport in muscle-specific insulin receptor knockout mice. *J Clin Invest* 1999; **104**: 1257–64.

56 Hayashi T, Hirshman MF, Kurth EJ, Winder WW, Goodyear LJ. Evidence for 5′ AMP-activated protein kinase mediation of the effect of muscle contraction on glucose transport. *Diabetes* 1998; **47**: 1369–73.

57 Kurth-Kraczek EJ, Hirshman MF, Goodyear LJ, Winder WW. 5′ AMP-activated protein kinase activation causes GLUT4 translocation in skeletal muscle. *Diabetes* 1999; **48**: 1667–71.

58 Derave W, Ai H, Ihlemann J *et al.* Dissociation of AMP-activated protein kinase activation and glucose transport in contracting slow-twitch muscle. *Diabetes* 2000; **49**: 1281–7.

59 Thorell A, Hirshman MF, Nygren J *et al.* Exercise and insulin cause GLUT-4 translocation in human skeletal muscle. *Am J Physiol* 1999; **277**: E733–E741.

60 Zierath JR, He L, Guma A, Odegoard WE, Klip A, Wallberg-Henriksson H. Insulin action on glucose transport and plasma membrane GLUT4 content in skeletal muscle from patients with NIDDM. *Diabetol* 1996; **39**: 1180–9.

61 Cusi K, Maezono K, Osman A *et al.* Insulin resistance differentially affects the PI3-kinase- and MAP kinase-mediated signaling in human muscle. *J Clin Invest* 2000; **105**: 311–20.

62 Dela F, Ploug T, Handberg A *et al.* Physical training increases muscle GLUT4 protein and mRNA in patients with NIDDM. *Diabetes* 1994; **43**: 862–5.

63 Houmard JA, Shaw CD, Hickey MS, Tanner CJ. Effect of short-term exercise training on insulin-stimulated PI3-kinase activity in human skeletal muscle. *Am J Physiol* 1999; **277**: E1055–E1060.

64 Veves A, Saouaf R, Donaghue VM *et al.* Aerobic exercise capacity remains normal despite impaired endothelial function in the micro- and macrocirculation of physically active IDDM patients. *Diabetes* 1997; **46**: 1846–52.

65 Schantz P. Capillary supply in heavy-resistance trained non-postural human skeletal muscle. *Acta Physiol Scand* 1983; **117**: 153–5.

66 Tesch PA. Skeletal muscle adaptations consequent to long-term heavy resistance exercise. *Med Sci Sports Exerc* 1988; **20**: S132–S134.

67 Tesch PA, Thorsson A, Essen-Gustavsson B. Enzyme activities of FT and ST muscle fibers in heavy-resistance trained athletes. *J Appl Physiol* 1989; **67**: 83–7.

68 Tesch PA, Thorsson A, Kaiser P. Muscle capillary supply and fiber type characteristics in weight and power lifters. *J Appl Physiol* 1984; **56**: 35–8.

69 Takala TO, Nuutila P, Knuuti J, Luotolahti M, Yki-Jarvinen H. Insulin action on heart and skeletal muscle glucose uptake in weight lifters and endurance athletes. *Am J Physiol* 1999; **276**: E706–E711.

70 Yki-Järvinen H, Koivisto VA. Effect of body composition on insulin sensitivity. *Diabetes* 1983; **32**: 965–9.

71 Kalkhoff R, Ferrou C. Metabolic differences between obese overweight and muscular overweight men. *N Engl J Med* 1971; **284**: 1236–9.

72 Ligtenberg PC, Blans M, Hoekstra JB, van der Tweel, Erkelens DW. No effect of long-term physical activity on the glycemic control in type 1 diabetes patients: a cross-sectional study. *Neth J Med* 1999; **55**: 59–63.

73 Wasserman DH, Zinman B. Exercise in individuals with IDDM. *Diabetes Care* 1994; **17**: 924–37.

74 Laaksonen DE, Atalay M, Niskanen LK *et al*. Aerobic exercise and the lipid profile in type 1 diabetic men: a randomized controlled trial. *Med Sci Sports Exerc* 2000; **32**: 1541–8.

75 Wallberg-Henriksson H, Gunnarson R, Henriksson J, Östman J, Wahren J. Influence of physical training on formation of muscle capillaries in type 1 diabetes. *Diabetes* 1984; **33**: 851–7.

76 Wallberg-Henriksson H, Gunnarsson R, Rossner S, Wahren J. Long-term physical training in female type 1 (insulin-dependent) diabetic patients: absence of significant effect on glycaemic control and lipoprotein levels. *Diabetol* 1986; **29**: 53–7.

77 Yki-Järvinen H, DeFronzo RA, Koivisto VA. Normalization of insulin sensitivity in type 1 diabetic subjects by physical training during insulin pump therapy. *Diabetes Care* 1984; **7**: 520–7.

78 Johnstone MT, Craeger SJ, Scales KM, Cusco JA, Lee BK, Craeger MA. Impaired endothelium-dependent vasodilation in patient with insulin-dependent diabetes mellitus. *Circulation* 1993; **88**: 2510–6.

79 McNally PG, Watt PAC, Rimmer T, Burden AC, Hearnshow JR, Thurston H. Impaired contraction and endothelium-dependent relaxation in isolated resistance vessels from patients with insulin-dependent diabetes mellitus. *Clin Sci* 1994; **87**: 31–6.

80 Mäkimattila S, Virkamäki A, Groop P-H *et al*. Chronic hyperglycemia impairs endothelial function and insulin sensitivity via different mechanisms in insulin-dependent diabetes mellitus. *Circulation* 1996; **94**: 1276–82.

81 Skyrme-Jones RA, O'Brien RC, Luo M, Meredith IT. Endothelial vasodilator function is related to low-density lipoprotein particle size and low-density lipoprotein vitamin E content in type 1 diabetes. *J Am Coll Cardiol* 2000; **35**: 292–9.

82 Calver A, Collier J, Vallance P. Inhibition and stimulation of nitric oxide synthesis in the human forearm arterial bed of patients with insulin-dependent diabetes. *J Clin Invest* 1992; **90**: 2548–54.

83 Elliott TG, Cockcroft JR, Groop PH, Viberti GC, Ritter JM. Inhibition of nitric oxide synthesis in forearm vasculature of insulin-dependent diabetic patients: blunted vasoconstriction in patients with microalbuminuria. *Clin Sci (Colch)* 1993; **85**: 687–93.

84 Mäkimattila S, Mäntysaari M, Groop P-H *et al*. Hyperreactivity to nitrovasodilators in forearm vasculature is related to autonomic dysfunction in IDDM. *Circulation* 1997, **95**: 618–25.

85 Pinkney JH, Downs L, Hopton M, Mackness MI, Bolton CH. Endothelial dysfunction in Type 1 diabetes mellitus. relationship with LDL oxidation and the effects of vitamin E. *Diabet Med* 1999; **16**: 993–9.

86 Smits P, Kapma J-A, Jacobs M-C, Lutterman J, Tien T. Endothelium-dependent vascular relaxation in patients with type 1 diabetes. *Diabetes* 1993; **42**: 148–53.

87 Gunnarsson R, Wallberg-Henriksson H, Rossner S, Wahren J. Serum lipid and lipoprotein levels in female type I diabetics: relationships to aerobic capacity and glycaemic control. *Diabetes Metab* 1987; **13**: 417–21.

88 Lehmann R, Kaplan V, Bingisser R, Bloch KE, Spinas GA. Impact of physical activity on cardiovascular risk factors in IDDM. *Diabetes Care* 1997; **20**: 1603–11.

89 Tsai EC, Hirsch IB, Brunzell JD, Chait A. Reduced plasma peroxyl radical trapping capacity and increased susceptibility of LDL to oxidation in poorly controlled IDDM. *Diabetes* 1994; **43**: 1010–4.

90 Makimattila S, Luoma JS, Yla-Herttuala S *et al*. Autoantibodies against oxidized LDL and endothelium-dependent vasodilation in insulin-dependent diabetes mellitus. *Atherosclerosis* 1999; **147**: 115–22.

91 Laaksonen DE, Atalay M, Niskanen L, Uusitupa M, Hanninen O, Sen CK. Increased resting and exercise-induced oxidative stress in young IDDM men. *Diabetes Care* 1996; **19**: 569–74.

92 Mosher PE, Nash MS, Perry AC, LaPerriere AR, Goldberg RB. Aerobic circuit exercise training: effect on adolescents with well-controlled insulin-dependent diabetes mellitus. *Arch Phys Med Rehab* 1998; **79**: 652–7.

93 Koivisto VA, Felig P. Effects of leg exercise on insulin absorption in diabetic patients. *N Engl J Med* 1978; **298**: 79–83.

94 Tamborlane WV, Sherwin RS, Koivisto V, Hendler R, Genel M, Felig P. Normalization of the growth hormone and catecholamine response to exercise in juvenile-onset diabetic subjects treated with a portable insulin infusion pump. *Diabetes* 1979; **28**: 785–8.

95 Tuominen JA, Karonen SL, Melamies L, Bolli G, Koivisto VA. Exercise-induced hypoglycaemia in IDDM patients treated with a short-acting insulin analogue. *Diabetol* 1995; **38**: 106–11.

96 Albright A, Franz M, Hornsby G *et al*. American College of Sports Medicine position stand. Exercise and type 2 diabetes. *Med Sci Sports Exerc* 2000; **32**: 1345–60.

97 Winder WW, Hardie DG. AMP-activated protein kinase, a metabolic master switch: possible roles in type 2 diabetes. *Am J Physiol* 1999; **277**: E1–E19.

98 Heath GW, Wilson RH, Smith J, Leonard BE. Community-based exercise and weight control: diabetes risk reduction and glycemic control in Zuni Indians. *Am J Clin Nutr* 1991; **53**: 1642S–1646S.

99 Vanninen E, Uusitupa M, Siitonen O, Laitinen J, Lansimies E. Habitual physical activity, aerobic capacity and metabolic control in patients with newly-diagnosed type 2 (non-insulin-dependent) diabetes mellitus: effect of 1-year diet and exercise intervention. *Diabetol* 1992; **35**: 340–6.

100 Lehmann R, Vokac A, Niedermann K, Agosti K, Spinas GA. Loss of abdominal fat and improvement of the cardiovascular risk profile by regular moderate exercise training in patients with NIDDM. *Diabetol* 1995; **38**: 1313–9.

101 Ligtenberg PC, Hoekstra JB, Bol E, Zonderland ML, Erkelens DW. Effects of physical training on metabolic control in elderly type 2 diabetes mellitus patients. *Clin Sci (Colch)* 1997; **93**: 127–35.

102 Dunstan DW, Mori TA, Puddey IB *et al.* The independent and combined effects of aerobic exercise and dietary fish intake on serum lipids and glycemic control in NIDDM. *Diabetes Care* 1997; **20**: 913–21.

103 Mourier A, Gautier JF, De Kerviler E *et al.* Mobilization of visceral adipose tissue related to the improvement in insulin sensitivity in response to physical training in NIDDM. Effects of branched-chain amino acid supplements. *Diabetes Care* 1997; **20**: 385–91.

104 Ruderman NB, Ganda OP, Johansen K. The effect of physical training on glucose tolerance and plasma lipids in maturity-onset diabetes. *Diabetes* 1979; **28** (Suppl. 1): 89–92.

105 Reitman JS, Vasquez B, Klimes I, Nagulesparan M. Improvement of glucose homeostasis after exercise training in non-insulin-dependent diabetes. *Diabetes Care* 1984; **7**: 434–41.

106 Trovati M, Carta Q, Cavalot F *et al.* Influence of physical training on blood glucose control, glucose tolerance, insulin secretion, and insulin action in non-insulin-dependent diabetic patients. *Diabetes Care* 1984; **7**: 416–20.

107 Allenberg K, Johansen K, Saltin B. Skeletal muscle adaptations to physical training in type II (non-insulin-dependent) diabetes mellitus. *Acta Med Scand* 1988; **223**: 365–73.

108 Schneider SH, Khachadurian AK, Amorosa LF, Clemow L, Ruderman NB. Ten-year experience with an exercise-based outpatient life-style modification program in the treatment of diabetes mellitus. *Diabetes Care* 1992; **15**: 1800–10.

109 Di GX, Teng WP, Zhang J, Fu PY. Exercise therapy of non-insulin dependent diabetes mellitus: a report of 10 year studies. The efficacy of exercise therapy. *Chin Med J* 1993; **106**: 757–9.

110 Barnard RJ, Jung T, Inkeles SB. Diet and exercise in the treatment of NIDDM. The need for early emphasis. *Diabetes Care* 1994; **17**: 1469–72.

111 Bourn DM, Mann JI, McSkimming BJ, Waldron MA, Wishart JD. Impaired glucose tolerance and NIDDM: does a lifestyle intervention program have an effect? *Diabetes Care* 1994; **17**: 1311–9.

112 Tarnow L, Cambien F, Rossing P *et al.* Insertion/deletion polymorphism in the angiotensin-I-converting enzyme gene is associated with coronary heart disease in IDDM patients with diabetic nephropathy. *Diabetol* 1995; **38**: 798–803.

113 Rigla M, Sanchez-Quesada JL, Ordonez-Llanos J *et al.* Effect of physical exercise on lipoprotein (a) and low-density lipoprotein modifications in type 1 and type 2 diabetic patients. *Metabolism* 2000; **49**: 640–7.

114 Ishii T, Yamakita T, Sato T, Tanaka S, Fujii S. Resistance training improves insulin sensitivity in NIDDM subjects without altering maximal oxygen uptake. *Diabetes Care* 1998; **21**: 1353–5.

115 Hurley BF, Hagberg JM, Goldberg AP *et al.* Resistive training can reduce coronary risk factors without altering $\dot{V}_{O_{2\,max}}$ or percent body fat. *Med Sci Sports Exerc* 1988; **20**: 150–4.

116 Craig BW, Everhart J, Brown R. The influence of high-resistance training on glucose tolerance in young and elderly subjects. *Mech Age Dev* 1989; **49**: 147–57.

117 Miller JP, Pratley RE, Goldberg AP *et al.* Strength training increases insulin action in healthy 50- to 65-yr-old men. *J Appl Physiol* 1994; **77**: 1122–7.

118 Honkola A, Forsen T, Eriksson J. Resistance training improves the metabolic profile in individuals with type 2 diabetes. *Acta Diabetol* 1997; **34**: 245–8.

119 Eriksson J, Tuominen J, Valle T *et al.* Aerobic endurance exercise or circuit-type resistance training for individuals with impaired glucose tolerance? *Hormone Metabol Res* 1998; **30**: 37–41.

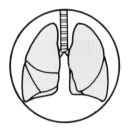

Chapter 4.5
Asthma and Chronic Airway Disease

MALCOLM SUE-CHU & LEIF BJERMER

Classical reference

Aretaeus of Cappadocia (81–131 AD)

Greek physician from Cappadocia who practiced in Rome and Alexandria, led a revival of Hippocrates' teachings and is thought to have ranked second only to the father of medicine himself in the application of keen observation and ethics to the art. In principle he adhered to the pneumatic school of medicine, which believed that health was maintained by 'vital air' or *pneuma*. Pneumatists felt that an imbalance of the four humours—blood, phlegm, choler (yellow bile) and melancholy (black bile)—disturbed the *pneuma*, a condition indicated by an abnormal pulse. In practice, however, Aretaeus was an eclectic physician, since he utilized the methods of several different schools. Aretaeus was the first to describe asthma as an airway disease. Asthma comes from the Greek word 'panting' and in 67 AD he wrote: 'If from running, gymnastic exercise or any other work, the breathing becomes difficult, it is asthma.'

After his death he was entirely forgotten until 1554, when two of his manuscripts, *On the Causes and Indications of Acute and Chronic Diseases* (4 volumes) and *On the Treatment of Acute and Chronic Diseases* (4 volumes) both written in the Ionic Greek dialect, were discovered (Fig. 4.5.1). In the first manuscript Aretaeus attributed asthma to 'thick and viscid phlegm caused by coldness and humidity suffered by the patient.' He also in the two books gave model descriptions of pleurisy, diphtheria, tetanus, pneumonia and epilepsy and was the first to distinguish between spinal and cerebral paralyses. He gave diabetes its name (from the Greek word for 'siphon', indicative of the diabetic's intense

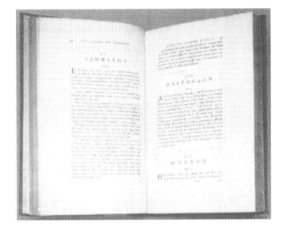

Fig. 4.5.1 Picture of the book: *De Causis et Signis Acutorum et Diuturnorum Morborum, Liber Primus* (Of the Causes and Signs of Acute and Morbid Disease) printed in Oxford 1723.

thirst and excessive emission of fluids) and rendered the earliest clear account of that disease now known.

Bronchial asthma

Definition

Asthma, which is derived from the Greek ασθμα, meaning short-drawn breath or panting, has until recently been defined as a disease characterized by an increased responsiveness of the trachea and bronchi to various stimuli and manifested by a widespread narrowing of the airways that changes in severity either spontaneously or as a result of therapy [1]. Although first highlighted in clinicopathologic studies of fatal asthma at the turn of the 20th century, it is only as a result of studies of bronchoalveolar lavage fluid, endobronchial biopsies and induced sputum over the past four decades that our appreciation and understanding of the inflammatory nature of the disease has increased [2,3]. This has resulted in a shift of emphasis away from airway smooth muscle dysfunction to a T-lymphocyte-modulated chronic desquamative eosinophilic bronchitis as the primary abnormality in asthma [4–6]. In the 1992 international consensus statement, asthma is now defined as 'a chronic inflammatory disorder of the airways in which many cells play a role, in particular mast cells, eosinophils, and T-lymphocytes. In susceptible individuals, this inflammation causes recurrent episodes of wheezing, breathlessness, chest tightness, and cough particularly at night and/or in the early morning. These symptoms are usually associated with widespread but variable airflow limitation that is at least partly reversible either spontaneously or with treatment. The inflammation also causes an associated increase in airway responsiveness to a variety of stimuli.'[7]

Exercise-induced bronchospasm (EIB)

It is well recognized that physical exercise has adverse effects in asthmatic subjects. In the 2nd century AD, Aretaeus of Cappadocia wrote: 'If from running, gymnastic exercise, or any other work the breathing becomes difficult, it is called asthma' [8], and the observation was repeated in the 17th century by the asthmatic physician, Sir John Floyer: 'All exercise makes the asthmatic to breathe short... and if the Exercise be continued it occasions a Fit' [9]. This phenomenon is described by the synonymous terms exercise-induced asthma (EIA) and exercise-induced bronchoconstriction (EIB).

The breathing difficulties are due to bronchospasm, which can be detected by changes in the forced expiratory volume in 1 s (FEV_1) on spirometry or in peak expiratory flow (PEF) using a peak flow meter. After a standardized bicycle ergometer or treadmill exercise protocol in the laboratory, the normal response in the postexercise period is a maximum fall in FEV_1 of less than 10% [10]. When exercise testing is conducted outside the laboratory, the normal fall in PEF is less than 15% [11].

In asthmatic individuals with entirely normal lung function or with a subclinical degree of obstruction at

baseline, an increase in resistance to airflow can be detected as early as 4 min after the start of prolonged strenuous exercise [12,13]. During or within the first 30 min after exercise, they have falls in lung function that are in excess of these limits, and commonly complain of wheeze, chest tightness, difficult breathing or cough, and may have difficulty in continuing or resuming exercise. An unusual complaint in children and adolescents may be chest pain on exercise [14]. The maximum fall in lung function occurs within 5–10 min of exercise, and the increased resistance to airflow is due to airway narrowing, which develops predominantly in the large airways. In severe cases, the small airways are involved [15], leading to pulmonary hyperinflation and arterial hypoxemia [16]. Asthmatic symptoms and airway obstruction resolve spontaneously within 60 min in most persons and, in approximately 40–50% of subjects, is accompanied by a refractory period of 2–4 h duration [17]. During this period, significantly less (less than 50%) bronchoconstriction is evoked on performance of an identical exercise task. The degree of this protection is independent of the severity of the preceding bronchoconstriction [18]. Moreover, Hahn *et al.* showed in adult asthmatics with documented refractoriness that the absence of bronchoconstriction after an exercise challenge did not protect against bronchoconstriction in a subsequent exercise challenge. In that study, a mean (SD) fall in FEV_1 of 3.1 (7.3)% was observed after a 6-min treadmill exercise challenge while breathing saturated air at 37 °C. However, a repeat challenge 20 min later at an inspired air temperature of 6 °C resulted in a mean (SD) fall in FEV_1 of 37.3 (17.3)% [19]. In some patients, the initial episode may be followed 3–10 h later by a second episode of bronchoconstriction [20], which is associated with increased neutrophil chemotactic activity [21] and is localized to the peripheral airways [22]. However, the existence of this late response has been disputed [23].

The severity of EIB is mainly dependent on the environmental conditions under which exercise is performed and the level of ventilation during exercise [24,25]. Environmental factors include the temperature and humidity of the inspired air, with an additive effect of inhalation of subfreezing air [26–28], and high levels of allergens and environmental pollutants

[29]. The level of ventilation is dependent on the nature, duration and intensity of the exercise. Swimming with high humidity of the inspired air is considered to be less asthmogenic than walking, running and cycling [30–32], while cross-country skiing, with inspiration of large volumes of cold, dry air, is considered to be the most asthmogenic. However, it has been suggested that, when controlled for temperature, humidity and accumulated ventilation, all forms of exercise are equally effective stimuli for EIB [33,34].

EIB is a sensitive indicator of asthma, being present in 80% of asthmatics not treated with inhaled corticosteroids [35] and in 50% of asthmatics despite current treatment with inhaled steroids [36], and absent in those asthmatics who become symptom free [37].

The stimulus for acute airway narrowing in sensitive subjects is the loss of water from the airways. Under resting conditions, full conditioning of the inspired air occurs in the nose and the upper airway. During exercise, ventilation, gas exchange, skeletal muscle activity and cardiac output increase in order to meet the increased aerobic demands. The increased minute ventilation is facilitated by an increase in the diameter of the lumen of the lower airways [38] and by a shift in ventilation from the nasal to the oronasal route, which forces the task of conditioning of the inspired air on to the lower airways. As the relationship between temperature and humidity is non-linear (Fig. 4.5.2), the colder the air the greater the loss of water from the airways during the conditioning process.

There are two main hypotheses regarding the mechanism of the bronchoconstriction: the hyperosmolarity and the vascular hypothesis. According to the hyperosmolarity hypothesis, airway narrowing is due to bronchial smooth muscle contraction in response to mediators released from mast cells, airway epithelial cells and nerve cells, secondary to the development of a hyperosmolar environment in the airways [39]. In contrast, the vascular hypothesis proposes that airway cooling and bronchoconstriction occur during exercise and that the increase in airway resistance after exercise is due to the reactive hyperemia in the bronchial vasculature and subsequent edema with subsequent airway narrowing [40]. In practical terms, the inhalation of cold air almost always means inhalation of dry air, especially as air at temperatures of −15 °C and lower is almost depleted of water [41].

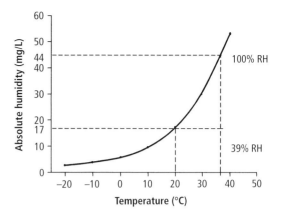

Fig. 4.5.2 Relationship between temperature and absolute humidity. For example, the relative humidity of a gas at 20 °C containing 17 mg/L water (its absolute humidity) is 100%; if the gas is then heated to 37 °C without the addition of water, its absolute humidity is the same but its relative humidity is only 39%. A saturated vapour at this temperature would hold 44 mg/L. Adapted from [28].

Training type and effects

Any kind of physical exercise can be safely performed by almost all asthmatics, as EIB can be prevented or attenuated by regular anti-inflammatory treatment and the prophylactic use of pre-exercise warm-ups and β_2-agonist or chromones [42–44]. Training programs should be based on the interval principle, as the airway response is less severe with intermittent than with continuous exercise [45]. Examples of useful activities are swimming, ball games, relay races and dancing. In addition to an amelioration of EIB, interval and endurance training result in significant improvements in the aerobic and anaerobic working capacities of asthmatics [46–49]. Minute ventilation is maintained under endurance training in asthmatics through a small increase in frequency with no change in tidal volume, which compensates for the airflow obstruction [50].

Protocol for exercise challenge test

Purpose

For diagnostic purposes, a free running test may be sufficient. It is important to instruct the subject to exercise to the extent of maximum effort for a period of at least 6 min. For scientific purposes, and when it is desirable to monitor effect by intervention, an exercise test preferably on a treadmill and under more controlled conditions of temperature and humidity is preferable.

Discontinuation of medication

Short-acting β_2-agonist	8 h
Long-acting β_2-agonist	24 h
Antihistamine	48 h
Antileukotrienes	48 h
Anticholinergics	8 h
Theophylline	24 h
Inhaled glucocorticosteroids (GCS)	Keep stable dose
Chromones	8 h

Exercise workload

In the free running test, it is important to instruct the subject to exercise to the extent of maximum effort for a period of at least 6 min.

In a treadmill or cycle ergometer test, a minimum provocation requires a minute ventilation of 40–60% of predicted maximum voluntary ventilation (FEV_1 predicted $\times$ 35) and a heart rate of more than 80% of maximum heart rate (220 – age [beats/min]) during the last 6 min of the exercise protocol. For optimal sensitivity in highly trained athletes, a greater exercise stimulus resulting in a heart rate of at least 85% maximum heart rate combined with inhalation of subfreezing air may be employed.

Evaluation of response

Spirometry or peak expiratory flow (PEF) is used to measure the effect of exercise on lung function. Measurements are taken at baseline and at 2, 5, 10, 15 and 30 min after the end of exercise. In some individuals, the fall in lung function may occur at 30 min after exercise. Exercise-induced bronchospasm is present if the fall in PEF exceeds 15% or in FEV_1 exceeds 10%.

Asthma in sports

After the disqualification of an asthmatic gold medallist in the 1972 Olympic Games for the use of a banned drug [51], there has been an increased focus on accurate diagnosis and treatment of asthma in Olympic team athletes, especially from the United States and Australia. This interest has since encompassed ath-

letes at other competitive levels, and was further intensified in the 1990s following the observation that 37% of cross-country skiers finishing in the top 15 places in short-distance competitive events in the 1991 World Championship used antiasthmatic medication (Videman Tapio, American College of Sports Medicine meeting, May 1992).

The relationship between asthma and sports appears to be dual in nature. It has long been recognized that asthmatics participating in sporting activities experience EIB. However, recent studies have highlighted high prevalences of chest tightness, cough, wheezing or prolonged shortness of breath and asthma in highly trained athletes, especially American football players, swimmers and cross-country skiers (Table 4.5.1), suggesting that exercise *per se* may cause normal individuals to develop asthma. In non-asthmatic subjects, inhalation of large volumes of cold air can cause a decrease in lung function [52]. Moreover, in a recent study, Langdeau *et al.* reported that 49% of elite athletes had bronchial hyperresponsiveness to methacholine, defined as $PC_{20} < 16$ mg/mL (provocative concentration causing 20% fall in FEV_1), with a greater prevalence in those athletes exposed to cold air and humid air [53]. In a case control study, Heir and Oseid observed that cross-country skiers with a diagnosis of asthma developed respiratory symptoms later in adolescence and early adulthood, compared to controls [54].

Possible risk factors

There are three possible risk factors for asthma in sport:
- allergy;
- air pollution/irritants; and
- exercise-induced immunosuppression.

Allergy

Inhalation of seasonal allergens should be considered as a substantial risk factor in summer sports. A recent survey of elite Australian athletes in Summer Olympic disciplines revealed a history of seasonal allergic rhinoconjunctivitis with a positive skinprick test in 29% [55]. In another study, Helenius *et al.* reported that atopic athletes had nearly a four-fold increased risk of developing bronchial hyperresponsiveness and more than a seven-fold risk of developing asthma,

Table 4.5.1 Asthma prevalence in highly trained athletes.

Study year	Athletic group	n	Method	Asthma prevalence (%)	Ref
1976	Australian Summer Olympic team	185	Physical examination	9.7	[68]
1980	Australian Summer Olympic team	106	Physical examination	8.5	[68]
1984	US Summer Olympic team	597	Questionnaire, treadmill exercise challenge in selected athletes	4.3	[69]
1986	Football players	156	Questionnaire, methacholine challenge	11.5	[70]
1986	Swiss athletes	2060	Questionnaire	3.7	[71]
1993	Swedish cross-country skiers	42	Questionnaire, methacholine challenge	54.8	[72]
1994	Norwegian cross-country skiers	153	Questionnaire	14.4	[54]
1994	Swedish cross-country skiers	299	Questionnaire	15	[73]
1994	Finnish runners	103	Questionnaire	15.5	[74]
1995	US swimmers	738	Questionnaire	13.4	[75]
1996	Norwegian cross-country skiers	118	Questionnaire, methacholine challenge	11.8	[76]
1996	Swedish cross-country skiers	53	Questionnaire, methacholine challenge	41.5	[76]
1996	US Summer Olympic team	699	Questionnaire	16.7 (50% in cyclists)	[77]
1998	US Winter Olympic team	196	Questionnaire	22.4	[78]
		170	Exercise challenge test	23% with EIB (50% in cross-country skiers, 43% in short-track speed skating)	[79]

EIB, exercise-induced bronchoconstriction.

compared to non-atopic athletes [56]. This increased risk may be due to an increased exposure of the lower airways to pollen as a result of an increase in nasal resistance and oral breathing, and of reduced nasal filtration of pollen.

Air pollution/irritants

Exposure to low levels of pollutants like sulfur dioxide and ozone during exercise causes a marked broncho-constriction and reduced ventilatory flow, compared to exposure at rest [29]. The airways are exposed to a much higher dose than at rest, because of a higher ventilatory rate and oronasal respiration. Cyclists are exposed to a wide spectrum of irritants, including road dust, diesel exhaust and ozone. Fifty per cent of cyclists in the 1996 US Olympic team reported that they had asthma or had taken an asthma medication in the

past [77]. Moreover, low-level exposure to ozone negatively affected exercise performance in elite cyclists [57].

Another group of athletes where exposure to irritants may be a significant factor is swimmers. Although the ambient chlorine concentration is well below the acceptable threshold levels, swimmers are exposed to high concentrations of chlorine in the course of a practice session because of the high minute ventilation achieved during training and competition, especially in indoor pools [58].

Immunosuppression

Physical training affects the function of the immune system. Although there is no apparent effect on the adaptive immune system, the level of exercise appears to have a differential effect on the innate immune

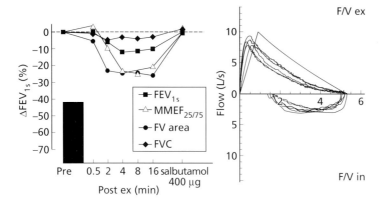

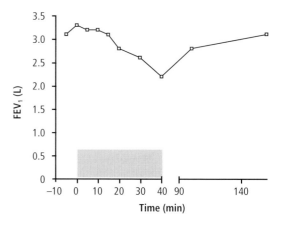

Fig. 4.5.3 Example of a positive exercise bronchoprovocation test. Following 6 min hard exercise, there was a significant fall in lung function parameters shortly after stopping exercise. A spontaneous recovery started to occur 10 min later. Complete reversibility was achieved after inhalation of salbutamol 400 µg.

system. Moderate exercise appears to enhance immune function, while prolonged endurance exercise appears to suppress immune function. Changes in immune function are discussed in detail in Chapter 4.2.

Differential diagnosis

Dyspnea in relation to strenuous exercise is common and there is always a risk of interpreting this as asthma. A carefully taken history is mandatory and an exercise challenge test to confirm the presence of EIB should be performed (Fig. 4.5.3). Typically, subjects with EIB report symptoms such as dyspnea and wheeze within the first 5–10 min after the start of the first bout of exercise. Some subjects are able to run through their symptoms, and after 20–30 min seem to attain a 'second wind' and become refractory to further episodes of bronchoconstriction. In the postexercise period, they usually complain of a worsening of dyspnea and cough within the first 5–10 min. Although commonly used to measure bronchial hyperresponsiveness in asthmatics, a positive response to methacholine or histamine challenge does not always imply the presence of EIB. Other important differential diagnostic aspects include vocal cord dysfunction, laryngotracheomalacia and vascular anomalies, which may also give symptoms early during exercise. While the typical subject with EIB experiences symptoms early in the course of exercise, a large proportion of subjects experience increasing dyspnea, sometimes associated with increased mucus production, at 20–40 min after the start of strenuous exercise. Lung function measurements in these subjects show a continuous decrease in FEV_1 without the typical dual pattern seen in EIB (Fig.

Fig. 4.5.4 Example of late-occurring obstruction in a ski athlete subject complaining of dyspnea and mucus production related to exercise. Exercise provocation test (▨) was negative but the patient experienced a continuous decline in lung function during endurance activity, measured by a pocket spirometer.

4.5.4). The reasons for this decline are unclear, but factors such as thoracic muscular fatigue, an uncoordinated breathing pattern and increased mucus secretion may be contributory. Finally, it is also necessary to state that dyspnea in relation to exercise may be related to overtraining, as well as to a limited capacity for improvement of physical fitness.

Treatment of EIB

Non-pharmacologic intervention

Non-pharmacologic measures are probably the most important, both to avoid the development of asthma in the healthy athlete and to prevent the occurrence of EIB in the asthmatic athlete. Prolonged endurance exercise should be avoided in the summer during periods and in areas with high pollen counts, and in the winter at temperatures lower than −15 °C. The same applies to exercise in areas with air pollution or other airway irritants, irrespective of the time of year. Moreover, strenuous exercise should not be commenced for at least 7 days after recovery from a recent upper respiratory tract infection. Athletes should be given a clear message that it is better to rest and stay in bed than to recommence training too early after such infections. Lastly, the use of heat–moisture exchange devices should be encouraged during training sessions to minimize heat and water loss from the airways. Inspiration of air at 15 °C and 50% relative humidity results in a loss to the environment of 25 mL water and 35 kcal/L of minute ventilation. The loss of heat and water can be considerable, especially in endurance athletes such as long-distance runners, swimmers and cross-country skiers, who can maintain minute ventilations up to 100 L/min for prolonged periods. Studies in dogs have shown that short periods of hyperventilation with inadequately conditioned air induce airway inflammatory changes that last for at least 24 h [59].

A carefully designed warm-up program is necessary in order to prevent the occurrence of EIB in the asthmatic athlete. The warm-up has two main purposes. Firstly, it accustoms the airways to changes in conditions in the ambient air. Rapid changes in temperature can cause changes in the tone of the bronchial vasculature and thus changes in airway calibre and resistance. Secondly, the warm-up program should be designed to provoke multiple episodes of a minor degree of bronchoconstriction in order to exploit refractoriness to the exercise stimulus later on in the competitive event. This can be achieved by multiple short bouts of exercise at submaximal intensity, preferably early in the warm-up period (Fig. 4.5.5).

Pharmacologic intervention

In some subjects, obstructive symptoms on exercise may be the only complaint, while in other subjects, they may be one of several expressions indicative of inadequately controlled asthma. In the latter case, treatment should be instituted in accordance with modern asthma treatment guidelines. The baseline therapy

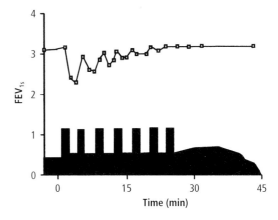

Fig. 4.5.5 Schematic illustration of a warm-up program aimed to induce refractoriness to exercise bronchoprovocative stimuli later during the competitive event.

should be anti-inflammatory, preferably with inhaled corticosteroids. Bronchodilator therapy with β_2-agonists should be given prophylactically prior to exercise. When inhaled corticosteroid therapy combined with short-acting β_2-agonists is inadequate, add-on therapy with other prophylactic agents, such as a long-acting β_2-agonist or a leukotriene receptor antagonist, is recommended. Leukotriene receptor antagonist treatment has a slight advantage over long-acting β_2-agonist therapy in that it does not appear to induce tolerance with regular treatment. However, large individual variations in response are present, and thus the best combination should be explored on an individual basis. Therapy with chromones, such as nedocromil and disodium chromoglycate, is an additional treatment option that may be used either regularly or prophylactically before exercise.

In those subjects with obstructive symptoms only on exercise, it is not clear at present whether long-term anti-inflammatory treatment is necessary or effective. They should be treated with inhaled β_2-agonists, either prophylactically prior to exercise or symptomatically after exercise. Exercise challenge testing should be performed and, if positive, regular anti-inflammatory treatment with either inhaled corticosteroids, chromones or oral antileukotriene receptor antagonists should be instituted on an individual basis.

Doping

In non-obstructed subjects, ventilation is never the limiting factor for athletic performance. Thus it is clear that medication that improves ventilation cannot be regarded as ergogenic. Studies of non-asthmatic, high-performance athletes using short- or long-acting β_2-agonists by inhalation have failed to show positive effects on aerobic capacity and performance [60–62]. On the contrary, inhaled β_2-agonists may even have a negative effect on performance, possibly due to an increase in ventilation–perfusion mismatch [63]. The short-acting β_2-agonists terbutaline and salbutamol, as well as the long-acting β_2-agonist salmeterol are approved for use by asthmatic athletes only when they are given by the inhaled route. There are several reasons for allowing the use of β_2-agonists only by inhalation. One reason is that β_2-agonists are far more effective when given by the inhaled route than by oral administration in preventing exercise-induced bronchoconstriction [64]. Another reason is that experiments carried out mainly in animals have suggested that orally administered β2-agonists, such as salbutamol and clenbuterol, may have an anabolic effect on and improve the strength of skeletal muscle tissue. However, recent studies suggest contradictory effects on exercise performance with a beneficial effect on intense submaximal exercise in recreational athletes after 3 weeks of oral salbutamol administration [65] and a deleterious effect on endurance and sprint exercise in rats after oral clenbuterol administration [66]. The leukotriene receptor antagonist, montelukast, when tested under similar conditions, has not been shown to have ergogenic effects [67], and at present, this class of drug is not included on the list of prohibited preparations. The use of inhaled corticosteroids and chromones by asthmatic athletes is allowed. In all circumstances, the use of antiasthmatic medication is reserved for athletes with clearly diagnosed asthma, and it is a prerequisite that the athlete can present medical documentation of the need for such treatment.

Summary

Asthma symptoms are common in athletes, with the highest prevalence figures seen in endurance sports athletes. Repeated hyperpnea may be stressful to the lower airways, with increased exposure to both allergens and irritants in the summer and to cold, dry air in the winter. Chronic endurance exercise activity suppresses both humoral and cellular immunity and is associated with an increased susceptibility to upper respiratory tract infections. With suitable attention to known risk factors, the development of asthma in the elite athlete may be prevented. Hard training should be avoided in an environment with high pollen counts and airway irritants during the summer months, and in a cold, dry environment with temperatures lower than $-15\,°C$ during the winter months. It is especially important not to recommence training soon after an upper respiratory tract infection. Medical treatment of asthma in athletes is very much the same as for asthma in non-athletes. Anti-inflammatory treatment with inhaled corticosteroids is baseline therapy, complemented with prophylactic and symptomatic bronchodilator therapy. Additional treatment with a long-acting β_2-agonist or leukotriene receptor antagonist may be considered as add-on options when baseline therapy is insufficient. When exercise symptoms are the only manifestation, regular anti-inflammatory therapy may not be needed. Non-pharmacologic treatment with a carefully designed warm-up program and use of a heat–moisture exchanger during winter training is equally important as medical treatment.

Although there are no data indicating that antiasthmatic medication taken by inhalation or orally administered leukotriene receptor antagonists have any ergogenic effect, both athletes and trainers should be aware of the regulations concerning the use of antiasthmatic medication to avoid disqualification or exclusion from competition.

Multiple choice questions

1 *What is the minimum required fall in lung function post exercise defining it as a positive test?*

a A $\Delta FEV_1 \geq 15\%$.

b A $\Delta FEV_1 \geq 10\%$.

c A $\Delta PEF \geq 10\%$.

2 *What is the expected prevalence of exercise-induced bronchoconstriction in previously untreated young asthmatics?*

a >90%.

b 70–80%.

c 50–60%.

3 *What is the most important trigger for exercise-induced bronchoconstriction in asthmatic subjects?*

a Hyperventilation.

b Anaerobic work with increase in blood lactate levels.

c Increased heart rate and adrenergic stimulation.

4 *What are the main risk factors for asthma development in skiers?*

a Hyperventilation of cold, dry air.

b Increased exposure to allergens.

c Both of the above.

5 *The target workload required to induce EIB in an exercise challenge test should be:*

a a pulse rate of 220 – age for 6 min

b a pulse rate > 80% of maximum pulse rate for 6 min

c an increase in blood lactate of more than 200%.

6 *The preferred treatment of persistent asthma with EIB should be:*

a a short-acting β_2-agonist before exercise

b chromones such as nedochromile or disodium chromoglycate before exercise

c regular inhaled glucocorticosteroid plus short-acting β_2-agonist before exercise.

References

1 American Thoracic Society Committee on Diagnostic Standards. Definition and classification of chronic bronchitis, and pulmonary emphysema. *Am Rev Respiratory Dis* 1962; **85**: 762–8.

2 Djukanovic R, Roche WR, Wilson JW, Beasley CR, Twentyman OP, Howarth RH *et al.* Mucosal inflammation in asthma. *Am Rev Respiratory Dis* 1990; **142**: 434–57.

3 Pin I, Gibson PG, Kolendowicz R, Girgis-Gabardo A, Denburg JA, Hargreave FE *et al.* Use of induced sputum cell counts to investigate airway inflammation in asthma. *Thorax* 1992; **47**: 25–9.

4 Reed CE. What I would like to learn about the pathogenesis of asthma. *Ann Allergy* 1989; **63**: 556–65.

5 Barnes PJ. New concepts in the pathogenesis of bronchial hyperresponsiveness and asthma. *J Allergy Clin Immunol* 1989; **83**: 1013–26.

6 Frigas E, Motojima S, Gleich GJ. The eosinophilic injury to the mucosa of the airways in the pathogenesis of bronchial asthma. *Eur Respir J (Suppl.)* 1991; **13**: 123s–35s.

7 Global initiative for asthma. Global strategy for asthma management and prevention. NHLBI/WHO workshop report. *Natl Instit Health* 1995; **3659**: 1–8.

8 Adams F. The extant works of Aretaeus, the Cappadocian. In: Brewis RAL, ed. *Classic Papers in Asthma.* London: Science Press 1990, 1–3.

9 Sakula A. Sir John Floyer's A treatise of the asthma (1698). *Thorax* 1984; **39**: 248.

10 Sterk PJ, Fabbri LM, Quanjer PH. Airway responsiveness: Standardised challenge testing with pharmacological, physical and sensitising stimuli in adults. *Eur Respir J* 1993; **6** (Suppl.): **16**: 53–83.

11 Kukafka DS, Lang DM, Porter S, Rogers J, Ciccolella D, Polansky M, D'Alonzo GE Jr. Exercise-induced bronchospasm in high school athletes via a free running test: incidence and epidemiology. *Chest* 1998; **114**: 1613–22.

12 Ghory JE. Exercise and asthma: overview and clinical impact. *Pediatrics* 1975; **56**: 844–60.

13 Suzuki S, Chonan T, Sasaki H, Takishima T. Time-course of response in exercise-induced bronchoconstriction. *Ann Allergy* 1984; **53**: 341–6.

14 Wiens L, Sabath R, Ewing L, Gowdamarajan R, Portnoy J, Scagliotti D. Chest pain in otherwise healthy children and adolescents is frequently caused by exercise-induced asthma. *Pediatrics* 1992; **90**: 350–3.

15 Cropp GJ. Grading, time course, and incidence of exercise-induced airway obstruction and hyperinflation in asthmatic children. *Pediatrics* 1975; **56**: 868–79.

16 Marotel C, Natali F, Heyraud JD, Vaylet F, L'Her P, Bonnet D *et al.* Severe forms of effort-induced asthma. *Allergy Immunol (Paris)* 1989; **21**: 61–4.

17 McNeill RS, Nairn JR, Millar JS, Ingram CG. Exercise-induced asthma. *Q J Med* 1966; **35**: 55–67.

18 Henriksen JM, Dahl R, Lundqvist GR. Influence of relative humidity and repeated exercise on exercise-induced bronchoconstriction. *Allergy* 1981; **36**: 463–70.

19 Hahn AG, Nogrady SG, Burton GR, Morton AR. Absence of refractoriness in asthmatic subjects after exercise with warm, humid inspirate. *Thorax* 1985; **40**: 418–21.

20 Belcher NG, O'Hickey S, Arm JP, Lee TH. Pathogenetic mechanisms of exercise-induced asthma and the refractory period. *N Engl Regional Allergy Proc* 1988; **9**: 199–201.

21 Lee TH, Nagakura T, Papageorgiou N, Iikura Y, Kay AB. Exercise-induced late asthmatic reactions with neutrophil chemotactic activity. *N Engl J Med* 1983; **308**: 1502–5.

22 Bierman CW, Spiro SG, Petheram I. Characterization of the late response in exercise-induced asthma. *J Allergy Clin Immunol* 1984; **74**: 701–6.

23 Zawadski DK, Lenner KA, McFadden ER Jr. Re-examination of the late asthmatic response to exercise. *Am Rev Respir Dis* 1988; **137**: 837–841.

24 Bar-Or O, Neuman I, Dotan R. Effects of dry and humid climates on exercise-induced asthma in children and pre-adolescents. *J Allergy Clin Immunol* 1977; **60**: 163–8.

25 Kilham H, Tooley M, Silverman M. Running, walking, and hyperventilation causing asthma in children. *Thorax* 1979; **34**: 582–6.

26 Fanta CH, McFadden ER Jr, Ingram RH Jr. Effects of cromolyn sodium on the response to respiratory heat loss in normal subjects. *Am Rev Respir Dis* 1981; **123**: 161–4.

27 McLaughlin FJ, Dozor AJ. Cold air inhalation challenge in the diagnosis of asthma in children. *Pediatrics* 1983; **72**: 503–9.

28 Shelly MP. *Humidification: Intensive Care Rounds*. Abingdon, UK: The Medicine Group (Education) Ltd, 1993.

29 Pierson WE, Covert DS, Koenig JQ, Namekata T, Kim YS. Implications of air pollution effects on athletic performance. *Med Sci Sports Exerc* 1986; **18**: 322–7.

30 Bar-Yishay E, Gur I, Inbar O, Neuman I, Dlin RA, Godfrey S. Differences between swimming and running as stimuli for exercise-induced asthma. *Eur J Appl Physiol* 1982; **48**: 387–97.

31 Inbar O, Dotan R, Dlin RA, Neuman I, Bar-Or O. Breathing dry or humid air and exercise-induced asthma during swimming. *Eur J Appl Physiol* 1980; **44**: 43–50.

32 Fitch KD. Comparative aspects of available exercise systems. *Pediatrics* 1975; **56**: 904–7.

33 Bundgaard A, Schmidt A, Ingemann-Hansen T, Halkjaer-Kristensen J. Exercise-induced asthma after swimming and bicycle exercise. *Eur J Respir Dis* 1982; **63**: 245–8.

34 Bundgaard A, Ingemann-Hansen T, Schmidt A, Halkjaer-Kristensen J. Exercise-induced asthma after walking, running and cycling. *Scand J Clin Lab Invest* 1982; **42**: 15–8.

35 Anderson SD, Silverman M, Konig P, Godfrey S. Exercise-induced asthma. *Br J Dis Chest* 1975; **69**: 1–39.

36 Waalkens HJ, van Essen-Zandvliet EE, Gerritsen J, Duiverman EJ, Kerrebijn KF, Knol K. The effect of an inhaled corticosteroid (budesonide) on exercise-induced asthma in children. Dutch CNSLD Study Group. *Eur Respir J* 1993; **6**: 652–6.

37 Balfour Lynn L, Tooley M, Godfrey S. Relationship of exercise-induced asthma to clinical asthma in childhood. *Arch Dis Child* 1981; **56**: 450–4.

38 Jones PS, Buston MH, Wharton MJ. The effect of exercise in ventilatory function of children with asthma. *Br J Dis Chest* 1962; **56**: 78–86.

39 Anderson SD. Is there a unifying hypothesis for exercise-induced asthma? *J Allergy Clin Immunol* 1984; **73**: 660–5.

40 McFadden ER Jr. Hypothesis: exercise-induced asthma as a vascular phenomenon. *Lancet* 1990; **335**: 880–3.

41 McFadden ER Jr. Heat and water exchange in human airways. *Am Rev Respir Dis* 1992; **146**: 8–10.

42 Bundgaard A. Exercise and the asthmatic. *Sports Med* 1985; **2**: 254–66.

43 Reiff DB, Choudry NB, Pride NB, Ind PW. The effect of prolonged submaximal warm-up exercise on exercise-induced asthma. *Am Rev Respir Dis* 1989; **139**: 479–84.

44 Weiler JM. Exercise-induced asthma: a practical guide to definitions, diagnosis, prevalence, and treatment. *Allergy Asthma Proc* 1996; **17**: 315–25.

45 Morton AR, Hahn AG, Fitch KD. Continuous and intermittent running in the provocation of asthma. *Ann Allergy* 1982; **48**: 123–9.

46 Svenonius E, Kautto R, Arborelius M Jr. Improvement after training of children with exercise-induced asthma. *Acta Paediatr Scand* 1983; **72**: 23–30.

47 Henriksen JM, Nielsen TT. Effect of physical training on exercise-induced bronchoconstriction. *Acta Paediatr Scand* 1983; **72**: 31–6.

48 Freeman W, Williams C, Nute MG. Endurance running performance in athletes with asthma. *J Sports Sci* 1990; **8**: 103–17.

49 Matsumoto I, Araki H, Tsuda K, Odajima H, Nishima S, Higaki Y *et al.* Effects of swimming training on aerobic capacity and exercise induced bronchoconstriction in children with bronchial asthma. *Thorax* 1999; **54**: 196–201.

50 Freeman W, Nute MG, Brooks S, Williams C. Responses of asthmatic and non-asthmatic athletes to prolonged treadmill running. *Br J Sports Med* 1990; **24**: 183–90.

51 Olympic MDs: win some, lose some. *Med World News* 1972; **13**: 27–35.

52 O'Cain CF, Dowling NB, Slutsky AS, Hensley MJ, Strohl KP, McFadden ER, Ingram RH. Airway effects of respiratory heat loss in normal subjects. *J Appl Physiol* 1980; **49**: 875–80.

53 Langdeau JB, Turcotte H, Bowie DM, Jobin J, Desgagne P, Boulet LP. Airway hyperresponsiveness in elite athletes. *Am J Respiratory Crit Care Med* 2000; **161**: 1479–84.

54 Heir T, Oseid S. Self-reported asthma and exercise-induced asthma symptoms in high-level competitive cross-country skiers. *Scand J Med Sci Sports* 1994; **4**: 128–33.

55 Katelaris CH, Carrozzi FM, Burke TV, Byth K. A springtime olympics demands special consideration for allergic athletes. *J Allergy Clin Immunol* 2000; **106**: 260–266.

56 Helenius IJ, Tikkanen HO, Sarna S, Haahtela T. Asthma and increased bronchial responsiveness in elite athletes: atopy and sport event as risk factors. *J Allergy Clin Immunol* 1998; **101**: 646–52.

57 Gong H Jr, Bradley PW, Simmons MS, Tashkin DP. Impaired exercise performance and pulmonary function in elite cyclists during low-level ozone exposure in a hot environment. *Am Rev Respir Dis* 1986; **134**: 726–33.

58 Drobnic F, Freixa A, Casan P, Sanchis J, Guardino X. Assessment of chlorine exposure in swimmers during training. *Med Sci Sports Exerc* 1996; **28**: 271–4.

59 Omori C, Schofield BH, Mitzner W, Freed AN. Hyperpnea with dry air causes time-dependent alterations in mucosal morphology and bronchovascular permeability. *J Appl Physiol* 1995; **78**: 1043–51.

60 Morton AR, Joyce K, Papalia SM, Carroll NG, Fitch KD. Is salmeterol ergogenic? *Clin J Sport Med* 1996; **6**: 220–5.

61 Sandsund M, Sue-Chu M, Helgerud J, Reinertsen RE, Bjermer L. Effect of cold exposure (−15 degrees C) and salbutamol treatment on physical performance in elite nonasthmatic cross-country skiers. *Eur J Appl Physiol* 1998; **77**: 297–304.

62 Sue-Chu M, Sandsund M, Helgerud J, Reinertsen RE, Bjermer L. Salmeterol and physical performance at −15 degrees C in highly trained nonasthmatic cross-country skiers. *Scand J Med Sci Sports* 1999; **9**: 48–52.

63 Carlsen KH, Ingjer F, Kirkegaard H, Thyness B. The effect of inhaled salbutamol and salmeterol on lung function and endurance performance in healthy well-trained athletes. *Scand J Med Sci Sports* 1997; **7**: 160–5.

64 Anderson SD, Seale JP, Rozea P, Bandler L, Theobald G, Lindsay DA. Inhaled and oral salbutamol in exercise-induced asthma. *Am Rev Respiratory Dis* 1976; **114**: 493–500.

65 Collomp K, Candau R, Lasne F, Labsy Z, Prefaut C, De Ceaurriz J. Effects of short-term oral salbutamol administration on exercise endurance and metabolism. *J Appl Physiol* 2000; **89**: 430–6.

66 Duncan ND, Williams DA, Lynch GS. Deleterious effects of chronic clenbuterol treatment on endurance and sprint exercise performance in rats. *Clin Sci* 2000; **98**: 339–47.

67 Sue-Chu M, Sandsund M, Holand B, Bjermer L. Montelukast does not affect exercise performance at sub-freezing temperature in highly-trained non-asthmatic endurance athletes. *Int J Sports Med* 2000; **2**: 424–428.

68 Fitch KD. Management of allergic Olympic athletes. *J Allergy Clin Immunol* 1984; **73**: 722–7.

69 Voy RO. The U.S. Olympic Committee experience with exercise-induced bronchospasm, 1984. *Med Sci Sports Exerc* 1986; **18**: 328–30.

70 Weiler JM, Metzger WJ, Donnelly AL, Crowley ET, Sharath MD. Prevalence of bronchial hyperresponsiveness in highly trained athletes. *Chest* 1986; **90**: 23–8.

71 Helbling A, Muller U. Asthma bronchiale bei Spitzensportlern. *Schweiz Z Sportmed* 1991; **39**: 77–81.

72 Larsson K, Ohlsen P, Larsson L, Malmberg P, Rydstrom PO, Ulriksen H. High prevalence of asthma in cross country skiers [see comments]. *Br Med J* 1993; **307**: 1326–9.

73 Larsson L, Hemmingsson P, Boethius G. Self-reported obstructive airway symptoms are common in young cross-country skiers. *Scand J Med Sci Sports* 1994; **4**: 124–7.

74 Tikkanen H, Helenius I. Asthma in runners. *Br Med J* 1994; **309**: 1087.

75 Potts JE. *Adverse respiratory health effects of competitive swimming. The prevalence of symptoms, illnesses, and bronchial responsiveness to methacholine and exercise.* Academic dissertation, The University of British Columbia, Vancouver, 1994.

76 Sue-Chu M, Larsson L, Bjermer L. Prevalence of asthma in young cross-country skiers in central Scandinavia: differences between Norway and Sweden. *Respir Med* 1996; **90**: 99–105.

77 Weiler JM, Layton T, Hunt M. Asthma in United States Olympic athletes who participated in the 1996 Summer Games. *J Allergy Clin Immunol* 1998; **102**: 722–6.

78 Weiler JM, Ryan EJ III. Asthma in United States Olympic athletes who participated in the 1998 Olympic Winter Games. *J Allergy Clin Immunol* 2000; **106**: 267–71.

79 Wilber RL, Rundell KW, Szmedra L, Jenkinson DM, Im J, Drake SD. Incidence of exercise-induced bronchospasm in Olympic winter sport athletes. *Med Sci Sports Exerc* 2000; **32**: 732–7.

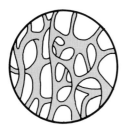

Chapter 4.6
Amenorrhea, Osteoporosis and Eating Disorders in Athletes

MICHELLE P. WARREN, JORUN
SUNDGOT-BORGEN & JOANNA L. FRIED

Classical reference

Drinkwater BL, Nilson K, Chesnut CH, Bremner WJ, Shainholtz S, Southworth MB. Bone mineral content of amenorrheic and eumenorrheic athletes. *N Engl J Med* 1984; **311**: 277–281.
The study was designed to determine whether the hypoestrogenic status of 14 amenorrheic athletes was associated with a decrease in regional bone mass relative to that of 14 eumenorrheic peers (Table 4.6.1). It was demonstrated that bone mass as measured by dual-photon and single-photon absorptiometry at the lumbar vertebrae (L1 to L4) was significantly lower in the amenorrheic group than in the eumenorrheic group. No difference was found at the radial site (Table 4.6.2).

This study was one of the first to demonstrate that amenorrhea observed in female athletes may be accompanied by a decrease in mineral density of the lumbar vertebrae.

Introduction

Women derive numerous short- and long-term benefits from regular physical activity. However, female athletes face a special health risk due to the sensitivity of the reproductive system to environmental stresses such as weight loss or exercise. The amenorrhea that may arise because of intensive exercise, insufficient energy intake, disordered eating or other stresses puts women at a greatly increased risk for stress fractures, osteopenia, osteoporosis and other bone complications. Many athletic women display what is known as the 'female athletic triad', which consists of amenorrhea, osteoporosis and eating disorders.

Amenorrhea

Introduction

Amenorrhea is most prevalent in exercise training which requires low body weight, such as ballet dancing or long-distance running. Women who participate in sports which do not place such a premium on low body weight, such as swimming or basketball, tend to experience menstrual dysfunction in other forms, such as irregular cycles [1]. Girls and women involved in sports such as gymnastics, long-distance running, skiing, ballet or figure skating are often pressured to keep their body fat below 10% of their total body weight [2].

Definitions

Amenorrhea is the lack of regular menstrual periods and may be classified as primary or secondary. Primary amenorrhea is a delay in menarche beyond the age of 16. Secondary amenorrhea is the absence of menstruation for more than 3–6 months in women who were previously cyclical [3]. Amenorrhea may occur in premenopausal women for a number of reasons, among them intensive physical training, premature ovarian failure, contraceptive use and nutritional restriction. We will focus here on hypothalamic amenorrhea, as it is the most relevant to the athlete. There are three types of hypothalamic amenorrhea.

Types of hypothalamic amenorrhea

Athletic amenorrhea
Women with low body weight and low body fat due to excessive exercise or disordered eating frequently

Table 4.6.1 Physical characteristics and training regimens of 14 amenorrheic and 14 eumenorrheic athletes.*

	Amenorrheic	Eumenorrheic	P value
Age (yr)	24.9±1.3	25.5±1.4	NS
Height (cm)	166.1±2.5	165.7±2.2	NS
Weight (kg)	54.4±2.3	57.9±2.2	NS
Body fat (%)	15.8±1.4	16.9±0.8	NS
Lean body mass	45.6±1.6	48.0±1.6	NS
Age at menarche (yr)	12.5±0.5	12.8±0.4	NS
Duration of amenorrhea (mo)	41.7±7.4		
Length of participation in sport (yr)	7.0±1.6	6.6±1.1	NS
Training			
Days/week	6.2±0.2	5.6±0.3	NS
Hours/day	1.6±0.2	1.8±0.3	NS
Time for 10-km race (min:sec)†	39:06±1:15	45:59±1:49	NS
Miles run/week‡	41.8±5.2	24.9±3.0	<0.01
Minutes/mile‡§	7:32±0:20	7:47±0:18	NS

* Plus–minus values are means ± S.E.M. NS denotes not significant.
† N = eight eumenorrheic and seven amenorrheic athletes.
‡ N = 12 eumenorrheic and 10 amenorrheic athletes.
§ Pace of long, slow distance run.

Table 4.6.2 Bone mineral content and density in 14 amenorrheic and 14 eumenorrheic athletes at two forearm sites and at the L1 through L4 lumbar vertebrae.*

Site	Amenorrheic	Eumenorrheic	P value
Radius			
S_1			
Mineral content (g/cm)	0.89±0.03	0.85±0.03	NS
Mineral density (g/cm^2)	0.53±0.02	0.54±0.01	NS
S_2			
Mineral content (g/cm)	0.91±0.02	0.88±0.03	NS
Mineral density (g/cm^2)	0.67±0.02	0.67±0.02	NS
Vertebrae (g/cm^2)	1.12±0.04	1.30±0.03	<0.01

* Plus–minus values are means ± S.E.M. NS denotes not significant.

develop hypothalamic amenorrhea [4]. In athletes, this may be due in part to some combination of heavy exercise, mental stress and the desire or pressure to maintain a certain body weight. The use of performance-enhancing drugs may also alter cycles, but the mechanism by which it does so is probably different. Menstrual irregularity is more common in female athletes than in non-athletic women [3]: in the general adult population, menstrual irregularities have an esti-

mated prevalence of 1.8–5% [5,6] while studies of adult athletes report a prevalence as high as 79% [7] (Table 4.6.3).

Eating disorder amenorrhea

The menstrual dysfunction seen in athletes in sports requiring low body weight is similar to that seen in women with eating disorders, particularly anorexia nervosa.

Table 4.6.3 Surveys of the prevalence of amenorrhea and oligomenorrhea in different athletic disciplines.

Activity	Study	n	Percentage with irregularities
General population	Petterson *et al.* [5]	1862	1.8
	Singh [6]	900	5.0
Weight-bearing sports			
Ballet	Abraham *et al.* [7]	29	79.0
	Brooks-Gunn *et al.* [8]	53	59.0
	Feicht *et al.* [9]	128	6–43
	Glass *et al.* [10]	67	34.0
Running	Shangold and Levine [11]	394	24.0
	Sanborn *et al.* [12]	237	26.0
Non-weight-bearing sports			
Cycling	Sanborn *et al.* [12]	33	12.0
Swimming	Sanborn *et al.* [12]	197	12.0

From [3].

Idiopathic/functional hypothalamic amenorrhea

Functional hypothalamic amenorrhea (FHA) is a diagnosis of exclusion; hypothalamic amenorrhea of unknown etiology in normal-weight, non-athletic women has long been thought to be psychogenic, caused by stress. However, mounting evidence suggests the possibility that this so-called idiopathic amenorrhea is actually caused by nutritional restriction and the resulting endocrine and metabolic response [13–16]. In a 1999 study, women with FHA were compared with normally menstruating controls of similar body mass index (BMI). In the amenorrheic women, body composition was significantly different from that of BMI-matched controls. The amenorrheic subjects had greater lean body mass and less body fat than the normal controls, and were also found to consume less fat and carbohydrates than the BMI-matched controls. Thus, FHA attributed to exercise or stress may actually be a response to nutritional disturbance [17]. Evidence of subclinical eating disorders have been found in weight-stable, non-athletic women with FHA as well as a significant restriction of dietary

fat intake [18]. While stress may contribute to the disordered eating which may cause amenorrhea, it is unlikely that the stress itself is directly responsible for menstrual dysfunction in women with FHA.

Etiology

The mechanism of the normal menstrual cycle is the result of a number of different endocrine systems working together. Puberty is initiated when the area of the brain called the hypothalamus is activated to secrete gonadotropin-releasing hormone (GnRH). Normally occurring every 60–90 min, the GnRH pulse signals the pituitary to release bursts of the gonadotropins (luteinizing hormone (LH) and follicle-stimulating hormone, FSH), which in turn stimulate the ovary to release the mature follicle. The rhythm of the pulse is controlled by a pulse generator located in the arcuate nucleus in the medial central area of the hypothalamus. GnRH pulses activate a sequence of events in the reproductive tract; the normal menstrual cycle is marked by a cyclic pattern of hormonal secretion. The ovaries primarily secrete estrogens (mostly estradiol), progestins (mostly progesterone) and androgens. These steroids regulate the hypothalamic–pituitary–ovarian axis through a feedback mechanism by acting directly on the pituitary or indirectly on the hypothalamic GnRH pulses [19].

The physiologic basis for hypothalamic amenorrhea is the disruption of the hypothalamus' pulsatile secretion of GnRH. The pulse generator appears to be very sensitive to environmental stresses and metabolic factors. GnRH inhibition seems to be caused by the decreased energy available when expenditure of exercise is greater than dietary intake [2]. GnRH inhibition then lowers the anterior pituitary's secretion of LH and FSH, which shuts down or limits ovarian stimulation and estradiol production. A prolonged follicular phase, or the absence of a critical LH or estradiol surge midcycle, results in the mild or intermittent suppression of menstrual cycles frequently observed in athletes. When levels of LH are very low, the result is delayed menarche, or primary or secondary amenorrhea [20,21].

Early research focused on body composition and the stress of exercise as possible causes of amenorrhea in athletes. However, more recent evidence suggests that the primary factor in exercise-induced reproductive dysfunction is the energy deficit athletic women incur when their daily caloric intake is insufficient for the level of their activity [16,22–24]. Moreover, a significant amount of recent research suggests that a decrease in resting metabolic rate (RMR) is associated with a negative energy balance and with menstrual dysfunction [25–27]. Even women who maintain a normal weight may suffer an energy deficit; their normal weight is probably maintained by a decrease in metabolic rate [24].

While GnRH inhibition clearly plays a major role in certain types of amenorrhea, the etiology of hypothalamic amenorrhea is not entirely understood. The role of the adipocyte hormone leptin, a protein product of the obesity gene, has been highlighted in recent research, some of which suggests that leptin may be an independent regulator of metabolic function [28]. The roles of dehydroepiandrosterone (DHEA), insulin-like growth factor (IGF) and cortisol are also being explored.

Leptin

New research on amenorrhea and body composition was prompted after the 1994 discovery of leptin, a hormone made by the adipocyte [28]. Leptin receptors were discovered on hypothalamic neurons thought to be involved in control of the GnRH pulse generator [29]. Studies have shown that rodents with an inactive form of leptin tend to be amenorrheic and infertile [30,31]. Low leptin levels have been associated with amenorrhea [16,32] and with disordered eating [16]; it appears that if leptin drops below a critical level, menstruation will not occur [33]. Because leptin regulates the basal metabolic rate, it is thought to be a particularly important indicator of nutritional status [34], and indeed, amenorrheic athletes typically have low metabolic rates. Leptin may be a significant mediator of reproductive function in that it responds to a negative energy balance found in women with exercise-induced amenorrhea [35].

Leptin also plays a role in thyroid function and the initiation of puberty. Research has shown that alterations in leptin levels are directly associated with thyroid hormone changes in the presence of nutritional deficiencies [16]. Thus, leptin may act not only as a regulator of metabolic rates but also as a mediator of menstrual status, responding to starvation by slowing metabolism, and may be involved in returning the woman to a prepubertal-like state.

Cortisol

Amenorrheic athletes often have slightly elevated cortisol levels, as do women with FHA or anorexia nervosa. Cortisol is a glucoregulatory hormone activated by low blood glucose levels [36]. Cortisol levels have found to be elevated in both FHA and exercise-associated amenorrhea.

Treatment

Management includes restoring ovulatory cycles if possible, replacing estrogen when necessary, reassurance and re-evaluation. In women with nutritional imbalances or disordered eating, one of the most important aspects of treatment is addressing and reversing unhealthy eating behaviors. Gonadotropin deficiency may be reversible in women with FHA upon the improvement of nutritional intake and body composition [17]. The treatment of amenorrhea should also take into account the likelihood of bone loss.

It is not clear whether hormone replacement therapy works (see Tables 4.6.5 & 4.6.6 below). Early studies on small numbers of treated subjects ($n=4$) suggest that oral contraceptives may be effective in athletic amenorrhea [37]. This subject will be addressed in greater depth below, in the section on osteoporosis.

Osteoporosis

Introduction

The effects of exercise on the skeleton are generally thought to be positive, and numerous studies have indicated that physical activity increases bone mass in humans. Particularly for women, physical activity is recommended for preventing the development of osteoporosis, and regular, vigorous, weight-bearing activity of 1 h or more each week is associated with an increase in bone mineral density (BMD) within a normal population [38]. However, research also indicates that too much physical activity in combination with inadequate energy intake may cause hormonal changes that ultimately increase the risk of bone loss [39].

While osteoporosis, or loss of bone mass, is a well-known effect of menopause and aging in adults, it is also a significant problem among younger individuals. Hypothalamic amenorrhea in young women is associated with reduced bone accretion or premature bone loss during adolescence [40–49], which places women at high risk for fractures, significant osteopenia (diminished bone mass) and severe osteoporosis at menopause. Amenorrhea in athletic women affects trabecular and cortical bone. Weight-bearing physical activity does not completely compensate for the side-effects of reduced estrogen levels even in weight-bearing bones in the lower extremities and the spine [50]. The most recent research suggests that poor nutrition or an energy deficit with an adaptation to large caloric needs is fundamentally linked not only with a prolonged amenorrheic state, but with osteopenia as well [51–54].

Definitions

Osteoporosis is a condition in which the rate of bone resorption exceeds the rate of bone formation. This imbalance leads to a progressive loss of bone mass, which in turn leads to a decrease in bone strength. It is a major public health concern and it often proceeds unnoticed until a stress fracture occurs. The World Health Organization formed a committee in 1994 to define osteoporosis. That committee created four diagnostic categories: Normal, Osteopenia, Osteoporosis and Established Osteoporosis. These diagnostic categories depend on bone density, and the presence of fractures. The committee set cut-off values that were relative to young healthy individuals. Osteopenia is a bone density between one standard deviation and 2.5 standard deviations below average for young people. Osteoporosis is a bone density lower than 2.5 standard deviations below young people [55].

Etiology

Like GnRH inhibition, osteopenia may also be an adaptive response to chronic low energy intake. Metabolic factors in response to nutritional insults might mediate reproductive and bone growth adaptations.

Two homeostatic mechanisms act on bone simultaneously: hormones and mechanical stress. In normal circumstances, these homeostatic mechanisms maintain both skeletal integrity and serum calcium levels. However, with aging or menstrual disturbance, factors such as diet, hormonal levels and mechanical strain cause bones to become more vulnerable to fracture and osteoporosis [56].

Recent studies suggest that at least 40% of bone mass is formed during adolescence and young adulthood, making this period critical to women's health [2,57–60]. The amount of bone attained during adolescence is a major determinant for fractures and osteoporosis later in life. As the skeleton enlarges in children and adolescents, bones are constantly growing; bones model as bone mass is added to areas of high loading or stress, and remodel as fatigue-damaged bone is resorbed and replaced by new bone [61]. Women who fail to reach peak bone mass (the maximal amount of bone tissue accrued in individual bones and the whole skeleton) are at an increased risk for osteoporosis later in life, and the reduction of bone mass accretion during adolescence may be a major cause of low bone density and fracture in old age [62]. After the age of 40, bone mass begins to decline [63].

Bone density is responsive to mechanical loading, and exercise is beneficial in preserving and increasing bone mass. In the mature, postmenopausal woman, exercise will offset the loss of bone mass associated with hypoestrogenism, and may even increase BMD above baseline. However, studies of hypoestrogenic ballet dancers suggest that they may not accumulate bone in response to mechanical stress [48] and amenorrheic athletes consistently exhibit spinal BMD 10–20% lower than their eumenorrheic counterparts [44,64–67]. When peak bone mass is not attained, the relative osteopenia in weight-bearing bones results in a higher risk for injury. A high incidence of stress fractures (61%), as directly related to delayed menarche, has been reported in young ballet dancers [49] and one study of ballet dancers found that the incidence of both scoliosis and stress fractures rose with each year of delayed menarche [68]. Studies have shown that spinal BMD is particularly affected in amenorrheic athletes [69] because high-impact activity appears to have a beneficial effect on BMD primarily at the hip [68]. One 1999 pilot study found the amenorrheic athlete's vertebral BMD to be up to 25% lower than normally cycling athletes [70].

It is unclear what changes in bone metabolism cause osteoporosis in women with hypothalamic amenorrhea. One 1999 study of women with anorexia nervosa suggested that bone formation is reduced while bone resorption remains normal [71], while another suggested that bone formation is decreased and bone resorption increased [72]. Further analyses of bone turnover indices in women with hypothalamic amenorrhea and anorexia nervosa have also produced inconsistent results, with some data suggesting normal bone turnover, while others suggesting low bone formation that is uncoupled from bone resorption [73,74]. Results of a 1998 study of amenorrheic long-distance runners demonstrated reductions in bone turnover and, in particular, bone formation [53]. The reduced bone formation was linked to a low BMI and an estrogen deficiency [54]. While the effects of prolonged estrogen deficiency on adolescents are not fully understood, recent research suggests that hypoestrogenism in young women decreases bone density and increases the risk of stress fractures and osteoporosis [2], causing serious bone loss similar to that which occurs after artificial or spontaneous menopause [47,75].

Nutrition and diet may be strongly predictive of stress fractures. A 1990 study found that dancers with restrictive eating patterns and eating disorders showed a much higher incidence of stress fractures than dancers without [76]. The diet of the dancers who sustained stress fractures was also much lower in fat and higher in the use of low caloric substitutes, such as saccharine, and nutritional supplements, such as vitamins. (Figs 4.6.1 & 4.6.2).

A recent study followed 111 subjects: 54 dancers (32 amenorrheic, 22 normal) and 57 controls (35 amenorrheic, 22 normal). Both exercising and non-exercising amenorrheics showed reduced BMD in the spine, wrist and foot. During the course of the study, seven of the amenorrheic women resumed menses, and while these seven showed an increase in spine and wrist BMD of 17%, they did not achieve normalization of BMD, suggesting that reduced bone accretion may result in a permanent failure to achieve peak bone mass. This underscores the importance of treatment, either preventative or therapeutic, for women with amenorrhea [77] (Table 4.6.4).

Early bone loss and osteoporosis are well documented and are common complications of anorexia nervosa [40,47,78–80]. Up to one-third of females who recovered from anorexia nervosa during adolescence were found to have persistent osteopenia [81]. Young women with anorexia nervosa may suffer irreversible developmental and growth retardation; older chronic

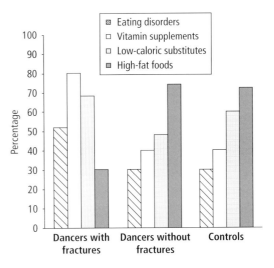

Fig. 4.6.1 Nutritional habits of dancers with and without stress fractures. From [76].

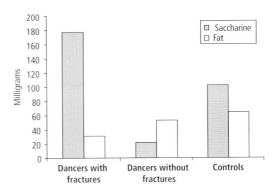

Fig. 4.6.2 Consumption of fat and saccharine. From [76].

anorectics are at a higher risk for pathologic fractures [82]. Multiple factors increase risk, including decreased body weight and fat content, elevated cortisol levels, inadequate vitamin D and calcium intake, and amenorrhea and hypoestrogenemia. Patients with bulimia nervosa or an eating disorder not otherwise specified may also be at risk for osteoporosis, particularly if they had an episode of anorexia nervosa at some point [83].

A 1990 study of ballet dancers with and without stress fractures found a strong correlation between certain dietary measures and the incidence of stress fractures [76]. When matched for age, weight and height, dancers who suffered fractures had much

Table 4.6.4 Bone density in amenorrhea in a 2-year longitudinal study.

Bone density (g/cm² ± SE)	Amenorrheic (n = 12)	Resumption of menses (n = 7)	Normal (n = 36)
Spine			
Baseline	1.16 ± 0.04	0.99 ± 0.05	1.27 ± 0.03
24 months	1.20 ± 0.04	1.16 ± 0.06	1.31 ± 0.02
% change	4.05 ± 1.95	17.47 ± 4.93*	4.01 ± 1.19
Wrist			
Baseline	0.61 ± 0.02	0.59 ± 0.05	0.66 ± 0.01
24 months	0.62 ± 0.03	0.67 ± 0.03	0.67 ± 0.01
% change	3.09 ± 2.37	17.54 ± 8.75*	2.85 ± 1.44
Foot			
Baseline	0.84 ± 0.03	0.76 ± 0.03	0.87 ± 0.02
24 months	0.83 ± 0.02	0.81 ± 0.03	0.86 ± 0.01
% change	−1.85 ± 2.88	7.05 ± 4.79	−0.74 ± 1.69

* $P < 0.001$. From [77].

more saccharin and much less fat in their diets than healthy dancers and normal controls, were significantly more likely to supplement their diets with vitamin supplements, and were far more likely to have eating disorders than their stress fracture-free counterparts (Figs 4.6.1 & 4.6.2). Thus, even in two athletes with similar weights and training regimens, it is possible that diet and nutrition are strongly predictive of osteopenia.

Other recent data also suggest that nutritionally regulated processes may underlie the osteopenia. Hypercortisolemia [20,84,85], hypoprogestinemia [85], insulin-like growth factor I (IGF-I) deficiency [52] or other metabolic adaptations seen in these athletes may contribute to the osteopenia. Undernutrition lowers bone formation markers, triiodothyronine (T3) and IGF-I in amenorrheic runners, but not in controls [52]. A 1986 study of ballet dancers showed normal vitamin D and parathyroid levels, suggesting that these may not be the causal factors in the bone loss [49]. In past studies of women with anorexia nervosa, levels of IGF-I and T3, two nutritionally dependent hormones, predicted the change in trabecular bone mass with estrogen–progestin therapy [86].

Leptin

Recently, leptin receptors were found on bone [87,88], suggesting that leptin may function as a physiologic regulator of bone mass. This presents the possibility of a mechanism other than hypoestrogenism that could

account for the low bone density and high stress fracture rates seen in women whose amenorrhea is associated with caloric deficiency, nutritional insults and exercise [13,16,73].

IGF-I

Levels of the bone trophic hormone insulin-like growth factor I (IGF-I) are closely correlated with certain indicators of nutritional status, such as BMI and leptin levels [71] and are also significantly reduced in patients with anorexia nervosa [53,71,89]. Results of a 1998 study of long-distance runners showed that IGF-I was one of the most powerful predictors of serum estrogen concentration [54]. It is hypothesized that IGF-I acts as a major contributor to the pathogenesis of osteopenia in hypothalamic amenorrhea. Deficiencies of the adrenal steroid dehydroepiandrosterone (DHEA) may inhibit secretions of IGF-I and other bone growth stimulators. Correcting DHEA deficiencies may prove to be a mechanism by which to increase secretions of IGF-I and other bone growth stimulators [90].

Cortisol

Subclinical hypercortisolism is prevalent in women with hypothalamic amenorrhea [91–93]. Hypercortisolism is associated with osteopenia, and may possibly contribute to bone loss via hypercortisolism-associated derangements in calcium and vitamin D metabolism including decreased osteoblastic activity, decreased intestinal absorption of calcium and increased urinary calcium losses [90].

Treatment

Ideally, female athletes should not develop long-term amenorrhea. In athletes with complete amenorrhea, a physical and pelvic examination is indicated to rule out androgenization, galactorrhea and hyperprolactinemia, as well as pregnancy. A careful history of weight loss and eating disorders should also be taken; eating disorders can often be missed, and often a standardized scale or diagnostic interview will be helpful in making the diagnosis [2].

Frequently, a weight gain of 1–2 kg or a 10% decrease in the duration or intensity of exercise is enough to reverse reproductive dysfunction [94,95]. Patients often resist this route, fearing weight gain may lead to decreased performance.

The most common treatment for young amenorrheic women has traditionally been estrogen therapy and oral contraceptives. Because of estrogen's antiresorptive effects on bone modelling, exogenous estrogen is often prescribed to prevent bone loss and/or increase overall bone accretion in women with hypothalamic amenorrhea, although clinical studies have not yet consistently demonstrated its efficacy in this group [72,96]. Preliminary studies on small numbers of subjects suggest that oral contraceptives may be effective in athletic amenorrhea [37], and another study showed that estrogen treatment produced increased spine and femoral BMD [90]. However, another investigation of estrogens and oral contraceptives indicated that the contraceptives prompted no change in BMD [97]. Research has not yet consistently demonstrated the efficacy of hormone replacement therapy or oral contraceptives in increasing the bone mass of women with hypothalamic amenorrhea [96] (Tables 4.6.5 & 4.6.6).

A lack of response to estrogen–progestin therapy in replacement doses has also been reported when given to anorectic women with hypothalamic amenorrhea [74,86]. Treatment of osteoporosis in anorexia nervosa includes weight normalization and supplemental calcium and vitamin D. Unlike postmenopausal osteoporosis, estrogen replacement does not prevent or correct the osteoporosis that occurs in anorexia nervosa [83]. Even after recovery, studies have found conflicting data about weight gain and changes in bone mineral density, and there is still uncertainty about the restoration of bone density with complete and sustained clinical recovery from anorexia nervosa [81,82,86,103,104]. The effect of estrogen supplementation differs from patient to patient. Further studies of different hormone replacement therapy regimens are needed, and the possibilities of other therapies aimed at increasing bone formation such as fluoride treatment, recombinant human insulin-like growth factor and recombinant human transforming growth factor β (TGF-β) are now being studied [72].

Eating disorders

Introduction

Some athletes and non-athletes do not consider train-

Table 4.6.5 Hormone replacement therapy (HRT) and its effect on bone mineral density (BMD).

Model	Study	Treatment (n)	BMD		
			Spine	Hip	Total
Hypothalamic amenorrhea (including eating disorders)	Hergenroeder[98]	Oral contraceptive, randomized, 12 months 0.035 mg ethinyl E_2 0.5–1.0 mg norethindrone (5)	↑	NS	↑
Exercise-induced amenorrhea	Cumming et al. [99]	HRT, observed 24–30 months (8)	↑	↑	–
Exercise-induced amenorrhea	Warren et al. [77]	HRT, randomized, 24 months (13)	NS	NS	–
Anorexia nervosa	Klibanski et al. [86]	HRT, randomized (22)	NS*	–	–

* Patients with the lowest BMD showed some increase. NS, not significant.

Table 4.6.6 Markers of bone turnover.

Model	Study (*n*)	Bone Formation	Resorption	Turnover
Postmenopausal estrogen deficiency	Manolagas [100] (review)	↑	↑	↑
Exercise-induced amenorrhea (runners)	Okano [101] (8)	↓	NA	?
Exercise-induced amenorrhea (runners)	Zanker [102] (9)	↓ (osteocalcin BAP*)	↓ (Dpyr†)	↓

* Bone-specific alkaline phosphate.
† Deoxypyridinoline.

ing or exercise sufficient to accomplish their idealized body weight or percentage body fat. Therefore, a significant number of them diet and use harmful, ineffective weight-loss practices such as restrictive eating, vomiting, laxatives and diuretics to meet their goals [105]. Eating disorders are the common denominator for such behaviors. Eating disorders can result in short- and long-term morbidity, poor recovery, impaired sports performance and mortality [106–108]. Signs and symptoms of eating disorders in athletes are often ignored. In some sports disordered eating seems to be regarded as a natural part of being an athlete [109]. It has been claimed that female athletes are at increased risk for developing eating disorders due to the focus on low body weight as a performance enhancer, comments from coaches or others and the pressure to perform [108,110,111].

Symptoms of eating disorders are more prevalent among elite athletes than non-athletes [108,112–114]. This section reviews the definitions, diagnostic criteria, prevalence and risk factors for the development of eating disorders in sport. Practical implications for the identification and treatment of eating disorders in athletes are also discussed.

Definitions

Eating disorders are characterized by disturbances in eating behavior, body image, emotions and relationships. Athletes constitute a unique population, and special diagnostic considerations should be made when working with this group [105,115,116]. Despite similar symptoms subclinical cases in athletes are easier to identify than in non-athletes [108]. Since

athletes, particularly at the elite level, are evaluated by their coach every day, changes in behavior and physical symptoms may be observed. However, symptoms of eating disorders in competitive athletes are too often ignored or not detected by coaches. Reasons for this include lack of knowledge of symptoms, feelings of guilt and the absence of strategies for approaching the eating-disordered athlete.

Tables 4.6.7 and 4.6.8 summarize the standard diagnostic criteria for anorexia nervosa and bulimia nervosa as defined by the fourth edition of the *Diagnostic and Statistical Manual of Mental Disorders* (DSM-IV) [117]. These criteria formalize overlapping conventions for subtyping anorexia nervosa into restricting and binge-eating/purging types on the basis of the presence or absence of bingeing and/or purging (i.e. self-induced vomiting or the misuse of laxatives or diuretics). Eating-disordered athletes often move between these two subtypes. However, it is the author's experience that chronicity leads to an accumulation of eating-disordered athletes in the binge-eating/purging subgroup.

The 'eating disorder not otherwise specified' category (EDNOS) [117] refers to disorders of eating that do not meet the criteria for any specific eating disorder. Examples of EDNOS are listed in Table 4.6.9, and the category acknowledges the existence and importance of a variety of eating disturbances. In the early phase of research on athletes and eating disorders the term 'anorexia athletica' was introduced [105]. Most of those athletes meeting the anorexia athletica criteria will also meet the criteria described in EDNOS.

Table 4.6.7 Diagnostic criteria for anorexia nervosa.

A Refusal to maintain body weight at or above a minimally normal weight for age and height (e.g. weight loss leading to maintenance of body weight less than 85% of that expected; or failure to make expected weight gain during period of growth, leading to body weight less than 85% of that expected)
B Intense fear of gaining weight or becoming fat, even though underweight
C Disturbance in the way in which one's body weight or shape is experienced, undue influence of body weight or shape on self-evaluation, or denial of the seriousness of the current low body weight
D In postmenarcheal females, amenorrhea, i.e. the absence of at least three consecutive menstrual cycles. (A woman is considered to have amenorrhea if her periods occur only following hormone (e.g. estrogen) administration.)

Specify type:
Restricting type: During the episode of anorexia nervosa, the person has not regularly engaged in binge-eating or purging behavior (i.e. self-induced vomiting or the misuse of laxatives, diuretics or enemas)
Binge-eating/purging type: During the current episode of anorexia nervosa, the person has regularly engaged in binge-eating or purging behavior (i.e. self-induced vomiting or the misuse of laxatives, diuretics or enemas)

From [117].

Prevalence of eating disorders among athletes

The epidemiology of eating disorders poses a particular challenge to investigators due to problems with case definition, and the tendency of eating-disordered subjects to conceal their illness and avoid professional help.

Estimates of the prevalence of the symptoms of eating disorders and clinical eating disorders among female athletes range from less than 1% to as high as 75% [108,118,119]. The prevalence of anorexia nervosa (2.2%), bulimia nervosa (7.2%) and subclinical eating disorders (10%) are more prevalent among female elite athletes than non-athletes [120]. Furthermore, this study showed that eating disorders are more frequent among female elite athletes competing in aesthetic and weight-class sports than among other sport groups where leanness is considered less important (Fig. 4.6.3).

Only two previous studies on male wrestlers [121,122] have based their results on the diagnostic criteria set forth by the *Diagnostic and Statistical*

Table 4.6.8 Diagnostic criteria for bulimia nervosa.

A Recurrent episodes of binge eating. An episode of binge eating is characterized by both of the following: (i) eating, in a discrete period of time (e.g. within any 2-h period), an amount of food that is definitely larger than most people would eat during a similar period of time in similar circumstances; and (ii) a sense of lack of control over eating during the episode (e.g. a feeling that one cannot stop eating or control what or how much one is eating)
B Recurrent inappropriate compensatory behavior in order to prevent weight gain, such as: self-induced vomiting; misuse of laxatives, diuretics or other medications; fasting; or excessive exercise
C The binge-eating and inappropriate compensatory behaviors both occur, on average, at least twice a week for 3 months
D Self-evaluation is unduly influenced by body shape and weight
E The disturbance does not occur exclusively during episodes of anorexia nervosa

Specify type:
Purging type: The person regularly engages in self-induced vomiting or the misuse of laxatives, diuretics or enemas
Non-purging type: The person uses other inappropriate compensatory behaviors, such as fasting or excessive exercise, but does not regularly engage in self-induced vomiting or the misuse of laxatives, diuretics or enemas

From [117].

Table 4.6.9 The 'eating disorder not otherwise specified' category.

1 All of the criteria for anorexia nervosa are met except the individual has regular menses.
2 All of the criteria for anorexia nervosa are met except, despite significant weight loss, the individual's current weight is in the normal range.
3 All of the criteria for bulimia nervosa are met except binges occur at a frequency of less than twice a week or for a duration of less than 3 months.
4 An individual of normal body weight regularly engages in inappropriate compensatory behavior after eating small amounts of food (e.g. self-induced vomiting after the consumption of two cookies).
5 An individual who repeatedly chews and spits out, but does not swallow, large amounts of food.
6 Binge-eating disorder: recurrent episodes of binge eating in the absence of inappropriate compensatory behaviors characteristic of bulimia nervosa.

From [117].

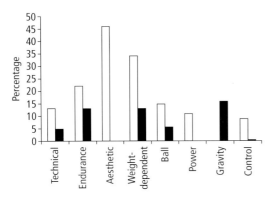

Fig. 4.6.3 Prevalence of eating disorders in female (*n* = 572) and male (*n* = 687) elite athletes. (None of the female athletes in the power and gravitation sports and none of the male athletes in the aesthetic or power sports met the DSM-IV criteria.) From [120].

Manual of Mental Disorders (DSM) [117]. They reported 1.7% and 1.4%, respectively, of male wrestlers with bulimia. A recent Norwegian study reported the prevalence of eating disorders to be as high as 8% among male elite athletes and 0.6% in age-matched controls. As many as 4.0%, 3.5% and 0.4% met the criteria for EDNOS, bulimia nervosa and anorexia nervosa, respectively [114,120]. The prevalence of clinical eating disorders in male elite athletes is highest among those competing in weight-class sports and gravitation sports [114].

Risk factors for the development of eating disorders

The etiology of eating disorders is multifactorial [123,124]. Because of additional stress associated with the athletic environment, however, female elite athletes appear to be more vulnerable to eating disorders than the general female population [111]. Furthermore, recent studies suggest that specific risk factors for the development of eating disorders occur in some sport settings; one retrospective study indicated that a sudden increase in training load may induce a caloric deprivation in endurance athletes, which in turn may elicit biologic and social reinforcements leading to the development of eating disorders [108]. However, longitudinal studies with close monitoring of a number of sports-specific factors (volume, type and intensity of training) are needed to answer questions about the role played by different sports in the development of eating disorders in athletes. Female athletes with eating disorders frequently start sport-specific training at an earlier age than healthy athletes [108]. Another factor to consider is that if female athletes start sport-specific training at a prepubertal age, they might not choose the sport that will be most suitable for their adult body type.

Many athletes report that they developed eating disorders as a result of traumatic events, such as the loss or change of a coach, injury, illness or overtraining [108,120,124]. An injury can curtail the athlete's exercise and training habits. As a result, the athlete may gain weight owing to less energy expenditure, which in some cases may develop into an irrational fear of further weight gain. Then the athlete may begin to diet to compensate for the lack of exercise [116].

Pressure to reduce weight has been a common explanation for the increased prevalence of eating-related problems among athletes. However, the important factor may not be dieting *per se*, but rather the situation in which the athlete is told to lose weight, the words used and whether the athlete receives guidance. In addition to the pressure to reduce weight, athletes are often pressed for time and must lose weight rapidly to make or stay on the team. As a result they often experience frequent periods of restrictive dieting or weight cycling [108]. Weight cycling has been suggested as an important risk or trigger factor for the development of eating disorders in athletes [108,125] and has been seen in men as well as women. Wrestlers have been characterized as high-risk athletes for developing eating disorders. A recent study on wrestlers concluded that although in-season wrestlers are more weight-conscious than non-wrestlers, these feelings and attitudes are transient [126]. Whether male athletes competing in weight-class sports have a transient condition or true clinical eating disorder may depend on the competitive level and the number of years of practicing weight loss techniques with weight fluctuation.

On the other hand, some authors argue that specific sports attract individuals who are anorectic before commencing their participation in sports, at least in attitude if not in behavior or weight [116,127]. It is possible that the attraction-to-sport hypothesis might be true for the general population, but athletes do not achieve the elite level if the only motivation is weight loss. Therefore, this hypothesis could probably rather be true for lower-level athletes. In most cases, the role of coaches in the development of eating disorders in athletes should be seen as part of a complex interplay of factors. Most researchers agree that coaches do not cause eating disorders in athletes, although inappropriate coaching may trigger or exacerbate the problem in vulnerable individuals [111]. There is a clear need for longitudinal quantitative and qualitative studies.

Medical issues

Eating disorders may cause serious medical problems and can even be fatal. Whereas most complications of anorexia nervosa occur as a direct or indirect result of starvation, complications of bulimia nervosa occur as a result of binge eating and purging [116]. Hsu [107], Johnson *et al.* [128], and Mitchell [129] provide information on the medical problems encountered in eating-disordered patients. Anorexia nervosa has a standard mortality rate up to six times higher than that of the general population [130]. Death in anorexia nervosa is usually attributable to fluid and electrolyte abnormalities, or suicide [131]. Mortality in bulimia nervosa is less well studied, but deaths do occur, usually secondary to the complications of the binge–purging cycle, such as gastric ruptures, or suicide.

Mortality rates of eating disorders among athletes are not known. However, a number of deaths of top-level female athletes in gymnastics, running, alpine skiing and cycling have been reported in the media. Of the female elite athletes diagnosed in the Norwegian study 5.4% reported suicide attempts [108].

Long-term health effects of eating disorders

The long-term effects of body-weight cycling and eating disorders in athletes are unclear. Biologic maturation and growth have been studied in girl gymnasts before and during puberty, suggesting that young female gymnasts are smaller and mature later than females from sports that do not require extreme leanness, such as swimming [132,133]. However, it is difficult to separate the effects of physical strain, energy restriction and genetic predisposition to delayed puberty.

Besides increasing the likelihood of amenorrhea and stress fractures, early bone loss may inhibit achievement of normal peak bone mass. Thus, athletes with frequent or longer periods of amenorrhea may be at high risk of sustaining fractures. Longitudinal data on fast and gradual body weight reduction and cycling in relation to health and performance parameters in different groups of athletes are clearly needed.

The nature and the magnitude of the effect of eating disorders on health and athletic performance are influenced by the severity and chronicity of the eating disorder and the physical and psychological demands of the sport. In addition to the negative health consequences, repeated or severe weight-loss attempts will result in poor recovery and impaired sports performance [106–108]. Norwegian female elite athletes reported increased fatigue, anger or anxiety when attempting to rapidly lose body weight [120].

Identifying athletes with eating disorders

Many individuals with eating disorders do not realize that they have a problem and therefore do not seek treatment on their own. Athletes might consider seeking help only if they experience that their performance level is leveling off.

In contrast to the athletes with anorectic symptoms most athletes suffering from bulimia nervosa are at or near normal weight, and therefore their disorder is difficult to detect. Hence the team staff must be able to recognize the physical symptoms and psychological characteristics listed in Table 4.6.10. It should be noted that the presence of some of these characteristics does not necessarily indicate the presence of the disorder. However, the likelihood of the disorder being present increases as the number of presenting characteristics increases [116].

Treatment of eating disorders

Eating-disordered athletes are more likely to accept the idea of going for a single consultation than the idea of committing themselves to prolonged treatment. Themes and questions that should be included in the first consultation with athletes possibly suffering from eating disorders are listed in Table 4.6.10. Included in Table 4.6.11 is also what should be included in the review of system, evaluation, lab tests and treatment.

At the Norwegian Olympic Training Center, athletes with eating problems have their first consultation without any medical examination, blood tests or nutrition evaluation. The first consultation focuses on the

Table 4.6.10 Physical symptoms, psychological and behavioral characteristics of athletes with eating disorders.

Physical	Psychological and behavioral
Significant weight loss beyond that necessary for adequate sport performance*	Claims of 'feeling fat' despite being thin
Frequent and often extreme weight fluctuations†	Resistance to weight gain or maintenance recommended
Low weight despite eating large volumes†	Dieting that is unnecessary for appearance, health or sport performance
Amenorrhea or menstrual irregularity	Binge eating†
Reduced bone mineral density	Agitation when bingeing is interrupted†
Stress fractures	Unusual weighing behavior (i.e. excessive weighing, refusal to weigh, negative reaction to being weighed)
Dehydration	Compulsiveness and rigidity, especially regarding eating and exercise*
Hyperactivity	Excessive or obligatory exercise beyond that required for a particular sport
Electrolyte abnormalities	Exercising while injured despite prohibitions by medical staff
Bradycardia	Restlessness
Fatigue beyond that normally expected in training or competition	Social withdrawal
Gastrointestinal problems (i.e. constipation, diarrhea, bloating, postprandial distress)	Depression and insomnia
Hypothermia*	Excessive use of the restroom†
Lanugo*	Self-critical, especially concerning body, weight and performance
Muscle cramps, weakness or both	Substance abuse
Swollen parotid glands†	Use of laxatives, diuretics (or both)
Anxiety, both related and unrelated to sport performance	
Avoidance of eating and eating situations	

* Anorexia nervosa.
† Bulimia nervosa.

athlete's presentation of her 'problem'. Then one of the members of the treatment team presents the treatment approach to athletes with one or more components of the triad.

In the Norwegian model, athletes with eating disorders receive individual therapy, a modified cognitive group therapy program and nutritional counselling. The first consultation with athletes with suspected or manifested eating disorders is extremely important. The goal is to create an alliance for treatment. Furthermore we define the roles and clarify who will make decisions about the athlete's training and health. For a number of athletes with eating disorders we also have to redefine their ambitions and clarify the therapist's involvement in training and competition programs.

Treatment, training and competition

The treatment of athletes with eating disorders should be undertaken by health care professionals. Coaches should never try to diagnose or treat eating disorders, but they should be specific about their suspicions. Furthermore, coaches should encourage medical evaluation and support the athlete during treatment.

Establishing a trusting relationship may be easier when the eating-disordered athlete feels that the therapist is familiar with the athlete's sport in addition to being trained in treating eating-disordered patients. Therapists who have good knowledge about eating disorders and know about various sports will better understand the athlete's training setting, daily demands and relationships that are specific to the sport, the types of events and the competitive level. Building such a relationship includes respecting the athlete's desire to be lean for athletic performance and expressing a willingness to work together to help the eating-disordered athlete to be lean and healthy. The treatment team needs to accept the athlete's fears and irrational thoughts about food and weight, and then present a rational approach for achieving self-management of healthy diet, weight and training program [134]. The various types of treatment strategies have been described in detail elsewhere [116].

A total suspension of training during treatment is not necessarily an appropriate solution. Unless there are severe medical complications, the athlete should be allowed to continue training at a lower volume and decreased intensity. For athletes with an eating disorder,

Table 4.6.11 History and medical examination of female elite athletes with disordered eating.

HISTORY RELATED TO EATING DISORDERS	REVIEW OF SYSTEMS, EVALUATION, LAB TESTS AND TREATMENT

Exercise
 Athlete's sport participation (is it fun, does she want to continue competing?)
 ?Hours spent training per week and intensity: aerobic and anaerobic training
 Time spent exercising outside of normal training regimen
 Continuing training in spite of injury
 	
 Nutrition
 Eating pattern
 24-h food recall/3-day weighing
 Number of meals/snacks per day
 List of foods avoided (e.g. meat, sweets)
 How does she feel about her present weight/percentage body fat?
 What does she consider her ideal weight/percentage body fat?
 Has she ever tried to control her weight using vomiting, laxatives, diuretics, other drugs, fasting or excessive exercise?
 	
 Menstrual history
 Age of menarche
 Frequency and duration of periods
 Date of last menstrual period
 Degree of regularity since menarche
 Use of hormonal therapy
 How does she feel about menstruating/not menstruating
 	
 Family, medical and psychological history
 Family including:
   weight history
   eating disorders or any other psychiatric disorders
 Medical:
   chronic disease
   infections
   previous surgery
   medications
   injuries (including stress fractures)
 Psychological:
   present stress factors in her life
   general mood, self-esteem and body image
	Symptoms of starvation and purging
	 Cold intolerance
	 Amenorrhea, delayed menarche
	 Light-headedness/lack of concentration
	 Abdominal bloating
	 Fatigue
	 Constipation/diarrhea
	 Sore throat and chest pain
	 Face and extremity edema
	
	 Physical examination
	 Dry skin, brittle hair and nails
	 Decreased subcutaneous fat
	 Hypothermia
	 Bradycardia
	 Lanugo
	 Cold and discolored hands and feet
	 Orthostatic blood pressure changes
	 Parotid gland enlargement
	 Erosion of dental enamel
	
	 Laboratory evaluation
	 Urine analysis
	 Complete blood count and sedimentation rate
	 Chemistry panel including electrolytes, calcium, magnesium and renal, thyroid and liver function tests
	 Indication for an electrocardiogram:
	   pulse is less than 50 b.p.m.* (depending on sport participation)
	 Electrolyte abnormality
	 Frequent purging behavior
	
	 Treatment
	 Multidisciplinary team approach
	 Physician
	 Nutritionist
	 Psychologist/mental health professional
	 Coach (?)†
	 Trainer (?)†
	 Criteria for hospitalization:
	   weight 30% below normal
	   hypotension/dehydration
	   electrolyte abnormalities

* Take into consideration that low pulse could be training induced.
† Dependent on the coach or trainer and athlete relationship. A good relationship is assumed to have a positive effect on treatment.

it is important to acknowledge that some aspects of their disregulated eating patterns may be the result of self-discipline and long-term goals. Moreover, it may be necessary for the athletes to continue with a dietary regimen or intensive training program that would automatically be targeted for elimination in a non-athlete. In general, to avoid reinforcing a message that sport performance is more important than health, it is recommended that athletes do not compete during treatment. Nevertheless, competitions during treatment might be considered for individuals with less severe eating disorders who are engaged in low-risk sports.

Prognosis

For most athletes, the reasons for the development of eating disorder seem to be related to extreme dieting, overtraining, injury or other more sports-specific factors. Data from a pilot study indicate that it may be easier to treat athletes, and that their prognoses should be better. However, this has not been fully investigated. When it comes to treatment, athletes may have some advantages compared to non-athletes; they are used to complying with rules and programs and few have personality disorders or clinical depression. However, there are a few possible negative factors that may delay the treatment progression in some athletes: lack of introspection, atypical psychological experiences and 'brainwashed' parents.

Prevention of eating disorders in athletes

It is likely that talking to athletes and coaches about eating disorders and related issues such as reproduction, bone health, nutrition, body composition and performance may help to prevent eating disorders in that population [120]. Therefore, coaches, trainers, administrators and parents should receive information about eating disorders and related issues. In addition, coaches should realize that they can strongly influence their athletes. Coaches or others involved with young athletes should not comment on an individual's body size, or require weight loss in young and still growing athletes. Without further guidance, dieting may result in unhealthy eating behavior or eating disorders in highly motivated and uninformed athletes [135]. Because of the importance that athletes ascribe to their coaches, the success of a prevention program tends to be related to the commitment and support of the coaches and others involved.

Early intervention is also important, since eating disorders are more difficult to treat the longer they progress. Therefore professionals working with athletes should be informed about: the possible risk factors for the development of eating disorders; early signs and symptoms of eating disorders; the medical, psychological and social consequences of these disorders; how to approach the problem if it occurs; and what treatment options are available.

Summary

Overall, exercise is extremely beneficial to women. It reduces adiposity while improving cardiovascular fitness, physical endurance, work capacity, muscle mass, muscle strength, flexibility, neuromuscular coordination and cognitive function. However, overtraining, energy deficit and/or disordered eating can result in reproductive dysfunction for athletes. Untreated amenorrhea may result in an increase in the incidence of stress fractures, scoliosis and thin body mass, and greatly increases the risk of osteopenia and osteoporosis. It is important to address amenorrhea as soon as possible, using the appropriate combination of weight normalization, nutritional evaluation, training reduction, behavior modification and/or in some cases oral contraceptives or hormone replacement therapy. The treatment of amenorrhea can frequently double as treatment for the accompanying osteoporosis. Many studies have shown an increased prevalence of eating disorders among athletes when compared with the general population. Eating disorders in athletes can easily be missed unless they are specifically targeted. If untreated, eating disorders can have long-lasting physiologic and psychological effects and may even be fatal. Treating athletes with eating disorders should be undertaken only by qualified health care professionals, ideally those who are familiar with the athlete's sport.

Multiple choice questions

1 *The inhibition of this hormone is speculated to cause athletic amenorrhea:*

a luteinizing hormone

b gonadotropin-releasing hormone

c follicle-stimulating hormone

d estradiol.

2 *With undernutrition leptin levels are seen to:*

a fall

b rise

c remain the same.

3 *Which of the following is/are thought to be predictive of loss of bone mass?*

a Leptin.

b Dehydroepiandrosterone.

c Parathyroid.

d Insulin-like growth factor I.

e Triiodothyronine.

4 *Which of the following types of athletes are more likely to develop an eating disorder and/or amenorrhea:*

a long-distance runner (female)

b swimmer (female)

c wrestler (male)

d figure skater

e gymnast.

5 *Which of the following are common symptoms of eating disorders?*

a Swollen parotid glands.

b Abdominal bloating.

c Increased bone density.

d Warm hands and feet.

e Bradycardia.

References

1 Al-Othman FN, Warren MP. Exercise, the menstrual cycle, and reproduction. *Infertility Reprod Med Clinics N Am* 1998; **9**: 667–87.

2 Warren MP, Shangold MM. *Sports Gynecology: Problems and Care of the Athletic Female*. Cambridge, MA: Blackwell Science, 1997.

3 Constantini NW, Warren MP. Physical activity, fitness, and reproductive health in women: clinical observations. In: Bouchard C, Shephard RJ, Stephens T, eds. *Physical Activity, Fitness and Health: International Proceedings and Consensus Statement*. Champaign: Human Kinetics, 1994: 955–66.

4 Locke RJ, Warren MP. How to prevent bone loss in women with hypothalamic amenorrhea. *Women's Health Primary Care* 2000; **3**: 270–8.

5 Pettersson F, Fries H, Nillius SJ. Epidemiology of secondary amenorrhea: incidence and prevalence rates. *Am J Obstet Gynecol* 1973; **7**: 80–6.

6 Singh KB. Menstrual disorders in college students. *Am J Obstet Gynecol* 1981; **1210**: 299–302.

7 Abraham SF, Beumont PJV, Fraser IS, Llewellyn-Jones D. Body weight, exercise and menstrual status among ballet dancers in training. *Br J Obstet Gynaecol* 1982; **89**: 507–10.

8 Brooks-Gunn J, Warren MP, Hamilton LH. The relationship of eating disorders to amenorrhea in ballet dancers. *Med Sci Sports Exerc* 1987; **19**(1): 41–4.

9 Feicht CB, Johnson TS, Martin BJ. Secondary amenorrhea in athletes. *Lancet* 1978; 1145–6.

10 Glass AR, Deuster PA, Kyle SB, Yahiro JA, Vigersky RA, Schoomaker EB. Amenorrhea in olympic marathon runners. *Fertil Steril* 1987; **48**: 740–5.

11 Shangold MM, Levine HS. The effect of marathon training upon menstrual function. *Am J Obstet Gynecol* 1982; **143**: 862–9.

12 Sanborn CF, Martin BJ, Wagner WW Jr. Is athletic amenorrhea specific to runners? *Am J Obstet Gynecol* 1982; **143**: 859–61.

13 Laughlin GA. The role of nutrition in the etiology of func-

tional hypothalamic amenorrhea. *Curr Opin Endocrin Diabet* 1999; **6**: 38–43.

14 Schweiger U. Menstrual function and luteal-phase deficiency in relation to weight changes and dieting. *Clin Obstet Gynecol* 1991; **34**(1): 191–7.

15 Warren MP, Holderness CC, Lesobre V, Tzen R, Vossoughian F, Brooks-Gunn J. Hypothalamic amenorrhea and hidden nutritional insults. *J Soc Gynecol Invest* 1994; **1**: 84–8.

16 Warren MP, Voussoughian F, Geer EB, Hyle EP, Adberg CL, Ramos RH. Functional hypothalamic amenorrhea: hypoleptinemia and disordered eating. *J Clin Endocrinol Metab* 1999; **84**: 873–7.

17 Couzinet B, Young J, Brailly S, Le Bouc Y, Chanson P, Schaison G. Functional hypothalamic amenorrhoea: a partial and reversible gonadotrophin deficiency of nutritional origin. *Clin Endocrinol (Oxf)* 1999; **50**: 229–35.

18 Laughlin GA, Yen SSC. Nutritional and endocrine-metabolic aberrations in amenorrheic athletes. *J Clin Endocrinol Metab* 1996; **81**: 4301–9.

19 Ferin M, Jewelewicz R, Warren MP. *The Menstrual Cycle*. New York: Oxford University Press, 1993.

20 Loucks AB, Mortola JF, Girton L, Yen SSC. Alterations in the hypothalamic-pituitary-ovarian and the hypothalamic-pituitary-adrenal axes in athletic women. *J Clin Endocrinol Metab* 1989; **68**: 402–11.

21 Warren MP. The effects of exercise on pubertal progression and reproductive function in girls. *J Clin Endocrinol Metab* 1980; **51**(5): 1150–7.

22 Loucks AB, Brown R, King K, Thuma JR, Verdun M. A combined regimen of moderate dietary restriction and exercise training alters luteinizing hormone pulsatility in regularly menstruating young women. *Endocrine Society Annual Meeting,* Washington DC, 1995: 558–558.

23 Loucks AB, Heath EM. Induction of low-T3 syndrome in exercising women occurs at a threshold of energy availability. *Am J Physiol* 1994; **266**: R817–R823.

24 Myerson M, Gutin B, Warren MP *et al.* Resting metabolic rate and energy balance in amenorrheic and eumenorrheic runners. *Med Sci Sports Exerc* 1991; **23**(1): 15–22.

25 Kaufman BA, Warren MP, Wang J, Heymsfield SB, Pierson RN. Bone density and amenorrhea in ballet dancers is related to a decreased resting metabolic rate. *J Clin Endocrinol Metab* 2002; **87**: in press.

26 Salisbury JJ, Levine AS, Crow SJ, Mitchell JE. Refeeding, metabolic rate, and weight gain in anorexia nervosa: a review. *Int J Eating Disord* 1995; **17**: 337–45.

27 Tuschl RJ, Platte P, Laessle RG, Stichler W, Pirke KM. Energy expenditure and every day eating behavior in healthy young women. *Am J Clin Nutr* 1990; **52**: 81–6.

28 Zhang Y, Proenca R, Maffei M, Barone M, Leopold L, Friedman JM. Positional cloning of the mouse *obese* gene and its human homolog. *Nature* 1994; **372**: 425–32.

29 Cheung CC, Clifton DK, Steiner RA. Proopiomelanocortin neurons are direct targets for leptin in the hypothalamus. *Endocrinology* 1997; **138**: 4489–92.

30 Legradi G, Emerson CH, Ahima RS, Flier JS, Lechan RM. Leptin prevents fasting-induced suppression of prothyrotropin-releasing hormone messenger ribonucleic acid in neurons of the hypothalamic paraventricular nucleus. *Endocrinology* 1997; **138**: 2569–76.

31 Legradi G, Emerson CH, Ahima RS, Rand WM, Flier JS, Lechan RM. Arcuate nucleus ablation prevents fasting-induced suppression of proTRH mRNA in the hypothalamic paraventricular nucleus. *Neuroendocrinology* 1998; **68**: 89–97.

32 Miller KK, Parulekar MS, Schoenfeld E *et al*. Decreased leptin levels in normal weight women with hypothalamic amenorrhea: the effects of body composition and nutritional insults. *J Clin Endocrinol Metab* 1998; **83**: 2309–12.

33 Kopp W, Blum WF, von Prittwitz S *et al*. Low leptin levels predict amenorrhea in underweight and eating disordered females. *Mol Psych* 1997; **2**: 335–40.

34 Maffei M, Halaas J, Ravussin E *et al*. Leptin levels in human and rodent: measurement of plasma leptin and ob RNA in obese and weight-reduced subjects. *Nat Med* 1995; **1**: 1155–61.

35 Laughlin GA, Yen SSC. Hypoleptinemia in women athletes: absence of a diurnal rhythm with amenorrhea. *J Clin Endocrinol Metab* 1997; **82**: 318–21.

36 Loucks AB. Exercise training in the normal female. In: Warren MP, Constantini NW, eds. *Sports Endocrinology*. Totowa: NJ Humana Press, Inc., 2000: 165–80.

37 DeCree C, Lewin R, Ostyn M. Suitability of cyproterone acetate in the treatment of osteoporosis associated with athletic amenorrhea. *Int J Sports Med* 1988; **9**: 187–92.

38 Etherington J, Harris PA, Nandra D *et al*. The effect of weight-bearing exercise on bone mineral density: a study of female ex-elite athletes and the general population. *J Bone Min Res* 1996; **11**: 1333–8.

39 Chilibeck PD. Hormonal regulations of the effects of exercise on bone. In: Warren MP, Constantini NW, eds. *Contemporary Endocrinology: Sports Endocrinology*. Totowa: NJ Humana Press, Inc., 2000: 239–52.

40 Biller BMK, Saxe V, Herzog DB, Rosenthal DI, Holzman S, Klibanski A. Mechanisms of osteoporosis in adult and adolescent women with anorexia nervosa. *J Clin Endocrinol Metab* 1989; **68**: 548–54.

41 Dhuper S, Warren MP, Brooks-Gunn J, Fox RP. Effects of hormonal status on bone density in adolescent girls. *J Clin Endocrinol Metab* 1990; **71**: 1083–8.

42 Drinkwater BL, Nilson K, Chesnut CH III, Bremner WJ, Shainholtz S, Southworth MB. Bone mineral content of amenorrheic and eumenorrheic athletes. *N Engl J Med* 1984; **311**(5): 277–81.

43 Jonnavithula S, Warren MP, Fox RP, Lazaro MI. Bone density is compromised in amenorrheic women despite return of menses: a 2-year study. *Obstet Gynecol* 1993; **81**: 669–74.

44 Lindberg JS, Fears WB, Hunt MM, Powell MR, Boll D, Wade CE. Exercise-induced amenorrhea and bone density. *Ann Intern Med* 1984; **101**: 647–8.

45 Marcus R, Cann CE, Madvig P *et al*. Menstrual function and bone mass in elite women distance runners. *Ann Intern Med* 1985; **102**: 158–63.

46 Rigotti NA, Neer RM, Skates SJ, Herzog DB, Nussbaum SR. The clinical course of osteoporosis in anorexia nervosa: a longitudinal study of cortical bone mass. *J Am Med Assoc* 1991; **265**: 1133–8.

47 Rigotti NA, Nussbaum SR, Herzog DB, Neer RM. Osteoporosis in women with anorexia nervosa. *N Engl J Med* 1984; **311**: 1601–6.

48 Warren MP, Brooks-Gunn J, Fox RP, Lancelot C, Newman D, Hamilton WG. Lack of bone accretion and amenorrhea: Evidence for a relative osteopenia in weight bearing bones. *J Clin Endocrinol Metab* 1991; **72**: 847–53.

49 Warren MP, Brooks-Gunn J, Hamilton LH, Warren LF, Hamilton WG. Scoliosis and fractures in young ballet dancers. Relation to delayed menarche and secondary amenorrhea. *N Engl J Med* 1986; **314**: 1348–53.

50 Pettersson U, Stalnacke B, Ahlenius G, Henriksson-Larsen K, Lorentzon R. Low bone mass density at multiple skeletal sites, including the appendicular skeleton in amenorrheic runners. *Calcified Tissue Int* 1999; **64**: 117–25.

51 Tsafriri A, Dekel N, Bar-Ami S. The role of oocyte maturation inhibitor in follicular regulation of oocyte maturation. *J Reprod Fert* 1982; **64**: 541–51.

52 Zanker CL. Bone metabolism in exercise associated amenorrhoea: the importance of nutrition. *Br J Sports Med* 1999; **33**: 228–9.

53 Zanker CL, Swaine IL. Bone turnover in amenorrhoeic and eumenorrhoeic distance runners. *Scand J Med Sci Sports* 1998; **8**: 20–6.

54 Zanker CL, Swaine IL. The relationship between bone turnover, oestradiol, and energy balance in women distance runners. *Br J Sports Med* 1998; **32**: 167–71.

55 World Health Organization. Assessment of fracture risk and its application to screening for postmenopausal osteoporosis. *Technical Report Series*. Geneva: WHO, 1994: 843.

56 Smith EL, Gilligan C. Bone concerns. In: Shangold MM, Mirkin G, eds. *Women and Exercise: Physiology and Sports Medicine*. Philadelphia: FA Davis Co., 1994: 89–101.

57 Kreipe RE. Bones of today, bones of tomorrow (editorial). *Am J Dis Child* 1992; **146**: 22–5.

58 Kreipe RE, Forbes GB. Osteoporosis: a 'new morbidity' for dieting female adolescents? *Pediatrics* 1990; **86**: 478–80.

59 Ott SM. Editorial: Attainment of peak bone mass. *J Clin Endocrinol Metab* 1990; **71**: 1082A–1082C.

60 Riggs BL, Eastell R. Exercise, hypogonadism and osteopenia. *J Am Med Assoc* 1986; **256**: 392–3.

61 Barr SI, McKay HA. Nutrition, exercise, and bone status in youth. *Int J Sports Med* 1998; **8**: 124–42.

62 Bass SL, Myburgh KH. The role of exercise in the attainment of peak bone mass and bone strength. In: Warren MP, Constantini NW, eds. *Contemporary Endocrinology: Sports Endocrinology*. Totowa: NJ Humana Press, Inc., 2000: 253–80.

63 Arnaud CD. Osteoporosis: Using 'bone markers' for diagnosis and monitoring. *Geriatrics* 1996; **51**: 24–30.

64 Bennell KL, Malcolm SA, Wark JD *et al*. Skeletal effects of

menstrual disturbances in athletes. *Scand J Med Sci Sports* 1997; **7**: 261–73.

65 Fisher EC, Nelson ME, Frontera WR *et al*. Bone mineral content and levels of gonadotropins and estrogen in amenorrheic running women. *J Clin Endocrinol Metab* 1986; **62**: 1232–6.

66 Lloyd SJ, Triantafyllou SJ, Baker ER *et al*. Women athletes with menstrual irregularity have increased musculoskeletal injuries. *Med Sci Sports Exerc* 1986; **18**(4): 374–9.

67 Wolman RL, Clark P, McNally E, Harries M, Reeve J. Menstrual state and exercise as determinants of spinal trabecular bone density in female athletes. *Br Med J* 1990; **301**: 516–8.

68 Khan KM, Warren MP, Stiehl A, McKay HA, Wark JD. Bone mineral density in active and retired ballet dancers. *J Dance Med Sci* 1999; **3**: 15–23.

69 Rutherford OM. Spine and total body bone mineral density in amenorrheic endurance athletes. *J Appl Physiol* 1993; **74**: 2904–8.

70 Gibson JH, Mitchell A, Reeve J, Harries MG. Treatment of reduced bone mineral density in athletic amenorrhea: a pilot study. *Osteoporos Int* 1999; **10**: 284–9.

71 Soyka LA, Grinspoon S, Levitsky LL, Herzog DB, Klibanski A. The effects of anorexia nervosa on bone metabolism in female adolescents. *J Clin Endocrinol Metab* 1999; **84**: 4489–96.

72 Bruni V, Dei M, Vicini I, Beninato L, Magnani L. Estrogen replacement therapy in the management of osteopenia related to eating disorders. *Ann New York Acad Sci* 2000; **900**: 416–21.

73 Grinspoon S, Miller KK, Coyle C. Severity of osteopenia in estrogen-deficient women with anorexia nervosa and hypothalamic amenorrhea. *J Clin Endocrinol Metab* 1999; **68**: 402–11.

74 Kreipe RE, Hicks DG, Rosier RN, Puzas JE. Preliminary findings on the effects of sex hormones on bone metabolism in anorexia nervosa. *J Adolesc Health* 1993; **14**: 319–24.

75 Cann CE, Martin MC, Genant HK, Jaffe RB. Decreased spinal mineral content in amenorrheic women. *J Am Med Assoc* 1984; **251**: 626–9.

76 Frusztajer NT, Dhuper S, Warren MP, Brooks-Gunn J, Fox RP. Nutrition and the incidence of stress fractures in ballet dancers. *Am J Clin Nutr* 1990; **51**: 779–83.

77 Warren MP, Brooks-Gunn J, Fox RP, Holderness CC, Hyle EP, Hamilton WG. Osteopenia in exercise-induced amenorrhea using ballet dancers as a model: a longitudinal study. *J Clin Endocrinol Metab* 2002; **87**: in press.

78 Brotman AW, Stern TA. Osteoporosis and pathological fractures in anorexia nervosa. *Am J Psychiatr* 1985; **142**: 495–6.

79 Hay P, Delahunt JW, Hall A, Mitchell AW, Harper G, Salmond C. Predictors of osteopenia in premenopausal women with anorexia nervosa. *Calcified Tissue Int* 1992; **50**: 498–501.

80 Salisbury JJ, Mitchell JE. Bone mineral density and anorexia nervosa in women. *Am J Psychiatr* 1991; **148**: 768–74.

81 Bachrach LK, Katzman DK, Litt IF, Guido D, Marcus R. Recovery from osteopenia in adolescent girls with anorexia nervosa. *J Clin Endocrinol Metab* 1991; **72**: 602–6.

82 Hartman D, Crisp A, Rooney B, Rackow C, Atkinson R, Patel S. Bone density of women who have recovered from anorexia nervosa. *Int J Eating Disord* 1999; **28**: 107–12.

83 Powers PS. Osteoporosis and eating disorders. *J Pediatr Adolesc Gynecol* 1999; **12**: 51–7.

84 Ding JH, Sheckter CB, Drinkwater BL, Soules MR, Bremner WJ. High serum cortisol levels in exercise-associated amenorrhea. *Ann Intern Med* 1988; **108**: 530–4.

85 Prior JC, Vigna YM, Schechter MT, Burgess AE. Spinal bone loss and ovulatory disturbances. *N Engl J Med* 1990; **323**: 1221–7.

86 Klibanski A, Biller BMK, Schoenfeld DA, Herzog DB, Saxe VC. The effects of estrogen administration on trabecular bone loss in young women with anorexia nervosa. *J Clin Endocrinol Metab* 1995; **80**: 898–904.

87 Steppan CM, Chidsey-Frink KL, Crawford DT *et al*. Leptin administration causes bone growth in ob/ob mice. *Regul Pept* 2000; **92**: 73–8.

88 Thomas T, Gori F, Burguera B *et al*. Leptin acts on human marrow stromal cells to enhance differentiation to osteoblasts and to inhibit adipocyte differentiation: *Endocrinology* 1999; **140**: 1630–8.

89 Grinspoon S, Baum H, Lee K, Anderson E, Herzog D, Klibanski A. Effects of short-term recombinant human insulin-like growth factor I administration on bone turnover in osteopenic women with anorexia nervosa. *J Clin Endocrinol Metab* 1996; **81**: 3864–70.

90 Miller KK, Klibanski A. Amenorrheic bone loss. *J Clin Endocrinol Metab* 1999; **84**: 1775–83.

91 Berga SL, Mortola JF, Girton L *et al*. Neuroendocrine aberrations in women with functional hypothalamic amenorrhea. *J Clin Endocrinol Metab* 1989; **68**: 301–8.

92 Biller BMK, Federoff HJ, Koenig JI, Klibanski A. Abnormal cortisol secretion and responses to corticotropin-releasing hormone in women with hypothalamic amenorrhea. *J Clin Endocrinol Metab* 1990; **70**: 311–7.

93 Suh B, Liu J, Berga S, Quigley M, Laughlin G, Yen S. Hypercortisolism in patients with functional hypothalamic amenorrhea. *J Clin Endocrinol Metab* 1988; **66**: 733–9.

94 Drinkwater BL, Bruemner B, Chesnut CH III. Menstrual history as a determinant of current bone density in young athletes. *J Am Med Assoc* 1990; **263**: 545–8.

95 Prior JC, Vigna YM. Gonadal steroids in athletic women: Contraception, complications and performance. *Sports Med* 1985; **2**: 287–95.

96 Robinson E, Bachrach LK, Katzman DK. Use of hormone replacement therapy to reduce the risk of osteopenia in adolescent girls with anorexia nervosa. *J Adolesc Health* 2000; **26**: 343–8.

97 Biller BMK, Schoenfeld D, Klibanski A. Premenopausal osteopenia: Effects of estrogen administration (#1616). *Endocrin Soc Annu Meeting* 1993; **75**: 454.

98 Hergenroeder AC, O'Brian Smith E, Shypailo R, *et al*. Bone mineral changes in young women with hypothalamic amen-

orrhea treated with oral contraceptives, medroxyproges-terone, or placebo over 12 months. *Am J Obstet Gynecol* 1997; **176**: 1017–25.

99 Cumming DC. Exercise-associated amenorrhea, low bone density, and estrogen replacement therapy. *Arch Intern Med* 1996; **156**(19): 2193–5.

100 Manolagas SC, Jilka RL. Bone marrow, cytokines, and bone remodeling. Emerging insights into the pathophysiology of osteoporosis. *N Engl J Med* 1995; **332**(5): 305–11.

101 Okano H, Mizunuma H, Soda M, Matsui H, Aoki I, Honjo S, Ibuki Y. Effects of exercise and amenorrhea on bone mineral density in teenage runners. *Endocrine Journal* 1995; **42**: 271–6.

102 Zanker CL, Swaine IL. Bone turnover in amenorrhoeic and eumenorrhoeic distance runners. *Scand J Med Sci Sports* 1998; 8: 20–6.

103 Baker D, Roberts R, Towell T. Factors predictive of bone mineral density in eating-disordered women: a longitudinal study. *Int J Eating Disord* 2000; **27**: 29–35.

104 Carruth BR, Skinner JD. Bone mineral status in adolescent girls. effects of eating disorders and exercise. *J Adolesc Health* 2000; **26**: 322–9.

105 Sundgot-Borgen J. Prevalence of eating disorders in elite female athletes. *Int J Sport Nutr* 1993; **3**: 29–40.

106 Fogelholm M, Hilloskopri H. Weight and diet concerns in Finnish female and male athletes. *Med Sci Sports Exerc* 1999; **21**: 229–35.

107 Hsu LKG. *Eating Disorders*. New York: Guilford Press, 1990.

108 Sundgot-Borgen J. Risk and trigger factors for the development of eating disorders in female elite athletes. *Med Sci Sports Exerc* 1994; **26**: 414–9.

109 Sundgot-Borgen J. Eating disorders, energy intake, training volume, and menstrual function in high-level modern rhythmic gymnasts. *Int J Sport Nutr* 1996; **6**: 100–9.

110 Otis CL, Drinkwater B, Johnson MD, Loucks AB, Wilmore JH. American College of Sports Medicine position stand. The female athlete triad. *Med Sci Sports Exerc* 1997; **29**: i–ix.

111 Wilmore JH. Eating and weight disorders in the female athlete. *Int J Sport Nutr* 1991; **1**: 104–17.

112 Dummer GM, Rosen LW, Heusner WW. Pathogenic weight control behaviors of young competitive swimmers. *Phys Sports Med* 1987; **15**: 75–86.

113 Rosen LW, McKeag DB, Hough DO, Curley V. Pathogenic weight-control behavior in female athletes. *Physician Sportsmed* 1986; **14**(1): 79–86.

114 Torstveit G, Rolland CG, Sundgot-Borgen J. Pathogenic weight control methods and self-reported eating disorders among male elite athletes. *Med Sci Sports Exerc* 1998; **5**: 181.

115 Szmukler G, Eisler I, Gillies C, Hayward M. The implications of anorexia nervosa in a ballet school. *J Psychiatr Res* 1985; **19**: 177–81.

116 Thompson RA, Trattner-Sherman R. *Helping Athletes With Eating Disorders*. Champaign, IL: Human Kinetics, 1993.

117 American Psychiatric Association. *Diagnostic and Statistical Manual of Mental Disorders*, 4th edn. Washington, DC: American Psychiatric Association, 1994.

118 Gadpaille WJ, Sanborn CF, Wagner WW Jr. Athletic amenorrhea, major affective disorders, and eating disorders. *Am J Psychiatr* 1987; **144**: 939–42.

119 Warren BJ, Stanton AL, Blessing DL. Disordered eating patterns in competitive female athletes. *Int J Eating Disord* 1990; **6**: 565–9.

120 Sundgot-Borgen J, Klungland M. The female athlete triad and the effect of preventive work. *Med Sci Sports Exerc* 1998; **30**: 181 (abstract).

121 Lakin JA, Steen SN, Oppliger RA. Eating behaviors, weight loss methods, and nutrition practices among high school wrestlers. *J Comm Health Nurs* 1990; **7**: 223–34.

122 Oppliger RA, Landry GL, Foster SW, Lambrecht AC. Bulimic behaviors among interscholastic wrestlers: a statewide survey. *Pediatrics* 1993; **91**: 826–31.

123 Garfinkel PE, Garner DM, Goldbloom DS. Eating disorders: implications for the 1990s. *Can J Psychiatr* 1987; **32**: 624–31.

124 Katz JL. Some reflections on the nature of eating disorders. *Int J Eating Disord* 1985; **4**: 617–26.

125 Brownell KD, Steen SN, Wilmore JH. Weight regulation practices in athletes: Analysis of metabolic and health effects. *Med Sci Sports Exerc* 1987; **19**: 546–56.

126 Dale KS, Landers DM. Weight control in wrestling: eating disorders or disordered eating? *Med Sci Sports Exerc* 1993; **31**: 1382–9.

127 Sacks MH. Psychiatry and sports. *Ann Sports Med* 1990; **5**: 47–52.

128 Johnson C, Connor SM. *The Etiology and Treatment of Bulimia Nervosa*. New York: Basic Books, 1987.

129 Mitchell JE. *Bulimia Nervosa*. Minneapolis: University of Minnesota Press, 1990.

130 Nielsen S, Moller-Madsen S, Isager T, Jorgensen J, Pagsberg K, Theander S. Standardized mortality in eating disorders—a quantitative summary of previously published and new evidence. *J Psychosom Res* 1998; **44**: 413–34.

131 Brownell KD, Rodin J. Prevalence of eating disorders in athletes. In: Brownell KD, Rodin J, Wilmore JH, eds. *Eating, Body Weight, and Performance in Athletes: Disorders in Modern Society*. Philadelphia: Lea & Febiger, 1992: 128–43.

132 Mansfield MJ, Emans SJ. Growth in female gymnasts. Should training decrease during puberty? *J Pediatr* 1993; **122**: 237–40.

133 Theintz G, Howald H, Weiss U, Sizonenko PC. Evidence for a reduction of growth potential in adolescent female gymnasts. *J Pediatr* 1993; **122**: 306–13.

134 Clark N. How to help the athlete with bulimia: practical tips and a case study. *Int J Sport Nutr* 1993; **3**: 450–60.

135 Eisenman PA, Johnson SC, Benson JE. *Coaches' Guide to Nutrition and Weight Control*, 2nd edn. Champaign, IL: Leisure Press, 1990.

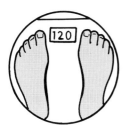

Chapter 4.7
Physical Activity and Obesity

PERTTI MUSTAJOKI, PER BJÖRNTORP &
ARNE ASTRUP

Classical reference

Prentice A, Jebb S. Obesity in Britain: gluttony or
sloth. *Br Med J* 1995; **311**: 437–439.
The paper describes the increased prevalence of
clinical obesity in Britain and demonstrates that this
has doubled over the decade from 1980 to 1990. It is
demonstrated that the cause for obesity cannot be
described as an increased absolute energy intake over
the years, but rather as a mismatch between food
intake and energy expenditure.

From Fig. 4.7.1 it can be seen that the increased
prevalence of obesity coincides with an increasing
amount of cars and hours of television viewing. Although no cause and effect relationship could definitively be stated from this paper, it is one of the first
papers to elegantly show that low levels of physical
activity play an important and perhaps dominating
role in the development of obesity by greatly reducing

energy needs.

The authors of the paper suggest that public health
strategies must be targeted both at a reduction in the fat
content of the diet and at avoidance of physical inactivity if they are to have any chance of reversing the current trend in obesity and of avoiding the associated
health consequences.

Introduction

There is a worldwide epidemic of obesity and because
it is followed by increased incidences of type 2 diabetes, heart disease and many other serious health
problems the WHO has given its prevention and
treatment the highest priority. Evidence suggests that
a major causal factor is increased physical inactivity.
The formulation of strategies to counteract this is
therefore highly topical. Physical activity and exercise
have many beneficial effects on health; among these are
increased energy expenditure, improved appetite

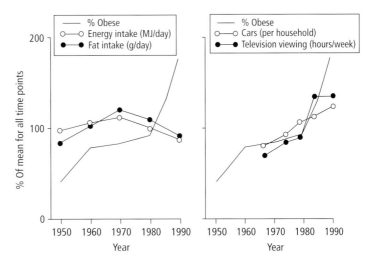

Fig. 4.7.1 Secular trends in diet (left)
and activity (right) in relation to obesity
in Britain. Data for diet from National
Food Survey; data for body mass index
from Office of Population Censuses and
Surveys and historical surveys; data for
television viewing and car ownership
from Central Statistical Office.

regulation and a lower risk of weight gain and obesity. Increased physical activity may be difficult to achieve in obese subjects and the impact on weight loss is minor. However, in normal-weight and slightly overweight populations, and in previously obese individuals after a dietary-induced weight loss, increased daily physical activity is an important component in the prevention of weight gain or regain, and obesity.

The role of physical inactivity in weight gain and obesity

The nature of physical activity

Physical activity is the increase of contraction of the muscles, particularly the large muscles in the leg, e.g. in walking or running. This costs energy and prevents the storage of too much lipid energy in adipose tissue, an essential part of the prevention of obesity. In the same way, the energy expended in physical activity can contribute to the creation of a negative energy balance, thus diminishing energy stores, and contribute to the treatment of obesity. A negative energy balance can also be accomplished by a decreased energy intake.

Physical activity is consequently a cornerstone in the prevention and treatment of obesity, but it must be acknowledged that a negative energy balance of thera-

Table 4.7.1 Different mechanisms by which increased physical activity and exercise can contribute to body weight control, and improve other health parameters.

 1 Increased energy expenditure
 2 Better aerobic fitness
 3 Improvement of body composition:
 • fat loss
 • preservation of lean body mass
 • reduction of visceral fat depot
 4 Increased capacity for fat mobilization and oxidation
 5 Control of food intake:
 • short-term reduction of appetite
 • reduction of fat intake
 6 Stimulation of thermogenic response:
 • resting metabolic rate
 • diet-induced thermogenesis
 7 Change in muscle morphology and biochemical capacity
 8 Increased insulin sensitivity
 9 Improved plasma lipid and lipoprotein profile
10 Reduced blood pressure
11 Positive psychological effects

peutic significance is more easily accomplished by dieting than by exercise. A decrease in daily food intake of 1000 kcal (4.2 MJ) is easily managed, but this corresponds to about 3 h of jogging, an activity which is impossible for most obese patients. Yet there is evidence that regular physical activity improves the possibility of maintaining energy balance, perhaps through an enhanced regulation of energy intake.

It is frequently forgotten that physical exercise exerts profound beneficial effects on the comorbidities associated with obesity (Table 4.7.1). The major action is the sensitization of muscle to insulin, and physical activity is thus the best available means to counteract insulin resistance, diminishing the risk of the development of type 2 diabetes mellitus, comorbidities such as dyslipidemia and hypertension, and other prevalent diseases.

Physical exercise appears to improve insulin sensitivity without necessarily creating a negative energy balance. This is seen as an acute effect after a bout of exercise and lasts for a day or two [1]. But, apparently, physical training also has more long-lasting effects. In a study by Björntorp *et al.* a group of obese subjects was submitted to a conventional physical training program whilst continuing with their habitual diet, i.e. they were asked not to diet during the experiment. In this way loss of body fat was prevented, but there was still a remarkable effect on insulin resistance [2]. This study showed that exercise training is a very efficient way to improve insulin resistance, and that this effect of training is independent of a decrease in body fat. However, as a rule body fat mass decreases with physical training, and this amplifies the sensitization to insulin. Lean, middle-aged men who exercise regularly have been found to dispose of 100 g oral glucose within 1 h of ingestion with a minimal increase in circulating insulin. In other words, they were markedly insulin sensitive [3]. This poses the question whether the effects of exercise on insulin resistance are not equally as important as the effects of loss of body fat mass in obesity, because obesity without its comorbidities should be a comparatively benign condition.

Assessment of physical activity

The amount of daily physical activity is very difficult to quantify, particularly over the prolonged period of time (years) involved in the development of obesity.

Typically an increase in weight of 10 kg occurs over a period of perhaps 2 years. This indicates that the individual has a positive energy balance of some 30–40 kcal/day, or the equivalent of 1–2% of total energy expenditure. This corresponds to an extra energy intake of less than half a sandwich per day or, on the output side, a walk of 15–30 min/day. In the short term these are such small changes in energy balance that they could perhaps correspond to differences in minor unconscious movements ('fidgeting') [4]. No method exists that can measure such differences over a sufficient period of time. The available methods, such as measurements of $\dot{V}o_{2\,max}$, step registration, Holter monitoring or activity history, are not very helpful at this low level of long-term change in energy balance. The problem is equally difficult for both energy intake and energy output, and such technical problems make obesity research very complicated. Free living energy expenditure can be measured with reasonable accuracy by the double-labeled water technique, and by subtracting resting metabolic rate from these readings a good estimate of the energetic cost of physical activity can be achieved. However, this method is very costly, which prohibits its use in population studies.

Epidemiologic evidence

Following the results of a survey by an expert group [5] of the global prevalence of obesity, the WHO has now declared obesity to be one of the major international health problems. The situation continues to worsen; for example, the prevalence of overweight and obesity in England has doubled over the past 10–15 years [5]. In this same period energy consumption, estimated on a national level, has been seen to be decreasing. This must mean that energy expenditure by physical exercise has diminished or, more accurately, that physical inactivity has been increasing. This is probably caused by a combination of the widespread availability of mechanized transportation, which requires no muscular activity, the increase in physically inactive jobs and production methods, and the increase in inactive leisure activities, such as watching television. The latter is a particular problem in children, where many age groups spend up to 5–6 h/day in front of the television [6]. The significance of these observations is, however, rather uncertain, as watching television is frequently associated with snacking, an indisputable contributor to the generation of obesity.

Because of the difficulties of assessment described above, most observations on physical inactivity are circumstantial. The available information does, however, suggest that physical inactivity is an important ingredient in the pathogenesis of the current obesity epidemic. If this interpretation is correct then the diminished physical inactivity is, of course, a highly important target priority in both prevention and therapy of obesity and its complications.

Prevention

Studies on the prevention of obesity by means of increased physical activity exclusively have not been performed, probably due to the practical difficulties inherent in such trials. The results of a few studies are available, showing some hopeful preventive results following a general change in lifestyle, including both dieting improvement and increased physical activity. The effects found are small. Even so, from a broader perspective they may be useful [7,8].

Physiologic mechanisms linking physical activity and energy balance

Increased physical activity and less physical inactivity raises total energy expenditure, allowing individuals to consume more calories without gaining weight. There are several lines of evidence to indicate that individuals with 'a low energy output syndrome' are at an increased risk of weight gain and obesity, irrespective of whether this is caused by a genetically determined low resting metabolic rate [9], by low levels of fidgeting or by an environmentally determined low level of physical activity [10]. Athletes with very high levels of physical activity may have the opposite problem: difficulty in ingesting enough calories to replenish and maintain body energy and fat stores.

Exercise bouts are followed by an acute suppression of hunger. This mechanism is short lived and it is more likely to occur after exercise of high intensity. Both physiologic and behavioral factors play a role in the maintenance of energy balance. Sedentary behavior allows more opportunity for food intake than a physically active lifestyle, e.g. children watching television are more likely to snack and drink than children engaged in sports activities.

The effect of exercise on energy intake

Does physical activity and exercise contribute to an improved appetite regulation? There is a public perception that exercise makes you eat more. This is most certainly true, but the important question is whether the resulting increase in energy intake fully, or only partially, compensates for the energetic cost of the physical activity. This may depend on the sizes of the fat stores and there is evidence to suggest that lean subjects fully compensate for the energy cost of exercise, while overweight and obese subjects are less likely to fully compensate. In a review, King *et al.* [11] conclude that exercise tends to normalize appetite response. It has also been suggested that exercise may help to regulate energy balance because of an asymmetry in appetite control, in which the hunger drive operates more powerfully and precisely than the satiety drive [12]. Overall, the available literature provides little evidence to suggest that exercise causes an increase in energy intake beyond compensation for the energy expended because of the exercise. There is usually a net energy deficit, which is more apparent in obese people, who appear to be less appetite responsive to exercise than normal-weight individuals.

Increased fat oxidation

The effect of exercise on substrate utilization may exert an impact on appetite regulation and energy intake, independent of the effect of exercise on energy expenditure. The contribution of fat oxidation to energy expenditure changes from nearly 100% at rest and during low-intensity exercise to very low levels during high-intensity exercise. However, the absolute oxidation of fat may be higher during high-intensity exercise than low-intensity exercise, because of the difference in total energy expenditure. It is known from studies in athletes that the body's capacity to store carbohydrate is very limited compared to its capacity to store fat. This has implications for the fuel mix that is oxidized, as well as for the ability of the overall regulatory system to counteract depletion of glycogen stores [13]. Consequently, variations in carbohydrate stores have a larger impact on appetite and satiety, and it is generally recognized that exercise that mainly utilizes fat as substrate is less likely to stimulate appetite. However, with regular high-intensity exercise training muscular fat oxidation capacity increases with increased fitness, and a larger proportion of the exercise-induced energy expenditure is covered by fat than in untrained individuals. Although these considerations suggest that fitness is an important independent factor in the regulation of body weight there is a need for more controlled studies with emphasis on identifying the optimal type of activity, i.e. endurance or strength, and optimal duration and frequency.

Interactions between dietary fat and physical activity

In a number of countries the prevalence of obesity has continued to rise despite a reduction in the proportion of calories from fat in the national diet. Having been observed in the USA, this phenomenon has been named 'The American Paradox' [14]. Among the explanations suggested for this apparent contradiction have been a concomitant overriding effect of decreasing physical activity, overconsumption of highly palatable, energy-dense, carbohydrate-rich, low-fat products, underreporting of fat consumed in dietary surveys, and obesity being an infectious disease caused by an adenovirus. It should be stressed, however, that a high dietary fat content is unlikely to be the only environmental factor responsible for obesity. A sedentary lifestyle with a low level of energy expended on physical activities is another causative factor, which interacts with dietary fat content. It has been demonstrated that dietary fat tolerance is greatly lowered by a sedentary lifestyle, even in non-obese individuals [15]. The result of this short-term study has been extended by a meta-analysis of intervention studies on the effect on weight loss of low-fat diets alone, and in combination with exercise [16]. Weight loss achieved by low-fat diet alone was 2.8 kg; with diet and exercise it was 5.7 kg. On a population basis the reduction of mean body weight by 5 kg could result in quite a dramatic change in the prevalence of obesity. The decrease in physical activity observed in population studies may therefore be responsible for the continuing increase in the prevalence of obesity. And the very modest, if any, decrease in dietary fat intake is insufficient to compensate for this development.

Physical activity in the treatment of obesity

Exercise and weight loss

The effect of exercise on body weight has been investigated in several studies. Wing systematically analysed investigations in which exercise without diet intervention had been studied in adults [17]. She found 10 randomized, controlled investigations which fulfilled the criteria set. Most of them included aerobic exercise (mostly walking). In six investigations statistically significant weight loss was observed, in four no change was seen. Thus, exercise without diet intervention seems to cause only minor weight loss, usually no more than 1–2 kg. The number of studies in children is too limited to evaluate the effect of exercise alone on weight reduction [18].

Weight reduction programs use a multidisciplinary approach. These include dietary counselling to decrease energy intake, exercise, and cognitive and behavioral therapy to promote permanent lifestyle changes. What are the effects of exercise in these programs? In Wing's review [17], 13 randomized, controlled trials addressing the treatment of adult obesity were evaluated. Interventions lasted from 4 to 6 months. Aerobic exercise was used in nine of the investigations, and strength exercise in four. In only two of the investigations did exercise cause statistically significant better weight loss than experiments with dietary intervention only. Thus, exercise seems to have only a weak, or even no, effect on weight loss, also in connection with dietary and behavioral interventions. Epstein and Goldfield [18] evaluated controlled trials in children and concluded that exercise increases the amount of weight lost in the short term. There were not enough trials to evaluate the long-term effect.

In weight reduction some three-quarters of the weight lost is comprised of adipose tissue and approximately one quarter is lean body mass. Does exercise during a weight reduction program preserve lean body mass better than dietary interventions without exercise? Garrow and Summerbell [19] evaluated this in a meta-analysis of studies in which exercise and non-exercise groups were compared. They found 28 studies from the years 1966–93 that fulfilled the criteria used. A regression analysis showed that for every 10 kg lost 2.9 kg in men and 2.2 kg in women was lean body mass when dietary intervention alone was used. When dietary intervention was combined with exercise the loss of lean body mass was 1.7 kg in both sexes. Thus exercise, especially strength exercise, may spare some 0.5–1 kg lean body mass for every 10 kg lost. This is probably advantageous although its clinical importance has not been demonstrated by investigation.

Exercise and maintenance after weight loss

Weight loss can generally be satisfactorily achieved through modern weight reduction programs but most people regain weight after concluding the weight loss programs. Weight maintenance after weight loss is a major challenge to obesity research. The effect of exercise on maintenance after weight loss has been evaluated in two recent reviews.

Wing [17] collected all randomized, controlled trials in which follow-up was 1 year or more. Six studies fulfilled the criteria used. In two studies exercise plus diet therapy was associated with significantly better maintenance than diet therapy alone. In four studies no significant effects were seen.

Fogelholm and Kukkonen-Harjula [20] evaluated all studies in which exercise was compared with non-exercise regimens and follow-up was 1 year or more. Seventeen non-randomized trials were included in the analysis. In 12 of these weight maintenance was associated with exercise during the intervention. Eighteen randomized, controlled trials were included and an association between weight maintenance and exercise was seen in four of these.

All in all, these results indicate some effect of exercise on weight maintenance, but the results vary. One reason for the variable results is that the investigation of long-term effects of exercise on weight maintenance is hampered by methodologic problems, such as how to measure the total amount of exercise, poor adherence to exercise programs, or a high dropout rate during long follow-up periods.

Weight gain is a consequence of an imbalance between energy intake and expenditure. Increased energy expenditure would certainly be an effective measure for weight maintenance, if people were willing to adopt a more active lifestyle. Variable and modest results in weight maintenance studies suggest that many obese people are not willing to do this. A key question is how obese individuals can be helped to adopt more active lifestyles.

A practical strategy for increasing physical activity in susceptible subjects

To increase physical activity it is necessary that individuals change their behavior. In planning a strategy for increasing physical activity in susceptible subjects general rules of behavior modification must be taken into consideration. These rules include the fact that most individuals are not motivated to change their habits when meeting a health care professional, admonition and advice is not usually effective, and changing an individual's habitual behavior is a complex process which takes time [21,22]. In addition there are specific problems attached to exercise for obese people: they are generally in worse physical condition and less motivated to exercise than normal-weight people.

If counselling is to be effective in increasing an individual's physical activity great attention must be paid to his or her motivation. Table 4.7.2 summarizes approaches that are likely to increase motivation for lifelong changes. Exercise 'prescribed' by a therapist is unlikely to be continued for the rest of a lifetime. Communication skills that include a client-centered approach are more likely to motivate sustained changes. In this approach the client determines the amount and quality of physical activity to be practised, and is responsible for planning the activity.

A multidisciplinary approach for increasing physi-

Table 4.7.2 Suggested practical strategies for counselling a client to increase physical activity for weight control.

Communication with the client
The counsellor does not give direct advice about how to exercise
The counsellor gives information and alternatives, the client makes choices
Minor changes are also reinforced, although they do not meet the expectations of the counsellor

Type of physical activity
Emphasis on low-intensity physical activity
Lifestyle activity as an alternative to structured exercise
The client selects a suitable type of physical activity in which he or she is interested

cal activity is recommended. This implies that preconceptions involving fixed pulse rate, specific types of exercise and whether the exercise is aerobic or not are not criteria of significance in the counselling of an obese individual about exercise. A client should be encouraged to select a type of exercise in which he or she is interested. Many obese people are not interested in formalized exercise programs and for them lifestyle activities are a useful alternative. Lifestyle activity includes taking the stairs instead of taking elevators or escalators, walking journeys of moderate distances instead of taking the car, using manual means to complete domestic tasks instead of using household machines, etc. In a randomized, controlled trial lifestyle activity has been shown to be as effective as aerobic exercise in weight maintenance after weight loss [23].

A recent clinical guideline for the treatment of obesity recommends that adults should set a long-term goal that they perform at least 30 min of moderate-intensity physical activity on most, and preferably all, days of the week [24]. This is a realistic goal for most obese people but in motivational communication minor changes, although they do not meet the expectations of the counsellor, should be reinforced.

Summary

Decreased levels of daily physical activity and exercise are important contributors to the increasing prevalence of overweight and obesity. The workplace and leisure-time-related inactivity which accompanies our modern lifestyle seems to be an additional factor. Lack of physical activity also increases the risk of type 2 diabetes, independent of the size of body fat mass. Increased daily physical activity level is therefore an important strategy for the prevention of weight gain and obesity.

Compared to energy restriction physical activity programs have only modest effects on weight loss in obese subjects. However, once a weight loss has been achieved through dietary restriction increased daily physical activity is important for long-term weight stability (Fig. 4.7.2).

Multiple choice questions

1 *To lose 1 kg body fat you have to jog for:*
a 2 h

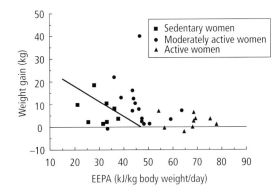

Fig. 4.7.2 Relationship between the free living energy expenditure produced by habitual physical activity and subsequent gain of body fat among a group of females with increased susceptibility to weight gain. The intercept with weight gain = 0 indicates that weight stability requires a daily energy expenditure of at least 47 kJ/kg body weight, which corresponds to an average of 80 min/day of moderate activity or 45 min/day of vigorous activity added to a sedentary lifestyle.

b 10 h

c 24 h

d 48 h

e 72 h.

2 *What is the definition of insulin resistance?*

a Increased insulin secretion.

b Increased secretion of hormones with effects antagonizing insulin effects.

c A diminished effect of insulin.

d Diabetes mellitus.

e Physical inactivity.

3 *Which one of the following statements is not correct? Insulin resistance is followed by:*

a hyperinsulinemia

b elevated very low density lipoproteins

c increased risk of the development of diabetes

d elevated cholesterol

e increased risk of developing cardiovascular disease.

4 *Physical activity may be useful for weight management because:*

a it represents a volume of energy expenditure under voluntary control

b it generates a large-scale energy deficit compared to energy restriction

c it has universal effects on individuals

d it only increases fat oxidation

e none of the above.

5 *In response to similar amounts of physical activity, which may be correct?*

a Males appear to lose more weight.

b Females appear to lose more fat weight.

c Males lose more fat-free mass compared to females.

d Males increase their fat mass.

e None of the above.

References

1 Fahlén M, Stenberg J, Björntorp P. Insulin secretion in obesity after exercise. *Diabetol* 1972; **8**: 141–4.

2 Björntorp P, deJounge K, Sjöström L, Sullivan L. The effects of physical training on insulin production in obesity. *Metabolism* 1970; **19**: 631–8.

3 Björntorp P, Grimby G, Sanne H, Sjöström L, Tibblin G, Wilhelmsen L. Adipose tissue fat cell size in relation to metabolism in weight-stabile, physically active men. *Hormone Metabol Res* 1972; **4**: 182–6.

4 Ainsworth BE. Compendium of physical activities: classification of energy costs of human physical activities. *Med Sci Sports Exerc* 1993; **25**: 71–80.

5 *Obesity. Preventing and Managing the Global Epidemic.* Report of a WHO Consultation on Obesity. Geneva, 3–5 June 1997. WHO/NUT/NCD/98.1, 1998.

6 Dietz WH, Gortmaker SL. Do we fatten our children at the televison set? Obesity and television viewing in children and adolescents. *Pediatrics* 1985; **75**: 807–12.

7 Jeffery RW, French SA. Preventing weight gain in adults. The Pound Prevention Study. *Am J Public Health* 1999; **89**: 747–51.

8 Taylor CB, Fortmann SP, Flora J *et al.* Effect of long-term community health education on body mass index. *Am J Epidemiol* 1991; **134**: 235–49.

9 Astrup A, Gotzsche PC, van de Werken K *et al.* Meta-analysis of resting metabolic rate in formerly obese subjects. *Am J Clin Nutr* 1999; **69**: 1117–22.

10 Thorburn AW, Proietto J. Biological determinants of spontaneous physical activity. *Obesity Rev* 2000; **1**: 87–94.

11 King AC, Tribble DL. Effects of exercise on appetite control: implications for energy balance. *Med Sci Sports Exerc* 1997; **11**: 331–49.

12 Blundell JE, King NA. Effects of exercise on appetite control: loose coupling between energy expenditure and energy intake. *Int J Obes Metabol Disord* 1998; **22** (Suppl. 2): S22–S29.

13 Saris WHM. Physical activity and body weight regulation. In: Bouchard C, Bray GA, eds. *Regulation of Body Weight: Biological and Behavioral Mechanisms.* Chichester, UK: John Wiley & Sons Ltd, 1996: 135–48.

14 Astrup A. The American paradox: the role of energy-dense fat-reduced food in the increasing prevalence of obesity. *Curr Opin Clin Nutr Metabol Care* 1998; **1**: 573–7.

15 Astrup A. Nutrition and diet for healthy lifestyles in Europe: obesity and diabetes. *Pub Health Nutr* 2001; **4**: 499–515.

16 Yu-Poth S, Zhao G, Etherton T, Naglak M, Jonnalagadda S, Kris-Etherton PM. Effects of the National Cholesterol Education Program's step I and step II dietary intervention programs on cardiovascular disease risk factors: a meta-analysis. *Am J Clin Nutr* 1999; **69**: 632–46.

17 Wing R. Physical activity in the treatment of the adulthood overweight and obesity: current evidence and research issues. *Med Sci Sports Exerc* 1999; **31** (Suppl.): S547–S552.

18 Epstein L, Goldfield GS. Physical activity in the treatment of childhood overweight and obesity: current evidence and research issues. *Med Sci Sports Exerc* 1999; **31** (Suppl.): S553–S559.

19 Garrow JS, Summerbell CD. Meta-analysis: effects of exercise, with or without dieting, on body composition of overweight subjects. *Eur J Clin Nutr* 1995; **49**: 1–10.

20 Fogelholm M, Kukkonen-Harjula K. Does physical activity prevent weight gain—a systematic review. *Obesity Rev* 2000; **2**: 85–112.

21 Rollnick S, Kinnersley P, Stott N. Methods of helping patient with behaviour change. *Br Med J* 1993; **307**: 188–90.

22 Biddle SJH, Fox KR. Motivation for physical activity and weight management. *Int J Obes Metabol Disord* 1998; **22** (Suppl. 2): S39–S47.

23 Andersen RE, Wadden TA, Barlett SJ, Zemel B, Verde TJ, Frankowiak SC. Effects of lifestyle activity vs. structured aerobic exercise in obese women. A randomized trial. *J Am Med Assoc* 1999; **281**: 335–40.

24 Clinical guidelines on the identification, evaluation and treatment of overweight and obesity in adults—the evidence report. *Obesity Res* 1998; **6** (Suppl. 2): 51S–209S.

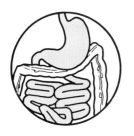

Chapter 4.8
Gastrointestinal Considerations

FRANK MOSES

Classical reference

Fordtran JS, Saltin B. Gastric emptying and intestinal absorption during prolonged severe exercise. *J Appl Physiol* 1967; **23**: 331–335.

Endurance exercise causes a loss of water, electrolytes and glycogen. Replacement of these is essential to avoid fatigue and impaired performance. This requires a functioning gastrointestinal (GI) tract and many athletes find it difficult to ingest enough to adequately replenish that which is lost. There are many factors that govern the rate of gastric emptying (GE) in the resting state. However, limited data existed regarding the effects of exercise on GE and results had been conflicting. In a landmark study Fordtran and Saltin performed one of the earliest and most rigorous evaluations of the effects of exercise on upper gastrointestinal function.

In their study GE was analysed by gastric aspiration of 750 mL of water and a test solution containing 13.3% glucose and 0.3% sodium chloride. Five healthy subjects were trained to the techniques and then tested at rest or with exercise on a treadmill for 1 h at 64–78% of $\dot{V}O_{2\,max}$. The subjects drank 150 mL of the test solution at the start and at 10-min intervals for 40 min. At 60 min a 20 French tube was placed and gastric contents were aspirated for analysis.

Furthermore, four subjects then were tested to determine the effects of exercise on intestinal absorption by a standard non-absorbable marker, constant perfusion technique. A small triple-lumen tube was placed in the jejunum and subsequently in the ileum and position verified by fluoroscopy. The authors measured net water, electrolyte and glucose (active) absorption, and (passive) absorption of L-xylose, urea-^{14}C and tritiated water in both the jejunum and ileum.

GE of water was more rapid than that of the saline–glucose test solution. However, exercise had minimal effect on GE (see Fig. 4.8.1), as measured by the remaining non-absorbable marker (polyethylene glycol) or residual gastric volume. Exercise did not alter absorption of the tested substances in either the jejunum or ileum. These results showed that rather intense exercise (71% of maximum) for 1 h had a very

Fig. 4.8.1 Effect of exercise on the recovery of polyethylene glycol (PEG) and on calculated volume of gastric contents 1 h after ingestion of 750-mL test solutions was started. Dotted lines refer to tests carried out with water, solid lines to those with a solution containing 13.3% glucose and 0.3% sodium chloride.

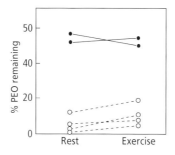
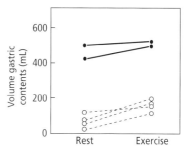

slight inhibition of liquid gastric emptying and no effect on intestinal absorption of water, electrolytes or glucose or passive intestinal absorption of L–xylose, urea–^{14}C or tritiated water.

The authors acknowledge prior studies demonstrating that exercise was associated with substantial reductions in splanchnic blood flow. However, they concluded that exercise to this degree did not alter intestinal blood flow sufficiently to significantly reduce GE or intestinal absorption. They felt that these data demonstrated that athletes should be capable of adequate rehydration and energy replacement during sustained heavy exercise, even during exercise in hot environments. The study was limited by the small number of young, asymptomatic, healthy subjects, but used rigorous methods of directly measuring GE and, in particular, intestinal absorption. The study demonstrated how successful these evaluations can be when performed by trained investigators. It opened up the field of GE with exercise that became of great interest to athletes, trainers, scientists and industry.

Introduction

Exercise influences gastrointestinal (GI) physiology in a variety of different ways and can alter GI function in healthy individuals and those who suffer underlying GI disorders. Some of these changes are beneficial. Exercise has been associated with improved gastric emptying, reduced constipation and reduced rates of GI malignancies. More commonly, the medical literature has linked exercise to unfortunate outcomes, such as ischemic bowel disease or GI bleeding following a marathon race. Over the past 20 years many investigators have contributed to the expanding literature of this topic. There has been extensive research to optimize oral rehydration during athletic events. Many case reports and series have demonstrated uncommon or untoward effects during exercise such as severe lower GI bleeding. However, much remains unknown or untested. This chapter will briefly review pertinent GI physiology associated with exercise and highlight the effect of exercise on healthy individuals and on those suffering from GI diseases.

GI physiology with exercise

Gastrointestinal physiology has traditionally been studied at rest and the methodology is typically vali-

dated for resting conditions. Experimental stress on the GI tract is more typically generated by drugs or disease. Evaluation of GI physiology under the stress of exercise often requires extensive modifications in experimental techniques and most GI physiologists are untrained in these methods. Intestinal motility, for example, is extremely sensitive to motion artifact. This has limited the published literature.

The most dramatic change associated with exercise is that cardiac output is diverted to exercising muscles and visceral blood flow falls by 50–80% of baseline values [1,2]. During prolonged events there is increased demand for absorption of water, electrolytes and nutrients. This relative hypovolemia may be compounded by hyperthermia, dehydration and, potentially, the use of non-steroidal anti-inflammatory drugs (NSAIDs). The stomach and colon seem particularly sensitive to ischemia induced by exercise.

The autonomic nervous system (ANS) is altered by acute and chronic exercise. During acute stress, the sympathetic nervous system predominates. However, with habitual exercise, the ANS adapts and parasympathetic effects predominate. These effects alter intestinal transit, blood flow and permeability. GI hormones are variably changed by exercise and these changes can also alter a variety of GI functions.

The mechanical effects of exercise on the GI tract are uncertain but could alter GI function by changing intra-abdominal pressure or facilitating trauma to more mobile sections of the GI tract.

Effects of exercise on GI function and symptoms in healthy individuals and athletes

GI symptoms: abdominal pain, cramps and diarrhea

Initial reports found that up to half of all marathon runners have occasional loose stools or three or more bowel movements per day. Furthermore, the urge to defecate, abdominal cramping and increased flatulence are common lower GI symptoms of runners. A small percentage of marathoners report bloody bowel movements with running. Upper GI symptoms such as heartburn are not infrequent, particularly during running. Other upper tract symptoms include increased eructations, abdominal pain, nausea and vomiting. Women, untrained athletes, younger athletes and competitors who 'give it all' more frequently reported GI symptoms. Symptoms such as abdominal pain, 'side stitch' [3], nausea and even vomiting are greater with hard runs or longer races such as the marathon and among athletes who suffer dehydration and hyperthermia [4]. While these may be infrequent causes of severe or lasting disability, they are common and may limit performance. GI symptoms with long-distance walking are less severe than during running but may limit performance and are also more severe in dehydrated or less experienced athletes [5].

A few of these surveys are based on large populations, which may limit the inherent reporting bias. However, many of these 'exercise-associated' symptoms are characteristic of the irritable bowel syndrome and the surveys are not generally controlled with a non-running group. Furthermore, these symptoms are non-specific and may be manifestations of dehydration, electrolyte disturbances or hyperthermia. Exercise may serve at times to be a 'disease detector', uncovering symptoms of underlying illness that are not symptomatic during non-strenuous normal daily activities [6]. This is most often seen in competitive athletes or others, such as soldiers, who are in a physically demanding occupation. Alternatively, the clinician can ask patients if they have recently chosen to avoid an active lifestyle for particular reasons. Clinical evaluation of these cases is difficult but is frequently most instructive if the athlete can be evaluated during or soon after a symptom-provoking event. Occasionally it may be necessary to recreate the athletic event in order to document the particular disorder. While abdominal pain is typically transient and of little clinical consequence, more severe outcomes may occur and should always be considered in appropriate circumstances [7]. (See Case Study 4.8.1)

GI bleeding

Gastrointestinal bleeding in athletes is an uncommon but dramatic and potentially serious complication that may manifest as acute upper or lower GI bleeding, as chronic bleeding or iron deficiency, or as incidentally noted occult positive stool tests. The term runners' (or sports) anemia was initially coined in 1970. While mean hemoglobin values of elite athletes may be lower than in the general population, the incidence of anemia

Case study 4.8.1: GI bleeding

A 30-year-old elite woman runner was admitted to hospital following completion of a marathon [8]. She had developed crampy lower quadrant abdominal pain followed by several episodes of bloody diarrhea at the 4-mile mark. Her symptoms improved transiently during the race but worsened near the end. Following the marathon she began passing frank blood per rectum and presented to an emergency room.

While her past GI history was unremarkable, she had noted abdominal pain and diarrhea during peak training 4–6 weeks previously while she was running 180 miles/week at a 10 000-foot elevation. She was on no pertinent medications and the remainder of her past history was unremarkable.

A sigmoidoscopy showed external hemorrhoids and severe hemorrhagic colitis of the sigmoid colon. The patient was admitted and treated with bowel rest, intravenous fluids and antibiotics. Her symptoms resolved within 24 h and she was discharged in 4 days. Further evaluation for other etiologies was unremarkable. A subsequent endoscopy at 6 weeks showed complete resolution and she resumed active running without recurrent symptoms over 24 months.

in athletes is difficult to determine but probably not different from age-matched controls [9]. The etiology of sports anemia is frequently multifactorial and may most commonly be artifactual due to plasma volume expansion. Alternatively, the anemia may be due to blood loss from GI bleeding which has the greatest potential to cause significant anemia. However, other causes are intravascular hemolysis, hematuria, increased iron loss in the sweat, or decreased dietary iron intake or intestinal absorption. Sports hematuria is generally felt to be a benign self-limited condition due

Table 4.8.1 Evaluations of GI bleeding in endurance events.

Distance	Subjects	Method	Results
Marathon	39	Postrace HemOccult	8% positive conversion
Marathon	707	Survey	1.2–2.4% report blood per rectum
Marathon	63	Pre/postrace HemOccult	13% positive conversion
Marathon	24	Pre/postrace HemQuant (Hb/g stool)	Pre: 0.99 mg Post: 2.25 mg
Marathon	125	Pre/postrace HemOccult	21% conversion
Marathon	32	Pre/postrace HemOccult	22% conversion
100-mile ultramarathon	34	Pre/postrace HemOccult	85% conversion

HemOccult is a guaiac-based qualitative test for fecal occult blood.
HemQuant is a quantitative measurement of hemoglobin in stool.

to repeated traumatic impact of the posterior bladder wall against the bladder base. However, renal causes of hematuria may exist and coexisting urinary pathology should be carefully excluded [10].

The incidence of clinically significant GI bleeding is difficult to determine but probably rare. Examples of acute upper or lower GI bleeding associated with exercise have been published as isolated case reports or small series. However, anemia and/or iron deficiency is not rare, particularly in women athletes where it may occur in up to a third. Occult GI blood loss prevalence has been generally found to range from 8 to 35% following marathons and to occur in the majority of ultramarathon competitors [11] (Table 4.8.1). The frequency and quantity of occult GI blood loss peaks 24–48 h following an event and may be proportional to athletic intensity as it is more prominent following competition than practice.

Hemorrhagic gastritis (HG) has been the most frequently reported endoscopic finding associated with exercise-associated GI bleeding. It is typically transient, spontaneously resolving within 72 h with rest and also when gastric acid is inhibited by cimetidine, a histamine receptor antagonist (H_2RA) [12]. Histologic changes of submucosal hemorrhage and edema in the gastric antrum immediately following running occur even in the absence of obvious endoscopic damage [13]. The prevalence of endoscopic changes with running has not been established but is likely common [14]. A recent endoscopic study found erosive gastritis in 11 and gastric ulcer in 1 of 16 runners completing a 10-km race [15]. Ischemia, mediated perhaps by gastric acid, has been the most frequently proposed etiol-

ogy. Prospective trials using prophylactic cimetidine to prevent GI bleeding in a group of recreational marathon runners have not been conclusive [16].

The second most commonly recognized site of exercise-associated GI bleeding is the colon. Several cases have been published of presumed ischemic colitis following strenuous running or other athletic events [8]. The cases may be associated with heat and ischemic damage to other organs and have led to diagnostic laparotomy and even subtotal colectomy [17]. Ischemic lesions develop in the right colon [18] and in the classic 'watershed' regions of the splenic flexure and sigmoid colon [8]. Generally hemorrhagic colitis is self-limited. If endoscopic evaluation is considered necessary, it should be performed within 48 h of the athletic stress. These lesions in the stomach and colon are typically transient and will resolve rapidly with rest.

NSAID medications, while inconsistently associated with GI blood loss in runners, may contribute to gastritis and gastric ulcers, and less commonly to small bowel or colon lesions and GI bleeding. Aspirin has been shown to enhance increased intestinal permeability associated with running [19]. It is always important to review the use of these medications in the athlete with gastrointestinal complaints.

Trauma has been proposed as an alternative etiology for GI bleeding. Athletes may be more prone to abdominal trauma. Cyclists can suffer abdominal trauma with falls that may be overlooked in the face of other injuries [20]. Runners are often thin and may have an increased incidence of redundant colon. This can lead to an increased susceptibility to cecal volvulus, which could also cause bleeding and abdominal pain. A recent case report of a man with recurrent abdominal pain with exertion was felt to be due to redundant colon and resolved after right hemicolectomy [21].

No instances of esophagitis, esophageal ulcers or small bowel ischemia causing bleeding have been observed to date. Exercise-associated mesenteric infarction has been reported [22]. Anorectal disorders, such as hemorrhoids or fissures, may be aggravated by local trauma, are common and may cause bleeding in some runners and cyclists, although the incidence is unknown.

Participation in exercise programs is part of a healthy lifestyle but does not confer immunity from underlying diseases that may manifest with GI bleeding. Evaluations for diseases such as colon cancer should be performed on individuals at risk for these conditions or in any athlete who develops recurrent GI bleeding of uncertain etiology.

The therapy of exercise-associated GI bleeding is dependent on the location and severity of the bleed. Most cases appear to be self-limited and spontaneously resolve. Abdominal pain associated with many of these injuries may limit damage in most athletes, although more severe injury has been seen in elite athletes who persist in the face of pain [8]. Some cases of HG may recur and these individuals may be treated with an H$_2$RA or perhaps a proton pump inhibitor. Treatment for hemorrhagic colitis is uncertain, though it appears not to generally recur.

Effects of exercise on patients with GI disorders

The esophagus

Exercise has been reported to cause heartburn associated with gastroesophageal reflux (GER) [23,24] and chest pain of esophageal origin. However, chest pain, whenever it occurs in the setting of exertion, demands an evaluation for cardiac cause prior to specific esophageal evaluation. Esophageal motility changes occur with exercise. However, it is difficult to quantify physiologic manometric changes in the face of movement artifact induced by running and many studies have used a cycling model. The clinical relevance of these exercise-induced motility changes is uncertain.

Heartburn is relatively common among athletes and

> ## Case study 4.8.2–The stomach
> A 37-year-old man was referred for recurrent vomiting during and following a run. He was employed as a military recruiter and did not participate in regular athletic activities. During rest and submaximal activities he was asymptomatic. However, during a physical fitness test, he was unable to complete a 2-mile run for time due to vomiting. His past history and physical examination were unremarkable. He was on no medications. An evaluation including an endoscopy, esophageal manometry and 24-h pH testing during exercise was normal. A graded exercise cardiac stress test did not show ischemic changes. A pulmonary exercise tolerance test showed poor exercise tolerance and his symptoms of nausea and vomiting were reproduced with supermaximal exercise efforts. He was placed on a retraining program, gradually improved his fitness level, and was able to complete his fitness testing successfully.

esophageal pH monitoring has demonstrated that GER occurs more frequently with exercise, notably running. Both the number of reflux episodes and the duration of acid exposure increase with running. Exercise-associated GER is increased postprandially vs. fasting and among those individuals who have an underlying predilection for GER [23]. The clinical relevance of these changes in uncertain. The symptoms are generally not severe and medical therapy for GER, including antacids, histamine receptor blockers and proton pump inhibitors, effectively reduces acid exposure in these circumstances. In rare cases exercise-associated regurgitation can lead to vomiting and impair athletic performance. (See Case Study 4.8.2)

The stomach

Exercise causes effort-dependent changes in gastric emptying (GE) and may lead to symptoms of nausea, bloating and vomiting. GE may fall significantly during intense ($\geq 75\%$ $\dot{V}_{O_{2\,max}}$) exercise but is generally unaffected or even increased with mild to moderate ($< 75\%$ $\dot{V}_{O_{2\,max}}$) intensity exercise. GE is the limiting factor in rehydration during and after endurance events and much research has been done to maximize GE in these settings [25,26]. Characteristics of the meals are the major factors controlling GE. Liquid meals empty quicker than solid meals. Larger gastric volumes are associated with accelerated GE. Increasing meal calories, osmolality and fat progressively delay GE. The athlete's hydration state, body temperature, sex, menstrual cycle and smoking status and even the time of day may all affect GE.

Liquid GE has been more thoroughly studied. Several studies have shown little change or even accelerated GE of water or glucose solutions at moderate or submaximal intensity levels [27–29]. GE rates of >2 L/h of water during exercise may be achieved in laboratory settings when gastric volumes are kept high. Thus GE rates are able to match sweat rates of many, but perhaps not all, athletes. Energy delivery is likewise more than sufficient to match requirements when fluids containing 6% glucose are used. Surveys have noted that runners are more troubled by gastric symptoms than cyclists or most other athletes. GE of solids is more complex and the literature is less robust. However, exercise appears to have similar effects on GE of solids. Studies have shown mild acceleration of GE of mixed solid meals with both low- and moderate-intensity cycling and walking [30,31]. Some have suggested that runners have significantly accelerated basal GE when compared to sedentary controls. Treatment for GE disorders is primarily preventative. Athletes should 'train their gut' to tolerate fluids and meals during training, and avoid fluids and foods in the diet known to adversely affect GE or historically to cause symptoms. Athletes should consume fluids early and often to avoid dehydration and hyperthermia. Once an athlete is dehydrated by $\geq 4\%$ of body weight, GE rates fall. In one study after 20 min exercise, euhydrated athletes had 81% GE compared to 70% in dehydrated athletes [32]. Performance levels will fall with dehydration and intensity may need to be reduced before oral rehydration can effectively proceed. Medications to accelerate gastric emptying are probably of limited value.

The colon

Symptoms attributed to the effects of exercise on the colon are the most commonly reported and seem to be most frequent among runners [33]. 'Nervous' diarrhea (43%), defecation with running (62%), diarrhea during racing (47%), diarrhea associated with severe cramps, rectal bleeding (16%) and even fecal incontinence (12%) were reported in a runners' club survey [34]. While symptoms are common, colonic physiology during exercise is obscure, conflicting and difficult to analyse. Probes are difficult to place and maintain during exercise. Motion artifact is more prominent and transit time is measured in many hours instead of minutes. No change in fecal transit time was found when measured by radioisotope markers in a controlled metabolic laboratory during a 9-week training period [35]. However, the training regimen was moderate, the subjects remained asymptomatic and inter- and intrasubject variability was high. In another study, no significant change was found in groups of varying degrees of athletic activity [36]. Others have found transit time to decrease with treadmill walking or riding a bicycle ergometer [37]. The mechanism of these changes, if any, is speculative at this time.

Colonic symptoms may be treated in various ways. 'Nervous' or prerace diarrhea is generally self-limited and may respond to low-residue diets. Some have used prophylactic antidiarrheal medications. Ultraendurance athletes report that it is possible to 'train the gut' by reducing exercise duration and intensity to subsymptomatic levels and gradually increasing effort. Prerace cathartics should be avoided due to the possibility of dehydration. Race-associated diarrhea generally responds to reduction in effort. However, severe watery diarrhea associated with racing has not been well studied and will require intensive investigation in symptomatic runners. Exercise is said to benefit patients with functional constipation. Acute graded exercise reversibly reduces colonic pressure waves which may explain some lower GI symptoms associated with exercise [38]. However, recent studies found no obvious effect [39–41] of exercise on bowel transit or delayed transit with inactivity [42]. Medications such as NSAIDs may also be associated with colonic mucosal damage.

Reduced GI malignancy rate

Epidemiologic studies have demonstrated that colon cancer is associated with a sedentary lifestyle and that those individuals who remain more active, ingest lower fat and higher fiber diets, and maintain a lower body mass index (BMI) are at a lower risk of colonic neoplasia [43,44]. Most of these studies have evaluated job-related physical activity. However, some have also shown that recreational activity may confer similar benefits. These epidemiologic findings are supported by several experimental findings. Shortened intestinal transit time, which has been noted in more active individuals, has been associated in several studies with a reduced rate of colonic cancer. Furthermore, active individuals frequently consume higher amounts of fiber, which may also accelerate GI transit. Increased fiber may also reduce the concentration of fecal bile acids and alter the ratio of secondary to primary bile acids. NSAID medications are often used by habitual exercisers. Some of these drugs have been shown to reduce colonic neoplasia in certain individuals with increased genetic risk and may alter cancer risk in selected cases.

Summary

Exercise can alter gastrointestinal (GI) function of athletes and also cause symptoms in patients with GI diseases. Exercise has been associated with improved gastric emptying, decreased rates of constipation and lower incidences of GI malignancy. More often exercise has been linked to abdominal pain, diarrhea, GI bleeding and ischemic bowel disease. Endurance athletes depend upon a functioning GI tract to sustain volume and energy requirements during competition. GI symptoms may adversely affect athletic performance or be associated with sustained morbidity or even mortality.

Gastroesophageal reflux (GER) is more common in runners than other athletes and is particularly frequent when exercise is performed after meals. GER symptoms are generally controlled by reducing gastric acid production. Chest pain of esophageal origin may also occur although the mechanism is uncertain. Lower GI symptoms are more commonly seen and have been reported in over half of runners in some series. In most instances, the etiology of exercise-associated GI

symptoms such as abdominal pain or diarrhea is uncertain. In severe cases, or when the exercise is sustained, GI bleeding secondary to ischemic bowel disease may occur in either the stomach or colon. Hemorrhagic gastritis may recur with repeated exercise and may be inhibited by gastric acid suppression. Hemorrhagic colitis is generally not recurrent but may be severe, leading to colon strictures or surgical exploration.

Multiple choice questions

For each question, please indicate which of the statements a–e is correct.

1 *Exercise-induced chest pain and heartburn:*
a are more common in weight lifters and swimmers than runners
b are difficult to manage medically
c require adequate evaluation to exclude a cardiac cause
d occur more often fasting than after meals
e are best treated with anticholinergic or sedative medications.

2 *Exercise-associated abdominal pain:*
a is generally worse during training than competition
b may be associated with diarrhea or a strong urge to have a bowel movement
c can be cured with cimetidine or fasting
d is often a marker of underlying GI pathology
e is generally worse if exercise is done fasting.

3 *GI bleeding associated with exercise:*
a may occur in one-third of runners after a marathon
b may be manifest as hematemesis, melena or chronic anemia
c is never a marker of underlying GI disease such as malignancy
d can be prevented by gastric acid blockade in some cases
e may be associated with ischemic lesions of the colon.

4 *Gastric emptying during exercise is important for rehydration during endurance events.*
a Liquids empty from the stomach faster than solids.
b Carbohydrates and salts may be added to liquids to promote quicker water absorption.
c Fat delays gastric emptying.
d The volume of ingested fluid does not affect the gastric emptying rate.

e Athletes should determine their personal preferences for fluid drinks prior to competition.

5 *Exercise may alter intestinal transit.*

a Intestinal transit is determined in part by the amount of fiber ingested.

b The majority of intestinal transit time is determined by the colonic transit.

c Exercise cures functional constipation.

d Running is frequently associated with diarrhea or increased urgency of bowel movements.

e Medications are of minimal value in managing symptoms caused by changes in intestinal transit during exercise.

References

1 Clausen JP. Effects of physical training on cardiovascular adjustments to exercise in man. *Physiol Rev* 1977; **57**: 779–815.

2 Qamar MI, Read AE. Effects of exercise on mesenteric blood flow in man. *Gut* 1987; **28**: 583–7.

3 Morton DP, Callister R. Characteristics and etiology of exercise-related transient abdominal pain. *Med Sci Sports Exerc* 2000; **32**: 432–8.

4 Rehrer NJ, Janssen GM, Brouns F, Saris WH. Fluid intake and gastrointestinal problems in runners competing in a 25-km race and a marathon. *Int J Sports Med* 1989; **10** (Suppl. 1): S22.

5 Peters HP, Zweers M, Backx FJ, Bol E, Hendriks ER, Mosterd WL, de Vries WR. Gastrointestinal symptoms during long-distance walking. *Med Sci Sports Exerc* 1999; **31**: 767–73.

6 Eichner RE, Scott WA. Exercise as Disease Detector. *Physician Sportsmed* 1998; **26**: 41–52.

7 Scobie BA. Gastrointestinal emergencies with marathon-type running: omental infarction with pancreatitis and liver failure with portal vein thrombosis. *N Z Med J* 1998; **111**: 211–2.

8 Lucas W, Schroy PC. Reversible ischemic colitis in a high endurance athlete. *Am J Gastroenterol* 1998; **93**: 2231–4.

9 Balaban EP. Sports Anemia. *Clin Sports Med* 1992; **11**: 313–25.

10 Abarbanel J, Benet AE, Lask D, Kimche D. Sports hematuria. *J Urol* 1990; **143**: 887–90.

11 Baska RS, Moses FM, Graeber G, Kearney G. Gastrointestinal bleeding during an ultramarathon. *Digestive Dis Sci* 1990; **35**: 276–9.

12 Cooper BT, Douglas SA, Firth LA, Hannagan JA, Chadwick VS. Erosive gastritis and gastrointestinal bleeding in a female runner. Prevention of the bleeding and healing of the gastritis with H$_2$-receptor antagonists. *Gastroenterology* 1987; **92**: 2019–23.

13 Gaudin C, Zerath E, Guezennec CY. Gastric lesions secondary to long-distance running. *Digestive Dis Sci* 1990; **35**: 1239–43.

14 Schwartz AE, Vanagunas A, Kamel PL. Endoscopy to evaluate gastrointestinal bleeding in marathon runners. *Ann Intern Med* 1990; **113**: 632–3.

15 Suck-Chei C, Kyoung-Hoon Y, Chang-Su C *et al.* Gastrointestinal endoscopy is helpful in long distance runner with gastrointestinal blood loss and/or anemia. *Gastrointest Endosc* 2000; **51**: AB84.

16 Moses FM, Baska RS, Peura DA, Deuster PA. Effect of cimetidine on marathon-associated gastrointestinal symptoms and bleeding. *Digestive Dis Sci* 1991; **36**: 1390–4.

17 Beaumont AC, Teare JP. Subtotal colectomy following marathon running in a female patient. *J Royal Soc Med* 1991; **84**: 439–40.

18 Moses FM, Brewer TG, Peura DA. Running-associated proximal hemorrhagic colitis. *Ann Intern Med* 1988; **108**: 385–6.

19 Ryan AJ, Chang RT, Gisolfi CV. Gastrointestinal permeability following aspirin intake and prolonged running. *Med Sci Sports Exerc* 1996; **28**: 698–705.

20 Lauder TD, Moses FM. Recurrent abdominal pain from abdominal adhesions in an endurance triathlete. *Med Sci Sports Exerc* 1995; **27**: 623–5.

21 McMahon JM, Underwood ES, Kirby WE. Colonic spasm and pseudo-obstruction in an elongated colon secondary to physical exertion: diagnosis by barium enema. *Am J Gastroenterol* 1999; **94**: 3362–4.

22 Kam LW, Pease WE, Thompson PD. Exercise-associated mesenteric infarction. *Am J Gastroenterol* 1994; **89**: 1899–900.

23 Kraus BB, Sinclair JW, Castell DO. Gastroesophageal reflux in runners. Characteristics and Treatment. *Ann Intern Med* 1990; **112**: 429–33.

24 Soffer EE, Merchant RK, Duethman G, Launspach J, Gisolfi C, Adrian TE. Effect of graded exercise on esophageal motility and gastroesophageal reflux in trained athletes. *Digestive Dis Sci* 1993; **38**: 220–4.

25 Murray R. The effect of consuming carbohydrate-electrolyte beverages on gastric emptying and fluid absorption during and following exercise. *Sports Med* 1987; **4**: 322–57.

26 Noakes TD, Rehrer NJ, Maughan RJ. The importance of volume in regulating gastric emptying. *Med Sci Sports Exerc* 1991; **23**: 307–13.

27 Fordtran JS, Saltin B. Gastric emptying and intestinal absorption during prolonged severe exercise. *J Appl Physiol* 1967; **23**: 331–5.

28 Neufer PD, Young AJ, Sawka MN. Gastric emptying during walking and running: effects of varied exercise intensity. *Eur J Appl Physiol* 1989; **58**: 440–5.

29 Marzio L, Formica P, Fabiani F, LaPenna D, Vecchiett L, Cuccurullo F. Influence of physical activity on gastric emptying of liquids in normal subjects. *Am J Gastroenterol* 1991; **86**: 1433–6.

30 Cammack J, Read NW, Cann PA, Greenwood D, Holgate

AM. Effect of prolonged exercise on the passage of a solid meal through the stomach and small intestine. *Gut* 1982; **23**: 957–61.

31 Moore JG, Datz FL, Christian PE. Exercise increases solid meal gastric emptying rates in men. *Digestive Dis Sci* 1990; **35**: 428–32.

32 Rehrer NJ, Beckers EG, Brouns F, Ten Hoor F, Saris WHM. Effects of dehydration on gastric emptying and gastrointestinal distress while running. *Med Sci Sports Exerc* 1990; **22**: 790–5.

33 Peters HPF, Bos M, Seebregts L, Akkermans LMA, Van Berge Henegouwen GP, Bol E, Mosterd WL, de Vries WR. Gastrointestinal symptoms in long-distance runners, cyclists, and triathletes: prevalence, medication, and etiology. *Am J Gastroenterol* 1999; **94**: 1570–81.

34 Sullivan SN, Wong C. Runner's diarrhea: different patterns and associated factors. *J Clin Gastroenterol* 1992; **14**: 101–4.

35 Bingham SA, Cummings JH. Effect of exercise and physical fitness on large intestinal function. *Gastroenterology* 1989; **97**: 1389–99.

36 Lampe JW, Slavin JL, Apple FS. Iron status of active women and the effect of running a marathon on bowel function and gastrointestinal blood loss. *Int J Sports Med* 1991; **12**: 173–9.

37 Oettle GJ. Effect of moderate exercise on bowel habit. *Gut* 1991; **32**: 941–4.

38 Rao SS, Beaty J, Chamberlain M, Lambert PG, Gisolfi C. Effects of acute graded exercise on human colonic motility. *Am J Physiol* 1999; **276** (5 Pt 1): G1221–6.

39 Sesboue B, Arhan P, Devroede G *et al*. Colonic transit in soccer players. *J Clin Gastroenterol* 1995; **20**: 211–4.

40 Meshkinpour H, Selod S, Movahedi H, Nami N, James N, Wilson A. Effects of regular exercise in management of chronic idiopathic constipation. *Digestive Dis Sci* 1998; **43**: 2379–83.

41 Robertson G, Meshkinpour H, Vandenberg K, James N, Cohen A, Wilson A. Effects of exercise on total and segmental colon transit. *J Clin Gastroenterol* 1993; **16**: 300–3.

42 Liu F, Kondo T, Toda Y. Brief physical inactivity prolongs colonic transit time in elderly active men. *Int J Sports Med* 1993; **14**: 465–7.

43 Bartram HP, Wynder EL. Physical activity and colon cancer risk? Physiological considerations. *Am J Gastroenterol* 1989; **84**: 109–12.

44 Giovannucci E, Ascherio A, Rimm EB, Colditz GA, Stampfer MJ, Willett WC. Physical activity, obesity, and risk for colon cancer. *Ann Intern Med* 1995; **122**: 327–34.

Part 5
Imaging in Sports Medicine

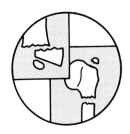

Chapter 5.1
Imaging of Sports Injuries

INGE-LIS KANSTRUP, HOLLIS G. POTTER &
WAYNE GIBBON

Classical reference

Glashow JL, Katz R, Schneider M, Scott WN.
    Double-blind assessment of the value of magnetic
    resonance imaging in the diagnosis of anterior
    cruciate and meniscal lesions. *J Bone Joint Surg
    (Am)* 1989; **71**(1):113–119.
A prospective double-blind study was undertaken to
evaluate the usefulness of magnetic resonance imaging
(MRI) in the accurate interpretation of pathologic
intra-articular changes in the knee. Forty-seven
patients who were scheduled to have arthroscopy and
three patients who were to have arthrotomy volun-
teered for magnetic resonance imaging preoperatively.
The radiologists had no clinical or roentgenographic
information about the patients before the evaluation of
the magnetic resonance images, and the radiologists'
interpretations were unknown to the surgeon before
the arthroscopy or arthrotomy was done. Our important observations were limited to the findings in the
menisci and in the anterior cruciate ligament. Magnetic resonance imaging had a positive predictive value of
75%, a negative predictive value of 90%, a sensitivity
of 83% and a specificity of 84% for pathologic findings
in the menisci. For complete tears of the anterior cruciate ligament, the positive predictive value was 74%,
the negative predictive value 70%, the sensitivity 61%
and the specificity 82%. We believe that magnetic
resonance imaging, when combined with clinical
and roentgenographic examination, provides the most
accurate non-invasive source of information that is
currently available for pathologic findings in the
menisci and in the anterior cruciate ligament. The authors further noted that since the interpretation of the
MR images were done in a 'blinded' fashion the results
will likely improve considerably when combined with
clinical history (Table 5.1.1).

Table 5.1.1 Correlation of the findings of the magnetic resonance imaging with the surgical findings. (From Glashow *et al.* Table II.)

	Surgical findings (no.)	Correctly interpreted in MRI (no.)	False positive (no.)	False negative (no.)	Positive predictive value (%)
Medial meniscus					
Normal	28	20	8		68
Torn	22	17		5	
Lateral meniscus					
Normal	36	34	2		87
Torn	14	13		1	
Anterior cruciate ligament					
Normal	27	22	5		74
Torn	23	14		9	

Introduction

Diagnostic imaging plays a great role in practical sports medicine today, as discrimination between related injuries may influence the decision about treatment and clarify the prognosis. Also, an exact staging is of importance in classification and evaluation of various treatments.

The clinician is offered different modalities for imaging, and when choosing between these not only must the question of which method is optimal be taken into account, but also accessibility, prices, waiting time, irradiation or other patient drawbacks must be considered. Furthermore, it is a great advantage if the clinician is familiar with the diagnostics in choice, as well as the imaging specialist. A good result is based on a dialogue between the clinician and the imaging specialist. A relevant patient history is a must, even on admissions to plain X-rays, so the imaging specialist can adjust the investigation to optimize it for the injury in question. It also optimizes the conditions for a relevant answer from the imaging specialist.

In addition, subsequent feedback to the imaging specialists about the final result of the diagnostic procedure or the consequences of the investigation is important in order to improve the learning experience for the future.

It is essential to remember that all imaging modalities have their pitfalls. All investigations are able to produce many irrelevant findings as their sensitivity and specificity are almost never 1.0. Therefore lots of irrelevant diagnoses can be made if there is not a dialogue between the clinician and the imaging specialist, and these will confuse, delay and increase the cost of the treatment.

Questions the clinician should ask when considering imaging:
- What is the problem to be solved?
- Is quantification/classification needed?
- Will the imaging result influence treatment?

A rough survey of the indications for using the various methods is given in Table 5.1.2.

New possibilities/techniques in the future—perspectives

When it comes to future possibilities, 'hot' research areas need to be considered.

While currently MR images anatomic disorders, in the future tools will also be developed for functional diagnostics of various conditions, perhaps even metabolic activity in selected tissues. As the number of MR scanners increases rapidly, access to this investigation will be facilitated and the costs reduced. This will increase the implementation dramatically.

Dynamic imaging with ultrasound (US) will expand—perhaps with small portable sound-heads for transmission of signals on line. Three-dimensional imaging with US is already possible, and this technique will be transferred to allow for dynamic movement analysis.

Scintigraphically, a new era has begun with the possibilities for quantitative flow and metabolism measurements with various positron-labeled markers (PET technique). The first results of muscle metabolism and selective muscle involvement in selected sports have been reported by use of the glucose-analog ^{18}F-fluorodeoxyglucose [1].

Conventional radiography

Conventional radiography
- Bone fractures
- Eliminates bone fractures
- Each film involves irradiation, but generally low dose
- Static images
- Cheap.

Conventional radiography is without doubt the most cost-effective and simple way of diagnosing acute fractures. It is also the most specific investigation. It is not, however, the most sensitive so that if a fracture is still clinically suspected in the presence of an apparently normal radiograph further investigation should be

Table 5.1.2 Survey of indications for diagnostic imaging.

	Ordinary X-ray	CT scan	MR scan	Ultrasound	Scintigraphy
Price	X	XX	XXXX	X	X
Waiting time	Low	Moderate	High	Low–moderate	Low–moderate
Bones					
Ordinary fractures	+++		If problems		+++(special)
Comminuted or complex fractures	++	+++			
Osteochondral fractures	+	+	+++		++
Stress fractures	+	(+)	+++		+++
Shin splints			++		+++
Vascularization			?		+++
Joints					
Arthritis	++		+++		++
Meniscus			+++	+	+
Collateral ligaments			+++	++	
Cruciate ligaments			+++	+	
Cartilage injury			++		
Osteochondritis	+	++	+++		++
Coalitio		++	+++		
Menisceal cyst			++	+++	
Ganglions			++	+++	
Baker's cyst			++	+++	
Inflammation			++(?)	++	++
Labral injuries		++	++	++	
Hill-Sachs lesions		++			+++
Muscle/tendon					
Sprain—acute			++	+++	
Sprain—chronic			+	+++	
Bursitis—acute			+++	+++	
Bursitis—chronic			++	+++	
Tendon ruptures			+++	+++	
Enthesopathies			?	?	++
Myotendinitis			+	+++	
Myositis ossificans	++	+	+	+++	+++

considered. The X-ray beam needs to be tangential to an abnormality for it to be visible. Conventionally only two radiographic views tend to be performed: usually a lateral and frontal projection (using an X-ray beam passing either from the front to the back of the patient, i.e. anteroposterior—AP, or from the back to the front, i.e. posteroanterior—PA). Using such orthogonal projections will normally demonstrate most fractures. If the bony anatomy is complex, as occurs in the spine and joints, then fractures may be obscured by overlying bone. Similarly if the structure is cylindrical, as is the case with many bones, small structures such as avulsed bone fragments may be missed as the beam may not be tangential to it if only two projections are used. In such circumstances additional oblique projections may be helpful or alternatively a tomographic technique may be successfully used, e.g. conventional linear tomography, computed tomography (CT), MRI or ultrasound imaging.

Conventional radiographs are also poor at demonstrating marrow pathology as they rely on alteration to cortices or a large area of spongiosa in order for the abnormality to be conspicuous. This inability to demonstrate bone marrow or periosteal edema means that radiographs are only able to demonstrate stress fractures or osteochondritis at a relatively late stage, i.e. when there is cortical breakdown or subchondral bone fragmentation or if sufficient time has occurred for an osteoblastic repair response to have taken place. Accordingly correctly tailored MR imaging is more appropriate for demonstrating these conditions early in their evolution.

Joint radiographs are able to demonstrate degenerative arthrosis but again usually only at a late stage in its evolution. The classical radiographic diagnostic signs are loss of joint space, subchondral cyst formation, marginal osteophytosis and subchondral sclerosis. All of these features when present usually reflect disease of reasonably long duration.

In cases of tarsal coalition specific oblique radiographic projections will often confirm the presence of bony (but not fibrous) bars. In many cases, however, CT or occasionally MR imaging is required for a definitive diagnosis.

Conventional radiographs are good at demonstrating established myositis ossificans but of limited use early in its evolution. The fact that US demonstrates the condition at an earlier phase may be helpful in terms of treatment. If myositis ossificans is present on US then a radiograph should be obtained. If the radiograph is positive then it confirms the diagnosis. If it is negative then the calcification is early and presumably more susceptible to benefit from therapies aimed at halting its progress.

Computed tomography (CT)

> **Computed tomography**
> • X-rays with higher radiation than conventional radiography
> • Tomography and three-dimensional reconstruction possible
> • Comminuted or complex fractures visualized
> • Less relevant in sports medicine.

Although contrast resolution is greater in computed tomography than conventional radiographs the spatial resolution is significantly less. The contrast resolution is higher as the provision of a nominal (Hounsfield) scale for radiographic densities produces a broader spectrum of densities even though in real terms it is still only fat, soft tissue, bone, air and metallic densities that are seen. The spatial resolution is lower due to the larger size of the pixels of CT scans, those of conventional radiographs being much smaller, i.e. reflecting the size of the silver crystals forming the film. Acquisition of a volume data set using a spiral scanner allows multiplanar reconstruction although even with modern reconstruction algorithms a much greater resolution occurs in the plane of acquisition.

There are only a few specific indications for CT imaging of sports injuries. Comminuted or complex fractures of the calcaneus, tibial plateau or proximal humerus whether due to athletic injury or not may require CT imaging to assess whether surgery is required and, if so, to plan the surgical technique. It may also be used to demonstrate significant but small fractures, e.g. bony Bankart-type glenoid fractures. Ostochondral fractures can be demonstrated on CT imaging in order to assess their presence and chronicity, e.g. talar dome osteochondral fractures, although MR imaging is probably preferable in most circumstances. Fractures are usually only seen on CT images where they are perpendicular rather than parallel to the acquisition plane. Stress fractures in long bones are usually transverse to the bone's axis and as such not well demonstrated. The exception is the relatively rare longitudinal stress fracture. Stress fractures to non-long bones, on the other hand, are often well demonstrated by CT. Tarsal bone fractures, for instance, run in a sagittal plane and are well demonstrated in the transverse axial plane. Similarly, stress fractures through the pars interarticularis of vertebrae are very well seen on transverse axial images, especially if the images are acquired using a 'reversed-angle' plane, i.e. not parallel to the disk but in a plane 45° coronal to the disk.

CT may be used to assess areas of osteochondritis, particularly to see if there is a 'free' fragment which may require removal. It is extremely good at 'untangling' complex bone anatomy such as tarsal fusions. It is also very good at confirming the diagnostic centrifugal nature of myositis ossificans circumscripta.

CT may also be performed following injection of intra-articular contrast, either positive contrast (iodinated contrast agent), negative contrast (air) or both (double-contrast study). CT arthrography is the best imaging method for demonstrating small intra-articular loose bodies and is good at demonstrating labral injuries, e.g. double-contrast CT arthrography of the glenohumeral joint performed with the patient in the prone-oblique position for demonstrating soft tissue (and bony) Bankart lesions in athletes with recurrent subluxation. Adsorption of contrast onto retropatellar articular cartilage and/or demonstration of surface irregularity on double-contrast CT-arthrography of the knee are diagnostic signs in athletes with chondromalacia patella.

Ultrasound

Ultrasound
- Sound waves, echo sounder
- Soft tissue: tendons, muscles, fluid accumulation in joints, bursae
- Real-time investigation: functional element
- Intervention possible (biopsy, local injections)
- Cheap
- Difficult, demands high skill
- Success dependent on investigator.

Introduction

The last two decades have seen spectacular developments in ultrasound equipment technology which has now resulted in production of ultrasound systems capable of high-resolution imaging of superficial structures, particularly superficial tendons. Initially problems arose due to the use of sector scanners with a narrow near field of view. Sector scanners also produced areas of artifactually low echogenicity at the extremes of the beam due to beam obliquity artifact (anisotropy, Fig. 5.1.1). Both of these problems have been overcome by production of high-quality linear array transducers and recognition of the necessity for the operator to maintain a perpendicular incident beam to the structure being examined. When tendons were originally examined they were thought to be hypoechoic relative to adjacent structures whereas now due to improvements in high-frequency transducer technology tendons are normally echogenic and exhibit an internal fibrillar pattern. The change in perception reflects the ability of a transducer to elicit separate collagen bundle interfaces within the tendon. If normal tendons are examined *in vitro* at different frequencies (7.5, 10, 13 and 15 MHz), the tendons will show an internal network of fine parallel and linear fibrillar echoes which become more numerous and thinner as the US frequency is increased. It is possible that our perception of the tendon internal architecture will change again as the spatial resolution continues to improve.

Symmetry of tendinopathy

The contralateral limb should always be scanned for comparison, but it cannot be assumed that the asymp-

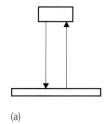 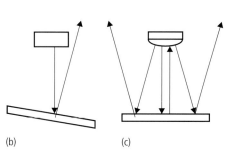

Fig. 5.1.1 Anisotropy—beam obliquity artifact. (a) Perpendicular beam; (b) oblique beam; (c) curved array.

(a) (b) (c)

tomatic side is normal. In a study of 31 patients with unilateral Achilles tendon rupture all patients had sonographic evidence of degeneration of the ipsilateral tendon remote from the rupture point and 90% had degenerative changes in the contralateral asymptomatic heel. The contralateral limb, however, may provide information with regard to the underlying disease mechanism, and particularly when changes on the symptomatic side are severe as it may be easier to assess the more subtle sonographic changes on the less severely involved side.

Tendon damage accumulation

Tendon is not a static tissue but appears to be constantly remodelling itself by a process of minor injury and repair. Normal asymptomatic tendons in non-athletic individuals will exhibit occasional small hypoechoic foci on sonographic examination which appear to reflect either microdefects or foci of altered collagen architecture. These presumably reflect a natural cycle of minor injury and repair.

The sonographic appearances of the asymptomatic Achilles, patellar and plantar aponeurotic tendons of all 46 members of the playing staff at a single professional soccer club were compared with 15 non-athletic controls [2]. Three soccer players and two control subjects were then excluded from the study due to previous tendon symptoms. Seventy per cent of soccer players demonstrated sonographic evidence of Achilles tendon disease compared to 7% of age- and sex-matched controls, 77% of players demonstrated patellar tendon disease compared to 26% of controls and 35% of players plantar fasciitis compared to no control subjects.

In the patellar tendon in elite volleyball players ultrasound changes were observed in 24% of the knees of athletes without symptoms. In addition, specific ultrasound findings such as paratenon changes, hypoechoic zones or pathologic tendon thickness proximally did not correlate significantly with the degree or the duration of symptoms [3]. Patellar tendon sonographic hypoechoic areas can resolve, remain unchanged, or expand in active athletes and are not directly related to symptoms. Therefore these sonographic changes should not in isolation be an indication for surgery [4].

Distribution of sonographic tendon changes

Achilles tendon

With ultrasound two distinct findings are seen, depending on whether the proximal two-thirds or the distal third of the Achilles tendon is involved.

In tendons exhibiting proximal/middle-third Achilles tendinosis with subtotal tendon cross-section involvement, over 90% exhibit changes in the medial segment, and isolated changes in the lateral segment are never seen. The medial distribution suggests that the tendinosis at least in part reflects increased tensile forces over the medial side of the tendon which in turn could reflect underlying hindfoot hyperpronation (see Fig. 5.1.2). Also, most tendons exhibit changes in the superficial segment and few in the deep segment. This may partially reflect the fact that the Achilles tendon's transverse axis is not transverse to the body axis, with the superficial segment being medial relative to the deep segment, which may increase the tensile forces along this superficial part of the tendon (Fig. 5.1.3).

In patients with mechanical symptoms in the distal Achilles tendon calcaneal insertion region the vast majority have distal Achilles tendon or paratenon changes associated with a retrocalcaneal bursitis, with predomination of changes in the deep portion of the tendon immediately adjacent to the posterior–superior calcaneal tuberosity. This is not surprising, as the retrocalcaneal bursa lies between the distal Achilles tendon and the posterior–superior calcaneal tuberosi-

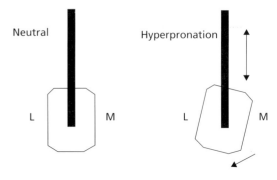

Fig. 5.1.2 Increased tensile forces on the medial side of the Achilles tendon in hyperpronation.

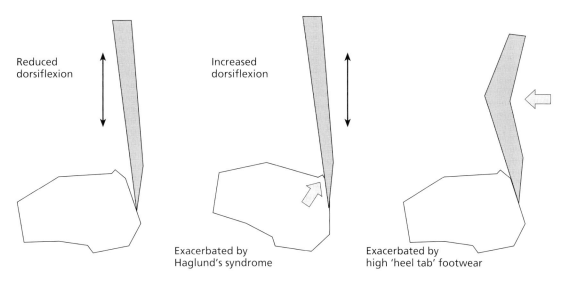

Fig. 5.1.3 Segmental distribution of changes.

ty. Ankle dorsiflexion produces compression of the retrocalcaneal bursa, protecting the distal tendon from direct contact with the calcaneal tuberosity. These compressive forces may be increased in excessive repetitive dorsiflexion, e.g. during running or jumping. In patients with severe retrocalcaneal bursitis there are usually also sonographic changes in the superficial segment of the proximal/middle-third of the tendon, which is not surprising as the posterior calcaneal impingement is likely to increase the tensile forces over the superficial portion of the tendon relative to the forces incident on its deep portion. This may be increased if a high 'heel-tab' is present on an athlete's footwear (Fig. 5.1.3). This phenomenon is well recognized by most elite track athletes who remove these ironically named 'Achilles tendon protectors' as soon as they purchase a new pair of running shoes!

Patellar tendon

The patellar tendon also exhibits characteristic patterns of change.

Jumper's knee. Focal tendon degeneration in the midline deep surface of the patellar tendon at the inferior pole of the patella with relative sparing of the medial, lateral and superficial portions of the proximal tendon. The distribution suggests an impingement phenome-

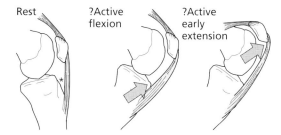

Fig. 5.1.4 Proximal and distal third patellar tendon changes. *Region of deep pretibial bursa.

non (Fig. 5.1.4) sometimes even resulting in a compression fracture or fragmentation of the inferior pole of the patella, i.e. Sinding–Larsen-type injury. Occasionally, changes occur slightly to the medial or lateral side of the midsagittal plane. Proximal tendon distribution is seen in 50–60% of cases.

Mid-tendon disease. Focal degeneration of the mid-tendon is usually localized to either the medial or lateral half of the patellar tendon and appears to reflect increased tensile forces to these areas, which may be due to patella maltracking (Fig. 5.1.5). This is an uncommon distribution and represents only approximately 2% of focal patellar tendinosis.

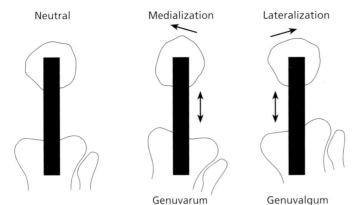

Neutral　　　Medialization　　　Lateralization

Genuvarum　　　Genuvalgum

Fig. 5.1.5 Middle third patellar tendon changes.

Distal tendon disease. These changes usually occur on the deep tendon surface and are almost inevitably associated with a deep pretibial bursitis. This is akin to the Haglund phenomenon with the tendon being impinged upon by the anterior tibial plateau during forced knee flexion. There are typical sonographic appearances in Osgood–Schlatter disease: distal patellar tendinitis, deep pretibial bursitis and osseocartilaginous fragmentation at the osseotendinous junction. Distal patellar tendon degeneration represents approximately 41% of focal tendinosis.

After removal of its central third for anterior cruciate ligament (ACL) reconstruction the ultrasonographic changes in the patellar tendon extend with time to involve the entire donor tendon. It becomes diffusely enlarged, hypoechoic and inhomogeneous compared with the presurgical state. The tendon thickening is maximal in the anteroposterior axis and peaks 2 months post surgery [5].

Tendon inflammation

Repair of tendon injury

Color Doppler imaging (CDI) may be helpful in assessing tendon disease activity. Under normal circumstances it is not possible sonographically to demonstrate flow in the paratenon vessels of the large tendons, i.e. Achilles and patellar tendons. In a severe tendinitis or acute exacerbation of tendinosis there may be marked hyperemia and dramatically increased

flow in these paratenon vessels which may be demonstrated extending deep into the tendon substance. In cases of the distal Achilles tendinitis hyperemia may also be demonstrated in the inferior portion of Kager's fatty triangle surrounding an inflamed retrocalcaneal bursa.

Tenosynovitis

Although vincula and synovial sheath vessel flow may not be seen on CDI or power Doppler imaging in normal tendons there may be markedly increased flow in an acute severe tenosynovitis whether due to inflammatory arthropathy or tendon sheath infection. The problem, however, with using CDI to monitor disease activity is the inability to demonstrate flow in nondiseased tendons and subsequently the difficulty in obtaining a baseline by which to assess hyperemia. The advent of inexpensive and reproducible ultrasound contrast agent studies may help to overcome this problem in the near future.

Muscle injury

Ultrasound investigation after muscle injury provides information useful for planning rehabilitation. If sonographically no abnormality is demonstrated in an athlete who clinically has an acute muscle tear, then significant muscle injury is unlikely and the athlete should be able to return rapidly to sporting activity.

Sonography may reveal a small hematoma dissecting between muscle groups or a small focus of heterogeneous muscle echogenicity occasionally with associated minor mass effect on adjacent connective tissue interfaces in more significant tears.

Partial or complete muscle discontinuity, or an area of muscle architecture disorganization involving a major portion of that muscle cross-section, usually means that the athlete will have to rest from sporting activity for 4–6 weeks and occasionally even longer depending on the precise anatomic site. Interestingly, partial tears often produce greater symptoms than full-thickness tears especially where other muscles in the same group are able to maintain muscle power, e.g. rectus femoris tears.

Occasionally a large intramuscular hematoma occurs following muscle tear and aspiration may readily be performed under ultrasound.

Ultrasound is the most sensitive method of imaging early soft tissue calcification whether in muscle or tendon. In its early stage myositis ossificans appears as an echogenic area within a heterogeneous area of muscle which subsequently produces acoustic shadowing as the calcification/ossification progresses. The calcification usually tends to be peripheral, i.e. centrifugal, but a herring bone pattern may be seen along the line of the injured muscle. In myositis ossificans US will usually demonstrate an echogenic focus at 7–10 days compared to 2–3 weeks on CT and slightly longer for conventional radiography. Isotope bone scans may demonstrate calcification as early as US but these appearances are non-specific. MR imaging will not usually show the calcification unless it is extremely large and appears as a very aggressive, possibly neoplastic, soft tissue abnormality.

Future

A number of technologic developments currently reaching fruition will help to further develop tendon US imaging. Manufacturers are now starting to produce inexpensive high-resolution systems dedicated for musculoskeletal ultrasound. These are being combined with very high frequency (12–20 MHz) linear array transducers with optimized near field for demonstration of very superficial structures such as the peripheral limb juxta-articular tendons. Finally hand-held US systems with the same imaging capabilities as the current top-of-the-range system will further expand the role of ultrasound in the clinical management of patients with tendinopathies.

Magnetic resonance imaging (MRI)

Magnetic resonance imaging
- Radio waves, magnetism
- Soft tissue, bones, cartilage
- Joint injuries
- Limited capacity
- Expensive
- Static images

Introduction

Due to its multiplanar capabilities, lack of ionizing radiation and superior soft tissue contrast, MR imaging is an important adjunct to conventional diagnostic examinations such as plain radiography, bone scintigraphy and ultrasound in assessing the magnitude and extent of soft tissue injury. Compared to bone scintigraphy, MR imaging has superior spatial resolution in localizing soft tissue injury, yet does not provide a direct measure of bone turnover. As such, these imaging tests are often complementary, rather than mutually exclusive.

Principles of MR imaging

MR imaging is founded on the principle that certain nuclear species, such as hydrogen, possess inherent magnetic properties. When placed in a high-strength external magnetic field these nuclei will precess, which is a resonance phenomenon, according to the axis of the external field. In order to obtain diagnostic information from these precessing protons, radiofrequency pulses are sent into the patient, which convert these nuclei to a higher energy state, by 'flipping' them from the longitudinal to the transverse plane. Once the disturbing radiofrequency (RF) pulse is turned off, thermal equilibrium is restored and the released electromagnetic energy induces a voltage in a receiver coil that is placed around the body part of interest. Based on the resistance of the imaging coil, this generates a current. This current, when sent through an analog to digital converter, creates digitized data that undergo a mathematical progression known as Fourier transformation, yielding an MR image.

Table 5.1.3 Simplified MR signal characteristics of joints.

	T$_1$-Weighted	T$_2$-Weighted
Cortical bone	Low	Low
Fat (marrow, subcutaneous)	High	High
Type I collagen (normal ligament, tendon, meniscus, labrum)	Low	Low
Fluid (normal joint)	Low	High
Muscle	Intermediate	Intermediate
Articular cartilage*	Intermediate	Slightly lower

* Signal characteristics are pulse-sequence and image-parameter dependent.

By varying the time between successive disturbing RF pulses (repetition time or TR) and the time between the disturbing RF pulses and the time at which echo information is recorded (echo time or TE), pulse sequences of varying soft tissue contrast may be generated. A simplified table of MR signal characteristics is provided in Table 5.1.3. T$_1$ relaxation time refers to the recovery of the initial magnetization following the disturbing RF pulse, which fat protons achieve quickly, thus yielding bright signal on a T$_1$-weighted sequence. T$_2$ relaxation time refers to the decay process which occurs in the transverse plane.

Commonly used MR pulse sequences for orthopedics include spin echo and fast or turbo spin echo, the latter of which yield rapid acquisition of images, often with superior soft tissue contrast. As the latter images are obtained more quickly, superior spatial resolution may be achieved by use of a higher resolution matrix. It should be remembered that all MR images are digitized; therefore, spatial resolution is dependent on the size of the picture element or pixel, which is in turn determined by the field of view, or area of study, divided by the imaging matrix. Maintaining an adequate field of view to cover diagnostic information may be performed with no sacrifice to spatial resolution, when an appropriate imaging matrix is chosen.

Gradient echo sequences are also commonly utilized, which provide a coarsened appearance to trabecular bone, as they have little correction for field inhomogeneities. Such pulse sequences typically have poor contrast between fat and muscle (in the absence of additional fat suppression techniques) and yield a phenomenon known as flow-related enhancement, which may be exploited for vascular MR pulse sequences.

Fat suppression techniques 'rescale' the contrast range, as fat is characteristically conspicuous on most MR pulse sequences. Such sequences are essential in orthopedic imaging to disclose subtle areas of trabecular microfracture or subchondral edema secondary to osteochondral impaction. They also accentuate the high signal from soft tissue fluid collections such as ganglion cysts of the menisci or shoulder labrum.

Imaging of specific injuries

Knee

MR imaging has been shown to be accurate in depiction of meniscal and ligament tears of the knee [6,7]. Meniscal tears are classified by an intrameniscal grading system for internal signal [8] or by the presence of abnormal meniscal pathology, in which the diagnosis of a radial split, displaced fragment or bucket-handle tear may be seen (Fig. 5.1.6). An awareness of normal meniscal vascularity is essential in order to aid in preoperative planning for potential meniscal repair. While a high prevalence of meniscal tears have been noted in asymptomatic patients, particularly those of middle to older age [9], this does not invalidate the utility of this same imaging test in a symptomatic patient. In older athletic patients, MR imaging will disclose the degree of cartilage degeneration, and assess for the presence of degenerative meniscal tears, as well as the potential for underlying osteonecrosis. Following meniscectomy, MR imaging is helpful in assessing for re-tears of a remnant [10] or an associated degenerative change. Following primary meniscal repair, fluid imbibition into the repair site can be distinguished from the fibrovascular response of the normal intact meniscus, and thus MRI may be efficacious in assessing the degree of meniscal healing or re-tear through the repair site [11,12]. Pulse sequences which are utilized to assess meniscal healing and evaluate the postoperative meniscus accentuate water, either through the use of frequency-selective fat suppression or by exploiting the inherent magnetization transfer found in fast spin echo sequences. This does not require prototype software and is available on all high field strength units.

Following ligamentous injury, MR is helpful in assessing the degree and location of cruciate ligament tear, as well as associated cartilage or meniscal injury (Fig. 5.1.7). Similar accuracies have been reported with mid- and high field strengths with regard to anterior cruciate ligament injuries [13]. While primary distal avulsion of the tibial eminence may be noted on the plain film, MR is helpful in determining the degree of displacement and may aid in determining whether surgical reduction of the eminence is warranted. It is important to remember that MRI is an anatomic test which assesses the anatomic continuity of ligaments and tendons at the time of imaging. Based on the signal characteristics, MR also reflects the histopathology of the tissue being excited. It is essential for the clinician to correlate those anatomic and histopathologic changes gleaned from the MR examination with their clinical assessment of joint function. For example, a high-grade partial cruciate ligament tear on MR examination of the knee may yield functional complete discontinuity at the time of exam under anesthesia, with a wide-based pivot shift. In addition, a discrete full-thickness tear of the medial collateral ligament of the knee, seen on one tomographic MR image, may not yield overt valgus instability on valgus stressing of the knee. Thus, global assessment of the injured extremity is best performed with a comprehensive physical examination to assess ligament function, as well as anatomic assessment of tissue continuity based on the MR examination.

Assessment of the multiple ligament injured knee is crucial, as MR may disclose the degree of posterolateral corner injury with concomitant cruciate tear, the severity of which may warrant a formal posterolateral corner reconstruction or, in some cases, primary repair [14]. Following ligament reconstruction, MR is helpful in assessing the position of the graft as well as the magnetic characteristics of the graft tissue which are a reflection of the status of the collagen, disclosing areas of either elastic deformation or traumatic disruption [15].

Stress fractures. Stress fractures are denoted as diminished signal intensity fracture lines surrounded by marrow edema, the latter of which are accentuated using fat suppression techniques. Due to its tomo-

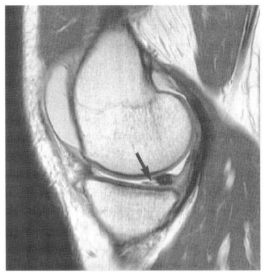

(a)

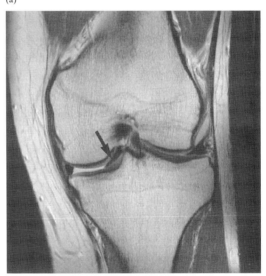

(b)

Fig. 5.1.6 Bucket-handle tear of the medial meniscus. (a) Sagittal fast spin echo sequence demonstrates foreshortening of the posterior horn of the medial meniscus, with fraying at the anterior edge (arrow). (b) Coronal image confirms the displaced bucket-handle fragment in the medial aspect of the intercondylar notch (arrow).

graphic nature and superior soft tissue contrast, MR imaging is more sensitive than plain film in disclosing stress fracture, and will disclose the continuum of stress-induced injury to bone, particularly that in competitive runners. This includes soft tissue periostitis

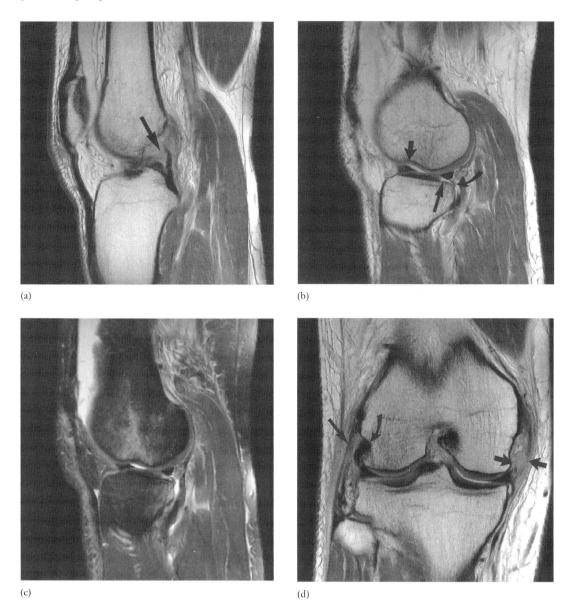

(a)

(b)

(c)

(d)

Fig. 5.1.7 Acute twisting injury to the right knee in a 32-year-old athlete. (a) Sagittal fast spin echo sequence through the intercondylar notch demonstrates complete disruption of the anterior cruciate ligament (arrows). (b) Sagittal fast spin echo sequence at the lateral aspect of the knee in the same patient demonstrates transchondral fracture to the posterior margin of the lateral tibial plateau with a full thickness cartilage defect (long straight arrow). Note the displaced chondral fragment in the meniscosynovial recess (curved arrow). Also note the additional osteochondral impaction of the lateral femoral condyle (small straight arrow). (c) The subchondral reaction is made more conspicuous using fat-suppression techniques, which 'rescale' the contrast range, thus making the edema in the subchondral bone more apparent. (d) Coronal fast spin echo sequence in the same patient discloses a high-grade partial tear of the medial collateral ligament at the femur, involving both deep and superficial components (short straight arrows). Also note the moderately high grade partial tear of the fibular collateral ligament (long straight arrow). The popliteus tendon is intact at the femur (curved arrow).

and endosteal callus as well as the presence of a frank cortical or medullary fracture. Bone scintigraphy is helpful in assessing for stress fracture; however, in older patients the presence of occult fracture may be more readily noted on MR imaging [16].

Cartilage imaging

One of the most recent developments of MR imaging has been the advent of dedicated cartilage pulse sequences [17,18]. These have been well validated in both the imaging and orthopedic literature, using either fat-suppressed T_1-weighted gradient echo techniques [17,19] or optimized fast spin echo techniques [18]. Using appropriate pulse sequences, the degree of transchondral fracture sustained during tibial translation in the presence of ACL insufficiency may be noted, as well as the appearance and status of the articular cartilage over osteochondritic lesions.

It is important to remember that the so-called 'bone bruise', seen in the setting of an ACL insufficiency, is indeed a transchondral fracture of varying severity. The importance of standardized cartilage pulse sequencing in every MR evaluation of the joint cannot be overstated, as seemingly innocuous bone bruises may in fact herald traumatic delamination of cartilage, yielding focal post-traumatic arthrosis of the knee which may have prognostic significance for the patient's outcome.

Following surgical manipulation of articular cartilage defects with mosaicplasty, autologous cartilage implantation or microfracture, MR imaging provides an objective measure of treatment outcome. Following cartilage transplantation, MR will assess the integrity of the periosteal flap, morphology of the transplant and interface with the native cartilage, as well as providing some tissue characterization of the substance 'filling the defect' [20]. With appropriate pulse sequencing, it is hoped that hyaline cartilage may be distinguished from reparative fibrocartilage [21].

Shoulder imaging

MR imaging is helpful in assessing the degree of rotator cuff tear, and has been proven accurate in distinguishing partial from full-thickness tears [22]. In addition to assessing the degree of rotator cuff deficiency, MR may also disclose the degree of osteoarthrosis, which may confound the clinical assessment of older athletes with cuff weakness [23]. In the presence of shoulder instability, MR is accurate using either optimized non-contrast techniques or MR arthrography in detecting labral detachment [24,25]. Following initial dislocation, MR imaging can distinguish labral lesions (Fig. 5.1.8) from primary capsular failure, thus aiding in the selection of those patients best suited for prompt arthroscopic debridement [26]. The diagnosis of isolated capsular tears requires high spatial resolution, in order to depict the glenohumeral ligaments as structures discrete from the adjacent capsule.

Superior labral anterior and posterior (SLAP) lesions may also be visualized either using MR arthrography or optimized non-contrast techniques [26]. In the setting of poorly defined shoulder pain without overt anterior instability, MR can be helpful in distinguishing isolated biceps lesions from superior labral lesions.

Elbow

Evaluation of the athlete's elbow is difficult, particularly in the throwing athlete, as flexor or pronator tendinopathy, medial collateral ligament pathology, and posteromedial cartilage injury may be difficult to distinguish as distinct clinical entities [27]. Using high spatial resolution and thin slice (1.5–2 mm) thickness, MR imaging may disclose subtle lesions of the medial collateral ligament (Fig. 5.1.9). Dedicated cartilage pulse sequencing is mandatory in these athletes as significant chondral wear may be seen, particularly of the posteromedial margin of the elbow in the throwing athlete, in the absence of plain radiographic change [28].

Posteromedial impingement, attributed to valgus extension overload, is denoted radiographically as a prominent posteromedial osteophyte [29]. Concomitant thickening of the posterior capsule and/or fracture of the osteophyte may be seen, as well as chondral wear over the posterior aspect of the trochlea [28].

Medial epicondylitis, or degeneration of the origin of the flexor and pronator tendons, is characterized by signal hyperintensity with variable amount of intratendinous disruption at the tendon origin. Similarly, lateral epicondylitis, or tennis elbow, is similarly diagnosed by degeneration and signal hyperintensity of the

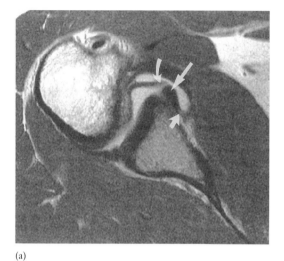

(a)

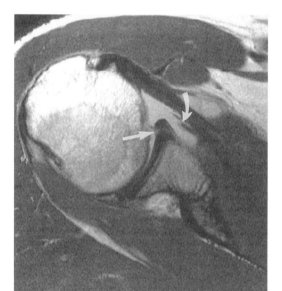

(b)

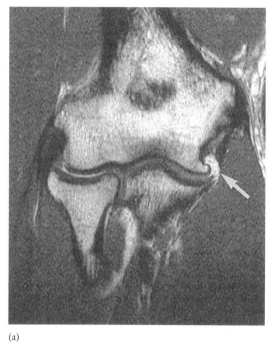

(a)

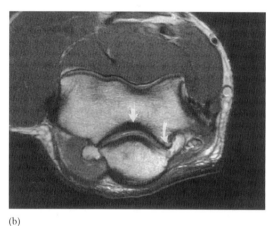

(b)

Fig. 5.1.8 (a) Axial fast spin echo sequence in the right shoulder in a 20-year-old collegiate athlete who sustained an anterior dislocation while skiing. There is displacement of the anteroinferior labrum (long arrow) in an inferomedial direction, with a partial tear of the anterior band of the inferior glenohumeral ligament (curved arrow). Note that the labrum is tethered medially by the stripped periosteum at the capsular attachment of the capsule (short straight arrow), indicating an anterior labral periosteal sleeve avulsion (ALPSA). (b) Axial fast spin echo sequence at a more cephalad level discloses a split (straight arrow) in the midanterior labrum. Note the frayed appearance of the middle glenohumeral ligament (curved arrow).

Fig. 5.1.9 (a) Medial elbow pain in a competitive throwing athlete. Coronal MR image discloses a non-acute high-grade tear at the ulnar attachment of the anterior band of the medial collateral ligament (arrow). Note the poor tissue remodeling, with residual signal hyperintensity. (b) Axial fast spin echo sequence in the same patient discloses an osteophyte (curved arrow) off the posteromedial margin of the elbow joint. Note the thinning of cartilage over the posterior margin of the trochlea with subchondral sclerosis (short arrow).

origin of the extensor carpi radialis brevis. The high signal intensity reflects the mucoid degeneration and vascular infiltration, without acute or chronic inflammatory response [30]. The utility of MR in the setting of elbow tendinosis lies in its ability to detect not only the degree of degeneration, but also the presence of associated partial or full-thickness disruption, the latter of which may warrant primary tendon reattachment. Associated chondral injuries may be noted, thus prompting preliminary MR arthroscopy prior to open tendon debridement. While MR imaging is also efficacious in assessing the degree of biceps rupture, these elbow tendinopathies may also be nicely disclosed by dedicated musculoskeletal ultrasound, where the biceps muscle may be loaded in a provocative measure to detect the degree of retraction. The use of ultrasound will obviate the need for potential surface coil repositioning in the setting of biceps retraction [28].

Bone scintigraphy

> **Bone scintigraphy**
> - Injection of radioactive pharmaceutical
> - Actual bone metabolism
> - Very sensitive, but not specific
> - Stress fractures, shin splints, vascularization
> - Can eliminate or localize skeletal involvement including joint disease
> - Static images, tomography possible
> - Semiquantification of local metabolism with uptake ratios.

Bone scintigraphy is an atraumatic, easily applied and relatively inexpensive technique. The method is very sensitive, reflecting the actual bone metabolism, and thus sites of rebuilding, mechanical stress, growth and reorganization are shown. In many cases, it is difficult or impossible to diagnose minor disturbances in bone metabolism by conventional radiography, whereas bone scintigraphy more easily detects these. Scintigraphy is abnormal within 48 h after even minor trauma (a

little longer in the elderly). Therefore it offers the advantage of wide availability and high sensitivity, but its lack of specificity means that it often only points out the areas where further diagnostics/treatment should be concentrated.

Method

Bone scintigraphy is performed 2–4 h after an intravenous injection of Tc-99m diphosphonate, a bone-seeking radionuclide, in an amount of 500–800 MBq, lower in children. Technetium-99m is a γ-emitting isotope with a half-life of 6 h. The radiation dose is 3–5 mSv, thus about twice the natural background radiation per year and comparable to the dose received by conventional X-ray pictures.

In principle, an investigation may be repeated after only 2–3 days, but the method is not suited to following a healing process as microstructural remodelling continues to take place long after clinical healing.

The uptake of the technetium phosphate complexes into the skeleton is related to the bone blood flow and especially the osteoblast activity. Increased blood flow leads to a certain, but not linearly increased, uptake, but of more importance is that compromised blood flow obstructs the supply of radionuclide, which leads to activity defects. The radionuclide is selectively localized below the laminar osteoid at the hydroxyapatite crystal surface, i.e. the actively bone-forming mineralizing layer. In addition, supplementary binding sites to, for example, immature or altered collagen or deposition in necrotic or otherwise damaged muscular tissue have been reported.

A focally increased uptake in bone scintigraphy most often reflects the osteoblastic response of bone to a local insult irrespective of the actual etiology, i.e. a reparative proces, but even in bone destruction with osteoclastic activity attempts at bone repair are involved, leading to 'hot spots'. Thus, bone scintigraphy is positive (shows focal increased uptake) in many diseases of the skeletal system, such as bone tumors, metastases, fractures including stress fractures, infections, etc. and is in this way unspecific. However, the scintigraphic findings in many of the frequent benign disorders in the skeletal system are typical, which is of interest to the sports physician.

Evaluation of the regional vascularity may be

valuable in patients with localized problems and may be obtained by a 'three-phase' scintigram, where sequential images are obtained for the first 30 s ('flow phase'), and a 'blood pool image' representing the bone extracellular fluid is obtained at 1 min in addition to the 3-h standard static views. In cases of avascularity (i.e. of the femoral head) no uptake is seen in any of the images.

Bone tomography, SPECT (single photon emission computed tomography), may be performed in order to obtain a more precise location in any area of the skeleton, e.g. in the spine where planar imaging is often normal, or to visualize the internal disturbances in a knee joint (Fig. 5.1.10).

Stress fractures

Suspicion of stress fractures (or fatigue fractures) is one of the main reasons for referral for bone scintigraphy in sports medicine. The most frequent localization for stress fractures has in several investigations been found to be the tibia (Fig. 5.1.11), accounting for about 50% of stress fractures [31,32]. Other frequent localizations are the tarsometatarsals (Figs 5.1.12 & 5.1.13), fibula and femur, but stress fractures have been described in almost all bones (Figs 5.1.14 and 5.1.15)—except the skull!

The typical finding in bone scintigraphy is an intense fusiform focus (Fig. 5.1.11), in the tibia often localized posteromedially. If an anterior margin stress fracture is (rarely) found, a much more serious and prognostic dubious condition exists [34]. A graduating system to classify the injury extension has been proposed among others by Matin [35] as a five-stage graduation, representing a continuous spectrum of injury from normal (minimal periosteal reaction, involving 0–20% of the bone) to stage V which is a full-thickness stress fracture. This differentiation demands scintigraphy in two projections. The less serious stages I and II will not be detected radiographically, while stages IV and V will most often show periosteal or endosteal thickening in X-rays 8–14 days after onset of symptoms. Scintigraphically, the minor injuries are normalized in 2–3 months, while the major ones are often visible for more than 6 months. The graduation thus gives a prognosis with regard to time for healing and guidance for loading.

A special problem is stress fractures in the femoral neck because of a potential risk for development of head necrosis. Spontaneous fractures here have been described in female athletes with long-lasting amenorrhea implying that bone scintigraphy should be performed with only a weak indication in athletes with

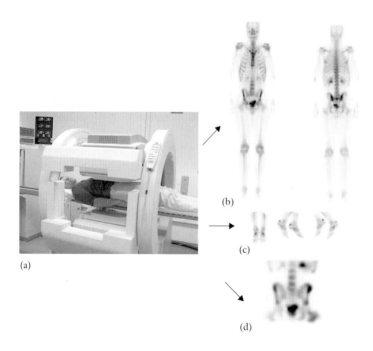

(a)

(b)

(c)

(d)

Fig. 5.1.10 Two-headed gamma camera (a) for (b) whole-body scintigraphy, (c) single acquisitions or (d) tomography (SPECT).

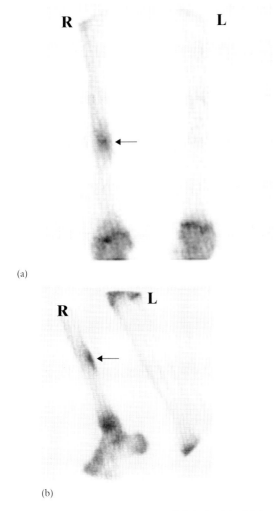

(a)

(b)

Fig. 5.1.11 Stress fracture posteromedially in the right tibia in a 17-year-old male soccer player.

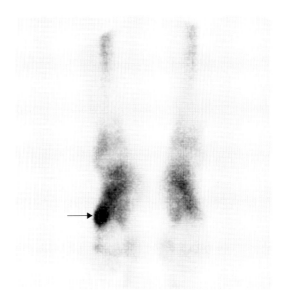

Fig. 5.1.12 Stress fracture in the fifth metatarsal, arising during a 1500-m run in a 23-year-old female elite runner.

pain in the pelvis, groin, femur and knee [36]. The bone scintigraphy shows activity accumulation at the location of the stress fracture, but concomitantly a defect in the femoral caput if the blood perfusion is interrupted (Fig. 5.1.16). Repeated stress fractures or stress fractures in female athletes with secondary amenorrhea and disordered eating may warrant an investigation of the general bone mineral content (Fig. 5.1.17).

Other fractures

Although bone scintigraphy is not the primary diag-

nostic tool applied for fractures, it may help in the evaluation of certain cases. It has been shown to be especially valuable in the investigation of wrist pain to exclude scaphoid ('navicular') fractures (Fig. 5.1.18) or to identify fractures in other carpal bones [37].

Tibial stress syndrome ('shin splints')

Scintigraphically, the condition presents as an elongated region of moderately increased activity in the periosteum, usually of the mid- or lower tibia, related to the insertion of the tibialis posterior or soleus (Fig. 5.1.19). We have found a similar condition in the ulna ('ulnar splint') in a kayak rower, performing intensive strength training of the wrists.

The condition may be differentiated scintigraphically from stress fractures or chronic compartment syndrome, other frequent causes of lower extremity pain, and is thought to result from increased stress from the muscles or connective tissues on the superficial portion of the bone cortex, leading to increased bone metabolism. Increased perfusion in the lesion is rare in contrast to stress fractures; thus a 'three-phase bone scan' may help to discriminate between the two conditions.

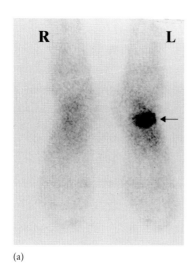

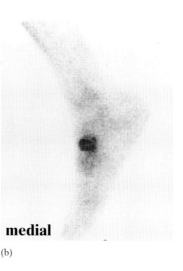

Fig. 5.1.13 Stress fracture of the left os naviculare pedis in a 24-year-old male elite runner. This is one of the few stress fractures that may demand total immobilization because of the risk of later necrosis.

(a)   (b)

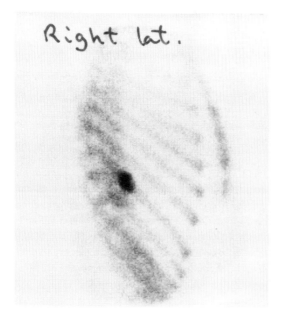

Fig. 5.1.14 Stress fracture in the ribs in a 24-year-old elite rower, following change of equipment to a new sweep-oar [33].

Other enthesopathies

The term 'enthesopathy' refers to calcification and bone formation due to aseptic inflammation at the site of tendon and ligament attachment. Scintigraphic changes appear earlier and are more sensitive than X-rays. Focal abnormal uptake is seen in the lateral epicondyle in cases of lateral epicondylitis ('tennis elbow'), and around the medial tuberosity of the calcaneus in the case of plantar fasciitis. Also, in Achilles tendinitis an increased uptake at the upper insertion of calcaneus as well as in the tendon may be found (Fig. 5.1.20). In athletes with groin pain, increased activity in the symphysis pubis, often with focal 'hot spots', is connected with inflammation of the symphysis, osteitis pubis (Fig. 5.1.21) [38].

Joint injuries

Bone scintigraphy may in many cases assist in the diagnostic evaluation of especially longer-lasting joint-related pain/problems. Being very unspecific, scintigraphy cannot discriminate between joint injury due to inflammatory or degenerative joint diseases. However, the investigation is so sensitive that it is well suited to determining whether a joint is affected or not [39]. In a prospective study of 44 younger patients referred for arthroscopy with a suspected meniscus tear, an accuracy of 0.92 was found for the bone scintigraphy in discriminating between potentially surgery-demanding lesions and minor injuries/healthy knees where arthroscopy and surgery could be avoided [39]. Thus, the investigation may be useful as a tool to ex-

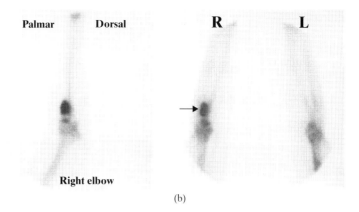

Palmar   **Dorsal**   **R**   **L**

Right elbow

(a)

(b)

Fig. 5.1.15 Radial stress fracture in a 37-year-old female from knitting.

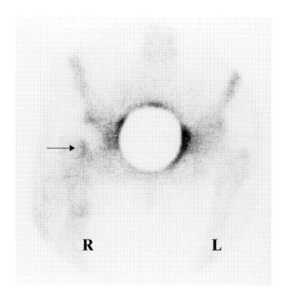

R   **L**

Fig. 5.1.16 Avascularity in the right caput femoris (arrow) after a collum femoris fracture illustrated in a 70-year-old female. (The big circular defect in the middle represents a lead shield covering the bladder.)

clude invasive diagnostics, but is not very valuable for obtaining a specific diagnosis in injured or degenerated joints (Fig. 5.1.22). Tomography may, however, improve this [40]. Bone scanning has been used in the follow-up after ligament reconstruction as an indicator of the mechanical stability of the joint [41].

In the shoulder, scintigraphy has been shown to be of no value in the detection of lesions caused by anterior shoulder dislocation apart from acute Hill–Sachs lesions [42]. Thus, labral injuries were not detected.

In very rare cases bone scintigrams have revealed severely decreased perfusion to joint-related parts of the long bones in the lower extremity as an explanation of long-lasting pain (Fig. 5.1.23) [43]. This points to the ability of the investigation to demonstrate viability (perfusion), an ability which is also utilized in the diagnosis of Calvé–Legg–Perthe's disease (Fig. 5.1.24) and avascular necrosis of the femoral head (Fig. 5.1.16). Although the latter investigation is mainly of interest in older patients, the possibility should be taken into account when dealing with young subjects with hip pains. In the case of osteochondritis dissecans, focal hyperemia and intense radionuclide accumulation is seen in the site of the subchondral lesion (Fig. 5.1.25), with no uptake in avascular bone fragments.

Back pain

Back pain is extremely common, even in athletes. Repetitive, vigorous exercise such as gymnastics or high dives induces considerable spinal torques and stress over the pars interarticularis which may develop into microfractures and subsequently a bone defect. This defect (spondylolysis) may persist and, being painful, limit activity. With SPECT spatial separation of overlapping bony structures is possible improving the diagnostics of the anatomic localization of abnormal findings [44].

With radiographic evidence of spondylolysis a

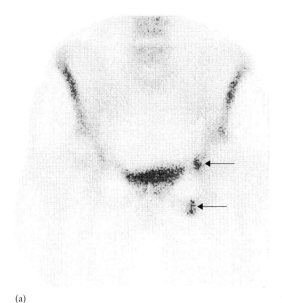

(a)

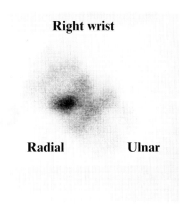

Right wrist

Radial   **Ulnar**

Fig. 5.1.18 Fracture of the scaphoid ('navicular') in the right wrist in a 19-year-old male ('pin-hole' acquisition).

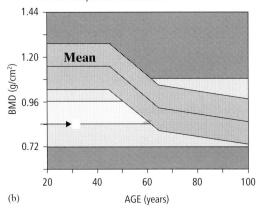

L2–L4 Comparison to Reference

(b)

Fig. 5.1.17 Pelvic stress fractures in a 32-year-old female with long-lasting secondary amenorrhea and markedly reduced bone mineral content, shown here in the lumbar spine.

scintigraphically active pars interarticularis defect is associated with a healing process which may be causing pain (Fig. 5.1.26), while a normal bone scan in the presence of a radiographically demonstrable pars defect is consistent with an old, healed process, not likely to explain the low back pain [44].

A semiquantification of the activity accumulation in the sacroiliac joints compared to the os sacrum by an 'activity profile' has been applied in the diagnostics of

Mb. Bechterew (sacroiliitis). However, other conditions such as rheumatoid arthritis, arthrosis and training overload may also lead to increased ratios.

Muscle uptake

A muscular focus may represent rhabdomyolysis, following unusual or excessive exertion leading to muscle injury. But abnormal muscle uptake is most frequently the result of heterotopic bone formation as in myositis ossificans. After a muscle lesion the initial inflammatory response probably leads to transformation of primitive mesenchymal-derived cells into bone-forming cells with subsequent ossification within the muscle (Fig. 5.1.27).

Bone tumors

Bone tumors, primary as well as metastases, will present in bone scintigrams as regions with focally increased uptake, often disseminated as in the case of prostate and breast cancer. However, single tumors may be difficult to discern from benign skeletal lesions and may demand further evaluation. Malignant tumors often appear irregular and 'invasive' centrally in the bone (Fig. 5.1.28), while benign lesions often involve the superficial bone tissues, and anamnestically are associated with overloading of the skeleton. Benign bone tumors (osteoid osteoma) are more well defined (Fig. 5.1.29). Scintigraphic suspicion of a bone tumor must always elicit a further diagnostic evaluation.

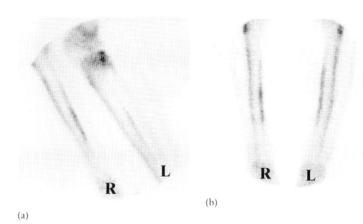

Fig. 5.1.19 Bilateral tibial 'shin splints' in a 19-year-old male runner.

(a)

(b)

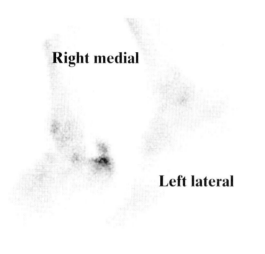

Fig. 5.1.20 Focal uptake on the upper part of the calcaneus and the adjacent Achilles tendon in a 40-year-old male runner, referred for uncharacteristic heel pains.

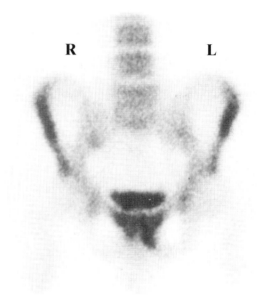

Fig. 5.1.21 Asymmetric especially left-sided increased pubic activity in a 23-year-old male football player with predominantly left-sided groin pains.

Summary

A number of modalities are available for diagnostic procedures in sports medicine and traumatology.

Conventional radiography is widely available and cheap. It is the first choice for fractures and is useful for demonstrating degenerative joint disease and calcifications. Computed tomography is useful for mapping comminuted fractures.

Ultrasound is a dynamic, real-time investigation with a high sensitivity for soft tissue pathologies, especially in tendons, muscles, bursae and joints. Biopsy and injection are possible under ultrasonographic guidance. It is cheap but demanding.

With appropriate pulse sequencing, MR imaging is efficacious in detecting the extent and location of most soft tissue injuries. Subchondral damage can be visualized (bone bruise), and dedicated cartilage pulse sequencing can demonstrate chondral injury. It is an important adjunct to bone scintigraphy, plain radiographs and, in some cases, musculoskeletal ultrasound.

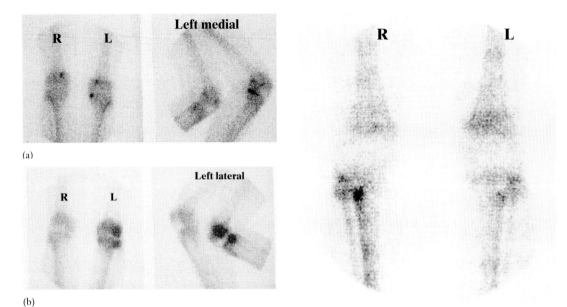

Fig. 5.1.22 (a) Focally increased uptake in the left medial tibial joint surface in a 25-year-old male with a bucket-handle medial meniscus tear (the focus marks the mechanical disorder and is not an uptake in the torn meniscus). Normal right knee scintigraphy. (b) Markedly increased irregular activity in the left knee, where arthroscopy showed ACL rupture and synovitis.

Fig. 5.1.23 Bilateral ischemia of the knee region in a 19-year-old male with knee pain of 4 months' duration. A core biopsy from the left distal femoral condyle verified avascular necrosis. Spontaneous recovery occurred after 26 months, and normalized bone scintigrams were obtained 6 months later [43].

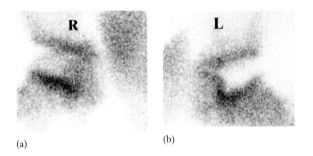

Fig. 5.1.24 Avascularity in the left caput femoris in an 11-year-old boy with Calvé–Legg–Perthe's diseaase. In the right hip a normal growth-zone is seen ('pin-hole' acquisitions).

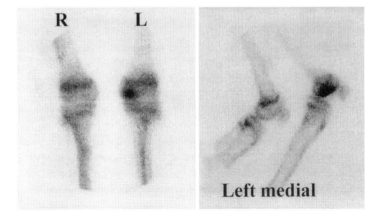

Fig. 5.1.25 Osteochondral lesion in the medial femoral condyle in the left knee in a 19-year-old male.

Bone scintigraphy is a cheap and very sensitive method for the evaluation of disorders in bone metabolism. A negative bone scintigram can exclude pathologic conditions. Stress fractures can be graded, allowing for prognostic interpretation. With back pain and radiographically demonstrated spondylolysis, tomography of bone scintigrams (SPECT) can distinguish between an active process, which may cause pain, and an inactive, healed process not likely to give back pain.

Multiple choice questions

One or several answers are correct.

1 *Stress fractures in athletes:*

a are best demonstrated with computed tomography

b are most commonly seen in the tibia but have been described in nearly all bones

c will show as diffuse activity of all of the posteriomedial border of the tibia in scintigrams

d of the femoral neck should be suspected and further investigated on a loose indication because of the risk for necrosis of the femoral head

e may only show on scintigraphy.

2 *A traumatic cartilage injury:*

a examined 2 weeks after injury will show as a narrowing of the joint space on X-rays

b can be demonstrated on standard T_1- and T_2-weighted MR sequences

c is not associated with bone bruise

d will show as subchondral activity on scintigrams

e repaired with a periosteal flap can be followed on MRI which can demonstrate filling of the defect with hyaline cartilage.

3 *On MRI:*

a meniscal lesions can be identified with high specificity and can be graded 1–3, but only grade 3 meniscal changes can be identified as tears by arthroscopy

b a healed meniscus lesion will not show

c multiple ligament injuries can be verified, enabling better planning of the acute treatment

d a ligamentous tear will always represent a clinical instability

e there are typical findings in the tennis elbow.

4 *Ultrasound:*

a is a very sensitive method for detecting tendinitis and tendinosis

b verified changes in Achilles and patella tendons are

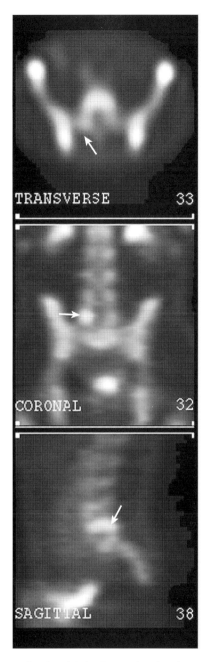

Fig. 5.1.26 SPECT of the lumbar vertebrae in a 28-year-old male soccer player, showing a focus in the right processus spinosus in L5.

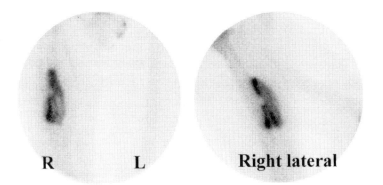

Fig. 5.1.27 Myositis ossificans in the right quadriceps in a 26-year-old male handball player after a blunt trauma.

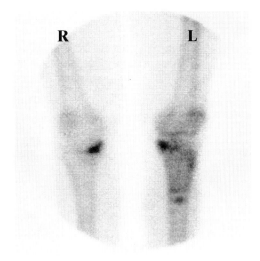

Fig. 5.1.28 Malignant tumor in upper left tibia. Note the irregular appearance and central location.

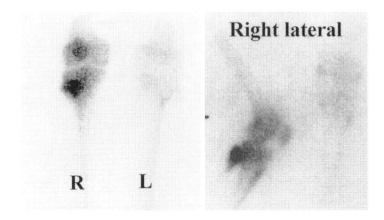

Fig. 5.1.29 Osteoid osteoma in the right fibula in a 23-year-old male.

closely associated to symptoms and should be an indication for surgical intervention

c is the most sensitive method for detecting calcifications in muscles and tendons

d can clearly distinguish between insertional Achilles tendinitis and tendinitis of the free tendon 4–7 cm above the insertion

e is cheap but examiner dependent.

5 *Regarding shoulder disorders:*

a X-rays can be used to distinguish between a traumatic (Bankart) and non-traumatic (multidirectional) instability of the shoulder.

b SLAP lesions and other labral lesions can nearly always be demonstrated on standard MRI.

c Clinically suspected partial or total rotator cuff tears are best verified with standard CT.

d Ultrasonography is the investigation of choice in rotator cuff tendinitis.

e Arthrography is never used in shoulder diagnostics.

References

1 Pappas GP, Olcott EU, Orace JE. Imaging of skeletal muscle function using ¹⁸FDG PET: force production, activation, and metabolism. *J Appl Physiol* 2001; **90**: 329–37.

2 Gibbon WW, Long G. US prevalence of lower limb tendon degeneration in professional soccer players. Presented at: *83rd Scientific Assembly and Annual Meeting of the Radiological Society of North America*, Chicago IL, USA, 1997.

3 Lian O, Holen KJ, Engebretsen L, Bahr R. Relationship between symptoms of jumper's knee and the ultrasound characteristics of the patellar tendon among high level male volleyball players. *Scand J Med Sci Sports* 1996; **6**: 291–6.

4 Khan KM, Cook JL, Kiss ZS *et al.* Patellar tendon ultrasonography and jumper's knee in female basketball players: a longitudinal study. *Clin J Sport Med* 1997; **7**: 199–206.

5 Wiley JP, Bray RC, Wiseman DA *et al.* Serial ultrasonographic imaging evaluation of the patellar tendon after harvesting its central one third for anterior cruciate ligament reconstruction. *J Ultrasound Med* 1997; **16**: 251–5.

6 Crues JV, Mink J, Levy TL, Lotysch M, Stoller DW. Meniscal tears of the knee: accuracy of MR imaging. *Radiology* 1987; **164**: 445–8.

7 Lee JK, Yao L, Phelps CT, Wirth CR, Czajka J, Lozman J. Anterior cruciate ligament tears: MR imaging compared with arthroscopy and clinical tests. *Radiology* 1988; **166**: 861–4.

8 Loytsch M, Mink J, Crues JV, Schwartz A. Magnetic resonance in the detection of meniscal injuries (abstract). *Magn Reson Imag* 1986; **4**: 185.

9 Kornick J, Trefelner E, McCarthy S, Lange R, Lynch K,

Jokl P. Meniscal abnormalities in the asymptomatic population at MR imaging. *Radiology* 1990; **177**: 463–5.

10 Smith DK, Totty WG. The knee after partial meniscectomy: MR imaging features. *Radiology* 1990; **176**: 141–4.

11 van Trommel MF, Potter HG, Ernberg LA, Simonian PT, Wickiewicz TL. The use of noncontrast magnetic resonance imaging in evaluation of meniscal repair: comparison with conventional arthrography. *Arthroscopy* 1998; **14**: 2–8.

12 van Trommel MF, Simonian PT, Potter HG, Wickiewicz TL. Different regional healing rates with the outside-in technique for meniscal repair. *Am J Sports Med* 1998; **26**: 446–52.

13 Vellet AD, Lee DH, Munk PL *et al.* Anterior cruciate ligament tear: prospective evaluation of diagnostic accuracy of middle- and high-field strength MR imaging at 1.5 and 0.5 T. *Radiology* 1995; **197**: 826–30.

14 Potter HG. Imaging of the multiple ligament injured knee. In: Johnson DL, ed. *Clinics in Sports Medicine*. Philadelphia: W.B. Saunders, in press.

15 Schatz JA, Potter HG, Rodeo SA, Hannafin JA, Wickiewicz TL. MR imaging of anterior cruciate ligament reconstruction. *Am J Roentgenol* 1997; **169**: 223–8.

16 Rizzo PF, Gould ES, Lyden JP, Asnis SE. Diagnosis of occult fractures about the hip. *J Bone Joint Surg* 1993; **75-A**: 395–401.

17 Disler DG, McCauley TR, Kelman CG *et al.* Fat-suppressed three-dimensional spoiled gradient-echo MR imaging of hyaline cartilage defects in the knee: Comparison with standard MR imaging and arthroscopy. *Am J Roentgenol* 1996; **167**: 127–32.

18 Potter HG, Linklater JM, Allen AA, Hannafin JA, Haas SB. Magnetic resonance imaging of articular cartilage in the knee. *J Bone Joint Surg (Am)* 1998; **80-A**: 1276–84.

19 Recht MP, Piraino DW, Paletta GA, Schils JP, Belhobek GH. Accuracy of fat-suppressed three-dimensional spoiled gradient-echo FLASH MR imaging in the detection of patellofemoral articular cartilage abnormalities. *Radiology* 1996; **198**: 209–12.

20 Potter HG. Imaging. In: Rosenberg AG, Mabrey JD, Woolson ST, Cole BJ, eds. *The Articular Knee* (CD-ROM). American Academy of Orthopaedic Surgeons: Rosemont, IL, 2000.

21 Bashir A, Gray ML, Hartke J, Burstein D. Nondestructive imaging of human cartilage glycosaminoglycan concentration by MRI. *Magn Reson Med* 1999; **41**: 857–65.

22 Iannotti JP, Zlatkin MB, Esterhai JL *et al.* Magnetic resonance imaging of the shoulder. *J Bone Joint Surg (Am)* 1991; **73-A**: 17–29.

23 Potter HG. Magnetic resonance imaging of the unstable shoulder. *Techniques Shoulder Elbow Surg* 2000; **1**: 25–38.

24 Gusmer PB, Potter HG, Schatz JA *et al.* Labral injuries: accuracy of detection with unenhanced MR imaging of the shoulder. *Radiology* 1996; **200**: 519–24.

25 Palmer WE, Caslowitz PL. Anterior shoulder instability.

Diagnostic criteria determined from prospective analysis of 121 MR arthrograms. *Radiology* 1995; **197**: 819–25.

26 Connell DA, Potter HG, Wickiewicz TL, Altchek DW, Warren RF. Noncontrast magnetic resonance imaging of superior labral lesions. 102 cases confirmed at arthroscopic surgery. *Am J Sports Med* 1999; **27**: 208–13.

27 Gaary EA, Potter HG, Altchek DW. Medial elbow pain in the throwing athlete: MR imaging evaluation. *Am J Roentgenol* 1997; **168**: 795–800.

28 Potter HG, Sofka CM. Imaging of the athlete's elbow. In: Altchek DW, Andrews J, eds. *The Athlete's Elbow*. Philadelphia: Lippincott-Raven, 2001: 59–80.

29 Wilson FD, Andrews JR, Blackburn TA, McCluskey G. Valgus extension overload in the pitching elbow. *Am J Sports Med* 1983; **11**: 83–7.

30 Potter HG, Hannafin JA, Morwessel RM, DeCarlo EF, O'Brien SJ, Altchek DW. Lateral epicondylitis: correlation of MR imaging, surgical, and histopathologic findings. *Radiology* 1995; **196**: 43–6.

31 Hulkko A, Orava S. Stress fractures in athletes. *Int J Sports Med* 1987; **8**: 221–6.

32 Matheson GO, Clement DB, McKenzie DC, Taunton JE, Lloyd-Smith DR, Macintyre JG. Stress fractures in athletes. *Am J Sports Med* 1987; **15**: 46–57.

33 Christiansen E, Kanstrup I-L. Increased risk of stress fractures of the ribs in elite rowers. *Scand J Med Sci Sports* 1997; **7**: 49–52.

34 Johansson C, Ekenmann I, Lewander R. Stress fractures of the tibia in athletes: diagnosis and natural course. *Scand J Med Sci Sports* 1992; **2**: 87–91.

35 Matin P. Basic principles of nuclear medicine techniques for detection and evaluation of trauma and sports medicine injuries. *Semin Nucl Med* 1988; **18**: 90–112.

36 Clement DB, Ammann W, Taunton JE *et al*. Exercise-induced stress injuries to the femur. *Int J Sports Med* 1993; **14**: 347–52.

37 Patel N, Collier BD, Carrera GF *et al*. High-resolution bone scintigraphy of the adult wrist. *Clin Nucl Med* 1992; **17**: 449–53.

38 Hölmich P, Uhrskou P, Ulnits L *et al*. Effectiveness of active physical training as treatment for longstanding adductor-related groin pain in athletes: randomised trial. *Lancet* 1999; **353**: 439–43.

39 Lohmann M, Kanstrup I-L, Gergvary I, Tollund C. Bone scintigraphy in patients suspected of having meniscus tears. *Scand J Med Sci Sports* 1991; **1**: 123–7.

40 Murray IPC, Dixon J, Kohan L. SPECT for acute knee pain. *Clin Nucl Med* 1990; **15**: 828–40.

41 Dye S, Chew MH. Restoration of osseous homeostasis after anterior cruciate ligament reconstruction. *Am J Sports Med* 1993; **21**: 748–50.

42 Schydlowsky P. *The value of non-invasive methods in the diagnosis of lesions caused by anterior shoulder dislocation. With special emphasis on labral lesions*. PhD thesis, University of Copenhagen, 1998.

43 Zerahn B, Kanstrup I-L, Lausten GS. Transient ischemia of the distal femur and proximal tibia in a 19-year-old male. *Clin Nucl Med* 1998; **23**: 190.

44 Bellah RD, Summerrilee DA, Treves ST, Micheli LJ. Low back pain in adolescent athletes: detection of stress injury to the pars interarticularis with SPECT. *Radiology* 1991; **180**: 509–12.

Part 6
Sports Injury: Regional Considerations. Diagnosis and Treatment

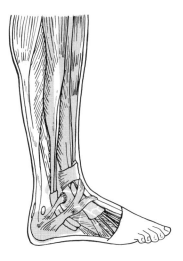

Chapter 6.1
Lower Leg, Ankle and Foot

JON KARLSSON, CHRISTER ROLF &
SAJKARI ORAVA

Classical reference

Freeman MAR. Treatment of ruptures of the lateral
ligament of the ankle. *J Bone Joint Surg (Brit)*
1965; **47-B**: 661–668.

Functional instability is the subjective symptom of
repeated giving way noted by the patient. Functional
instability is the most common and serious residual
disability after ligament injuries of the ankle joint. The
term functional instability was described by Freeman
in 1965. He found a high incidence of functional instability after rupture of the lateral ankle joint ligaments.
He stated that increased mechanical laxity was not a
primary decisive factor in ankle joint function. Subsequently it has been shown that functional instability
is the most important subjective symptom and can be
caused by a combination of mechanical laxity, proprioceptive deficit and peroneal muscle weakness.

Soft tissue overuse injuries of
the lower leg in athletes

Introduction

Lower leg (Fig. 6.1.1) pain in athletes has several different etiologic factors. Clinical conditions causing
lower leg symptoms include chronic compartment
syndrome, tendinitis, medial tibial stress syndrome,
stress fractures, periostitis, fascial defects, musculotendinous injuries (ruptures, partial tears, scars) such
as 'tennis leg', popliteal artery entrapment syndrome,
claudication, effort-induced venous thrombosis, nerve
injuries, entrapments and radiculopathies [1]. The
proper treatment requires that an accurate diagnosis is
made. Diagnosis can be established by a thorough history and by performing a physical examination with
reference to the underlying anatomic structures. In
order to make an exact diagnosis, radiologic and isotope
examinations, ultrasonography, magnetic resonance
imaging (MRI), neurophysiologic and tissue pressure
measurements can be used. Clinicians should be familiar with the problems causing leg pain in order to pre-
scribe specific treatment for each athlete.

The frequency of lower leg injuries

Lower leg overuse injuries comprise approximately
10% of all overuse injuries in athletes. In younger athletes, the incidence is lower than in older. In runners,
lower leg injuries account for approximately 20% of all
injuries [2,3]. James *et al.* [4] evaluated 232 lower leg
pain conditions in 180 runners, of which 13% were
lower leg overuse injuries. Some of these (6%) were
stress fractures of the tibia and/or fibula.

   The frequency of different pain syndromes of the
lower leg varies according to different studies. Medial

tibial syndrome was the most common lower leg overuse pain in athletes in the study of Puranen and Alavaikko [5] in Finland. In other reports anterior tibial syndrome has been seen more often [6,7]. Posterior calf muscle pain, tennis leg and other pain syndromes are seen less frequently.

The incidence of stress fractures of the lower leg is less than half the incidence of soft tissue leg pain [8], but the clinical symptoms are often very similar.

The term 'shin splints' has been used as a general name for overuse injuries of the lower leg, except stress fractures and compartmental syndrome [1,4]. The pain is induced by physical exercise and is located anterolaterally or medially on the leg. Rather than the diffuse term shin splints, the exact diagnoses of lower leg injuries in athletes with lower leg pain should be used. These include the medial tibial syndrome, anterior, lateral and posterior compartment syndromes, fascial defects, the tennis leg, the popliteal artery entrapment syndrome and effort-induced venous thrombosis in addition to stress fractures (see Table 6.1.1, p. 536).

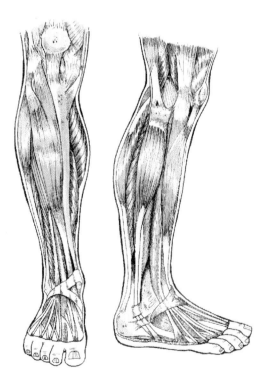

Fig. 6.1.1 Muscles of the lower leg and foot.

Medial tibial stress syndrome

Pain at the medial and posterior aspect of the distal leg is called 'medial tibial syndrome' or 'medial tibial stress syndrome' [9,10]. This is caused by overuse and is seen especially in endurance athletes as runners, triathlonists, cross-country skiers, orienteers and joggers. It is seen also in athletes participating in jumping sports, such as basketball, volleyball and other indoor ball games.

Some authors state that medial tibial (stress) syndrome begins as a tendinitis, but progresses to a periostitis. During the midstance phase of running the foot pronates and the tibia rotates internally, pulling the posterior tibial tendon and muscle at their attachments to both tibia and the interosseus membrane, which by means of powerful and frequent repetitions may result in overloading of these structures. Others, however, believe that the soleus muscle rather than the posterior tibial muscle is involved in medial tibial stress syndrome. Michael and Holder [11] demonstrated in their anatomic study how the posterior tibial muscle originates a considerable distance from the medial border of the posterior tibia (the pain site) and that the muscle belly is higher in location than the usual site of pain. The soleus muscle has a tough aponeurotic covering, which extends directly to the posterior medial border of the tibia for three-quarters of its length where it attaches at the muscle's origin. The insertion is complex, but its tendinous portion inserts on the medial third of the calcaneus. Biomechanically, this insertion makes the soleus vulnerable to excessive elongation when the heel is pronated [11], and overloading may result in tibial leg pain. But there is great variation in the tibial origin of the plantar flexor musculature, and separate fascial compartments have been identified in the posterior tibial muscle and other medial flexors [12], which may explain the variation in symptoms.

Patients with medial tibial syndrome usually complain of exertional pain located at the medial (posterior) aspect of the leg. Usually the most painful area is the proximal part of the distal third of the tibial border, where palpation tenderness is also felt. There is some variation as to the location of pain [1,10,11]. In addition, 'medial tibial stress syndrome' has been classified by Detmer [9] into three subclasses: (i) bone stress reaction or stress fracture; (ii) periostitis from traction at the periosteal–fascial junction of the soleus muscle; and (iii) chronic posterior compartment syndrome. Clement has introduced the term 'posterior tibial syndrome' [2], characterized by pain and tenderness along the posterior medial aspect of the tibia over the posterior tibialis muscle and tendon.

To establish the diagnosis of medial tibial stress syndrome, radiographic evaluation, bone scintigraphy and compartmental pressure measurements can be used. Radiographs are usually negative, but they help to exclude other pathologic processes. Technetium pyrophosphate bone scanning can be very helpful in differentiating a stress fracture from 'periostitis' or 'bone stress' (Fig. 6.1.2). In the latter, the uptake of the tracer is longitudinal and diffuse along the posteromedial tibia, and not local as in the case of a stress fracture [11]. MRI has been found to be helpful in defining the degree and extent of bone involvement in tibial stress reaction. It also helps in follow-up of the patients.

Elevated intracompartmental pressure in the deep posterior compartment has been noticed in some patients with medial tibial syndrome during exercise [5]. After fasciotomy the pressure levels during exercise did not rise above pressure during rest in some series [5] but others have not been able to demonstrate elevated pressure values in patients with medial tibial syndrome [10].

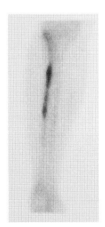 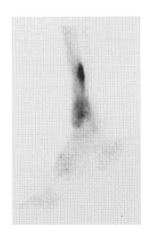

Fig. 6.1.2 Scintigram of 'shin splints' (left) with disperse accumulation of activity along the medial border of tibia, and of a stress fracture of tibia (right) with distinct activity at the fracture. From Department of Clinical Physiology, Copenhagen University Hospital at Bispebjerg, Denmark.

Treatment of medial tibial syndrome is primarily non-surgical. In addition to reduction in the amount of impact activity, massage, stretching and aerobic training with cycling or rowing can have a positive effect on early medial tibial syndrome [1]. Insoles with an antipronation effect may also reduce symptoms. If these conservative measures fail, surgical intervention with fasciotomy is probably the best treatment. Fasciotomy for medial tibial syndrome was first done in 1971. The results have been excellent or good in 70–90% [9,10,12]. During fasciotomy, the common crural fascia covering the deep posterior compartment should be opened, as well as the separate fascia of the posterior tibial muscle. The distal medial soleus muscle insertion can be freed from the medial tibial border at the same time and the soleus fascia opened proximally [11]. Recovery time to full training is approximately 6 weeks, but there seems to be a longer recovery time and somewhat poorer results in female athletes after fasciotomy [13].

Complications related to the surgical treatment include injuries to saphenous nerve branches or the vein, postoperative hematoma and infection. The risk of complications can be reduced using careful operation technique.

Anterior tibial compartment syndrome

Anterior tibial syndrome exists in both an acute and a chronic form, both caused by overuse [6].

The acute anterior tibial syndrome is an exertional pain syndrome with dramatic symptoms including pain and major swelling and should be treated by early fasciotomy. Ischemia and muscle necrosis may develop if the diagnosis is missed and treatment is delayed. The subcutaneous fasciotomy should not be used, in order to avoid the tourniquet effect by intact skin in the distal leg and ankle.

Chronic anterior compartment syndrome is a typical chronic exertional compartment syndrome. The muscles of the anterior compartment of the leg are involved, causing burning pain in dorsiflexion of the ankle, especially during running, walking and jumping. The compartment is usually painful during palpation and the muscle mass may be hypertrophic. An elevated intracompartmental pressure has been found in several studies, during both rest and exercise [1,6,7,14,15]. It is generally agreed that a pre-exercise pressure of 15 mmHg or more, a 1-min postexercise pressure of 30 mmHg or more and a 5-min postexercise pressure of 20 mmHg or more is pathologic and proof of chronic compartmental syndrome [1]. During exertion the intracompartmental pressure can be higher than 100 mmHg. Some non-invasive tests for the detection of chronic compartmental syndrome have been developed. These include radioisotope scintigraphy associated with emission tomography for regional muscle perfusion defects in the calf musculature.

Fasciotomy of the affected compartment is the only definitive treatment, as rest and other conservative treatments affect the chronic form of this syndrome relatively little. The results after fasciotomy are good in more than 90% of cases [6,14,16]. Patients are usually able to train normally 3–6 weeks after surgery. Surgical failures can be associated with too short fasciotomy, injury to the superficial peroneal nerve, postoperative hematoma and infection.

Lateral (peroneal) compartment syndrome

Isolated chronic compartment syndrome in the peroneal muscles is rarely seen. But several authors state that when there is an anterior compartment syndrome, the lateral peroneal compartment is simultaneously affected. Therefore standard surgery has been fasciotomy of both the anterior and lateral compartments of the leg [6]. The necessity of the strategy has been questioned, and one study [15] has shown that the results after fasciotomy of the anterior compartment alone were as good as when fasciotomy of both compartments were performed.

Posterior compartment syndrome

This pain syndrome is mainly seen in middle-distance and endurance runners as well as in orienteers. Symptoms appear during and after running and may progress to a chronic compartment syndrome located at the gastrocnemius–soleus muscle complex. Intracompartmental pressure measurements can confirm the diagnosis, and in case of elevated pressure, fasciotomy is the ultimate treatment. The common crural fascia can be opened posteriorly at one or both sides.

In some cases pain of the posterior compartment is caused by a partial calf muscle rupture. In these pa-

tients, massage, stretching and reduced intensity of training is usually effective treatment.

Fascial defects

Fascial defects can be symptomatic in association with chronic compartment syndromes. Increased intracompartmental pressure may result in herniation of muscle through an attenuated fascial defect [1,6]. Reneman [6] observed fascial defects in approximately 60% of patients with chronic compartment syndrome. Usually the herniation occurs in the distal third of the anterolateral leg, often at the fascial opening for the cutaneous branch of the superficial peroneal nerve. Not all fascial defects are symptomatic, though. If there is pain, local tenderness, compression neuropathy or ischemia of herniated muscle tissue, fasciotomy is recommended, avoiding damage to the nerve branches [6,7]. Closure of the defect is contraindicated as it can lead to increased symptoms and, in the worst case, to an acute compartment syndrome.

Tibialis posterior tendon dysfunction/rupture

Tibialis posterior tendinopathy is most often seen as an overuse tendon injury. This condition is not an inflammatory tendinitis, but a degenerative tendinosis.

The typical clinical sign is pain of the medial aspect of the ankle behind the medial malleolus. This pain may radiate along the tendon to the naviculare bone. The tibialis posterior tendinopathy is often associated with excessive pronation of the hindfoot.

On examination there is pain on palpation of the tendon. The pain is increased by passive eversion and resisted inversion of the foot. In rare cases crepitation may be present. In the case of a total rupture of the tibialis posterior tendon a collapse of the medial arc of the foot is seen (Fig. 6.1.3). The patient is unable to increase the weight-bearing of the foot and there is marked valgus of the heel; the so-called 'too many toes sign' is present.

Primary treatment is aimed at reduction of pain as well as strengthening of the tendon. Excessive tightness of the proximal tibialis posterior muscle should always be looked for and treated if present. As tibialis posterior tendinopathy is frequently associated with excessive pronation, a shoe correction and an insole should be used.

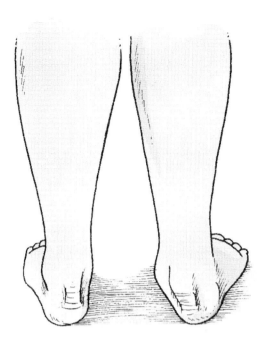

Fig. 6.1.3 Valgus foot. At weight-bearing the heel is in valgus position compared to the normal foot.

In athletes with rupture of the tibialis posterior tendon, examination may reveal thickening of the tendon and/or absence of the tendon. There is inability to raise the heel. MRI and/or ultrasonography should be used in order to establish the diagnosis.

Surgical repair is indicated in patients with subtotal or total rupture of the tendon. Direct suture of the tendon will usually not produce satisfactory results; instead transposition of either flexor hallucis longus or flexor digitorum longus is indicated. Rupture of the posterior tibialis posterior tendon in athletes is infrequent, but is, however, a serious injury.

Tennis leg

The term 'tennis leg' is used for a partial rupture of the medial head of the gastrocnemius muscle, not to be clinically confused with a tear of the plantaris tendon [1]. Often the tear occurs at the musculotendinous junction. The injury occurs most frequently during running, jumping or ball games and usually results from an eccentric load placed across the ankle with the knee in extension. The injury mechanism is thus indi-rect, but the patient may describe a direct trauma to the calf region, such as a kick or hit by the ball or bat to the calf. In physical examination of the painful calf swelling can be seen. A maximal point of tenderness with a palpable defect in the medial head of the gastrocnemius muscle can be recognized at examination. Ankle plantar flexion is weakened and painful. Sometimes deep venous thrombosis may exist simultaneously.

Ultrasonographic or venographic investigation can be performed to establish the diagnosis and to exclude deep venous thrombosis. With MRI the location and extent of muscle injury can be visualized.

Treatment of the tennis leg is non-surgical, including elevation, ice, compressive wrapping and partial weight-bearing. Heel lifts in the shoes may be used during the first week. A progressive calf stretching and strengthening program is undertaken as pain and swelling resolve. Usually full recovery occurs in a few weeks. However, some of the ruptures are so large that a permanent defect and muscle weakness remains. However, the results of late repair of the musculo-tendinous defect are not good, and operative treatment should be avoided.

Popliteal artery entrapment syndrome (PAES)

Partial or complete compression of the popliteal artery as a result of aberrant anatomy in the popliteal fossa causes the popliteal artery entrapment syndrome, which is an uncommon reason for exertional leg pain. Usually the compression is caused by the gastrocnemius muscle. The various anatomic anomalies causing PAES include:
1 the popliteal artery passing medial to the medial head of the gastrocnemius;
2 an abnormal origin of the medial head of the gastrocnemius;
3 the presence of an accessory band of the medial head of the gastrocnemius; and
4 the popliteal artery passing deep to the popliteal muscle [17].

Popliteal artery entrapment syndrome usually affects younger male athletes, inducing calf pain during strenuous exercise. The symptoms are bilateral in more than 50% of patients [17]. Leg weakness and paresthesias may be associated with PAES. The pain appears after a certain amount of exercise, just as vascular claudication. Reduction of activity relieves the symptoms, whereas elevation of the leg makes them worse. The symptoms resemble posterior compartment syndrome, but there are normal intracompartmental pressures. In physical examination distal pulses can be weak or absent during maximal isometric ankle dorsiflexion and hyperextension of the knee. With non-invasive vascular investigations such as ankle/brachial index and Doppler ultrasound the diagnosis can usually be established. However, angiography directly after exercise is the most precise diagnostic investigation.

PAES is a progressive disease with increasing vascular occlusion over time. Treatment is surgical decompression of all constricting structures. The surgical procedure can range from musculotendinous sectioning and thrombectomy to resection of the damaged arterial section with saphenous vein graft interposition [17]. The prognosis is usually good, but is dependent on the extent of arterial damage and the vascular intervention required.

Effort-induced venous thrombosis

The etiology of effort-induced venous thrombosis is unknown, but it has been described in connection with the 'tennis leg', repetitive muscular use during jogging and kick boxing, in which intimal venous damage may occur as a result of knee hyperextension. There are also case reports of this syndrome occurring in American football and skiing [1]. Anatomic variations of the popliteal fossa veins may be an etiologic factor.

The typical patient is the well-conditioned athlete who experiences a sudden calf pain unilaterally without any direct trauma. Swelling develops later. The symptoms and physical signs often mimic gastrocnemius muscle tear. However, there swelling is more pronounced and Homan's sign is positive. The diagnosis is confirmed by ultrasonography. In the case of grave symptoms and negative ultrasound, venography should be performed.

Immediate treatment with low molecular heparin and oral anticoagulants is important to prevent the development of serious complications such as clot propagation and pulmonary embolism. Initial treatment also includes bed rest and leg elevation.

Stress fractures of the tibia

Occurrence of stress fractures

Breithaupt reported in 1855 metatarsal stress fractures in soldiers after long marches. A stress fracture is a dynamic, metabolic process of bone, in which remodelling dominates over repair, and is related to overuse impact. The character of the load and the degree of training seems to be of importance for the occurrence of stress fractures. Of 324 consecutive patients with stress fractures 84% were athletes at district or national elite level, while the remaining 15% were sedentary individuals [8]. The incidence of stress fractures has been reported to be 5–15% of all sports injuries in different populations, with a higher incidence among runners [18,19]. The tibia is the most common location of stress fractures. The incidence of stress fractures in the tibia among track and field athletes has been reported to be 10%, and among young elite orienteers lower than 1% during 1 year, whereas among elite soccer players there were no stress fractures.

Predisposing factors

Extrinsic factors, such as sudden changes in training or running surface, have been reported to cause stress fractures [8,19]. Previously relatively untrained recruits, committed to intensive military training, equipped with new military boots, carrying weapons and other equipment, running and jumping excessively daily, are at high risk of sustaining stress fractures.

Intrinsic factors, such as leg length discrepancy, cavus foot, overpronation during running [19] and osteopenia are referred to in the literature as contributing factors for stress fractures. Despite the fact that we often claim that these stress fractures are related to fatigue, we do not know whether good muscular function can decrease the local deformation of the bone. Many clinically important questions remain unanswered.

Clinical presentation, diagnosis and management

There are two types of stress fractures in the tibia, classified in relation to their location as posteromedial or anterior stress fractures [20].

The diagnosis is based on clinical findings and verified by technetium-99 bone scan, radiography, computed tomography (CT) or MRI. The bone scan typically shows an increased bone turnover at the injury site a few days after injury and as X-rays are often normal for several weeks, bone scan may be the first examination to verify a clinical suspicion of a stress fracture.

The *anterior stress fracture* is connected with an excessive cortical and fibrous formation and heals slowly. This injury was initially described by Burrows [21] in ballet dancers. Three of these underwent biopsies of the lesion, showing 'dense cortical bone with some evidence of granulation tissue'. The delay in healing has been suggested to be caused by the fibrous ingrowths which prevent bone-to-bone contact [21–23]. A low vascularity of the anterior cortex may also be an important pathophysiologic factor [24]. This injury is serious for the elite athlete, for in addition to the very slow healing, complete fracture may occur [24]. Athletes performing frequent jumps such as long-jumpers, basketball players, runners and dancers are at high risk of sustaining this type of stress fracture [21–26]. The diagnosis is often delayed because of the slow onset of symptoms. At later stages radiography shows a typical V-shaped cut into the cortical bone and also cortical hypertrophy as a consequence of the long-term excessive load.

The treatment of this injury is still controversial. Despite long immobilization periods these fractures have a low healing potential. Various operative techniques including stabilization with plating, drilling proximal and distal of the fracture or intramedullary nailing have shown good results with healing of the fracture and resumption of sport activities [22,27]. Pulsating electromagnetic field therapy also seems to be effective [25].

The *posteromedial stress fracture* (Fig. 6.1.4) is located close to the site of the deep plantar flexor muscle attachments of the flexor digitorum longus, tibialis posterior and soleus muscles at the mid-diaphysis of the tibia. It has been debated whether this injury is a true stress fracture, periostitis, or a rupture of the musculotendinous attachment on tibia [28]. There is great variation in anatomy related to the deep plantar flexor

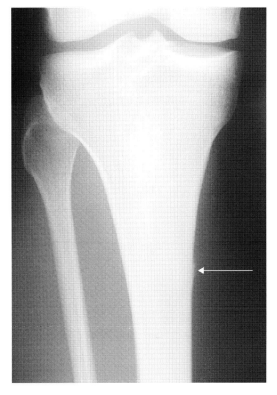

Fig. 6.1.4 X-ray of stress fracture of tibia. The only indication of a fracture is a little callus formation on the medial side of the tibia (arrow).

attachments [28], which to some extent may explain different clinical presentations depending on anatomic predisposition in each individual (Table 6.1.1).

The medial tibial stress fracture usually heals easily with reduction in load and training intensity.

Achilles tendon injuries

Chronic Achilles tendon disorders
Chronic Achilles tendon pain is a common clinical feature [29,30]. Most acute Achilles tendon conditions heal with non-surgical and symptomatic treatment, but some patients do complain of longstanding pain and swelling of the Achilles tendon, stiffness and dysfunction, which makes it difficult for them to retain a desired level of activity. A chronic condition is defined as symptoms lasting more than 2–3 months. Even

Table 6.1.1 Characteristics of and differences between tibial stress syndrome, compartment syndrome and stress fractures.

	Tibial stress syndrome	Chronic compartment syndrome	Stress fracture
History	Running on hard surface. Hyperpronation? Quite diffuse pain during weight-bearing and activity, but pain may decrease during activity	Increase or change of training No pain at rest Increasing pain with increasing activity. Paresthesia may occur	Huge increase of activity and load Can be progression of tibial stress syndrome Sudden onset Localized pain even during small load
Findings	Tenderness of tibial edges, small tender swellings on tibia	Tenderness of musculature	Localized tenderness of the bone
Investigations	Basically clinical examination Bone scan may show periosteal activity, and may be normal	Compartment pressure measurements: > 15 mmHg pre-exercise > 30 mmHg 1 min after exercise > 20 mmHg 5 min after exercise	Bone scan: activity in the bone X-rays MRI
Treatment	Conservative: Medial stress: antipronation support, muscle training, reduction of training load Anterior stress: shock absorption (shoes, surface) Operative treatment?	Surgical: Fasciotomy	Conservative: Medial fracture: reduce load and training for 3 months Anterior stress: full reduction of load Surgery: osteosynthesis

though reported as an overuse injury in the literature, up to 30% of cases with chronic Achilles tendon disorders are not related to sports or excessive loading. Rheumatologic disorders, immunologic and infectious diseases as well as adverse drug effects are also reasons to be considered.

'Tendinitis' is a term often used by clinicians to describe a painful Achilles tendon. An inflammatory reaction in the tendon, characteristic for acute tendinitis, is seldom found in chronic situations, however, even though an initial inflammation may have induced the condition, which later becomes chronic [31–33].

'Tendinosis' is often used to describe chronic changes of the Achilles tendon. Tendinosis means that only degenerative, but no inflammatory, changes are found in the tendon. The etiology of tendinosis is unknown. It may pass through various stages of structural changes, clinical symptoms, weakening and finally microrupture. On the other hand, tendinosis may start with microruptures of the tendon and develop through a failed healing process. The processes of

inflammation, degeneration, and regeneration/repair form a functional spectrum of cell matrix responses, and the predominance of any of these responses depends on the mechanism of injury and the hemostatic balance of the tendon tissue. When tissue breakdown exceeds repair, the tendinosis cycle is initiated. In the development of Achilles tendinosis, it is likely that tissue microtrauma and dysfunction precede the moment of the first perception of pain, stiffness, tenderness, or discomfort. In other words, the tissue damage may have started to accumulate long before the first symptoms [34–36].

Kvist *et al.* [37] carried out histopathologic and biochemical studies on chronic paratendinosis and suggested that it is caused by hypoxia, neovascularization and degeneration in interrelation, and that an inadequate circulation in the critical zones in the tendon could be the reason for subsequent ruptures. On the other hand, Åström and Rausing [38] found only minor changes in the paratendinous tissue, but noted mucoid degeneration, neovascularization and disorganization of the collagen in the tendon itself. They observed with laser Doppler technique that chronic tendinosis was associated with an increased blood circulation. Leadbetter[39] has suggested that a failure of the cell matrix to adapt to excessive changes in load could be one explanation for tendinosis, stimulating the local release of cytokines, resulting in both autocrine and paracrine modulation of further cell activity including cell deaths. However, an increased number of hyperactive cells in tendinosis tissue has also been described.

Ultrasound imaging of chronic Achilles tendon disorders shows widening of the tendon and low echogenicity and correlates well with the histopathologic changes. Pathologic findings are often localized 1.5–5 cm proximal of the distal insertion, mostly on the medial side of the tendon (Fig. 6.1.5). MRI with gadolinium contrast enhances the imaging further and shows a greater intratendinous volume than ultrasonography, indicating a more widespread pathology.

Management

Chronic Achilles tendon disorders should be divided into conditions affecting the tendon insertion, the free tendon, the proximal tendon–muscle transition, and the paratenon. In clinical practice, there is often a combination of paratenon and tendon involvement. It is logical that there is some degree of relationship between paratenon and tendon disorders.

There is a lack of controlled studies on operative and non-operative treatment of chronic Achilles tendon disorders.

Clement *et al.* [40] treated 109 patients with rehabilitation including calf muscle training, medical treatment of inflammation and correction of various biomechanical dysfunctions and found good or excellent results in the majority of the cases. A program of hard eccentric muscle training has been found to have excellent short-term effect on the symptoms of chronic Achilles tendinosis [41,42], but the long-term effect is not known.

Topical treatment has always interested athletes, but the scientific evidence for its effect is vague. Topically applied ketoprofen penetrates through the skin, the paratenon and into the tendon, where it is present in high concentrations, when compared to oral treatment. This treatment should probably only be

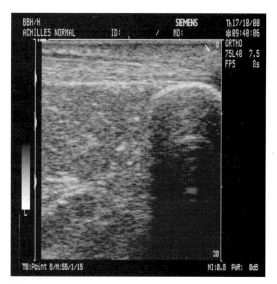

(a)

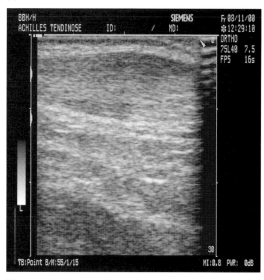

(b)

Fig. 6.1.5 Ultrasound investigation of (a) a normal Achilles tendon and (b) a painful, swollen tendon of a runner. Tendinosis is visible as hypoechoic areas inside the tendon, and the dark area at the top represents peritendinosis.

used for acute, inflammatory tendon conditions. Since chronic tendinosis is not an inflammation, it is not surprising that no study has been able to show any reliable clinical effect of anti-inflammatory preparations.

Corticosteroid injection around the Achilles tendon is a common but controversial treatment for chronic

Achilles tendon problems. In one study it has been reported that 30% of 215 outpatients and 60% of 298 inpatients with chronic Achilles tendon pain had received one or more cortisone injections, and this is in agreement with earlier published data of a frequency of around 50–75%. During the 1950s the first report on Achilles rupture after cortisone injection was published. Corticosteroid-induced changes in the tendon's vicinity such as pigment changes and atrophy of the skin and subcutaneous tissue are probably more common than tendon ruptures. In Malmö, Sweden, two groups of patients with chronic achillodynia have been studied to assess the frequency of corticosteroid-related complications; 298 consecutive patients operated on during 1972–1990; and 215 consecutive cases who were evaluated as outpatients during 1988–1989. In the surgically treated group, partial ruptures of the tendon were found in 23%, but the frequency was doubled in those patients who had previously had corticosteroid injections. In the outpatient group, an annual incidence of total Achilles rupture was found to be 2.4% and 0.2% for patients with and without earlier corticosteroid injections, respectively, compared to an incidence of 0.016% for Malmö's general population [43].

Two surgical methods have been described as treatment for problems at the tendon insertion: resection of the posterosuperior angle of the calcaneus (Fig. 6.1.6), and wedge osteotomy of the calcaneus. Some studies

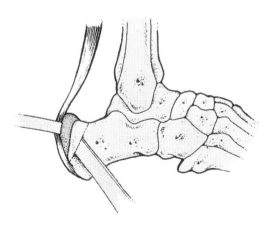

Fig. 6.1.6 Removal of the superior–posterior edge of calcaneus in chronic bursitis/tendinosis due to prominent bone.

have described good clinical results from these procedures while others find poorer results [44].

Chronic paratendinitis and tendinitis of the free tendon can be treated with excision, which has an excellent effect on the symptoms in large series. The tendon is incised longitudinally, followed by removal of the adhesions between the skin and paratenon, and those between the paratenon and the tendon. Ljungqvist [45] operated on 24 cases with partial ruptures and all these cases became free of symptoms, in 12 cases after more than 6 months. Nelen *et al.* [46] studied 50 cases of chronic tendinopathy who were operated with resection of macroscopic unhealthy tissue and half of the cases with a turndown flap. They found good results in 73% of the cases not operated with reinforcement, and in 87% of cases who had reinforcement, at follow-up more than 2 years after the operation. The majority of these patients were operated on with excision of the macroscopically damaged tissue without any reinforcement. The operation can be performed under local anesthesia without the use of a tourniquet [16].

Postoperative treatment is individualized depending on the intraoperative findings. Below-the-knee cast or an individually produced brace can preferably be used during the wound healing period. Full weight-bearing is allowed, with limited dorsal flexion, directly after the operation in most cases. Controlled studies of different rehabilitation protocols are lacking.

Complications after surgery are seen in 2–10%.

Achilles tendon ruptures

The incidence of Achilles tendon rupture is approximately 10/100 000 population per year. The incidence has increased 3–5 times during the last 30–40 years. The male dominance is from 2/1 to 20/1 in different studies. The average age of the patients is 35–40 years. Sports activity is the triggering factor in 75%. In Scandinavia, Achilles tendon ruptures most often occur during badminton. In the USA, Achilles tendon ruptures are related to basketball and tennis. In the elderly, underlying systemic disease or long-term corticosteroid medication are common contributing causes. Chronic degeneration of the tendon may be a predisposing factor. A number of studies have shown degenerative changes in the ruptured tendon, but in most cases the patient did not have any symptoms before the rupture occurred. An uncontrolled and strong contraction leads to the rupture. It is remarkable that the group which is most often affected is people who were physically active when they were younger. When they take up their sports activities again, they suffer an Achilles tendon rupture.

The diagnosis is easily assessed in cases with complete rupture of the tendon. The history is typical: the patient feels as though something snaps in the calf, sometimes associated with a burning pain and is not able to continue with the ongoing activity. Despite this the diagnosis is primarily missed and detected later in up to 25% of the patients. A positive Thompson's (Simmonds) test is present (Fig. 6.1.7). The patient lies in the prone position with bare legs and flexed knees. The examiner firmly squeezes the calf from side to side and observes the movement in the foot. If the tendon is intact, a plantar flexion movement is observed. By applying resistance to the plantar flexion, the absence of force is obvious. A defect in the tendon is also palpable.

Traditionally, Achilles tendon ruptures have been operated on in the majority of cases. A number of studies were published where the surgical methods were described, etiology investigated and the operated persons were evaluated by clinical follow-up. Following studies in the 1970s showing good results with immobilization in a cast without operation, this treatment has also been used in many cases. However, in a recent prospective randomized multicenter study [43], non-operative treatment with 8 weeks of cast immobilization was compared with surgical treatment with early graded mobilization using brace. Surgical treatment combined with early mobilization produced better results in terms of lower rerupture rate, and the patients reported a high quality of life during the treatment with fewer complications.

At surgery, the tendon ends are adapted by sutures anchored in the firm parts of the tendon and the paratenon is closed. The operation can favorably be performed under local anesthesia without the use of a tourniquet in an outpatient clinic. After surgery, the active rehabilitation phase is 6 months. An early return to work and sporting activity has been reported to give better functional results especially in terms of muscle strength and endurance. Early mobilization is advantageous and has not given rise to higher risk of complica-

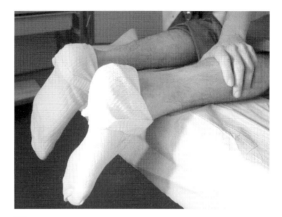

(a)

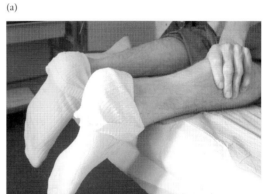

(b)

Fig. 6.1.7 Thompson's test: With the patient lying with the back facing up and the foot placed over the edge of the investigation couch (a), the investigator compresses the calf muscles side to side (b). With an intact Achilles tendon, the foot plantar flexes, whereas nothing happens if the Achilles tendon is ruptured.

tions. Lower leg braces that inhibit dorsal extension can be used. Stirrup casts can also be used, allowing loading and movement in the ankle to a certain level. Normally, the patients function well in their daily activity in terms of walking without limping after 1–2 months of rehabilitation. The prognosis with regard to function is good, and most patients have relatively few subjective problems from the Achilles tendon. The majority can return to preinjury activity including sports.

Suture of the Achilles tendon can also be performed percutanously. The short-term results are encouraging.

Complications after non-surgical treatment are unsatisfactory healing with pain and reduced strength, healing with lengthening of the tendon giving rise to increased dorsal extension, decreased flexibility, inability to walk on tiptoe, problems with balance, and frequent tripping. Rerupture is the most dreaded complication. The frequency of rerupture varies in different studies between 10% and 35%, but is lower after surgical treatment. After surgery, the most common complication is superficial infection, requiring antibiotic treatment.

Ankle joint injuries

Ankle arthroscopy

Ankle arthroscopy is a valuable tool in the diagnosis and treatment of various intra-articular ankle disorders. Visualization of intra-articular pathology without arthrotomy is possible, thus reducing the risk of surgical complications. Indications for ankle arthroscopy are osteochondral fractures, chondral lesions, soft tissue impingement, bony impingement, post-traumatic osteoarthritis and loose bodies. Chronic pain at the anterior aspect of the ankle joint is rather frequent in athletes, e.g. soccer players, and is often referred to as 'footballer's ankle', and is also a frequent indication for arthroscopy [47].

Patients with recurrent ankle pain, chondral and osteochondral lesions, anterior tibial spurs and soft tissue pathology such as synovitis and 'meniscoid' lesion are those who are most often in need of arthroscopic intervention. Although the risk of complications after arthroscopic surgery of the ankle is low, it should be kept in mind that numerous anatomic structures are at risk. The frequency of neurovascular complications in some reports is as high as 10%. It has been shown that the anteromedial, anterolateral and posterolateral portals give nearly complete access to all parts of the ankle joint.

Acute ligament injuries

A sprained ankle is the most common sport-related injury, mainly in the younger age groups [48–50]. The injury may occur as an athletic trauma or during activities of daily living. The reported incidence of ankle ligament injuries varies, mainly due to the profile of sporting activities in the population (Figs 6.1.8 and 6.1.9). The incidence in a high-risk sports population is

between 2 and 6 per 100 participants per season. It has been estimated that these injuries constitute approximately 25% of all time loss due to sports injuries to the ankle, especially in sports that involve running and jumping, e.g. soccer, basketball and volleyball. Although many of these injuries are not serious *per se*, they are very costly to society due to their high incidence.

Ligament injuries to the ankle are divided into acute and chronic. In most cases lateral ligament injury

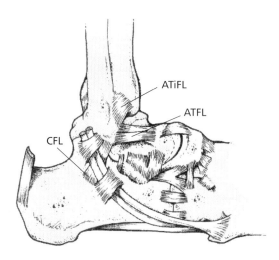

Fig. 6.1.8 Ligaments at the lateral aspect of the ankle and foot. ATFL, anterior talofibular ligament; CFL, calcaneofibular ligament; ATiFL, anterior tibiofibular ligament.

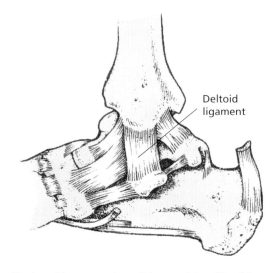

Fig. 6.1.9 Ligaments at the medial aspect of the ankle and foot.

occurs with the foot rotating inwards in plantar flexion when the tibia is simultaneously rotating outwards, giving rise to anterolateral rotational movement. The medial malleolus acts as a fulcrum when the ankle moves into increased inversion, losing its stabilizing function and increasing the strain on the lateral side.

Ankle ligament injuries are classified as Grade I (mild), Grade II (moderate) and Grade III (severe). Grade I injuries include stretching of the ligaments without macroscopic rupture. There is minor swelling and tenderness and no increase in laxity. The loss of function is minimal and the recovery is usually quick. In Grade II injuries there is a partial macroscopic rupture of the ligaments, with moderate swelling, tenderness and pain. There is a mild to moderate increase of laxity, some loss of motion and moderate functional disability. These lesions have a low frequency ($<5\%$). Grade III injuries always include complete rupture of the ligaments and the joint capsule, with severe bruising, swelling and pain. There is a major loss of function, reduction of motion and increased laxity due to the ligament rupture. The injured subject is often unable to bear weight because of pain. Radiographs are often needed to rule out fracture.

Over 90% of all ankle ligament injuries involve the lateral ligaments (Fig. 6.1.8). The anterior talofibular ligament (ATFL) is the most vulnerable of the lateral ankle ligaments. Further, rupture of the ATFL occurs as an isolated injury in approximately two-thirds of all ankle ligament injuries. With an increasing force, the calcaneofibular ligament (CFL) is also damaged. A rupture of both the ATFL and the CFL occurs in 15–25%. Isolated rupture of the CFL happens in approximately 1%, and injury to the posterior talofibular ligament (PTFL) is extremely rare. Individuals with generalized hypermobility of the joints or a previous history of ankle ligament injury are at greater risk of ankle injuries.

Isolated ligament injuries of the deltoid ligament are infrequent (Fig. 6.1.9). The frequency has been estimated as approximately 2.5% of all ankle ligament injuries. The injury mechanism is an excessive outward rotation of the foot during simultaneous inwards rotation of the tibia. This type of injury usually takes several weeks to heal, and more often gives rise to chronic anteromedial pain rather than recurrent medial instability. Pain and swelling are present for a longer period of time than for a corresponding injury on the lateral side.

Injury of the anterior tibiofibular ligament (anterior syndesmosis ligament) is sometimes seen in soccer players after external rotation of the foot, in dancers after forced dorsiflexion of the foot or in alpine skiers after combined external rotation, axial compression and forced dorsiflexion. When this injury is suspected, a complete radiographic examination of the lower leg should be performed to rule out a fracture of the proximal fibula. This ligament injury is painful, and heals slowly, but residual disability with recurrent instability episodes is not frequent.

A supination trauma is associated with a distraction force on the lateral side and compression force on the medial side of the joint. Apart from anterolateral pain and swelling, 60% of patients experience pain on palpation of the anteromedial ankle joint structures, indicating that damage has happened to the anterior rim of the tibia, to the cartilage or the joint capsule. Depending on the degree of damage, a repair reaction with cartilage proliferation, scar tissue formation and calcification will follow. Additional damage due to recurrent instability or forced ankle movement, especially forced dorsiflexion, will enhance this process. It has been shown that in patients with anteromedial osteophytes 75% had a history of supination trauma or had participated in soccer. Presence of osteophytes is not always associated with serious complaints. Removal of these spurs is important to create normal movement and prevent recurrence of the impingement. Arthroscopic removal of these osteophytes produces a good or excellent result in over 90% of cases. Grading the degree of osteoarthritis in patients with an anterior impingement syndrome is important for the prognosis.

Although ruptures of the ankle ligaments are very common, treatment remains controversial. In a recent systematic review of the orthopedic literature, it was found that treatment of too short a duration or which did not include sufficient support of the ankle joint tended to result in more residual symptoms. It was concluded that a 'no treatment' strategy for ruptures of the lateral ankle ligaments led to more residual symptoms. After a supination trauma it is therefore important to distinguish a simple distorsion from an acute ankle ligament rupture since adequate treatment is associated with a better prognosis. The reliability of physical examination can be enhanced when the investigation is repeated a few days after the trauma. The accuracy of physical examination has been determined in a series of 160 patients, comparing physical examination within 48 h of the injury and 5 days after injury. All patients underwent arthrography. The specificity and sensitivity of delayed physical examination for the presence or absence of a lateral ankle ligament rupture were 84% and 96%, respectively. The most important features of physical examination are swelling, hematoma, discoloration, pain on palpation and the anterior drawer test. Physical examination is unreliable in the acute situation, since the anterior drawer test cannot be performed due to pain. A few days after the trauma, the swelling and pain have subsided and it becomes obvious whether the cause of swelling was edema or hematoma. The pain on palpation has become more localized and the anterior drawer test can now be performed. The site of pain on palpation is important. If there is no pain on palpation over the ATFL, there is no acute lateral ligament rupture. Pain on palpation over the ATFL itself cannot distinguish between a rupture or a distorsion. Pain on palpation in combination with hematoma discoloration means, however, a 90% chance of acute lateral ligament rupture. A positive anterior drawer test has a sensitivity of 73% and a specificity of 97%. A positive anterior drawer test in combination with pain on palpation over the ATFL and hematoma discoloration has a sensitivity of 100% and a specificity of 77%. Delayed physical examination provides a diagnostic modality with a high sensitivity and specificity.

If there is ankle pain after ligament injury, a number of concomitant lesions should be looked for: cartilage damage (especially on the joint surface of the talus); synovitis/impingement (inflammation and entrapment); entrapment of the tibialis posterior nerve (tarsal tunnel syndrome); partial rupture of the short peroneal tendon; bony outgrowths (osteophytes) in the joint; and loose bodies in the joint. Arthroscopy of the ankle is often of great value in establishing the diagnosis.

Treatment of acute ligament injuries

All Grade I and Grade II ligament injuries are safely treated non-surgically. Functional treatment with a very short period of *r*est, cooling (*i*ce), *c*ompression and *e*levation to reduce the edema (the RICE principle) during the first 1–3 days, depending upon the amount of swelling, bruising and pain, should always be recommended. Early weight-bearing without crutches, if possible, is encouraged. Active range of motion training should be started after the acute phase treatment is completed, followed by neuromuscular coordination training using balance boards and peroneal strengthening exercises [51].

The injured ligaments should be protected from new injuries during the healing phase by using external support (ankle tape or a brace) to control the range of motion and to reduce the symptoms of functional instability. Both ankle tape and ankle braces, e.g. the air-stirrup, are easy to apply, versatile and effective in stimulating the proprioceptive system. The results of functional treatment of Grade I and Grade II ligament injuries are good in the majority of cases, and most athletes are able to return to sporting activities within 1–3 weeks. It has been shown that costs are significantly lower and ankle function is significantly better following early functional treatment (supervised rehabilitation program) or air-stirrup brace than immobilization in a plaster cast.

On the other hand, there is still some controversy as to whether grade III ligament ruptures should be treated non-surgically by active functional treatment and early mobilization, or by primary surgical repair followed by immobilization using a plaster cast or a brace. Unfortunately, there are only a few prospective, randomized and controlled studies in the literature. These studies have mostly shown that the medium- and long-term results are satisfactory in the majority of these patients regardless of the primary choice of treatment, i.e. surgical repair, cast immobilization alone for 3–6 weeks, or functional treatment based on the principle of early mobilization. In a recent prospective, randomized trial comparing early mobilization with plaster cast immobilization, it was shown that these treatment modalities prevented late residual symptoms and persistent ankle instability equally well, but patients treated with early mobilization had significantly less pain at 3 weeks (57% vs. 87%) and were more likely to be back at work after 1 week (54% vs. 13%). Taken together, at least 80–90% of patients with grade III injuries will regain satisfactory functional stability after non-surgical treatment. This is, however, not uncontroversial and a recent meta-analysis has suggested early repair as the best treatment.

Functional treatment includes a short period of relative immobilization using an ankle tape, elastic bandage or ankle brace. Absolute immobilization using plaster cast is not advantageous. Training of range of motion, peroneal muscle strength, and coordination is started as soon as pain and swelling have subsided. Weight-bearing should be encouraged as soon as possible. The functional treatment does not increase the risk of residual laxity and complications are less frequent than with surgical repair followed by cast immobilization. It should also be borne in mind that secondary reconstructive procedures usually produce satisfactory results, even several years after the index injury. This makes the argument in favor of early surgical repair weaker. Also, the cost and the length of sick-leave have been shown to be lower after functional treatment. Thus, there are fairly strong arguments that functional treatment is the treatment of choice for all grades of acute ligament injuries to the ankle joint, providing the syndesmosis is stable.

Chronic ankle joint instability

Functional instability is the most common residual disability after acute, lateral ligament ruptures and is a description of the subjective symptoms of the patient, e.g. repeated giving way, in some cases combined with pain. Laxity, on the other hand, refers to an objective measurement, e.g. standardized stress radiographs or clinical measurement of anterior drawer sign.

Functional instability is a complex syndrome, in which mechanical, neurologic, muscular and constitutional factors interact. The etiologic factors are not exactly known and in several cases there is a combination of factors. Elongation of the ruptured ligaments, i.e. increased laxity, proprioceptive deficit, peroneal muscle weakness and subtalar instability, are all documented etiologic factors of functional instability, either alone or in combination [52–54].

A correlation between functional instability and isometric peroneal muscle weakness has been shown. Correlation between functional instability and decreased postural control has also been shown using stabilometric measurements, indicating a proprioceptive

deficit after ligament injury. In these studies, however, no correlation has been found between functional instability and increased laxity.

The reaction time of the peroneal muscles, measured during sudden inversion using electromyography (EMG), has been shown to be significantly longer in unstable ankles than in stable ones. This difference in the reaction time is due to the time that elapses between the start of the inversion of the ankle and the stimulation of the mechanoreceptors in the ligaments and the joint capsule. Delayed proprioceptive response to sudden angular displacement of the ankle may be one of the most important causes of functional instability of the ankle joint [55,56].

Taken together, functional instability is caused by increased laxity, inhibition of proprioceptive function, peroneal muscle weakness or a combination of these factors. The specific cause of functional instability in each individual case has to be analyzed separately.

Chronic functional ankle joint instability develops in approximately 10–20% of patients after acute ligament rupture. This ligament instability does not always require surgical reconstruction. Non-surgical treatment is always recommended before operative management should be considered. Surgical reconstruction is probably more often needed in athletes with high demands of ankle function. There is no absolute indication for surgical intervention, but relative indication for surgical treatment is recurrent giving way in spite of proprioceptive training.

Several different surgical procedures have been described to correct chronic ankle joint instability. These surgical procedures can be classified as either non-anatomic, using some of the tendons around the ankle joint, or anatomic reconstruction, using either direct suture of the torn ligaments, or imbrication and reinsertion to bone, and in some instances reinforcement with local tissue, such as the inferior extensor retinaculum or a local periosteal flap.

The clinical evaluation of chronic ankle joint instability is primarily based on the assessment of anterior drawer sign (Fig. 6.1.10) and the inversion (supination) test, always in comparison with the contralateral side. Increased anterior translation of the talus in the talocrural joint is due to rupture or elongation of the ATFL. Increased inversion is due to rupture or elongation of the CFL, or a combination of ATFL and

CFL insufficiency, which is more common. Increased inversion may also imply increased laxity between talus and calcaneus (subtalar instability). Subtalar instability has been suggested to be one of the factors behind the development of functional instability. However, no definition of subtalar instability exists in the literature.

A correlation between chronic functional instability and prolonged peroneal reaction time has been shown, indicating that a proprioceptive deficit can be at least partly responsible for ankle instability.

Good knowledge of the laxity of the ankle joint ligaments in both the sagittal and the frontal plane can give valuable information during the diagnostic assessment of chronic functional instability. Radiographic measurements of ankle joint stability are sometimes used before deciding upon the treatment of chronic lateral instability. Standardized stress radiographs can be used in both differential diagnostic evaluation and assessment of therapy. Their main drawback is the limited correlation between functional instability and increased laxity [57,58].

The two radiographic tests which are used are the lateral instability/laxity test (talar tilt, TT) and the anterior instability/laxity test (anterior talar translation, ATT) (Fig. 6.1.10). Increased laxity can be defined either as a single value of ATT > 10 mm or as TT > 9°. Another way of defining increased laxity is a difference of ATT > 3 mm, i.e. the difference in ATT between the functionally unstable ankle and the contralateral ankle and/or TT > 3° in patients with unilateral instability. A good correlation between functional and mechanical instability has been shown in some studies, but this correlation is highly variable, since several factors other than mechanical instability can be responsible for the development of functional instability. Several studies have questioned the reliability of stress radiographs, especially the measurements of TT, and it must be borne in mind that radiographs alone can never be used to establish an indication for surgery (Fig. 6.1.10).

Ultrasonography (US) and magnetic resonance imaging (MRI) have been used to delineate injuries such as partial or total ruptures of the ankle ligaments. MRI in particular can provide useful information in patients with chronic pain after ligament injury to the ankle. MRI is both sensitive and specific, although it cannot replace stress radiographs. US can be useful as a screening modality, especially when there is a discrepancy between clinical and radiologic examinations after trauma. US is cheap and non-invasive. However, like MRI, it cannot replace stress radiographs.

Treatment of chronic ankle instability

Non-surgical treatment

Less than 10% of all subjects who have sustained acute ligament injuries will need stabilizing surgery. Before deciding upon surgical treatment in a patient with chronic ligament insufficiency, a supervised rehabilitation program based on peroneal muscle strengthening and coordination training should always be carried out. More than half of all these patients will regain satisfactory functional stability after such a program. The goals of the program are to strengthen the peroneal muscles, to regain normal proprioceptive function, and to re-establish normal protective reflexes. It is of major importance to make the rehabilitation program as complete as possible to regain full ankle function, i.e. full range of motion, improved balance and coordination (proprioceptive reflexes), and full strength and endurance of the injured limb. The training of the calf muscles should be both eccentric and concentric. Patients with high-grade mechanical laxity have less favorable prospects in regaining satisfactory function by physiotherapy. In these patients surgical treatment should be considered at an earlier stage. The aim of the rehabilitation program is to normalize the range of motion, balance, coordination, strength and endurance. The estimated rehabilitation time is at least 12 weeks [59].

Surgical treatment

Several different surgical procedures to stabilize the unstable ankle have been described. Most of these are either tenodeses or anatomic reconstructions. Increased laxity only, without giving way episodes, is not an indication for surgical stabilization of the ankle. It is also questionable whether repeated episodes of giving way predispose to osteoarthrosis of the ankle. Therefore, the indication for surgical intervention must always be based on the functional status of the ankle.

Tenodeses have previously been the most widely used

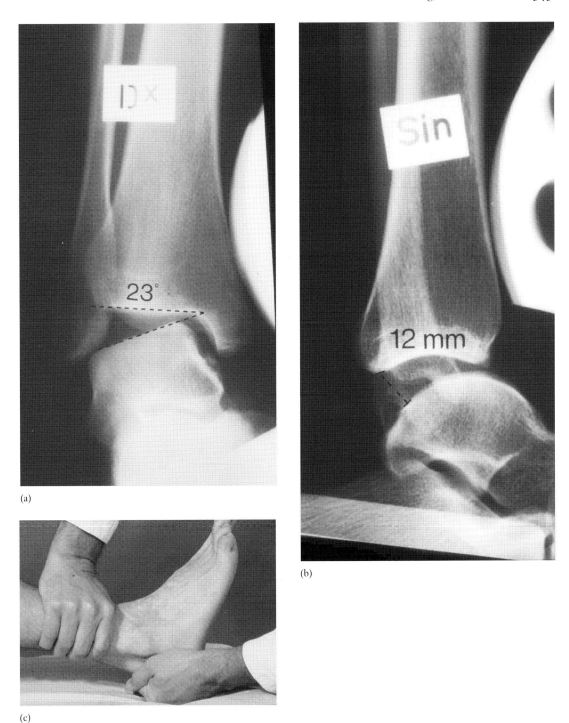

(a)

(b)

(c)

Fig. 6.1.10 Stress radiographs of the ankle with lateral instability and test for it. (a) Lateral talar tilt (TT) in AP projection (23°). (b) Anterior talar translation (ATT), 12 mm. (c) Testing for the anterior drawer sign: while stabilizing the tibia with one hand, the examiner with the other hand posterior to the subject's heel, applies an anterior draw to the foot.

principle of surgical reconstruction. All tenodeses sacrifice normal, and in most cases, well-functioning anatomic structures around the ankle joint, either the peroneus brevis or the peroneus longus tendons. The plantaris tendon, part of the Achilles tendon, or even a free fascia lata graft may also be used. None of the tenodeses in common use can be considered anatomic reconstructions and they nearly always result in altered kinematics, with limitation of joint motion and gradual deterioration of the reconstructed ligament function. This might cause degenerative changes of the ankle in the long run, leading to osteoarthrosis. All of these procedures also restrict the subtalar motion. Biomechanical analysis of non-anatomic reconstructions have shown that normal ankle biomechanics are not restored.

The four classic tenodeses—Elmslie, Evans, Watson–Jones and Chrisman–Snook—are all well known, and the short- and long-term results are well reported. The Evans tenodesis is technically the least demanding of these tenodeses (Fig. 6.1.11). However, the Evans tenodesis reconstructs neither the ATFL nor the CFL, as the tendon is positioned in a plane between these two ligaments [60–62]. Several authors have reported good short-term results after this reconstruction and its modifications, but the long-term re-

sults have been less encouraging. Many patients with satisfactory early results have deteriorated after a few years, resulting in unsatisfactory function in the long run. In one study it was shown that less than 50% of subjects had satisfactory results after a mean follow-up period of 14 years. This reconstruction is therefore not recommended as the primary choice.

The Watson–Jones tenodesis reconstructs the ATFL, but not the CFL. Thus, patients with insufficiency of the CFL will not benefit from this procedure. Several good short-term results have been reported, but long-term follow-up studies have shown disappointing functional results in approximately two-thirds of the patients. Late deterioration is common, with increased laxity and reduction of ankle function, as well as pain [63].

The Chrisman–Snook tenodesis restores both the ATFL and the CFL (Fig. 6.1.12), and is probably the most widely used non-anatomic reconstruction today [64]. The peroneus brevis tendon is split longitudinally, and half of the tendon is used to reconstruct both ligaments. Satisfactory long-term results have been reported in 94% of patients in one study. Stress provocation has also shown less residual laxity after the Chrisman–Snook reconstruction than after the Evans reconstruction. This procedure is technically more

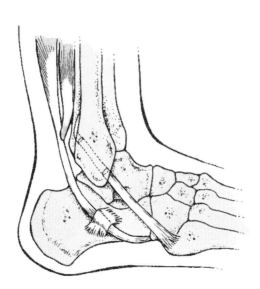

Fig. 6.1.11 Evans operation for chronic lateral ankle instability.

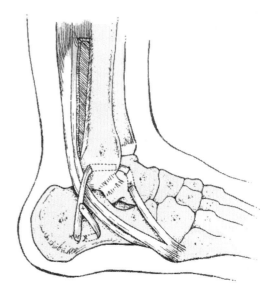

Fig. 6.1.12 Chrisman–Snook operation for chronic lateral ankle instability.

demanding than the other tenodeses. The majority of the complications reported after using this procedure are related to the long skin incision needed for harvesting the peroneus brevis tendon. Problems with delayed wound healing and sural nerve injuries have also been described. Nevertheless, this procedure is a sound alternative, at least in patients where anatomic reconstruction cannot be performed or has failed. This procedure should probably also be considered in case a reoperation is needed.

The *anatomic reconstruction* is the second main principle of stabilization of the unstable ankle. The remaining tissues of the injured ligaments are used, thus permitting a reconstruction without sacrificing any normal anatomic structure, such as the peroneal tendons. Broström, who described this procedure in detail, found that direct suture (repair) of the ruptured and elongated ligaments was possible, even several years after the primary injury (Fig. 6.1.13). The combination of shortening, imbrication and reinsertion to the bony attachment of the injured ligaments has been successful [62,65,66].

Good or excellent functional results after anatomic reconstruction of the lateral ankle ligaments have been described in many studies. The surgical technique is simple and easily performed. The damaged remnants of the ATFL and CFL are divided, shortened 3–5 mm, imbricated and reinserted into bone using sutures tied over bony bridges. Satisfactory functional results have been reported in approximately 90% of patients, with radiographic evidence of less residual laxity. The results are, however, less satisfactory in patients with generalized hypermobility of the joints, in very long-standing ligamentous insufficiency (over 10 years) and in patients who have undergone previous ankle joint ligament surgery. These patients should probably be treated with tenodesis; the Chrisman–Snook tenodesis has been especially recommended in these cases. Simultaneous reconstruction of both the ATFL and the CFL gives better results than reconstruction of the ATFL alone. After surgery, an air-stirrup ankle brace can be safely employed for early range of motion training without any risk of compromising the reconstructed ankle. Full weight-bearing is allowed.

These procedures are technically simple with few complications, producing satisfactory functional results in both the short and long run. Until recently, no

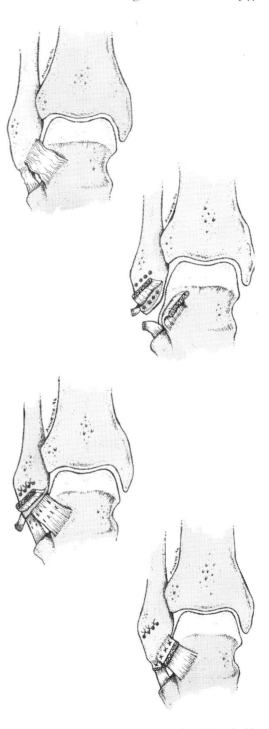

Fig. 6.1.13 Anatomical reconstruction for chronic lateral ankle instability.

long-term results in athletes with very high demands on ankle stability have been found, but recent studies have indicated good functional results in these patients even after a long observation period. Anatomic reconstruction, rather than the more complex tenodeses, should therefore be the primary choice in patients with chronic ankle instability. Normal range of motion is most often regained during the postoperative rehabilitation after anatomic reconstruction. The loss of motion which is common after the tenodeses is a major drawback for the athlete who is in need of full functional range of motion of the ankle and this speaks in favor of anatomic reconstructions.

Modifications of anatomic reconstructions have been described, mainly in order to reinforce the local structures when the ligaments are badly damaged or weak [67]. These modifications include using a periosteal flap from the lateral aspect of the fibula and the inferior extensor retinaculum and reinforcement of the CFL repair with the lateral talocalcaneal ligament. This procedure was primarily designed for correction of combined ankle and subtalar instability. Tensioning of the lateral ligaments and capsular tissue has also been described. The use of fresh frozen allografts in the reconstruction of the lateral ankle ligaments has also been reported to give satisfactory results in one study. Neither immunologic rejections nor complaints of late instability were reported. As no normal tissues are sacrificed, this procedure can be considered as an alternative to anatomic reconstructions if the quality of the ligamentous tissue is poor. All of these modified procedures have produced results in the range of 90% satisfied patients, without any significant difference between the various procedures.

Prevention

Two different methods for preventing ligament injuries of the ankle exist: coordination training and external ankle support.

Proprioceptive training improves both postural control and functional stability. Balance board training can reduce the incidence of ankle ligament injuries among athletes with a history of previous injury, as well as in those with previously uninjured ankles.

External ankle support theoretically reduces the ligamentous laxity. Both ankle taping and semirigid braces are much used to prevent ankle ligament in-

juries, both during the rehabilitation phase after injury and to prevent the previously injured ankle joint from further injury. The mechanism behind the function of ankle tape is not fully understood. There are three possible theories: (i) reduction of the ligamentous laxity; (ii) limitation of the extremes of ankle motion; and (iii) shortening of the reaction time of the peroneal muscles by affecting the proprioceptive function of the ligaments and joint capsule.

Ligamentous laxity
Laxity in both the sagittal plane (ATT) and the frontal plane (TT) has been shown in several studies to be reduced by the use of ankle tape. The frontal plane (TT) laxity is more effectively controlled than sagittal laxity. A significant reduction of TT has been shown after ankle taping. The highest degree of protection is found in ankles with the highest degree of laxity. In contrast to this, some authors have found insignificant reduction of laxity using ankle tape, analyzed as ATT and TT measured with standardized stress radiographs. The reduction of laxity is thus debated.

Limitation of ankle motion
Ankle tape significantly affects the pattern of ankle motion. Tape effectively limits the extreme ranges of ankle motion. In spite of the fact that tape becomes looser after exercise, the partial reduction of laxity gained by limiting the extremes of ankle motion is possibly a major factor behind the function of ankle tape.

Functional instability
Shortening the reaction time of the peroneus brevis and longus muscles by enhancing the proprioceptive function of the ankle ligaments and joint capsule might explain the mechanism behind the function of ankle tape. Ankle tape has in some studies been found to have a stimulating effect on the peroneus brevis muscle in unstable ankles, measured using EMG. A significantly slower reaction time of both the peroneus longus and peroneus brevis muscles has been found in unstable ankles than in stable ones using a trap-door mechanism and EMG measurements of the reaction time. These changes were, however, only found in ankles with increased laxity as a sign of residual ligament injury. The reaction time of the peroneal muscles in stable ankles is not shortened using ankle tape. This

mechanism is not uniform in all studies and is therefore debated.

Indications and use of ankle tape

1 Prophylactic: prevention of ligament injury in previously uninjured ankles.
2 After injury: prevention of further ligament injury in previously injured ankles.
3 During the rehabilitation phase as a part of the rehabilitation program, to bridge the time gap between acute injury and full recovery.
4 Treatment of chronic ligament instability, either temporarily or permanently instead of surgery.

The role of ankle tape in uninjured ankles is not well proven scientifically. The tape loses at least a part of its stabilizing effect after a short period of exercise.

Ankle tape or brace?

Ankle tape is not a substitute for normal soft tissue function. Ankle tape must always be used as a part of a rehabilitation program aimed at restoring normal range of motion, muscular strength and neuromuscular coordination. Some studies have shown that ankle tape is effective in the prevention of ankle ligament injuries. The effect of prophylactic ankle taping is roughly equivalent to coordination training of the ankle. A negative factor in the use of ankle taping is the loss of mechanical support after a short period of exercise, leaving the ankle with only partial protection. In one study it was shown that approximately 40% of the supporting force of the tape was lost after 10 min of exercise. Other researchers have found that after exercise most of the adhesive bandages are loose and the tape is mostly acting as canvas boots. The cost–benefit of tape used as a general prophylaxis can therefore be questioned.

Several different methods of ankle taping have been described. Alternative methods include rigid or semirigid ankle braces, some of which give good external support to prevent ankle sprain and to protect ligament reconstruction. An effective and functional alternative to ankle tape is the air-stirrup, a non-rigid prefabricated shell with an inner lining of air bags. It has been shown to provide good protection by reducing the range of ankle motion. The air-stirrup can be recommended, especially during early tissue healing and full functional recovery (1–12 weeks after injury).

Ankle tape and braces are effective in protecting the ankle joint during the rehabilitation phase after acute ligament injuries. These methods can also be used for the prevention of ankle distorsions or as treatment in chronic cases. The best stabilizing effect is generally obtained in ankles with the highest degree of laxity. If an external support is required during physical exercise, a brace of good quality should be chosen, due to lower cost.

Subtalar instability

Subtalar instability lacks clinical and scientific definition. In spite of this, ligament insufficiency of the subtalar joints is now recognized as one of the important factors behind the development of chronic functional instability, and it is probably frequently overlooked. The incidence of subtalar instability is unknown, but the estimated prevalence is 10% in patients with chronic lateral ankle instability, although this is not documented. Using subtalar arthrography, injuries to the subtalar joints have been found in a high proportion of patients who have sustained acute lateral ligament injuries. The clinical diagnosis of subtalar instability is difficult and unreliable. The diagnosis can be supported by using subtalar arthrography, subtalar stress view or stress tomography. The value of MRI, CT and ultrasonography is unknown.

In patients with symptomatic chronic instability of subtalar joints not responding to a supervised rehabilitation program anatomic reconstruction or tenodesis may be recommended. The short-term results of these procedures are promising, but further studies are needed to evaluate their long-lasting function. No comparative studies exist, and the optimal treatment is not known.

Deltoid ligament rupture

The deltoid ligament is located on the inside of the ankle. This ligament is thick and strong and, in addition, is in both superficial and deep planes. Damage to this ligament is therefore much more uncommon than to the lateral ligaments. The injury arises following outward rotation of the foot. There can be partial or total rupture of the ligament depending on the amount of force and the direction. Ligament injury can occur in isolation, but is more common in association with a fracture of the ankle.

There is pain and swelling at the inside of the ankle. The pain is most pronounced at the front of the ligament. A test of stability is difficult to perform, even for an experienced examiner. Definite instability can therefore often not be established. Radiographic examination is often necessary, in order to rule out fracture.

Treatment

Acute treatment is according to the RICE principle, with pressure dressing and possibly ice-packs. After the pressure dressing has been removed, a compression bandage is applied. As soon as the pain allows rehabilitation with agility, balance and weight training can be begun. There are no studies which show that immobilization or surgery in the acute phase improve results, in either the short or long term.

Healing time is significantly longer and the discomfort greater than with acute ligament damage to the lateral ankle ligaments. Swelling and pain often persist for several weeks or months. It is important to give the injury a chance to heal without forcing treatment, to reduce the risk of prolonged inflammation together with pain and a reduction in function. There is very little need for surgery in the long run.

Syndesmosis rupture

Rupture of syndesmosis ligaments is uncommon. The injury generally occurs in association with a fracture, but can in rare cases also arise as an isolated injury. Damage to syndesmosis ligaments occurs upon forced outward rotation of the ankle (Fig. 6.1.14). In most cases it is the anterior syndesmosis ligament (anterior tibiofibular ligament) which is damaged. Acute surgery is generally necessary to prevent future reduction of functions. There can be a fracture of the fibula directly below the knee joint. Careful examination with palpation of the whole fibula is therefore necessary, if there is suspected rupture of syndesmosis ligaments. Rupture of syndesmosis ligaments can be difficult to detect. Careful clinical examination is therefore important. There is swelling and pain over the ligament, which is further forward and higher up the lower leg than with a normal acute ligament injury.

Severe pain occurs upon provocation of the syndesmosis ligaments during forced outward rotation of the foot in relation to the lower leg. This test can, how-

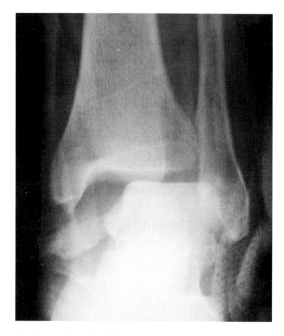

Fig. 6.1.14 Rupture of the syndesmosis with widening of the medial joint space.

ever, be difficult to carry out in acute cases. It should therefore be complemented with radiographic examination to rule out a fracture and examination for instability by means of fluoroscopy. The provocation test reveals instability between the tibia and fibula upon maximum outward rotation of the foot if the syndesmosis ligaments are damaged.

Treatment

Acute surgery to stabilize the syndesmosis by osteosynthesis and suturing of the ligament is recommended. Early rehabilitation training is possible if surgery achieves good stability. Chronic pain may follow damage of the syndesmosis, which has not been detected in the acute phase. Healing time is approximately 10–12 weeks. With early active training, a return to play can take place slightly more quickly.

Dislocation of the peroneal tendons

Dislocation of one of the peroneal tendons, in most cases the short peroneal tendon, occurs when the tendon moves or dislocates out of the shallow groove located behind the lateral malleolus. The retinaculum, which holds the tendon in place, tears. The injury arises during inward rotation and simultaneous inward twisting of the foot.

The acute symptoms are almost identical to those of acute ligament damage, i.e. pain and swelling around the lateral malleolus. Clinical diagnosis is generally difficult and the injury is therefore not always detected. With suspected dislocation of the peroneal tendon, the foot is rotated inward at the same time as the peroneal muscles on the outside of the lower leg are activated. Movement of the peroneal tendon over the lateral malleolus can then be seen and felt. If there is recurrent instability, the tendon can dislocate over the lateral malleolus; this causes a perceptible clicking and is clearly visible. The condition is often painful.

Treatment

Initial treatment of acute dislocation of the peroneal tendon is a compression dressing and ice-packs. Immobilization using a plaster cast or a brace is recommended for 4–6 weeks and is then followed by active rehabilitation, weight-bearing and balance training. If the acute damage heals spontaneously, sports activity can be started after 8–10 weeks. With recurrent instability surgical stabilization of the tendon is necessary. Several different methods can be used. Recent studies have shown that simple reconstruction of the ligament and ligament reinforcement in the rear of the ankle give good results. The prognosis is good in most cases. Results following surgery are generally good. The majority of sports active people regain normal flexibility and strength in the ankle and can return to the same level of activity as before the injury.

Os trigonum

One of the accessory bones in the foot which can give rise to problems is the os trigonum, which is located behind the ankle joint, between the talus and the Achilles tendon. Upon plantar flexion of the foot, the bone can become trapped and produce pain. This bone is normally found in approximately 10% of the population, but only causes problems if the area is subjected to high stress or pinching.

The diagnosis is clinical, based on the occurrence of pain in the posterior part of the ankle joint during stress, such as running on uneven ground or stepping on tiptoe. Radiographic examination corroborates the diagnosis. The diagnosis can be confirmed if injection of a small amount of local anesthetic around the bone makes the pain during loading of the foot disappear. Further examination, e.g. MRI, is not necessary.

Treatment

Initial treatment consists of correction of external training factors, such as changes in the amount of training and training surface. Tape, which reduces movement of the ankle—especially on downward bending, can also be used. If the player has pronounced, persistent pain which prevents training or play, surgical removal of the bone is appropriate. Prognosis following surgery is generally good. Return to full activity after approximately 4 weeks can be expected.

Footballer's ankle

Footballer's ankle ('anterior impingement') arises relatively often in footballers, especially at the end of their career. The injury occurs after repeated minor injuries to the front of the ankle. In tearing of the joint capsule attachment to the tibia and talus, small bone fragments become detached, initiating outgrowth of bone osteophytes, which gradually build up on the edges of the joint surface (Fig. 6.1.15).

During examination there is pain upon palpation in the front of the ankle joint and pain upon provocation when the foot is dorsally extended. Further, dorsal extension is often reduced. Footballer's ankle is not uncommonly combined with chronic ligament instability.

Initially the injury can be treated with anti-inflammatory drugs and stabilizing ankle support such as tape, to prevent pain. However, surgery is often necessary. During the operation, the anterior osteophytes are removed. The surgery can be performed very well arthroscopically. The damage is benign, but often bothersome and painful. Results following surgery are generally good and the sports active can return to the same level of activity as before, after approximately 4 weeks.

Osteochondritis dissecans

The cause of osteochondritis dissecans is unknown. The pathologic condition is in the talus, generally on the posteromedial corner (Fig. 6.1.16), but anterolat-

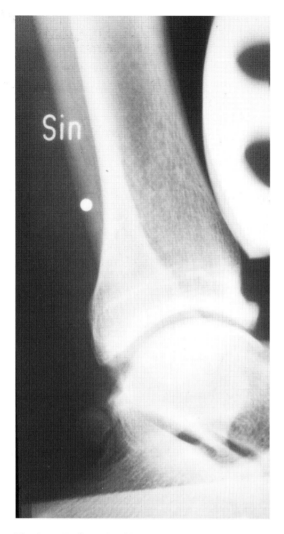

Fig. 6.1.15 Radiography of footballer's ankle.

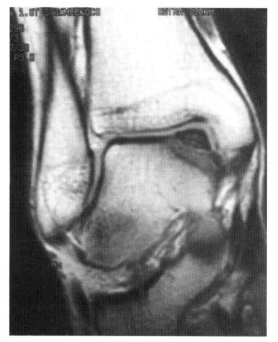

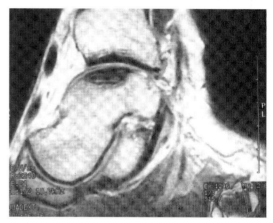

Fig. 6.1.16 Medial osteochondritis of the talus as seen on MRI.

erally related to ligament damage to the lateral aspect of the ankle joint. The condition is most common in young people, but does not often produce symptoms until adulthood. There is either a bony fragment covered by cartilage, or detachment of the bone fragment which moves freely in the joint and can cause catching, locking and pain. Symptoms are either pain during exertion or recurring catching and/or locking, if a loose body has formed in the joint. The first symptoms are often pain on movement and reduced range of motion.

In order to establish a diagnosis radiographic examination is always necessary. In certain cases, arthroscopic inspection can be of great value in assessment, especially if surgical treatment becomes necessary. Sometimes osteochondritis dissecans is detected on radiographs taken for other reasons.

Treatment depends on the findings made during direct examination. If the bony fragment is loose, removal of this is recommended, if possible by arthro-scopic surgery. This results in a bony surface which is not covered with cartilage in the joint surface of the talus. If, on the other hand, the surface of the cartilage is intact, an attempt is made to induce healing of the bone fragment by drilling or pinning. Prognosis is best in children and young people, especially if the cartilage joint surface is intact. If a free body has formed in the joint, the prognosis is worse with a risk of cartilage damage from wear, giving rise to osteoarthrosis.

Injuries to the foot

The foot is divided into three functional units—the forefoot, the midfoot and the hindfoot. The foot is composed of 26 bones, not including the two sesamoid bones under the first metatarsophalangeal joint. There are additional 10 named accessory bones in the foot. Some of these, such as the os trigonum in the rear of the ankle, can give rise to problems.

In all, there are 57 named joints in the foot and over 100 ligaments which keep these joints together.

Problems in the foot in connection with sport are either acute injuries or strain injuries. Fractures of the toes or the metatarsal bones are the most common acute injuries. Many of these fractures are not greatly dislocated and can be treated simply by temporary non-weight-bearing and in severe cases immobiliza-tion in a cast, and will heal in 2–3 weeks. Healing time, before full-scale sports activity can be resumed, is gen-erally roughly twice that. The prognosis for fractures of the toes and bones in the metatarsus is, with a few exceptions, good.

Serious injuries involving fractures or dislocations of the foot are rare during sports activity. In rare cases there are for example compound fractures and disloca-tions in the joint between the forefoot and the midfoot. Diagnosis can be difficult to make. If such an injury is suspected with pain upon provocation, radiographic examination should be carried out. In certain cases, this must be complemented with CT. It is then often revealed that the injury is more serious than was originally estimated.

Haglund's disease

Haglund's disease is similar to Osgood–Schlatter's disease in the knee joint as far as symptoms and origin are concerned. This disease occurs particularly in

young people between 12 and 14, and the problem disappears during late puberty. The Achilles tendon attachment is strained where the tendon attaches to the heel bone, probably after running on a hard surface, when the Achilles tendon attachment is subject to repeated tension. Fragmentation of bone then occurs and can be seen on radiographs. There is pain and a painful protuberance in the back of the heel, as well as soreness on palpation. The pain increases particularly before and after physical activity.

It is a clinical diagnosis which can be confirmed by radiographic examination, which shows a fragmenta-tion of the bone.

Treatment is focused on symptoms. Footwear adjustment and a soft insole, such as a heel cup, with a slight heel lift, which reduces symptoms, can be ap-propriate. In certain cases temporary rest combined with alternative exercise can be necessary. It is com-pletely safe to continue sports activities despite the discomfort. Prognosis is practically always good and the condition is self-healing. A large, protruding lump can be left on the calcaneus, which in isolated cases leads to later problems in connection with exercise and sport.

Plantar fasciitis (calcaneal spur)

This condition is a stress injury in the tendon aponeu-rosis (plantar fascia) on the underside of the foot (Fig. 6.1.17). Athletes are at particular risk if they are play-ing on a hard surface, especially if they use shoes with insufficient shock absorption. Partial rupture with inflammation in the plantar fascia attachment to the calcaneus, or tendinosis (degenerative changes) in-creases the pain. Athletes with a high (pes excavatus) or low (pes planus) foot arch are considered more vulnerable than others.

The most common symptom is pain, which corre-lates to strain, especially during running or jumping, in particular when the heel strikes the ground or upon tension of the plantar fascia. There is generally pain after training and stiffness is pronounced.

Radiographs generally show no specific changes, but sometimes a 'calcaneal spur' can be seen. It is not the cause of the problem, but rather a result of it. Radiographic examination is recommended most of all to exclude or confirm other diagnoses, such as stress fracture of the calcaneus.

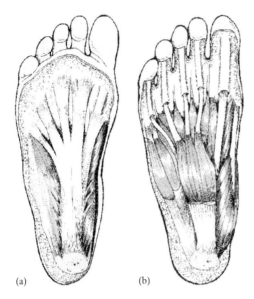

(a)   (b)

Fig. 6.1.17 The structures of the foot: (a) the plantar aponeurosis (fascia plantaris); (b) flexor muscles deep to the aponeurosis.

Treatment

Correction of external factors, such as unsuitable footwear, excessively hard training surface and internal factors, such as malalignment of the foot, is necessary. Activities should be modified; e.g. running on the forefoot/toes should be avoided. Even running which involves mainly starting, stopping and/or changes in direction should be kept to a minimum. Temporary rest, combined with alternative exercise, can be necessary. Stretching of the plantar fascia is recommended, along with an insole to correct high or low foot arch. Anti-inflammatory drugs can produce good results in the acute phase.

Corticosteroid injections can also produce good results. Surgery with tenotomy of the plantar fascia at the calcaneus is only indicated in exceptional cases.

The healing period is often very long, but the prognosis is good and the condition normally heals on its own, although it can take several months until the athlete is completely free from pain.

Stress fracture

A stress fracture can occur in any bone of the foot, but is most common in the second metatarsal (known as a march fracture). This type of stress fracture generally arises in long-distance runners. Stress fractures also occur with lower incidence in the fifth metatarsal, in the navicular bone, talus and calcaneus. Women are more vulnerable than men.

The injury mechanism in a stress fracture is always excessive strain, i.e. the strain is greater than the bone can withstand. External factors, such as inappropriate footwear, too much training or excessively hard ground are often contributing factors.

In the initial stage, there is stress-related pain during exertion, such as running on a hard surface, but no pain at rest. The pain increases gradually. Although training is possible in this phase, it eventually becomes too painful. Upon examination there is localized pain when pressure is applied and on provocation. There is rarely any swelling. Radiographs initially reveal no fracture. Radiographic examination should be repeated after 2–3 weeks. The fracture is then often visible. In cases where there is strong suspicion of a stress fracture, an isotope scan (scintigraphy) should be carried out. This shows the fracture within a day of the injury.

Diagnosis of a stress fracture of the navicular bone, talus and calcaneus can be difficult. The fracture is often invisible on plain radiographs. When there is a high suspicion of fracture of these bones, isotope scans, CT or MRI should be performed. Delayed diagnosis can lead to impaired results of treatment.

Treatment varies depending on which bone is injured. Keeping weight off the foot, combined with alternative training, e.g. wet-vest training, until the athlete is free from pain, is important. In certain cases immobilization by means of plaster or a brace can be necessary.

The general treatment of a metatarsal stress fracture is keeping weight off the foot for 3 weeks, either with or without a plaster. With other stress fractures, such as the navicular bone, talus or calcaneus, longer immobilization is generally necessary (8–12 weeks). In spite of this, healing complications are not infrequent, but surgery is rarely necessary.

A stress fracture in the metatarsal generally heals without persisting problems, but the healing period varies. The healing period for a stress fracture in the navicular, talus and calcaneus is long and rehabilitation can also be very long, often as much as 6 months. However, with correct diagnosis, treatment and rehabilitation, the prognosis for healing is generally good.

Jones fracture

Jones fracture is a stress fracture to the proximal part of the fifth metatarsal. The fracture has a slightly worse healing prognosis than other stress fractures in the metatarsus. The reason for this is that the peroneal brevis tendon attaches to the proximal part of the bone. This leads to increased risk of delayed healing or formation of a false joint (pseudoarthrosis).

There is pain over the proximal part of the fifth metatarsal upon direct pressure and provocation, and there can be slight swelling. If there is suspected fracture, radiographic examination is recommended. If disturbances in healing and a false joint are suspected, CT or MRI can be necessary to confirm the diagnosis.

Treatment

The fracture should be treated with immobilization, using plaster cast or a brace, for 4–6 weeks. Despite this, the risk of healing complications is relatively large. With delayed healing or development of a false joint, osteosynthesis with an intramedullary screw is recommended.

Healing complications are relatively common. Following surgery, however, prognosis is generally good. Return to sports activity is possible in approximately 6–8 weeks.

Fracture of the sesamoid bone

Under the metatarsal of the big toe there are two sesamoid bones in the flexor tendon. Damage to these bones is relatively common in sports, especially when training on a hard surface. Fracture of the sesamoid bone can occur as a stress injury and a false joint can develop.

Persistent problems with pain often arise. The damaged sesamoid bone causes pain upon direct pressure. Radiographs, which are not always necessary, however, show that the bone is in two pieces (false joint).

This fracture is treated by keeping weight off the foot, using an insole and reducing the amount of training. Surgery is indicated only in exceptional cases and involves removal of the damaged sesamoid bone. This is especially appropriate when the damage is to the

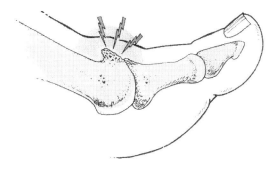

Fig. 6.1.18 Hallux rigidus with dorsal, bony impingement.

medial sesamoid bone. Prognosis is good in the majority of cases.

Hallux rigidus

Hallux rigidus is caused by degenerative changes (arthrosis) in the metatarsophalangeal joint of the big toe.

There is pain and increasing stiffness in the metatarsophalangeal joint of the big toe. Upon examination movement is reduced, especially in dorsal extension. In addition, there is a painful bony outgrowth, which is mainly felt on top of the metatarsophalangeal joint (Fig. 6.1.18).

Radiographic examination provides the diagnosis. It shows bony spurs at the dorsal aspect of the joint or reduced joint space in the whole joint.

Treatment

Taping of the big toe avoids the extremes of motion, in particular dorsal flexion, and relieves symptoms. A relatively stiff insole is often used, although with varying success.

Surgery often becomes necessary. Excision of the bony growth on the top of the joint is recommended. Freedom from pain is achieved if movement can be restored. Other operations, such Keller's operation or fusion, are rarely successful in athletes.

The condition can be very painful and lead to protracted problems. Surgery generally only gives temporary success.

Morton's metatarsalgia (interdigital neuroma)

Morton's neuroma has recently been defined as a nerve entrapment of one of the interdigital nerves in the forefoot, in most cases between the third and fourth metatarsal heads. The older term neuroma is not correct and should accordingly be replaced.

The typical complaint is a radiating pain into the toes. The pain is also often associated with numbness. The pain is elicited and increased by narrow-fitting footwear and weight-bearing activities such as running or skiing. Localized tenderness and an audible click during compression of the metatarsal heads is usually present. This click is most often painful. In several cases excessive pronation of the hindfoot is found, leading to metarsal hypermobility and increased risk of interdigital nerve entrapment.

Primary treatment is aimed at reduction of acute pain with a metatarsal padding and shoe insole, in order to spread the load of the metatarsals during weight-bearing. Foot muscle strengthening may be indicated to improve balance and foot strength. In chronic cases little improvement is seen with non-surgical treatment. Corticosteroid injection in the interdigital space can be used and in case of excessive pronation corrective insoles should be used.

If all other treatment fails, surgical excision of the entrapped nerve through either a plantar or dorsal excision usually gives good pain relief.

Summary

Overuse injuries of the lower leg are most commonly seen in runners and include medial tibial stress syndrome, stress fracture of anterior or posterior tibia and compartment syndromes. The diagnostic considerations and treatments have been discussed. Achilles tendon problems are common, most often as tendinosis in the tendon or paratendon, and sometimes as acute tendinitis/peritendinitis. The various treatment options, correction of biomechanical dysfunction, hard eccentric muscle training, corticosteroid injections and surgery, are generally not evidence based, but the prognosis is usually good. Dysfunction or rupture of the tibialis posterior tendon can result in collapse of the medial arc of the foot.

Ninety per cent of acute ankle ligament injuries are lateral and most often the anterior talofibular ligament is ruptured. Grade I and II injuries are treated non-surgically with functional rehabilitation. Treatment of Grade III injuries can be surgical or non-surgical. Ten to 20% suffer from chronic functional ankle instability after an acute injury. The primary treatment is strengthening of peroneal muscles, regain of proprioception and re-establishment of the normal protective reflexes by functional training. With continuous instability surgical stabilization is indicated. Anatomic procedures have better long-term results than tenodeses. Prevention has been discussed.

Footballer's ankle with tibial osteophytes, loose bodies in the ankle joint, ligament tears and cartilage injury can be treated with arthroscopic house-cleaning.

Stress fractures of the middle foot or metatarsal bones are not unusual in the athletic population. Plantar fasciitis is also common in runners and jumpers, and responds well to correction of mechanical dysfunction.

Case story 6.1

A 32-year-old-soccer player with a history of ankle problems for more than 5 years initially sustained a serious inversion trauma of the ankle. The ankle was swollen and he was unable to bear weight. Radiographic examination did not reveal any skeletal injuries. The patient was treated with compression bandaging and range of motion exercises. He was allowed to return to sports (soccer) after 4 weeks.

He did not, however, recover fully. His ankle repeatedly gave way, combined with swelling and pain. In spite of this he was able to continue playing soccer using an ankle tape. The problem has increased and he has now been forced to quit playing soccer.

1 Why did he not recover and why did his ankle keep giving way? How should he be evaluated and treated?

The most important factor at this stage is the almost total lack of rehabilitation. The player was allowed to return to sports without a proper rehabilitation, and furthermore there was a delay in returning to sport of several weeks. With a well-conducted rehabilitation program, most players are able to return to sports such as soccer after approximately 1 week. However, the rehabilitation program should be continued for at least 12 weeks. Therefore, the most probable reason why the player did not recover was the lack of rehabilitation. This is regretfully a rather frequent occurrence.

This player is probably suffering from ligamentous insufficiency of the lateral ankle ligaments, a rather common sequela after acute injury. At this stage the patient should be evaluated for ligamentous insufficiency, but also for secondary bony or cartilage changes. It should be remembered that ligament instability alone does usually not lead to repeated swelling and pain. Besides a thorough clinical evaluation, the first investigation should be plain radiographs in order to evaluate the ankle joint for skeletal changes, such as anterior tibia or talus osteophytes, loose bodies or even osteoarthrosis. Secondary changes at the joint line, such as osteophytes, are common, but arthrosis is not.

At clinical investigation, the ankle displayed increased laxity, i.e. increased anterior drawer sign and inversion, indicating ligament injury. The ankle was slightly swollen, with distinct tenderness and swelling behind the lateral malleolus. The plain radiographs were negative.

At this stage it should be decided whether the patient is to be treated surgically or non-

surgically or even investigated further. The retromalleolar pain and swelling could be investigated using either ultrasonography of the peroneal tendons or MRI.

It was decided to treat the patient with a prolonged and well-supervised rehabilitation program. After 4 months, the patient still had problems, with giving way and pain. MRI of the ankle with special emphasis on the peroneal tendons was therefore performed. This imaging study showed a longitudinal rupture of the peroneus brevis tendon behind the lateral malleolus.

2 How should the patient be treated?
It was decided to treat the patient with a ligament reconstruction of the ankle joint. Anatomic reconstruction of both the anterior talofibular and the calcaneofibular ligaments was performed. At the same time the injury of the peroneus brevis tendon was repaired after excision of the partial rupture using side-to-side sutures and furthermore the superior peroneal retinaculum was reconstructed using drill holes through the posterior edge of the fibula. The ankle was immobilized in a below-the-knee plaster for 3 weeks and thereafter in an air-cast brace for a further 3 weeks. The rehabilitation was uneventful and the patient recovered well.

What we can learn from this is that all patients who sustain an ankle ligament injury should undergo a well-planned and supervised rehabilitation program and further that ankle ligament injuries may be more serious than anticipated. In this case a serious tendon injury was present and needed to be addressed before the patient eventually became free of symptoms.

Multiple choice questions

1 *The most important investigation which should be performed within 2 days in case of a suspected stress fracture of the navicular bone of the foot is:*
a anterior–posterior and lateral radiographs
b computed tomography (CT)
c bone mineral content investigation
d magnetic resonance imaging (MRI)
e none of the above.

2 *The healing time of deltoid ligament injuries of the ankle is:*

a approximately the same as for lateral ligament injuries

b approximately two to three times longer than for lateral ligament injuries

c approximately five to ten times longer than for lateral ligament injuries

d likely to result in surgery in more than 50% of cases

e none of the above.

3 *Stress fractures of the tibia are:*

a the most common stress fractures of the lower extremity

b connected with more healing problems when located in the anterior aspect (cortex) of the tibia than the posterior

c connected with more healing problems when located in the posterior aspect (cortex) of the tibia than the anterior

d likely to result in surgery in more than 50% of cases

e none of the above.

4 *Total (complete) rupture of the Achilles tendon:*

a is always associated with chronic degeneration of the tendon

b is never associated with chronic degeneration of the tendon

c will always need surgical treatment

d will never need surgical treatment

e none of the above.

5 *Partial rupture of the Achilles tendon:*

a is equivalent to Achilles tendinitis

b is equivalent to tendinosis of the Achilles tendon

c never needs surgical treatment

d always needs surgical treatment

e none of the above.

References

1 Touliopolous S, Hershman EB. Lower leg pain: diagnosis and treatment of compartment syndromes and other pain syndromes of the lower leg. *Sports Med* 1999; **27**: 193–204.

2 Clement DB, Taunton JE, Smart GW, McNicol KL. A survey of overuse running injuries. *Physician Sportsmed* 1981; **9**: 47–58.

3 Lysholm J, Wiklander J. Injuries to runners. *Am J Sports Med* 1987; **15**: 168–71.

4 James SL, Bates BT, Osternig LR. Injuries to runners. *Am J Sports Med* 1978; **6**: 40–50.

5 Puranen J, Alavaikko A. Intracompartmental pressure increase on exertion in patients with chronic compartment syndrome in the leg. *J Bone Joint Surg (Am)* 1981; **63-A**: 1304–9.

6 Reneman RS. The anterior and lateral compartment syndrome of the leg due to intensive use of muscles. *Clin Orth Rel Res* 1975; **113**: 69–80.

7 Styf J. Diagnosis of exercise-induced pain in the anterior aspect of the lower leg. *Am J Sports Med* 1988; **16**: 165–9.

8 Hulkko A. *Stress fractures in athletes*. Doctoral thesis, University of Oulu, Finland, 1988.

9 Detmer DE. Chronic shin splints: classification and management of medial tibial stress syndrome. *Sports Med* 1986; **3**: 436–46.

10 Mubarak SJ, Gould RN, Lee YF, Schmidt DA, Hargens AR. The medial tibial stress syndrome (a cause of medial shin splints). *Am J Sports Med* 1982; **10**: 201–5.

11 Michael RH, Holder LE. The soleus syndrome: a cause of medial tibial stress (shin splints). *Am J Sports Med* 1985; **13**: 87–94.

12 Davey JR, Rorabeck CH, Fowler PJ. The tibialis posterior muscle compartment: an unrecognized cause of exertional compartment syndrome. *Am J Sports Med* 1984; **12**: 391–7.

13 Micheli LJ, Solomon R, Solomon J, Plasschaert VF, Mitchell R. Surgical treatment for chronic lower-leg compartment syndrome in young female athletes. *Am J Sports Med* 1999; **27**: 197–201.

14 Rorabeck CH, Fowler PJ, Nott L. The results of fasciotomy in the management of chronic exertional compartment syndrome. *Am J Sports Med* 1988; **16**: 224–7.

15 Schepsis AA, Gill SS, Foster TA. Fasciotomy for exertional anterior compartment syndrome: is lateral compartment release necessary? *Am J Sports Med* 1999; **27**: 430–5.

16 Schepsis AA, Leach RE. Surgical management of Achilles tendinitis. *Am J Sports Med* 1987; **15**: 308–15.

17 Collins PS, McDonald PT, Lim RC. Popliteal artery entrapment: an evolving syndrome. *J Vasc Surg* 1989; **10**: 484–90.

18 Brubaker CE, James SL. Injuries to runners. *Sports Med* 1974; **2**: 189–98.

19 Matheson G, Clement D, McKenzie D, Taunton J, Lloyd-Smith D, McIntyre J. Stress fractures in athletes. A study of 320 cases. *Am J Sports Med* 1987; **15**: 46–58.

20 Johansson C, Ekenman I, Lewander R. Stress fractures of the tibia in athletes: diagnosis and natural course. *Scand J Med Sci Sports* 1992; **2**: 87–91.

21 Burrows J. Fatigue infraction of the middle of the tibia in ballet dancers. *J Bone Joint Surg (Brit)* 1956; **38-B**: 83–94.

22 Rolf C, Ekenman I, Gad A, Törnqvist H. The anterior stress fracture of the tibia—an atrophic pseudarthrosis? *Scand J Med Sci Sports* 1997; **7**: 249–53.

23 Stanitski CL, McMaster JH, Scranton PE. On the nature of stress fractures. *Am J Sports Med* 1978; **6**: 391–6.

24 Green N, Rogers R, Libscomb A. Nonunions of stress fractures of the tibia. *Am J Sports Med* 1985; **13**: 171–6.

25 Rettig A, Shelbourne D, McCaroll J, Bisesi M, Watts J. The natural history and treatment of delayed union stress

fractures of the anterior cortex of the tibia. *Am J Sports Med* 1988; **3**: 250–5.

26 Rolf C. Overuse injuries in the lower extremity in runners. *Scand J Med Sci Sports* 1995; **5**: 181–90.

27 Orava S, Karpakka J, Hulkko A, Vahanen K, Takala T, Kallinen M, Alen M. Diagnosis and treatment of stress fractures located at the mid-tibial shaft in athletes. *Int J Sports Med* 1991; **12**: 419–22.

28 Ekenman I, Tsai-Felländer L, Westblad P, Turan I, Rolf C. A study of intrinsic factors in patients with stress fractures of the tibia. *Foot Ankle* 1996; **17**: 477–82.

29 Morberg P, Jerre R, Swärd L, Karlsson J. Long-term results after surgical management of partial Achilles tendon ruptures. *Scand J Med Sci Sports* 1997; **7**: 299–303.

30 Sandmeier R, Renström PAFH. Diagnosis and treatment of chronic tendon disorders in sports. *Scand J Med Sci Sports* 1997; **7**: 96–106.

31 Józsa L, Reffy A, Kannus P, Demel S, Elek E. Pathological alterations in human tendons. *Arch Orthop Trauma Surg* 1990; **110**: 15–21.

32 Józsa L, Kannus P. *Human Tendons: Anatomy, Physiology and Pathology*. Champaign, IL: Human Kinetics, 1997.

33 Järvinen M, Józsa L, Kannus P, Järvinen TLN, Kvist M, Leadbetter W. Histopathological findings in chronic tendon disorders. *Scand J Med Sci Sports* 1997; **7**: 86–95.

34 Kannus P, Józsa L. Histopathological changes preceding spontaneous rupture of a tendon. A controlled study of 891 patients. *J Bone Joint Surg (Am)* 1991; **73-A**: 1507–25.

35 Kannus P, Józsa L, Natri A, Järvinen M. Effects of training, immobilization and remobilization on tendons. *Scand J Med Sci Sports* 1997; **7**: 67–71.

36 Kannus P, Natri A. Etiology and pathophysiology of tendon ruptures in sports. *Scand J Med Sci Sports* 1997; **7**: 107–12.

37 Kvist M, Józsa L, Järvinen MJ, Kvist H. Chronic Achilles paratenonitis in athletes: a histological and histochemical study. *Pathology* 1987; **19**: 1–11.

38 Åström M, Rausing A. Chronic Achilles tendinopathy. A survey of surgical and histopathologic findings. *Clin Orth Rel Res* 1995; **316**: 151–64.

39 Leadbetter WB. Cell-matrix response in tendon injury. *Clin Sports Med* 1992; **11**: 533–78.

40 Clement DB, Taunton JE, Smart GW. Achilles tendinitis and peritendinitis: etiology and treatment. *Am J Sports Med* 1984; **12**: 179–84.

41 Alfredsson H, Pietilä T, Lorentzon R. Chronic Achilles tendinitis and calf muscle strength. *Am J Sports Med* 1996; **24**: 829–33.

42 Curwin SL, Stanish WD. *Tendinitis: Its Etiology and Treatment*. Lexington, MA: Collamore Press, DC Heath, 1984.

43 Möller M, Movin T, Granhed H, Lind K, Faxen E, Karlsson J. Acute rupture of tendon Achilles. A prospective randomised study of comparison between surgical and nonsurgical treatment. *J Bone Joint Surg (Brit)* 2001; **83**: 843–8.

44 Clancy WG Jr, Neidhart D, Brand RL. Achilles tendonitis in runners: a report of five cases. *Am J Sports Med* 1976; **4**: 46–57.

45 Ljungqvist R. Subcutaneous partial rupture of the Achilles tendon. *Acta Orthop Scand Suppl* 1968; 113–20.

46 Nelen G, Martens M, Burssens A. Surgical treatment of chronic Achilles tendinitis. *Am J Sports Med* 1989; **17**: 754–9.

47 Ferkel RD, Karzel RP, Del Pizzo W, Friedman MJ, Fischer SC. Arthroscopic treatment of anterolateral impingement of the ankle. *Am J Sports Med* 1991; **19**: 440–8.

48 Balduini FC, Vegso JJ, Torg JS, Torg E. Management and rehabilitation of ligamentous injuries of the ankle. *Sports Med* 1987; **4**: 364–404.

49 Broström L. *Sprained ankles: a pathologic, arthrographic and clinical study*. Dissertation, Karolinska Institute, Stockholm, Sweden, 1966.

50 Kannus P, Renström P. Treatment for acute tears of the lateral ligaments of the ankle. Current concepts review. *J Bone Joint Surg (Am)* 1991; **73-A**: 305–12.

51 Karlsson J, Bergsten T, Peterson L, Zachrisson BE. Radiographic evaluation of ankle joint stability. *Clin J Sports Med* 1991; **1**: 166–76.

52 Freeman MAR, Dean MRE, Hanham IWF. The etiology and prevention of functional instability of the foot. *J Bone Joint Surg (Brit)* 1965; **47-B**: 678–87.

53 Freeman MAR. Instability of the foot after injuries to the lateral ligament of the ankle. *J Bone Joint Surg (Brit)* 1965; **47-B**: 669–77.

54 Freeman MAR. Treatment of ruptures of the lateral ligament of the ankle. *J Bone Joint Surg (Brit)* 1965; **47-B**: 661–8.

55 Karlsson J, Andreasson GO. The effect of external ankle support in chronic lateral ankle joint instability. An electromyographic study. *Am J Sports Med* 1992; **20**: 257–62.

56 Karlsson J, Peterson L, Andreasson GO, Högfors C. The unstable ankle: a combined EMG and biomechanical modeling study. *Int J Sports Biomech* 1992; **8**: 129–52.

57 Johansen A. Radiological diagnosis of lateral ligament lesion of the ankle: a comparison between talar tilt and anterior drawer sign. *Acta Orthop Scand* 1978; **49**: 295–301.

58 Karlsson J, Lansinger O, Faxen E. Conservative treatment of chronic lateral instability of the ankle. *Swedish Med J* 1991; **88**: 1404–8.

59 Karlsson J, Lansinger O. Lateral instability of the ankle joint. *Clin Orth Rel Res* 1992; **276**: 253–61.

60 Evans DL. Recurrent instability of the ankle: a method of surgical treatment. *Proc Roy Soc Med* 1953; **46**: 343.

61 Karlsson J, Bergsten T, Lansinger O, Peterson L. Lateral instability of the ankle treated by the Evans procedure: a long-term clinical and radiological follow-up. *J Bone Joint Surg (Brit)* 1988; **70-B**: 476–82.

62 Karlsson J, Bergsten T, Lansinger O, Peterson L. Recon-

struction of the lateral ligaments of the ankle for chronic lateral instability. *J Bone Joint Surg (Am)* 1988; **70-A**: 581–8.

63 Rijt AJ, Evans GA. The long-term results of Watson–Jones tenodesis. *J Bone Joint Surg (Brit)* 1984; **66-B**: 371–8.

64 Chrisman OD, Snook GA. Reconstruction of lateral ligament tears of the ankle. An experimental study and clinical evaluation of seven patients treated by a new modification of the Elmslie procedure. *J Bone Joint Surg (Am)* 1969; **51-A**: 904–11.

65 Karlsson J, Bergsten T, Lansinger O, Peterson L. Surgical treatment of chronic lateral instability of the ankle joint: a new procedure. *Am J Sports Med* 1989; **17**: 268–74.

66 Löfvenberg R, Kärrholm J, Ahlgren O. Ligament reconstruction for ankle instability. A 5-year prospective RSA follow-up of 30 cases. *Acta Orthop Scand* 1994; **65**: 401–8.

67 Sjölin SU, Dons-Jensen H, Simonsen O. Reinforced anatomic reconstruction of the anterior talofibular ligament in chronic anterolateral instability using a periosteal flap. *Foot Ankle Int* 1991; **12**: 15–20.

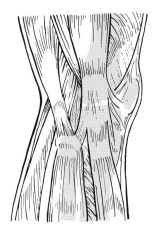

Chapter 6.2
Knee

LARS ENGEBRETSEN, THOMAS MUELLNER,
ROBERT LAPRADE, FRED WENTORF,
RANA TARIQ , JAMES H-C. WANG, DAVID STONE
& SAVIO L.-Y. WOO

Classical reference

Palmer I. Primary repair of ruptures of the anterior cruciate ligament. *Acta Chir Scand Suppl* 1938; LIII Vol LXXXI.

Even though several authors had published on the injury and repair of the anterior cruciate ligament in the early 1900s, the father of modern treatment of cruciate ligament injuries is thought to be the Swedish professor Ivar Palmer. His publication of the repair technique of the anterior cruciate ligament (ACL; Fig. 6.2.1) led to renewed interest in the biology and mechanics of ACL injury as well as to a number of animal and clinical studies on its subsequent repair.

Palmer describes his interest in the knee ligament in the preface of his thesis: 'My interest in injuries to the ligaments of the knee joint dates back to 1930, when two cases of crucial band injury came under my care practically simultaneously while I was working in a

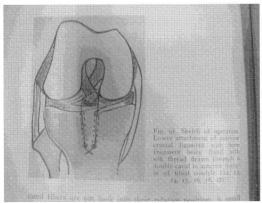

(a)

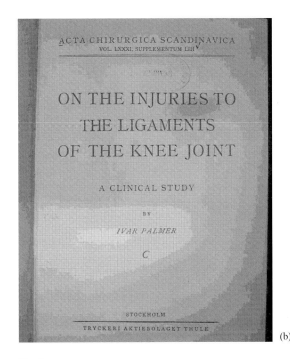

(b)

Fig. 6.2.1

country town. During my four years of service at the Sabbatsberg Hospital, Surgical Clinic II, very extensive material has been placed at my disposal. Throughout this period, the chief of the clinic, Med. Dr. K.H. Giertzhas, with his encouragement and confidence and never failing interest, stimulated me in my attempts to solve the problem of the diagnosis of ligament injuries and to evolve new methods for their treatment. It is therefore a pleasant duty to express to him my respectful and profound gratitude.'

'No large series of reliably diagnosed, uniformly treated and sufficiently followed up cases of ligamentous injury has been published. The presentation of the therapy of lesions of the bands is therefore mainly based on my own experience. In some respects, the operative procedure may be claimed to be relatively new, for example as regards the treatment of recent and longstanding injuries to the posterior cruciate ligament and of the recent injuries to the tibia collateral ligament. However, the clinical observations are based on too few cases to be considered incontestable, and, in most of the cases, the follow-up period is too short. Therefore, in this paper no claims are made to import any established clinical truths or definitive therapeutic rules, but is rather intended to arouse more interest in this branch of surgery—the surgery of the ligaments. What can chiefly be attained hereby is more general recognition of these lesions and greater uniformity in their diagnosis. In this way, material will gradually be collected which can be used for a conclusive investigation on the value of various therapeutic methods and the prognosis in cases of ligamentous injuries. To achieve this end, large series and long follow-up periods are necessary.'

Since 1938, more than 20 000 papers regarding the cruciate ligaments have been published. Not all of them have used Ivar Palmer's careful approach. His words of caution on the interpretation of scientific data are still very much valid!

Introduction: knee problems in sports

Knee problems are among the most common sports injuries [1–3]. The fact that knee ligament injuries are the most common sports injury leading to medical disability compensation from insurance companies shows the seriousness of these injuries. The diagnosis of an

Table 6.2.1 Differential diagnoses in acute knee injury.

Most common	Less common	Must not be missed
Injury leading to hemarthosis		
Rupture of the anterior cruciate ligament	Avulsion of the anterior cruciate ligament in children	Knee dislocation
Peripheral meniscal tear	Osteochondral fracture	Rupture of the extensor apparatus
Fracture of the tibial plateau		
Patellar dislocation		
Injury without hemarthosis		
Central meniscal tear	Cartilage injury	Epiphyseal-injury
Rupture of the medial collateral ligament	Rupture of the posterior cruciate ligament	Rupture of the lateral ligament and postero-lateral corner

acute knee injury is difficult and necessitates knowledge of anatomy and biomechanics as well as good clinical skills. In addition, a good overview of imaging techniques is necessary.

Table 6.2.1 shows the most common diagnoses in the acute situation. The incidences of these injuries is well known. The incidence of meniscal injuries is 1/1000, and of ACL injuries 2–5/10 000 depending on the population at risk [2]. In Europe, team handball has a much higher incidence (4–8/1000 h play/year) of ACL injuries with women 3–6 times more at risk than men [4]. To get an impression of what physicians will be exposed to in a Scandinavian capital, the numbers from the Emergency Department at Oslo University may be representative. Of 50 000 acute musculoskeletal injuries treated at the main emergency room at Oslo University in 1998, 2597 were knee injuries. Of these 271 were classified as serious (Table 6.2.2).

Table 6.2.2 Main diagnosis in 271 cases of serious knee injuries treated at the emergency room at Oslo University Hospital in 1998.

Diagnosis	n	%
ACL total tear	87	32
PCL total tear	6	2
Medial meniscal tear	105	39
Lateral meniscal tear	20	7
Patellar dislocation	39	14
MCL tear grade III	13	5
LCL tear grade III	1	0

ACL, anterior cruciate ligament; LCL, lateral collateral ligament; MCL, medial collateral ligament; PCL, posterior cruciate ligament.

Following the introduction of magnetic resonance imaging (MRI) as a possible diagnostic tool, the detection of serious knee injuries has become easier. At the Emergency Department in Oslo it led to an increase in the detection rate of serious knee injuries during the first 2 weeks after injury of 50% (Frihagen, personal communication). In addition to this, clinical skills in detecting posterior and posterolateral knee ligament injuries have improved. This has led to an improved diagnosis. Also, treatment options for knee injuries have changed both for conservative as well as for surgical treatment. In the most recent years we have seen a surge in treatment options for traumatic and degenerative cartilage injuries. Only good clinical science can tell us which methods will become standard in the near future. The present chapter deals with the most common injuries to the knee after an introduction covering recent discoveries in anatomy and biomechanics.

Anatomy and biomechanics

Introduction

Knee mechanics is the understanding of how the bones, ligaments, muscles and tendons combine to produce knee stability both statically and dynamically. The knee is composed of four different bones, four major ligaments, two menisci and 11 muscles that cross the joint. An understanding of anatomy is therefore required in order to better understand the mechanics.

With this in mind, we will first describe the anatomy of each individual structure and then demonstrate the mechanics and function. The description will be kept simple and will just focus on passive mechanics of the knee.

Bones of the knee

The knee joint is composed of four bones: the tibia, femur, patella and fibula. The tibia is a long triangular bone beginning proximally at the tibial plateau and extending distally to articulate at the ankle. The femur is a long cylindrical bone, which begins at the femoral head, which articulates with the acetabulum to form the hip joint, and ends distally at the femoral condyles. The patella is a sesamoid bone that articulates anterior to the femur and tibia. The fibula extends proximally to its fibular styloid and distally to articulate at the ankle.

These bones come together to form individual joints that combined form the knee joint. The tibiofemoral joint is the most important individual joint. The tibiofemoral joint dictates the possible range of motion or kinematics of the knee. The articulating surfaces of the femur and the tibia are shaped in such a way as to allow for motion in all six degrees of freedom: flexion–extension, internal–external rotation, varus–valgus angulation, anterior–posterior translation, medial–lateral translation, and joint compression–distraction. The femoral condyles are obviously designed to allow a large range of motion and this is seen in the rotation about the flexion–extension axis, but the knee cannot be thought of having only this motion. This flexion–extension axis changes as the knee is flexed and extended and can be thought of as an axis through the intersection of the ACL and posterior cruciate ligament (PCL). This intersection moves anteriorly with extension and posteriorly with flexion, and so does the flexion–extension axis. The remaining axes are simple and can be thought of as fixed.

There are three other joints involved in the knee, the tibofibular, the patellofemoral and the patellotibial. The tibia and fibula come together proximally to form a syndesmosis. There is very little motion at this joint and it thus has little influence on the knee joint's mechanics as a whole. The patella's articulation in and out of the trochlear groove comprises the patellofemoral joint. This joint's mechanics are highly dependent on whether the patella is in or out of the groove and on the level of activation of the quadriceps muscle. The patellotibial joint only comes to mind when trying to understand or calculate the mechanical advantage created by the patella for the quadriceps mechanics. This joint does not have any articulations in the usual meaning. Only the tibiofemoral joint affects the overall static stability of the knee and it will be the focus of the remaining part of the chapter.

Meniscus

The menisci can be thought of as extensions of the tibia. They increase the joint congruency with the femoral condyles. The peripheral of each meniscus is thick and convex, and attaches to the inside of the joint capsule. The medial meniscus is semicircular in shape and is wider posteriorly than anteriorly (Fig. 6.2.2). The anterior horn is attached to a tibial plateau near the intercondylar fossa anterior to the ACL. The transverse ligament attaches the medial and lateral menisci. The posterior horn of the meniscus is attached to the posterior intercondylar fossa of the tibia. The lateral meniscus is almost circular and covers more of the tibial plateau than does the medial meniscus. The lateral meniscus is approximately the same width from front to back. The anterior horn attaches to the tibia anterior to the intercondylar eminence, and the posterior horn attaches posterior to the intercondylar eminence. There are also femoral attachments to the posterior horn of the lateral meniscus, the ligament of Humphrey and the ligament of Wrisberg.

Ligament mechanics

The most basic definition of a ligament is a structure that attaches bone to bone. From this definition, it can be deduced that the ligament's mechanical properties will affect the ability for the two attached bones to move with respect to each other. Thus to understand joint kinematics you need to understand ligament mechanics.

The effect of a load along the long axis of a ligament will displace the attachment sites in a similar pattern, no matter which ligament or location. The easiest way to understand the ligament's ability to resist load is by studying the load–elongation curve (Fig. 6.2.3).

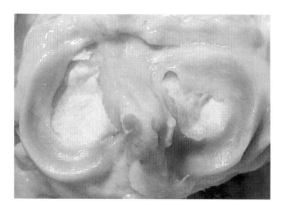

Fig. 6.2.2 Anatomy of the menisci.

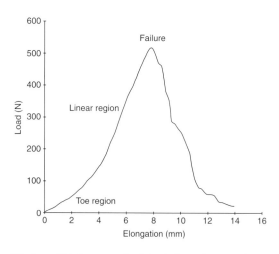

Fig. 6.2.3 This is an example of a load–elongation curve that was recorded during a tensile failure test of a goat ACL. The regions of interest are: (1) the non-linear toe region, that corresponds to the aligning of the collagen fibers to the axis of load; (2) the linear region, this is when all the collagen fibers are aligned and the corresponding slope is the stiffness of the structure being tested; (3) failure, this corresponds to the breaking of the collagen fibers.

The load–elongation curve is generated during a mechanical tensile failure test. When load is applied along the long axis of the ligament the ligament elongates. The first part of the curve is non-linear and is referred to as the toe of the load–elongation curve. During this portion of the loading the collagen fibers of the ligament are aligned along the axis of load. When all the fibers are aligned along the long axis of the ligament, the loading curve reaches a portion that is approximately linear. The stiffness of a ligament is quantified from a linear assumption from this portion of the curve. The curve remains the same until the yield point is reached. This yield point is where the ligament loses its ability to transmit load. If loading continues a maximum load will be reached and then a sudden drop in load will signal total failure of the ligament.

Several different criteria can affect the properties of the load–elongation curve, such as age, loading orientation and loading rate [5,6]. Younger ACLs were found to have a maximum load of $2160 \pm 157 \, N$ and a stiffness of $242 \pm 28 \, N/mm$, which was a threefold increase from the older ACLs. Orienting the load along the tibial axis for an ACL test will give you a maximum load of $1600 \, N$, but applying the load along the ACL axis will produce a maximum load of $2200 \, N$. The change of loading rates from a slow $0.01\%/s$ to $200\%/s$ increases the maximum load by 2.3 times.

Autografts and allografts have different properties from the structures that they are used to replace. Both grafts are known to have low stiffness and maximum loads soon after implantation, but these increase with time. The autografts on average are expected to reach 40% of the original ACL maximum load at 1 year post surgery. The properties of allografts vary according to the preparation procedure, but have been shown to be anywhere from 15 to 29% of the maximum load of the native ACL at 1 year after implantation.

Knee ligaments

Anterior cruciate ligament

The anterior cruciate ligament is the most researched ligament in the body. It has its proximal attachment in a fossa on the posterior portion of the medial side of the lateral condyle of the femur and terminates distally on the tibial plateau in front of and lateral to the anterior tibial spine. The ACL can be broken down into two bands, the anteromedial and posterolateral. The anteromedial attaches on the proximal aspect of the femoral attachment and inserts on the anteromedial portion of the tibial insertion. The posterolateral band comprises the remaining fibers that attach to the posterolateral portion of the tibial attachment.

It is this multiple-bundled make-up that allows the ACL to function throughout all angles of flexion.

The anteromedial bundle is tight in flexion and the fibers of the posterolateral bundle are lax. When the knee goes into extension the reverse happens: the posterolateral bundle tightens and the anteromedial bundle loosens. The posterolateral bundle also prevents hyperextension.

The ACL's primary function is to restrain anterior motion of the tibia with respect to the femur. It was found by Butler *et al.* that the ACL produced 85.1% and 87.2% of the restraining force for anterior translation at $90°$ and $30°$ of knee flexion, respectively [7].

Posterior cruciate ligament

The posterior cruciate ligament is made up of two distinct bands, the anterolateral and posteromedial. The anterolateral is the larger of the two bundles and attaches to the lateral side of the medial condyle on the anterior portion of the femoral notch and terminates on the lateral side of the PCL facet on the tibia. The posteromedial bundle attaches posterior to the anterolateral bundle on the medial condyle and ends distally on the medial side of the PCL facet. The ligaments of Humphrey and Wrisberg are meniscofemoral ligaments that are sometimes grouped with the PCL. Both attach to the posterior horn of the lateral meniscus, with the Humphrey ligament running anterior to the PCL and the Wrisberg posterior.

Like the ACL, the PCL is composed of several bands, allowing it to function through the whole flexion–extension arc. The different bands of the PCL function independently. The anterolateral band becomes taut in flexion and the posteromedial band tightens with the knee in extension.

The primary function of the PCL is to resist posterior translation of the tibia with respect to the femur. Butler *et al.* found that the PCL provided 94.3% of the restraining force to an applied posterior drawer at $90°$ and 96.0% at $30°$ of knee flexion [7].

Medial collateral ligament

The medial collateral ligament (MCL) is a combination of several different structures and is sometimes referred to as the medial collateral ligament complex. The largest component is the tibial collateral ligament (TCL) or superficial MCL. This structure attaches proximally at the medial epicondyle of the femur and runs distally to attach to several places on the tibia. The first is 2 cm distal to the joint line anterior to the posteromedial border of the tibia, and then continues distally to attach further down the tibia just past the pes anserine tendon insertions. The next components are thickenings of the medial joint capsule and are also called the deep MCL. The meniscofemoral attaches proximally just distal to the medial epicondyle on the femur and terminates distally in the middle of the medial meniscus. The meniscotibial begins at the bottom of the medial meniscus and runs just 4–5 mm past the proximal edge of the tibia to terminate. The posterior oblique ligament attaches to the posterior edge of the previously mentioned meniscofemoral portions, the medial capsule and adductor tubercle.

The primary function of the MCL complex is to restrain valgus rotation of the tibia with respect to the femur and secondarily to restrain anterior translation in an ACL-deficient knee. Grood *et al.* [58a] measured the percentage of valgus restraining moment contributed by the different portions of the MCL. It was found that at 5° of knee flexion the TCL was 57.4% and the deep MCL was 25.2% of the valgus restraining moment. At 25° the TCL contributed 78.2% and the deep MCL only 7.6%. The remaining percentage of restraining moment was found to be contributed by the ACL and PCL.

Fibular collateral ligament

The fibular collateral ligament (FCL) and the popliteus complex are commonly grouped together and referred to as the posterolateral complex (Fig. 6.2.4). The FCL attaches posteriorly and proximally to the lateral epicondyle on the femur and travels distally to attach to the fibular head. The popliteus complex consists of the popliteus tendon, popliteofibular ligament and popliteomeniscal fascicles. The popliteus tendon begins at the termination of the popliteus muscle body and runs deep to the FCL and attaches to the anterior and superior portions of the popliteal sulcus. The popliteofibular ligament begins at the musculotendinous junction of the popliteus and attaches to the fibular styloid [8–10].

The posterolateral complex resists varus opening and external rotation. Grood *et al.* [58a] also studied the effect of structures to restrain varus opening. The FCL was found to add 57.4% resistance at 5° and 78.2% at 25°. The popliteus complex contributed

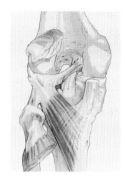

Fig. 6.2.4 The popliteofibular complex.

25.2% at 5° and 7.6% at 25°. Again the ACL and PCL contributed the remaining resistance. A study by Gollehon *et al.* [11] demonstrated that sectioning of the FCL and the popliteus complex increased external rotation at 0°, 30°, 60° and 90°.

In recent studies it has been found that the absence or deficiency of the posterolateral structures can significantly increase the force on ACL and PCL reconstruction grafts [12]. LaPrade *et al.* found that after sectioning the FCL, popliteus tendon and popliteofibular ligament, the ACL graft force increased over 200% at 0° and over 300% at 30° of knee flexion with an applied varus moment. Simply tensioning the ACL graft was found to externally rotate the tibia up to 10° with respect to the tibia (Wentorf *et al.*, personal communication). In an unpublished study by LaPrade, it was found that the PCL graft force increases with posterolateral deficiency. Varus loading was found to increase the PCL graft force significantly with the posterolateral structures sectioned at 30°, 60° and 90° of knee flexion, with the highest being a 200% increase at 90°.

The anatomy of the patellofemoral joint

The patellofemoral joint is difficult to examine because it functions as a dynamic joint and static loading thus provides limited information. However, a thorough knowledge of the anatomy and the different dynamic interactions that occurs in this joint, is necessary to understand its complexity.

The patellofemoral joint has a rather unique anatomy because it relies on a combination of both static and dynamic stabilizers to have normal function. Imbalances in any of these can lead to patellofemoral dysfunction and pain. This can include the lack of dynamic stability due to muscle weakness or hamstring tightness or a lack of static stabilizers due to injury or to intrinsic anatomic bony abnormalities. It is important to understand the anatomy of both the dynamic and the static portions of the patellofemoral joint in order to understand both its function and how to treat its dysfunction.

The patella is a sesamoid bone which sits within the confines of the quadriceps and patellar tendon and articulates in the trochlear groove of the femur. Normally, the patella sits within the confines of the trochlear groove at approximately 45° of knee flexion. In most knees, the confines of the trochlear groove provide significant inherent stability to the knee past 45° of knee flexion. In those patients who have dysplastic trochleas, there is a loss of this normal inherent bony stability.

The two main facets of the patella are the medial and lateral facets. The Wiberg classification notes three types of these facets, with type 1 having equal sized medial and lateral facets, type 2 having a slightly larger lateral facet than the medial facet, and type 3 having essentially a minimal medial facet with the majority of the patellar articular surface being the lateral facet.

Dynamic stability of the patellofemoral joint is provided by the quadriceps muscles consisting of the vastus medialis obliquus, vastus medialis, rectus femoris, rectus intermedius, vastus lateralis, genu articularis and vastus lateralis obliquus. Forty to 50% of the total thigh muscular volume is provided by the vastus lateralis muscle [13]. It is important to recognize this so that one does not release this muscle when performing a lateral release. A significant release of this portion of the quadriceps musculature can result in permanent thigh atrophy.

Static stability of the patellofemoral joint is provided by several thickenings of the joint capsule and extra-articular expansions around the patellofemoral joint. The medial patellofemoral ligament, which runs from the medial border of the patella to the adductor tubercle, is thought to provide the most stability to the patellofemoral joint in preventing lateral translation. This structure is the most commonly torn structure in acute lateral patellar dislocations (Fig. 6.2.5).

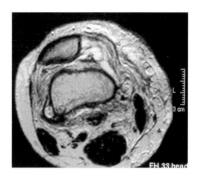

Fig. 6.2.5 Axial MR scan of a patella after dislocation with tearing of the medial patellofemoral ligament.

In addition, the medial patellotibial and patellomeniscal ligaments provide stability to lateral translation of the patella. The function of these two ligaments is not well understood.

On the lateral side of the knee, the lateral patellofemoral ligament runs from the lateral border of the patella down to the iliotibial band and lateral intramuscular septum at its attachment on the femur. The lateral patellotibial ligament runs from the distal lateral border of the patella down to Gerdy's tubercle. This ligament is the distal edge of the distal margin of the iliopatellar ligament. This ligament is found to be extremely important in preventing medial patellar subluxation. However, a patellomeniscal ligament also exists on the lateral aspect of the knee.

The patellar tendon runs from the inferior pole of the patella to the tibial tubercle. It is trapezoid shaped, with the average width approximately being 38 mm and the average width distally being 28 mm. At its more proximal aspect, it is intimately attached to the retropatellar fat pad, while distally the deep infrapatellar bursa is present between the patella tendon and the proximal anterior tibia prior to its insertion on the tibial tubercle.

The medial suprapatellar plica is a fold of synovial tissue which is separate from the medial retinaculum in the knee. It extends from the genu articularis muscle in the suprapatella pouch down to the retropatellar fat pad along the anterior medial aspect of the medial meniscus. This structure has been found to have many pain fibers and can become fibrotic in some instances. In addition, in some patients, this fibrotic band can impinge and erode on the articular cartilage of the medial femoral condyle.

While not actually part of the patellofemoral joint, the hamstring muscles are included in the assessment of the patellofemoral joint, due to their interactions with it. On the medial side of the knee, the direct arm of the semimembranosus is known to attach on the proximal aspect of the posterior medial tibia. There is a large semicircular bursa just proximal to this attachment site. The sartorius, gracilis and semitendinosis tendons attach at the anterior medial aspect of the tibia approximately two finger breadths medial to the tibial tubercle. Just proximal and medial to this attachment site, there is a bursa between the tendons and the proximal tibia. On the lateral aspect of the knee, the short and long heads of the biceps femoris attach to the posterior lateral aspect of the fibular styloid. In addition to this attachment site, the anterior arm of the long head of the biceps femoris continues laterally to the fibular head where a bursa is formed when it crosses the fibular collateral ligament [14]. This bursa, which has an average length of 18 mm, is also commonly found to be irritated in patients with tight hamstrings and patellofemoral dysfunction.

Knowledge of the anatomy of all these particular structures of the patellofemoral joint will greatly assist the clinician in helping to make a diagnosis and arrive at the proper treatment protocol for these patients. It is important to understand how all of these structures interact in order to formulate the proper treatment protocols.

History and physical examination

A thorough and detailed physical examination of the knee is more useful than any other diagnostic test to aid the examining physician in determining the etiology of a patient's presenting complaints. The presenting complaints for the majority of knee injuries are fairly specific in the majority of cases and a clinician should have a general idea of what to expect on physical examination after reviewing a thorough history on a patient.

The initial part of the history should start with the etiology of the patient's initial presentation. It is important to determine whether it was a traumatic or a non-traumatic event that caused the onset of symp-

toms. In addition, it is useful to have the patient describe what type of problems they have with their knee. It is also helpful to have them point to the area where their knee hurts. This helps to determine whether pain is located in their patellofemoral joint or in their tibiofemoral joint. Patellofemoral joint symptoms are most commonly located over the anterior aspect of the knee, while tibiofemoral joint problems are usually associated with pain localized to the joint line or feelings of instability.

Mechanism of injury

It is extremely helpful to review the mechanism of injury with the patient to assist in understanding their knee pathology. Injuries to the patellofemoral joint are usually caused by direct trauma or a contact valgus injury. In this instance, a direct blow to the patella, retinaculum or fat pad could result in a contusion, hemorrhage and effusion. In addition, a sudden twist or pivot could result in a lateral patellar subluxation or dislocation event.

Injuries to the tibiofemoral joint can be either contact or non-contact. Non-contact injuries are usually associated with a sudden twist, turn or pivot, with the athlete feeling a pop inside the knee. The most common finding in this type of presentation, especially when there is a large knee effusion that develops rapidly, is an anterior cruciate ligament tear. Other things to suspect are a meniscal tear or a bone bruise.

In the evaluation of contact injuries to the knee, it is important to recognize that the structures most commonly injured occur on the side opposite to the contact to the knee. When a patient has a valgus contact injury, then generally the most common finding will be an MCL complex injury, followed by medial meniscal pathology, patellar subluxations or dislocations, ACL tears, and lateral compartment bone bruises. Varus contact injuries usually cause an injury to the posterolateral corner of the knee and may injure the common peroneal nerve as part of this mechanism. Pure hyperextension contact injuries are rare, with the usual blow being anteromedial or anterolateral. Either cruciate ligament may be injured in this type of mechanism, with a high suspicion of a posterolateral corner injury with an anteromedial blow to an extended knee and a medial collateral ligament complex injury with an anterolateral blow to an extended knee.

Which structures are injured with a direct blow to a flexed knee usually depends upon the ankle position. In the case of a dorsiflexed ankle, a direct blow to a flexed knee may cause an injury to the patellofemoral joint. Likewise, in a plantar flexed ankle, a blow to the anterior aspect of a flexed knee may result in an injury to the PCL, because the force is transmitted to the intra-articular structures via the tibial tubercle (rather than by the patella).

Physical examination of the patellofemoral joint

The examination of the patello-femoral joint[15] starts with an overview of the mechanical axis of the extremity compared with the non-affected side. The q-angle (the intersection of the center line of the patellar tendon and the line from the center of the patella to the anterior superior iliac spine) is measured. The normal q-angle is reported to range between 10 and 15° with the knee in full extension. An increase in the q-angle may cause an increase in the peak patellofemoral pressure and may be associated with unpredictable patterns of cartilage loading. In the examination of the patellofemoral joint, it is helpful to be thorough in evaluating all potential sources of pain and the examiner should strive to examine the structure which the patient states hurts the most last to eliminate any potential guarding by the examiner. An overall assessment of the quadriceps tone is helpful to determine the patient's overall strength. This is of course difficult to assess clinically, and is therefore usually done with isokinetic devices such as Cybex, Biodex, Kinkom, etc. In addition, measurement of the thigh circumference may help to assess whether there is any underlying thigh atrophy. It is recommended that the thigh circumference be measured at a point 15 cm proximal to the superior pole of the patella. Thigh atrophy of greater than 1 cm on the affected side compared to the contralateral side is generally considered significant. A number of functional tests have been developed to assess the functional strength of the patient, such as one-leg jump and triple jump tests [16]. The next assessment performed is to evaluate the amount of hamstring tightness. Hamstring tightness can be evaluated by measuring the hamstring–popliteal angle and comparing it to the contralateral side. In general, males tend to have tighter hamstrings than females. Next, palpation of the hamstring tendon attachments on the tibia and fibular head is performed to determine whether there is any irritation at these attachment sites which may indicate an amount of underlying bursitis. The pes anserine, semimembranosus and the FCL–biceps bursae are palpated to assess them for any underlying bursal irritation. In addition, we palpate the quadriceps attachment on the superior pole of the patella and the patellar tendon attachment on the distal pole of the patella to determine whether there is any quadriceps insertional tendinopathy or patellar tendinitis, respectively. We also palpate the patellar tendon just proximal to its attachment on the tibial tubercle and distal to its insertion on the patella to determine whether there are any symptoms of Osgood–Schlatter's or Sinding–Larsen–Johansson's irritation or irritation of the deep infrapatella bursa.

The next evaluation of the patellofemoral joint is to determine whether there is any plical irritation (medial retinacular synovium). The examiner can roll the fingers over the medial suprapatellar plica about two finger breadths medial to the medial border of the patella to see if there is any plical irritation in this location. The plica can be felt as a band of tissue in the area. If there is any pain present with palpation, it is important to ask the patient if this duplicates their symptoms, because some patients may have some normal irritation to palpation of their plica. The plica on the lateral side can also be assessed for any associated pain to palpation. Concurrent with this evaluation, the patellomeniscal and patellotibial ligaments and the retropatellar fat pad should be palpated to determine whether there is any associated pain, which may be indicative of scarring or injury to these structures.

Next, we evaluate any potential subluxation or dislocation of the patellofemoral joint. Medial patellar subluxation is assessed in the initial 0–35° of knee flexion. A gentle medial push to the lateral aspect of the patella is applied when the knee is in full extension and then the knee is slowly flexed. If the patella subluxes medially, there is usually a catch which is felt upon reduction when it enters the bony confines of the trochlear groove at approximately 35–40°. Medial patellar subluxation rarely occurs due to trauma and

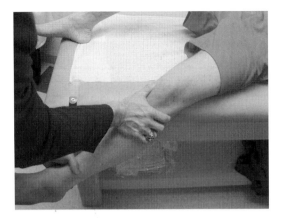

Fig. 6.2.6 Lateral patellar apprehension test.

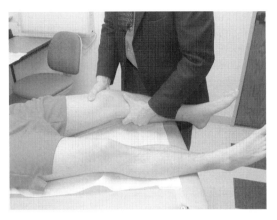

Fig. 6.2.7 The Lachman test for anterior knee instability.

usually is due to iatrogenic causes such as an overzealous lateral release. It is important to compare the symptomatic side to the contralateral normal side to determine whether there is any increase in subluxation on the symptomatic knee.

Lateral patellar subluxation is assessed by the lateral patellar apprehension test. This test is usually performed with the knee flexed to 45° and over the side of the examination table (Fig. 6.2.6). It is important in this test to make sure that the patient is totally relaxed. The examiner then applies a gentle lateral force on the patella to assess for any increase in translation. It is important in performing the test for the examiner not to apply the lateral force through an irritated medial plica. During the course of this test, the examiner can also get an assessment of any underlying crepitation in the patellofemoral joint which can be felt with the fingers, which may be indication of chondromalacia of the patella or trochlear articular surfaces. If a patient expresses pain or apprehension with a lateral force, the test is considered positive.

Physical examination of the tibiofemoral joint

When considering examination of the tibiofemoral joint, the examiner should think in terms of both intra-articular pathology and potential ligamentous instability. Examination of any potential intra-articular pathology can be easily assessed during the evaluation of any joint line instability and we prefer to measure it in this manner.

Examination of anterior translational abnormalities

The primary structure that resists anterior translational abnormalities of the knee is the ACL. Since the ACL is most isolated in terms of its contribution to resisting anterior translation of the knee at approximately 30° of knee flexion Lachman's test is an extremely useful tool to assess for the integrity of the ACL.

Lachman's test is performed with the knee flexed to approximately 25–30°. In this test, the examiner uses one hand around the distal thigh, which attempts to stabilize the distal thigh against resisting motion. The other hand of the examiner is utilized to apply a gentle anterior translation force anteriorly in neutral rotation (Fig. 6.2.7). It is essential that the examiner gets the patient to totally relax while performing Lachman's test. With an intact ACL present, the examiner should feel a good solid endpoint when performing this test. However, when the ACL is torn, either no endpoint or a soft endpoint will be felt at the end of the examiner's translation of the tibia on the distal femur. It is also important to make sure that pure anterior translation is being measured because a posterolateral corner injury can give the false impression of increased anterior translation in some instances. In this circumstance, the increase in motion should be felt as due to posterolateral rotation and there should be a good endpoint to Lachman's test.

Instrumented mechanical testing has also been successful in determining the integrity of the ACL.

The KT-1000, KT-2000, Rolimeter and Stryker mechanical devices have all proved useful in determining the integrity of the native ACL and have been used as an assessment of the success of an ACL reconstruction in restoring normal anterior translation stability to the knee. With all of these devices, it is felt that the difference in anterior stability between the tested knee and the contralateral normal knee should be ≤3mm. Increased translation stability of greater than this amount would indicate either a torn native ACL or an ACL reconstruction graft which is slightly lax or potentially non-functional. The limitations of these mechanical devices are such that they are still user specific and it is most ideal to have a limited number of personnel using these devices on patients to eliminate the potential variability among examiners.

The pivot-shift tests produce anterior subluxation and internal axial rotation in early flexion in ACL-deficient knees. The posterior pull of the iliotibial tract then reduces the tibia subluxation at 20–40° flexion. The tests (McIntosh, Slocum or flexion rotation drawer test) are consistently positive in the relaxed patient with a chronic ACL deficiency and in the acutely injured anesthetized patient with an ACL tear.

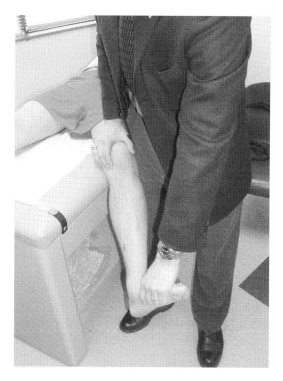

Fig. 6.2.8 Test for medial knee instability.

Examination of medial-sided knee injuries

The tibial collateral ligament and associated medial collateral ligament complex is the primary stabilizer to valgus instability of the knee [17,18]. Since it is primarily isolated when the knee is flexed to 30°, this is the best position to perform stability testing for MCL complex injuries.

In performing the valgus stress test at 30° of knee flexion, the patient is placed on the examination table such that one hand of the examiner is placed with the fingers over the medial joint line to measure the amount of medial compartment joint line opening, while the other hand is used to apply a valgus force through the leg. We recommend that the hand applying the valgus force be placed on the foot, and not the tibial shaft, to apply this force so that the true amount of valgus and coupled valgus rotational instability can be assessed (Fig. 6.2.8). Concurrent with measuring the amount of medial compartment opening, the examiner's fingers assess for any underlying joint line crepitation. This may indicate any associated meniscal or chondral pathology in the medial compartment of the knee. If a large 'clunk' is felt, we have found it to be consistent with a detached peripheral medial meniscal tear.

Assessment of medial joint line opening can also be performed with the knee in full extension. When there is increased medial joint line opening to a valgus stress with the knee in full extension, it is usually due to a significant injury involving the entire MCL complex as well as both cruciate ligaments. In this instance, the examiner needs to be cognizant of the fact that there may have been a tibiofemoral dislocation.

The one thing to be careful of in assessing this situation is in a patient with open physes. In any patient who has open physes, consideration should be given to obtaining valgus stress AP radiographs when there is apparent MCL complex instability. This is because there is a potential for an underlying physeal fracture which could appear to be a MCL complex injury on clinical examination.

Assessment of posterior instability of the knee

The posterior cruciate ligament (PCL) is the main structure responsible for preventing posterior translation of the knee [7,11,19,20]. The PCL has two main portions, the anterolateral and posteromedial bundles. The anterolateral bundle is the strongest and is the primary stabilizer against posterior translation of the knee when the knee is at 90° of knee flexion. In this position, it is in its most isolated state. For this reason, the majority of assessment tests for posterior instability of the knee are performed at 90° knee flexion. The posteromedial bundle protects against posterior tibial displacement near full knee extension.

The posterior sag sign should be one of the first tests performed to assess for the integrity of the PCL. In this test, both knees are flexed to 90°. In the PCL-deficient knee, a posterior sag of the proximal tibia on the distal femur will occur such that there is a visible difference in the posterior step-off of the affected knee (Fig. 6.2.9). Concurrent with assessment of the posterior step-off, the quadriceps active test is next performed. In this test, the patient's knee is flexed to 90° and the examiner uses one of his hands to hold down the ankle of the patient. The patient is then asked to try to extend or straighten out their leg. In the process of doing this, the quadriceps muscle contracts and by pulling through the patella and patellar tendon on the tibial tubercle, the posteriorly translated proximal tibia is pulled back into a more reduced position (Fig. 6.2.9). This is something that can be seen graphically by the examiner. We have found the quadriceps active test to be very effective for helping to determine whether the patient has an ACL tear, an ACL tear with a partial PCL tear, or a partial PCL tear when it is not possible to be certain as to the amount of anterior to posterior translation in a knee during the physical examination.

After the quadriceps active test, the posterior drawer test is next performed. It is important to make sure that this test is performed with the knee in neutral rotation. In this test, the knee is flexed to 90° and we recommend that the examiner sits on the foot, or stabilizes the foot by other means, such that the foot is in neutral rotation. It is important to obtain complete relaxation of the patient's hamstrings to be able to best perform this test. A gentle to and from force is then applied to

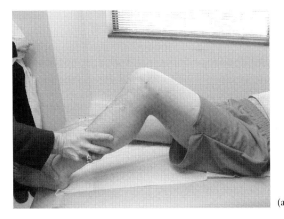
(a)

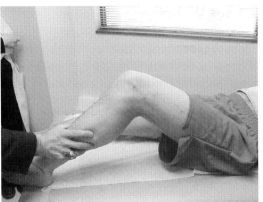
(b)

Fig. 6.2.9 The posterior sag sign test (a) and the quadriceps active test (b) for posterior ligament instability. The tibia excursion is reduced when the patient tries to extend the knee (b).

the knee by pushing gently on the proximal tibia with the examiner's hands to determine the amount of anterior to posterior translation that is present. The grading of the posterior drawer is usually done in relation to the amount of step-off that occurs in relation to the proximal tibia and the distal femur. A I+ posterior drawer test is present when there is some increase in posterior translation, but the proximal tibia remains anterior to a line drawn parallel to the femoral condyles and the anterior aspect of the tibia. A II+ posterior drawer test occurs when there is increased posterior translation and the line drawn parallel with the femoral condyles is in line with the anterior aspect of the tibial plateau. A III+ posterior drawer test occurs when the posterior tibia falls posterior to this parallel line and the anterior tibial plateau is posterior to the anterior aspect of the femoral condyles.

Assessment of posterolateral instability of the knee

The main function of the many structures of the posterolateral aspect of the knee is to prevent excessive recurvatum, varus opening of the knee, and posterolateral rotation of the knee [9,12,14,17,18,21–23]. Assessment of potential injury to the posterolateral structures of the knee primarily requires an assessment of abnormalities in motion testing for these motion and translation tests.

The external rotation recurvatum test is one of the first tests that should be performed when examining a knee. In this test, the examiner lifts the patient's great toe to determine whether there is any increase in relative varus and recurvatum of the knee (Fig. 6.2.10) [21,22]. It is important to compare this finding to the patient's normal contralateral knee to see if there is any increase in instability present. Any increase in recurvatum is considered abnormal and may be indicative of a significant knee injury involving one or both cruciate ligaments. Measurement of heel height differences off the examination table is a potential means of quantifying this examination.

The varus stress test at 30° knee flexion is performed in the same way as a valgus stress test at 30° knee flexion. In this test, one of the examiner's hands is placed with the fingers in the lateral compartment to assess the amount of joint space opening which occurs with application of a varus stress. The varus stress is applied to the leg by the other hand, which holds the foot and applies a varus stress. It is especially important to compare the amount of lateral-sided joint line opening to the contralateral normal knee as there is a wide variation of varus opening among individuals. This has been quantified to vary between 2 and 12 mm among asymptomatic patients in the general population [21].

The dial test assesses the amount of external rotation, which occurs in the tibia compared to the femur. In laboratory studies, it has been shown to be one of the most accurate methods of assessing the integrity of the posterolateral corner structures of the knee [23]. While this test has been described primarily as being performed with the patient prone, we prefer to have it

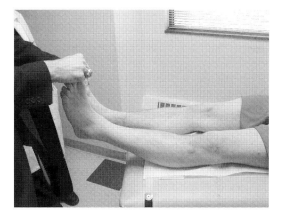

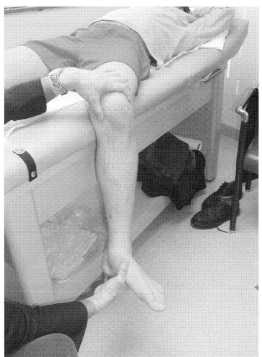

Fig. 6.2.10 The external rotation recurvatum test, and the dial test for rotational instability of the knee.

performed with the patient supine. The dial test is performed at both 30 and 90° knee flexion. One of the examiner's hands is used to stabilize the distal thigh while the other hand is placed around the patient's foot and an external rotation force is performed (Fig. 6.2.10). The amount of rotation of the tibial tubercle is then compared to the normal contralateral knee. At 30°

knee flexion, any increase in external rotation is indicative of any injury to the posterolateral corner structures with a greater than 15° rotational difference considered a severe injury. After testing at 30° knee flexion, the test is then repeated at 90° knee flexion. In the knee with an isolated posterolateral corner injury, there should be a slight decrease in external rotation of the tibia on the femur at 90° knee flexion compared to 30° knee flexion. However, if there is a concurrent PCL injury in the knee, there will be an increase in external rotation at 90° compared to 30° knee flexion.

The posterolateral drawer test assesses the amount of coupled posterior translation and external rotation due to a posterolateral corner injury of the knee. In this test, the knee is flexed to 90° knee flexion and the foot is externally rotated to about 15°. We choose to sit on the foot to make sure that we know how much external rotation is actually present. It is very important to make sure that the examiner understands the difference in this test compared to the posterior drawer test. With the patient's knee totally relaxed, we then apply a gentle posterior force to the knee with a coupled external rotation torque (Fig. 6.2.11). It is important to compare the amount of posterolateral rotation that occurs in the injured knee to the contralateral uninjured knee to determine the amount of pathologic increase in motion that may be present. An increase in posterolateral rotation of the knee compared to the normal knee is indicative of an injury to the posterolateral structures of the knee.

The reverse pivot-shift test derives its name from the fact that it is almost the reverse of the normal pivot-shift test which assesses anterolateral rotation of the knee. This test starts out with the knee flexed, with the foot externally rotated, and a valgus force applied. In this position, the lateral tibial plateau may be subluxated posterolaterally under the lateral femoral condyle. The knee is then extended and the examiner looks for any signs of a reduction of the subluxed joint between 35 and 45° knee flexion when the iliotibial band goes from a flexor to an extender of the knee (Fig. 6.2.12). If this subluxation reduction occurs, the reverse pivot-shift test is considered positive. This reduction in the posterolateral subluxation is very similar to what is seen with a reduction of an anterolat-

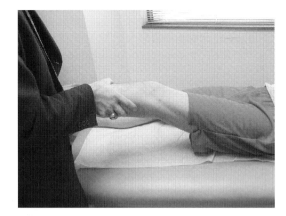

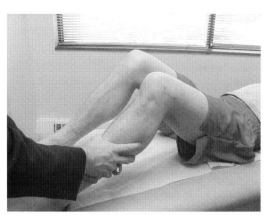

Fig. 6.2.11 The posterolateral drawer test for posterolateral instability.

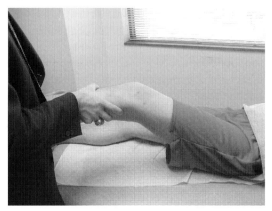

Fig. 6.2.12 The reverse pivot-shift test for posterior rotational instability of the knee.

Table 6.2.3 A number of clinical tests for knee examination, and the diagnostic possibilities in relation to the results of the tests.

Test	Diagnosis	Be aware of
Varus/valgus stress at 30° flexion (Fig. 6.2.6)	MCL or LCL injury (grade I < 5 mm side difference, grade II 5–10 mm side difference, grade III > 10 mm side difference)	Physeal injury in children may mimic the collateral ligament injury laxity
Lachman's test 30° flexion (Fig. 6.2.7)		
Pivot-shift test	Anterior cruciate ligament injury	Describes the lateral tibial plateau subluxation on the femur
		Feeling of the endpoint
Posterior drawer at 90° flexion	Posterior cruciate ligament injury	Often partial injury
Sag test (Fig. 6.2.9)	Posterior cruciate ligament injury	
Posterolateral Lachman at 30° (Fig. 6.2.11)	Posterolateral injury often to LCL, popliteal tendon, popliteofibular tendon	
Recurvatum test (Fig. 6.2.10)	Posterolateral injury often in combination with ACL or PCL injury	Be aware of side difference
McMurray meniscal test	Medial or lateral meniscal injury	Pain in the joint space and often a small click against your fingertip

eral subluxed knee during the pivot-shift test. The reverse pivot-shift test has the most variability among all motion tests. Up to 35% of normal subjects may have a reverse pivot-shift test when tested under general anesthesia. The majority of these patients were also noted to have some degree of recurvatum in their knee.

There are a number of meniscal tests described in the literature. Usually, three relatively simple tests are sufficient. In the McMurray test for the medial meniscus, the tibia is externally rotated on the femur, a small valgus stress is put on the knee, and the knee joint is flexed and extended during the test. The examiner has the pulp of the long finger in the medial joint space. When testing the lateral meniscus, a varus stress is carried out and the tibia is internally rotated. In doing this, the meniscus is rotated toward the finger of the examiner and the patient with a meniscal tear may express pain. In the original McMurray test a click should be felt when the meniscus is torn—this is, however, unusual. Apply's test is carried out with the patient in the prone position. The knee is flexed to 90°. The tibia is distracted from the femur and rotated. The test is then repeated, this time with compression and rotation of the tibia on the femur. Pain on compression suggests meniscal tear, pain on distraction suggests ligament pathology. The final test done by the authors is the hyperextension test where the knee is simply hyperextended thereby compressing the meniscus which will elicit pain if the meniscus is not stable.

In Table 6.2.3, the most common tests and their possible results are listed.

Imaging of the knee

Diagnostic imaging of sports-related injuries of the knee (Table 6.2.4) is an area that is currently undergoing rapid evolution. Specifically, the imaging techniques of cartilage injuries as well as dynamic techniques of ligament injuries are developing. This short section gives the reader an overview of current techniques available and follows this with a proposed use of the techniques in the most common diagnosis of the knee. It is important for the examiner to order scans or radiographs that should either result in significant decision-making in patient management or prognosis alteration, or give information not available from the history, physical examination or routine X-rays.

Understanding the basis of the imaging modalities available for diagnosis of many commonly encountered disorders of the bones and joints is of utmost importance. It may help determine the most effective radiologic technique, minimizing the cost of examination as well as the exposure of patients to radiation. It is important to choose the modality appropriate for specific types of orthopedic abnormalities and, when using routine X-ray techniques, to be familiar with the views and the techniques that best demonstrate the abnormality. Routine radiography remains the most effective means of demonstrating a bone and joint abnormality.

Use of imaging techniques differs in evaluating the presence, type and extent of various bone, joint and soft tissue abnormalities. Therefore, both the radiologist and orthopedic surgeon must know the indications for use of each technique, the limitations of a particular modality, and the appropriate imaging approaches for abnormalities at specific sites (Table 6.2.4). The choice of techniques for imaging bone and soft tissue abnormalities is dictated not only by clinical presentation, but also by equipment availability, expertise and cost.

No matter what ancillary technique is used, conventional radiography should be available for comparison. Most of the time, the choice of imaging technique is dictated by the type of suspected abnormality. For instance, if osteonecrosis is suspected after obtaining routine X-ray, the next examination should be MRI, which detects necrotic changes in bone long before plain films, tomography, CT or scintigraphy become positive. In evaluation of internal derangement of the knee, conventional films should be obtained first, and if the abnormality is not obvious, should again be followed by MRI, since this modality provides exquisite contrast resolution of the bone marrow, articular cartilage, ligaments, menisci and soft tissue.

Radiographs (routine X-ray)

Routine X-ray remains the mainstay for diagnostic evaluation of orthopedic problems, and often it is sufficient for evaluating many traumatic conditions of the knee joint.

AP (anteroposterior) and lateral radiographs fulfil the minimum requirement for the knee following trauma. In addition, tunnel views are routinely obtained. Evaluation of condyles requires both oblique projections [24]. For adequate evaluation of the patellofemoral joint axial views beside the lateral view is necessary [25]. An anteroposterior radiograph of the knee is obtained with the beam directed 5–7° toward the head, and a lateral radiograph is obtained with the knee flexed 20–35°. A 45° oblique view is

usually necessary in a patient who has knee trauma. An angulated posteroanterior projection with the knee flexed 40–50°, the tunnel view, is used to visualize the intercondylar notch. In such a patient, a cross-table lateral projection should also be added to the examination, allowing demonstration of fat–fluid levels, indicative of fractures with release of medullar fat into the articular cavity. Upright standing views are required to accurately access the femurotibial joint. Several techniques can be used in patients who are able to bear weight for this procedure. Typically a 14×17 inch cassette is positioned posterior to the knee so that the lower femur and upper tibia and fibulas are included on the film. The tube is parallel to the floor or angled slightly (tibia plateau 10° caudal posteriorly) toward the feet. A 45° weight-bearing view has been described by Rosenberg *et al.* [26]. The knees are flexed 45° and the tube angled 10° off the horizontal. The tube is positioned 100 cm from the cassette. This method was more accurate than conventional extension weight-bearing views in evaluating cartilage lesions.

Conventional tomography

Conventional tomography is a useful adjunct to plain film radiography, may compare with CT in the evaluation of certain musculoskeletal problems, and should be used when standard and specialized views fail to provide needed information for correct diagnosis and treatment. Tomography has been recommended to evaluate the amount of articular surface depression or displacement, the site of the fracture, and extent of comminution. Tomography is especially useful in differentiating split-depression fractures from fractures in which depression of the articular surface alone is present. Tomography, through its ability to demonstrate the integrity of the anterior cortex, is also helpful in planning a surgical treatment of tibial plateau fractures. This technique is now being replaced by reconstructed CT scans (spiral T) and magnetic resonance.

Arthrography

This technique uses injection of radiopaque contrast material into the knee to outline articular cartilage, menisci and cruciates with multiple X-rays recorded to visualize structures. MRI has now predominantly replaced the technique. The advantage is its relatively low cost, but its disadvantage is the fact that it is invasive and visualizes structures with far less accuracy than MRI or other techniques. The sensitivity and specificity for meniscal tears, for example, in an arthrogram is only approximately 50%.

Scintigraphy (radionuclide bone scan)

Scintigraphy is a modality that detects the distribution in the body of a radioactive agent injected into the vascular system. Following an intravenous injection of radiopharmaceutical agent, the patient is placed under a scintillation camera, which detects the distribution of radioactivity in the body by measuring the interaction of γ rays emitted from the body with sodium iodide crystals in the head of the camera. The photoscans are obtained in multiple projections and may include either the entire body or selected parts. One major advantage of skeletal scintigraphy over all other imaging techniques is its ability to image the entire skeleton at once.

As in most procedures in nuclear medicine, the bone scan is an extremely sensitive but relatively non-specific method. Any process that disturbs the normal balance of bone production and resorption can produce an abnormality on the bone scan. These abnormalities may be manifested as regions of increased or decreased activity. The great majority of lesions appear as focal areas of increased activity. The amount of radiopharmaceutical agent accumulated in any region of bone depends on two major factors, the rate of bone turnover and the integrity of the blood supply. Of these two factors, the intactness of the vascular supply appears to have a more important influence on the bone scan; when blood perfusion is absent, a photon-deficient or 'cold' region is evident on the scan. Although there are many indications for the use of bone scanning in clinical practice, the most common use is in oncology for detection and follow-up of metastatic bone disease primarily from prostate, breast and lung cancer or primary bone tumors. The orthopedic uses of bone scanning primarily include diagnosis of trauma and infection, determination of vascularity, compartmental evaluation of degenerative arthritis of the joints, and evaluation of patients with painful prostheses [27]. Secondary uses include evaluation of elevated alkaline phosphates and diagnosis of patients who present with bone pain of undetermined etiology [28].

The bone scan may be helpful in imaging either fatigue or insufficiency fractures, especially when radiography is unrevealing. This technique is also useful in the diagnosis of shin splint syndrome. On bone scan shin splint pain is associated with periosteal deposition of the radiopharmaceutical, with the appearance of a 'double stripe' sign, similar to that reported in hypertrophic osteoarthropathy.

The role of the radionuclide study in the evaluation of infection includes early detection, differentiation of osteomyelitis from cellulitis and identification of renewed activity in cases of chronic osteomyelitis. The differentiation between osteomyelitis and cellulitis may be a difficult clinical problem. The three-phase or four-phase bone scan is widely used for these purposes.

In chronic osteomyelitis, comparison of Tc-99m phosphate bone imaging and Ga-67 citrate imaging suggests greater accuracy of the gallium scan in detecting the response or lack of response of the infection to therapy [29].

Despite the recent emphases on the role of MR imaging in the assessment of osteonecrosis, bone scintigraphy remains an effective diagnostic technique. Initially, on the bone scan, if a substantial interruption of blood supply has occurred, the radiopharmaceutical cannot reach the involved area and decreased activity may be evident on the scan. As the bone reacts to the insult with revascularization and reossification, scintigraphy may show increased activity in the involved area.

Computed tomography

In this technique computer-generated X-ray images are used in surgical, coronal and axial planes providing exceptional detail as to bone location, comminution and displacement. Currently 3-D constructions are being used which are very helpful in certain fracture circumstances. The indications are tibial plateau fractures, osteochondritis dissecans, bone tumors and occasionally, in the patella, femoral tracking. Computed tomography (CT) is often able to define soft tissue and bone alterations that are undetectable with conventional radiography because of its cross-sectional display, excellent contrast resolution, and ability to measure specific attenuation values. CT has matured into a reliable and prominent tool for study of the musculoskeletal system. Like conventional tomography, CT is planar, but CT images are transaxial and unobscured by overlying tissue. This technique has superior contrast resolution with a capacity to provide quantitative measures of the skeleton. In a dramatic departure from film methods, the CT images are produced in a computer that allows manipulation of the display.

CT can be used to evaluate many anatomic regions of the body and a variety of musculoskeletal disorders. The specific musculoskeletal disorders are trauma, infection and neoplasm. The role of CT in evaluation of tibial plateau has been well established; CT provides optimal visualization of the plateau depression, defects and split fragments. It has also proved more accurate than conventional tomography in assessing depressed and split fractures when they involve the anterior and posterior border of the plateau, and in demonstrating the extent of fracture comminution. The degree of fracture depressions and separation as measured by the computerized technique is often more accurate than measurements obtained from conventional tomograms. Particularly useful are reformatted images in various planes and three-dimensional reformation [30]. Kode and coworkers [31] have suggested that MRI was equivalent or superior to two-dimensional CT reformation for depiction of tibial plateau fracture configuration. The multiplanar capabilities of MRI may facilitate three-dimensional perception, and in addition, this technique permits assessment of the associated injuries to the ligaments and menisci that are not visible on CT scans. The early diagnosis of osteomyelitis is best left to scintigraphy or MR imaging, but defining the intraosseous extent of disease can be accomplished with CT, owing to a change in attenuation values as normal marrowfat is replaced. In cases of chronic osteomyelitis, CT may be used to identify sequestra, bone abscess and soft tissue abscesses as well as sinus tracts.

The role of CT in the evaluation of musculoskeletal neoplasm is best described by considering separately the neoplasms arising in bone and those originating in soft tissue. CT has not replaced conventional radiography in the diagnosis of primary and secondary bone tumors; however, it is better able to delineate the osseous and soft tissue extent of the process. Intraosseous extension of the neoplasm leads to the conversion of fatty marrow, with its negative CT numbers, to marrow containing tumorous tissue, with higher CT numbers. The ability of CT to delineate the soft tissue extent of the bone neoplasm is a consequence of its excellent contrast resolution.

Ultrasound

The term ultrasound refers to mechanical vibrations whose frequencies are above the limit of human audible perception. Medical ultrasonography utilizes frequencies in the range of 2–10 MHz. A central component of any ultrasound instrument is the transducer, which contains a small piezoelectric crystal. It serves as both the transmitter of sound waves into the body and the receiver of the returning echoes. When a brief alternating current is applied to the crystal, it vibrates at a characteristic frequency. By applying this vibrating transducer to the skin surface (through an acoustic coupling medium such as mineral oil or gel), the mechanical energy is transmitted into the body as a brief pulse of high-frequency sound waves. The advancing wave front interacts with tissues in various poorly understood ways and generates small reflected waves that return to the transducer. These cause the crystal to vibrate again, thereby generating an electrical signal that is conducted back to the machine where it is processed and displayed. Perhaps the most severe limitation of diagnostic ultrasound imaging is due to the inability of sound waves to penetrate gas and bone. The applications of this modality to orthopedics are generally limited to the soft tissues [32].

Ultasonography is non-invasive and painless to the patient. Furthermore, it is less expensive, safer, and performed more rapidly than most alternative imaging methods. Because it allows localization of lesions in three dimensions, sonography is a useful technique for guiding percutaneous aspiration or biopsy and for mapping radiation portals.

The use of ultrasound for evaluating various swellings in the popliteal space gained acceptance early. Because the fluid–solid distinction was accomplished easily even by early instruments and because popliteal cysts and popliteal artery aneurysms constitute the majority of masses in this area, sonography has been used frequently in diagnosing these lesions [33].

Ultrasound has been recommended as a screening procedure for patients with rheumatoid arthritis who have painful or asymptomatic swelling of the popliteal space. Moreover, ultrasound is a particularly attractive means of performing serial non-invasive studies to monitor response to various forms of therapy [34].

MR imaging has diminished the role of ultrasound in the evaluation of the knee. However, sonography has been shown to be capable of measuring the thickness of articular cartilage and of assessing its surface characteristics [35]. Real-time ultrasound can show the posterior horn of the medial and lateral menisci. The normal meniscus appears as a triangular hyperechoic structure. Meniscal cysts are also easily identified sonographically as fluid-containing spaces superficial to the menisci and ligaments. Ultrasound is also useful in diagnosing tendinitis and bursitis around the knee [36–38]. At the knee, tendinitis is frequently observed in the quadricipital, patellar, bicipital and per anserinus tendon. Tendinitis is seen as a swelling and hypo-echoic appearance of the tendon. Calcifications are rare, but are pathognomonic of a chronic stage. Ultrasound is the only method that can show tendon fibers. In contrast to MRI, ultrasound is able to show microruptures, due to its high resolution. In MRI, a hyperintense signal is seen in tendinitis, as well as in partial rupture.

Magnetic resonance imaging

The phenomenon of nuclear magnetic resonance (NMR) was first investigated nearly 50 years ago [39]; since then it has become a standard tool in chemistry and in the last two decades it has served as the basis for a remarkably powerful and flexible medical imaging technique [40]. The intense enthusiasm for and the rapid introduction of MRI into the clinical environment stem from the abundance of diagnostic information present in MR images. Although the image format is similar to CT, the fundamental principles are quite different; in fact, an entirely different part of the atom is responsible for the image formation. In MRI, it is the nucleus that provides the signal used in generating an image. We note that this differs from conventional diagnostic radiology in which the electrons are responsible for the imaging signal. Furthermore, it is not only the nucleus of the atom but also its structural

and biochemical environment that influence the signal.

The musculoskeletal system is ideally suited for evaluation by MRI since different tissues display different signal intensities on T_1- and T_2-weighted images. The images displayed may have low signal intensity, intermediate signal intensity or high signal intensity. Low signal intensity may be subdivided into: (i) signal void (black); and (ii) signal lower than that of normal muscle (dark). Intermediate signal intensity may be subdivided into: (i) signal equal to that of normal muscle; and (ii) signal higher than muscle but lower than subcutaneous fat (bright). High signal intensity may be subdivided into: (i) signal equal to normal subcutaneous fat (bright); and (ii) signal higher than subcutaneous fat (extremely bright). High signal intensity of fat planes and differences in signal intensity of various structures allow separation of the different tissue components including muscles, tendons, ligaments, vessels, nerves, hyaline cartilage, fibrocartilage, cortical bone and trabecular bone. For instance, fat and yellow (fatty) bone marrow display high signal intensity on T_1- and intermediate signal on T_2-weighted images; hematoma displays relatively high signal intensity on both T_1 and T_2 sequences. Cortical bone, air, ligaments, tendons and fibrocartilage display low signal intensity on T_1- and T_2-weighted images; muscle, nerves and hyaline cartilage display intermediate signal intensity on T_1- and T_2-weighted images. Red (hematopoietic) marrow displays low signal on T_1- and low-to-intermediate signal on T_2-weighted images. Fluid displays intermediate signal on T_1- and high signal on T_2-weighting. Most tumors display low-to-intermediate signal intensity on T_1-weighted images and high signal intensity on T_2-weighted images. Lipomas display high signal intensity on T_1- and intermediate signal on T_2-weighted images.

Traumatic conditions of the bones and tissues are particularly well suited to diagnosis and evaluation by MRI. Some abnormalities, such as bone contusion or trabecular microfractures not seen on radiography and CT, are well demonstrated by this technique. Occult fractures, which can be missed on conventional X-ray films, become obvious on MR imaging.

The value of MRI for the imaging of musculoskele-

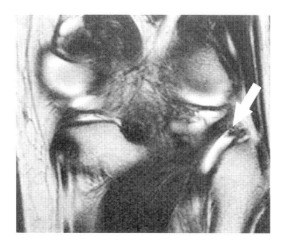

Fig. 6.2.13 MRI of an injured popliteofibular ligament.

tal conditions such as tumors and osteonecrosis became apparent almost immediately after the introduction of this modality in the early 1980s. Many advances have been made in MRI of the knee since its initial application, in 1984, for evaluation of the meniscus, and MR examination is now routinely used to assess a wide spectrum of internal knee derangement and articular disorders (Fig. 6.2.13) [41]. A non-invasive modality, MR has replaced conventional arthrography in the evaluation of the menisci and the cruciate ligaments and has decreased both the morbidity and the cost associated with arthroscopic examinations that yield negative results [42,43]. The decrease in the cost of MR knee studies has also contributed to their acceptance by the orthopedic community as a non-invasive replacement for arthrography and non-therapeutic arthroscopy. With MR imaging, the anatomic and pathologic definition of soft tissue, ligaments, fibrocartilage and articular cartilage is superior to that seen with CT. Fast spin echo imaging, used in conjunction with fat suppression MR techniques, has extended the sensitivity and specificity of MR for the detection of articular cartilage injuries. Additional advantages of MR imaging are multiplanar and thin-section capability and the ability to evaluate subchondral bone and marrow. As a result, MR imaging is recommended instead of CT for the evaluation of bone contusion and occult knee fractures, including tibial plateau fractures of the knee. MR has supplanted

nuclear scintigraphy in the characterization of osteonecrosis and, furthermore, can be used to assess the integrity of the overlying articular cartilage surfaces. MR imaging is unique in its ability to evaluate the internal structure as well as the surface of the meniscus. With conventional arthrography, intra-articular injection of contrast media permits visualization of surface anatomy but does not allow delineation of fibrocartilage structure or subchondral bone.

MR arthrography

Despite the challenge presented by arthroscopy and newer imaging techniques such as CT and MR imaging, the role of arthrography is most established for abnormalities of the knee [44]. Single-contrast examination using air and oxygen or radiopaque substances [45] has been replaced, in large part, by double-contrast examination using air and radiopaque contrast material [46]. In recent years computed arthrotomography (or CT alone) has been introduced in the evaluation of chondromalacia of the patella, cruciate ligament injuries and even meniscal abnormalities.

The postoperative evaluation of partial meniscectomies and primary repair offers unique challenges for MR imaging. Correlation of MR findings with preoperative MR studies or details of the arthroscopic surgery is useful in increasing the accuracy of MR diagnosis of a retear, persistent tear or a normal healing response in the meniscal fibrocartilage. It may be difficult to identify tears in the meniscal remnants after a partial meniscectomy. Even in the absence of a retear, the meniscal remnant may demonstrate a residual grade 3 signal intensity. Long TE or T_2-weighted spin echo images or T_2^* gradient echo images can be used to identify fluid directly extending into the cleavage plane of a tear in a meniscal remnant. This finding is more specific than the presence of grade 3 signal intensity on short TE or T_1-weighted images. Applegate and colleagues [47] have reported an 88% accuracy for the diagnosis of recurrent tears in the postoperative meniscus with MR arthrography compared with an overall accuracy of 66% when conventional MR imaging was used. MR arthrography was particularly useful in characterizing small meniscal remnants.

MR arthrography has become popular in recent

Table 6.2.4 Imaging of acute knee injuries.

Test	Interpretation	Be aware of
Plain radiograph AP and lateral	Will diagnose a fracture	Stress radiograph if epiphyseal injury is suspected
MRI	Will diagnose ACL, PCL, MCL, LCL and posterolateral ligament injuries, meniscal tears, bone bruise and extensor apparatus tears	The newer extremity MRI machines do not usually image the entire extensor apparatus — a tear may be missed
Ultrasonography	May diagnose tears of the extensor apparatus	Operator dependent
CT scan	Reconstruction CTs are useful in tibial plateau fractures	

ACL, anterior cruciate ligament; AP, anteroposterior; LCL, lateral collateral ligament; MCL, medial collateral ligament; PCL, posterior cruciate ligament.

years. The diagnostic accuracy of this technique may exceed that of conventional MRI because the intra-articular structures are better demonstrated if they are separated by means of capsular distension. Such distension can be achieved with intra-articular injection of contrast material such as diluted gadolinium or saline. The generated images are very similar to those obtained of the joint with pre-existing joint effusion. In clinical practice MR arthrography is predominantly used in the evaluation of shoulder abnormalities. An indication in the knee joint is the imaging of postoperative menisci. There are many studies that indicate the difficulty encountered in the MR imaging analysis of the repaired or partially resected meniscus. The diagnostic value of standard arthrography in this clinical setting is based primarily on the intrameniscal extension of fluid after an iatrogenic effusion produced by the injection of contrast material into the joint. MR arthrography using gadolinium compound or saline solution shares many of the advantages of standard arthrography in the diagnosis (or exclusion) of a retorn meniscus. With MR arthrography, the most definite sign of a retorn meniscus is the presence of contrast material within the meniscus. The absence of such contrast material is consistent with (but not diagnostic of) the absence of a new tear [47–49].

Fractures and chondral injuries

Fractures of the femoral or tibial part of the knee are relatively common in sports. The usual fractures are located on the proximal part of the tibia, primarily as tibial plateau fractures, often in conjunction with cruciate ligament injuries. It is beyond the scope of this book to review the typical intra-articular fractures.

Cartilage injuries have become quite frequent in the athletic population. In a Norwegian study, 11% of patients in 1000 consecutive arthroscopies had cartilage damage suitable for treatment [50]. Cartilage injuries can be acute or chronic. The so-called bone bruise which occurs with rotational injuries and may lead to secondary cartilage damage occurs in as many as 90% of rotational injuries to the knee [51,52]. Recent studies, both basic science and clinical, suggest that bruising of the subchondral bone changes the environment for the cartilage in the area. Follow-up MRI studies of patients with bone bruise suggest that this may lead to degeneration of the cartilage and early arthritis [51,52]. In addition it has been shown that isolated cartilage injuries may lead to degeneration of the adjacent cartilage [53]. These changes may be caused by the abnormally high stresses acting on the rim of the defect [54]. The cartilage surface opposing an isolated cartilage injury often shows fibrillation caused by mechanical irritation [55]. Thus there is evidence that rotational injury to the knee with bone bruise and additional cartilage changes may develop into degenerative arthritis. Twyman *et al.* [56] prospectively followed 22 knees in which osteochondritis dissecans (OCD) had been diagnosed before skeletal maturity. At an average of 34 years, 32% had radiographic evidence of moderate or severe osteoarthritis. Only 50% had a good or excellent functional result.

In the prospective study of 1000 consecutive arthroscopies, three main cartilage injury patterns were detected [50,57]: cartilage injuries in conjunction with bone bruise as mentioned above; osteochondral fractures caused by a traumatic incident; and osteo-chondroses representing the typical osteochondritis dissecans or the subtler avascular necrosis. After an acute traumatic event, an osteochondral injury will lead to hemarthrosis and pain. Some patients will even experience locking. The injury will not usually be picked up on a plain radiograph, but will be detected on a MRI arthrogram. Symptoms from OCD are usually pain and swelling with occasional locking. The majority of patients will be adolescents. Even though the cause of an OCD is presently unknown, the symptoms often occur after a sports event. Consequently the patient feels that the injury has occurred during sport.

It is well established that damaged articular cartilage has a very limited potential for healing. The literature suggests that defects larger than 2–4 mm in diameter in particular rarely heal. Articular cartilage in adults possesses neither a blood supply nor lymphatic drainage. Although the cells continue to produce new extracellular matrix throughout life, they are ineffective in responding to injury [58]. Not until the subchondral bone is penetrated is the usual inflammatory wound healing response observed. Cells recruited from the bone marrow then attempt to fill the defect with new tissue. To date, no one has been able to fill the defects with normal hyaline cartilage regardless of methodology.

According to O'Driscoll the options for operative treatment of damaged cartilage can be grouped according to four concepts [58,59]. The articular cartilage can be restored, replaced, relieved or resected. In the following an overview of the current status in this field is presented.

Osteochondritis dissecans

Review of the literature of ostechondritis dissecans (OCD) is quite confusing. There is little agreement among investigators concerning the etiology of OCD. The most widely accepted theories include trauma, ischemia, abnormal ossification within the epiphyses, or a combination of these. Regardless of cause, the symptoms and signs are identical, with pain, stiffness and swelling the most common. The diagnosis is confirmed with a plain radiograph, preferably a tunnel view. A more dynamic approach is through a scintigraphic or MRI arthrographic evaluation. Currently, MRI arthrogram seems to give the best information on the degree of ingrowth of the OCD in the surrounding bone. After the diagnosis is confirmed, treatment in the child and adolescent will involve non-weight-bearing with motion for 4–6 weeks if the piece is still in its bed. In most patients below the age of 16, this leads to ingrowth of the OCD with good long-term results. If the patient continues to have pain after a period of non-weight-bearing, an arthroscopic examination is recommended. If the bone piece is still in place, but loose, it should if at all possible be fixed. This can be done as an arthroscopic procedure with either a metal screw or synthetic screws or pegs. Many authors have also published good results using an open procedure with bony pegs. If the bone piece is either impossible to retain or in many small pieces, it should be removed. During the same procedure a microfracture technique to obtain the so-called 'super clot' may be carried out. This procedure followed by continuous passive motion daily for 4 weeks has been shown to produce hyaline-like cartilage in rabbits and good clinical results in humans [59–61]. If this procedure fails and the lesion is on the weight-bearing surface of the femoral condyle, a number of procedures are available currently. These will be described briefly in the next paragraph.

Osteochondral or chondral fractures

These fractures occur during a traumatic event, often in combination with major ligament injuries or bony fractures. The patient will complain of stiffness and pain and the examiner will often note swelling. The diagnosis is confirmed through either a MRI arthrogram or an arthroscopic examination. The natural history of these injuries is not well documented. The literature shows that ACL tears with additional cartilage or meniscal injuries do worse than the isolated ACL tear. In addition there is indirect evidence through animal studies that isolated cartilage injuries in the knee leads to development of degenerative arthritis. Because the natural history in humans is not well documented, a number of treatment options exist. Currently, there seems to be consensus on the fact that defects less than $2\,cm^2$ can be treated conservatively even when they are located on weight-bearing surfaces. This is based on retrospective studies showing these patients to do reasonably well short term. This concept has been accepted, although no science exists regarding this problem. In patients with defects larger than $2\,cm^2$ on weight-bearing surface of femur, a large number of well-proven and new techniques are currently undergoing tests.

Subchondral drilling or microfracture

These techniques have in common the goal of recruiting pluripotential stem cells from the marrow by penetrating the subchondral bone. According to Steadman [60,61], the penetration must be done with specific awls to avoid the heating that occurs with drilling. The Steadman technique has been shown to produce hyalin-like cartilage in small defects in rabbits and in larger defects in horses. Human studies have not as yet had a control group, but several publications have suggested good efficacy in reducing pain. The method is currently being used as a first choice in patients with untreated cartilage defects. Salter introduced and investigated the biologic concept of continuous passive motion (CPM) of joint for the postoperative treatment of articular cartilage injuries [59]. His group found a good effect of CPM in rabbits with small cartilage defects, with much smaller effect on larger defects. CPM has subsequently been used by Steadman in his microfracture technique with good success. The present use of CPM in several of the new cartilage repair techniques is controversial. To date, no controlled, randomized studies have been published on the microfracture technique.

Periosteal transplant

Periosteum has been used alone for biologic resurfacing arthroplasty in humans for more than a decade. In Scandinavia, the Swedish Umeå group has published long-term results of their technique for resurfacing patellar cartilage defects (Fig. 6.2.1). Their clinical use of periosteum is built on animal data predominantly from rabbits where short-term results are encouraging, showing a majority of hyalin-like cartilage. O'-

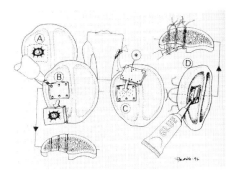

Fig. 6.2.14 Periosteal transplantation for a patellar cartilage defect.

Driscoll [58] has published extensively on the animal side and has reported encouraging clinical results. As he and the Umeå group point out, the technique is demanding and relies on meticulous surgical procedure.

Transplantation of autogenous chondrocytes

Many investigators have chosen to use chondrocytes for cell transplantation for the regeneration of cartilage [62–65]. Other possibilities include undifferentiated stem cells or even allogene cells. Bone marrow as well as periosteum can be used as sources for such cells. The fully differentiated chondrocytes have the capacity to produce cartilage matrix and may be suitable for chondral defects only. Most defects, however, involve a bony part as well, and chondrocytes cannot produce bone. Periosteal and bone marrow cells do have the capacity to regenerate both the cartilage and the subchondral bone. In many instances the osteochondral defects are several mm deep and an isolated chondrocyte transplant will not be able to fill the gap. Many clinicians have therefore now moved to a combination of bone graft followed by chondrocyte transplantation, or use periosteal transplantation alone. Another trend is to use a carrier, that is, a scaffold or matrix upon which the cells are grown. The ideal material has not been identified, and to date biodegradable matrices seem to have the most promise. Carriers have already been marketed and development will continue also with regard to growth factor stimulation attached to the scaffolds.

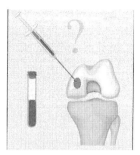

Fig. 6.2.15 Autogenous chondrocyte transplantation for a cartilage defect of the medial femoral condyle.

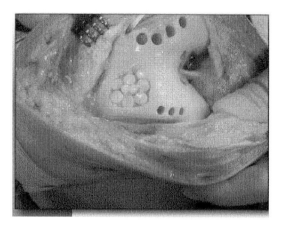

Fig. 6.2.16 A 35-year-old patient treated with mosaicplasty because of a major cartilage injury during skiing.

So far animal results of chondrocytes transplants have varied from excellent in rabbit studies [62,63] to mediocre in dog studies [66]. A remaining problem is the incomplete incorporation of the healing tissue into the cartilage defect. On the experimental side much research remains to be done to confirm the scientific validity of transplantation of chondrocytes using the currently advocated technique.

Several clinical studies have reported promising results with chondrocyte transplantation in femoral cartilage defects [62,63,65] (Fig 6.2.15). The procedure involves the patient having to undergo harvesting through an arthroscopic procedure, followed 4–8 weeks later by an arthrotomy where the cells are injected under a cover of periosteum. Clinical results from femoral defects have ranged from 60 to 85% excellent and good in different studies. So far no controlled studies are available. At the moment the procedure is reserved for patients with large defects on the weight-bearing surface of the femur. The defects should not be deeper than approximately 5 mm without being bone grafted. Currently, the procedure is generally carried out on the femur. Chondral transplantation onto the tibia and patella is being done in centers for research purposes only for the time being. So far no randomized, controlled studies have been published on this technique.

Mosaicplasty and osteochondral autogenous grafts

An alternative to biologic regeneration of a defect is to replace it with a substitute. This can be done either partly using special equipment where available, or completely with a matched osteochondral transplant (Fig. 6.2.16). Several orthopedic companies have produced coring drills, which will harvest plug from areas that are relatively less weight-bearing such as the intercondylar notch or the most lateral part of the femoral condyle (Fig. 6.2.16). The plugs are then placed in the defect in predrilled cylinders. Studies have shown that no part of the femoral condyle is non-weight-bearing and the long-term results of the harvesting procedure are not known. So far there is limited animal data on the procedure. The first clinical data were published by Hangody and Bobic [67–69] and match those of chondrocyte transplantation by Brittberg *et al.* [62,63]. As for chondrocyte transplantation, no controlled studies exist. The procedure is much cheaper than cell transplantation and can be used in defects that are deeper without bone grafting. The use is limited only by the size of the defect due to the necessity of harvesting from relatively less weight-bearing areas.

Osteochondral allografts

Because large, symptomatic cartilage defects are difficult to fill with autologous osteochondral plugs, allografts have been used. So far, the use of osteochondral allografts has primarily been after fracture sequela of the femur or tibial plateau or large OCD lesions [70]. The viability of chondrocytes has been demonstrated both after refrigerated allografts and in retrieved specimens after as long as 12 years. There seems to be a larger immune response to fresh vs. frozen allografts, but the bottom line is that the technique seems to work well. The use of the technique is currently only limited by allograft availability.

Osteotomy

None of the techniques mentioned so far will be successful if the knee is malaligned. Consequently, one must consider an osteotomy if the knee is valgus or varus compared to the normal knee. The most common is a varus knee in conjunction with injuries to the ACL and/or PCL and posterolateral structures. Some of these patients will have a so-called 'varus thrust' gait and are candidates for an opening wedge osteotomy. Patients with normal ligament function, but with a knee in varus malalignment, may need a closing wedge osteotomy to decrease the load on the medial part of the joint [71].

Conclusion

Cartilage lesions or injuries are common in sports. There are indications that the damaged articular cartilage can be restored through cell or periosteal transplantation, microfracturing be replaced through an osteochondral auto- or allografts, and/or relieved through an osteotomy that unloads the injured joint compartment and decreases the stress. Currently, efforts to induce healing and regeneration of cartilage are being directed toward enhancing the natural healing potential of cartilage or replacing the damaged cartilage with tissues or cells that can grow cartilage. These procedures have shown promise but are not yet at a stage where they should be used indiscriminately. So far, no controlled, randomized studies have been published in this field. It remains to be seen which, if any, of these procedures will survive after good, controlled studies have been carried out.

Meniscal injuries

Injuries to the menisci are common in sports, with an incidence between 6 and 10/10 000 per year [50]. They are frequently the culprits for keeping athletes out of activity and for creating early osteoarthritis.

The menisci are known to serve a crucial role in the complex biomechanics of knee joint function. The fact that meniscal injury and meniscectomy may result in early osteoarthritis of the knee serves as an impetus to advance our knowledge of this structure with regard to basic biomechanics, kinematics and reparative qualities. There has been great development in meniscal repair devices over the last few years. Efforts are also being made to substitute the meniscus with allografts or prosthetic replacements. Two aspects of the treatment of lesions of the meniscus are currently the subject of much discussion and research: repair of the tears in the 'avascular zone' and meniscal transplant. Histologic examination of adult cadaveric specimens has suggested that the inner 70–90% of the meniscus is avascular. Tears in the so-called 'white zone' have been thought to have little or no potential for healing and consequently have led to resection of large parts of the injured meniscus. The avascular part of the meniscus may be given access to a blood supply by making vascular access channels and placing a fibrin clot between the edges of a meniscal tear. Other investigators have covered the meniscus with synovial flaps to encourage vascularization. Both these techniques have expanded the indications for meniscal repair, which now can be carried out with a number of different devices.

Diagnosis

A knee sprain followed by immediate swelling usually points toward a cruciate ligament injury. However, an acute tear of the red–red or red–white zone of the meniscus will lead to intra-articular bleeding and pain. If the patient is unable to extend the knee, further suspicion of a meniscal tear results. Acute swelling of the knee, however, caused by bleeding will lead to decreased range of motion. It is often difficult to discern between a meniscal, osteocartilage or ligament injury. The usual meniscal tests may be difficult to carry out due to pain. In a more chronic case, the diagnosis can usually be made based on the clinical examination using the McMurray test and hyperextension test. Most patients will also have pain on palpation in the joint line close to the meniscal tear. If the clinical diagnosis is difficult, the final diagnosis may be made through MRI which has high sensitivity and specificity for meniscal tears.

Treatment

Meniscal injuries leading to symptoms should be arthroscopically examined and treated. A small radial tear can easily be removed by basket forceps, whereas a peripheral injury may be suitable for a repair. Today these are carried out with the use of the arthroscope and additional devices. The repair is carried out either in the inside-out fashion with transmeniscal sutures tied through an incision outside the knee, or with an all-inside approach using meniscal arrows or tacs which are absorbable. The best results of a meniscal repair are achieved when the repair is done in conjunction with an ACL reconstruction within 8 weeks after the injury, and the injury is located close to the periphery. Repairs in a stable knee approach 90% good results, whereas repairs in an unstable knee are associated with a 30–40% rate of retear. The choice between bioabsorbable tacs or arrows and suture repair is not easy. The tacs are easy to use and have shown good results, although there have been reports of the tacs creating temporary synovitis in the joint and not being resorbed for a long time resulting in migration to the skin. The authors prefer inside-out suture repair in large tears. In small tears in the posterior part of the lateral meniscus, arrows or tacs may be the technique of choice. No randomized controlled studies are available to date on the different techniques.

In patients with total or subtotal meniscectomies and chronic pain, osteoarthritis is often found in one compartment. The joint angle is usually changed from neutral to varus or valgus based on radiographs. These are the patients who have been operated on with a combination of osteotomies and meniscal allografts. A few studies have been published on the long-term effectiveness of meniscal allografts, and the results have varied considerably [72]. For the treatment of partial meniscectomies and osteoarthritis, collagen-based templates have been sutured to the meniscal remnants in a limited number of patients. No controlled studies are available on any of these techniques.

Meniscal cysts

Meniscal cysts are uncommon lesions usually found in the lateral meniscus. They are usually associated with a degenerative tear. The patient commonly has lateral joint line pain and 60% will have a palpable mass. Other patients have pain, but the cyst can only be detected on MRI or by ultrasound. The cysts will usually not disappear once the meniscus injury is established and will usually need surgical removal. This should always be preceded by an arthroscopy examination since these patients always have a meniscal tear with connection to the cyst. The tear can be debrided arthroscopically and the cyst emptied. However, the cyst itself will often need removal through a separate skin incision.

Ligament injuries

Isolated ligament injuries of the knee

Medial collateral ligament

The medial collateral ligament complex of the knee is the main stabilizer to a valgus force applied to the knee. Isolated MCL complex injuries are usually secondary to a valgus contact injury [7,73].

In addition to diagnosing the severity of the MCL complex injury by performing the valgus stress test at 30° knee flexion, the medial epicondyle, the meniscofemoral portion of the complex, the joint line, the meniscotibial portion of the complex and the MCL complex attachment sites on the proximal tibia are palpated to determine the potential location of injury. While this may not be as important for incomplete MCL injuries, it is very important for complete tears of the MCL complex. This is because it is believed that tears of the meniscofemoral portion of the MCL complex are inherently more stable and have a lesser likelihood of needing surgical intervention and repair than meniscotibial lesions, because of the inherent bony stability of the medial side of the knee. The convex surface of the medial femoral condyle articulates well on the concave surface of the medial tibial plateau. Complete tears of the meniscofemoral portion of the MCL complex do not usually result in any significant instability to this. However, tears of the meniscotibial portion of the complex tend to give more rotational laxity, which may not heal completely over time.

Grade I or II MCL complex injuries [1] (incomplete) are primarily diagnosed by the physical examination. Acute injuries will have pain over a portion of the MCL complex with an endpoint present on the valgus stress test at 30° knee flexion. If there is joint line opening > 1 cm, it is considered that the MCL complex is completely torn. If the physical examination does not suggest any evidence of other ligament injury, meniscal pathology or lateral-sided joint line pain (which could be due to either a bone bruise or a meniscal tear), the patient is started on a program of physical therapy to address their pathology and to return them back to function as soon as possible [74,75]. After the initial swelling and pain has been addressed in these injuries, these patients start a functional program of rehabilitation soon after injury. Patients are allowed to weight bear as tolerated and may come off crutches when they can walk without a limp. They start to perform quadriceps setting exercises and straight-leg raises immediately. Once range of motion allows, they are started on an exercise biking program and progressed in both time and level of effort based upon their symptomatology. Utilizing this program, athletes are usually back to full participation within 1–2 weeks for a grade I MCL tear, and 4–6 weeks for a grade II MCL tear.

In the evaluation of isolated grade III (complete) MCL complex tears, it is especially important to make sure that there is no associated concurrent injury present. In this regard, it is important to check the patellofemoral joint for evidence of any lateral patellar dislocation and to check for the integrity of the anterior cruciate ligament to make sure that it is not torn. While performing the valgus stress test, the examiner can also assess for any significant meniscal pathology, which is usually felt as a clunk or crepitation by one's fingers over the joint line of the medial compartment.

Grade III MCL tears require closer follow-up and more individualized treatment than grade I or II tears do. We do not use a brace for meniscofemoral-based tears, but will use a hinged knee brace for 6 weeks for meniscotibial-based lesions to make sure that there is no significant abnormal motion of the tibia as the patient progresses in rehabilitation. After pain and swelling have subsided, the patient is enrolled in a program of rehabilitation. First, the patient is allowed to weight bear as tolerated with the use of crutches. Crutches are used for 3–4 weeks with these tears to ensure that the athlete does not significantly stress the knee. They are allowed to come off the crutches at this point if the physical examination indicates that the MCL complex is healing well and they are making good progress in their rehabilitation program.

Patients will begin a program of quadriceps sets and straight-leg raises immediately. Once their range of motion allows, they are also started on an exercise bike. The goal is to have them working on increasing amounts of time and levels of intensity with the exercise bike based on the symptomatology of their knee. The patients are followed closely at approximately 1–2-week intervals to ensure that their MCL complex is healing and no residual laxity is present. For those patients who do show good evidence of healing, our goal is to increase their functional activities as tolerated at approximately 3–4 weeks after injury with a goal of return to full activities by 5–6 weeks after injury. This clinical program is based on the animal studies of Frank and Woo [76] who noted that early motion improved the overall strength of a ruptured MCL. This may be true in the human clinical situation and athletes are encouraged to use an exercise bike as much as possible both to build up their overall strength and to put some beneficial stress on the healing MCL complex.

In those rare instances where there is still no evidence of healing of the MCL complex at approximately 3–4 weeks after injury, consideration is given to performing a primary repair or surgical augmentation of the torn structures.

Anterior cruciate ligament tears

As mentioned previously, the ACL is the primary stabilizer to anterior translation of the knee. Functional limitations caused by ACL tears include difficulty with cutting, pivoting and twisting due to anterolateral subluxation of the lateral tibial plateau on the lateral femoral condyle. Lack of an ACL does not usually hinder function with level jogging in a straight line, ice skating or in-line skating.

Partial ACL tears are not common. When they do occur, they are usually due to a tear of either the posterolateral or anteromedial bundles of the ACL rather than a partial intrasubstance stretch of the ligament. When these partial ACL tears do occur, the basic principles are to decrease the effusion in the knee, minimize quadriceps atrophy, and regain full range of motion as soon as possible. It is also important to make sure that there are no concurrent intra-articular injuries present, such as an osteochondral fracture or a meniscus tear, which could hinder subsequent rehabilitation. Patients with perceived partial ACL tears are entered into a rehabilitation program as soon as their pain and effusion will permit. Patients are instructed to work on range of motion of their affected knee several times daily. In addition, they are instructed in quadriceps sets, straight-leg raises, and other closed-chain kinetic exercises. This would include the use of an exercise bike, leg presses and minisquats, or the use of a squat rack as tolerated. The amount of weight used initially is approximately one-quarter body weight (if tolerated). Progressive strengthening is then performed, based upon the patient's symptomatology. The patient is also instructed to initiate a walking program, with progression to jogging at approximately 3–4 weeks after injury, as tolerated. Once the patient is able to perform sports-specific functional activities without limitations, he or she is allowed to participate in sports. Many centers are using isokinetic muscle testing or specific functional tests as guidelines for return to sport [16,77,78].

It is believed that patients who have a partial ACL tear may in some instances have an unrecognized complete ACL tear or they may be at higher risk for a resultant complete ACL tear with minimal trauma. For this reason, these patients should be counselled to look for signs of instability with function and to seek treatment if this should occur.

Complete tears of the ACL may be diagnosed either by physical examination or by other diagnostic methods. Evidence of functional limitations in the patient with activity, a positive Lachman's test and a positive pivot-shift test is evidence enough of a complete ACL tear and further diagnostic testing, such as an MRI scan, is probably unnecessary. We recommend that obtaining an MRI scan for purposes of diagnosing an ACL tear be reserved for those patients in which the diagnosis is in doubt based on the clinical picture. This would include those patients who present acutely with a knee effusion and who have evidence of a potential mechanical block or a substantial decrease in the range of motion of their knee (especially with an inability to extend their knee). In these instances, the examiner needs to be cognizant of the fact that the patient could potentially have a displaced bucket-handle tear of their meniscus, which could be amenable to repair. The use of an MRI scan for diagnosis in this instance would be considered good use of health care resources. It would also be considered useful to perform an MRI scan in either acute or chronic cases in which it is difficult to determine whether the increased translation that is seen is due to an isolated ACL tear or whether there is a component of other ligamentous instability present which makes the physical examination somewhat inconclusive.

Complete isolated anterior cruciate ligament tears

After diagnosis has been made of a complete tear of the ACL in a patient, it is important to consider the patient's age, activity level and expectations. An important decision needs to be made in terms of whether to proceed with non-operative or operative treatment.

In those patients who are relatively young with open physes or in patients whose activity levels may not justify an ACL reconstruction, a trial of rehabilitation and activity modification, possibly supplemented with the use of an ACL functional brace, may be indicated. Due to the fact that most patients who have an acute ACL tear have a significant intra-articular hemarthrosis, it is important for the patient to resolve the pain, swelling and decrease in range of motion that is normally seen with an acute ACL tear prior to working on an aggressive rehabilitation program. Once the effusion has diminished and the patient has achieved full range of motion, they may initiate a rehabilitation or exercise program which does not cause any significant irritation or symptomatology in their affected knee. This would primarily consist of a closed-chain kinetic exercise program for the quadriceps and hamstrings with an emphasis on low-impact activities, such as the use of an exercise bike, leg presses and squats. The usual time for a patient to return to full activities after an acute ACL tear is 4–6 weeks. In those patients who wish to return to sports, they should be counselled as to the fact that they are at increased risk for meniscal tears and chondral injuries with subsequent subluxation episodes. The overall functional benefits from the use of an ACL brace are still unknown. While some braces have been shown to be effective at reducing anterolateral subluxation of the tibia on the distal femur at low applied loads in *in vitro* testing in the lab, this has not been demonstrated for the higher loads that a patient's knee would see functionally [78]. However, it is recognized that many patients do obtain some benefit from wearing these braces. It still remains to be seen whether this benefit is due to actual prevention of subluxation episodes or the potential improved proprioception that a patient may have while using the brace.

For those patients who choose to return to cutting, pivoting and contact sports, we currently recommend that they strongly consider an ACL reconstruction to prevent resubluxation events in the future. While there are many choices with varying arguments for the type of graft utilized for an ACL reconstruction, it is currently accepted that anatomically placed reconstruction tunnels of the ACL have the best functional results [79]. One way to visualize and understand where to place these tunnels correctly is to look at an MRI scan of a normal ACL on the sagittal view (Fig. 6.2.17). It becomes especially obvious that the normal femoral attachment for the ACL is at the very far posterior aspect of the intercondylar notch. The authors' current recommended tunnel positions for an ACL reconstruction on the tibia are at a point approximately 7–8 mm anterior to the ligament of Humphrey/PCL, at the bottom of the medial tibial spine, and in line with the anterior horn of the lateral meniscus. Due to distortion from the 30° arthroscope, the anatomic landmark of the anterior horn of the lateral meniscus is not very useful in arthroscopic reconstructions. However, it is especially useful in open reconstructions,

especially in knee dislocations where there is a combined ACL and PCL tear with loss of the normal ACL reference off the PCL. In this anatomic reconstruction point on the tibia, there should be either no or only minimal impingement of the ACL graft on the intercondylar roof. Anterior tibial tunnel placement usually results in an extension deficit to the knee unless an aggressive roofplasty of the intercondylar notch is performed. Knee extension deficits are not well tolerated by patients and usually lead to functional limitations. It can also lead to a cyclops lesion (Fig. 6.2.18) as the fibers of the ACL graft become sloughed with the formation of an anterior nodule on the graft.

Malplacement of the femoral tunnel is still believed to be one of the most common causes of a failed ACL reconstruction. Anterior tunnel placement of the femoral tunnel results in the knee being overconstrained in flexion. Invariably, either these patients have a loss of full knee flexion, or over time they gradually stretch out their ACL reconstruction grafts when they do achieve full flexion. The current recommended tunnel position is to put the ACL graft as far

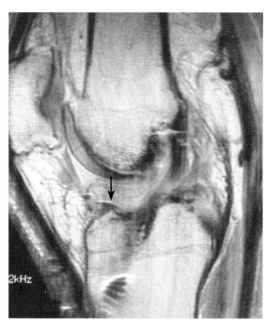

Fig. 6.2.18 Cyclops nodule of fibrous tissue (arrowed) anterior to an ACL reconstruction, blocking full extension of the knee.

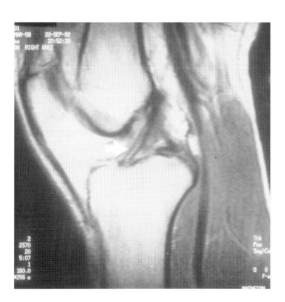

Fig. 6.2.17 MRI of a normal anterior cruciate ligament.

posterior on the intercondylar notch as possible. This usually means that only a 1-mm back wall is present after the femoral tunnel has been drilled. In addition, the normal ACL is located at approximately 10:30 on the right knee and 1:30 on the left knee so this is where the tunnels are recommended to be placed rather than centrally in the intercondylar notch. Because of this, it is important to make sure that the tibial entry site is positioned properly during a one-incision ACL reconstruction so that the graft is not malpositioned and placed centrally rather than in the correct position. Two-incision ACL reconstructions also need to follow these tunnel placement positions.

The surgical technique of ACL reconstruction using an autogenous central third patellar tendon graft or four-bundle hamstrings is considered the best technique for ACL reconstruction [26,80].

Posterior cruciate ligament tears

In the discussion of the treatment of PCL tears, it is important to know whether it is an isolated tear or one with a combined concurrent ligament injury. This is because it is felt that the natural history of isolated PCL tears is very different from that of combined ligament injuries. Parolie and Bergfeld [81] have reported that about 2% of American collegiate senior football players at a National Football League predraft examination were found to have chronic PCL-deficient knees. Fowler and Messieh [82] reported that 13 athletes, with arthroscopically diagnosed isolated PCL tears who were followed for an average of 2.6 years were able to return to their previous activities without limitation. More recently a prospective study of 133 athletes with isolated PCL tears treated non-operatively for the mean follow-up of 5.4 years has been reported. In this group of patients, regardless of the amount of residual laxity they had from their PCL tear, half the patients were able to resume sports at the same or higher level.

In light of this information, which demonstrates that the natural history of isolated PCL tears in many instances may result in little functional loss to the patient in the short term, a course of non-operative treatment of acute PCL tears may be indicated. Some centers splint an acute isolated PCL tear with the knee in full extension. In this position, posterior translation of the knee is minimized and there is little tension on the anterolateral bundle of a PCL. Splinting from anywhere from 3 to 6 weeks may allow the PCL tear to heal and result in little instability over the long term. Once the period of initial splinting has been followed, the patient is then placed in a rehabilitative program to work on regaining their range of motion and rehabilitating their quadriceps mechanism. The importance of the quadriceps mechanism is especially important in PCL-deficient knees. This is because of its protective role in preventing posterior tibial translation. A strong quadriceps muscle group pulls through the quadriceps tendon, patella and patellar tendon anteriorly on the tibial tubercle to reduce the posteriorly subluxed tibial plateau to a normal position. Patients who undergo this form of rehabilitation program can usually return to activity by 3 months. In patients who continue to have functional limitations at 4 months after injury, PCL reconstruction is considered. In addition, it is important to investigate whether there are any other associated ligamentous injuries, which are initially not recognized, in this patient group.

Avulsion fractures

We believe that acute intervention may be indicated when there is a displaced avulsion fracture of the PCL. These avulsion fractures are usually from the PCL facet on the posterior proximal tibia. In those cases where there is a large bony avulsion fragment, we first perform a diagnostic arthroscopy of the knee to determine whether there is any concurrent structural damage (such as a meniscal tear or chondral injury). The avulsion is then fixed with a screw through a posterior, curved incision. Postoperative care for this type of treatment usually involves placing a patient into an immobilizer for 3–6 weeks and then starting a program of range of motion. The aggressiveness of this technique will depend upon the intra-articular appearance of the PCL. If there is a stretch component of the PCL in addition to the ligament avulsion fracture, or if intrasubstance necrosis has started because of the time from injury to surgical treatment (we prefer to treat these within the first 1–2 weeks after injuries), then the length of time in the immobilizer may be increased to nearer 6 weeks rather than 3 weeks. Once the avulsion fracture has healed, we will initiate the patient on a program of rehabilitation similar to the treatment of an isolated PCL tear.

Posterior cruciate ligament reconstructions

The authors' preferred technique is to use a single-bundle reconstruction of the anterolateral bundle of the PCL. Our preferred graft source is an Achilles tendon allograft, although a quadruple-bundle hamstring allograft may be indicated in those places where an Achilles allograft may not be available.

Posterior cruciate ligament onlay technique

The tibial onlay technique for a PCL reconstruction relies on the principle that passing a tendon graft over the posterior aspect of the knee and through a PCL tibial tunnel can result in fraying of the graft and possible loosening over time. In attempts to avoid this 'killer turn' of the PCL reconstruction graft, some authors have advocated a direct onlay on the posterior tibia with a bone block to achieve fixation of the graft. We have found this technique to have some use in patients in revision PCL cases where there may be osteolysis of the tibial tunnel and attempting a primary revision reconstruction, as opposed to a two-stage reconstruction with bone grafting of the tibial tunnel performed, would be difficult. One of the limitations that we have found with this technique is in using patellar tendon allografts. In some of our cases, we found that there was a second 'killer turn' created by using this technique. While we were able to obtain excellent placement of the PCL tibial bone plug, when the patellar tendon graft was passed intra-articularly and out through the femur, there was frequently graft tunnel mismatch and the entire bone plug on the femoral side exited the femoral tunnel (Fig. 6.2.19). We have utilized bone staples to fix the graft under the vastus medialis obliquus (VMO) and obtain fixation. In all of our cases, patients have had irritation of their vastus medialis obliquus from utilization of this technique. For this reason, we have reserved this reconstructive technique using patellar tendon grafts for revision PCL reconstructions with previous tibial tunnel osteolysis present.

Double-bundle posterior cruciate ligament reconstructive technique

A newer technique for reconstructing both the anterolateral and the posteromedial bundle of the PCL has been advocated by some centers [8,19]. The rationale behind this is to totally anatomically reconstruct the PCL. While the anterolateral bundle of the PCL is

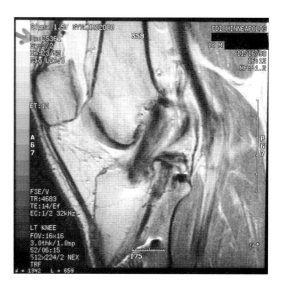

Fig. 6.2.19 Graft tunnel mismatch in reconstruction of the PCL.

important in preventing posterior translation of the tibia on the femur at 90° knee flexion, the posteromedial bundle helps to provide stability against posterior translation close to extension. The importance of recreating the posteromedial bundle is probably of greater significance when there is a concurrent posterolateral corner injury present.

In performing the double-bundle PCL reconstructive technique, the methods of preparing the PCL tibial tunnel are the same. Either a tunnel is drilled or an onlay technique with a bone plug is utilized. The difference lies in that instead of one large graft which recreates the anterolateral bundle of the PCL, smaller bundles are utilized which recreate both anterolateral and posteromedial bundles of the PCL. The femoral tunnels are placed at the normal anatomic positions of the anterolateral and posteromedial bundles of the PCL, respectively.

Usually with this technique, the femoral tunnel position is the same as in the single-bundle PCL reconstruction. The difference is that instead of the usual 12-mm PCL femoral tunnel, a 10- or 11-mm tunnel is drilled. Once this is in place, a second femoral tunnel is then drilled slightly distal and posterior to this, which has an entry point slightly proximal and parallel to the anterolateral bundle's femoral tunnel. The size of this tunnel is usually 7–8 mm in diameter.

The usual graft used to reconstruct these two-bundle PCLs is either hamstring tendons or Achilles allografts. The usual method of fixation on the femur is either with soft tissue interference screw or bone staples. The same technique in positioning of the knee for fixation of the anterolateral bundle is followed. However, there is some disagreement among different centers about how the posteromedial bundle should be fixed. The general consensus is to fix this bundle with the knee in full extension.

Rehabilitation principles for posterior cruciate ligament reconstructions

The general concepts behind a PCL reconstruction are that these reconstructions must be rehabilitated differently from ACL reconstructions. The grafts are generally larger and probably take longer to revascularize, and are considered to stretch out if an overly aggressive initial rehabilitation program is performed. With these general concepts in mind, it is still recognized that no prospective studies have demonstrated that this occurs with a more aggressive rehabilitation program. In many centers, a less aggressive rehabilitation program for the PCLs is utilized. For the initial 2 weeks after surgery, we splint the patient's knee in full extension for isolated PCL reconstructions for 2 weeks. At 2 weeks, the patient's surgical subcuticular stitches are removed and a program of range of motion is initiated. In the initial 2-week interval, attention is turned towards obtaining pain control and attempting to minimize the postoperative effusion. Cold compression devices are utilized routinely to attempt to achieve this. In addition, patients are allowed to perform quadriceps sets and straight-leg raises in their immobilizer. This is performed because the quadriceps mechanism is protective to a PCL reconstruction. Aggressive hamstring exercises should be avoided for 3 months after a PCL reconstruction to avoid putting any potential significant increased stress on the healing graft.

At weeks 4–6, the patient is initiated on a program of range of motion. Immobilizers are still worn for protection whenever the patient is up and out of bed. We continue to work on active and active assisted range of motion to 90° during this time period. The patient works on performing straight-leg raises (done in the immobilizer), quadriceps sets, hip extension and hip abduction exercises. After 6 weeks, the patient works on weaning themselves off crutches and achieving a normal gait pattern. By 3 months postoperatively, the patient should have achieved 125° flexion. The use of a stationary bicycle is initiated once 115° knee flexion is achieved. At 3 months postoperatively, the patient may initiate a walking program as well as the use of a stairmaster. Patients may progress functionally in activities with attempts to avoid patellofemoral irritation by 4 months postoperatively. They may progress to a jogging program between months 3 and 4 based on their overall quadriceps strength. Pivoting sports are avoided for 6 months, with no contact sports allowed for 9 months.

Posterolateral knee injuries

Treatment of isolated posterolateral knee injuries

The recommended treatment protocol for partial posterolateral knee injuries, which includes grade I and grade II instabilities, is primarily non-surgical. The program of immobilization of the knee in full extension and either an immobilizer or a plaster of Paris cast for 3 weeks may be followed by a progressive functional rehabilitation program similar to that which would be performed for an MCL complex injury. Those patients who have functional limitations after this treatment program should be carefully evaluated to determine whether they have residual varus instability or rotational abnormalities, which are contributing to their lack of function. In this instance, surgical repair of the torn structures may be indicated [14].

The treatment of grade III posterolateral knee complex injuries is almost uniformly surgical. Patients who do have grade III posterolateral knee corner injuries treated non-surgically, or with a cast, have been shown to do poorly [75]. Surgical repair is recommended as soon as possible after injuries to enhance the identification of the torn structures, prior to the onset of scar tissue planes. This handling also provides good structures to hold the sutures. After the initial 2 weeks, scar tissue planes develop which make it more difficult to identify the normal anatomy. In addition, identification of the peroneal nerve would be greatly complicated by these scar tissue planes which could add time to the surgical repair. It is helpful to break down the zone of injury for posterolateral knee injuries in attempts to determine where to perform the repair. Avulsions of either the popliteus tendon or the fibular collateral ligament off the femur are best repaired with a recess procedure. The popliteal recess procedure may be more useful than attempted direct suturing to bone or suture anchors, as these repairs tend to get more lax over time. In the recess procedure, a small tunnel is drilled at the anatomic location of the attachment site of the injured structure with an eyelet pin threaded out which exits on the medial aspect of the femur, proximal to the adductor tubercle region. A whipstitch-type repair is then placed into the avulsed structure, the sutures are then placed into the eyelet and the guide pin is then pulled out medially on the femur. The sutures can then be tied medially on the femur with the use of a surgical button. It is important to aim proximally when drilling this guide pin to exit on the anteromedial aspect of the distal femur such that the guide pin does not enter through the intercondylar notch. Tears of the mid-third lateral capsular ligament or the lateral gastrocnemius tendon off the femur can be repaired with suture anchors.

Tears of the meniscotibial portion of the mid-third lateral capsular ligament or the anterior arm of the short head of the biceps femoris, or the components of the iliotibial band off the lateral aspect of the tibia, can easily be repaired either directly to bone or with suture anchors in this location. It is important to attempt to put these structures back into their anatomic position prior to repair. We have found the bone to be relatively soft in this area and often the needle can be placed directly through the bone for purposes of repair such that suture anchors are not necessary.

The other type of common anatomic injury is avulsion of structures off the fibular head and styloid. This would include the popliteofibular ligament, direct arms of the long and short head of the biceps femoris, and the fibular collateral ligament. Due to the hard cortical bone of the fibula in this location, we have found that suture anchors allow for anatomic replacement of the structures and good secure repair. In those cases where the fibular styloid has an avulsion fracture (arcuate avulsion), it can be repaired by either an open reduction and internal fixation or a cerclage nonabsorbable suture or wire.

The repair of the structures should be sufficient to ensure that early range of motion (ROM) can be initiated without compromise of the postoperative stability. Occasionally, a period of cast immobilization is necessary in those patients in whom the structures that have been sutured have tenuous fixation. In those patients who need cast immobilization, we recommend that casting be performed at 60° knee flexion with the tibia internally rotated. In other words, in order to make sure that there is no external rotation of the tibia on the femur in the cast during this period of immobilization, we place a dowel rod at the foot of the cast, which is positioned to prevent external rotation. Weight-bearing is not allowed for the first 6 weeks after surgical repair and work with these patients primarily involves a program of ROM. In addition, they are allowed to perform straight-leg raises in the knee immobilizer during this period. Their progressive strengthening exercises are slowly progressed after the tissues have healed at 6 weeks if the clinical examination seems to indicate that repair has healed. In addition, the use of the hamstrings is minimized for the first 4 months after surgery due to the perceived deleterious effect of hamstring firing on posterolateral corner repairs.

The treatment of chronic isolated grade III posterolateral corner injuries requires a more thorough workup than the acute situation. First, it is recognized that patients who have underlying genu varus alignment with grade III chronic posterolateral rotatory terrain instability need a full-length standing radiograph of the affected extremity to make sure that there is no varus malalignment. If there is, we recommend that a proximal tibial opening wedge osteotomy be performed to restore the mechanical access to the downslope of the lateral tibial spine. It is well recognized that the failure of the clinician to recognize the genu varus and to perform an osteotomy in these cases often results in a failure of the repair or reconstruction because the resultant varus thrust gait will cause the tissues to stretch over time.

Although chronic injuries to the posterolateral corner structures can occasionally have an anatomic repair, it has been recognized that there is frequently a return of instability in joint laxity in many of these patients over time. Therefore, reconstructions of these posterolateral knee complex injuries have been devised to attempt to restore stability for these injured anatomic structures.

A primary repair cannot be performed in the chronic situation if the posterolateral structures are deficient. In such cases a biceps tenodesis or an allograft reconstruction have been utilized in attempt to reproduce the normal function of the fibular collateral ligament in the popliteus–popliteofibular ligament complex. Most of the current procedures used attempt to create a soft tissue sling to inhibit varus opening and/or external rotation. However, it must be recognized that this is an extremely difficult knee instability problem with a large learning curve for the individual surgeon. Therefore, there is no clear-cut answer as to which technique would work best in the individual patient.

The biceps tenodesis procedure [19] attempts to reconstruct a portion of the fibular collateral ligament by taking all or a portion of the common biceps tendon and transferring it just proximally and anterior to the lateral epicondyle. The biceps tenodesis procedure has been shown to overconstrain the knee somewhat in external rotation and then there is some concern as to its long-term effect on the knee. In addition, it has been recommended that this procedure only be performed in those cases in which the capsular arm and the capsulosseous confluence layers of the short head of the biceps femoris have not been injured. Since this occurs in less than 25% of cases other options for surgical reconstruction should be thought out in advance.

Some authors have advocated an osteotomy of the femoral attachments of the lateral head, gastrocnemius, fibular collateral ligament, mid-third lateral capsular ligament and popliteus tendon origin in attempt to perform an advancement of these structures and restore normal tension of these structures on the posterolateral aspect of the knee. In this technique, a square or rectangular-shaped piece of bone is osteotomized off the distal lateral femur with the above-noted attachments and advanced proximally and anteriorly and then held in place with some type of internal fixation (usually a four-pronged bone staple).

Allograft reconstruction of chronic posterolateral corner knee injuries is often necessary to reconstruct the deficient native injured anatomic structures. There are a large variety of these techniques which attempt to duplicate the normal function of the popliteus ten-

don complex and/or the fibular collateral ligament (R. F. LaPrade, personal communication). One or both of these structures may be reconstructed depending upon whether the patient's primary instability problem is varus and/or external rotation. The main goal behind all of these reconstructions is to provide an increased tissue mass of appropriate strength to make up for the poor quality of the injured native structures.

Treatment of combined grade III posterolateral knee injuries and other ligament ruptures of the knee

In the acute injury situation, it is recommended that a primary repair of the injured grade III posterolateral corner structures be performed at the same time as a repair or reconstruction of the other ligamentous structures within the first 1–2 weeks after injury. All structures should be either repaired or reconstructed in one sitting rather than using a staged surgical technique. While a period of immobilization may be necessary in some instances because of the poor quality of tissues repaired with sutures, in the majority of cases an early ROM program is instituted to prevent the onset of arthrofibrosis which can commonly occur in multiligament knee injuries. This is especially important when there are concurrent medial collateral ligament complex injuries present. The majority of chronic posterolateral corner injuries occur in combination with an ACL or PCL tear. Once it has been determined that these patients do not have underlying varus alignment, the decision must be made to proceed with either a repair or reconstruction of the injured posterolateral corner structures at the same time as the cruciate ligament reconstruction procedures. It has been demonstrated that a failure to repair the posterolateral corner structures at the time of the cruciate ligament reconstruction results in a significant increase in a force on the cruciate ligament graft which could potentially lead to its failure [12,23]. In addition, an examination under anesthesia must be performed prior to the fixation of the cruciate ligament grafts. The grafts will overconstrain the knee and hide any potential residual posterolateral instability if the knees are examined immediately after cruciate ligament fixation. In these instances, the examiner may be misled into believing that the posterolateral reconstruction may not need to be performed. The type of primary repair or surgical reconstruction is similar to that described in the previous section.

The rehabilitation principles that are followed with combined posterolateral and other ligament repairs of the knee depend on the overall quality of the tissue repair. It is desirable to start a program of early ROM in these knees. Commonly, the knee is put through a full ROM prior to skin closure to determine the point at which there may be increasing tension on the posterolateral corner repair. If the patient cannot achieve a full ROM, or is limited in deep flexion, the patient will then be placed into a hinged knee brace which would be locked within the limits of the patient's ROM. In addition, a program may be instituted using a continuous passive motion (CPM) machine for these patients. In these instances, the patient is placed into a hinged knee brace such that the CPM does not stretch out the repair when we feel that the repair may be stretched out past a certain range of motion. If the motion needs to be limited, the CPM is commonly utilized for 3 weeks in attempt to increase the program of ROM such that full motion is achieved by 6 weeks after surgery. The patients are kept non-weight-bearing for the first 6–8 weeks after surgery to allow time for the posterolateral corner structures to heal. Patients are initiated in a program of quadriceps sets and straight-leg raises in their knee immobilizer (only) for the first 6 weeks. An exercise bike program may be initiated at weeks 6–8 if their ROM allows it. Commonly a patient will be instructed to start by simply cycling and not trying to put any resistance on the exercise bike. Patients are allowed to initiate gentle leg presses at 2 months after surgery. Active hamstring exercises are avoided for the first 3 months postoperatively because of the potential deleterious effects of the hamstring muscles firing on the posterolateral corner repairs or reconstructions. At approximately 2 months after surgery, patients are allowed to progress to the rehabilitation protocol according to the principles of the other combined ligament reconstructions in the knee.

Overuse injuries

Introduction

Tendon overuse injury, often called tendinitis, is a common problem in both sports and industry. Data

from the Bureau of Labor Statistics (1988) indicate that tendon overuse injuries account for 48% of reported occupational illness. Also, in a large European sports clinic, a quarter of all athletes treated for knee disorders were diagnosed with tendon overuse injury [83]. Clinically, the treatment of tendon disease has been largely empirical. Typical treatment protocols include combination of relative rest, therapeutic exercise, modalities such as electrical stimulation and ultrasound and non-steroidal anti-inflammatory drugs (NSAIDs). Guidelines have been published in an attempt to direct treatment, but with little scientific data to support them [84]. In this section, current understanding of the etiology and pathology of tendon overuse injury will be reviewed with a focus on the patellar tendon. This will be followed by a discussion of non-invasive imaging techniques for diagnosis of tendon overuse injuries. Then, both the *in vivo* and *in vitro* studies that have attempted to elucidate cellular mechanism of tendon overuse injury will be presented. Finally, future directions of research on tendon overuse injury will be suggested.

Etiology of tendon overuse injury

In spite of the high incidence of tendon overuse injury, the etiology of this disease is unclear. The incidence of patellar tendon overuse injury also varies within the tendon. In the order of frequency, the incidence has by some authors been found to be 81% in the infrapatellar insertion, 13% in the tuberosity and 6% in the quadriceps patellar insertion site [85]. It has been generally believed that tendon overuse injury is related to cumulative trauma on tendons by repetitive mechanical loading. In addition, the effect of mechanical loading on tendons can be adversely impacted by intrinsic factors, including malalignment, inflexibility and muscle weakness or imbalance. The combination of these factors can cause a large magnitude of load, a high frequency of load, or both, on tendons during normal activities. Other etiologic factors include age-related degeneration of the tendon and decreased vascular supply to the tendon [86]. In patients with chronic tendon problems, histologic examination reveals degenerative tendons without apparent inflammatory changes within the tendons. Nevertheless, it is possible that the tendons may have undergone inflammation when they are first injured. This is because most biopsy specimens were obtained only after the tendon failed to heal after a prolonged non-surgical treatment; the phase of the tendon inflammation may have already passed.

Therefore, it seems that the etiology in chronic tendon injuries is multifactorial. However, these factors may not play an equal role in different individuals. For example, in young athletes with healthy tendons, repetitive mechanical loading of the patellar tendon may be the major factor for tendon overuse injury, whereas in aging patients a sedentary lifestyle combined with pre-existing tendon degeneration may contribute to the tendon becoming symptomatic. On the other hand, all explosive start–stop or jump sports, such as basketball, volleyball and soccer, predispose the participants to tendon overuse injury in the knee. Deceleration and jumping entail eccentric muscle contraction, which results in tension that would be much greater than with concentric muscle contraction. As a result, if the large contraction is repeated, tendon microstructure damages are likely to occur.

Pathologies of tendon overuse injury

Many researchers have tried to distinguish the pathology between the acute traumatic inflammatory response and the more insidious process of chronic tendon degeneration. Consistent findings include mucoid degeneration and fibrinoid necrosis within the tendon. Microtearing and areas of repair with proliferation of the tendon fibroblasts and thin-walled vessels can also be observed [85]. Leadbetter [86] reported the following features of specimens from many types of tendons including the patellar tendon: (i) hyperplasia of tendon fibroblasts; (ii) morphologic change of the tendon fibroblasts from the linelike to blastlike; (iii) small vessel ingrowth with accompanying mesenchymal cells; (iv) perivascular collections of macrophage-like cells; (v) endothelial hyperplasia and microvascular thrombosis; (vi) collagen fiber disorganization with mixed reparation and degenerative change; and (vii) collagen fiber microtear and separation. In addition, there are other changes. For example, quadriceps atrophy occurs as a secondary effect of the tendon overuse injury [85].

Diagnosis of tendon overuse injuries with imaging techniques

Magnetic resonance imaging (MRI), ultrasonography and computerized tomography (CT) are non-invasive techniques able to visualize tendon structures. Therefore, it is possible to use these tools to identify the location of tendon overuse injury. MRI offers clear soft tissue contrast and direct sagittal imaging [87]. Hence, patellar tendon structures can also be clearly imaged with MRI. Ultrasonography is one of the most efficient and effective ways of imaging the tendons. It provides an accurate anatomic picture that allows for greater specificity in treating patellar tendon overuse injury [88]. Hence, this technique makes it possible for clinicians to determine where tendinosis, a degenerative change in extracellular matrix of a tendon, or partial tears are present in persistently symptomatic tendons not responding to non-surgical intervention.

NSAIDs for treatment of tendon overuse injury

An early study showed that NSAIDs were able to inhibit the production of prostaglandins [89]. It is now thought that the mechanism of action by NSAIDs is through inhibiting cyclooxygenase (COX), which is the key enzyme for the formation of prostaglandins from arachidonic acid. Recently, two COX isoforms have been discovered. These are COX-1 and COX-2, which are variably expressed in different tissues. COX-1 is expressed constitutively in most tissues throughout the body, including the gastrointestinal mucosa [90], whereas COX-2 is induced mainly at inflammation sites. Furthermore, unlike COX-1, COX-2 can be up-regulated at inflammatory sites by cytokines and bacterial products such as lipopolysaccharides [91].

There are three types of NSAIDs: (i) COX-1 selective; (ii) COX-2 selective; and (iii) non-selective. Clinically, there is an enormous interest in using COX-2 selective NSAIDs to treat inflammatory conditions, particularly because COX-1 selective and non-selective NSAIDs often result in gastric and intestinal ulcers. Studies have shown that NS-398, rofecoxib and celecoxib, which are recently developed COX-2 selective NSAIDs, can achieve an anti-inflammatory effect on gastric biopsies [90], and an analgesic effect on postdental surgery pain [92] and on pain from

Table 6.2.5 Overview of common overuse problems of the knee.

Most common	Less common	Do not miss
Anterior knee pain including PFSS		Malignant tumors
Cartilage lesions including degenerative arthritis	Fat pad syndrome	
Jumper's knee	Osteochondritis dissecans	
Quadriceps tendinitis	Popliteus tendinitis	
Biceps tendinitis		
Meniscal tears	Runner's knee/iliotibial band friction syndrome	
Bursitis		
Plica syndrome		
Mb. Osgood–Schlatter–Johansson		
Mb. Sinding–Larsen		
Popliteal artery entrapment		
Saphenous nerve entrapment		

PFSS, patellofemoral pain syndrome; Mb, morbus.

osteoarthritis [93]. However, the efficacy of these drugs for the treatment of tendon overuse injuries is yet to be determined.

Differential diagnoses

An overview of the usual diagnoses is seen in Table 6.2.5. Most common are meniscal injuries, jumper's knee and patellofemoral arthralgia. Meniscal injuries and patellofemoral pain syndrome (PFPS) are covered in other parts of this chapter.

Patellar tendinitis (jumper's knee)

Jumper's knee, as an adult form of the Sinding–Larsen-Johansson disease, may occur due to an acute partial tear or overuse, but usually a good medical history will detect one specific event leading to later pain. The syndrome is characterized by tenderness at the inferior pole of the patella. This problem usually occurs in sports characterized by a high number of maximal jumps and sprints. Out of 47 elite division volleyball players, 25 players fulfilled the diagnostic criteria of jumper's knee [94]. The histopathologic changes described include tearing of tendon fibers, myxomatous degeneration and capillary proliferation [49,95,96]. Clinically, jumper's knee can be classified into four grades, originally described by Roels *et al.* [96] and modified by Lian *et al.* [94] (Table 6.2.6). According to Ferretti [95], the insertional tendinopathy affects, in order of frequency, the insertion of the patellar tendon into the patella in 65% of cases, the at-

Table 6.2.6 Classification of jumper's knee according to symptoms as outlined by Roels *et al.* [96] and current classification system.

Roels *et al.*	Current classification
Grade I	
Pain at the infrapatellar or suprapatellar region after practice or after an event	Same
Grade II	
Pain at the beginning of the activity, disappearing after warm-up and reappearing after completion of activity	Same
Grade III	
Pain remains during and after activity and the patient is unable to participate in sports	IIIa: Pain during and after activity, but the patient is able to participate in sports at the same level
	IIIb: Pain during and after activity and the patient is unable to participate in sports at the same level
Grade IV	
Complete rupture of the tendon	Same

tachment of the quadriceps tendon into the patella in 25%, and the insertion into the tibial tubercle in 15%.

Symptoms and signs

The athlete often has a small, but significant acute trauma in the history. An epidemiologic study of volleyball players showed that half the players had had symptoms of the syndrome. The study also suggested that the players with the highest jumps were the ones most susceptible to the problem. Typical symptoms are pain when reducing speed or trying to make a quick stop, landing after a jump and walking downstairs, and ultimately it becomes difficult to run and play. Most patients do well in biking and swimming. The history can be classified according to Lian *et al.* [94] (Table 6.2.6).

Diagnosis

The diagnosis is based on the history and clinical findings. During physical examination, marked tenderness is detected at the insertion site of the patellar tendon on the patella. This finding is furthermore reinforced if the patella is pushed in the distal direction with the finger of the examiner palpating the insertion site of the tendon on the distal pole of the patella. Ultrasonography and MRI strengthen the diagnosis. As recently shown, however, the correlation between ultrasonography and clinical findings is not good [94,97].

Treatment options

Treatment is conservative, including eccentric exercises for at least 3 months. If a well-supervised conservative treatment program fails, surgical excision of the necrotic part of the patellar tendon is indicated. However, only 30–60% [98] of competitive athletes return to their original sporting level. Both arthroscopic and open patellar tenotomy provide symptomatic pain relief in most patients with end-stage patellar tendinopathy. After open patellar tenotomy, MRI and ultrasound findings remain abnormal despite clinical recovery. Thus, clinicians should base postoperative management of patients undergoing patellar tenotomy on clinical grounds rather than imaging findings (Fig. 6.2.20).

No consensus exists on the treatment of jumper's knee. The consensus at the moment seems to be that a

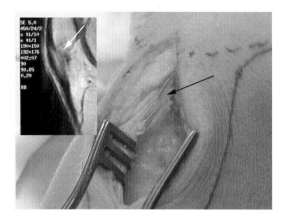

Fig. 6.2.20 Intraoperative appearance of the necrotic patellar tendon in an 18-year-old handball player who had had jumper's knee for 2 years and in whom conservative treatment had failed. Appearance of the granuloma on MRI inserted.

small tear in collagen fibers is followed by a short inflammatory phase. Theoretically, NSAIDs should be effective in the acute phase, but there are no clinical studies confirming this. The inflammatory phase is followed by a degenerative phase where there are very few inflammatory cells in the injured area. In this phase the goal is to rebuild the tendon, and recent literature suggest that eccentric training over a period of 12 weeks or more may be efficient. So far, good studies comparing a rehabilitation program with eccentric exercises to surgery have not been published.

The prognosis for returning to sport is not favorable, as mentioned above. However, patellar tendinitis does not lead to major arthritis or disability. On the other hand, it may lead to the retirement of the player from sports involving jumping and fast running.

Quadriceps tendinitis

Tendinitis at the quadriceps tendon insertion into the proximal pole of the patella might seem to be a situation similar to that of patellar tendinitis, although much less frequent. This author has seen this primarily in volleyball players, hockey goalies, cyclists and weight lifters. In each case, the player has developed a major eccentric force leading to a partial tear at the insertion site of the tendon. This leads to an inflammatory reaction followed by a repair phase.

Diagnosis

Tenderness to direct palpation is the only clinical finding. This finding can be substantiated by ultrasonography or MRI which often needs contrast to reveal a small tendon tear.

Treatment options

Treatment should follow the same protocol as jumper's knee. In the acute phase NSAIDs and RICE (Rest, Ice, Compression, Elevation) should reduce the inflammation. In the chronic phase the goal is to rebuild collagen fibers. This seems to be successfully achieved with an eccentric training protocol in the majority of cases. If the pain is still there after 12–26 weeks, surgical excision of the degenerative area may be chosen. There is only one study available (four patients) on the results after surgical treatment [95] and no conclusions can be drawn based on this. The general feeling is that recovery is faster than after surgery for patellar tendinitis and probably more successful.

Popliteal tendinitis

The muscle and tendon of the popliteal complex is both an active structure involved in tibia inward and forward rotation and a passive restraint preventing posterolateral instability. The tendon is most often irritated and injured in athletes involved in downhill running such as marathoners or cross-country racers.

Diagnosis

This is a clinical diagnosis, although increased signals due to inflammation may be picked up on MRI. Pain is usually localized to the insertion site of the tendon on the popliteal groove on the femur, which is easiest to palpate in the figure-of-four position. It occurs mainly during weight-bearing with the knee flexed between 15 and 30° or during the early part of the swing phase of gait. The onset is usually insidious with no history of acute injury. Typically, the distance runner will report pain after 4–5 km preventing him or her from continuing the run. The main diagnostic task is to differentiate popliteal tendinitis from biceps tendinitis, iliotibial friction syndrome, lateral meniscal tears or lateral cartilage tears.

Treatment options

No studies have shown structural damage to the popliteal tendon with tendinitis. Consequently anti-inflammatory medication should theoretically be effective, as should a corticosteroid injection. The main treatment modality is, however, training modification. In first few 2–3 weeks the athlete should use alternative training methods on the bike or in the pool; he or she should make training changes such as running uphill or changing the side of the road or the direction run on a track.

Runner's knee — iliotibial band syndrome

Iliotibial band (ITB) syndrome is an overuse injury caused by excessive friction between the ITB and the lateral femoral epicondyle as the knee is flexed and extended. In extension the ITB lies anterior to the lateral epicondyle of the femur. As the knee flexes, the tendon passes over the condyle. Due to the excessive friction here, a bursa is often developed which secondarily gets inflamed. The ITB is often described as tight in affected athletes. Many of these athletes also have increased pronation, genu varum and increased tibial torsion.

The clinical findings are pain on palpation, and often crepitation and aggravation on running downhill or downstairs. A diagnostic anesthesia blockade will help in pinpointing the area of maximum tenderness. A radiograph should be obtained to rule out other causes of pain. Treatment consists of advice on alternative training and stretching. Orthoses are usually prescribed based on the form of the foot. A cortisone injection is often carried out and is documented to achieve good results in this diagnosis. If no improvement occurs after 6 months of conservative treatment, surgery is sometimes resorted to [99]. The procedure is simple and consists of decreasing the friction between the tendon and the condyle by making a 'window' in the tendon and removing the inflamed bursa. The reported results have been encouraging.

Bursitis

A bursa is a sac with a synovial-like lining that functions to reduce friction and protect structures from pressure. These sacs may be inflamed, infected or traumatized, with a hematoma as a frequent result.

The most frequent bursitis is that of the prepatellar bursa located anterior to the distal half of the patella. This is seen frequently in wrestlers and team handball players when the fronts of their knees hit the floor during matches. The other frequent bursitis around the knee is pes anserinus bursitis. The bursa is located between the aponeurosis of the three-hamstring tendon insertion and the medial collateral ligament, approximately 5 cm below the joint line. Treatment consists of training guidance, anti-inflammatory medication including corticosteroid injections, and occasionally surgical removal of the inflamed bursa.

Future directions

To help understand the biologic mechanisms of tendon overuse injury, several lines of future research are suggested. With the advent of gene-chip technologies [100], the differential expression of multiple genes in the tendon fibroblasts when subjected to repetitive mechanical loading could be examined. This approach has the potential to identify specific genes, and their products (proteins) that are involved in the onset and progression of tendon overuse injury. With this knowledge, novel targets for intervention of the disease can then be developed. Another approach involves the development of an organ culture system, in which tendons from experimental animals are placed in growth medium and are cyclically stretched. In this way, the biologic responses of the tendons can be studied in a well-controlled environment. The organ culture system can also potentially be used to evaluate the effects of various NSAIDs and steroids on tendon structure and function, and provide a scientific basis for evaluation of the efficacy of NSAIDs in the treatment of tendon overuse injuries. Once the mechanisms of the tendon overuse injury are better understood, the creation of animal models of tendon overuse injury would become more useful and realistic. In the final analysis, the treatment protocol for tendon overuse injuries can be developed and optimized on a scientific basis.

The patellofemoral joint

Patellofemoral pain syndrome (PFPS)—anterior knee pain

Symptoms and signs
See Table 6.2.7.

Diagnosis
The diagnosis of PFPS is made if the patient has three of the symptoms listed in Table 6.2.7. The diagnosis is clinical; a radiograph, CT scan or MRI will not give further information. The diagnosis of chondromalacia during an arthroscopic procedure is inconclusive. Many patients without any symptoms from the patellofemoral joint may have chondromalacia on their patella and patients with major patellofemoral pain may have normal cartilage under arthroscopic examination.

Treatment
The patient will be referred to a physical therapist for a program of strength and proprioceptive training.

Table 6.2.7 Overview of typical history of patients with patellofemoral (PF) pain syndrome.

Usual history	Mechanism	Comments
Pain on stair climbing (usually downwards)	Eccentric use of the extensor apparatus results in creation of high forces in the PF joint	Most painful in patients with established osteoarthritis in the PF joint
Pain on squatting	May be able to go down, but cannot rise without help	
Pain when driving a car	Increased pressure in the PF joint?	
Pain when sitting at a movie		
Pain on deceleration	Increased forces on the PF joint	Most usual in patients with pathology in the patellar tendon

The basic rehabilitation principles for the patellofemoral joint are to restore the normal balance between the quadriceps and hamstring muscle groups. This must be done in balance with how the joint responds to a particular exercise program.

One of the first basic principles in addressing rehabilitation for the quadriceps mechanism is to make sure that the patient is on an appropriate hamstring stretching program. The role that tight hamstrings can play in increasing the force on the anterior aspect of the knee, and thus causing anterior knee pain, is often not given appropriate recognition by physicians and therapists alike. When a patient shows signs of hamstring bursal irritation, it is important that they be placed on an appropriate hamstring stretching program. This includes stretching several times daily. In the more severe cases, we often recommend an hourly stretching program. Patients must be taught that they can stretch in almost any environment, as long as they keep their ankle dorsiflexed, their knee straight, and their back straight.

Rehabilitation of the quadriceps mechanism primarily involves the use of closed-chain quadriceps exercises. In the majority of cases, even when patients participate in a regular physical therapy exercise program, patients need to engage in a regular exercise program for maintenance at home. Patients should work on quadriceps setting exercises, straight-leg raises, leg presses (preferably with the knees not bent past 70° knee flexion), squats and the use of an exercise bike. The patients are recommended to set the seat height of their exercise slightly higher than normal in their initial usage of the bike if they have any patellofemoral discomfort. The preferred seat height is to have the lower leg flexed to approximately 15° when the foot is on the pedal. It is recommended to start cycling for 5 min with no resistance on alternating days. If there is no patellofemoral discomfort created with this, patients can proceed to a cycling program on a daily basis. The amount of time on the bike can be increased in 5-min increments every few days or weeks, depending on the patient's symptoms. Once the patient is able to tolerate 20 min on the exercise bike, we recommend that they return to 5 min biking and increase the resistance. The amount of time on the bike is then increased up to 20 min again and the cycle is repeated. Patients should strive to achieve a workout whereby they can use the exercise bike for 20 min at a tolerable resistance several times a week [15].

Another form of treatment recommended for patients with significant patellofemoral discomfort and atrophy is a hydrotherapy program. While this may not be available to many patients, pool walking is an excellent form of low-impact energy exercising for these patients. Patients can start out by walking pool lengths in waist-high water, and then can progress to deeper lengths as tolerated. In addition, if the patient can wear a personal flotation device, they can work on walking or jogging on the spot at the deep end of the pool as an excellent source of low-impact exercises.

Open-chain quadriceps exercises are seldom recommended because of the added pressure that they place on the anterior aspect of the knee. Knee extension exercises can cause significant irritation of the patellofemoral joint. The preference is to avoid them in these patients. These exercises should be reserved for the terminal phases of rehabilitation and elite-level athletes, or for sports participants who have no evidence of any patellofemoral arthritis or other abnormalities.

Many of these patients experience major feelings of pain at the start of their rehabilitation program. Often it is difficult for the patient even to step down from a height. The majority of these patients will have developed hip, especially abductor muscle, weakness and rehabilitation on this is needed in addition. These patients are often aided by the use of a special tape that may improve patellar alignment. A special program emphasizing this technique is used by many therapists although the science behind it is limited.

Patellar dislocation

Patellar dislocations are usually caused by a traumatic event. Typically, the patella is hit on the medial side by a pole in skiing or by an opponent in contact sports. The patella always dislocates laterally. At the time of dislocation, the patella may hit the lateral femoral epicondyle resulting in a small fracture of most often the medial facet of the patella. The dislocation is painful and frequently requires anesthesia for relocation. Due to extensive tears of the medial ligament stabilizing the patella, a large hemarthrosis is usually seen. Treatment consists of relocating the patella and immobilizing it in a brace for 4–6 weeks. If the patient is young (<25), recurrent dislocations may occur. A patellofemoral brace may reduce the number of redislocations, as will proper strength in the extensor apparatus, specifically the vastus medialis obliquus, but only surgery has been shown to prevent redislocations. Today the torn structures are usually repaired. In cases where malalignment of the extensor apparatus is found, a distal–proximal realignment may be the surgery of choice.

Knee pain in adolescents

The structures in and around the knee are frequently injured in children in athletics as a result of chronic overuse and the special anatomic and morphologic situations in the growing adolescent. This section will focus on common causes of knee pain in the adolescent, but will also emphasize the importance of tumors and referred pain in the diagnostic approach. Traumatic, acute disorders have been covered in the previous sections.

Knee pain in adolescents has many etiologies and the clinician must also rule out rare entities (e.g. tumor, referred pain) to establish a thorough diagnosis. Although meniscal injuries are less common in children than in adults, several recent reports indicate an increasing incidence of meniscal lesions in children and adolescents, especially those in competitive sports. De Inocencio [101] investigated the distribution of musculoskeletal pain in children. The knee was the most affected joint (33%), followed by other joints (e.g. ankle, wrist, elbow, in 28%), soft tissue pain (18%), heel pain (8%), hip pain (6%) and back pain (6%). Symptoms were caused by trauma in 30%; overuse syndromes in 28% (e.g. chondromalacia patellae, mechanical plantar fasciitis, overuse muscle pain); and normal skeletal growth variants (e.g. Osgood–Schlatter syndrome, hypermobility, Sever's disease) in 18% of patients. Sources of chronic pain about the knee may include tendinitis, apophysitis, patellofemoral malalignment and maltracking, quadriceps dysfunction, hamstring contracture, neural dysfunction, vascular dysfunction, pathologic plica, cartilage degeneration, meniscal tears, and also benign and malign tumors around the knee. Special consideration must be given to the possibility of referred knee pain, e.g. from slipped capital femoral epiphysis.

Compared to adults the long bones in children are able to absorb more energy before breaking, and the presence of growth plates and apophyses for the attachment of musculotendinous structures leads to a different spectrum of injuries compared with those in adults. Both epiphyses and apophyses have physes that grow and develop by enchondral ossification. Apophyses have physes similar to epiphyses, but in contrast to epiphyses do not participate in longitudinal growth, are usually not perpendicular to the long axis of bone, are not articular, and are subjected to tension forces rather than to compression.

The reason for knee pain in children is often difficult to establish and depends on an experienced physician. The history and clinical examination are crucial, as is the correct choice of additional diagnostic investigations. This section discusses the most frequent causes of knee pain in children.

Extensor apparatus

Osgood–Schlatter disease

According to Sponseller and Beaty, Paget described in 1891 the clinical symptoms which later became known as Osgood–Schlatter disease (OS). In 1903, Osgood [102] and Schlatter published separate papers on the avulsion phenomena of the tibial tubercle. OS is thought to result from submaximal, repetitive, tensile stresses acting on the immature junction of the patellar tendon, tibial tubercle and tibia, causing mild avulsion injuries followed by attempts of osseous repair. The symptoms usually start during a rapid growth phase. In girls, the condition tends to appear at an earlier age—11–13 years—than in boys who usually present 1–2 years later [103]. Boys are more commonly affected than girls, but the prevalence in girls is increasing because of their increased participation in sports activity. In a group of athletic adolescents, Kujala *et al.* [103] found a 21% prevalence of OS, while in a group of non-athletes the prevalence was only 4.5%. Usually one side is more symptomatic and the tibial tubercle may become prominent. In 20–30% of patients both sides are symptomatic. Swelling and prominence of the tibial tubercle can be found on clinical examination, accompanied by exquisite local tenderness. The pain is usually made worse by climbing stairs, running and jumping. Radiographs are essential to rule out a bone tumor or other rare disorders. Approximately

50% show a discrete, separate ossicle at the tibial tubercle [104]. This fragment is cartilaginous initially and may ossify later. Krause *et al.* [104] described patients who presented with fragmentation of or an abnormally shaped apophysis, and had abnormal tibial tubercles on follow-up examination after an average of 9 years. These patients were much more likely to have chronic symptoms.

Treatment should be based on the symptoms. Immature athletes with open physes should be treated with guided activity limitations and in a few cases with partial immobilization (no casting) for a period of 6 weeks or until the tubercle apophysis is no longer tender. Be aware that this group may have a physeal injury in the area — a so-called Ogden lysis [105,106]. In these acute traumatic avulsions of the tibial tuberosity, pain and swelling occur immediately and standing or walking is impossible. However, open reduction and internal fixation may be necessary, depending on the displacement and type of avulsion fracture (Fig. 6.2.21).

For the skeletally mature patient with OS disease a treatment regimen consisting of rest, training modification, ice and oral anti-inflammatory drugs will be helpful. Tenderness is a sign of inflammation, and with pain relief strengthening and flexibility exercises are started. Surgery may be indicated for the adult patient with chronic OS disease, multiple ossicles and failed conservative treatment, when excision of symptomatic ossicles may lead to pain relief. This ossi-

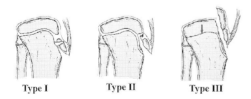

Type I   Type II   Type III

Fig. 6.2.21 Traumatic avulsions of the tibial tuberosity. In type I the avulsion fracture involves the secondary ossification center, in type II the proximal tibial epiphysis, and in type III the fracture passes proximally and posteriorly accross the epiphyseal plate and proximal articular surface of the tibia. (From Roberts JM. Fractures and dislocations of the knee. In: Rockwood CA Jr, Wilkins KE, King RE (eds). *Fractures in Children.* Philadelphia: J.B. Lippincott Co., 1984, used with permission.)

cle resection can also be performed endoscopically [107].

Sinding–Larsen–Johansson disease

Sinding–Larsen-Johansson disease is usually seen in an active preteen boy with activity-related pain. Persistent traction on the cartilaginous junction of the patella and the patella tendon is thought to be the cause of this condition. Sometimes similar symptoms can be found at the insertion site of the quadriceps tendon into the patella. The main symptom is usually tenderness at the involved site. Radiographs may show varying amounts and shapes of calcification or ossification near the patellar apex. Medlar and Lyne [108] identified four radiographic stages of the disease process. Differential diagnosis includes a stress fracture of the patella, a sleeve fracture and a type I bipartite patella. In the older adolescent, an adult type of jumper's knee must be considered [109]. The symptoms usually resolve with progressive skeletal maturation. As in OS disease, adult patients who do not respond to conservative treatment may benefit from surgical debridement of the necrotic intratendinous tissue.

Patellofemoral pain syndrome — patellar overload syndrome

Many of the most difficult management problems in the adult knee are a result of ill-advised surgical interventions during youth [110]. Inappropriate surgery in patients diagnosed with patellofemoral malalignment is often the first episode in a series of surgical disasters. Fairbank *et al.* [111] found no correlation of an abnormality of q-angle, patellar height and patellar tilt in adolescents with and without knee pain. They concluded that chronic overloading, rather than faulty mechanics, is the dominant factor in the genesis of anterior knee pain in adolescent patients. Patellofemoral crepitus does not indicate knee pathology in adolescents. Abernethy *et al.* [112] found asymptomatic patellofemoral crepitus in more than 60%, only four (3%) having true chronic anterior knee discomfort. However, the treatment of 'patellofemoral dysfunction' requires patience. More than 90% of patients can be spared a surgical procedure by using conservative treatment, and 67% of patients will have no limitations and 25% only minimal limitations by 6 months to 2 years [113]. A directed isometric progressive resistance quadriceps program with iliotibial band and hamstring stretching exercises improved patients consistently in a study of O'Neill *et al.* [114]. The patellofemoral pain syndrome can also be caused by a deficiency in motor control. The vastus medialis muscle has been implicated because it is often underdeveloped in patients suffering anterior knee pain. Further support for a neural component derives from the observation that the deficit in torque production is seen only during eccentric exercises, and that training relieves pain [115].

Extensor apparatus overload is perhaps the most common cause of anterior knee pain. Pain is aggravated by activity and accompanied by mild swelling. The pain is more troubling because of its chronicity than because of its severity. Activities requiring increased hamstring contractions cause the characteristic anterior knee pain. Synovial thickening may be detected which was described by Eilert [116] as the 'silk' sign of synovitis. Growth is a common factor in anterior knee pain, because rapid increase of the extremity length is not always a balanced pattern. There are no correlations between mechanical disturbances and knee pain in children. In 90% the adolescent will recover within a year and should be encouraged to live a normal life. If the patient has developed strength deficit in the knee and hip, a rehabilitation program similar to the one outlined for adults should be instigated.

Bipartite patella
The frequency rate of bipartite patella has been reported to be as low as 0.05% to as high as 1.66%. Anatomically, bipartite patella is indistinguishable from a pseudarthrosis, with a cartilaginous bridge uniting the two fragments. In many respects it is similar to a synchondrosis. According to Saupe, three types of bipartite patella can be distinguished: in type I the second part is located at the inferior pole (5%), in type II at the lateral patellar margin (20%), and in type III at the superolateral pole (75%) [117]. Acute or chronic stress may make the junction site symptomatic. When the diagnosis of an acute fracture, a stress fracture and a dorsal patellar defect has been ruled out, the treatment depends on the severity of the symptoms. When symptoms persist despite conservative treatment, the entire fragment may be excised to eliminate the painful

pseudoarticulation [106,118,119]. Before such excision arthroscopic examination of the joint is appropriate. If the articular cartilage is normal, the fragment may be fixed.

Intra-articular disease

Osteochondritis dissecans (OD)
The disease was given its present name by König in 1877 in the belief that an inflammatory reaction to an injury is the underlying pathologic process. However, Paget called this disease 'quiet necrosis' and reported on it in 1870. Four main theoretical explanations of OD exist: (i) ischemia; (ii) endogenous trauma; (iii) exogenous trauma; and (iv) the constitutional theory. OD is a process whereby a segment of hyaline cartilage, together with subchondral bone, separates from the articular surface, and is most common in the knee. It occurs specifically in athletic boys between the ages of 10 and 20. The medial femoral condyle is affected in 85%, and the 'classic site' (i.e. lateroposterior position of the medial femoral condyle) in 69%. The patella is involved in approximately 5% [120] (Fig. 6.2.22). The early presentation is often inconclusive with knee pain, joint effusion and thigh atrophy. Giving way, catching or locking suggest separation of the fragment. OD can be diagnosed on routine radiographs, but MRI can detect whether the lesion is loose. A diagnostic test described by Wilson [121] produces pain when the knee is extended from 90° of flexion and thereby internally rotated. The reaction is explained by abutment of the ACL from its tibial attachment with the lesion on the medial femoral condyle. The goal of treatment should be to prevent partial or complete detachment of the lesion. Important factors in the natural history of OD include among others the patient's age and the status of physis. The natural history of OD is different in children and adults, and different in the medial and lateral femoral condyles [70]. Based on these variables patients with OD may be placed into three groups. Linden [122] found no complications of OD that could be related to the original condition in 23 patients who had the condition in childhood, and were re-examined an average of 33 years later. A more recent study of another 22 knees diagnosed before skeletal maturity was not quite so positive; the follow-up was

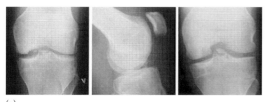

(a)

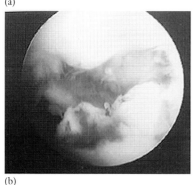

(b)

Fig. 6.2.22 Osteochondritis dissecans of the medial femoral condyle in an 18-year-old patient whose main problems were pain, catching and locking. (a) Plain radiographs (AP, lateral and tunnel view). (b) Arthroscopic appearance of a loose osteochondritis fragment.

33 years, and 32% showed moderate or severe arthritis [56]. The results were less favourable if the lesion was large and/or involved the lateral femoral condyle. Lesions in the classic area of the non-weight-bearing portion of the medial femoral condyle did well with simple excision. However, there is no published evidence at present to warrant an aggressive surgical or arthroscopic approach to OD in children, with the exception of large lesions involving the lateral femoral condyle.

The OD of the patella is less likely to heal than in other locations, and fixation has to be considered before total separation occurs. Separation of the fragment yields a poorer prognosis [123]. These lesions are described to be more common in males and in patients with open epiphysis and in the lateral patellofemoral compartment [124]. In approximately 30% the trochlea is involved, while in the other 60% the OD is located on the patella. At the follow-up examination 62% out of 25 patients achieved fair or poor results [123]. In children with a mean age of 11.4 years, de Ganzy *et al.* reported [125] that, without any treat-

ment, in all 31 cases of OD pain had disappeared and that in 30 of the 31 the OD was not detectable on a follow-up radiograph. Therefore they recommend no treatment for an osteochondritis dissecans in children.

Plica

The plicae are normal synovial folds whose function is probably to assist in lubrication of the femoral condyle, in the same way that an eyelid spreads tears over the eyeball. The symptomatic plica usually presents with a snapping or catching sensation and localized tenderness at the involved site. Synovial plicae of the knee have been suggested to be a cause of anterior pain in children and adolescents [126]. Flexion of the knee to 60° brings the plica into prominence. Inflammation and fibrosis, either from a single major incident or from repetitive microtrauma, causes thickening of the plica. According to Tindel *et al.* the plica syndrome is an uncommon pathologic entity diagnosed far too often in the setting of concomitant pathology [127]. Dorchak *et al.* [128] found 76 of nearly 2000 patients (4%) who underwent diagnostic arthroscopies to have thickened and/or fibrotic plicae. The diagnosis of the plica as the cause of knee pain is difficult and often one of exclusion. Conservative measures are very effective and must be emphasized before operative treatment. When arthroscopy is indicated, a thorough examination of the entire knee joint is necessary. When a pathologic plica is found, reports are available on success after their removal [127], but again no controlled studies exist.

Synovitis

Persistent swelling of the knee and generalized tenderness are signs of inflammatory synovitis. In the majority of cases, the cause of the synovitis is unknown and it is therefore characterized as reactive, often after a traumatic event. In pigmented villonodular synovitis and other types of synovitis, arthroscopic synovectomy has proved to be superior to open synovectomy in adolescents because of its lower incidence of postoperative stiffness. However, pigmented villonodular synovitis which is characterized by pain, swelling and hemarthrosis, recurs in approximately 50%. The test for rheumatoid factor is notoriously negative in children even with confirmed juvenile rheumatoid arthritis. There is no specific laboratory test diagnostic for rheumatoid arthritis. Positive antinuclear antibodies are found in 25% of children with juvenile rheumatoid arthritis, and rheumatoid factor is detected in less than 80%. Slit lamp examination of the eye for iridocyclitis is indicated if monarticular rheumatoid arthritis is suspected, as iridocyclitis is treatable and potentially very damaging. Iridocyclitis, the most severe extra-articular manifestation of juvenile rheumatoid arthritis, occurs in 10–15% of patients. A popliteal cyst (Baker's cyst) may also be an early manifestation of juvenile rheumatoid arthritis.

Meniscal injuries—discoid meniscus

Meniscus injuries occur in children at a much reduced rate compared to adults. The menisci assume their adult semilunar form by the 10th fetal week. During the remainder of growth, the menisci change in size but not in shape. Especially in the peripheral, the child's meniscus is more vascular, and blood vessels have been demonstrated to penetrate the inner zones even at the age of 13 years. Most reports on the meniscus in the adolescent deal with the discoid lateral meniscus [129–132]. When a congenital discoid lateral meniscus becomes symptomatic during childhood, the symptoms are variable and inconsistent. The classification of Watanabe in describing the discoid meniscus is widely accepted. There are three classes: an incomplete discoid meniscus, a complete discoid meniscus and the Wrisberg type. In a Wrisberg type of discoid meniscus total excision is indicated [133]. If a peripheral attachment is present, then a peripheral rim may be left. Hayashi *et al.* recommend a residual rim of 6–8 mm. A torn discoid meniscus may be excised and the meniscus reshaped to 'normal' anatomy. Meniscal injuries may also occur in children and adolescents (Fig. 6.2.23). Out of 166 arthroscopies 17% of the patients had a meniscal injury, while cartilage lesions were found in most patients [134]. In 92 knee arthroscopies, Maffulli *et al.* [135] found 10 meniscal tears in children with a mean age of 14.6 years. There is only a 56% chance of making a correct diagnosis on clinical grounds, which contrasts with an accuracy in excess of 90% of MRI and 99% with arthroscopy [136]. The treatment of meniscal tears in adolescents is similar to adults, with a tendency for increased frequency of

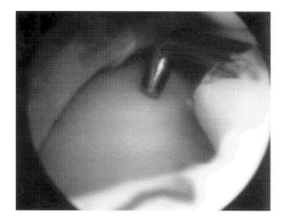

Fig. 6.2.23 Medial meniscus tear.

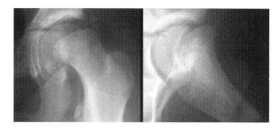

Fig. 6.2.24 Referred pain of the knee: slipped capital femoral epiphysis in a 12-year-old boy.

repair. The potential for osteoarthritis after meniscectomy in children is discussed in Chapter 4.3.

Referred pain

Slipped capital femoral epiphysis is a relatively common disorder in late childhood and adolescence (Fig. 6.2.24). It is more common in blacks and males and there seems to be a relationship to geographical location. If the slippage is slow and more chronic, clinical findings may be minimal and subtle. Referred pain to the medial knee via the obturator nerve is a common reason for delayed diagnosis. As many as 30% of patients diagnosed with a slipped capital femoral epiphysis have onset of symptoms for week to months before diagnosis. Left untreated the slip will often progress and stabilize when the physis closes. Thus severe slips will result in severe deformity and significant early arthritis. Also an avascular necrosis of the femoral head—Legg–Calvé–Perthes disease—

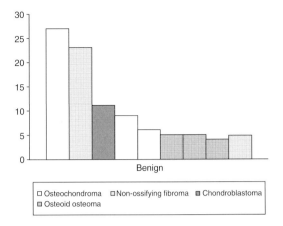

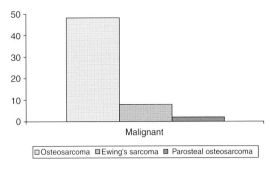

Fig. 6.2.26 Malignant bone tumors around the knee in children [138].

Fig. 6.2.25 Benign bone tumors around the knee in children [138].

plastic problem. Most young patients seeking treatment for knee pain will have a traumatic, infectious or developmental cause for the symptom [138]. Differential diagnoses are seen in Figs 6.2.25 and 6.2.26. Unilateral knee pain exceeding 2 weeks should lead to a radiograph to prevent doctor's delay in this patient group.

Tumor

The incidence of most musculoskeletal neoplasms is highest around the knee. Nevertheless Dickinson *et al.* report that a majority of patients with knee tumors had symptoms for around 6 months prior to initial radiographs. It is fortunate that tumors make up a small fraction of the many causes of pain and mass around the knee, but suspicion must be maintained in order to avoid making an error in diagnosis that could lead to loss of a limb or even life [138]. Malignant bone tumors and soft tissue sarcomas are the sixth and seventh most common causes of childhood cancer, respectively. Gebhardt *et al.* reported on 199 patients, of whom 114 had bone lesions and 77 soft tissue lesions (Figs 6.2.25 & 6.2.26) [138]. The knee is the most frequent site for osteosarcoma, probably related to the rapid growth at this location. Approximately 50% of osteosarcomas are located in the knee region (34%: distal femur; 17%: proximal tibia) [138]. As a cause for recurrent hemarthrosis, an intra-articular hemangioma may be found and mechanical instrumentation during arthroscopy may result in significant bleeding. Evaluation of a child with a suspected bone neoplasm is a complex process, but initially the most important thing is to recognize that one is dealing with a neo-

Conclusion

The vast majority of the sources of knee pain in adolescents are benign and treatable. Keep in mind those chronic cases in which the pain may sometimes be due 'only' to a physical expression of unhappiness. But the pain of adolescence must not be underestimated, since serious diseases such as tumors could be the reason. An error in diagnosis could lead to loss of limb or even life. One should remember that the incidence of most musculoskeletal neoplasms is highest around the knee. It has been reported that the majority of patients had symptoms for around 6 months prior to the initial radiograph, irrespective of age or the grade of malignancy. The evaluation of history and the clinical examination are crucial in the establishment of the diagnosis and should always be performed. Radiographic imaging is the most appropriate supplemental test to be done after examination and should be done in the majority of patients with longstanding pain. The standard views of the knee (anteroposterior, lateral, tunnel and tangential) usually provide sufficient information. To finalize the diagnosis additional tests and investigations such as MRI, CT or bone scan may be necessary and should be performed when they

can be the reason for knee pain and is diagnosed through decreased rotation of the hip as well as radiographically [137].

are appropriate and needed to establish the correct diagnosis.

Rehabilitation of knee injuries

Goals of rehabilitation

Phase 1 Normal and pain-free range of motion.
Phase 2 Normal strength in quadriceps and hamstrings compared to normal side.
Phase 3 Normal proprioceptive function.

The rehabilitation program after knee injuries will differ according to the injury the patient has. However, injuries to cartilage, menisci and ligaments may benefit from a general database of exercises provided the therapist takes into consideration special aspects of each injury. This differentiation is especially important when it comes to starting time for the different exercise activities, frequency, intensity and speed of the exercises. The most important steering variables for the therapist are *pain and function*. If the patient reacts with pain and/or swelling and thereby decreased function, the program must be adjusted accordingly until the knee has settled down. The therapist then should return to exercises tolerated by the patient previously. A good tip is to only change one exercise at a time to judge the effect of each individual exercise.

In the general program it is important to emphasize proprioceptive training as well as motion and strength exercises. Knee injuries reduce the proprioceptive sense and it takes time to return to normal. Consequently, one must encourage the patient to train daily to re-establish proprioceptive function as early as possible.

Return to sport

After surgery, patients are usually given an approximate time for return to sport. After ACL surgery, the patient may return after 6–12 months depending on the sport and additional injuries. After meniscal surgery this varies considerably. While a repair may require 4–6 months, a simple resection may enable the player to return after 2 weeks. Collateral ligament injuries usually require a rehabilitation period of at least 6 weeks—if surgery is needed, longer.

There are tests available to aid the physician in predicting return to sports. A strength test in an isokinetic testing device may be of help. The usual goal before training is 80% strength compared to the normal side and 90% for full return. Functional tests such as one-leg-jump and triple jumps have been shown to correlate well with isokinetic strength testing and may be more functional [16,77,78]. The most important aspect in judging when to return to sports is for the physician and therapist to create sports-specific testing programs, preferably with a control population consisting of baseline data of players including the injured player. One key issue in rehabilitation of knee injuries is the prevention of re-injuries. Unfortunately, there is little evidence that current braces or orthoses are able to unload meniscus, cartilage or ligaments under healing, and consequently few athletes use braces to prevent re-injuries.

After ACL injuries and surgery, patients are usually hospitalized for a day or two. Prior to discharge from the hospital or outpatient clinic, the physical therapist (PT) must instruct the patient in activities needed to restore range of motion. After ACL surgery, the motion is usually normalized after 12 weeks. The patient is then usually equipped with devices for cryotherapy to prevent swelling and given an appointment with a PT after 5–7 days. The first few days will emphasize circulatory exercises with many repetitions and little resistance (typical are series of 4×20–30 repetitions). After approximately a week, more active quadriceps and hamstring exercises will start and full weight-bearing may be commenced. Controversy still exists on the issue of closed- vs. open-chain exercises. Most PTs recommend closed-chain exercise to reduce loading of the healing ligament or tendon. However, recent studies have challenged this view and feel that exercises emphasizing open-chain exercises are more effective without compromising the healing of the ligaments.

In patients with meniscal repairs, the rehabilitation program is affected only if the repair is done without a concomitant ACL reconstruction. A repair in conjunction with an ACL reconstruction will give priority to the important rehabilitation protocol for the ACL with the exception of preventing hyperflexion for 4 weeks. In isolated repairs, the patient will usually have restrictions on weight-bearing and flexion based on the perceived motion of the meniscus when the knee is flexed beyond 90°.

Patients with cartilage surgery will usually be allowed full range of motion and in fact be on a CPM machine for 2 h 2 times a day for a week or more. However, their weight-bearing will be restricted to approximately 20 kg for 4–6 weeks.

For ACL rehabilitation a few randomized controlled studies exist on early 'aggressive' rehabilitation compared to a more restricted protocol. No differences have been detected on later laxity of the ACL after an early and aggressive protocol has been followed. There are no randomized controlled trials (RCTs) on different protocols for meniscus or cartilage rehabilitation.

Summary

Knee injuries are among the most common traumas in athletes. The history and mechanism of injury is helpful to establish the correct diagnosis. Clinical tests for instability, meniscus lesions and patellofemoral disorders are described in this chapter. Their individual indications are discussed as well as the use of imaging techniques. The use of MRI and ultrasound has increased the diagnostic accuracy.

The natural course of osteochondral lesions of the knee is not known. The best treatment of these lesions in athletes with persistent symptoms has not been established, despite the development of several different techniques: drilling, microfracture, periosteal transplantation, mosaicplasty and autogene chondrocyte implantation.

Lesions of the medial collateral ligament are treated non-operatively with active rehabilitation. Ligament reconstruction is often necessary in active athletes after anterior or posterior cruciate ligament lesions to prevent subluxation and giving way. Complete (grade III) posterolateral lesions, either isolated or combined with other ligament lesions, should be repaired subacutely to assure optimal function.

Overuse problems with degenerative changes of the tendon structure are most common in the inferior patellar ligament and are primarily treated conservatively with eccentric training. Surgery is rarely indicated. Anterior knee pain is treated with rehabilitation of the extensor mechanism.

Case story 6.2.1

A 19-year-old-team handball player injures her knee when performing a two-step fake. She immediately falls to the ground in great pain. Within the next 24 h she develops a large swelling and decreased range of motion. Which are the four most typical differential diagnoses?

Answer: Swelling within 24 h in a young female handball player must mean hemarthrosis which narrows the diagnoses down to ACL injury, peripheral meniscal tear, patellar dislocation and intra-articular fracture.

The patient is seen again by you after 7 days. The swelling is receding, but she still has an extension deficit with a solid stop when you are approaching full extension. What is your thinking?

Answer: The extension stop is probably caused by either a meniscal or cartilage tear.

How will you improve your diagnostic accuracy?

Answer: An MRI will detect a meniscal bucket-handle tear. Only an MRI arthrogram will be able to find a possible large cartilage tear.

A bucket-handle tear is detected; furthermore the patient is found to have an ACL tear as well as extensive bone bruise in the lateral femoral epicondyle and tibia. What are your treatment options?

Answer: The bucket handle tear in the meniscus may be repairable and as such should have surgery within the next 2 weeks. Some surgeons will do this alone and wait to perform the ACL surgery, whereas others will do everything at the same time. The healing ability for the meniscal repair is improved when the knee is stabilized and the repair is done at the same time as the ligament reconstruction. Although the bone bruise is extensive, no controlled studies exist on whether reduced weight-bearing on the extremity will be beneficial.

Knee pain in adolescents is most often a problem of overload in bone (Osgood–Schlatter), tendons or cartilage (osteochondritis) and is generally treated with decrease of load and active rehabilitation. Referred pain from the hip or pain from tumors must always be kept in mind.

Rehabilitation of the knee has been discussed.

Multiple choice questions

1 *Which of the following is the most accurate clinical test to assess for an anterior cruciate ligament tear?*

a Reverse pivot-shift test.

b Varus stress test at 30° of knee flexion.

c Anterior drawer test at 90° of knee flexion.

d Lachman's test.

e Quadriceps active test.

2 *In the evaluation of a chronic grade III posterolateral corner injury, the most appropriate initial diagnostic test to order would be which of the following?*

a Anteroposterior standing radiograph of the knee.

b KT-1000 testing.

c Varus thrust standing radiographs.

d Full-length standing (hip to ankle) anteroposterior radiographs.

e Ultrasound of the knee.

3 *The main structure injured in a traumatic lateral patellar dislocation is which of the following?*

a Chondral fracture of the lateral trochlea.

b Tear of the lateral patellotibial ligament.

c Tear of the medial patellofemoral ligament.

d Medial patellomeniscal ligament tear.

e Vastus medialis obliquus tendon tear off patella.

4 *A positive dial test at 30° of knee flexion is indicative of a tear of which structure / complex?*

a Anterior cruciate ligament.

b Posterior cruciate ligament.

c Ligament of Wrinsberg.

d Tibiocollateral ligament.

e Posterolateral knee structure.

5 *A team handball player makes a sudden stop and twisting valgus maneuver with the knee near extension, where she notices her knee buckle and she hears a pop inside her knee. Within the next 1–2 h, a large knee effusion develops. The most likely diagnosis for the injury sustained to the athlete is:*

a medial meniscal tear

b medial collateral ligament tear

c ACL tear

d lateral patellar subluxation

e osteochondral fracture.

6 *Which of the following is true when the knee is in full extension?*

a The posterolateral band of the anterior cruciate ligament and posteromedial band of the posterior cruciate ligament are tight.

b The anteromedial band of the anterior cruciate ligament and anterolateral band of the posterior cruciate ligament are tight.

c The anteromedial and posterolateral bands of the anterior cruciate ligament are lax.

d The posteromedial and anterolateral bundles of the posterior cruciate ligament are tight.

7 *What external load and what knee flexion angle increase the anterior cruciate ligament graft force the most with a deficient posterolateral corner?*

a Posterior drawer at 90°.

b Anterior drawer at 0°.

c Varus moment at 30°.

d External rotation moment at 90°.

e Varus moment at 0°.

8 *Which of the following is true of the kinematics of the tibiofemoral joint?*

a The tibia rotates about the femur about one fixed axis.

b The tibia can only rotate and cannot translate with respect to the femur.

c The tibiofemoral joint can be assumed to be a simple hinge joint.

d The tibia flexes and extends with respect to the femur along a moving axis.

e The tibia can only translate with respect to the femur, not rotate.

9 *The medial collateral ligament is:*

a a ligament that restrains tibofibular distraction

b a ligament that is composed of the tibial collateral ligament and deep medial collateral ligament structures

c a ligament that attaches the patella to the medial proximal tibia

d a ligament that is composed of an anterolateral and posteromedial bundles

e a ligament whose primary function is to restrain varus opening of the joint.

10 *Which of the following factors does not affect ligament properties?*

a Age.

b Load.

c Orientation.

d Loading rate.

e Sex.

References

1 American Medical Association. *Standard Nomenclature of Athletic Injuries.* Chicago: AMA Committee on Medical Aspects of Sports, 1968.

2 Daniel DM, Stone ML, Dobson BE, Fithian DC, Rossman DJ. Fate of the ACL-injured patient. A prospective outcome study. *Am J Sports Med* 1994; **22**: 632–44.

3 Dye SF. The knee as a biologic transmission with an envelope of function theory. *Clin Orth Rel Res* 1996; **325**: 10–8.

4 Myklebust G, Mæhlum S, Holm I, Bahr R. A prospective cohort study of ACL ligament tears in elite Norwegian team handball. *Scand J Sci Med Sports* 1998; 8: 149–53.

5 Woo SL, Peterson RH, Ohland KJ *et al.* The effects of strain rate on the properties of the medial collateral ligament in skeletally mature rabbits: a biomechanical and histological study. *J Orth Res* 1990; 8: 712–21.

6 Woo SL, Hollis JM, Adams DJ *et al.* Tensile properties of the human femur–anterior cruciate ligament–tibia complex: the effect of specimen age and orientation. *Am J Sports Med* 1991; **19**: 217–25.

7 Butler DL, Noyes FR, Grood ES. Ligamentous restraints to anterior–posterior drawer in the human knee: a biomechanical study. *J Bone Joint Surg (Am)* 1980; **62-A**: 259–70.

8 Harner CD, Xerogeanes JW, Livesay GA, Carlin GJ, Smith BA, Kusayama T, Kashiwaguchi S, Woo SL. The human posterior cruciate ligament complex: an interdisciplinary study. Ligament morphology and biomechanical evaluation. *Am J Sports Med* 1995; **23**: 736–45.

9 Terry GC, LaPrade RF. The posterolateral aspect of the knee: anatomy and surgical approach. *Am J Sports Med* 1996; **24**: 732–9.

10 Veltri DM, Deng XH, Torzilli PA, Warren RF, Maynard MJ. The role of the cruciate and posterolateral ligaments in stability of the knee: a biomechanical study. *Am J Sports Med* 1995; **23**: 436–43.

11 Gollehon DL, Torzilli PA, Warren RF. The role of the posterolateral and cruciate ligaments in the stability of the human knee: a biomechanical study. *J Bone Joint Surg (Am)* 1987; **69-A**: 233–42.

12 LaPrade RF, Resig S, Wentorf FA, Lewis JL. The effects of Grade III posterolateral complex injuries on force in an ACL reconstruction graft: a biomechanical analysis. *Am J Sports Med* 1999; **27**: 469–75.

13 Fulkerson JP, Buuck DA, Post WR. *Disorders of the Patellofemoral Joint*, Vol. 1, 3rd edn. Baltimore: Williams & Wilkins.

14 LaPrade RF, Hamilton CD, Engebretsen L. Treatment of acute and chronic combined anterior cruciate ligament and posterolateral knee ligament injuries. *Sports Med Arthroscopy Rev* 1997; **5**: 91–9.

15 Fulkerson JP, Arendt EA. Anterior knee pain in females. *Clin Orth Rel Res* 2000; **372**: 69–73.

16 Risberg MA, Holm I, Tjomsland O, Ljunggren E, Ekeland A. Prospective study of changes in impairments and disabilities after ACL reconstruction. *J Orth Sports Phys Ther* 1999; **29**: 400–12.

17a Busch MT. Meniscal injuries in children and adolescents. *Clin Sports Med* 1990; **9**: 661–80.

17 Hughston JC, Andrews JR, Cross MJ *et al.* Classification of knee ligament instabilities. Part II. The lateral compartment. *J Bone Joint Surg (Am)* 1976; **58-A**: 173–9.

18 Hughston JC, Norwood LA. The posterolateral drawer test and external rotation recurvatum test for posterolateral rotatory instability of the knee. *Clin Orth Rel Res* 1980; **147**: 82–7.

19 Clancy WG, Shelbourne KD, Zoellner GB *et al.* Treatment of knee joint instability secondary to rupture of the PCL. *J Bone Joint Surg* 1983; **65-A**: 310–22.

20 Grood ES, Stowers SF, Noyes FR. Limits of movement in the human knee. Effect of sectioning the posterior cruciate ligament and posterolateral structures. *J Bone Joint Surg (Am)* 1988; **70-A**: 88–97.

21 LaPrade RF, Terry GC. Injuries to the posterolateral aspect of the knee: Association of anatomic injury patterns with clinical instability. *Am J Sports Med* 1997; **25**: 433–8.

22 LaPrade RF. Arthroscopic evaluation of the lateral compartment of knees with Grade III posterolateral knee complex injuries. *Am J Sports Med* 1997; **25**: 596–602.

23 LaPrade RF, Bollom TF, Gilbert TF *et al.* The magnetic resonance imaging appearance of individual structures of the posterolateral knee. A prospective study of normal knees and knees with surgically verified grade III injuries. *Am J Sports Med* 2000; **28**: 191–9.

24 Daffner Rh, Tabas JH. Trauma oblique radiographs of the knee. *J Bone Joint Surg (Am)* 1987; **69-A**: 568–72.

25 Egund N. The axial view of the patellofemoral joint. *Acta Radiol Diagnosis* 1986; **27**: 101–4.

26 Rosenberg TD, Paulos LE, Parter RD, Coward DB, Scott SM. The 45° posteroanterior flexion weight-bearing radiograph of the knee. *J Bone Joint Surg (Am)* 1988; **70-A**: 1479–82.

27 Thomas RH, Resnick D, Naomi PA, Alazraki NP, Danel D, Greenfield R. Compartmental evaluation of osteoarthritis of the knee. A comparative study of available diagnostic modalities. *Radiology* 1975; **116**: 585–94.

28 Collier BD, Johnson RP, Carrera GF *et al.* Chronic knee pain assessed by SPECT. Comparison with other modalities. *Radiology* 1985; **157**: 795–802.

29 Alazraki NP, Fierer J, Resnick D. Chronic osteomyelitis; Monitoring by 99mTc phosphate and 67Ga-citrate imaging. *Am J Roentgenol* 1985; **145**: 767.

30 Raffi M, Lamont JG, Firooznia H. Tibial plateau fractures.

CT evaluation and classification. *Crit Rev Diagnostic Imaging* 1987; **27**: 91–112.

31 Kode L, Lieberman JM, Motta AO, Wilber JH, Vasen A, Yagan R. Evaluation of tibial plateau fractures: efficacy of MR imaging compared with CT. *Am J Roentgenol* 1994; **163**: 141–7.

32 Hentz VR, Green PS, Arditi M. Imaging studies of the cadaver hand using transmission ultrasound. *Skeletal Radiol* 1987; **16**: 474–80.

33 McDonald DG, Leopold GR. Ultrasound B-scanning in the differentiation of Baker's cyst and thrombophlebitis. *Br J Radiol* 1972; **45**: 729.

34 Ambanelli U, Manganelli P, Nervetti A, Ugolotti U. Demonstration of articular effusions and popliteal cysts with ultrasound. *J Rheumatol* 1976; **3**: 134–9.

35 Aisen AM, McCune WJ, MacGuire A, Carson PL, Silver TM, Jafri SZ, Martel W. Sonographic evaluation of the cartilage of the knee. *Radiology* 1984; **153**: 781–4.

36 De Flaviis L, Nessi R, Scaglione P, Balconi G, Albisetti W, Derchi LE. Ultrasonic diagnosis of Osgood–Schlatter and Sinding–Larsen–Johansson disease of the knee. *Skeletal Radiol* 1989; **18**: 193–7.

37 Kelly DW, Carter VS, Jobe FW, Kerlan RK. Patellar and quadriceps tendon ruptures—jumper's knee. *Am J Sports Med* 1984; **12**: 375–80.

38 Kälebo P, Swärd L, Karlsson J, Peterson L. Ultrasonography in the detection of partial patellar ligament ruptures—jumper's knee. *Skeletal Radiol* 1991; **29**: 285–9.

39 Purcell EM, Torrey HC, Pound RV. Resonance absorption by nuclear magnetic moments in a solid. *Phys Rev* 1946; **69**: 37.

40a Engebretsen L, Svenningsen S, Benum P. Poor results of ACL ligament repair in children. *Acta Orthop Scand* 1988; **59**: 684–6.

40 Lauterbur PC. Image formation in induced local interaction: Examples employing nuclear magnetic resonance. *Nature* 1973; **242**: 190.

41 Burk DL Jr, Mitchell DG, Rifkin MD, Vinitski S. Recent advances in magnetic resonance imaging of the knee. *Radiol Clinics N Am* 1990; **28**: 379–93.

42 Ruwe PA, Wright J, Randall RL, Lynch JK, Jokl P, McCarthry S. Can MR imaging effectively replace diagnostic arthroscopy? *Radiology* 1992; **183**: 335–9.

43a Ferretti A, Puddu G, Mariani PP, Neri M. Jumper's knee: An epidemiological study of volleyball players. *Physician Sportsmed* 1984; **12**: 97–103.

43 Spiers AS, Meagher T, Ostlere SJ, Wilson DJ, Dodd DA. Can MRI of the knee affect arthroscopic practice? A prospective of 58 patients. *J Bone Joint Surg (Brit)* 1993; **75-B**: 49–52.

44 Langer JE, Meyer SJF, Dalinka MK. Imaging of the knee. *Radiol Clinics N Am* 1990; **28**: 975.

45 Lindblom K. The arthrographic appearance of the ligaments of the knee joint. *Acta Radiol* 1938; **19**: 582.

46 Tegtmeyer CJ, McCue FC, Higgins SM, Ball DW. Arthrography of the knee: a comparative study of the accuracy of single and double contrast techniques. *Radiology* 1979; **132**: 37–41.

47 Applegate GR, Flanningan BD, Tolin BS, Fox JM. MR diagnosis of recurrent tears in the knee: value of intraarticular contrast material. *Am J Roentgenol* 1993; **161**: 821–5.

48 Deutsch AL, Mink JH, Fox JM, Arnoczky SV, Rothman BJ, Stoller DW. Peripheral meniscal tears: MR findings after conservative treatment or arthroscopic repair. *Radiology* 1990; **176**: 485–8.

49 Karlsson J, Lundin O, Lossing IW, Peterson L. Partial rupture of the patellar ligament. Results after operative treatment. *Am J Sports Med* 1991; **19**: 403–8.

50 Årøen A, Løken S, Heir S, Alvik E, Granlund OG, Ekeland A, Engebretsen E. Leddbruskskader i kneet. En prospektiv registrering ved kneartroskopier. In: Hofgaard H, ed. *Kirurgisk Hostmote.* Holmenkollen Park Hotel: de Norske Kirurgers Foreninger, 1999: 245.

51 Engebretsen L, Arendt E, Fritts HM. Osteochondral lesions and cruciate ligament injuries. *Acta Orthop Scand* 1993; **64**: 434–6.

52 Faber KJ, Dill JR, Amendola A, Thain L, Spouge A, Fowle PJ. Ocult osteochondral lesions after ACL rupture. Six-year MRI follow up. *Am J Sports Med* 1999; **27**: 489–94.

53 Wei X, Gao J, Messner C. Maturation-dependent repair of untreated osteochondral defects in the rabbit. *J Biomed Materials Res* 1997; **34**: 63–72.

54 Brown TD, Pope DF, Hale JE, Buckwalter JR, Brand RA. Effect of ostechondral defect size on cartilage contact stresses. *J Orth Res* 1991; **9**: 559–67.

55 Messner K, Maletius W. The long-term prognosis for severe damage to weight-bearing cartilage in the knee: a 14-year clinical and radiographic follow-up in 28 young athletes. *Acta Orthop Scand* 1996; **67**: 165–8.

56 Twyman RS, Desai K, Aicroth PM. OCD of the knee. A long-term study. *J Bone Joint Surg (Brit)* 1991; **75-B**: 461.

57 Aarseth L, Strand T, Solheim E. Symptomer og funksjon ved fokale leddbruskskader i kneet. In: Hofgaard H, ed. *Kirurgisk Hostmote.* Holmenkollen Park Hotel: de Norske Kirurgiske Foreninger, 1999: 247.

58a Grood ES, Noyes FR, Butler DL, Suntay WJ. Ligamentous and capsular restraints preventing straight medial and lateral laxity in intact human cadaver knees. *J Bone Joint Surg (Am)* 1981; **63-A**: 1257–69.

58 O'Driscoll SW. Articular cartilage regeneration using periosteum. *Clin Orth Rel Res* 1999; **367**: 186–203.

59 O'Driscoll SW, Giori NJ. Continuous passive motion (CPM): a theory and principles of application. *J Rehabil Res Dev* 2000; **37**: 179–88.

60 Steadman JR, Rodkey WG, Singleton SB *et al.* Microfracture technic for full-thickness chondral defects. Technique and clinical results. *Op Tech Orthop* 1997; **7**: 300–4.

61 Steadman JR, Rodkey WG, Briggs KK *et al.* The microfracture technic in the management of complete

cartilage defects in the knee joint. *Orthopade* 1999; **28**: 26–32.

62 Brittberg M, Lindahl A, Nilsson A *et al*. Treatment of deep cartilage defects in the knee with autologous chondrocyte transplantation. *N Engl J Med* 1994; **331**: 889–95.

63 Brittberg M, Nilsson A, Lindahl A *et al*. Rabbit articular cartilage defects treated with autologous cultured chondrocytes. *Clin Orth Rel Res* 1996; **326**: 270–83.

64 Chu CR, Convery FR, Akeson WH *et al*. Articular cartilage transplantation. Clinical results in the knee. *Clin Orth Rel Res* 1999; **360**: 159–68.

65 Minas T. The role of cartilage repair techniques, including chondrocyte transplantation, in focal chondral knee damage. *Instruct Course Lect* 1999; **48**: 629–43.

66 Breinan HA, Matin SD, Hsu HP, Pector M. Healing of canine articular cartilage defects treated with microfracture, a type II collagen matrix, or cultured autologous chondrocytes. *J Orth Res* 2000; **18**: 781–9.

67 Bobic V. Arthroscopic osteochondral autograft transplantation in anterior cruciate ligament reconstruction: a preliminary clinical study. *Knee Surg Sports Traum Arthrosc* 1997; **3**: 262–4.

68 Hangody L, Kish G, Karpati Z *et al*. Arthroscopic autogenous osteochondral mosaicplasty for the treatment of femoral condylar articular defects. A preliminary report. *Knee Surg Sports Traum Arthrosc* 1997; **5**: 262–7.

69 Hangody L, Kish G, Karpati Z *et al*. Mosaicplasty for the treatment of articular cartilage defects: application in clinical practice. *Orthopedics* 1998; **21**: 751–6.

70 Garrett JC. Osteochondritis dissecans. *Clin Sports Med* 1991; **10**: 569–93.

71 Noyes FR, Barber-Westin SD, Hewett TE. High tibial osteotomy and ligament reconstruction for varus angulated anterior cruciate ligament-deficient knees. *Am J Sports Med* 2000; **20**: 282–96.

72 Goble EM, Verdonk R, Kohn D. Arthroscopic and open surgical techniques for meniscus replacement. *Scand J Med Sci Sports* 1999; **9**: 168–76.

73 Gomez MA, Woo SL-Y, Inoue M, Amiel D, Harwood FL, Kitabayashi L. Medial collateral ligament healing subsequent to different treatment regimens. *J Appl Physiol* 1989; **66**: 245–52.

73a Kent RH, Pope CF, Lynch JK *et al*. Magnetic resonance imaging of the surgically repaired meniscus: Six month follow-up. *Magn Reson Imag* 1991; **9**: 335.

74 Indelicato PA. Nonoperative treatment of complete tears of the medial collateral ligament of the knee. *J Bone Joint Surg (Am)* 1983; **65-A**: 323–9.

74a Kirkley A, Webster-Bogart S, Litcfield R, Amendola A, MacDonald S, McCalden R, Fowler P. The effect of bracing on varus gonarthrosis. *J Bone Joint Surg (Am)* 1999; **81-A**: 539–48.

75 Kannus P. Nonoperative treatment of Grade II and III sprains of the lateral ligament compartment of the knee. *Am J Sports Med* 1989; **17**: 83–8.

76 Frank C, Woo SL-Y, Amiel D, Harwood F, Gomez M,

Akeson W. Medial collateral ligament healing. A multidisciplinary assessment in rabbits. *Am J Sports Med* 1983; **11**: 379–89.

77 Risberg MA, Beynnon BD, Peura GD. Proprioception after ACL reconstruction with and without bracing. *Knee Surg Sports Traum Arthrosc* 1999; **7**: 303–9.

78 Risberg MA, Holm I, Seen H, Eriksson J, Ekeland A. The effect of knee bracing after ACL reconstruction. A prospective, randomized study with 2 years followup. *Am J Sports Med* 1999; **27**: 76–83.

79 Grøntvedt T, Pena F, Engebretsen L. Accuracy of femoral tunnel placement and resulting graft force using drill guides. A cadaver study on ten paired knees. *Arthroscopy* 1996; **12**: 187–92.

80 Grøntvedt T, Heir S, Rossvoll I, Engebretsen L. Five-year outcome of 13 patients with an initially undiagnosed anterior cruciate rupture. *Scand J Med Sci Sports* 1999; **9**: 62–4.

81 Parolie JM, Bergfeld JA. Long term results of nonoperative treatment of isolated PCL in the athlete. *Am J Sports Med* 1986; **14**: 35–8.

82 Fowler PJ, Messieh SS. Isolated PCL injuries in the athlete. *Am J Sports Med* 1987; **15**: 553–7.

83 Kujala UM, Kvist M, Osterman K. Knee injuries in athletes. Review of exertion injuries and retrospective study of outpatient sports clinic material. *Sports Med* 1986; **3**: 447–56.

84 Fredberg U. Local corticosteroid injection in sport. Review of literature and guidelines for treatment. *Scand J Med Sci Sports* 1997; **7**: 131–9.

85 Martens M, Wouters P, Burssens A, Mulier JC. Patellar tendinitis: pathology and results of treatment. *Acta Orthop Scand* 1982; **53**: 445–50.

86 Leadbetter WB. Cell matrix response in tendon injury. *Clin Sports Med* 1992; **11**: 533–78.

87 Davies SG, Baudouin CJ, King JB, Perry JD. Ultrasound, computed tomography and magnetic resonance imaging in patellar tendinitis. *Clin Radiol* 1991; **43**: 52–6.

88 Fritschy D, de Gautard R. Jumper's knee and ultrasonography. *Am J Sports Med* 1988; **16**: 637–40.

89 Vane JR. Inhibition of prostaglandin synthesis as a mechanism of action for aspirin-like drugs. *Nature New Biol* 1971; **231**: 232–5.

90 Cryer B, Feldman M. Cyclo-oxygenase-1 and cyclo-oxygenase-2 selectivity of widely used non steroidal anti-inflammatory drugs. *Am J Med* 1998; **104**: 413–21.

91 Tsujii M, Kawano S, Tsuji S, Sawaoka H, Hori M, DuBois RN. Cyclooxygenase regulates angiogenesis induced by colon cancer cells. *Cell* 1998; **93**: 705–16.

92 Morrison BW, Christensen S, Yuan W, Brown J, Amlani S, Seidenberg B. Analgesic efficacy of the cyclooxygenase-2-specific inhibitor rofecoxib in post-dental surgery pain: a randomized, controlled trial. *Clin Therapeut* 1999; **21**: 943–53.

93 Fort J. Celecoxib, a COX-2 specific inhibitor: the clinical data. *Am J Orthop* 1999; **28**: 13–8.

94 Lian Ø, Holen KJ, Engebretsen L, Bahr R. Relationship

between symptoms of jumper's knee and the ultrasound characteristics of the patellar tendon among high level male volleyball players. *Scand J Med Sci Sports* 1996; **6**: 291–6.

95 Ferretti A, Puddu G, Mariani PP, Neri M. The natural history of jumper's knee. Patellar and quadriceps tendonitis. *Int Orthop* 1985; 8: 239–42.

96 Roels J, Martens M, Mulier JC, Burssens A. Patellar tendinitis (jumper's knee). *Am J Sports Med* 1978; **6**: 362–8.

97 Lian Ø, Engebretsen L, Øvrebo RV, Bahr R. Characteristics of leg extensors in male volleyball players with jumper's knee. *Am J Sports Med* 1996; **24**: 380–5.

98 Pierets K, Verdonk R, DeMuynck M, Lagast J. Jumper's knee: postoperative assessment. A retrospective clinical study. *Knee Surg Sports Traum Arthrosc* 1999; **7**: 239–42.

98a Messner K, Gilquist J. Synthetic implants for the repair of osteochondral defects of the MCL. *Biomaterials* 1993; **14**: 513–21.

99 Drogset JO, Rossvoll I, Grøntvedt T. Surgical treatment of iliotibial band friction syndrome. A retrospective study of 45 patients. *Scand J Med Sci Sports* 1999; **9**: 296–8.

100 Lockhart DJ, Dong H, Byrne MC *et al.* Expression monitoring by hybridization to high-density oligonucleotide arrays. *Nature Biotechnol* 1996; **14**: 1675–80.

100a Mikkelsen C, Werner S, Eriksson E. Closed kinetic chain alone compared to combined open and closed kinetic chain exercises for quadriceps strengthening after an ACL reconstruction. *Knee Surg Sports Traum Arthrosc* 2000; **8**: 337–42.

101 de Inocencio J. Musculoskeletal pain in primary paediatric care: analysis of 1000 consecutive general pediatric clinic visits. *Pediatrics* 1998; **102**: E63.

102 Osgood RB. Lesions of the tibial tubercle occurring during adolescence. *Boston Med Surg* 1903; **148**: 114–7.

103 Kujala UM, Kvist M, Heinonen O. Osgood–Schlatter's disease in adolescent athletes. Retrospective study of incidence and duration. *Am J Sports Med* 1985; **13**: 236–41.

104 Krause BL, Williams JP, Catterall A. Natural history of Osgood–Schlatter disease. *J Pediatr Orthop* 1990; **10**: 65–8.

105 Ogden JA. *Skeletal Injury in the Child*, 2nd edn. Philadelphia: Lea & Febiger, 1990.

106 Ogden JA, McCarthy SM, Jokl P. The painful bipartite patella. *J Pediatr Orthop* 1982; **2**: 263–9.

107 Klein W. Endoscopy of the deep infraparellar bursa. *Arthroscopy* 1996; **12**: 127–31.

108 Medlar RC, Lyne ED. Sinding–Larsen–Johansson disease. Its etiology and natural history. *J Bone Joint Surg (Am)* 1978; **60-A**: 1113–6.

109 Blazina ME, Kerlan RK, Jobe FW, Carter VS, Carlson GJ. Jumper's knee. *Orthop Clinics N Am* 1973; **4**: 665–78.

110 Day B. The management of anterior knee pain in the adolescent. *Am J Knee Surg* 1997; **10**: 184–7.

111 Fairbank JC, Pynsent PB, van Poortvliet JA, Phillips H.

Mechanical factors in the incidence of knee pain in adolescents and young adults. *J Bone Joint Surg (Brit)* 1984; **66**: 685–93.

112 Abernethy PJ, Townsend PR, Rose RM, Radin EL. Is chondromalacia patellae a separate clinical entity. *J Bone Joint Surg (Brit)* 1978; **60-B**: 205–10.

113 Goldberg B. Patellofemoral malalignment. *Pediatr Ann* 1997; **26**: 32–5.

114 O'Neill DB, Micheli LJ, Warner JP. Patellofemoral stress. A prospective analysis of exercise treatment in adolescents and adults. *Am J Sports Med* 1992; **20**: 151–6.

115 Bennet JG, Stauber WT. Evaluation and treatment of anterior knee pain using eccentric exercise. *Med Sci Sports Exerc* 1986; **18**: 526–30.

116 Eilert RE. Adolescent anterior knee pain. *Instruct Course Lect* 1993; **42**: 497–516.

117 Green WT Jr. Painful bipartite patellae. A report of three cases. *Clin Orth Rel Res* 1975; **110**: 197–200.

118 Bourne MH, Bianco AJJ. Bipartite patella in the adolescent: results of surgical excision. *J Pediatr Orthop* 1990; **10**: 69–73.

119 Weaver JK. Bipartite patella as a cause of disability in the athlete. *Am J Sports Med* 1977; **5**: 137–43.

120 Aichroth PM. Osteochondritis dissecans of the knee. In: *International Cartilage Repair Society, 3rd Symposium*. Gothenburg, Sweden: International Cartilage Repair Society, 2000: Keynote Lectures 6A.

121 Wilson JN. A diagnostic sign in osteochondritis dissecans. *J Bone Joint Surg* 1967; **49**: 477–80.

122 Linden B. Osteochondritis dissecans of the femoral condyles: a long-term follow-up study. *J Bone Joint Surg (Am)* 1977; **59-A**: 1340–8.

122a Safran MR, Fu FH. Uncommon causes of knee pain in the athlete. *Orthop Clinics N Am* 1995; **26**: 547–59.

123 Schwarz CMEB, Sisto DJ, Hirsh LC. The results of operative treatment of osteochondritis dissecans of the patella. *Am J Sports Med* 1988; **16**: 522–9.

124 Peters TA, McLean ID. Osteochondritis dissecans of the patellofemoral joint. *Am J Sports Med* 2000; **28**: 63–7.

125 de Ganzy S, Mousat C, Darodes PH, Cahuzac JP. Natural course of osteochondritis in children. *J Pediatr Orthop* 1999; **8-B**: 26–8.

126 Johnson DP, Eastwood DM, Witherow PJ. Symptomatic synovial plicae of the knee. *J Bone Joint Surg (Am)* 1993; **75**: 1485–96.

127 Tindel NL, Nisonson B. The plica syndrome. *Orthop Clinics N Am* 1992; **23**: 613–8.

128 Dorchak JD, Barrack RL, Kneisl JS, Alexander AH. Arthroscopic treatment of symptomatic synovial plica of the knee. Long-term follow-up. *Am J Sports Med* 1991; **19**: 503–7.

129 Aglietti P, Bertini FA, Buzzi R, Beraldi R. Arthroscopic meniscectomy for discoid lateral meniscus in children and adolescents: 10-year follow-up. *Am J Knee Surg* 1999; **12**: 83–7.

130 Connolly B, Babyn PS, Wright JG, Thorner PS. Discoid

meniscus in children: magnetic resonance imaging characteristics. *Can Assoc Radiol J* 1996; **47**: 347–54.

131 Stark JE, Siegel MJ, Weinberger E, Shaw DW. Discoid menisci in children: MR features. *J Computer Assisted Tomogr* 1995; **19**: 608–11.

132 Washington ER III, Root L, Liener UC. Discoid lateral meniscus in children. Long-term follow-up after excision. *J Bone Joint Surg (Am)* 1995; **77-A**: 1357–61.

133 Aichroth PMPD, Marx CL. Congenital discoid meniscus in children; a longterm follow-up study and evolution of management. In: Aichroth PM, Cannon DC, eds. *Knee Surgery. Current Practice*. New York: Raven Press, 1992: 530–9.

134 Lauterburg MT, Segantini P. Post-traumatic knee joint arthroscopy in children and adolescents. *Schweiz Z Medizin Traumatol* 1994; **3**: 25–34.

135 Maffulli N, Chan KM, Bundoc RC, Cheng JC. Knee arthroscopy in Chinese children and adolescents: an eight year prospective study. *Arthroscopy* 1997; **13**: 18–23.

136 Angel KR, Hall DJ. The role of arthroscopy in children and adolescents. *Arthroscopy* 1989; **5**: 192–6.

137 Tippett SR. Referred knee pain in a young athlete: a case study. *J Orth Sports Phys Ther* 1994; **19**: 117–20.

138a Gebhardt MC, Ready JE, Mankin HJ. Tumors about the knee in children. *Clin Orth Rel Res* 1990; **255**: 86–110.

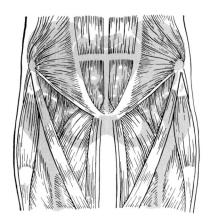

Chapter 6.3
Hip, Groin and Pelvis

PER HÖLMICH, PER A.F.H. RENSTRÖM &
TÖNU SAARTOK

Classical reference

Renström P, Peterson L. Groin injuries in athletes. *Br J Sports Med* 1980; **14**: 30–36.
This paper was one of the first to discuss the problem of groin injuries in athletes in a systematic way. It tried to define some diagnoses and discuss the epidemiology and treatment of these, and for many years was the most frequently quoted paper regarding this subject.

Introduction

Groin pain in association with sports activities continues to be a major problem in sports medicine. The incidence of groin pain among, for example, soccer players is 5–18% per year [1–5]. The pain may originate from various anatomic structures such as muscle, tendon, ligament or bone, but abdominal or gynecologic disorders, referred pain and nerve entrapment can also cause groin pain. The majority of papers concerning groin problems in the athletic population are empiric in nature. One major problem is the lack of consensus regarding definitions of diagnosis, examination techniques or treatment. When reviewing and comparing the papers concerning this difficult problem it is imperative that definitions and terminology are agreed upon. The prerequisite for a successful treatment is to set a correct diagnosis, and the examining therapist needs to have knowledge about the differential diagnoses.

Anatomy

The pelvic region is an essential part of the functional anatomy in most sports activities. The pelvis needs to be stable and well controlled for the athlete to perform with skill. The pelvis is the turning point between the upper and the lower part of the body. Multiple muscles and ligaments originate from and/or insert onto the pelvis, and to control and stabilize the pelvis a delicate balance exists between these structures to coordinate the movements passing through this region. Two of the most important ligaments in the pelvis are the sacrotuberal and the sacrospinal ligaments (Fig. 6.3.1). They both control the retroversion of the sacrum and are prone to overuse conditions. They are both phylogenetic new ligaments representing transformed parts of the hamstrings and the coccygeus muscle, respectively.

The hip joints are the meeting points between the lower extremities and the pelvis, whereas the sacrum is the meeting point between the trunk and pelvis. The hip joint is one of the most stable joints in the body. Both the bony parts of the joint as well as the capsule and ligaments contribute to the stability. The iliofemoral, pubofemoral and ischiofemoral ligaments are the three main ligaments protecting the hip joint. They are very strong ligaments, especially the iliofemoral ligament which is one of the strongest ligaments in the body. The ligaments run spirally from the pelvis to the femur. When the hip joint is extended the

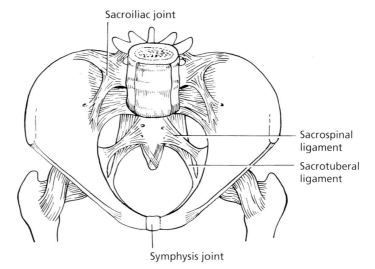

Fig. 6.3.1 Male pelvis with its ligaments.

Labels on figure: Sacroiliac joint; Sacrospinal ligament; Sacrotuberal ligament; Symphysis joint

ligaments are tightened, thus protecting the joint from dislocation.

The femur consists of a single bone and some very powerful muscles. These are:

the quadriceps muscles: knee extensors and a hip flexor (the rectus femoris);

the sartorius muscle: a hip flexor and external rotator as well as a knee flexor and internal rotator;

the hamstring muscles (biceps femoris, semitendinosis and semimembranosis): hip extensors, knee flexors and knee rotators;

the adductors (adductor magnus, adductor longus, adductor brevis, gracilis and pectineus): hip adductors, hip flexors and hip external rotators depending on the position of the hip joint; the posterior part of the adductor magnus can even extend the hip joint. The gracilis can also flex and internally rotate the knee joint;

the abductors and gluteal muscles (tensor fasciae latae, gluteus maximus, medius and minimus): hip abductors, hip extensors, hip external and internal rotators and hip flexors;

the external hip rotators (piriformis, gemelli, obturatorius externus and internus and quadratus femoris): external hip rotators and hip abductors when the hip is flexed;

the iliopsoas muscle: primarily a hip flexor but also a hip external rotator and a flexor of the lumbar spine.

Muscle actions are usually defined according to the way they move the leg when the leg is non-weight-bearing and the muscle is contracting concentrically. It is, however, important to realize that these muscles also function as stabilizers of the hip joints and the pelvis, and thereby the trunk. This function is especially evident in eccentric actions. Using this approach, it is easier to understand the importance of the adductors as a major stabilizing muscle group and not only as 'adductors' of the femur in the non-weight-bearing situation.

The abdominal muscles, including the rectus abdominis, external oblique, internal oblique and transversus abdominis, are important in the stabilization of the pelvis and in the control of the movements of the trunk in relation to the pelvis and the legs. They work in synergy with the muscles of the back (described elsewhere) and the above-mentioned muscles. As an example, the synergy between the transversus abdominis and the multifidus muscles seems to be of particular importance [6,7]. The tendons of the internal oblique and the transversus abdominis muscles blend to create the conjoined tendon (the falx inguinalis) and a close anatomic relationship seems to exist between the conjoined tendon, the rectus abdominis sheath and the common adductor origin [8,9] (Fig. 6.3.2). This relationship could explain the close connection often found between adductor-related groin pain and incipient hernia (see below).

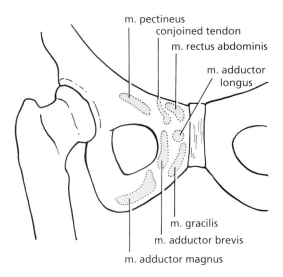

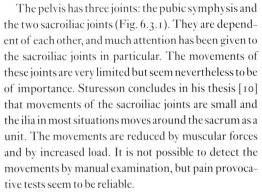

Fig. 6.3.2 Tendon insertions on the pubic bone close to the symphysis joint.

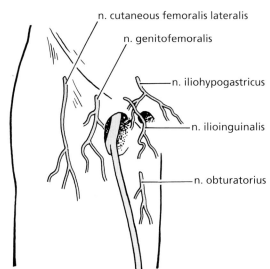

Fig. 6.3.3 The important nerves of the groin region.

The pelvis has three joints: the pubic symphysis and the two sacroiliac joints (Fig. 6.3.1). They are dependent of each other, and much attention has been given to the sacroiliac joints in particular. The movements of these joints are very limited but seem nevertheless to be of importance. Sturesson concludes in his thesis [10] that movements of the sacroiliac joints are small and the ilia in most situations moves around the sacrum as a unit. The movements are reduced by muscular forces and by increased load. It is not possible to detect the movements by manual examination, but pain provocative tests seem to be reliable.

The nerves of the region represent both the lumbar and sacral plexuses. Important nerves are *the ischial nerve* to the posterior and lateral side of the leg and *the femoral nerve* to the anterior side. The clinically important cutaneous nerves are the obturator nerve, the ilioinguinal nerve, the genitofemoral nerve, the lateral cutaneous nerve and the iliohypogastric nerve (Fig. 6.3.3).

History and physical examination

The history is extremely important. It will frequently give a good indication of the pathoanatomic site of the diagnosis. It is important to realize that even when dealing with otherwise healthy and often young persons, more serious diseases (e.g. infection, cancer and systemic disease) are possibilities that should always be considered.

If an *acute episode* was the start of the injury, a thorough description of the precise injury mechanism can be very helpful (see box).

Important questions to be asked in the case of an *acute* groin injury

Was the trauma violent or was it just a minor episode?

How did the patient move when the injury happened (e.g. speed, direction)?

Was it a non-contact or a contact injury?

Was a snap, click, pop or similar sensation felt or even heard?

Could the sports activities be continued?

What treatment has been given until now?

If *no acute episode* can be recalled, an analysis of the athletic activities in the time preceding the injury can be especially helpful as well as a description of the development of symptoms (see box).

Important questions to be asked in the case of a *chronic groin injury*

Any changes in the amount of sports activity (frequency, intensity and load)?

Any changes in training methods, surface or equipment?

Previous overuse injuries (underlying biomechanical abnormality)?

What were the first symptoms and how have they changed?

What treatment has been given until now?

A history of systemic, urogenital, abdominal or low-back symptoms should be taken as well.

The present symptoms should be investigated (box).

Important questions to be asked about the present symptoms in athletes with groin pain

What is the precise location?

What are the symptoms?

Does the pain radiate anywhere?

What can provoke the symptoms?

When does it happen?

The present activity level is also important, including not only sports-related activities but also work and leisure time activities.

In some cases the history and the present symptoms leave very little doubt and a direct examination of the relevant region will promptly reveal the diagnosis. But in other cases, such as painful conditions involving the groin or the gluteal region, a rather comprehensive examination is required. In such cases a systematic approach is imperative.

It is important to realize that most examination methods are not evaluated scientifically and reproducibility might be a problem [11]. Another point to be aware of is the lack of consensus in the scientific literature on definitions and diagnostic criteria. It is a prerequisite for the correct evaluation of different treatment methods that the same definitions are used. An approach to solving this problem in the case of athletes with groin pain has recently been suggested [11].

The physical examination (box) should of course be focused on the region indicated by the history. However one should be aware of the possibility of pain radiating to this region from, for example, nerve entrapment, abdominal or genital organs, sacroiliac joints and the spine.

An assessment of the patient's *gait and posture* is a useful start of the examination. The region should be *inspected* for swelling, discoloration and other abnormalities.

Various *functional tests* to evaluate the balance and the pelvic stability can be performed. These could include a one-leg balance test evaluating the ability to maintain balance (e.g. for 30s standing on one leg), exercises on a soft surface evaluating the athlete's ability to adjust body posture to sudden changes in the surface, a lunge test to evaluate dynamic stability and others.

The physical examination should include *systematic palpation* for tenderness and abnormalities and functional testing of the muscles and ligaments based on the anatomy and biomechanics. An evaluation of the *range of motion* and the musculoskeletal flexibility including the lumbar spine and the hip and knee joints should be included.

The bony landmarks should be palpated systematically for tenderness and abnormalities, including the symphysis joint, the sacrum, the ischial tuberosity, the greater trochanter and the iliac crest.

The main points of the physical examination of athletes with groin pain

Gait and posture
Functional tests
Inspection
Systematic palpation
Range of motion
Sensibility
Abdominal palpation
Laboratory testing when indicated

The *neurologic investigation* should include sensibility of the relevant regions and an examination of the deep tendon reflexes may be indicated.

The *abdomen should be palpated*, and especially in male patients, an examination of the hernial orifices is often indicated. If urogenital diseases are suspected from the history, relevant examinations (e.g. rectal palpation) should be performed.

If infections or rheumatic and other relevant systemic diseases are suspected *laboratory testing* is indicated.

Imaging

Plain radiographs are usually the first choice in most conditions involving the pelvis and the hip joints (Fig. 6.3.4). When osseous involvement is suspected a stan-

dard radiologic examination should include an antero-posterior projection of the pelvis with the pubic symphysis visible and an anteroposterior and lateral projection of the hip joints. Depending on the symptoms and the findings of the physical examination, additional projections might be relevant.

Tomography and computed tomography (CT) are an important supplement in the case of fractures and can be very helpful in preoperative planning.

Technetium-99m triple-phase bone scan can in some cases be very helpful. Increased uptake can be seen in the case of e.g. stress fracture, bone neoplasm, bone infection and arthrosis. In the case of enthesopathy also, as seen at the adductor insertions and the rectus femoris insertion, a bone scan will often show increased uptake (Fig. 6.3.5) [11,12].

Ultrasound is another possibility in many cases of soft tissue-related problems in the pelvic region. The method is cheap and fast and has a major advantage in the possibility of dynamic real-time scanning. Muscles and tendons can be visualized using linear high-resolution transducers (Fig. 6.3.6). These can also visualize bursae, cysts, excessive fluid in the hip joints, and pathology of the viscera, genitourinary tissues and blood vessels that might be related to the region.

The visualization is real time and can be performed dynamically. The patient can perform the movements that provoke the pain during simultaneous ultrasound scanning, thus helping to identify the structures causing the pain. The pressure of the transducer against the injured site might also help to identify the injured structure. In the case of a palpable unidentified structure or clicking, the ultrasound can be helpful in identifying the nature of this. Ultrasound is also very useful as a guide for biopsies, punctures and steroid injections.

Magnetic resonance imaging (MRI) has some obvious advantages: the lack of ionizing radiation, the high sensitivity, the capability to show soft tissue and the multiplanar capability. T_2-weighted images in particular can reveal muscular and musculotendinous injuries as increased signals in muscle strains. *Short tau inversion recovery* (STIR) images are useful to show edema and hemorrhage in both soft tissues and bone marrow (Fig. 6.3.5). In the case of calcifications, plain radiographs or CT scan may be superior to MRI. MRI still

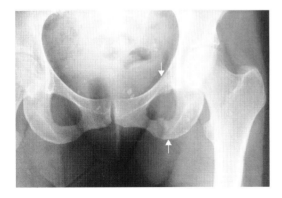

Fig. 6.3.4 X-ray of a female long-distance runner with groin pain. The X-ray shows a stress fracture in the pubic bone (arrows).

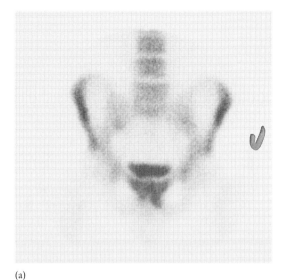

(a)

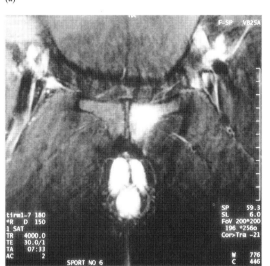

(b)

Fig. 6.3.5 (a) Technetium-99m triple-phase bone scan of the pelvis showing increased uptake around the symphysis joint and down the inferior rami of the pubic bone indicating enthesopathy of the adductor longus insertion. (b) MRI of the symphysis region in a male patient suffering from longstanding adductor-related groin pain, showing increased signal from the pubic bone on one side of the symphysis joint indicating enthesopathy of the adductor longus insertion.

has the disadvantages of limited availability and cost and the indication for MRI is often the presence of a doubtful clinical diagnosis or the wish to eliminate the possibility of a neoplasm.

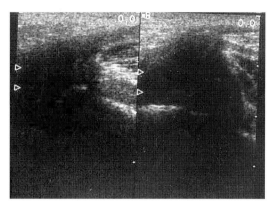

Fig. 6.3.6 Ultrasound examination of the insertion into the pubic bone of a normal adductor longus tendon (left). In the case of longstanding enthesopathy the insertion is thickened and the signals close to the bone are hypoechoic (right, indicated by arrows). Courtesy of Michael Bachmann Nielsen.

Groin — muscles and tendons

Acute myotendinous groin injuries

Etiology
The iliopsoas can be strained by a forceful flexion against resistance as occurs when the ground is mistakenly kicked instead of the ball, or in eccentric contraction, e.g. when the thigh is forced into extension. *The adductor muscles* are usually strained in eccentric contraction, e.g. in a forceful abduction, often with some degree of hip joint rotation, as in a sliding tackle in soccer.

The injury usually occurs in the myotendinous junction but can also occur in the tendon itself or at the bony insertion. Fatigue, lack of concentration or insufficient muscle coordination seems to be important etiologic factors.

Other muscles in the groin region such as *rectus femoris, sartorius, the abdominal muscles and the conjoined tendon* can also be injured by a hyperextension of the muscle and tendon.

Clinical presentation
Muscle lesions can be divided into three grades [13].
Grade I — a mild strain with only a minimal tear of the muscle.

Grade II—damage of more muscle fibers but not a complete disruption. There is a definite loss of strength.

Grade III—a total tear of the muscle–tendon unit with a total lack of function of the muscle.

Grade I and II lesions are painful and often disabling. Except for the iliopsoas lesion a discoloration and swelling can frequently be found representing local hematoma and edema. Usually a 'pull' has been felt in the muscle with a sudden sharp pain and the athlete is often unable to continue the activity. Complete muscle tear (grade III) is rare and is in most instances located to the distal insertion [14,15].

At clinical examination the swelling can be palpated, and sometimes a localized defect in the muscle can be felt. There is pain at palpation, and usually pain at the injury site on both passive and resisted active functional testing of the injured muscle(s). An anteroposterior radiographic projection of the pelvis, sometimes in combination with other projections depending on the location of the injury, may be very helpful to exclude fractures or avulsions. Ultrasound examination can be very helpful to visualize the precise location and size of the injury, especially when an iliopsoas strain is suspected.

When the lesion is a grade III rupture a retraction of the injured muscle can be seen. If the patient is examined at a late stage, the injured muscle often appears as a mass in the groin region and needs to be distinguished from a hernia or a tumor; additional examination with imaging techniques like ultrasound, CT or MRI is usually indicated.

With a typical history of an acute myotendinous lesion and clinical findings to support it, further investigations are seldom necessary. But in doubtful cases the entire groin region should be examined carefully and a neurologic examination of the limb and an examination of the low back including the thoracolumbar region and the sacroiliac joints should be made.

Treatment—acute injuries

The initial management of acute myotendinous strain consists of rest, elevation, compression and ice. Massage, active stretching, heat and ultrasound should be avoided the first 2–3 days to prevent rebleeding. Early passive range of motion exercises and the use of crutches during the first few days are recommended. Careful muscle exercises consisting of isometric contractions without resistance progressing to isometric resistance exercises and eventually dynamic exercises may be started when possible. Moderate pain may be tolerated as long as the exercises are controlled. Proprioceptive exercises carefully re-establishing the muscle strength and pelvic balance and coordination, combined with a careful stretching program, are recommended. An aquatic training program can be helpful in the initial training period. Analgesics may be used for the first days. Non-steroidal anti-inflammatory drugs (NSAIDs) are sometimes recommended, but the widespread use of these has, however, been questioned.

When the initial exercise program can be performed without pain, and the muscle coordination is good, the sport-specific exercises can be initiated before a gradual return to sport. It may take 4–8 weeks or even longer before return to sport depending on the nature and degree of injury. When the adductor muscles are injured, it is the authors' experience that re-establishing the muscular strength and balance around the pelvis is extremely important to avoid relapse or development of chronic injury.

Chronic myotendinous groin injuries

In the athlete with longstanding groin pain the symptoms are often more diffuse. In some cases the symptoms even seem to be contradictory and confusing. The athlete describes the pain as 'moving around' and the examiner will have to be aware of the possibility that more than one cause for the chronic groin pain very often can be found [11,16]. The multiple clinical entities responsible for the chronic groin pain are probably the result of the 'first' injury causing an imbalance and altered function affecting the pelvic stability, thus stressing other structures related to the pelvis. Pain from the sacroiliac joints, the low back or the sacrotuberal ligaments are not uncommonly found in combination with myotendinous groin injuries.

In the literature the three most frequently mentioned causes for chronic groin pain in athletes are (i) adductor-related groin pain, (ii) lesions to the inguinal canal and associated structures and (iii) iliopsoas-related groin pain.

Etiology

Adductor-related pain is a frequent cause of groin pain [5,17]. Fatigue, overuse or acute overload of the adductor muscles during sports activities may lead to injuries. The adductor muscles act as very important stabilizers of the hip joint [18], and as such are at risk if the load on the hip joints and the pelvis is no longer balanced. Injuries influencing the stability of the hip joints and the pelvis might thus precipitate overuse problems of the adductor muscles.

The iliopsoas muscle (Fig. 6.3.7) is a very important contributor to the pelvic stability constantly involved in most sports activities. The precise functions of the iliopsoas muscle apart from hip flexion are not yet fully understood, but the muscle seems to work as a pelvic stabilizer as well as a stabilizer for the lumbar spine [19]. One reason why the muscle is at risk could be that the workload on the muscle includes a considerable amount of both eccentric and concentric work and fast changes between these work forms. Another reason

could be that this muscle is 'hidden' to the athlete's knowledge and is difficult to examine clinically. Knowledge of the preventive measures usually practiced for other muscles at risk such as strength training and stretching is thus sparse, and both strains and overuse injuries in the iliopsoas muscle might develop into a chronic problem.

Lesions to the inguinal canal and associated structures are probably in most cases of a myotendinous nature as well. In some cases a predisposition to hernia development might be present. In other cases an acute trauma or a period of overuse as a result of a misbalanced pelvis combined with a period of strenuous athletic activity can result in a chronic lesion. The primary lesion can be in the rectus abdominis muscle or insertion, the external oblique, internal oblique and/or transversalis muscle(s) or aponeurosis, and the conjoined tendon [8]. The nature of the lesion is not clear, since it may be a strain or tear, an inflammation or degeneration of certain points of excessive stress, or an avulsion, a

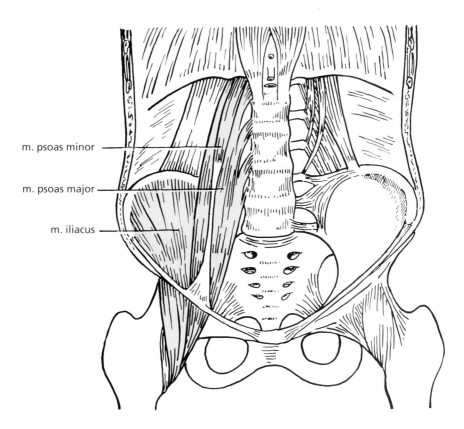

Fig. 6.3.7 The pelvis with the iliopsoas muscle complex.

m. psoas minor

m. psoas major

m. iliacus

hemorrhage or an edema. The problem is discussed further in the section on 'Sports hernia'.

Clinical presentation

The typical complaints from an athlete with myotendinous-related chronic groin injury are pain and stiffness in this region in the morning and at the beginning of athletic activity. This pain and stiffness decreases and sometimes disappears after a period of warming up, but may reappear when the athlete gets fatigued or after the sports activity has ceased. Pain when coughing and sneezing and when standing on one leg to pull on socks or pants is a frequent complaint. The athlete can usually run forward and straight without pain at a moderate speed, but with increasing speed and/or sudden changes of direction the groin pain reappears. Characteristic activities causing pain include sprinting, making cutting movements, kicking the ball and making a sliding tackle.

When the pain is *adductor related* it is localized medially in the groin and may radiate down along the adductor group on the medial side of the thigh, whereas when the injury is *iliopsoas related*, the pain is localized to the central anterior part of the proximal thigh, and thus more laterally in the groin. It sometimes radiates down the anterior thigh and sometimes involves an element of lower abdominal pain lateral to the rectus abdominis muscle.

Myotendinous pain localized to the *lower abdomen* is most prominent around the conjoined tendon insertion at the pubic bone and may radiate into the adductor region and in males to the scrotum.

Chronic injuries related to the *rectus femoris* or the *sartorius* are more rare. They are usually located at the proximal end of the muscle and tendon close to the insertion.

Chronic groin injuries are in some cases preceded by an acute episode, but more frequently the athlete has no recollection of this. A pattern of a sudden increase in training, including the intensity, the training methods or the total amount, in the period before the appearance of injury is typical. For example, an iliopsoas-related overuse problem can typically be sustained by increased repetitive hip flexion as when running uphill or by intensive kicking exercises in soccer or football.

Stress fracture is an important differential diagnosis including stress fracture of the femoral neck, the sacrum, the pubis and the ischium (see below). When there is a sudden onset of pain without an adequate trauma, when weight bearing is painful and when the pain is persistent without a corresponding palpation pain, a stress fracture should be considered.

When *clinically examining* the athlete with long-standing groin pain, it is important that the palpation and functional testing is very accurate, as the muscle insertions as well as other potentially injured structures are closely located (Fig. 6.3.2), and the functions of the muscle groups are somewhat similar.

Using a set of precisely defined and reproducible examination techniques, it has been suggested that a number of diagnostic entities concerning athletes with groin pain should be defined [11]. It is recommended that the term 'diagnostic entities' is used instead of the term 'diagnosis' since the evidence-based data needed to define a precise diagnosis are not yet available. Terms such as adductor tendinitis, osteitis pubis, symphysitis and others in relation to these patients are so far without scientific basis.

Tenderness of the origin of the adductor longus and/or the gracilis at the inferior pubic ramus, and groin pain on resisted adduction are typical findings in what has been suggested to be defined as *'adductor-related groin pain'* (Fig. 6.3.8). Decreased adductor muscle strength and groin pain on full passive abduction often with a decreased range of abduction are also frequent signs. Tenderness over the pubic symphysis

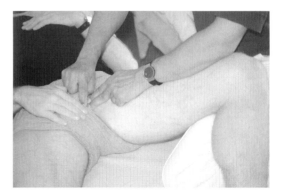

Fig. 6.3.8 Palpation of the adductor longus and gracilis insertions. The painful site is usually found at the bony part of the insertion into the pubic bone. Pain at the tendon itself is a more rare finding indicating a tendinosis inside the tendon.

Table 6.3.1 Clinical signs of the three most common musculotendinous groin injuries in athletes.

	Adductor-related groin pain	Iliopsoas-related groin pain	Inguinal canal-related groin pain
Tenderness at the adductor tendon insertion	***		
Pain at adduction against resistance	***		
Decreased muscle strength of the adductors	**		
Pain with passive stretching of the adductors	*		
Tenderness of the iliopsoas in the lower abdomen		***	
Pain with passive stretching of the iliopsoas		***	
Tightness of the iliopsoas		**	
Tenderness at the symphysis joint	**	**	**
Tenderness at the conjoined tendon			***
Tenderness of the inguinal canal			***

***, Most common presenting sign; **, common presenting sign; *, less common presenting sign.

and sometimes also of the insertion of the rectus abdominis muscle on the pubic bone are findings often seen with adductor-related groin pain (Table 6.3.1). Examination techniques for these finding have proven to be reproducible [11].

The definition of '*iliopsoas-related groin pain*' includes pain when palpating the muscle through the lower abdominal wall combined with pain at passive stretching of the muscle using the Thomas test position [21]. Frequently the iliopsoas muscle is also tight and palpating it just distal to the inguinal ligament is often painful (Table 6.3.1). The palpation of the muscle is done above the inguinal ligament and lateral to the rectus abdominis. It can also be palpated in the area just below the inguinal ligament lateral to the femoral artery and medial to the sartorius muscle (the only area where the iliopsoas is directly palpable). The Thomas test should be performed to assess the tightness of the iliopsoas, and if passive stretching of the muscle is painful. The test is done in the supine position: both knees are brought to the chest and then one leg is held in this position while the other leg is allowed to return to extension; the patient might lift the head and shoulders in order to straighten the lumbar lordosis (Fig. 6.3.9). Incomplete extension is a sign of a tight iliopsoas muscle. Pressure by the examiner's hand to extend the hip further is a test for pain on passive stretching. The above-mentioned tests for the iliopsoas were all found to be reproducible [11].

Muscle weakness and pain when flexing the hip joint

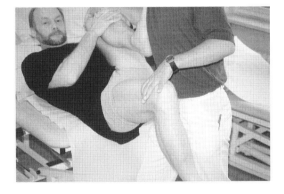

Fig. 6.3.9 The Thomas test is very useful for evaluating the flexibility of the iliopsoas muscle and the rectus femoris muscle. The position is also valuable in order to passively stretch the iliopsoas muscle and in testing it for pain during passive stretching.

against resistance at 90° is often found. Sitting with the legs stretched and then elevating the heels might result in pain since only the active hip flexor in this position is the iliopsoas: this is known as Ludloff's sign [22].

Imaging techniques can sometimes be helpful in the diagnosis of musculotendinous groin pain. Osteitis pubis-like radiologic changes around the symphysis joint are frequently found but are not specific enough (see elsewhere in this chapter). Calcified spurs can in some instances be seen along the adductor insertions. Increased uptake on the affected side in a bone scan seems to be correlated with adductor-related groin

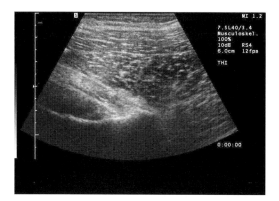

Fig. 6.3.10 Ultrasound examination of the iliopsoas tendon (indicated by arrows) near the insertion at the trochanter minor of the femur (indicated by asterisk). The tendon is thickened and the signals from this part of the tendon are more hypoechoic than in the normal tendon. Courtesy of Michael Bachmann Nielsen.

pain [11,12]. MRI also seems to show increased uptake in the same region (Fig. 6.3.5). Ultrasonography can visualize the enthesopathy of the adductors, and is also useful in detecting pathology in the lower part of the iliopsoas muscle and tendon (Fig. 6.3.10). At the time of writing all three imaging techniques lack scientific documentation for these conditions.

Treatment—chronic injuries

Various treatment modalities for chronic groin pain have been suggested in the literature. Most modalities are based on the experiences of clinical practice, lacking randomized trials.

Adductor-related pain

One clinical randomized trial [11] has described a specific exercise program found to be highly effective in the treatment of adductor-related groin pain. The trial included 68 male athletes. Seventy-five per cent of the patients trained at least 3 times a week in the period before they sustained the injury. On average they had had their symptoms for 9 months, and 75% had ceased to participate in sport. The control group was randomized to receive physiotherapy without training. The exercise group received a training program including static and dynamic exercises aimed at improving the muscles stabilizing the pelvis and the hip joints, in particular the adductor muscles. Both groups received the same amount of physiotherapy, and after the treatment period they received identical instructions about sport-related rehabilitation before returning to sports participation.

At follow-up 4 months after the end of the treatment period, 79% of the patients in the exercise group vs. 14% in the physiotherapy group were without pain at clinical examination and could participate in sport at the same or a higher level of activity without any groin pain. The patients' subjective assessment accorded with the objective outcome measures.

The exercise program consisted of two modules. The first module was a period of 2 weeks with careful static and dynamic exercises to teach the patient to reactivate the adductor muscles (Fig. 6.3.11). In most cases the athlete with adductor-related groin pain has difficulties activating these muscles, probably as a result of negative feedback caused by the pain. In the second module the exercises were gradually more demanding; heavier resistance training as well as challenging balance and coordination exercises were added (Fig. 6.3.12). The groin exercise program was performed three times a week and the exercises from module 1 were done on the days in between the treatment days. The total length of the exercise training period was between 8 and 12 weeks. Sports activities were not allowed in the treatment period. Riding a bicycle was allowed if it did not cause any pain. After 6 weeks of the treatment period jogging was allowed as long as it did not provoke any groin pain. The exercise rehabilitation program stopped when neither the treatment nor the jogging caused any pain. The athletes were then allowed to increasingly progress to demanding sports-specific training towards final sports participation.

No stretching of the adductor muscles was allowed during this 2–3-month exercise training period. However, stretching of the other lower extremity muscles was recommended, in particular stretching of the iliopsoas muscle. The iliopsoas muscle is often affected in patients with longstanding groin pain and it is the experience that proper stretching is a good treatment and prevention of *iliopsoas-related pain*.

We do not recommend steroid injections to athletes with *adductor-related groin pain*. In our experience

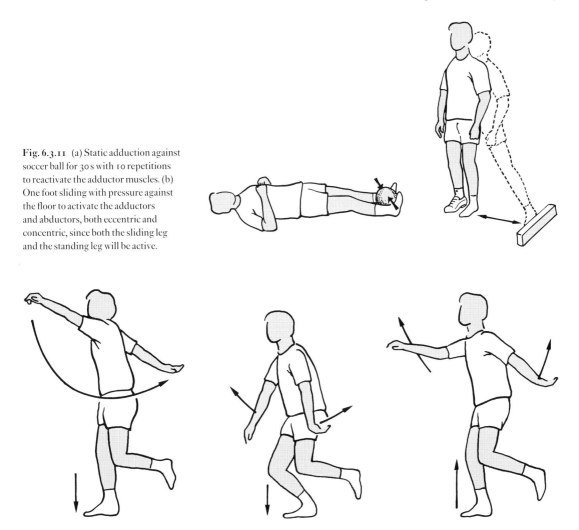

Fig. 6.3.11 (a) Static adduction against soccer ball for 30 s with 10 repetitions to reactivate the adductor muscles. (b) One foot sliding with pressure against the floor to activate the adductors and abductors, both eccentric and concentric, since both the sliding leg and the standing leg will be active.

Fig. 6.3.12 One-leg coordination exercise flexing and extending the knee and swinging the arms in the same rhythm and at the same time keeping the truncus stable (cross-country skiing on one leg); five series of 1 min for each leg.

there is no long-term beneficial effect in these patients, and if the injections affect the pain temporarily, it only makes it more difficult to monitor the training program needed to cure the groin pain [11].

There are a limited number of scientific studies supporting surgery in the treatment of adductor-related chronic groin pain. A number of papers concerning adductor tenotomy have been published. Åkermark and Rolf [24] suggest an adductor longus tenotomy 1 cm from the insertion, and Neuhaus [23] suggests that the tendon be cut at the insertion. Meyers *et al.*

[25] suggest that the adductor longus tendon be released 2–3 cm from the insertion and that multiple longitudinal incisions are made into the tendinous insertion. On the other hand Martens *et al.* [26] suggest a tenotomy of the gracilis tendon close to the insertion combined with a rectus abdominis plasty.

It is the experience of the authors that a tenotomy of the adductors *is seldom indicated*. Most patients can probably be treated successfully with the above-mentioned training program combined with sufficient treatment of concomitant injuries.

Iliopsoas-related groin pain

The authors' preferred treatment of this pain entity consists of stretching and careful dynamic strengthening — both concentric and eccentric — combined with a series of pelvic stabilization and balance exercises. Supplementary physiotherapy including massage and trigger point stimulation might also be helpful. If the treatment regimen is not progressing satisfactorily a steroid injection may be considered. The injection seems to alleviate the pain and the tension of the muscle thereby making it easier to stretch and strengthen the muscle. The injection can be technically difficult. It is placed just under the muscle fascia and along the tendon. Preferably the injection is done guided by real-time ultrasound. If ultrasound is not available the injection should be placed in the area just distal to the inguinal ligament, lateral to the femoral vessels and nerve and medial to the sartorius muscle.

The inguinal canal and associated structures

A number of *lower abdominal lesions* giving rise to groin pain in connection with athletic activities have been described. They have been named sports hernia, sportsman's hernia, incipient hernia, Gilmore's groin, pubic pain, athletic pubalgia and others. The lesions seem to be non-specific and difficult to describe pathoanatomically. The pathologic findings at surgery have been described in subjective terms as: 'loose-feeling inguinal floor', 'thinning of the fascia', 'tendency to bulge', 'weakening of the transversalis fascia', etc. [25,27–29]. Bias could be a relevant problem.

To clarify these problems a scientific approach is necessary. No consensus regarding the clinical diagnosis, the use of imaging techniques, the surgical findings and the treatment of these lesions can be found in the scientific literature. Until now very few papers have dealt with these problems scientifically [30]. No randomized trials have so far been reported considering surgery to clarify the contribution of rehabilitation, placebo, denervation and time itself.

Sports hernia

The term 'sports hernia' refers to a condition of chronic groin pain caused by a weakness of the posterior inguinal wall without a clinically obvious hernia. Because of the insidious onset and non-specific nature of the symptoms, there is often a prolonged course prior to diagnosis. In one study, the average duration of symptoms was 20 months, with a range of 6 weeks to 5 years [27].

The *etiology* to these lesions is sometimes a traumatic episode where the athlete overstretches the front of the groin and lower abdomen, as in a forceful sliding tackle in soccer. In other cases the athlete cannot recall any single episode precipitating the pain but recalls it as developing gradually, often in connection with overuse over a period of time. The patient will often have multiple diagnoses contributing to the groin pain. Adductor-related pain, iliopsoas-related pain, sacroiliac pain and low back pain are typically concomitant findings in these patients [11,16]. Which lesion was the primary lesion resulting in the other(s) is seldom clear: it is often a question of 'the chicken or the egg'.

The pain in sports hernia is experienced 'deep' in the groin, slightly more proximal than the adductor-related pain. Kicking and endurance running tend to increase the symptoms. The pain tends to be diffuse, with radiation along the inguinal ligament, the perineum, the rectus muscles, adductor muscles, and sometimes also to the opposite side. Scrotal pain may also be a component. Maneuvers that cause increased intra-abdominal pressure, such as coughing, sneezing or bowel movements, will usually cause increased pain.

The most specific signs are tenderness at the conjoined tendon towards the pubic tubercle, tenderness and enlargement of the external ring of the inguinal canal, and tenderness of the posterior wall of the inguinal canal (Table 6.3.1). The posterior wall tenderness is usually worse and sometimes a bulge can be felt with increased intra-abdominal pressure from e.g. coughing. The pain may be exacerbated during coughing. An examination after vigorous exercise may be helpful in difficult cases. The examination of the inguinal canal must be performed through the scrotum, or in women through the labia majores, to be able to evaluate most structures. In addition, in males a scrotal and testicular examination are necessary to exclude tumors. If gastrointestinal or gynecologic diseases are suspected further examination must be undertaken.

The diagnosis of a clinically apparent hernia is straightforward, with obvious clinical signs and symptoms. However, this is usually not the case for sports hernias, and in those athletes with continued groin pain despite adequate rest and no obvious hernia, herniography and/or ultrasonography can be helpful. Both methods have been described in the literature [31,32] but better scientific evaluation is needed.

Treatment of sports hernias

Since the sports hernia by nature is an incipient hernia, rehabilitation should always be tried as a first step. A regular hernia has not yet developed, and a training program improving pelvic stabilization by training the strength, balance and coordination of the involved muscles may give the abdominal wall lesion a chance to heal. This strategy would allow simultaneous treatment of the other diagnostic entities causing groin pain often found at the same time as a sports hernia. The suggested treatment is, however, not yet supported by scientific evidence.

If the pain continues despite this regimen, and examination or other tests detect no other pathoanatomic explanation, surgical treatment may be considered.

Surgical treatment of painful sports hernia is aimed at repair and reinforcement of the weak posterior inguinal wall. A variety of open surgical procedures have been described to reinforce the posterior wall, either by plication and tightening of the existing tissue or by reinforcement with an artificial mesh graft. It has also been reported that a simple repair of small tears in the external oblique aponeurosis and/or the conjoined tendon will give good results [33]. Recently, laparoscopic procedures have been developed for hernia repair. This usually involves placement of synthetic mesh over the defect superficial to the peritoneum. Early results have been relatively encouraging, with recurrence rates near the level of open procedures [34]. However, the procedure is technically difficult with a significant learning curve, and the procedure is more costly than open procedures.

After surgery rehabilitation before returning to sport is imperative. The rehabilitation program based on the experience of the authors is shown in the box.

Week 1—walking and lifting up to 10 kg.
Week 2—faster walking, careful jogging and normal day-to-day activities.
Week 3—running carefully and gentle groin-related strength training.
Week 4—full participation in the pelvis-stabilizing rehabilitation program performed before the operation.
When running and rehabilitation program can be done pain free—careful gradual return to sport.

Symphysis joint-related pain

Osteitis pubis is a term that was originally used to describe an infection in the pubic bone around the symphysis joint. This infection was seen especially in connection with suprapubic abdominal surgery [35]. The characteristic radiologic findings—bone resorption, widening of the symphysis and sclerosis along the rami (Fig. 6.3.13)—were in the 60s reported to appear on X-rays from athletes with chronic groin pain. However, it was soon evident that no bone or joint infection was present, and that this X-ray appearance was the result of a biomechanical problem applying stress on the symphysis joint and leading to the radiographic changes. Harris and Murray [20] found that

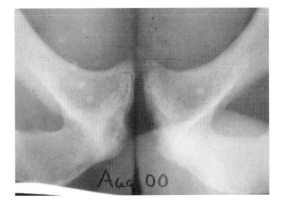

Fig. 6.3.13 The characteristic radiologic findings of longstanding stress to the symphysis joint (often seen without any symptoms)—bone resorption, widening of the symphysis and sclerosis—characterized as 'osteitis pubis-like' changes.

these 'osteitis pubis-like' changes seemed to be correlated to the amount of physical activity — in particular soccer — undertaken and as such were a poor indication of groin pain in athletes. Groin straining activities such as soccer increase the shearing forces in the symphysis joint. The stress on this joint might thus lead to these radiologic signs, merely indicating an increased load of the joint rather than pathology.

Some authors consider 'osteitis pubis' as a diagnosis based on vaguely defined findings and symptoms, that in most cases is covered by other diagnostic entities. It is described as a condition with a gradual onset of pain that may radiate to the sides and distally. The condition is considered to be self-limiting and sometimes a cortisone injection may be given under fluoroscopic control.

It seems that, when a specific anatomic and pathologic diagnosis for chronic groin pain cannot be made, the term 'osteitis pubis' is often used as the diagnosis. McCarthy *et al.*[36] described osteitis pubis in athletes as: '. . . a broader diagnostic category, that encompasses several different etiologic entities in or near the symphysis.' The characteristic radiologic changes are often found in athletes without groin problems as well as in athletes with a specific groin-related diagnosis. In a study of adductor-related groin pain radiologic signs of osteitis pubis were found in 66% of the patients and scintigraphic changes in the bone in 85%[11].

It is the view of the present authors that 'osteitis pubis' should not be used as a specific diagnosis in the case of athletes with groin pain, unless an infection is present in the pubic bone. The term should be reserved to describe 'osteitis pubis-like' radiologic changes around the symphysis joint.

Inflammation in pelvic joints

Inflammatory conditions may be seen in the joints of the symphysis and sacroiliac joints. Sacroiliitis is not uncommon in outdoor winter sports. Sacroiliitis can also be a symptom in a generalized disease such as rheumatoid arthritis or Bechterew's disease. Pain and/or discomfort may radiate to the groin, to the hip joint, or to the thigh. Changes in the sacroiliac joints may be present without the athlete feeling any pain. The symptoms may be vague and most pronounced in the morning. Long intervals without symptoms may be present. The diagnoses are made by clinical examination and with the aid of CT scan. The treatment consists of anti-inflammatory medication and physical therapy.

Fractures

Fractures of the pelvis, femoral neck and trochanteric region are common in the elderly but can also appear in adolescence and active adult athletes, in this case being a result of major trauma such as traffic accidents but also high-energy impact in sports.

In sports the most common fractures in this region are stress fractures and avulsion fractures.

Stress fractures

Many stress fractures probably remain unrecognized because the patients treat themselves by resting until the pain improves. Stress fractures are considered to occur from a repetitive cyclic load by submaximal forces leading to overload of the bone tissue, but the exact etiology is still unknown. The common factor is that cyclic forces cause breakdown of the bone that occurs faster than the bone's remodeling capacity. The tibia is the most commonly affected bone, but stress fractures may appear in apparently all bones of the weight-bearing lower extremities. Stress fractures of the pubic rami seem to be particularly common among long-distance running athletes. These fractures appear to be associated with anorexia and amenorrhea among female athletes (Fig. 6.3.4). Barrow and Saha reported that stress fractures occurred in 49% of collegiate female distance runners that had less than five menses per year. In addition, of those athletes that were amenorrheic, 47% had an eating disorder.

Stress fractures *of the pubic rami* present as an insidious onset of lower pelvic and groin pain that is worsened with pounding-type activities. The pain is often worse immediately after running, and will gradually improve with rest. Stress fractures are often related to a sudden increase in the intensity of the athlete's training. Stress fractures are often not evident on plain radiographs until the formation of callus. Therefore, if early stress fracture is suspected, a bone scan or MRI is most sensitive in the early phases.

Treatment of stress fractures in the pelvis, except for femoral neck fractures, is relatively straightforward. This involves a period of 4–6 weeks' rest from the activities responsible. When the athlete is pain free, a graduated program of return to activities can begin. Any dietary or hormonal contributions to this diagnosis must be addressed to assist in healing and prevention of recurrence.

The most serious stress fracture in the pelvis region is that to *the femoral neck*. An unrecognized stress fracture of the femoral neck can proceed to complete fracture with the high risk of avascular necrosis. This is a potentially devastating problem, so early recognition and treatment is the key. One study reported on 23 athletes with femoral neck stress fractures. Of the seven patients that developed complications, five had a displaced fracture. This stresses the importance of early recognition and treatment of these injuries to prevent displacement and necrosis.

Treatment of femoral neck stress fractures is based on the displacement and location of the fracture at diagnosis. All displaced fractures require surgery to anatomically reduce the fracture supported with internal fixation. Non-displaced fractures can be divided into two categories: (i) fractures that occur on the compression side of the bone, the inferior femoral neck; and (ii) fractures that occur on the tension side of the bone, the superior femoral neck. The compression-sided fractures have a good healing potential and they can be treated non-surgically. Activities should be restricted by pain and this usually requires a short period of crutch walking to prevent progression into a complete fracture. This is followed by a gradual return to normal pain-free activities. It is important to stress that no pain should occur either during or after the activity. Progression of healing should be monitored with serial plain radiographs. Return to light running cannot usually begin until 2–3 months after appearance, and only as long as there is no pain and the radiographs show healing of the fracture.

Tension-side fractures are best treated with surgical internal fixation, e.g. using screws or pins. The tension-side fractures have a poor healing capacity and are more prone to proceed to complete fracture. For non-displaced fractures treated surgically as described above, return to pain-free light running can begin at about 2–3 months.

Avulsion fractures

Avulsion fractures about the pelvis occur almost exclusively in the adolescent population. The apophyses make a relatively weak connection to the central bony skeleton through the zone of provisional calcification of the growth plate. Powerful muscle contractions from the muscles around the hip and pelvis are occasionally able to overpower the stability of the growth plate and cause avulsion fractures.

There are three typical locations for avulsion fractures of the pelvis: (i) anterior superior iliac spine (ASIS); (ii) anterior inferior iliac spine (AIIS); and (iii) ischial tuberosity. Avulsions from the ASIS typically occur from a strong contraction of the sartorius muscle during jumping in sports such as basketball. AIIS avulsions occur in kicking sports such as soccer, resulting from a violent contraction of the rectus femoris muscle. Avulsions of the ischial tuberosity occur from hamstring contractions and are most frequently seen in running and hurdling sports. For avulsion fractures of the ASIS and AIIS, most authors recommend non-operative treatment. This includes symptomatic activity restriction until the fracture heals. Although there are no large series in the literature, it does not appear that operative fixation results in either earlier return to activity or better return of strength than non-operative treatment.

The treatment of the ischial tuberosity avulsion remains controversial. Although again there are no randomized studies reported, some authors have indicated no functional deficits following non-operative treatment, while others have reported a decrease in strength and function resulting from 'widely displaced' fractures. These fractures can sometimes cause massive callus formation that can cause pain and may occasionally mimic an osteosarcoma. Therefore, in these cases, some reports have advocated early surgical fixations, while others have pointed out that late excision of the massive callus can be performed to relieve symptoms. We presently recommend that large fragments that are displaced more than 1–1.5 cm need surgical reduction and fixation.

Rehabilitation after an avulsion fracture depends on the stability of the fracture. If it is operated on and evaluated as stable, range of motion exercises can start immediately with increasing strength training. If it is not stable exercises may be delayed for 3–6 weeks depending on the location. If the avulsion fracture is not operated on, the patient can often start mobilizing activities fairly early and let pain decide the level of these. Physiotherapy should be used.

Hip joint changes

As with the groin region, with pain in the hip it must be ascertained what tissues are involved. According to Cailliet four specific structures about the hip joint may cause pain:

1 the fibrous capsule and its ligaments;
2 the surrounding muscles;
3 the bony periosteum; and
4 the synovial lining of the joint.

The most painful condition of the hip joint is degenerative joint disease—osteoarthrosis. In athletes late degenerative changes in the hip joint is probably a risk. In runners some papers have not been able to find any increased risk for developing arthrosis. There are however, increasing indications that extensive top-level running may be a risk factor in causing late degenerative changes in the hip joints. The same may be true for top-level soccer, but the scientific evidence is not yet conclusive. Top-level sport of the highest intensity is probably a risk factor for developing late degenerative changes in the hip.

Pain in the hip joint may be an early symptom of localized changes in the joint such as low-grade arthrosis–arthritis, osteochondritis dissecans, or loose bodies. In rare cases the outer rim of the joint labrum or limbus can be avulsed, and the torn end can rotate into the joint. These injuries may produce a sharp and catching pain during exercise and often persistent pain after exercise.

Pain elicited by rotation in the hip joint *may* indicate an intra-articular lesion and requires radiographic examination. If a plain X-ray is negative, sometimes a CT scan, an MRI or an MRI arthroscan is necessary to establish a diagnosis. Arthroscopy is of less diagnostic help but can be of value, especially in the management of loose bodies.

The most common cause of painful hip in children is transient synovitis or capsulitis. This is assumed to be a benign self-limited condition seen in children younger than 10 years of age. This condition should be differentiated from serious lesions such as congenital dislocation of the hip, Legg–Calvé–Perthes disease, osteomyelitis, bone disorders, osteoid osteoma, tuber-culosis and rheumatoid arthritis. Two significant hip conditions in adolescents are slipped capital femoral epiphysis and osteochondritis dissecans, both of which will cause pain in the groin area.

Bursitis

There are at least 13 permanent bursae present in the hip region, and they are often localized between tendons and muscles and over bony prominences.

The pathologic conditions involving the bursae can be divided into traumatic and inflammatory conditions. Traumatic bursitis can be called *hemorrhagic bursitis,* or *hemobursa.* The most common cause of hemorrhagic bursitis is either a direct trauma, e.g. a fall against the bursa, or an indirect trauma through a strain in a passing tendon with hemorrhage. In a hemorrhagic bursa, the hemorrhage can be extensive and if it is not treated adequately, the blood will coagulate, and eventually fibrinous adhesive tissue of fibrin bodies will be formed in the bursa. These adhesions or free bodies will produce a chronic inflammatory bursitis with recurrent problems. The treatment of acute hemorrhagic bursitis should be evacuation of the hematoma. A fluctuation over the bursa may be palpated; a common example is the superficial trochanteric bursa, which is often subject to direct trauma. In acute cases the hematoma may be aspirated. Ultrasound-guided puncture can sometimes be helpful and endoscopically assisted lavage has been proposed. If the condition becomes chronic, surgical excision of the bursa is often the treatment of choice.

Inflammatory bursitis may be divided into friction bursitis, chemical bursitis and infection bursitis. Friction bursitis may be caused by repeated frequent movements of a muscle tendon against a bursa, e.g. iliopsoas against the iliopectineal bursa. The iliopectineal bursa is the largest synovial bursa in the whole body and it is located anterior to the hip joint and dorsal to the iliopsoas tendon. This bursa communicates with the hip joint in about 15% of adults. This bursa may be the location for inflammation, whether isolated or combined with iliopsoas pathology. *Iliopectineal bursitis* may give a feeling of tenderness and swelling in the middle of the groin, which may spread across the inguinal ligament.

On the lateral proximal femur, deep to the iliotibial band, there is a superficial bursa. Between the tendons to the gluteus medius and tensor fascia latae and behind the greater trochanter there is a deeper-located bursa. Both these bursae may be the location for an inflammation, e.g. because of untreated hemorrhage. Malalignment with increased pronation and compensatory internal leg rotation can cause overload in this region. Trochanteric bursitis will cause pain and tenderness just lateral and posterior to the greater trochanter. The pain can radiate down along the outside of the thigh and be erroneously diagnosed as referred pain from herniated disk lesions in the lumbar spine. Pain may be elicited by rotation of the hip joint at 90° of flexion. Careful palpation around the lateral posterior aspect of the trochanter region may reveal localized tenderness. Ultrasonographic examination is very helpful in localizing and diagnosing the bursitis. Initial treatment consists of cold packs, NSAIDs and rest. After the acute phase cortisone injection — preferably ultrasound guided — may give relief. Foot orthotics are sometimes of value to address any malalignment of the leg. This condition can be long lasting and therapy resistant, and surgery may therefore sometimes be indicated.

The chemical bursitis that is sustained after a chemical irritation from products and seen after inflammation or degeneration in tendon tissue is not common in the groin. Bursitis due to infection may be septic or caused by a bacterial immigration through lacerated skin, and can occasionally be seen over the trochanteric region.

The snapping hip

This condition can be ascribed to a number of very different causes. The snapping sensation is audible but not always associated with pain. When the snapping is just associated with the sound of the snapping and no discomfort or pain is felt, the condition can usually be ignored and considered to be without any pathologic importance.

The snapping can be located externally, that is on the lateral side of the hip, or internally on the medial side.

The external snapping hip is normally easily palpated on the lateral side of the hip, often in the area of the greater trochanter. The condition is in most cases caused by a thickened border of the iliotibial band or by the anterior border of the gluteus maximus. In both cases they are tight in relationship to the bone prominence and the friction produces a bursitis. The problem is most prominent in female athletes, perhaps as a result of their broader pelvis and/or hyperpronation. The treatment consists of correction of any malalignment that might have caused the problem combined with stretching of the affected muscle. NSAID or steroid injections into the bursa may occasionally give long-term relief. In rare cases surgical treatment releasing the tight part of the tendon and excising the bursa can be necessary.

The internal snapping hip can be either an intra-articular problem in the hip joint or a snapping iliopsoas tendon. Intra-articular loose bodies in the hip joint caused by a trauma, osteochondritis dissecans or osteochondromatosis can result in intra-articular locking, clicking and pain. A labral tear might also result in a painful snapping internal hip. A more common cause is a tight and/or fibrotic iliopsoas tendon snapping over the iliopectineal eminence or over the femoral joint. The tendon lies in a groove between the iliopectineal eminence and the anterior inferior iliac spine; it crosses over the femoral head and capsule and inserts into the lesser trochanter (Fig. 6.3.7). When the hip is extended, especially from the flexed and externally rotated position, an audible and sometimes painful snap is felt. Palpation over the hip joint can often reveal a snapping sensation against the fingers. An iliopsoas bursography can demonstrate the snapping of the iliopsoas tendon, but real-time ultrasound examination with a small 5 MHz convex array transducer can show more clearly in a fast, cheap and non-invasive way the snapping of the iliopsoas tendon.

The intra-articular lesions can be diagnosed with MRI or CT scan combined with an arthrography. Hip arthroscopy can also be indicated, both as a diagnostic method and as the method of choice for extracting loose bodies or debriding a labral lesion.

The painful snapping iliopsoas can in most cases be treated non-surgically with a combination of stretching and careful dynamic strengthening exercises. Sometimes a steroid injection (see iliopsoas injury) may be tried. If the non-surgical treatment fails, a surgical release of the tendon in some form of a lengthening procedure can be effective [37].

Nerve entrapment

Peripheral nerves may become entrapped after direct trauma or inflammatory conditions. Nerves most commonly affected are the ilioinguinal, genitofemoral and lateral cutaneous femoral nerves. The obturatorial and iliohypogastric nerves may also be involved (Fig. 6.3.3).

The ilioinguinal nerve transmits sensations from the proximal part of the external genitals and parts of the medial thigh. Pain in these areas should lead to suspicion of engagement of the nerve. These sensations may be elicited by e.g. intensive abdominal muscle training leading to entrapment of the nerve where it passes through the different layers of the abdominal muscles and their fasciae. The intensity and character of the pain vary. Hyperextension of the hip joint might augment the pain. It is usually possible to detect skin hyperesthesia, which is demonstrated by drawing a needle across the skin from a non-painful area to a painful area. The diagnosis is confirmed by a block of the nerve with local anesthetics that will promptly relieve the pain. If the pain is severe, surgical treatment may be considered.

The genitofemoral nerve is divided into two parts: (i) the ramus genitalia, which transmits sensations from the labium major/scrotum; and (ii) the ramus femoralis, which gives sensations from the skin of the thigh just distal to the ilioinguinal ligament. The symptoms are similar to those mentioned for the ilioinguinal nerve.

Westman has reported on seven cases of entrapment of the ilioinguinal and genitofemoral nerves, which were operated on. He considers a lasting cure to be obtained only by local nerve resection.

A sensory mononeuritis of the lateral cutaneous nerve of the thigh is called meralgia paresthetica. The posterior branch of the nerve transmits cutaneous sensations from the superior lateral part of the buttock. The anterior branch, which is the most important clinically, passes through the fascia lata through a small canal and transmits sensations, and occasionally causes skin hyperesthesia. Usually there is no history of any trauma, but factors such as tight belts or corsets or long periods of acute hip flexion may cause the condition.

Posture exercises that decrease lordosis are considered valuable. Anti-inflammatory medicine may be tried, but most often surgical decompression is the treatment of choice.

Tumors

Tumors are not uncommon in the groin area, and we have seen several cases in which the pain was first experienced in the groin area in connection with a soccer game or similar sports activity. The pain was often considered to be caused by strain in the groin muscles and tendons. After a couple of months, the patients are often referred to surgical or orthopedic departments because of persistent pain or tumor-suspicious findings on X-ray. Osteosarcomas, chondrosarcomas, malignant schwannomas and other tumors have been diagnosed often at a late stage, due to both patient's and doctor's delay. Persistent pain or an unexplained 'mass' in the groin region should be carefully investigated to exclude a tumor, and a radiology examination should always be included at an early stage in patients with diffuse groin pain. Ultrasound, MR imaging or CT scan will secure the diagnosis.

Summary

Injuries and pain in the groin and pelvic area remain one of the more difficult areas in sports medicine due to their highly variable pathoanatomy. The incidence of these injuries seems to be increasing. Earlier, such injuries mostly occurred, or were at least diagnosed, in soccer and ice hockey. As a result, top-level athletes in soccer and ice hockey have recently been participating in preventive groin exercise programs, and the incidence of groin pain seems to be leveling off. These injuries are, however, now being recognized in sports such as basketball, American football and baseball, and also in long-distance runners and other athletes. Some of these groin injuries are apparently secondary to acute strains that have been neglected or not treated properly. Others are often caused by muscle imbalances and poor biomechanics resulting in chronic conditions, when proper rehabilitation and treatment is lacking. The dilemma remains that there are many different causes, from many organs and tissues, of groin pain.

The only way to successfully treat groin injury and pain is to base the treatment and rehabilitation protocol on a correct diagnosis, even though this may be highly challenging. It is imperative that the athlete, the coach, the trainer and the physician have great respect for groin problems and do not neglect these symptoms. If the athlete experiences groin pain, he/she should limit activities to those that are pain free until a probable diagnosis is secured. If these injuries are mismanaged or, more commonly, ignored, there is a high risk of developing a chronic groin pain condition. If there is any difficulty or doubt about the diagnosis, then these athletes should be referred to specialists in this area, who have often developed a multidisciplinary approach to groin injuries.

Even if knowledge in this area is developing, information about chronic groin pain problems is still limited, being mostly based on clinical experience. There remains a need for much more research in this area.

In conclusion, groin injuries may not in themselves be serious injuries. However, they may lead to chronic pain and impair athletic ability and performance, especially if not correctly diagnosed, and promptly adequately treated. Groin injuries and pain may prevent an athlete from participating in sport activities over a long period of time—or even end his or her career—something bound to distress the dedicated athlete.

Case story 6.3.1

A male football (soccer) player, 27 years old, has played at elite level for 9 months. He is suffering from pain in the right groin and remembers one painful episode of hyperextension of the right hip during a match 3 months ago.

The physiotherapist in the club has treated him with ultrasound, stretching, massage and some abdominal and back exercises.

Six weeks after the groin pain started, he was examined at our sports medicine center. Clinical signs of adductor-related pain, iliopsoas-related pain and incipient hernia were found. These findings were confirmed by ultrasonography.

Treatment was initiated. It consisted of the exercise program for adductor-related groin pain, combined with exercises to stimulate and stretch the iliopsoas. A combination of abdominal and back exercises was added to improve pelvic and lumbar stability.

The program was performed 3 times a week and jogging was allowed after 6 weeks.

At clinical control after 8 weeks of treatment *no* pain from the adductors or the iliopsoas was found any more.

With regard to the lower abdominal pain there are *two possible endings* to this case story: A or B.

A The previous treatment had only slightly reduced the abdominal pain. The patient still had lower abdominal pain both at palpation and at functional testing. It was still painful to sprint, make fast turns and do resisted sit-ups.

The patient was operated on and a small rupture of the external oblique aponeurosis was seen and repaired. A soft posterior wall was repaired with a mesh onlay. No hernia sac was found.

Four weeks after surgery he was able to run fast and make fast turns, and during the next 3 weeks he was allowed to sprint and participate in football training. Seven weeks after surgery he played his first match and had no groin pain.

B The pain in the lower abdomen was reduced considerably and he was able to run straight without pain. The treatment program was continued and after 15 weeks he returned to football 3 times a week without any groin pain. At clinical examination no pain was found at the adductors, the iliopsoas, the conjoint tendon or in the inguinal canal. At follow-up 10 months after the first symptoms the patient was without any groin problems.

Both scenarios are commonly found and our problem is that it is not possible from the clinic to decide which treatment is the best. Which patient should have surgery right away and which patient needs no operation but can be managed solely with the exercise treatment?

Multiple choice questions

1 *Ultrasound examination is of value in diagnosing groin injuries because:*

a it is pain free

b it can be done on the sports field

c it is real-time and can be performed dynamically

d it is easy to visualize cartilage

e it can show bone edema around the symphysis joint.

2 *Among the three most common causes of groin pain in athletes are:*

a adductor-related pain

b stress fracture of the femoral neck

c lateral hernia

d snapping iliopsoas

e incipient hernia.

3 *Typical findings in the athlete with adductor-related groin pain are:*

a pain when jogging

b tenderness at the insertion of the adductor longus muscle insertion at the pubic bone

c tight lower leg muscles

d increased range of abduction

e groin pain on resisted adduction.

4 *The most serious stress fracture in the pelvis region is:*

a the superior pubic bone

b the inferior pubic bone

c the sacrum

d tension side femoral neck fracture

e compression side femoral neck fracture.

5 *Treatment of adductor-related groin pain should include:*

a strengthening exercises of the adductor muscles

b steroid injection

c balance and coordination exercises for the pelvis

d stretching of the adductor muscles

e transverse friction massage.

References

1 Ekstrand J, Gillquist J. Soccer injuries and their mechanisms: a prospective study. *Med Sci Sports Exerc* 1983; **15**: 267–70.

2 Ekstrand J, Hilding J. The incidence and differential diagnosis of acute groin injuries in male soccer players. *Scand J Med Sci Sports* 1999; **9**: 98–103.

3 Engström B, Forssblad M, Johansson C, Törnkvist H. Does a major knee injury definitely sideline an elite soccer player? *Am J Sports Med* 1990; **18**: 101–5.

4 Nielsen AB, Yde J. Epidemiology and traumatology of injuries in soccer. *Am J Sports Med* 1989; **17**: 803–7.

5 Renström P, Peterson L. Groin injuries in athletes. *Br J Sports Med* 1980; **14**: 30–6.

6 Hides JA, Richardson CA, Jull GA. Multifidus muscle recovery is not automatic following resolution of acute first episode low back pain. *Spine* 1996; **21**: 2763–9.

7 Wilke HJ, Wolf S, Claes LE. Stability increase of the lumbar spine with different muscle groups: a biomechanical in vitro study. *Spine* 1995; **20**: 192–8.

8 Gibbon WW. Groin pain in athletes (letter). *Lancet* 1999; **353**: 1444–5.

9 Gibbon WW, Jenkins CN, Crowe MTI, Freeman SJ. Groin pain in soccer players; MRI appearences. *Br J Sports Med* 1999; **33**: 57.

10 Stureson B. *Load and movement of the sacroiliac joint*. Lund University, Sweden, 2000.

11 Hölmich P, Uhrskou P, Ulnits L, Kanstrup I, Nielsen MB, Bjerg AM *et al.* Effectiveness of active physical training as treatment for long-standing adductor-related groin pain in athletes: randomised trial. *Lancet* 2001; **353**: 439–43.

12 Le Jeune JJ, Rochcongar P, Vazelle F, Bernard AM, Herry JY, Ramée A. Pubic pain syndrome in sportsmen: comparison of radiographic and scintigraphic findings. *Eur J Nuclear Med* 1984; **9**: 250–3.

13 O'Donoghue DH. Principles in the management of specific injuries. In: O'Donoghue DH, ed. *Treatment of Injuries to Athletes*. Philadelphia: W.B. Saunders, 1970: 43–100.

14 Peterson L, Stener B. Old total rupture of the adductor longus muscle. *Acta Orthop Scand* 1976; **47**: 653–7.

15 Symeonides PP. Isolated traumatic rupture of the adductor longus muscle of the thigh. *Clin Orth Rel Res* 1972; **88**: 64–6.

16 Lovell G. The diagnosis of chronic groin pain in athletes: a review of 189 cases. *Aust J Sci Med Sport* 1995; **27**: 76–9.

17 Gibbon WW. Groin pain in professional soccer players: a comparison of England and the rest of Western Europe. *Br J Sports Med* 1999; **33**: 435.

18 Morrenhof JW. *Stabilization of the human hip-joint*. Thesis: Rijksuniversiteit of Leiden, Holland, 1989.

19 Andersson E, Oddsson L, Grundström H, Thorstensson A. The role of the psoas and iliacus muscles for stability and movement of the lumbar spine, pelvis and hip. *Scand J Med Sci Sports* 1995; **5**: 10–6.

20 Harris NH, Murray RO. Lesions of the symphysis in athletes. *Br Med J* 1974; **4**: 211–4.

21 Hölmich P. Adductor-related groin pain in athletes. *Sport Med Arthrosc Rev* 1997; **5**: 285–91.

22 Mozes M, Papa MZ, Zweig A, Horoszowski H, Adar R. Iliopsoas injury in soccer players. *Br J Sports Med* 1985; **19**: 168–70.

23 Neuhaus P, Gabriel T, Maureo W. Adduktoren-insertionstenopathie, operative therapie und resultate. *Helv Chir Acta* 1982; **49**: 667–70.

24 Åkermark C, Johansson C. Tenotomy of the adductor longus tendon in the treatment of chronic groin pain in athletes. *Am J Sports Med* 1992; **20**: 640–3.

25 Meyers WC, Foley DP, Garrett WE, Lohnes JH,

Mandlebaum BR. Management of severe lower abdominal inguinal pain in high-performance athletes. *Am J Sports Med* 2000; **28**: 2–8.

26 Martens MA, Hansen L, Mulier JC. Adductor tendinitis and musculus rectus abdominis tendopathy. *Am J Sports Med* 1987; **15**: 353–6.

27 Hackney RG. The sports hernia: a cause of chronic groin pain. *Br J Sports Med* 1993; **27**: 58–62.

28 Polglase AL, Frydman GM, Farmer KC. Inguinal surgery for debilitating chronic groin pain in athletes. *Med J Aust* 1991; **155**: 674–7.

29 Taylor DC, Meyers WC, Moylan JA, Lohnes J, Bassett FH, Garrett WE. Abdominal musculature abnormalities as a cause of groin pain in athletes. *Am J Sports Med* 1991; **19**: 239–42.

30 Lovell G, Malycha P, Pieterse S. Biopsy of the conjoint tendon in athletes with chronic groin pain. *Aust J Sci Med Sport* 1990; **22**: 102–3.

31 Orchard JW, Read JW, Neophyton J, Garlick D. Groin pain associated with ultrasound finding of inguinal canal posterior wall deficiency in Australian Rules Football. *Br J Sports Med* 1998; **32**: 134–9.

32 Smedberg SGG, Broome AEA, Gullmo Å, Roos H. Herniography in athletes with groin pain. *Am J Surg* 1985; **149**: 378–82.

33 Williams P, Foster ME. 'Gilmore's groin'—or is it? *Br J Sports Med* 1995; **29**: 206–8.

34 Ingoldby CJH. Laparoscopic and conventional repair of groin disruption in sportsmen. *Br J Surg* 1997; **84**: 213–5.

35 Adams RJ, Chandler FA. Osteitis pubis of traumatic etiology. *J Bone Joint Surg* 1953; **35**: 685–96.

36 McCarthy B, Dorfman HD. Pubic osteolysis—a benign lesion of the pelvis closely mimicking a malignant neoplasm. *Clin Orth Rel Res* 1990; **251**: 300–7.

37 Jacobson T, Allen WC. Surgical correction of the snapping iliopsoas tendon. *Am J Sports Med* 1990; **18**: 470–4.

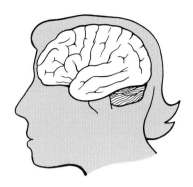

Chapter 6.4
Head

LIYING ZHANG, KING H. YANG,
ALBERT I. KING & LARS ENGEBRETSEN

Classical reference

Lissner H, Lebow M, Evans F. Experimental studies
    on the relation between acceleration and
    intracranial changes in man. *Surg Gynecol Obstetr*
    1960; 11: 329–338.

In the United States, Wayne State University initiated
fundamental research in biomechanics in 1939.
Biomechanics is defined as the application of the
principles of mechanics to living biologic material.
Specifically, the study of head injury, initiated jointly
by a neurosurgeon, Dr E. Stephen Gurdjian, and an
engineer, Prof. Herbert R. Lissner, was the earliest
known collaborative effort in biomechanics. From
1939 to 1963, the Wayne State group pioneered a long
series of head injury experiments. These included the
dropping of metal balls onto dry human skulls, impacts to the foreheads of embalmed cadavers against
rigid and padded surfaces and the application of an air
pressure pulse directly onto the dura of anesthetized
animals. Based on clinical observations that moderate
levels of concussion were usually accompanied by a
linear skull fracture in 80% of the patients, they
hypothesized that head accelerations causing cadaveric skull fracture could be used to infer the onset of
concussion. Their work led to the development of a
concussion tolerance curve in 1960. It is now known as
the Wayne State tolerance curve (WSTC) (see Fig.
6.4.1). It basically states that the brain can tolerate a
larger magnitude of translational acceleration if the
acceleration duration is shorter, and that there is
an acceleration limit for the occurrence of concussive

injury due to frontal impact over a range of impact
durations.

The complete WSTC was constructed by combining data from cadaveric skull fracture tests, animal intracranial pressure studies and the voluntary sled ride
of Col. John Paul Stapp. In the cadaveric tests, linear
fractures of the frontal bone were associated with
an effective acceleration of 112 G, with peaks of up to
200 G and with an intracranial pressure build-up of
206 kPa. The average impact duration was 0.004 s.
Other data in the range of 0.001–0.006 s were obtained
by dropping a group of intact cadavers and decapitated
heads onto a rigid slab. These skull fracture data anchor the short-duration end of the curve, up to 0.006 s.
For longer durations of up to 0.01 s, concussion data
from animal experiments along with head acceleration
and pressure data obtained from cadaver head impacts

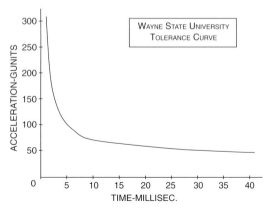

Fig. 6.4.1 Wayne State University Tolerance Curve.

638

with automobile dash panels were used to plot that part of the WSTC. The asymptotic tolerance level for durations of 0.040 s and longer was based on the sled ride of Col. Stapp. He experienced an estimated peak deceleration of 45 G and sustained a detached retina in one eye. This level was later raised to 80 G because the injury was not related to the brain. There was a lot of scatter in the data but a tolerance curve in the form of a hyperbola was drawn through the data points. The WSTC is a plot of effective head acceleration vs. impact duration and is an assessment of injury potential of the head due to impact.

Later, the WSTC was used by Gadd[1] to arrive at a weighted impulse criterion, known as the Gadd Severity Index. It was further modified by Versace[2] who proposed the Head Injury Criterion (HIC). This acceleration–time function, derived from the WSTC, is currently used by the US Government as a safety standard for automobile crashes. This standard has now been adopted in many other parts of the world as well. In real-world collisions, however, head injury occurs when there is combination of translational and rotational acceleration, both of which do not need to be extremely high. It is recommended that any new criterion should reflect the contribution of both forms of acceleration.

Introduction

Injury to the head is a major cause of serious disability and fatality and tends to have a greater long-term effect than injuries to the extremities. Acute head injury is also commonly referred to as traumatic brain injury (TBI). The most common causes of TBI are automotive and contact sports-related accidents. Head and facial injuries in contact sports have been around since the first pugilists and wrestlers began competing thousands of years ago. The specter of serious head injury in athletes leading to death, permanent brain damage or quadriplegia, although infrequent, has been consistently associated with American football, ice hockey, boxing, water sports, motorcycling and gymnastics.

The most common head injury in sports is minor traumatic brain injury (MTBI) or concussion. According to the National Health Interview Survey (NHIS), there are more than 300 000 MTBIs attributed to sports or recreational activities each year in the US[3]. American football alone is responsible for more than 100 000 concussions. Estimates regarding the likelihood of an athlete in a contact sport experiencing a concussion vary, but may be as high as 19%. Furthermore, the effects of concussions are now known to be cumulative, even when the concussive blows are relatively minor. Recent data suggests that college football players who have experienced two or more prior concussions perform more poorly on tests of cognitive functioning (speed and problem solving) relative to those who have experienced one or zero previous concussions.

In boxing, the MTBI rate for amateurs has been set at 5% while for professionals this figure rises to 6.3%. While many concussions are minor, some can be quite serious with long-term brain dysfunction. One serious issue in sports is the frequency and cumulative neurologic damage of repeated concussions. It is also recognized that a second concussion occurring while an individual is still symptomatic from an earlier concussion can be catastrophic or fatal. This phenomenon, termed second impact syndrome, is now being reported more frequently in sports medicine with a mortality rate as high as 50% in the most severe cases [4]. Public awareness of the severity of repeated concussion has only started to increase because career-threatening concussions have affected some well-known players.

Although head injury has been a serious problem since the dawn of mankind, little is known about the basic mechanism of head injury. The discipline of biomechanics studies the effects of forces and motion on the body, and the strength of biologic tissues. Head injury biomechanics research started in 1939 at Wayne State University when Professor H. R. Lissner, a professor in engineering, and Dr E. S. Gurdjian, a neurosurgeon, started working on a joint project to study the mechanism of skull fracture. Their work, outlining the first human cerebral concussion tolerance curve, was published by Lissner *et al.*[5]. This tolerance curve, as replotted by Gadd[1] and further modified by Versace [2], is used to determine the safety characteristics of automobiles, sports helmets, etc., to this day.

Biomechanics of head injury

A number of studies have been performed to provide and improve our understanding of brain injury. They point to brain deformation or strain as a principal cause of injury. Unfortunately, direct measurements of tissue deformation are almost impossible during an *in vivo* impact. Therefore, input variables, such as head acceleration, are used as alternate parameters to characterize the injury mechanism. Currently, impacts with head contact (translational acceleration) and inertial loading without head contact (rotational acceleration) have been postulated as the two major mechanisms that cause head injury. Rotational acceleration can produce both focal and diffuse brain injuries, while translational acceleration is considered to produce mainly focal brain injuries. These two major theories of brain injury are discussed below. Note that in real-world injury events, the head sustains a combination of both translational and rotational accelerations because the resultant force does not pass through the center of gravity and the force system is not a couple. At the beginning of a head impact, translation is frequently predominant. Eventually, rotational acceleration takes over as the effect of neck restraint comes into play. In addition to these two mechanisms, hypotheses for the mechanism of concussion are also presented under a separate heading.

Translational acceleration theory

The translational acceleration theory hypothesized that intracranial damage is mainly caused by injurious pressure gradients developed in the brain due to brain motion and skull deformation [6,7]. Studies included the use of embalmed cadavers and anesthetized animals. Focal injuries such as cerebral contusions and intracerebral hematomas are considered to be the consequence of translation of the head in the horizontal plane [8]. Concussion can be produced in experimental monkeys solely by translational acceleration from a direct impact while no correlation exists between the occurrence of concussion and rotational acceleration [9].

Rotational acceleration theory

The rotational head injury concept was formulated by Holburn [10] using a photoelastic model of the head. This theory hypothesized that shear deformation generated by rotational acceleration could produce shear strain throughout the brain, resulting in diffuse injury, cerebral concussion and rupture of the bridging veins.

Later experimental studies using live subhuman primates and physical models [11,12] suggest that rotational acceleration is the most injurious in the production of concussive injuries, diffuse axonal injuries and subdural hematomas. They claimed that virtually every known type of head injury could be produced by angular acceleration. However, the level of angular acceleration used was inordinately high.

Concussion mechanisms

Concussion, a common result of a blow to the head, has been studied the most of all types of head injury. Various injury mechanisms were proposed by researchers to explain their experimental results. Several injury mechanisms hypothesized for cerebral concussions are: (i) shear strains generated by rotation [10]; (ii) relative displacement between the brain and the skull producing coup/contrecoup cavitation [13]; (iii) shear deformation or mass movement in the brainstem principally caused by pressure gradients due to impact loading and translational acceleration [6,7]; and (iv) disturbance of consciousness caused by strains affecting the brain in a centripetal sequence of disruptive effect on function and structure. The effects of this sequence always begin at the surface of the brain in the mild cases and extend inwards to affect the core at the most severe levels of trauma [14].

Considerable controversy exists within the biomechanics community regarding the validity of competing hypotheses because they do not always correlate with clinical and pathologic observations. Although both translational and rotational acceleration can individually cause brain injuries in test animals, the severity of impact needed to produce these injuries is much higher than that experienced by humans involved in vehicular crashes or sports collisions. As a matter of fact, there is rarely an impact that is purely rotational or translational in the real world. Because there is no direct way of verifying these hypotheses on living humans, experiments using laboratory animals and computer models will be needed in order to advance knowledge on head injury mechanisms.

Types of acute head and maxillofacial injuries

The extent of sports-related head injury can range from minor concussion to fatal injury. Generally, acute head injuries are classified as open head injury or closed head injury. Open head injuries are caused by objects impacting the head leading to damage to the skull, such as scalp injury and skull fracture, dural tear and sometimes laceration of the brain. Closed head injuries, which may take place without skull fracture, are classified as focal and diffuse. The face is particularly vulnerable because major sense organs are housed inside the fragile facial bones. Maxillofacial injuries can occur in all kinds of sports, particularly in contact sports. All of these injuries can occur separately or in combination.

Scalp injuries

The scalp is 5–7 mm thick and consists of five layers of tissue, namely, the skin, the connective tissue layer, the aponeurosis epicranialis, the loose connective tissue and finally, the periosteum of the skull. The scalp is susceptible to all types of injury, particularly lacerations, as it is readily crushed and split against the underlying bone. Such lacerations are often linear due to the convexity of the underlying skull. Upon impact, the scalp often swells markedly due to edema or hematoma above or below the galeal layer.

Maxillofacial injuries

Maxillofacial injuries refer to damage to the soft tissues and bones of the face. There are 14 bones in the face. Complex midfacial fractures are routinely observed in sports injury. Usually, fractures with upper facial involvement are at greater risk for serious craniocerebral injuries while midface and mandibular traumas are associated with mild closed head injuries. Le Fort classified maxillary fractures into three types. Most maxillary fractures are severely commuted and consist of a combination of Le Fort fractures.

A Le Fort I fracture is horizontal and segmented across the maxilla. The teeth are often contained in the detached bony portion, thereby shearing off the hard plate and upper dental alveolus. This fracture responds well to intramaxillary fixation. Le Fort II is also a fracture of the maxilla. The body of the maxilla is separated from the facial skeleton, across and through the infraorbital foramen, and across the dorsum of the nose. The fractured portion is a pyramid-shaped section of the facial bone. Surgical fixation is required. Le Fort III is a fracture causing craniofacial dissociation. The entire maxilla and one or more bones are completely separated from the cranium through the front zygomatic region, the orbital floor, and across the nasal pyramid. Sufficient force to produce a Le Fort III fracture usually results in Le Fort II and I fracture as well ('total facial smash').

Skull fractures

The head is composed of eight cranial bones, each of which is made up of an outer and an inner table of compact bone and a diploë layer of spongy bone. When the head is directly impacted by an object, skull fracture occurs if the force and deformation is over the tolerance level of the skull. Fracture of the skull may be linear, depressed or comminuted depending upon the geometry and stiffness of the object the head collides with. Skull fracture may result in no signs or symptoms of neural injury. Conversely, severe neural injury may occur in the absence of skull fracture.

Linear skull fractures occur when a blunt object impacts the head. The fracture initiates from the point of impact to the nearest weaker portion of the skull, such as a suture line. Linear fractures comprise approximately 80% of fractures of the skull, with a low fatality rate. Clinically, linear fractures are not indicative of the extent of brain injury. A depressed skull fracture occurs when cranial bones are depressed or driven inward into the vault of the skull. It happens when the head collides with sufficient force against a blunt surface of small area and with a sharp radius of curvature, such as a cylindrical or hemispheric rigid surface. The concentrated stress could produce circumferential cracks about the impact site resulting in local failure of the bone.

Another type of skull fracture is the basal (basilar) skull fracture, defined as fractures involving the floor of the anterior, middle or posterior cranial fossae. They can be fatal, causing direct brainstem damage or placing the central nervous system in contact with the contaminated paranasal sinuses, predisposing patients to meningitis.

Focal brain injuries

Focal brain injuries usually involve some noticeable localized damage to cranial tissues and blood vessels. These include epidural hematoma, subdural hematoma, intracerebral hematoma and cerebral contusion.

A hematoma is a blood clot within the brain or on its surface. Epidural hematoma is an infrequently occurring sequel to head trauma (0.2–6%). It occurs as a result of tears of the middle meningeal artery and is not due to a brain injury. Due to pressure cased by the hematoma on the brain, this is an extreme medical emergency. Be aware that there may be an interval of several hours between the blow to the head and emergence of symptoms followed by signs of increased brain pressure.

Subdural hematomas are the most common acute pathologic brain injury in boxing and are the leading cause of boxing and American football fatalities. Acute subdural hematoma is mainly caused by direct lacerations of cortical arteries and veins, large contusion bleeding into the subdural space, or tearing of veins bridging the brain surface to various dural sinuses. Subdural hematoma is often associated with relative motion between the skull and the brain causing stretch (strain) of vessels. Intracranial hematomas occur primarily in the parasagittal regions of the cortex and subcortical white matter as well as in the deep white matter. Some cases of hematoma extend to the corpus callosum and cerebellar peduncles [15]. A severe headache usually presents if the patient remains conscious.

A contusion may be thought of as an area of bruised brain. Contusions may accompany concussion but need not do so. Contusions generally occur at the site of impact (coup contusions), as a result of increased pressure due to either local deformation of the bone or caused by skull fracture, and at the opposite site from the impact due to pressure wave propagation (contrecoup contusions). It is well established in both the clinical and neuropathologic literature that contusions occur predominantly at the frontal and temporal poles. It has been hypothesized that the responsible agents are the rough and irregular anterior fossae and the knife-like edge of the sphenoid ridge. Contusions are most often multiple and are frequently associated with cerebral hemorrhage, subdural hematoma and epidural hematoma.

Diffuse brain injuries

Diffuse brain injuries are fundamentally different and associated with widespread tissue damage. They involve damage to the neuronal, axonal, neurovascular and dendritic structures. This damage may only involve physiologic disruption of brain function as in the case of concussion, or cause sufficiently severe damage to the cerebral hemispheres or the brainstem to induce prolonged coma. This form of injury is called diffuse axonal injury (DAI).

Diffuse axonal injury (DAI) is characterized by widespread, microscopic damage to axons, macroscopic hemorrhages and overt tissue tears. It involves anatomic disruption of the white matter of brain tissue, generally associated with immediate loss of consciousness. It is caused by a sudden stretching or shearing of axons at the moment of impact [16]. Diffuse damage to axons exemplified by the presence of hemorrhagic foci is commonly found in the cerebral hemispheric subcortical lobar white matter, the cerebrum semiovale, the corpus callosum, the basal ganglia, the dorsolateral part of the rostral brainstem and the cerebrum. The outcome depends largely upon the severity of the impact sustained by the brain. Microscopic evidence of axonal damage takes the form of axonal balloonings in short survival cases (from 12–24 h to several days) [17], long tract degeneration in long survivals (several weeks to months), or diffuse gliosis of white matter in survivals of several years. A milder form of DAI in the chronic phase may cause neuropsychiatric problems, including cognitive deficits.

Concussion is the most common head injury in sports. Historically, concussion was described as traumatic paralysis of nervous function with a tendency to recover without deficit and revealing no anatomic abnormality. There are many definitions of concussion in the literature. Most recently, the American Orthopaedic Society for Sports Medicine Concussion Workshop Group has defined cerebral concussions as any alteration in cerebral function caused by a direct or indirect force transmitted to the head resulting in one or more of the following acute signs or symptoms: a brief loss of consciousness, light-headedness, vertigo, cognitive and memory dysfunction, blurred vision, difficulty concentrating, amnesia, headache, nausea, vomiting, photophobia or a balance disturbance. In 1983, Gerberich *et al.* surveyed the head coaches and players of 103 secondary school football teams in Minnesota. The incidence of cerebral concussion in football was 19 per 100 participants, and 24% of all football injuries were listed as concussions. In 1999 Powell and Barber-Foss in their study on high school contact sports found a much reduced incidence of concussions—the figure was reduced from 200 000 per year to approximately 40 000 per 1.1 million high school football players.

Management guidelines

Many grading systems have been developed in sports medicine to assess the severity of brain injury. None of the current guidelines for concussion and return to play has been developed on the basis of specific scientific knowledge regarding the process of recovery from concussion. All of the guidelines with the exception of one assume that traumatic loss of consciousness is associated with greater morbidity and poorer outcomes. This assumption seems to be based on the concept that injuries that result in traumatic loss of consciousness require a greater deal of mechanical force than do blows to the head that do not result in loss of consciousness. Lovell *et al.* [18] recently evaluated the importance of loss of consciousness for 383 patients with mild head injuries who were admitted to a major trauma service. The *a priori* assumption was that the patients who had experienced a loss of consciousness would perform worse on neuropsychologic tests known to be sensitive to MTBI. In a comparison of concussed patients who did and did not experience loss of consciousness, however, those authors found no support for weighting the loss of consciousness more

heavily than other factors such as amnesia or confusion, in making decisions regarding the return to previous activities.

Recently, one of the classifications of such brain injury, Standardized Assessment of Concussion (SAC), has been developed by the Quality Standards Subcommittee of the American Academy of Neurology (Table 6.4.1). It is used on the sideline to assess the orientation, memory and concentration as a mental status examination of athletes who are suspected of having suffered concussion [19]. The SAC is used by the American football league and the National Hockey League (NHL) to manage concussion on the field.

In 1973, Schneider [20] described two young athletes who experienced initial concussive syndromes and subsequently died after relatively minor second impacts. Since then 19 deaths from second impact syndrome (SIS) have been documented in the US. Furthermore, successive concussive impacts may also lead to milder but still significant impairment of cognitive processes (attention, memory), personality, language functioning and somatic concerns (sensitivity to light, dizziness), commonly referred to as 'postconcussion syndrome'. Based on the perception that MTBI still has a high incidence and may cause late problems, renewed interest in neuropsychologic testing of athletes has occurred. While neuropsychologic tests were used in the early seventies [21], it was first in 1989 that Barth *et al.* [22] published their results on more than 2350 college athletes participating in football. The study

Table 6.4.1 American Academy of Neurology Guidelines for Concussion Grading and Management.

Grade	Grade 1 concussion	Grade 2 concussion	Grade 3 concussion
Definition	Transient confusion, no loss of consciousness. Concussion symptoms or mental status abnormalities resolve in less than 15 min	Transient confusion, no loss of consciousness. Concussion symptoms or mental status abnormalities last more than 15 min	Any loss of consciousness, either brief (seconds) or prolonged (minutes)
Management recommendations	May return to play the same day if normal sideline assessments at rest and with exertion	Defer contact until 1 full week without symptoms at rest and with exertion	If brief (seconds), defer contact for 1 week without symptoms; if prolonged (minutes), defer for 2 weeks without symptoms (minimum)

showed that effects of mild head injuries can be assessed by neuropsychologic tests and that the majority of players typically returned to their baseline score within 10 days after injury. In soccer, Mastser *et al.* [23] recently suggested that participation in amateur soccer might be associated with chronic MTBI based on impaired scores in memory and planning tests compared to a control group. Lovell *et al.* [18] and Maroon *et al.* [24] based on their own preliminary work developed specific protocols for testing US professional athletes. These tests are currently being used in all teams in the National Hockey League and most teams in the National Football League. The test is based on a baseline neuropsychologic computer-guided assessment. The group based in the University of Pittsburgh Medical Center for Sports Medicine has emphasized the importance of baseline data. Individual players vary tremendously with respect to their levels of performance on tests on memory, attention/concentration, mental processing speed and motor speed. Without prior knowledge it is difficult to know whether any defects detected during testing may be attributed to the effects of the concussion or to previous unrelated factors. In addition to the evaluation of cognitive defects, the Pittsburgh group stresses the importance of evaluating players' reports of postconcussive symptoms. They divide these symptoms into three general categories: (i) somatic symptoms such as headaches, dizziness, balance problems or nausea; (ii) neuropsychiatric symptoms such as anxiety, depression or irritability; and (iii) cognitive complaints, such as impairment of attention, memory or processing speed.

Future directions

Current research is working in part on head injury modelling to predict impact and impact tolerance in head injuries, and in part on developing neuropsychologic tests that will be able to measure the injury to the patient and prevent the second impact problem. The Pittsburgh group has developed the Immediate Measurement of Performance and Cognitive Testing (IMPACT). This test battery has been designed to evaluate multiple aspects of neuropsychologic functioning among athletes, including attention span, sustained and selective attention, reaction time and several dimensions of memory. The test battery can be administered using a microcomputer and may involve the kind

of tests where the sports physician will be able to differentiate between a player with mild head trauma with no symptoms who can return to sport early vs. a player with a mild head trauma who may on the basis of the test results have to sit out until the test results are normal. It remains to be seen whether this will reduce the number of players with postconcussion problems.

Summary

The most common head injury in sports is concussion, which is a diffuse brain injury. The effects of repeated concussions are cumulative, and secondary minor impacts to the head shortly after a concussion can be fatal (secondary impact syndrome). Focal brain injuries include epidural, subdural and intracerebral hematomas and cerebral contusion. Mechanisms of brain trauma are theoretically divided into acceleration and rotational forces, but most injuries are probably created by a combination. An established human cerebral concussion tolerance curve is described. As neuropsychologic performance varies individually it has recently been suggested that all athletes register a baseline neuropsychologic assessment to enable comparison after a concussion. The time till recovery after concussion is unknown.

Maxillofacial injuries are classified according to Le Fort and surgical intervention is often necessary.

Multiple choice questions

1 *When an impact force acts on a rigid sphere, the sphere has only translational acceleration, if the force passes through the center of the sphere. What motion will the sphere undergo if the line of action of this force impacts it at some distance away from the center of the sphere?*

a Rotational acceleration only.

b Higher translational acceleration plus rotational acceleration.

c Same translational acceleration plus rotational acceleration.

d Lower translational acceleration plus rotational acceleration.

e Translational acceleration only.

2 *How does a helmet protect the brain during impact?*

a By absorbing the impact energy.

b By distributing the impact loading over a large surface area.

c By prolonging the loading time on the head.

d By reducing the acceleration transferred to the head.

e All of the above.

3 *Which of the following statements is correct?*

a A collision between two bodies of different size and mass results in an equal and opposite time varying force, which acts on each body during the period of contact.

b Given two moving objects with the same energy ($E = 1/2\,mv^2$), proportionately more of the energy of the smaller, faster-moving object will be spent in producing local deformation at the impact site, than that of the heavier, slower-moving body which will tend to cause more head acceleration.

c By increasing the area of impact, an increased amount of energy can be absorbed.

d Skull fractures are the result of tensile strains that exceed the strength of the compact bone of the skull.

e All of the above.

4 *Cranial and facial injuries resulting from a collision depend on the following:*

a force and direction of the collision

b area of load distribution

c impact interface geometry

d stiffness and energy absorption characteristics of the head and opposing object

e all of the above.

5 *When a water-filled oval-shaped rigid shell is subjected to a force which passes through the center of the shell as shown in the Fig. 6.4.2 a pressure gradient is developed across the water. Which pressure distribution is correct?*

a The pressure is highest (positive) at A and lowest (negative) at B.

b The pressure is highest at A and lowest at C.

c The pressure is highest at B and lowest at A.

d The pressure is highest at B and lowest at C.

e The pressure is highest at C and lowest at A.

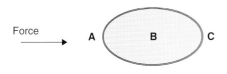

Fig. 6.4.2 A water-filled oval-shaped rigid shell is impacted by the force acting at location A.

Case story 6.4.1

A 24-year-old-male fell during alpine skiing and hit his head on a tree. He was unconscious for 80–90 s, woke up but was a bit dizzy. After 30 min he felt well, except for a minor headache, and he returned home.

1 If the period following this is uneventful, how should he be treated? When can he return to skiing? If he was a boxer, when could he return to boxing?

Because he also injured his arm, he went to the emergency room. When he arrived — 4 h after the injury — he was alert. On examination a possible forearm fracture was discovered and he was admitted for X-ray investigation. While waiting he suddenly became drowsy. There were no other neurologic findings.

2 What would you do as the emergency room doctor? What has most likely happened?

References

1 Gadd C. Use of a weighted impulse criterion for estimating injury hazard. *Proc 10th Stapp Car Crash Conf* 1966; SAE paper no. 660793.

2 Versace J. A review of the severity index. *Proc 15th Stapp Car Crash Conf* 1971; SAE Paper no. 710881.

3 Thurman D, Branche C, Sniezek J. The epidemiology of sports-related traumatic brain injuries in the United States: recent developments. *J Head Trauma Rehabil* 1998; **13** (2): 1–8.

4 Saunders R, Harbaugh R. The second impact in catastrophic contact-sports head trauma. *J Am Med Assoc* 1984; **252**: 538–9.

5 Lissner H, Lebow M, Evans F. Experimental studies on the relation between acceleration and intracranial changes in man. *Surg Gynecol Obstetr* 1960; **11**: 329–38.

6 Gurdjian ES, Lissner HR, Patrick LM. Concussion — mechanism and pathology. *Proc 7th Stapp Car Crash Conf* 1963; **35**: 470–82.

7 Gurdjian E, Lissner H. Photoelastic confirmation of the presence of shear strains at the conjunction in closed head injury. *J Neurosurg* 1961; **18**: 58–60.

8 Gennarelli T, Ommaya A, Thibault L. Comparison of translational and rotational head motions in experimental

cerebral concussion. *Proc 15th Stapp Car Crash Conf* 1971; SAE P-39: 797–803.

9 Ono K, Kikuchi A, Nakamura M, Kobayashi H, Nakamura H. Human head tolerance to sagittal impact: reliable estimation deduced from experimental head injury using sub-human primates and human cadaver skulls. *Proc 24th Stapp Car Crash Conf* 1980; SAE Paper no. 801303.

10 Holburn A. Mechanics of head injuries. *Lancet* 1943; 2: 438–41.

11 Gennarelli T, Thibault L, Adams J, Graham D, Thompson C, Marcincin R. Diffuse axonal injury and traumatic coma in the primate. *Ann Neurol* 1982; 12: 564–74.

12 Thibault L, Gennarelli T. Biomechanics of diffuse brain injuries. *Proc 29th Stapp Car Crash Conf* 1985; SAE Paper no. 856022.

13 Gross AG. Impact thresholds of brain concussion. *J Aviation Med* 1958; 29: 725–32.

14 Ommaya A, Gennarelli A. Cerebral concussion and traumatic unconsciousness: Correlation of experimental and clinical observations on blunt head injuries. *Brain* 1974; 97: 633–54.

15 Lampert P, Hardman J. Morphological changes in brains of boxers. *J Am Med Assoc* 1984; 251: 2676–9.

16 Strich S. Shearing of nerve fibres as a cause of brain damage due to head injury. *Lancet* 1961: 443–8.

17 Povlishock J, Becker D, Cheng C, Vaughan G. Axonal change in minor head injury. *J Neuropathol Exp Neurol* 1983; 42(3): 225–42.

18 Lovell MR, Iverson GL, Collins W, McKeag D, Maroon C. Does loss of consciousness predict neuropsychological decrements after concussion? *Clin J Sports Med* 1999; 9: 193–8.

19 Report of the Quality Standards Subcommittee of the American Academy of Neurology. Practice parameter: The management of concussion in sports. *Neurology* 1997; 48: 581–5.

20 Schneider R. Mechanisms of injury. In: Schneider R, ed. *Head and Neck Injuries in Football: Mechanisms, Treatment and Prevention.* Baltimore: Williams & Wilkins, 1973: 77–126.

21 Yarnell PR, Lynch S. Retrograde memory immediately after concussion. *Lancet* 1970; 1: 863–4.

22 Barth JT, Alves WA, Ryan TV, Macciocchi SN, Rimel RW, Jane JA, Nelson WE. Mild head injuries in sports: neuropsychological sequel and recovery of function. In: Levin HS, Eisenberg HM, Benton AL, eds. *Mild Head Injury.* New York: Oxford University Press, 1989: 257–275.

23 Mastser EJ, Kessels AG, Lezak MO, Jordan BD, Troost J. Neurophysiological impairment in amateur soccer players. *JAMA* 1999; 282(10): 971–3.

24 Maroon JC, Lovell MR, Norwig J, Podell K, Powell JW, Hartl R. Cerebral concussion in athletes. *Eval Neuropsychol Test Neurosurg* 2000; 47: 659–72.

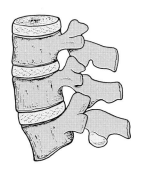

Chapter 6.5
Spine

JENS IVAR BROX

Classical reference

Indahl AA, Velund L, Reikeraas O. Good prognosis
for low back pain when left untampered. *Spine*
1995; **20**: 473–477.
It has been suggested that the more seriously low back
pain has been treated, the worse it has become.

In this study Indahl *et al.* reported that low back pain
treated as a benign, self-limiting condition with recommended light mobilization gives superior results
with regard to return to work compared to conventional medical treatment. At 200 days 60% were still on
sickness leave in the control group compared with 30%
in the intervention group. The study included 975 patients on sickness leave from work for at least 8 weeks.
Patients were randomized into either a control or an intervention group. The control group was not called in
for examination, but was treated within the conventional medical system which includes rest, medication,
restricted activity, physiotherapy or chiropractic treatment. The intervention group was given a standardized examination, physical tests, plain radiographs and
computed tomography scans.

In addition they were told that involvement of the
disk could cause a reflex activation in the paraspinal
muscles. Then they were given assurance that light
activity would not further injure the disk or any other
structure that could be involved. It was emphasized
that the worst thing they could do to their backs was to
be too careful. The therapist set no fixed exercise goals,
but rather the patients were given the guidelines and
encouraged to set their own goals. Information was
reinforced after 3 months.

The new intervention is very different from conventional treatment. The results oppose some of the
myths concerning low back pain. This study has inspired a future paradigm shift in the treatment of low
back pain (Fig. 6.5.1).

Anatomy and biomechanics

The spine or vertebral column consists of 33 vertebrae: seven cervical, 12 thoracic connected with the
ribs, five lumbar, five sacral fused together, and three or
four rudimentary vertebrae forming the coccyx. A
typical vertebra consists of a body with paired pedicles
upon its posterior surface to support the laminae,
paired transverse processes for attachment of muscles
(and, in the thoracic region for attachment of the ribs),
and a spinous process, also for the attachment of muscles. The laminae and the pedicles together form an
arch; between the arch and body is the vertebral foramen (Fig. 6.5.2). Successive vertebral foramina form
the vertebral canal. The intervertebral foramen is
formed by a notch in the upper surface of the pedicle.
The lateral recess is the entrance portion of the intervertebral foramen. Articular processes or zygapo-
physes make up the facet joints (Fig. 6.5.3). Synovial
joints formed by the articular processes, cartilaginous
connections between the bodies and fibrous bands
between other parts of the arches, connect most of the
vertebrae.

Two vertebrae and their connections are termed a
motion segment. Normally, the two lower segments
have to absorb the heaviest load. Correspondingly,
degenerative changes commonly occur in these segments. Only a weak association is found between degenerative disks and back pain. The concepts hyper-
and hypomobility, albeit not documented by radiologic

647

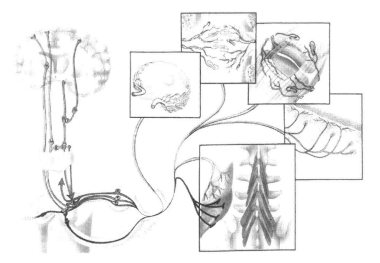

Fig. 6.5.1 Neuromuscular network connecting the central nervous system to peripheral structures (shown in boxes): intervertebral disk, ligament, zygapophysal joint, skin and spinal muscles. In low back pain where no specific pathoanatomic findings can be demonstrated, the cause of pain may be mainly a functional disturbance. Overload of specific parts can be detected by high-threshold nerve endings, and in due course, inhibit muscle actions responsible for the increased loading, and thereby prevent injury. This may be the reason why heavy physical loading does not seem to have the impact on degeneration of the spine that was earlier assumed. The common clinical findings of decreased range of motion in low back pain patients point to increased muscle activity, which therefore points to an alteration in the recruitment system. For example an irritation of the nerve endings surrounding the annulus fibrosus may cause increased activation of the paraspinal muscles in a bracing pattern and subject the muscles to static work, which is thought to be responsible for muscle pain. Original drawing by Ane Reppe. Reprinted with permission from Aage Indahl. *Low back pain—a functional disturbance*. Thesis. University of Oslo, Norway, 1999.

methods, are often used to describe abnormal load-displacement behavior of motion segments.

The vertebral column serves two main purposes: supporting the trunk and protecting the spinal cord. In addition to this, the back must be prepared to stabilize the upper body in movements of the head and the limbs. The stability of the spine depends on a number of factors. When weight is properly balanced and the spine is close to the center of gravity, minimal muscular activity is needed for stabilization. Only human beings habitually use the vertebral column in an upright position. The two lordotic curves (cervical and lumbar) characterize the regions with the greatest mobility and enhance the ability of the vertebral column in weight-bearing (Fig. 6.5.4). The two kyphotic curves (thoracic and sacral) are present at birth and are dictated largely by the shape of the constituent vertebrae.

Spinal motion is usually described in three planes: the frontal plane, the sagittal plane and the coronal plane. In the thoracic spine the normal frontal

(kyphotic) curve is 15–30°. Abnormal kyphosis is observed in congenital disorders, fractures, Scheuermann's disease and ankylosing spondylitis. Thoracic motion in the sagittal and coronal planes is limited by the facet joint orientation and the ribs. Normally approximately 5° flexion/extension, lateral flexion and axial rotation takes place at each vertebral segment.

Lordosis is the normal sagittal plane alignment of the lumbar spine. The normal lumbosacral angle is 120–130°. Excessive lordosis may stress the posterior elements and the anterior longitudinal ligament considerably. Normally, the lumbar spine range of motion from maximal flexion to maximal extension is approximately 80°. In athletes the length of the hamstring muscle/tendon complex may limit the range of motion. Extension is limited by the orientation of the facet joints. Movements that force the spine to exceed this limitation, for example in gymnastics, will stress the vertebrae, disks and ligaments in this region considerably.

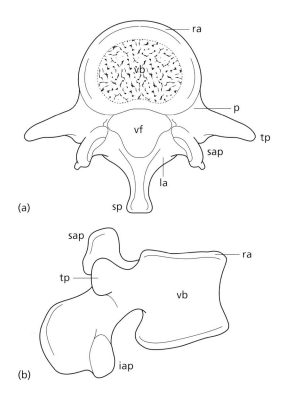

Fig. 6.5.2 Lumbar vertebra. Top (a) and side (b) view of a lumbar vertebra. vb, vertebral body; ra, ring apophysis; p, pedicle; la, lamina; sp, spinous process; tp, transverse process; sap, superior articular process; iap, inferior articular process; vf, vertebral foramen.

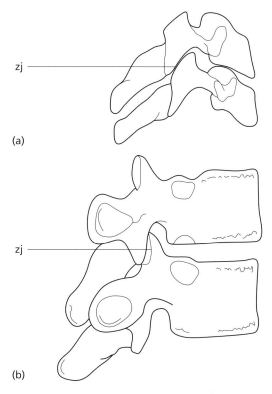

Fig. 6.5.3 Two vertebrae and their connections are termed a motion segment. Regional differences in the orientation of the zygoapophyseal joints as seen in lateral views.

Scoliosis is the lateral curvature of the spine (Fig. 6.5.5). Scoliosis may be structural or non-structural. In structural scoliosis the deformity cannot be corrected by alteration of posture. In idiopathic scoliosis, several vertebrae at one or two levels (primary curve) demonstrate a rotational deformity (the spinous processes rotate into the concavity and the bodies which carry the ribs rotate into the convexity). Above and below the relatively fixed primary curve, more mobile secondary curves develop to maintain the normal position of the head and pelvis. Thoracic curves do not appear to be associated with pain, but limited curves may interfere with shoulder function in athletes.

Superficial and deep layers of muscles work in a complex synergy with the support offered by the lumbosacral fascia and spinal ligaments. Their activity is often peculiar to an individual — and thus postural advice should be given with this point in mind. The deep muscles (multifidi) run from one segment to another (Fig. 6.5.6). They act as a functional unit together with the deep abdominal muscles, the diaphragm and the pelvic muscles. Their main function is segmental stabilization of the spine in movements of the arms and legs. Back muscles become inactive in a maximal forward bending position (Fig. 6.5.7). The muscle relaxation phenomenon describes how the electromyographic activity of the erectores spinae is decreased just when the load has been lifted off the ground contrary to the increased activity in the midrange of forward flexion. This phenomenon presented a challenge to schools that promote the role of the lumbar muscles in lifting. Recent models propose that the force necessary to perform a lift is generated by

(a)

(b)

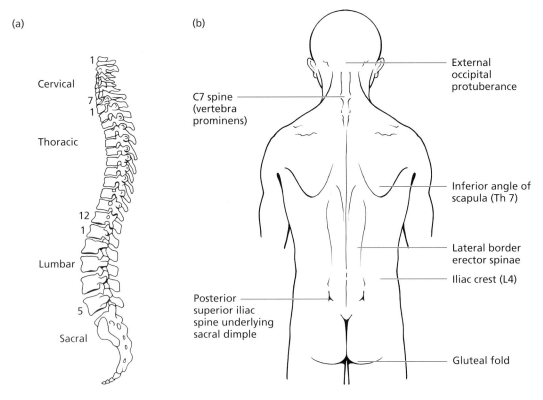

Cervical

1

7
1

Thoracic

12
1

Lumbar

5

Sacral

C7 spine
(vertebra
prominens)

Posterior
superior iliac
spine underlying
sacral dimple

External
occipital
protuberance

Inferior angle of
scapula (Th 7)

Lateral border
erector spinae

Iliac crest (L4)

Gluteal fold

Fig. 6.5.4 (a) The vertebral column and its curves (cervical and lumbar lordosis and thoracic kyphosis) viewed from the lateral side with the vertebrae numbered. (b) Anatomical landmarks.

the hip extensors and then transmitted from the ileum to the upper extremities through the lumbosacral fascia portion of the posterior ligamentous system [1]. Prolonged isometric muscle activity in the midrange forward bending position is often painful. Also pain can inhibit flexion relaxation. The absence of this phenomenon discriminates patients with low back pain from controls [2]. In addition, muscular activity is influenced by emotional distress—therefore back muscles have been called our largest 'mimic muscles'.

Neural structures at the L3–4 level are schematically described in Fig. 6.5.8. For each lumbar vertebra there is an associated lumbar spinal nerve. The spinal nerves divides into a dorsal and ventral ramus which innervate various passive and active structures. Free nerve endings and mechanoreceptors are located in these structures and are potential pain sensors and proprioceptive transducers for monitoring the position

and movements in the motion segment. The neurologic feedback from passive structures provides sensory information needed to regulate muscle tension, and hence the stability of the spine. Normal locomotion requires multiple levels of neural control. An example of a functional disturbance of this control is the lack of flexion relaxation in chronic low back pain patients described above.

The intervertebral disks make up about 25% of the total height of the vertebral column. They connect the bodies, allow motion, and absorb and distribute the load acting on the vertebral column. They receive nutrition by diffusion from the vertebral endplates and surrounding soft tissue. Only the outer part, termed the annulus fibrosus, is innervated. The annulus fibrosus consists of collagen lamellae organized in different directions. It provides strength to the disk in bending and twisting. The inner part, termed the nucleus pulposus, consists of 90% water into the third decade of

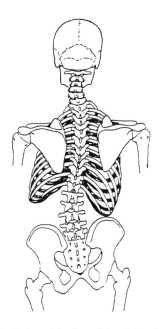

Fig. 6.5.5 Scoliosis resulting from tilting of the pelvis through shortening of the left leg. Note the convexity of the lumbar curve pointing at the shortening leg. Compensatory thoracic and cervical curves and an apparent difference in shoulder height are shown.

life. Compressive load on a healthy disk is mainly borne by the nucleus pulposus. The hydration depends on the amount of proteoglycan present and over the next four decades the water content gradually diminishes to 60–65%. Sufficient dehydration can occur during a day's activity to result in a loss of height of 2 cm in an adult man. Dehydration is visualized as black disks on magnetic resonance imaging (MRI). This is often recognized as an early sign of degeneration and is observed in asymptomatic and symptomatic individuals. The intradiscal pressure may be increased about tenfold from the supine position if 20 kg is lifted without compensatory use of the quadriceps muscles. On the other hand, the intradiscal pressure may be higher while sitting compared to jumping. The load is reduced by increasing the intra-abdominal pressure. Stimulation of the intervertebral disk activates the deep back muscles. This may elict a functional disturbance, for example the protective scoliosis observed in patients with acute low back pain.

Acute injuries of the spine

Epidemiology

Traffic accidents are the single most common cause of spinal cord injury, followed by sports activities. The 1-year prevalence of spinal cord injury in sports in

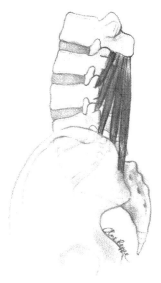
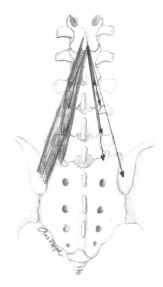

Fig. 6.5.6 Schematic showing the polysegmental attachments of the multifidus fascicles originating from L1 vertebrae. Their function is that of fine adjustment of loads of polysegmental spinal structures. Original drawing by Ane Reppe. Reprinted with permission from Aage Indahl. *Low back pain—a functional disturbance*. Thesis. University of Oslo, Norway, 1999.

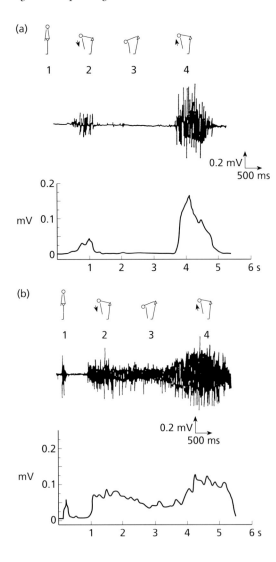

Fig. 6.5.7 Flexion/relaxation phenomenon. Reprinted with permission from [2].

parachute jumping, hang gliding, paragliding, climbing, ice hockey, biking, snowboarding, downhill skiing and ski-jumping. In a recent study from Canada, the prevalence of vertebral fractures was 0.01 and 0.04 per 1000 skiing days for downhill skiing and snowboarding, respectively [3]. Most snowboard injuries resulted from jumps, while most skiing injuries were related to falls. About 70% are burst fractures, most commonly located to Th12 and L1. Nine per cent of the injured snowboarders and 24% of the skiers had a neurologic injury, about half of them a spinal cord injury. American football and ice hockey have become increasingly more popular. The incidence of non-fatal catastrophic injuries was 0.7 injuries per 100 000 in American football and 2.6 injuries per 100 000 injuries in ice hockey. The number of spinal cord injuries in American football peaked at 32 in 1976 [4]. In Canadian ice hockey, the number of spinal cord injuries was about 15 per year through the 1980s [5]. More than 60% of these injuries occurred in the 11–20-year-old group. In Finnish ice hockey there were eight spinal cord injuries in the 1980s and 1990s [6]. Burst fractures and dislocations are the most common fractures of the cervical spine and about half of these fractures result in spinal cord involvement. Biomechanically the greatest forces are applied to the cervical spine, in slight flexion. This injury position is consistent with actual injury situations in ice hockey and football. Most injuries in ice hockey result from head-first contact with the boards after a check from behind.

There is today a general acceptance of the importance of injury prevention through education, personal safety routines, more stringent competition rules and improved equipment. Research to improve knowledge about injury frequency and injury-specific mechanisms should be given a high priority within sports organizations and sports medicine.

North America is about 30 per million. About 50% of all sports-related spinal cord injuries result in complete quadriplegia. This is one of the most serious sequelae after injury in sports with major consequences for the injured athlete and society. More than 30% of all vertebral fractures and about 50% of all fractures/luxations of the cervical spine result from diving accidents. Major spinal injuries are also reported in riding, motor vehicle sports (including snowscooter driving),

Diagnostic thinking

Direct back trauma most commonly causes muscular contusions associated with acute intense pain and hematoma. Fall injuries may cause a muscular rupture, ligamentous injury, fracture, and occasionally a disk herniation.

For a proper differential diagnostic evaluation, it is essential to consider the injury mechanism and the forces involved according to what is required to cause a

Active structures

Passive structures

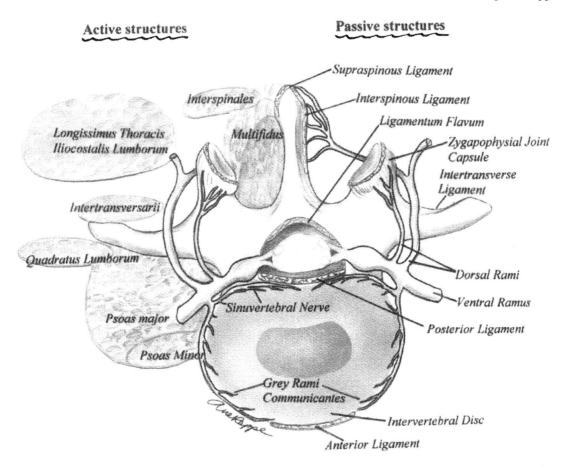

Supraspinous Ligament

Interspinous Ligament

Ligamentum Flavum

Zygapophysial Joint Capsule

Intertransverse Ligament

Interspinales

Longissimus Thoracis Iliocostalis Lumborum

Multifidus

Intertransversarii

Quadratus Lumborum

Dorsal Rami

Ventral Ramus

Posterior Ligament

Sinuvertebral Nerve

Psoas major

Psoas Minor

Grey Rami Communicantes

Intervertebral Disc

Anterior Ligament

Fig. 6.5.8 Active and passive structures and sensory innervation at the L3–4 level. Original drawing by Ane Reppe. Reprinted with permission from Aage Indahl. *Low back pain—a functional disturbance*. Thesis. University of Oslo, Norway, 1999.

particular injury, and to consider its possible progression and consequences. A vertebral fracture may result in a spinal cord injury. There may be no signs of spinal cord injury at the primary examination at the sports arena. The patient should not be moved until a neurologic examination has been completed and a spinal cord injury or an unstable fracture has been ruled out. Dysesthesia and lower extremity numbness should be interpreted as symptoms indicating a spinal cord injury. In a conscious patient, a reflectory spasm or scoliosis of the cervical spine may reflect a protective mechanism and therefore should not be corrected. The unconscious patient should not be moved until the cervical spine has been stabilized. Unexpected movements may result in permanent neural damage in a patient without symptoms and signs indicating spinal cord injury. Proper knowledge about the consequences of an injury and practical skills for handling the patient with an acute spinal injury are important to prevent neural damage resulting from incorrect transportation of the patient. Guidelines for emergency management of patients with a suspected spinal cord injury are described in Table 6.5.1.

In contact sports, associated injuries of the kidney, spleen and liver should be excluded. These injuries may be acutely life-threatening because of major intra-abdominal bleeding and drop in blood pressure.

Patients with vertebral fractures should be eva-

Table 6.5.1 Emergency management of patients with a suspected spinal cord injury.

Establish free airways and stop bleeding
Most experienced person takes command
Stabilize head—do not correct position if the patient is
    conscious
Carry out primary examination
Call for ambulance
Organize turning—the neck should be stabilized in an
    unconscious patient
Check if adequately stabilized—the ambulance should be
    driven carefully

Table 6.5.2 Mechanisms of neck injury.

Direct compression injury of the head/neck
Fall with opponent's body weight superimposed
Fall from height
Equipment failure, illegal procedure
Attempting maneuvers beyond skill
Direct violence
Forced excessive range of motion

luated at an orthopedic or neurosurgical department. When the diagnostic evaluation is completed less serious injuries are treated by the primary health care physician.

History

Knowledge about the various sports makes it easier to understand the injury mechanism. It is important to discriminate between injuries that result from a simple fall to the ground or collision on the track, or more complex mechanisms like a simultaneous twisting and collision. Acute back pain in throwing suggests a fracture of the transverse process or vertebral arch or a muscular rupture.

Cervical injury mechanisms are outlined in Table 6.5.2. Forceful extension associated with a sudden force applied to the forehead may result in a rupture of the anterior spinal ligament, avulsion fracture or spondylolysis. The intervertebral disk and posterior structures are vulnerable in compression/rotation injuries.

Classification systems for thoracolumbar fractures are based on history and on particular knowledge about the injury mechanism—and may improve the understanding of the consequences for various injuries. The most common classification systems are by Denis, Gaines and the AO group (Magerl/Aebi) [7]. Denis introduced the concept of three columns [8]. According to this system, an unstable fracture requires that at least two columns are injured (Fig. 6.5.9). Gaines' system and indications for surgery are mainly based on the degree of contusion of the vertebrae. Fractures are classified (A, B, C) according to history and radiologically evaluated injury mechanism (Figs 6.5.10–6.5.12).
A Compressive forces (burst fracture without ligamentous injury, e.g., by a fall on the buttocks or landing on the feet in paragliding or parachute jumping).

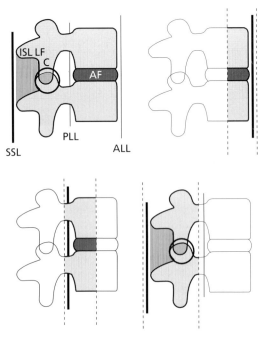

Fig. 6.5.9 Vertebral fractures. The three column concept. The anterior, middle and posterior column are illustrated. SSL, superior spinous ligament; ISL, intraspinous ligament; LF, ligamentum flavum; PLL, posterior longitudinal ligament; ALL, anterior longitudinal ligament.

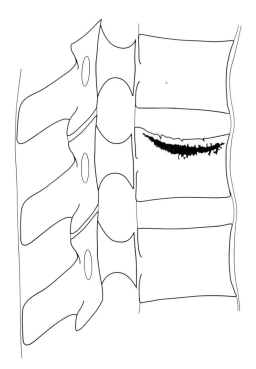

Fig. 6.5.10 Compressive forces resulting in an endplate impaction. This is a common fracture in juvenile and osteoporotic bone.

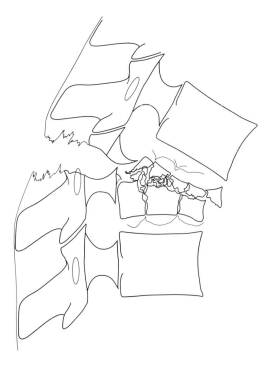

Fig. 6.5.11 Tension forces in flexion. Anterior subluxation with fracture of articular processes and an associated complete burst fracture.

B Tension forces in flexion or extension (discoligamentous injuries or **A** combined with an injury of the posterior ligament).

C Isolated rotational injuries or in combination with **B** and **C**.

Injuries are then subclassified according to how serious they are (degree of neurologic injury). The highest percentage of neurologic injury is found in rotational injuries.

Group A: 14% neurologic injury.
Group B: 32% neurologic injury.
Group C: 55% neurologic injury.

Clinical examination
If a serious spinal injury is suspected, it is important to evaluate the level of consciousness, circulation and respiration and then perform a neurologic examina-

tion. Fractures, luxations, and discoligamentous injuries with malalignment and instability that may affect the spinal cord during transportation may be present without neurologic signs at clinical examination. Occasionally, numbness and dysesthesia may be the only symptoms that suggest a spinal cord injury. The spinal shock may mask hyperreflexia. Table 6.5.3 describes neurologic injury by level, function, reflex and sensibility.

Imaging
If an acute traumatic cervical injury is suspected, flexion and extension views should be omitted until screening lateral views are done. A negative lateral screening does not exclude an unstable neck injury, and bilateral symptoms in association with an acute trauma indicate that further evaluation is necessary. This

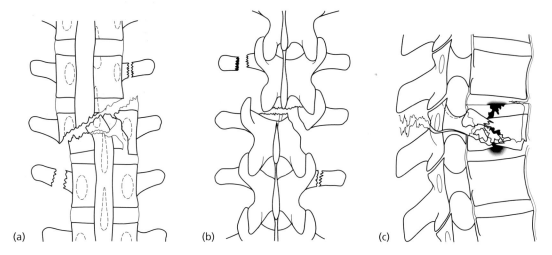

Fig. 6.5.12 Rotational injury with complete burst fracture: (a) vertebral body; (b) posterior elements; (c) lateral view.

Table 6.5.3 Level of spinal cord or nerve root injury.

Level	Function	Reflex	Sensibility
C3–5	Respiration (diaphragm)		
C5	Shoulder abduction (deltoid)	Biceps	Lateral shoulder
C6	Elbow flexion	Brachiorad.	Lateral arm
C7	Elbow extension	Triceps	Index finger
C8	Finger flexion		Little/ring finger
Th1	Finger abduction		Medial arm
L1–2	Hip flexion		
L3–4	Knee extension	Patellar	Medial thigh
L5	Hallux extension	Achilles	Basis hallux
S1	Plantar flexion and toe flexion	Achilles	Lateral foot
S2–4	Sphincter function at rectal expl.		

includes extension and flexion views conducted by a skilled person in a specialized radiological department. The unconscious patient should be examined to exclude cervical injury. MRI is the best method for evaluation of soft tissue structures including the spinal cord and nerve roots. In discoligamentous injuries this is the only method for detailed description of the injury, while instability is assessed by plain films.

Radiologic assessment of burst fractures includes an evaluation of the eventual reduction of the diameter of the spinal foramen and the degree of vertebral body collapse. An isolated burst fracture without major col-

lapse is stable, but an associated rupture of the interspinous ligament indicates instability and requires surgical stabilization.

Spinal cord injury

Symptoms and signs. Neck pain, numbness and dysesthesia. Inability to move the hands and feet. The level of injury should be established by neurologic examination (Table 6.5.3).

Diagnosis. According to clinical symptoms and signs and injury mechanism. It is important to remember that neurologic symptoms and signs may be absent in a person with an unstable vertebral fracture.

Treatment. Transportation to hospital (Table 6.5.1). Methylprednisolone 30 mg/kg body weight should be started within 8 h and continued with a dose of 5.4 mg/kg for 24–48 h to reduce the degree of a permanent paralysis [9]. Surgical treatment consists of decompression and eventual fusion of at least two contiguous vertebrae. Decompression is always recommended in a patient with a partial spinal cord injury if CT or MRI indicates compression of the spinal cord. This surgical procedure may reduce the extent of pareses even in patients without progressive neurologic signs. In patients with a complete injury of the spinal cord, a decompression may be effective only if it is performed in the acute phase.

Unstable fractures

Symptoms and signs. Muscular spasm and crooked neck may reflect a protective mechanism in a patient with an unstable fracture or spinal cord injury. A palpable defect may reflect a rupture of the posterior ligaments.

Diagnosis. Radiologic evaluation including plain films and MRI.

Treatment. Skull traction or surgical treatment in unstable cervical fractures. Surgical treatment of unstable thoracolumbar fractures.

Stable fractures

Vertebral body fractures

Symptoms and signs. Depends on the mechanism and localization of the injury. A localized muscular spasm and pain at the fracture site with a dermatomal radiation corresponding to the fracture and on palpation of the spinous process of the affected vertebra is common.

Diagnosis. Radiologic evaluation. Exclusion of unstable fracture and tumor.

Treatment. Surgical treatment of thoracolumbar frac-

tures is usually recommended if the anterior part of the vertebral body is reduced by more than 40% of the average height of the vertebral bodies above and below [8]. The rationale for this strategy is that surgical treatment stabilizes the fractures, makes it possible to mobilize the patient within a short time and prevents further collapse of the vertebral body. However, recent literature debates the indication for surgery and claims the prognosis is good without surgical treatment [10]. There is a poor correlation between the degree of kyphosis resulting from the fracture and complaints. According to the present view, there is a need for randomized studies to compare the effectiveness of surgical and conservative treatment. It seems important to mobilize the patient as soon as a proper diagnostic evaluation is complete [11]. Early mobilization will reduce the risk for venous thrombosis and does not seem to increase the degree of kyphosis. It is not documented that specific back muscle exercise is more effective than simple mobilization. Return to competition should not be expected until the fracture is radiologically healed. A corset limits large movements of the upper body, but does not limit segmental motion. Even a hyperextension corset does not affect stabilization or the degree of vertebral body collapse. A corset may be indicated if pain makes it impossible to mobilize the patient. In a few patients, pain becomes chronic and interferes with return to previous sports activities.

Fractures of the spinous and transverse process

Isolated fractures of the spinous processes are rare. Specific treatment of an isolated fracture of the spinous process is not indicated. It is important to exclude a simultaneously occurring and more serious injury. An isolated fracture of the transverse process is more common. The fracture is commonly located to the lumbar spine, and is related to the insertion of the iliopsoas and the quadratus lumborum muscles.

Symptoms and signs. Intense acute pain that is worsened by hip flexion, lateral bending and rotation. Distinct unilateral pain upon paravertebral and abdominal palpation. Bleeding from the fracture and the muscle may result in a drop in hemoglobin rate.

Diagnosis. Plain films will reveal the fracture, but CT is the best method for detailed evaluation.

Treatment. The patient should be sent to hospital for a complete evaluation, but the treatment is conservative. A corset may be useful for the first weeks and makes it possible to maintain general physical fitness. The fracture will normally heal within 6–8 weeks, but full contact sports are not recommended until 12 weeks.

Prevention

A group of neurosurgeons in the USA have claimed to have reduced the incidence of spinal cord injury by 40% by an educational campaign aimed at teenagers. The campaign used a 'feet first—first time' slogan. The results from this preventive intervention indicate that it is cost-effective when it is successful (Table 6.5.4).

In ice hockey, the introduction of helmets and facial masks has dramatically reduced the number of ocular injuries resulting in blindness. The helmet, however, adds mass to the head and may shift the head mass anteriorly sufficiently to result in flexion of the neck on impact [5]. The sense of invulnerability by players when wearing a helmet may cause them to engage in more aggressive play [6]. Rules have been introduced to reduce the number of spinal cord injuries, including major penalties for checking from behind. However, rules are only helpful if they are enforced. It seems reasonable to increase the severity of penalty for dangerous play in contact sports like ice hockey.

High and acrobatic jumps are some of the various challenges in snowboarding. The jumps increase the risk for serious injuries, but at the same time there is no reason to believe that signs like 'jumps not allowed' are effective. Well-prepared jumps and improved skills may reduce the number and consequences of injuries.

Table 6.5.4 Guidelines for reducing diving injuries.

Do not dive into water shallower than twice your height
Do not dive into unfamiliar water
Check out first what is underneath the surface
Do not assume the water is deep enough
Remember the influence of tides on water depth
Do not dive near dredging or construction work, as water levels change and dangerous objects may be underneath the surface
Do not dive until area is clear of other swimmers
Do not drink and dive
Limit horseplay to safe areas, do not include as part of diving

Neck pain

Epidemiology

Neck pain is a commonly occurring complaint. Its yearly prevalence is comparable with low back pain and is about 50% in the adult population. Neck pain is the main complaint in about 3% of those who consult a physician. The yearly prevalence of cervical radiculopathy is 40–80 per 100 000 [12]. Repeated collision injuries in contact sports not resulting in fractures or spinal cord injuries are associated with neck pain and paresthesia. The symptoms are commonly recurrent, existing just for seconds during a match, and result from traction of the brachial plexus or nerve root irritation. In a large Finnish survey the neck and head accounted for 9% of all soccer injuries [13]. A heading in soccer involves hyperextension and compression of the cervical spine and may affect the vertebrae, intervertebral joints, disks, ligaments and muscles. Chronic complaints of pain and limited range of motion of the cervical spine were found in about 30% of former players from the Norwegian national soccer team [14]. Degenerative changes of the cervical spine were significantly more frequent and present about 10–20 years earlier as compared with a control group. Disk herniation with radicular symptoms and signs has been reported in conjunction with heading in soccer.

Neck pain associated with traffic accidents has been epidemic for the last two to three decades in Western societies. The complaint is usually difficult to explain from a biomechanical point of view, and there are no particular pathophysiologic changes or clinical signs. These complaints seem to be less frequent in athletes who frequently are exposed to similar or more pronounced biomechanical forces during sports. By unduly focusing on the injury mechanism, somatic symptoms, imaging and prolonged treatment and rest, physicians, physiotherapists and chiropractors may actually have reinforced symptoms [15,16]. Thus, this epidemic in Western societies may be at least partly iatrogenic. The patient may become overcautious and complain about diffuse symptoms of tiredness, dizziness and pulsation in the neck together with chronic pain and disability.

Diagnostic thinking

Neck pain may be classified according to etiology, pathophysiology and biomechanics, or symptom localization. Commonly neck pain radiating to the arm (cervicobrachialgia) is discriminated from neck pain (cervicalgia). The pain may radiate in a nerve root pattern (cervical radiculopathy), or may be aggravated on elevation of the arm and palpation of the brachial plexus (thoracic outlet syndrome) or result from entrapment by peripheral nerves. A common clinical challenge is to discriminate primary neck pain radiating to the shoulder and arm from primary shoulder pain associated with secondary cervical myalgia. Neck pain may also result from collar tumors or infections. In the elderly population, a vertebral artery stenosis may result in dizziness and neck pain.

Acute neck pain and reflectory muscle spasm may be frightening. The emotional security represented by a careful and confident primary consultation is therefore of utmost importance. Most patients with acute neck pain improve within a short time without specific treatment. In patients with chronic pain the clinician should screen for somatization symptoms. Imaging is indicated in patients with radicular symptoms or atypical pain. For evaluation of neck pain associated with traffic accidents most patients will benefit from a careful primary evaluation. The efficacy of physiotherapy and chiropractic treatment is undocumented, and prolonged manipulation or soft tissue or exercise therapy is not indicated.

History

Did the complaints start following trauma or gradually? It is important to get a precise description of pain localization: is the pain distinct or widespread? Does it radiate to the upper extremity? Is the pain aggravated by coughing? Are there associated symptoms like headache, fatigue, dizziness or nausea?

Clinical examination

Inspection. Torticollis may reflect a serious injury, involvement of the facet joints or cervical disks, a congenital disorder, inflammatory, malignant or infectious pathology, or psychological stress. General muscular tension and shoulder shrugging should be noted. Look for collar tumors.

Neurologic examination. This is indicated in patients with radiating pain.

Range of motion. Examine active and passive range of motion. Normal passive range of motion is $55°$ extension, $45°$ flexion and side bending and $70°$ bilateral rotation. In patients with muscular pain the reduced range of motion observed in the sitting or forward-flexed position is commonly recovered when assessed in the supine and relaxed position. Specific segmental examination includes palpation of the spinous and transverse processes and particular techniques to assess segmental motion.

Stress tests. A positive Spurling maneuver suggests nerve root involvement, but the test may give a false negative (Fig. 6.5.13). The test has a good inter-

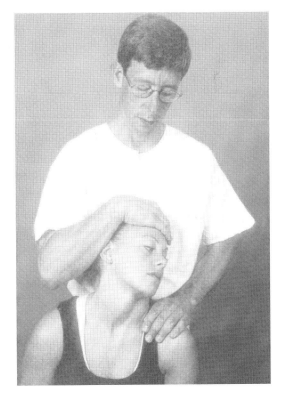

Fig. 6.5.13 The Spurling test is applied to detect radiculopathy. The neck is first laterally flexed, rotated and extended. Then an axial compression is applied. Reprinted with permission from *Norsk Fysikalisk Medisin*. Niels Gunner Juel (editor). Fagbokforlaget, Bergen, Norway, 1999.

examiner reliability [17]. The test may accentuate limb pain or paresthesia because neck extension causes posterior disk bulging, whereas lateral flexion and rotation narrow the ipsilateral neural foramina. The Spurling maneuver is performed by extending the neck and rotating to the side of the pain and then applying downward pressure on the head. When radiating pain or extremity numbness is produced, the test is positive and should be stopped.

Roos' test for thoracic outlet syndrome is performed with the arm abducted and externally rotated. The patient is then instructed to repetitively clench his fist for 3 min. The test is positive if the patient's symptoms are reproduced or aggravated.

Palpation. Palpate upper neck muscles, the trapezius bilaterally and in the supraclavicular fossa. Sore neck muscles are common, but localized sharp pain should be noted.

Imaging

An anterior–posterior cervical radiograph including flexion and extension views should be performed as they may detect unsuspected fractures or tumors. Evaluate the intervertebral foramina. Current radiologic opinion is that MRI is the technique of choice in patients with radicular pain. Electromyography (EMG) is useful to differentiate between central and peripheral involvement and entrapments and nerve root pain.

Acute torticollis

Acute neck pain associated with side flexion and rotation.

Symptoms and signs. Frequently athletes are awakened from sleep by the pain, or when they wake up in the morning the neck is stiff and sore.

Diagnosis. History will usually rule out differential diagnoses. In non-traumatic torticollis, search for underlying malignant, inflammatory or infectious pathology if the condition does not resolve within a short time.

Treatment. Muscle relaxants, anti-inflammatory medication or paracetamol. Inform the patient that the condition usually resolves within a few days. Manual

therapists or chiropractors claim that the muscle spasm results from subluxations of the facet joints, and that the patient will benefit from gentle mobilization.

Cervicalgia

Repeated monotonous activity, prolonged unfamiliar activity, degenerative changes and psychosocial factors may contribute to pain.

Symptoms and signs. Neck pain that may radiate to the shoulder or upper extremity. In patients with pain-inhibited active range of motion a full range of motion is commonly found by passive examination with the patient in a relaxed supine position. Typical stress-related symptoms such as tiredness, concentration difficulties, dizziness and nausea may predominate.

Diagnosis. Radicular symptoms and referred pain should be excluded by clinical examination. Imaging is normally not indicated at the primary consultation.

Treatment. Anti-inflammatory medication or paracetamol for 1–7 days and information for patients with acute pain. The patient should be told not to be over-cautious, and that the symptoms will normally resolve within 1–2 weeks. The effectiveness of various modalities including ergonomic interventions and rest is not well documented, but if acute pain is not reduced, short-term mobilization may improve symptoms [18]. Treatment should attempt to reinforce active coping strategies. Rest may not relieve symptoms if the stressor is not identified. Manipulation of the neck is not recommended because of potential complications. Athletes should continue general training, but in some athletes with chronic neck pain, contact sports may need to be discontinued permanently.

Cervical radiculopathy

The most common cause of cervical radiculopathy is the herniated disk. In patients older than 40 years, symptoms may result from hypertrophic facet and uncovertebral joints and reduced disk height. The prevalence of disk herniations and protrusions is about 30% in the asymptomatic population. Compared to the prevalence of radicular pain 'pathologic' changes such as disk herniation and protrusion most commonly are not recognized by the patient.

Symptoms and signs. Pain in the neck often lasting a few weeks and radicular distribution of symptoms in one or both upper extremities. The pain may at times be atypical and present as chest, breast or facial pain. Paresthesia, hyperesthesia or dysesthesia, and muscle weakness usually interfere with daily activities. Concomitant sensory changes, weakness, atrophy and unilateral diminished tendon reflexes or MRI correlating with radicular symptoms are definite diagnostic criteria. Despite the variations in clinical findings, single nerve root involvement can be diagnosed by manual muscle testing 75–80% of the time. The neck compression test first described by Spurling has a high specificity, but the sensitivity is low. It is performed by extending the neck and rotating to the side of the pain and then applying downward pressure on the head. When cervical myelopathy is present, pain is described in the back and the legs. Other important signs include balance and walking difficulties, and bowel or bladder complaints.

Diagnosis. The diagnosis is mainly clinical. An anterior–posterior cervical radiograph including flexion and extension views should be performed as this may detect unsuspected fractures or tumors. Current radiologic opinion is that MRI is the technique of choice.

Treatment. Corticosteroids and anti-inflammatory medication is the first choice. Epidural steroids can be administered in experienced hands as an alternative where surgery may otherwise be indicated. Usually most patients recover without surgical treatment. A recommendation of a specific treatment strategy including surgery cannot be based on present randomized studies [19]. A rigid collar restricts extension and can be used intermittently until extremity pain has disappeared. These collars may be uncomfortable to wear, which is reported to reduce compliance. Manipulation is contraindicated [20]. Bladder and bowel paralysis or progressive walking difficulties require admission to a neurologic or neurosurgical department. Athletes can normally maintain general training activities with some modifications. Recovery may be long term and, depending on the type of sports activity, many athletes have to take a long break from competitions and plan for the next season.

Thoracic outlet syndrome

The term is used to describe several disorders attributed to mechanical compression of neural and/or vascular structures between the base of the neck and axilla.

Symptoms and signs. Aggravation of symptoms with the arm in the elevated position, paresthesia corresponding to segments C8–T1, tenderness over the brachial plexus supraclavicularly, and a positive Roos' test.

Diagnosis. When at least three of the four criteria listed above are positive.

Treatment. Good results after surgery are achieved in less than 40% of patients, and complications after surgery for thoracic outlet syndrome may be severe. Thus, a proper evaluation of symptoms and disability is important to rule out differential diagnoses and initiate the best conservative treatment. The evaluation should include measurements of range of motion and muscle strength, and a screen for somatization symptoms. According to a large recent study, most patients seem to recover with a conservative model that is based on the functional findings in each patient. Therapy includes exercises emphasizing stretching and strengthening (Figs 6.5.14–6.5.17) [21]. The program seeks to restore the function of the cervical spine and thoracic aperture.

Transient pain and paresthesia of the upper extremity

Frequently reported in contact sports like American football and rugby [22].

Symptoms and signs. Burning pain and numbness in the upper extremity. Symptoms are commonly more circular than dermatomal. May be present as short-term recurrent complaints or chronic paresthesia and muscle weakness.

Diagnosis. Exclude cervical radiculopathy and thoracic outlet syndrome. The risk for chronic complaints is increased in patients with a ratio of the sagittal diameter of the spinal foramen to vertebral body diameter of <0.7.

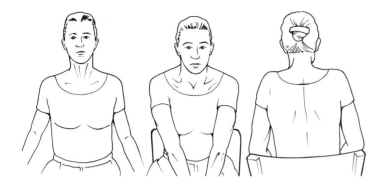

Fig. 6.5.14 Shoulder girdle exercises. Reproduced with permission from [21].

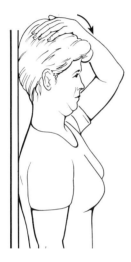

Fig. 6.5.15 Exercise for the upper cervical spine. Reproduced with permission from [21].

Treatment. Prevent development of complaints by recommending to athletes with an increased risk for relapse and chronic pain that they discontinue their sports career.

Rehabilitation

Strengthening and stretching exercises are illustrated in Figs 6.5.14–6.5.17. Recovery is normally not shortened by exercise therapy in the acute stage. The athlete should be able to perform his or her ordinary training schedule before returning to competition.

Prevention

A correctly performed heading in soccer demands technical skills that should be aimed for in organized training of younger players. Improper heading tech-

nique or associated collisions with an opponent may result in long-term complaints. Soccer seems to include more close contact, and it is reasonable to enforce standing rules and increased severity of penalty for dangerous play. The mass of the football is about 400 g and it may hit the head at speeds exceeding 100 km/h. Based on various assumptions, the calculated force against the head may exceed 2000 N. The forces that have to be counteracted by the neck muscles can thus be far beyond the forces occurring in common car collisions.

Low back pain

Epidemiology

The lifetime, 1-year and point prevalence of low back pain in the adult general population is reduced in persons who are physically active for at least 3 h/week [23]. Back pain is more common in the general population than in former elite athletes [24]. Weight-lifting is associated with degeneration of the entire spine, and soccer with degeneration in the lower lumbar region. The prevalence of back pain and degeneration is low in runners. The incidence of chronic low back pain varied from 50 to 85% in a Swedish epidemiologic study including soccer and tennis players, wrestlers and gymnasts [25]. In 36–55% of the athletes, the radiologic examination was interpreted as abnormal. Low back pain is reported to interfere with sports activity at least once a year in about 30–40% of elite swimmers and more than 60% of elite cross-country skiers. The complaints in cross-country skiing are more related to the double-poling and diagonal stride techniques than to skating techniques [26].

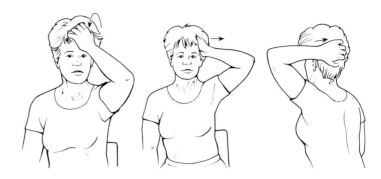

Fig. 6.5.16 Exercise for the scalene muscles. Reproduced with permission from [21].

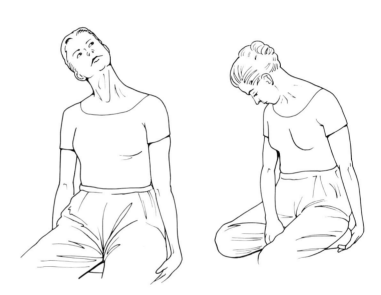

Fig. 6.5.17 Stretching of the anterior muscles of the cervical spine. Reproduced with permission from [21].

Several epidemiologic studies report the prevalence of spondylolysis in athletes being three to four times higher in athletes than among the general population, which varies between 3% and 7%. Its prevalence in a large epidemiologic study in elite Spanish athletes was 8%, with the highest percentages occurring in throwing (27%), rowing (17%) and gymnastics (16%) [27]. Although the prevalence of spondylolysis among wrestlers is reported to be 3–5 times higher than in the normal population and the prevalence of back pain in former wrestlers is about twice as high as that in the normal population, absence from work due to illness is lower. Low back pain is the second most frequent site for pain in dancers. The prevalence is about the same in dancers with and without spondylolysis. Thus, spondylolysis frequently appears incidentally in radiologic examinations, and it is considered that only about 10% have pain.

The cumulative prevalence of low back pain in adolescence is about 30% [28]. Watching television or performing vigorous exercise for more than 2 h daily are associated with increased back pain in the growth period [23]. The majority report mild complaints and only 8% of those with pain seek medical treatment. It is reported that radiologic examinations demonstrate spondylolysis in about 50% of young athletes with back pain who consult an orthopedic surgeon.

Diagnostic thinking

In most athletes, low back pain resolves within 1–2 weeks even without the seeking of medical care. The physician or therapist should acknowledge this observation and not institute unnecessary imaging or treatment at this stage.

Often those who seek advice have tried to continue for weeks despite significant pain, and therefore present with a chronic problem. At this stage, an understanding of differential diagnosis, careful history and physical examination is obligatory to pinpoint the problem. Based on this evaluation, simple advice or a functional rehabilitation program will help most athletes to return to their sport. Imaging procedures are only supplementary and cannot replace the clinical examination. Sensitive procedures like MRI may describe abnormalities that are not specific because of their high prevalence in the asymptomatic population. In adults radiologic spondylolysis/spondylolisthesis correlates poorly with low back pain. In young athletes, an isthmic stress fracture may explain acute low back pain. Low back pain and walking difficulties in the elderly that are relieved by forward bending suggest spinal stenosis; alternatively, coxarthrosis or cardiovascular disease may give similar symptoms and can occur at the same time. Most people with back pain do not (and probably should not!) visit a physician, a physiotherapist or a chiropractor. The challenge is to perform or request the right procedures and to give the right information to the right patient. Table 6.5.5 outlines the most common reasons for back pain in various age groups.

In athletes with radiculopathy, the physician has to consider surgery and inform the patient about the alternatives according to short- and long-term consequences associated with continued sports activity. Lack of bladder or rectal control may indicate the need for immediate surgery—thus the patient should be sent to hospital as an emergency because the prognosis may be worsened after a delay of more than 12 h. Intraspinal tumors, mononeuritis caused by entrapment of peripheral nerves or neurologic disease, a pelvic stress fracture, or the sacroiliac joint syndrome may present as radiating pain. Entrapment of the fibularis nerve as it passes the fibular head usually presents with drop-foot or paresis of dorsal flexion of the ankle and leg pain. Pain referred from the gluteal muscles (including the hip rotators) may radiate below the knee.

In patients with chronic pain the examiner should make an effort to pinpoint why pain has become

Table 6.5.5 Age-related spinal diagnoses.

Young child
Genetic (structural) disturbances, such as unsegmented vertebrae and scoliosis
Spondylolysis
In severe low back pain, neoplasm, discitis or juvenile disk herniation should be excluded
Adolescent
Structural disturbances affected by growth spurt: idiopathic scoliosis, Scheuermann's kyphosis, spondylolysis
Osteomyelitis
Osteoid osteoma
Juvenile disk herniation
Extreme loading in weight-lifting or gymnastics
Young adult
Fractures in high-risk sports
Soft tissue injury
Stress fractures in anorexia or hormonal disturbances
Middle age
Disk and facet joint degeneration
Ankylosing spondylitis and other inflammatory diseases
Elderly
Spinal stenosis
Neoplasm or secondary tumor

chronic. Key questions are as follows. Have diagnostic procedures failed in the acute stage? Should a prolonged course be expected according to the natural course of a specific disorder? Did the patient return to sports too early? Has previous treatment been adequate? Are there other factors influencing complaints?

The diagnostic evaluation in patients with chronic pain should include psychological and social factors (Table 6.5.8). Elite athletes who usually tolerate psychological stress well may be vulnerable and demonstrate fear of avoidance, muscular defence and even abnormal illness behavior if their career or goals for the season are threatened.

History

The chief complaint should be clearly established. Most commonly it is pain, but occasionally the main complaint is stiffness, specific functional loss or structural abnormality. Pain localization and disability should be clarified precisely. Pain may be absent or not disabling in normal activity, but triggered by certain

Table 6.5.6 Common mechanisms of back pain.

Mechanism of injury	Sport
Repetitive loading	Roller skiing, rowing, kayaking
Repetitive loading in contact sports	Soccer, European handball, ice hockey, wrestling, judo, karate
Lifting human bodies	Ballet, dance, figure skating
Loading an immature spine	Weight training, gymnastics
Sudden violent muscle contraction	Throwing sports
Hyperextension/torsion	Throwing sports, gymnastics

Table 6.5.7 Red flags in the evaluation of back pain.

First-time back pain in patients <20 and >55 years
Constant, progressive, non-mechanical pain
History: drug abuse, cancer, human immunodeficiency virus
Weight loss
Widespread neurologic signs and symptoms
Structural deformity
Thoracic pain or chronic cough
Intermenstrual bleeding
Violent trauma
Altered bladder control
Associated visual disturbance
Balance problems or upper limb dysesthesia
Persisting severe restriction of lumbar flexion

sport-specific movements—thereby suggesting functional overload of a specific structure. It is important to know whether the patient suffers from back pain, leg pain, or both. An acute disk herniation may present as unilateral leg pain without back pain. Isolated back pain is usually not discogenic in young individuals. Pain in young athletes that is worsened by trunk hyperextension (but not forward bending) suggests spondylolysis/spondylolisthesis. The nature of the onset and the association with trauma may point towards muscular strain, contusion or discogenic involvement. Muscular pain may be localized and provoked by specific exercise, or present as diffuse widespread pain worsened by physical and psychological stress.

The degree of disability should be clarified. The level of activity and the degree to which pain is aggravated by or interferes with training or competition should be noted, along with the goals of the athlete. A detailed history is required to pinpoint the level of discomfort during each of the activities. This may help to explain why pain has developed. In throwing, skiing and weight-lifting, inflammation and/or partial muscle/tendon ruptures may be caused by acute or repetitive loading. For example, pain located at the iliac crest, groin and leg that is worsened by side flexion, extension and rotation may be referred from the quadratus lumborum muscle. Common mechanisms of back pain in sports are outlined in Table 6.5.6.

Significant chronic back pain and disability in patients under the age of 10 should raise the question of tumor or discitis. Spinal tumors in this age group commonly have a 1–2-year delay in diagnosis. Similarly, a first-time history of back pain in anyone over the age of

60 should introduce the possibility of tumor. Red flags are outlined in Table 6.5.7. If responses to these possibilities are negative, one can focus on expanding the history of the presenting complaint.

Severe pain and disability are commonly associated with fear. Athletes, like other patients with acute pain, may demonstrate helplessness and fear which may be more related to the consequences of pain than the pain itself. If a careful history and examination do not suggest serious back pain or specific treatment, the evaluation should focus on the functional limitations, and the athlete should be encouraged to gradually return to former activity. Sometimes the athlete for various reasons may not want to return to former sports activity (Table 6.5.8). It is therefore important to explore what beliefs and expectations the patient has about pain, treatment and sports.

For evaluation of chronic back pain, it is important to reassess the patient with an open mind. Let the patient tell his history in his own words, and then re-examine him before previous reports including imaging are considered. Ask the patient if he has experienced similar complaints previously, and what kind of explanations, advice and treatment he has previously received.

Clinical examination

Acute pain
The purpose of the clinical examination is to discriminate between patients who need further examination

Table 6.5.8 Yellow flags or risk factors for chronicity.

Previous history of low back pain
Total absence from sports or work over the last year
Radicular pain
Reduced trunk muscle strength, endurance and flexibility in
    relation to sport-specific demands
Disproportionate illness behavior
Psychological distress, depressive symptoms, disturbed sleep
    and social isolation
Dissatisfaction
Personal problems: alcohol, marital, financial
Adversarial medicolegal proceedings
Belief that back pain is dangerous
Fear of physical activity
Expectation of passive treatment

or hospitalization and patients who do best with simple advice and analgesics. Nerve root signs assessed by conventional neurologic examination are reliable, but palpation of tenderness in the lumbar spine is highly unreliable [29].

If rectal or bladder function is disturbed, sensitivity in the saddle area and sphincter function should be examined.

Weakness in patients with sciatic pain is rapidly assessed by asking the patient to walk on toes (S1) and heels (L5), and bend the knees (L4).

Does the patient present a limited range of motion or a protective scoliosis? Are all movements painful or is pain provoked by one leg extension only (spondylolisthesis)?

Examination of the abdomen and peripheral pulses should be performed. Rectal or vaginal examination may be required where indicated by the history.

Does palpation confirm the pain reported on history? Is pain localized or widespread?

Chronic pain

Gait (rolling, limping, functional) should be assessed when the patient enters the room and on demand when undressed. A systematic examination should then be performed in as few positions as possible.

Standing. Important landmarks are the prominent vertebra (C7 or Th1), the inferior angle of the scapula (Th7), the lowest rib (Th12) and the tops of the iliac crest (L4) (Fig. 6.5.4).

Leg length differences >1 cm and scoliosis can be observed. In patients with a protective scoliosis, apparent spasm of paravertebral muscles is confirmed by gentle palpation.

If the lateral curve remains on forward flexion, this suggests that the scoliosis is fixed or structural. A rib hump confirms the diagnosis (Fig. 6.5.18). Is the range of forward flexion limited? Measure fingertip–floor distance. What is the cause of the limitation: thoracic kyphosis, low back pain or short hamstring muscles? In a patient with a complaint of sciatica, forward flexion may provoke pain down the leg by increasing tension of the ischiadic nerve, the hamstring muscles or the deep gluteal muscles. Patients with low back pain often present with a dysfunctional movement pattern clearly demonstrated as they assist by using their arms and legs to straighten up from the forward flexed position. It should be kept in mind that measurements of range of motion as well as muscle strength in patients are always affected by the patient's pain and motivation. Therefore assessment of pain intensity and psychological tests can add information that assists interpretation of the results from physical tests in patients.

Assess lateral flexion. Record the point reached from the floor. Note whether there is an asymmetric movement pattern or a sharp break in the curve that may suggest segmental pain. Assess rotation. Then ask the patient to keep his hands firmly at his sides and repeat. The major part of the motion will now take place in the legs and not interfere with back pain (Fig. 6.5.19d).

A series of heel raises with either leg is the best way to test S1 function. The examiner may look for evidence of a Trendelenburg sign and gluteus medius atrophy while the heel raise is being performed.

Supine. Muscle strength of the tibialis anterior and toe extensors (L5), and peroneal muscles and triceps surae (S1) are examined with the knees flexed. Weakness of knee extension (L4) and hip flexion (L2) indicate that the femoral nerve is affected. Widespread weakness suggests overlay or pain-inhibited weakness (Fig. 6.5.19e).

Deep tendon reflexes (patellar, Achilles and plantar) are examined with the knees in 90° flexion. All reflexes may be augmented by having the patient 'clench' their

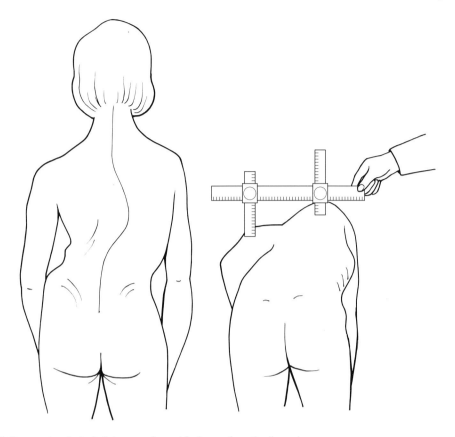

Fig. 6.5.18 Structural scoliosis. A rib hump on forward flexion confirms the diagnosis.

teeth, lock the fingers and tense the upper limb muscles (Fig. 6.5.20).

Straight-leg raising should be examined with and without reinforcement (bending the neck and dorsiflexion of the ankle). This test is positive if pain radiates beyond the knee at 45° elevation (Fig. 6.5.21). This test is false positive if the patient (while the examiner uses the pretext of examining the back from behind) is able to sit up on a bench without spontaneously flexing his knees (Fig. 6.5.19a).

Test sensation to pinprick for nerve roots L4, L5 and S1 and finally for peripheral nerves. Diminution of sensation at the side of the foot is the most common finding (S1). Stocking anesthesia indicates that sensory loss is not radicular (Fig. 6.5.22).

Hip flexion is evaluated with the knees flexed. The examiner should limit sacral tilting and lumbar lordo-sis. A positive Faber test (passive *f*lexion/*ab*duction/*ex*ternal *r*otation) (Fig. 6.5.23, p. 673) suggests involvement of the sacroiliac joint or coxarthrosis.

The quadratus lumborum muscle is assessed with the patient lying on their side with the arms upright and a pillow underneath the lumbar spine. The muscle is assessed by palpation as the patient contracts the quadratus lumborum by performing a combined abduction/retraction maneuver of the lower extremity.

Prone. The femoral nerve stretch test is performed by passive hip extension with knee flexion and produces pain on the anterolateral part of the thigh (L3–4). If this maneuver triggers sciatic pain, it suggests L5 root irritation.

Osteoarthritis of the hip and low back pain are

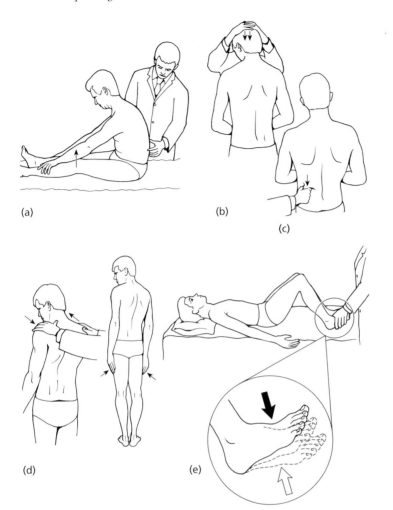

Fig. 6.5.19 Waddel signs: (a) straight-leg raising; (b) pressure to the head; (c) superficial stimulation; (d) pelvic rotation; (e) widespread weakness or cogwheel compliance on motor examination.

frequently confused. A full range of hip rotation with the absence of pain at the extremes is generally required to eliminate the former.

If pain is provoked by the combined motion of hip flexion/external rotation/adduction, pain referred from the external hip rotators is suspected.

The paravertebral muscles, the spinous processes, the sacroiliac area with the gluteal muscles, the insertion of the hamstring muscles on the ischial tubercle, and the great trochanter are palpated for pain. Is pain localized or widespread? Is paravertebral palpation more painful than palpation of each spinous process? Does the patient scream or withdraw on light palpation?

Imaging

Based on a proper clinical examination, appropriate imaging investigations may be ordered. History, main symptoms and clinical signs should be precisely described. Unless a fracture or serious back pain is suspected or neurologic signs are demonstrated at the clinical examination, imaging is usually not requested in a patient presenting with back pain for the first time. Routine X-rays are indicated if a fracture is suspected, and in elderly patients without sciatic pain. A lateral thoracic view is taken in patients with kyphosis. In cases of suspected spondylolysis, an oblique view or a CT scan through the vertebral arch gives additional information. CT is the first choice in patients with

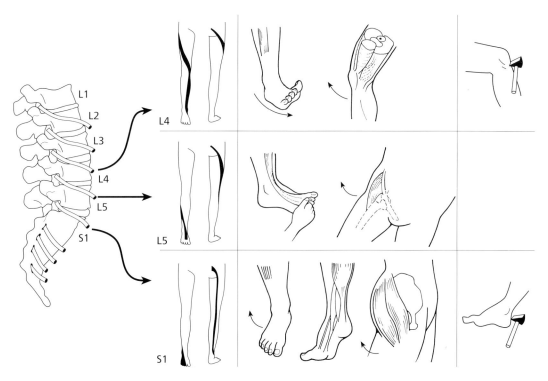

Fig. 6.5.20 Neurologic examination in patients with L4–S1 radiculopathy. Reproduced with permission from *Norsk Fysibalisk Medisin*, Niels Gunner Juel (editor), Fagbokforlaget, Bergen, Norway, 1999.

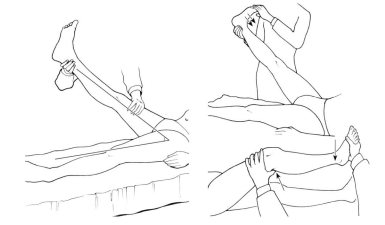

Fig. 6.5.21 Straight-leg raising test. Pain must be below the knee if the roots of the sciatic nerve are involved. Passive dorsiflexion of the foot or palpation of the stretched tibial nerve aggravates pain.

sciatic pain. CT is also the best method of visualizing the facet and sacroiliac joints. Scintigraphy is indicated if history and clinical examination indicate spondylo–lysis in a patient with acute pain. MRI is the first choice if an infection (discitis or vertebral abscess) or tumor is suspected. MRI is also the best method to discriminate between scar tissue and a disk herniation in patients with back and leg pain who have had previous disk surgery. Discography may be used preoperatively to evaluate discogenic pain. This evaluation is positive if pain

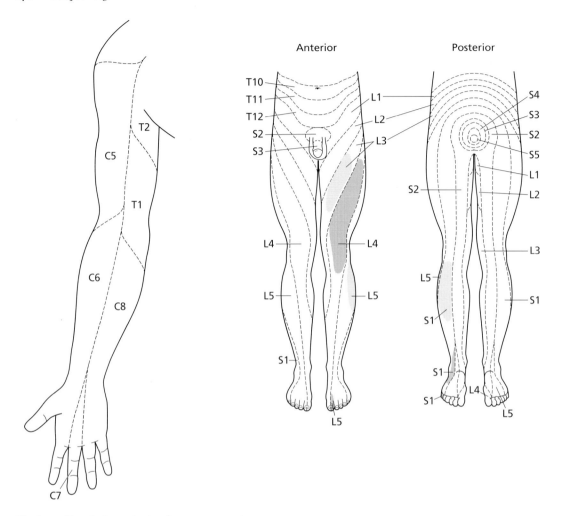

Fig. 6.5.22 Neurologic examination. Sensory assessment.

is concordant, but the number of false-positive ratings is high. The recent opinion therefore is that it is difficult to interpret the information from a positive discography. Facet joint anesthesia should reduce pain intensity by at least 50% and be supplemented by a negative placebo injection to be considered positive. The expense of a procedure and its therapeutic consequences should be considered before ordering an investigation [30,31]. Limited imaging is recommended, particularly in patients with low back pain without objective clinical findings. Repeated radiologic investigations should be limited because of radiation exposure.

Muscle contusion

Muscular contusions are common in many collision sports.

Diagnosis. History and exclusion of other diagnoses by clinical examination, imaging if a fracture is suspected.

Treatment. Ice, compression and anti-inflammatory medication. Disability is short-lived, and return to sports activity is usually possible within a few days.

Muscle rupture

Muscular ruptures are common in sports with rapid movements including torsion and twisting. Occasionally there is an associated avulsion fracture of the transverse process by the quadratus lumborum or the iliac crest by the external oblique.

Diagnosis. Distinct unilateral pain on palpation. Pain is usually associated with muscle spasms during the first 2 weeks.

Treatment. As for muscle contusion. Alternate exercise for endurance and exercise for muscular strength after a few days. Additionally, a thoracolumbar orthosis may be helpful during the first 2–3 weeks. Gradual progression in activity that allows for competitive training after 3–8 weeks. In the case of an avulsion of the transverse process or the iliac crest up to 3 months may be required before the athlete can return to competition that involves contact activity or rapid movements through a full range or sudden twisting or deceleration.

Ligament strain

Diagnosis. Acute localized pain not provoked by isometric contraction. Usually located to the cervical, interscapular or lumbosacral area.

Treatment. As for muscular contusion. Manual mobilization may be indicated in patients with chronic pain.

Radiculopathy

Radicular pain in athletes is most commonly related to disk herniation. Recent research has found only a weak correlation between disk degeneration and herniation. In the middle-aged or elderly athlete reduced disk height and facet joint degeneration contribute to radicular pain. Inhibited motor function indicates nerve root compression. The association between pain or a positive Lasegue's test and nerve root compression is more uncertain [32]. Current knowledge indicates that acute radicular pain is caused by an inflammation induced by an autoimmunologic process involving the herniated disk and irritation of the dorsal root ganglion [33,34]. Under chronic conditions ischemic, inflammatory, metabolic and neurophysiologic changes affecting the nerve root or the dorsal root ganglion and central inhibiting or enhancing mechanisms may contribute to the pain-producing process.

Symptoms and signs. Pain radiation below the knee that is provoked by coughing. Prolonged standing and sitting is difficult. At consultation the patient may present with a limp, the upper body forward flexed, and a protective scoliosis. The diagnosis is supported by positive neurologic signs in a nerve root pattern and a positive straight-leg raising test.

Diagnosis. The diagnosis is based mainly on clinical symptoms. CT is indicated if the complaints do not improve within 2 weeks or in patients with progressive paresis.

Treatment. A patient with a large central herniation producing bladder disturbance, diminished perineal sensation and even paraplegia is a surgical emergency, and immediate exploration is imperative.

All other patients are first treated with conservative methods. Anti-inflammatory medication is recommended. Corticosteroids, 40–60 mg prednisolone for 3–7 days is usually well tolerated. Analgesics (including opiates) are indicated in patients with pain-related sleep difficulties. The patient should be informed that the prognosis is good without surgery, and that improvement is not delayed by ordinary activities or improved by bed rest. In the long term extrusion of disk material leads to narrowing of the disk space.

Participation in competition should normally be delayed until the athlete is able to conduct his normal training program although this may sometimes be controversial. Recently a Norwegian cross-country skier won the World Championship title despite sciatica with motor disturbances.

Reduced activity is recommended in patients with unaltered or progressive complaints. Twisting and bending when lifting should be avoided. The physiotherapist should motivate the athlete to remain active, to use and flex his back in order to maintain general physical fitness, and to maintain a positive attitude. In general there is no reason to be overcautious. The effect of traction is limited at best to short-term pain relief, and has no documented effect on recovery. Exercises to improve the function of the deep stabilizing trunk muscles have no documented effect on recovery, but may reduce the risk of relapse. In dancers and in athletes in other sports that include lifting a partner, a corset or a stabilizing belt can make it possible to maintain performance.

Progressive pareses or muscle weakness and radicular pain for 6–12 weeks indicate surgery. The effect of extirpation of the herniation with or without arcotomy or laminectomy improves radicular pain and muscle weakness in about 80% of the patients, but the effect on back pain is more variable. Therefore, the indication for surgery in patients with a disk herniation and back pain (but no radicular pain) is more controversial. Percutaneous nucleotomy is not indicated.

There is no consensus about rehabilitation after surgery. A recent study suggests that the patient should resume ordinary activities as soon as the operative wound is healed [35]. From this baseline, the athlete should gradually increase his training volume and intensity.

Absence from sports in athletes with radiculopathy is highly variable. In patients without muscle weakness we expect a setback of 6–12 weeks; in patients with objective neurologic signs the setback is commonly 12–24 weeks or longer. Therefore, long-term planning is an important part of the rehabilitation process, preferably in agreement with the physiotherapist, coach and athlete. In some cases it may be wise to recommend reduction of ambitions and eventually giving up the sports career in order to set new, more realistic goals in another arena.

Spinal stenosis

Encroachment of the spinal canal, usually by hypertrophic bone, produces signs of neural claudication, and is particularly problematic in the elderly runner or orienteering athlete (>60 years). Symptoms may present at an earlier age when associated with previous fracture or spinal surgery.

Symptoms and signs. Leg aching and numbness with or without back pain and morning stiffness. Reduced walking or running distance. Pain is normally reduced by forward flexion. In patients with a central spinal stenosis symptoms are almost always bilateral. Muscle weakness and loss of the patellar reflex is common. The patient may present with a foot drop.

Diagnosis. According to clinical symptoms and signs described above and confirmation of decreased canal size based on CT scan. MRI is used preoperatively. Myelography is used if more than one level is affected or if patients have scar tissue after previous surgery. It is important to exclude other diagnoses that can produce signs of claudication: compartment syndrome, diabetic neuropathy, disk herniation, vascular claudication and tumor.

Treatment. Anti-inflammatory medication. The athlete should possibly change activity from running to swimming or cycling. Group exercise (e.g. aerobics) is recommended in inactive patients to improve general flexibility, strength and endurance, and to reduce depressive symptoms. Analgesics (including opiates) may be indicated if sleep is disturbed by pain. The effectiveness of surgical treatment is uncertain in patients with back pain, but surgery is indicated in patients with progressive claudication and muscle weakness.

Spondylolysis/spondylolisthesis

Spondylolysis is defined as a defect in the vertebral isthmus (lysis) or most commonly the pars interarticularis. Multiple factors may be involved in its genesis. In athletes, a stress fracture is considered to cause the defect, predominantly located at the L5 level. Biomechanically, torsion against resistance, hyperextension and rotation are possible causative movements. Previous studies have described that spondylolisthesis is found in about 80% of spondylolytic lesions, but the frequency was only about 30% in a large current study. Spondylolisthesis is classified into five grades: grade I is defined as a 25% forward slip of L5 in relation to S1, whereas grade V is a 100% slip (opthosis) (Fig. 6.5.24). Grades I–II are most frequent. Instability is usually minimal because the vertebrae are anchored by ligaments and stabilized actively by trunk muscles. The slip rarely increases after growth is complete.

Symptoms and signs. Low back pain that may be referred to the buttock. Activity usually aggravates pain. May present with associated spasms of the erector spinae or hamstring muscles. Sciatica in the young patient is sometimes observed in grades III and IV.

Sciatica from disk and facet joint degeneration or hypertrophic tissue in the pseudarthrotic defect is sometimes observed in adult patients.

Diagnosis. Distinct back pain aggravated by one leg extension and a positive bone scan indicate that the defect is the source of discomfort (Fig. 6.5.25). Radiologic examination with front and side projections will usually reveal the lysis; diagnosis is confirmed by an oblique view (Fig. 6.5.26). Instability is assessed by comparison of measurements of the slip in forward flexion and extension. CT is the best method to describe the defect in detail. Spondylolysis appears frequently incidentally in radiologic examinations. It is considered that only about 10% of those with a positive radiologic examination have pain.

Treatment. It is not documented that a corset is effective for pain relief or healing of the lytic defect in patients with acute pain and a positive bone scan. Treatment involves training modification, anti-inflammatory medication and proprioceptive exercises to activate the transversus and multifidus muscles (Figs 6.5.27 & 6.5.28) [36]. The physiotherapist should instruct, give feedback and supervise treatment over a few sessions. Progression is made not so much by increasing the number of repetitions as by integration of the stabilizing activation of the deep trunk muscles in more complex motions (from four-foot kneeling to the soccer kick) (Fig. 6.5.28). Surgery is indicated in grades III and IV and in grade II if conservative treatment does not improve function.

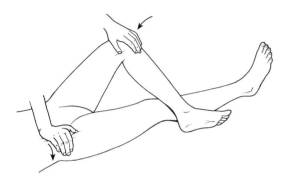

Fig. 6.5.23 Patrick or FABER test to detect pelvic or hip pain. Combined *f*lexion, *ab*duction, *ex*ternal *r*otation of the hip with the patient supine, the knee flexed and the foot placed on the opposite patella. The flexed knee is then pushed laterally.

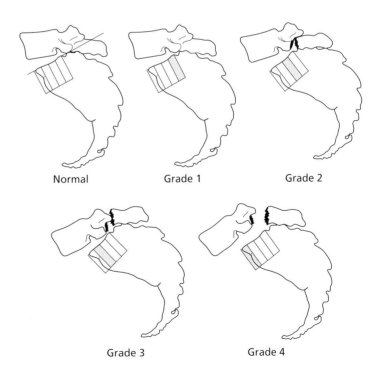

Normal   Grade 1   Grade 2

Grade 3   Grade 4

Fig. 6.5.24 Classification of spondylolisthesis.

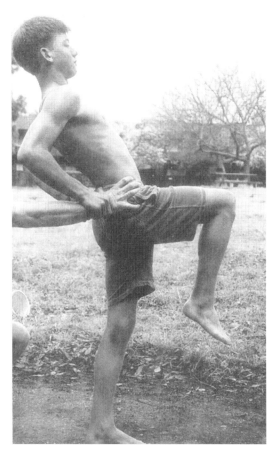

Fig. 6.5.25 Spondylolisthesis: one-leg hyperextension test. Reprinted with permission.

Scoliosis

Scoliosis is a lateral curvature of the spine (Fig. 6.5.5). Scoliosis may be structural (idiopathic, congenital, neuromuscular, iatrogenic or due to rare syndromes) or non-structural (tilting of the pelvis, apparent shortening of one leg or due to unilateral protective muscle spasm—particularly that accompanying a prolapsed intervertebral disk). Non-structural scoliosis disappears when the patient is bending forward. The prevalence of structural scoliosis is 3%. About 3‰ of the population should be offered specific treatment according to current guidelines. The prevalence ratio of idiopathic scoliosis in girls compared with boys is 7/1. Structural scoliosis is a multifactorial inherited disorder characterized by either dominant inheritance or

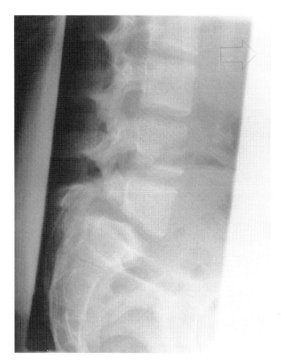

Fig. 6.5.26 Spondylolisthesis grade II–III in a 19-year-old soccer player and snowboarder. He has performed his sports without any restrictions for 4 years.

reduced penetration. There is a tendency for increasing curves until growth is finished.

Symptoms and signs. Patients with a structural scoliosis do not usually seek treatment because of pain. A simple screening examination can be conducted by the gymnastics teacher by asking the children to bend forward at yearly examinations. A marked asymmetrical curve with the shape of a boatkeel corresponding to the rib girdle on the convex side will appear in scoliosis (see Fig. 6.5.18). The muscular activity on the concave and the convex side of a curve will be different, and the patient may sometimes complain about fatigue associated with monotonous activities.

Diagnosis. Admission to an orthopedic department for evaluation. The diagnosis is verified and classified by radiologic examination.

Treatment. Natural course, brace or surgery. Treatment should be started and controlled regularly at an orthopedic department which can offer both conservative and surgical treatment. The patient should be

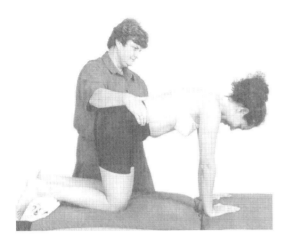

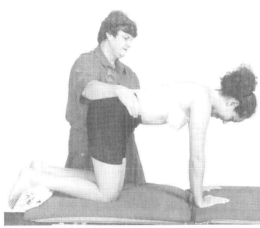

Fig. 6.5.27 Teaching the test action in the four-point kneeling position: (a) with the abdomen relaxed; (b) following the abdominal drawing-in action. Reproduced with permission from [49].

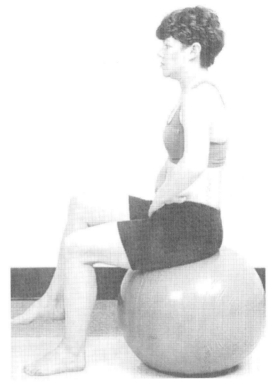

Fig. 6.5.28 Integrative exercise for back stabilization.

encouraged to participate in physical activity. A brace is generally recommended if the curve increases and exceeds 25°. The brace should be worn day and night, but can usually be taken off during physical activity. The patient is advised against carrying a heavy bag; therefore it is recommended that these patients have two separate sets of school books.

Scheuermann's disease

Originates during the growth spurt, and is more common among boys than girls. The prevalence is about 5%. In 70% of patients, the disorder is localized in the thoracic spine. An aseptic necrosis of the thoracic vertebral bodies caused by ischemia of the growth zone is the most likely pathophysiologic mechanism. The necrosis is most pronounced in front, giving the vertebrae their characteristic wedge shape (Fig. 6.5.29). Repetitive traumatization during the growth spurt may increase the risk. A high prevalence of radiologic changes, but with mild or no symptoms, have been observed in cross-country skiers. Excessive rollerskiing during the growth spurt has been suggested as a possible mechanism.

Symptoms and signs. The kyphosis of the thoracic spine is usually obvious when the patient is viewed from the side. When mobility is normal in the kyphotic spine the deformity is most frequently postural in origin. Thoracolumbar curves are more frequently associated with pain than thoracic curves.

Diagnosis. The radiologic definition is at least three adjacent vertebral bodies showing 5° or more anterior wedging. The epiphyses of the vertebral bodies are often irregular, and may be disturbed by herniations of the nuclear pulposus.

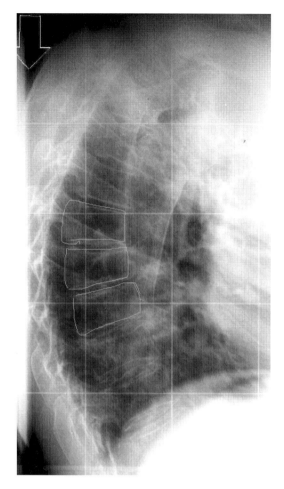

Fig. 6.5.29 Mb. Scheuermann. The radiologic definition is at least three adjacent vertebral bodies showing 5° or more anterior wedging.

Treatment. Physiotherapy, exercises, or breaststroke swimming to strengthen back and interscapular muscles. If the curve reaches 50° in adolescence, a brace should be worn for 12–18 months. The prognosis is good. Surgical treatment is rare.

Ankylosing spondylitis

The prevalence is about 1–2‰ with a yearly incidence of 300–400 patients in Norway. The incidence is greatest during the third and fourth decade and, unlike rheumatoid arthritis, it is rare in women. The disorder is characterized by progressive ossification of the joints of the spine and sacroiliac joints. Its etiology is unknown, but a hereditary tendency is reported.

Symptoms and signs. Increasing pain and stiffness in the thoracic and lumbar spine and the sacroiliac joints. Occasionally, hip, knee and shoulder pain, and/or pain at the insertion of the Achilles tendon or the plantar fascia, is the presenting symptom. Night pain and morning stiffness is common. Symptoms usually improve during the day and by physical activity. Palpation of the spinous processes, the sacroiliac joints, and the insertion of the Achilles tendon and the hamstring tendon is usually painful. In a late stage the thoracic kyphosis may be pronounced with associated neck pain because of stiffness and difficulties in keeping forward vision. A characteristic gait is normally seen at this stage.

Diagnosis. The diagnosis is clinical according to the symptoms and signs described above. The thoracic excursion may be reduced (<2.5 cm) in the early stage. Radiologic examination of the spine may demonstrate characteristic features (bambooing spine), but subchondral sclerosis and arthritis of the sacroiliac joints are found on CT at an earlier stage. The sedimentation rate may be high. HLA-B27 is not diagnostic.

Treatment. Regular physical activity is an important part of the treatment. Anti-inflammatory medication is given periodically. Manual mobilization may help to postpone deformation in a forward flexed position. When kyphotic deformity is gross, a thoracic wedge osteotomy can improve the erect posture and normalize forward vision.

Unspecific low back pain

Low back pain may be caused by a variety of spinal structures, and may be inhibited or reinforced by the human mind [37]. Disorders discriminated by either characteristic history, symptoms, signs or pathophysiologic features are described above. Clinical techniques developed by chiropractors, manual therapists and osteopaths, and various imaging procedures are widely used, but the diagnostic specificity of these procedures is either low or poorly documented with regard to the asymptomatic population. Furthermore, facet joint injections and discography may be used to discriminate pain elicited from these structures from muscular pain. However, the number of false-positive tests and the modest effectiveness of specific treatments have turned the focus to interaction of the various structures. Experimental studies have demonstrated the existence of neural pathways between various spinal structures and also between the sacroiliac joint and the spinal and gluteal muscles (Fig. 6.5.1). Regardless of the cause of low back pain, free nerve endings and mechanoreceptors located in the outer annulus of the intervertebral disk, the zygapophyseal joints, the ligaments, the muscles and the tendons provide sensory information needed to regulate muscle tension. Reflex activity, that is, an involuntary response to a specific stimulus, may interfere with previously programmed movement patterns. At the same time, pain and fear of pain influence muscle activity. Low back pain may therefore be regarded as a functional disturbance. Of particular interest is the activation of postural muscles prior to lifting and pulling (or actually any motion of the arms and legs), to maintain equilibrium before the movements are executed.

Muscular insufficiency may also occur in extremely well-trained athletes. Increased fatigability of the multifidus muscles verified by EMG was associated with chronic low back pain in a study including elite rowers [38].

Disk injuries in the adolescent athlete are observed in sports that involve a large training volume and particular stress of the spinal structures during growth, for example in gymnastics (Fig. 6.5.30). Efforts are continuously made to prevent such injuries, but the volume of training needed to achieve a high level of performance at a young age makes these athletes particularly vulnerable.

Symptoms and signs. Low back pain with or without radiation to the hip, groin and buttocks. Occasionally the patient presents with a protective scoliosis. All movements may be painful and the range of motion limited.

Diagnosis. A thorough clinical examination is important to eliminate differential diagnoses and gain confidence. In patients with subacute or chronic pain, a CT scan and a clinical evaluation of inorganic signs are recommended if symptoms have lasted longer than 2–4 weeks (Fig. 6.5.28).

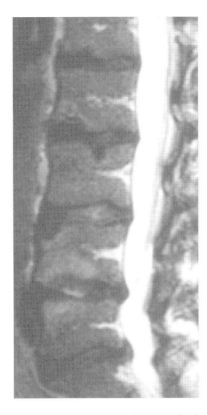

Fig. 6.5.30 MRI — disk herniation and degenerative signs suggesting injuries at the vertebral endplates during adolesence.

Treatment

Acute pain. Inform the patient that he or she should attempt to continue with ordinary activities — including general physical activity. Analgesics or anti-inflammatory medication for 3–5 days shortens the recovery period. Opiates are rarely indicated. The effectiveness of manipulation and exercise regimens in the acute phase is not documented and is therefore rarely indicated [39]. General physical activity can usually be continued, at times after a rest period for a couple of days. The athlete can return to competition when he or she is able to continue ordinary training activity. The prognosis is good. About 90% of patients have recovered within a week after their first episode of low back pain [40]. The physician and physiotherapist should acknowledge this information. The patient should be treated with empathy, but overcautiousness may reinforce fear and functional complaints.

Chronic pain. Information about the nature of the problem, emphasizing reduction of fear, will give the patient confidence to resume light activity. Guidelines recommending avoiding twisting and bending when lifting and excess carrying that involves prolonged isometric activity, and encouraging use of the thighs when lifting heavy objects can be given. The patient should be instructed to use the back and flex it [37]. Information may be reinforced at repeated appointments. It is documented that patients with chronic low back pain will benefit from exercise therapy. A recent study indicates that low-impact aerobics is the most cost-effective physiotherapy method [41]. A variety of other methods have also been offered.

The effect of disk surgery in patients with a disk herniation and low back pain is controversial [42]. Surgery is the ultimate treatment, with the drama of preparation, contact with the surgical team, anesthesia and invasion of the body. Surgery carries strong implications of success. For example, relief of sciatica and back pain has been reported in at least one-third of back surgery patients who proved to have no disk herniation [43]. On the other hand it is estimated that the concept of failed back surgery contributes to as much as 20% of all patients with chronic pain. The effectiveness of fusion surgery or disk prosthesis is, with the exception of one study, not documented by randomized, prospective studies and should at present be considered as experimental treatment for only a few patients.

Rehabilitation

The main goals are to help the athlete to return to previous sports activity and to prevent relapse. Some athletes with recurrent or chronic pain may need advice and support in order to reduce activity or to turn to another sport, while other patients with chronic pain should be encouraged to be more active. A careful evaluation, reassurance, simple advice and reduction in competitive activity, followed by a graded increase in training intensity and volume, will enable most patients to return to their previous sports level.

Treatment in the acute phase is described above. Considering the efficacy of anti-inflammatory medication as compiled from randomized trials with various pain conditions, the number needed to treat (NNT) was about 2–3 [44]. This means that of every two to three patients who receive the drug at clinical

doses, one patient will report at least 50% pain relief. In contrast the NNT for codeine (60 mg) was 16–17. Also, opiates like codeine are associated with abuse and are illegal to use while driving. The consumption of these drugs should preferably be limited. The analgesic action of anti-inflammatory medication remains a controversial subject, but recent studies support the view that both a direct peripheral and a spinal effect of inhibition of cyclooxygenase contribute to pain relief. Anti-inflammatory medication as analgesic treatment over 1–7 days for relief of mild to moderate pain is well tolerated and equivalent to paracetamol, and is recommended because of the potential risk of paracetamol overdose [45].

In patients with recurrent or chronic complaints a functional evaluation by a physiotherapist with sport-specific knowledge is recommended. For example, gymnastics requires a full range of motion at the shoulder and the hips. In gymnasts with limitations of these movements, acceptable skills may be achieved to compensate for the limited range of motion by increasing the lumbar lordosis. Therefore, a thorough functional evaluation includes observation of the athlete during competition and exercise, tests for muscle strength and range of motion and finally analysis by high-speed video camera and measurement of EMG activity. The rehabilitation program should be individualized, based on the findings from the functional evaluation and sport-specific demands. According to this some athletes may benefit from stretching exercises while others may need specific strengthening exercises. The use of passive therapies such as soft tissue treatment, electrotherapy and corsets should be kept at a low level. Despite the widespread use of manual therapy for millennia, evidence of its effectiveness from clinical trials is still controversial. The mechanism by which it produces pain relief—according to a recent postulated model based on experimental studies—is probably by involvement of a supraspinal control center [46].

Most athletes have to modify training activity, and it may not be possible to enter forthcoming competitions. It is therefore important to maintain long-term goals. Relatively minor injuries can turn into a personal catastrophic experience for the athlete if they disqualify him or her from major competitive events. In this situation, the major duty of the medical team is to support the athlete and to set new goals. Clinicians should strive to understand how their patients view the world and should provide a rational explanation about their disease and its treatment within this framework. Treatment will be most effective if time is spent searching for the best possible treatment and then administering it with utmost confidence.

Psychosocial factors should be recognized in patients with chronic pain (Table 6.5.8). Questionnaires can be helpful as a screening procedure for somatization symptoms, fear-avoidance beliefs and depression. Most patients with symptoms of somatization and depression will benefit from participation in exercise groups by improved coping skills and reduction of symptoms. Some patients may need to consult a psychologist or a psychiatrist. The screening questionnaires are helpful for use in athletes who demonstrate inappropriate symptoms and signs or an abnormal treatment response.

The commonly used principle 'let pain be your guide' is a misleading approach to use in the rehabilitation of patients with chronic low back pain. Exercise regimens should be based on a dose–contingency principle and not on pain [47,48]. This is particularly important in patients who prefer passive treatment regimens because of pain. It is advisable to set the quotas (doses) from baseline observations. This includes results of 6–10 functional tests in which the patient has to perform each exercise until fatigue or pain limits activity. The exercise dose is normally set to 50% of the baseline result and the dose is increased by 1–5 repetitions every other day. When the patient is able to do 30 repetitions a more demanding exercise is chosen. Exercise is always to be followed by rest. The main indication for this program is pain restricting participation in exercise programs founded on exercise physiologic principles.

Group exercise such as low-impact aerobics is the most cost-effective type of physiotherapy [41]. Specific exercises or training with devices may be equally effective but at a higher cost, at least when physiotherapy regimens are applied to patients with low back pain in the general population. The main effect of exercise therapy may be to reduce fear of avoidance. In athletes, results from the functional evaluation should be considered because of specific demands in each sport. The volume of competition-specific train-ing should be gradually increased before entering a competition.

Recent studies indicate that activation, size and fatigability of the deep stabilizing trunk muscles are different in asymptomatic individuals and patients [49]. In back pain caused by a disk herniation, ligament injury or muscle strain, the stabilizing trunk muscles are normally inhibited while other muscles such as the iliopsoas and the erector spina are activated. Atrophy of the deep muscles and increased activity of the outer muscle may in turn increase the functional disturbance. Proprioceptive exercises emphasizing the function of the trunk may therefore be included at all stages in the rehabilitation process. The principles may easily be applied to group exercise as well as to training for specific sports. Treatment normally starts with certain movements (e.g. 'draw in your navel') (Fig. 6.5.27) supervised by a physiotherapist, and these movements are then gradually incorporated in more complex activities including specific sports (Fig. 6.5.28).

Summary

A steady rise in the rates of consultations, disability sickness and invalidity payments for low back pain has been observed in the Western world since the 1950s despite advances in imaging procedures and surgical techniques. The focus of research has gradually shifted from the intervertebral disk to more integrative models including neural mechanisms, fear-avoidance beliefs and 'yellow flags'.

About 90% of patients will have recovered within a week after their first episode of low back pain. The patient should be encouraged to continue with ordinary activities and limit bed rest. In subacute and chronic low back pain, low-impact aerobics is the most cost-effective physiotherapy method. This suggests that physical activity to improve fitness and reduce fear-avoidance beliefs may become a key factor for reversal of the exponential growth in disability caused by low back pain.

Sport is the second most common cause of spinal cord injury. Knowledge about primary diagnostics, treatment and proper stabilization before transportation, can reduce the number of patients with life-long quadriplegia after spinal sports injury. In risk sports like ice hockey, the rules should be reinforced, in particular the penalty for checking from behind.

An understanding of differential diagnosis, careful history and physical examination is obligatory to pinpoint the neck or back problem. Pain localization and disability should be clarified precisely. An acute disk herniation commonly presents as unilateral leg pain. Isolated back pain is usually not discogenic in young individuals. Pain in young athletes that is worsened by trunk hyperextension suggests spondylolisthesis.

For evaluation of chronic low back pain it is impor-
tant to reassess the patient with an open mind. Severe pain and disability are commonly associated with fear, and athletes, like other patients, may demonstrate helplessness and fear-avoidance.

Imaging procedures for neck and back pain are only supplementary and cannot replace the clinical examination. Sensitive procedures like MRI may describe abnormalities that are not specific because of their high prevalence in the asymptomatic population.

Case story 6.5.1

The patient is a 32-year-old semiprofessional soccer goalkeeper. He has previously been treated for a complicated fracture of the distal phalanx of the right thumb and minor finger injuries, had resected an exostosis of the lateral region of the right distal femur and glenoid labral lesions in both shoulders, and has had surgical treatment of both Achilles tendons because of tendinopathy.

He has played 120 compulsory matches in a row without missing one single match because of injury.

During his 14-year-long soccer career he has been manipulated 1–2 times yearly because of slight to moderate low back pain, but never missed a soccer game until January 1999. He was periodically moderately impaired by pain, but his impairment did not make him disabled and did not interfere with his participation in soccer games at an outstanding level. In 1997 he had a CT scan which showed a central protrusion at the L5–S1 level not affecting the S1 nerve roots. Considering the activity patterns of a goalkeeper struggling for the ball in various positions, he had an excellent performance level and the protrusion appearing on the CT scan was most likely an incidental, asymptomatic finding. He had no back pain during the summer and spring season in 1998, periodically low back pain during the autumn season, but played all the matches for his team.

In a soccer exercise session in the beginning of 1999 he slipped and experienced severe low back pain radiating below the knee. He was recommended bed rest for 3 days. At the clinical examination after 3 days he had a protective muscle spasm, scoliosis and marked reduced flexibility of his back, but negative radicular signs. Magnetic resonance imaging (MRI) revealed both degenerative findings and a lateral herniation (Fig. 6.5.30). Recent scientific opinion states that the process leading to herniations may be somewhat different from that leading to degenerative findings [50]. As previously, a central protrusion was observed at the L5–S1 level, and in addition a left-positioned disk herniation was revealed at the L4–L5 level. Schmorl's nodels in the endplates of the upper lumbar vertebral bodies suggesting injuries during the growth period were also visualized. The abnormalities of the vertebral bodies on the MRI scan could be an outcome of torsional forces reflecting the biomechanics of the soccer keeper, including bending, twisting and jumping, combined with collisions against other players. In particular the endplate irregularities may reflect this type of activity during adolescence [51].

The patient had cortisone tablets for two 5-day periods, and some physiotherapy including massage and traction. He gradually increased his

Case story 6.5.1 (continued)

activity level and managed to perform ordinary activities. Clinically he developed moderate signs of radiculopathy with paresis of dorsiflexion of the foot and a positive Lasegues sign. Three different consultant surgeons did not recommend surgery.

During the spring he increased his activity level to regularly exercising 4–6 times a week, and the radiating pain and weakness of the calf muscles in the left leg gradually disappeared. He was not able to return to soccer and missed matches in the European Cup. By the beginning of June he had returned to office work. He continued to exercise regularly, and in November he tried to perform specific goalkeeper sessions including jumping, twisting and fighting for the

ball. He was not able to finish the training sessions because of increasing pain.

He eventually retired from soccer, but returned to full-time work. At the clinical examination 2 years after the injury the flexibility of his lower back was still markedly reduced for lateral bending and forward flexion and backward bending. The lumbar lordosis was straightened and he had a minor left scoliosis and protective muscle spasm. The fingertip to floor distance was about 40 cm. He had no muscle atrophy. The neurologic examination revealed normal findings except for dorsiflexion of the left ankle. Lasegues test and Waddel signs were negative.

He is permanently disabled as a soccer goalkeeper, but not for regular work.

Multiple choice questions

1 *Scheuermann's disease is:*

a a congenital structural deformity

b an aseptic necrosis of the (thoracic) vertebral bodies caused by ischemia of the growth zone during the growth spurt

c associated with progressive ossification of the joints of the spine

d a defect in the vertebral isthmus or pars interarticularis

e encroachment of the spinal canal, usually by hypertrophic bone.

2 *A spinal cord injury:*

a is always associated with a vertebral fracture

b can be excluded if no signs of neurologic injury have been detected at the primary examination

c occurs less frequently where helmets have been obligatory in ice hockey

d is commonly not detected in the multitrauma patient, and is often caused by inproper stabilization of the neck in the injured athlete during transportation to hospital

e is usually complete in younger patients.

3 *Cervical radiculopathy:*

a is characterized by neck pain and a disk herniation on MRI

b is associated with balance and walking difficulties, and bowel and bladder complaints

c describes pain in the neck and radicular distribution of symptoms in one or both upper extremities, concomitant sensory changes, weakness, atrophy and unilateral diminished tendon reflexes or MRI correlating with radicular symptoms

d usually demands surgical treatment

e requires complete rest from physical activity for 12 weeks.

4 *Spondylolysis/spondylolisthesis:*

a is a stress fracture of the vertebral isthmus or pars interarticularis that is always treated by corset or surgery

b appears rarely in radiologic examinations in asymptomatic individuals

c is a congenital deformity predominately located at the L_5 level

d describes a bony defect associated with pain and segmental instability that is not altered by proprioceptive exercises to improve the stabilizing function of the truncus muscles in sports and daily activity

e is associated with hyperextension/torsion injury in athletes and is most frequently observed in javelin throwers.

5 *Patients with unspecific low back pain:*

a should be recommended bed rest until an MRI examination has been conducted

b should be informed that exercises and activities such as aerobics will increase the risk for reinjury

c can effectively be treated with instrumental fusion surgery

d should have an MRI examination in order to get a correct, specific diagnosis

e should be treated with empathy but not overcautiousness which may reinforce fear and functional complaints. Information about the nature of the problem, emphasizing reduction of fear, will give the patient confidence to resume light activity and gradually return to former sports activity.

References

1 Bogduk N, Macintosch JE, Pearcy MJ. A universal model of the lumbar back muscles in the upright position. *Spine* 1992; **17**: 897–900.

2 Sihvonen T, Partanen J, Hänninen O, Soimakallio S. Electric behavior of low back muscles during lumbar pelvic rhythm in low back pain patients and healthy controls. *Arch Phys Med Rehab* 1991; **72**: 1080–7.

3 Tarazi Dvorak MFC, Wing PC. Spinal injuries in skiers and snowboarders. *Am J Sports Med* 1999; **27**: 177–9.

4 Cantu RC. Catastrophic injuries of high school and collegiate athletes. *Surg Rounds Orthop* 1988; **2**: 62–6.

5 Reynen PD, Clancy WG. Cervical spine injury, hockey helmets, and face masks. *Am J Sports Med* 1994; **22**: 167–70.

6 Mölsä J, Kujala U, Näsman O, Lehtipuu T-P, Airaksinen O. Injury profile in ice hockey from the 1970s through the 1990s in Finland. *Am J Sports Med* 2000; **28**: 322–7.

7 Aebi M, Thalgott JS, Webb JK. *AO ASIF Principles in Spine Surgery*. Berlin, Heidelberg: Springer, 1998.

8 Denis F. The three column spine and its significance in the classification of acute thoracolumbar spinal injuries. *Spine* 1983; **8**: 817–31.

9 Bracken MB. Pharmacological interventions for acute spinal injury. *Cochrane Database Syst Rev* 2[CD001046], 2000.

10 Seybold EA, Sweeny CA, Fredrickson BE, Warhold LG, Bernini PM. Functional outcome of low lumbar burst fractures. *Spine* 1999; **24**: 2154–61.

11 Kraemer WJ, Schemitsch EH, Lever J. Functional outcome of thoracolumbar burst fractures without neurologic deficit. *J Orth Trauma* 1996; **10**: 541–4.

12 Radhakrishan K, Litchy WJ, O'Fallon M, Kurland LT. Epidemiology of cervical radiculopathy. *Brain* 1994; **117**: 325–35.

13 Lüthje P *et al.* Epidemiology and traumatology of injuries in elite soccer: a prospective study in Finland. *Scand J Med Sci Sports* 1996; **6**: 180–5.

14 Tysvær AT, Sortland O, Storli O-V, Løchen EA. Hode- og nakkeskader blant norske fotballspillere. *Tidsskrift for Den Norske Laegeforening* 1988; **108**: 2471–3.

15 Cassidy JD, Carroll LJ, Cote P, Lemstra M, Berglund A, Nygren A. Effect of eliminating compensation for pain and suffering or outcome of insurance claims for whiplash injury. *N Engl J Med* 2000; **342**: 1179–86.

16 Linton S. A review of psychological risk factors in back and neck pain. *Spine* 2000; **25**: 1148–56.

17 Viikari-Juntura E. Interexaminer reliability of observations in physical examinations of the neck. *Phys Ther* 1987; **67**: 1526–32.

18 Aker PD. GAGCPP: conservative management of mechanical neck pain: systematic overview and meta-analysis. *Br Med J* 1996; **313**: 1291–6.

19 Persson LCG, Carlsson CA, Carlsson JY. Long-lasting cervical radicular pain managed with surgery, physiotherapy or a cervical collar. *Spine* 1997; **22**: 751–8.

20 Powell FC, Hanigan WC, Olivero WC. A risk/benefit analysis of spinal manipulation therapy for relief of lumbar and cervical pain. *Neurosurgery* 1993; **33**: 73–9.

21 Lingren K-A. Conservative treatment of thoracic outlet syndrome: a 2-year follow-up. *Arch Phys Med Rehab* 1997; **78**: 373–8.

22 Meyer SA, Sculte KR, Callghan JJ, Albright JP, Powell JW, Crowley ET, El-Khoury GY. Cervical spinal stenosis and stingers in collegiate football players. *Am J Sports Med* 1994; **22**: 158–66.

23 Harreby M, Hesselsø G, Kjær J, Neergaard K. Low back pain and physical exercise in leisure time in 38-year-old men and women: a 25-year prospective cohort study of 640 school children. *Eur Spine J* 1997; **6**: 181–6.

24 Videman T, Sarna S, Battie M, Koskinen SK, Gill K, Paananen H, Gibbons L. The long-term effects of physical loading and exercise lifestyles on back-related symptoms, disability, and spinal pathology among men. *Spine* 1995; **20**: 699–709.

25 Swärd L, Hellström M, Jacobsson B, Peterson L. Back pain and radiologic changes in the thoraco-lumbar spine in athletes. *Spine* 1990; **15**: 124–9.

26 Eriksson K, Nemeth G, Eriksson E. Low back pain in elite cross-country skiers. *Scand J Med Sci Sports* 1996; **6**: 31–5.

27 Soler T, Calderon C. The prevalence of spondylolysis in the Spanish elite athlete. *Spine* 2000; **28**: 57–62.

28 Kujala UM, Taimela S, Erkintalo M, Salminen JJ, Kaprio J. Low-back pain in adolescent athletes. *Med Sci Sports Exerc* 1996; **28**: 165–70.

29 Waddel G, Main CJ, Morris RW *et al.* Normality and reliability in the clinical assessment of backache. *Br Med J* 1982; **284**: 1519–23.

30 Buirski G, Silberstein M. The symptomatic lumbar disc in patients with low back pain. *Spine* 1993; **13**: 1808–11.

31 vanTulder M, Assendelft WJ, Koes BW, Bouter LM. Spinal radiographic findings and nonspecific low back pain. *Spine* 1997; **22**: 427–34.

32 Takahashi K, Shima I, Porter RW. Nerve root pressure in lumbar disc herniation. *Spine* 1999; **24**: 2003–6.

33 Rydevik B, Brown MD, Lundborg G. Pathoanatomy and

pathophysiology of nerve root compression. *Spine* 1984; **9**: 7–15.

34 Satoh K, Konno S, Nishiyama K, Olmarker K, Kikuchi S. Presence and distribution of antigen–antibody complexes in the herniated nucleus pulposus. *Spine* 1999; **24**: 1980–4.

35 Carragee EJ, Han MY, Yang B, Kim DH, Kraemer H, Billys J. Activity restrictions after posterior lumbar discectomy. *Spine* 1999; **24**: 2346–51.

36 O'Sullivan PB, Twomey LT, Allison GT. Evaluation of specific stabilizing exercise in the treatment of chronic low back pain with radiologic diagnosis of spondylosis or spondylolisthesis. *Spine* 1997; **22**: 2959–67.

37 Indahl A. *Low back pain – a functional disturbance.* Thesis. University of Oslo, Norway, 1999 .

38 Roy SH, DeLuca CJ, Snyder-Mackler L, Emley MS, Crenshaw RL, Lyons JP. Fatigue, recovery, and low back pain in varsity rowers. *Med Sci Sports Exerc* 1990; **22**: 463–9.

39 Brox JI, Storheim K, Juel NG, Hagen KB. Har treningsterapi og manipulasjon effekt ved korsryggsmerter? *Tidsskrift for Den Norske Laegeforening* 1999; **14**: 2042–50.

40 Coste J, Delecoeuillerie G, Cohen DL, Le PJ, Paolaggi JB. Clinical course and prognostic factors in acute low back pain: an inception cohort study in primary care practice. *Br Med J* 1994; **308**: 577–80.

41 Mannion AF, Müntener M, Taimela S, Dvorak J. A randomised clinical trial of three active therapies for chronic low back pain. *Spine* 1999; **24**: 2435–48.

42 Turner JA, Deyo RA, Loeser JD, Von Korff M, Fordyce WE. The importance of placebo effects in pain treatment and research. *J Am Med Assoc* 1994; **271**: 1609–14.

43 Spangford EV. The lumbar disc herniation: a computer-aided analysis of 2504 operations. *Acta Orthop Scand* 1972; **342** (Suppl): 1–95.

44 McQuay H, Moore A. *An Evidence-Based Source for Pain Relief.* Oxford: Oxford University Press, 1999.

45 Moore N, van Ganse E, Le Parc J-M *et al.* The PAIN study: paracetamol, aspirin and ibuprofen new tolerability study. *Clin Drug Invest* 1999; **18**: 89–98.

46 Vicenzino B, Collins D, Wright A. The initial effects of a cervical spine manipulative physiotherapy treatment on pain and dysfunction of lateral epicondyalgia. *Pain* 1996; **68**: 69–74.

47 Fordyce WE, Fowler R, Lehman J, DeLateur B, Sand PL, Trieshmann RB. Operant conditioning in the treatment of chronic clinical pain. *Arch Phys Med Rehab* 1973; **54**: 399–408.

48 Lindstrom I, Öhlund C, Eek C, Wallin L, Peterson L-E, Nachemson A. Mobility, strength, and fitness after a graded activity program for patients with subacute low back pain. *Spine* 1992; **17**: 641–9.

49 Richardson CA, Jull GA, Hodges PW, Hides JA. *Therapeutic Exercise for Spinal Segmental Stabilization in Low Back Pain.* Edinburgh: Churchill Livingstone, 1999.

50 Videman T, Battie M, Gill K, Manninen H, Gibbons L, Fischer LD. Magnetic resonance imaging findings and their relationship in the thoracic and lumbar spine. *Spine* 1995; **20**: 928–35.

51 Hamanishi C, Kawabata T, Yosii T, Tanaka S. Schmorl's nodes on magnetic resonance imaging: their incidence and clinical relevance. *Spine* 1994; **19**: 450–4.

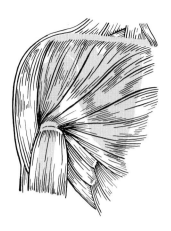

Chapter 6.6
Shoulder

MICHAEL R. KROGSGAARD, RICHARD E. DEBSKI,
ROLF NORLIN & LENA RYDQVIST

Classical reference

Bankart AS. Recurrent or habitual dislocation of the
    shoulder joint. *Br Med J* 1923; **2**: 1132–1133.
    (Reprinted in *Clin Orth Rel Res* 1993; **291**: 3–6.)
Bankart AS. The pathology and treatment of
    recurrent dislocation of the shoulder joint. *Br J
    Surg* 1938; **26**: 23–29.

Sir A.S. Blundell Bankart was the first to recognize the
pathology of the shoulder after traumatic, anterior
dislocations. In his first article from 1923 he described
four cases he had operated on. They all had a typical lesion, which now bears his name. He wrote: 'The head
of the humerus is forced out of the joint, not by lever-
age, but by a direct drive from behind forewards. In
its passage forward the head shears off the fibrous
capsule of the joint from its attachment to the fibrocartilaginous glenoid ligament. The detachment occurs over practically the whole of the anterior half of
the glenoid rim. The reason why the dislocation recurs
after reduction is that, whereas a rent in the fibrous
capsule heals rapidly and soundly, there is no tendency
whatever for the detached capsule to unite spontaneously with the fibro-cartilage'.

Bankart was also aware that recurrent dislocation is
closely connected to forceful motion and activity,
and he stated that it 'may almost be said to be peculiar
to athletes and epileptics—a rather curious association, which, as I shall show, is not without etiological
significance'.

He presented his classic open operation to repair
this condition (Fig. 6.6.1). His operation differed basically from standard operations of the time in two ways.
First, by osteotomizing the coracoid process and de-

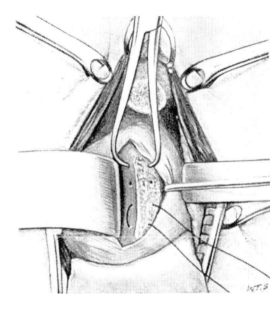

Fig. 6.6.1 A thin shaving of bone has been raised from the
anterior margin of the glenoid cavity and the neck of the
scapula. Three holes have been made in the glenoid margin, and
a pair of vulsellum forceps is seen in the act of making a fourth
hole. A suture has been passed through the two holes in the
lower half of the glenoid margin, and the two ends of this suture
are seen emerging from the raw surface on the front of the neck
of the scapula. Original drawing from Bankart AS [16].

taching it, and dividing the subscapularis tendon he gained very good access to the anterior portion of the glenoid, which enabled him to recognize the typical lesion. Second, he reattached the stripped-off capsule and ligaments to the glenoid with sutures (Fig. 6.6.1).

His first article from 1923 reported 4 patients and his second 27. All recovered full range of motion after the operation, and there were no re-dislocations.

Bankart's operation is still widely used, and it has even been adapted as an arthroscopic procedure.

Introduction: shoulder problems in sports

Shoulder problems are common in sports, and are the result of either relative overuse or trauma. The spectrum of problems is broad, because the shoulder more than any other joint is dependent on the soft tissues and a very precise neuromuscular coordination during movement.

The risk of developing shoulder problems among athletes is closely connected to the sport, the activity level and the age of the athlete. Even though shoulder problems are common in overhead activities, they are rare in other sports, and the overall risk of shoulder problems in athletes is 3–8% [1,2]. Up to 60% of athletes performing overhead throwing sports or swimming have experienced significant shoulder problems which have influenced their sporting activity [3]. Overhead activities are performed repetitively and with great force, mainly by younger athletes, and put enormous demands on shoulder stability and muscle coordination. These athletes are therefore at high risk of overusing tendons and muscles, of stretching or deteriorating soft tissues and bone and of being involved in traumatic episodes.

It is well documented that the frequency of shoulder problems—in particular shoulder pain—increases with increasing activity level [3–5], competitive athletes having most problems.

Pain, muscle fatigue, stiffness and reduced range of motion because of degenerative disease of bone, joint cartilage, tendons and ligaments are results of either age-related changes in the tissues, repeated episodes of minor trauma, or long-term overuse. They are rare among young athletes and mainly seen in older athletes who have performed forceful or repetitive motions for longer periods.

The understanding of normal function and pathologic conditions in the shoulder has increased dramatically during the past 30 years. In the 1990s, arthroscopy revealed pathologies such as the superior labrum anterior to posterior (SLAP) lesion [6], and arthroscopy and MRI have refined the diagnostic process to much greater detail. Intensive studies of the coordination of muscle activity during shoulder movements have shed some light on muscular imbalance and the symptoms this elicits in the athlete. Several conditions are recognized in clinical experience but not fully explained scientifically yet, such as secondary impingement and scapular instability. Many treatments still lack solid documentation.

So, just as this chapter would have been very different (and much shorter) if written 25 years ago, it will probably end up very different if revised 10 years from now. That is what makes the shoulder complicated, but also extremely interesting.

Anatomy, dynamic function and neuromuscular coordination

Anatomy
A large range of mobility is essential at the shoulder to enable the prehensile hand to be placed in all of the positions required for everyday life. As a consequence, the shoulder has less bony stability than other diarthrodial joints. The shoulder complex has evolved such that mechanisms exist to guide and limit joint motion. Normal function of the shoulder requires the coordinated function of four joints and over 30 muscles as well as the contributions of the joint capsules, ligaments and tendons comprising the shoulder complex [7].

Glenoid and humeral version
The geometric relationship between the humeral head and glenoid articular surface allows for the large range of motion at the normal glenohumeral joint. Radiographic, computed tomographic [8,9] and anthropometric studies have been used to characterize this relationship but its relative importance to glenohumeral stability still remains controversial. With the arm at the side, the scapula faces 30° anteriorly on the chest wall and is tilted 3° upward relative to the transverse plane and 20° forward relative to the sagittal

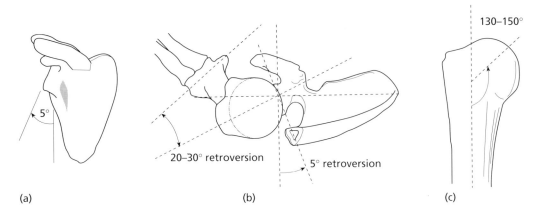

(a)   (b)   (c)

Fig. 6.6.2 Glenoid and humeral version. (a) 5° superior tilt of the glenoid; (b) 20–30° retroversion of the humeral head relative to the axis between the humeral condyles. Version of the glenoid is widely variable between 7° retroversion and 10° anteversion. (c) 130–150° angle between humeral neck and shaft.

plane [7]. In general the glenoid has a superior tilt of 5° [10] and a range of version in the transverse plane from 7° retroversion to 10° anteversion [10]; however, a wide range of variability exists. The humeral head articular surface is inclined dorsally and retroverted relative to the humeral shaft [7]. The angle between the neck and shaft ranges from 130 to 140° [10] while the humeral head is retroverted approximately 30° relative to the axis determined by the humeral condyles [11] (Fig. 6.6.2).

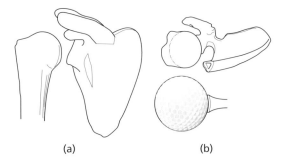

(a)   (b)

Fig. 6.6.3 Geometric relationships of the humeral head and glenoid which provide joint stability. (a) Anterior view of a right glenohumeral joint. (b) Superior view of a left glenohumeral joint showing the comparison between the humeral head–glenoid and a golf ball sitting on a tee.

Articular conformity

The surface area mismatch between the humeral head and glenoid, expressed as a ratio of the maximum glenoid diameter to the maximum humeral head diameter (glenohumeral index), has been determined by Saha and others [10,12] and found to be 0.75 and 0.76 in the sagittal and transverse planes, respectively. The traditional comparison to this mismatch has been a golf ball sitting on a tee (Fig. 6.6.3), but it has been shown that the articular surfaces of the glenoid and humeral head are almost perfectly congruent, within 3 mm, when the cartilage layer is included in the analysis [13].

Labrum

The glenoid labrum has been studied extensively [14,15] and its contribution to stability of the glenohumeral joint can be described in terms of three mech-

anisms. First, it acts as a fibrocartilaginous ring around the glenoid to which the capsuloligamentous structures are secured [14,16,17]. The labrum also deepens the concavity of the glenoid socket approximately 9 mm in the superior–inferior plane and 5 mm in the anterior–posterior plane [18–20]. Finally, the labrum increases the surface area of contact for the humeral head, thereby enhancing joint stability [18–20].

Capsuloligamentous structures

The glenohumeral joint capsule is composed of a variably thick layer of tissue with discrete thickenings that constitute the glenohumeral ligaments [15,21].

Cadaver dissections [15,22] and observations during surgery [23–25] have been the tools used to elucidate the anatomy of these structures. DePalma and coworkers [15] described the marked variability of the capsuloligamentous components and noted six types of anatomic arrangements which they believed could be correlated with the risk for joint instability. More recently, arthroscopy has confirmed the high variability in size and appearance of the glenohumeral ligaments [26].

Superior glenohumeral, coracohumeral, middle glenohumeral and inferior glenohumeral ligaments and the posterior capsule (Fig. 6.6.4)

The superior glenohumeral (SGHL) and coracohumeral (CHL) ligaments are usually described together because their anatomic courses are parallel. These ligaments form the region of the glenohumeral capsule referred to as the 'rotator interval' which constitutes the triangular space between the anterior

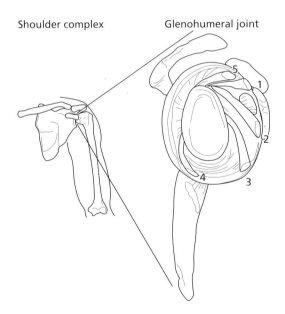

Fig. 6.6.4 Capsuloligamentous anatomy viewed from the side with the anterior aspect to the right and the posterior aspect to the left. The humeral head has been removed, leaving the glenoid. 1: SGHL, superior glenohumeral ligament; 2: MGHL, middle glenohumeral ligament; 3: AB-IGHL, anterior band of the inferior glenohumeral ligament; 4: PB-IGHL, posterior band of the inferior glenohumeral ligament; 5: LBT, long head of the biceps tendon.

border of the supraspinatus tendon and the superior border of the subscapularis tendon [21,24,27–29]. The SGHL originates from the superior glenoid rim, just inferior to the long head of the biceps tendon, and inserts into the lesser tuberosity of the humerus just medial to the bicipital groove. Although quite variable in size, it is the most consistently present of the glenohumeral ligaments and found in more than 90% of individuals [15,21,26,30].

The CHL courses from the lateral surface of the coracoid process to the lesser and greater tuberosities of the humerus. Patel and associates [31] described the CHL as consisting of two bands, anterior and posterior, with the anterior band inserting on the lesser tuberosity and the posterior band inserting on the greater tuberosity. Gross and histologic work by Cooper and associates [30] demonstrated that the CHL is usually a thin capsular fold which does not demonstrate the typical ligamentous form. Boardman and coworkers [27] established that the CHL's cross-sectional area at the midsubstance was approximately four times greater than that of the SGHL.

The middle glenohumeral ligament (MGHL) is the most variable of the glenohumeral ligaments, being found in only 70–90% of individuals and poorly defined in 10% of the joints where it was found [15,26,32]. It originates from the superior glenoid just below the SGHL, slightly medial to the glenoid labrum, and above the anterior band (AB) of the inferior glenohumeral ligament (IGHL) complex. The MGHL usually manifests itself in two morphologic variations: (i) sheet-like and confluent with the AB-IGHL; or (ii) cord-like, with a foraminal separation between it and the AB-IGHL.

The IGHL was originally described by Depalma and coworkers [15] as a triangular-shaped structure running from the labrum to the neck of the humerus between the subscapularis and triceps. This anatomic description was then modified by Turkel and associates [33] who found a thickening in its anterior edge termed the superior band. Others have confirmed that this structure appears consistently from specimen to specimen [22]. O'Brien and coworkers [21], using arthroscopy and gross and histologic dissection, redefined this component as the IGHL complex which has three distinct components. Discrete anterior (AB-IGHL) and posterior (PB-IGHL) bands bounded a thin axillary pouch. Bigliani and associates [34] also found the superior or AB-IGHL to be consistently present and to represent the thickest portion of the complex (~2.8mm); however, they did not find any posterior ligamentous bands.

The region of the capsule located posteriorly and superiorly to the PB-IGHL [21,35] is called the posterior capsule (PC). There is little anatomic information available on this region, although many people have described it as the thinnest portion of the joint capsule [35,36].

Ligament dynamization

The glenohumeral ligaments and capsule are relatively lax in the midranges of joint rotation and seem to function only at the end ranges to limit excessive translations and prevent further rotation of the humerus with respect to the scapula [18,26,33,37]. Studies have demonstrated that the rotator cuff tendons attach directly to the various capsuloligamentous components [38]. Therefore, it is possible that the glenohumeral capsule and ligaments may be loaded during contraction of the rotator cuff muscles.

Dynamic function

Rotator cuff muscles (Fig. 6.6.5)

Four muscles comprise the rotator cuff: the supraspinatus, subscapularis, infraspinatus and teres minor. The supraspinatus has its origin on the posterior/superior scapula, superior to the scapular spine. It passes under the acromion, through the supraspinatus fossa, and inserts on the greater tuberosity. The supraspinatus is active during the entire range of scapular plane abduction, and a suprascapular nerve block results in a loss of abduction torque of approximately 50% [39,40]. The supraspinatus muscle can abduct the joint without the action of the deltoid.

The infraspinatus and teres minor muscles originate on the posterior scapula, inferior to the scapular spine, and insert on the posterior aspect of the greater tuberosity. Their tendinous insertions are not separate from each other or from the insertion of the supraspinatus tendon. These muscles function together to externally rotate and extend the humerus [41].

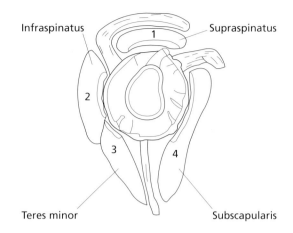

Fig. 6.6.5 Rotator cuff muscles viewed from the side with the anterior aspect to the right. The humeral head has been removed.

The subscapularis muscle arises from the anterior scapula and is the only muscle to insert on the lesser tuberosity. It is the sole component of the anterior rotator cuff and functions to internally rotate and flex the humerus [7,42]. The tendinous insertion of the subscapularis tendon is continuous with the anterior capsule; therefore it is considered to be responsible for anterior stability [33].

The deltoid is the largest of the glenohumeral muscles and covers the proximal humerus on a path from its tripennate origin at the clavicle, acromion and scapular spine to its insertion midway down the humerus at the deltoid tubercle. Each of the three sections of the deltoid has a different function. The anterior portion is primarily a forward flexor of the glenohumeral joint, the middle portion is an abductor, and the posterior portion extends the joint [43]. The deltoid is active throughout the entire arc of glenohumeral abduction and an axillary nerve block results in a loss of abduction torque of 50% [39].

Long head of the biceps tendon

The long head of the biceps has its origin just superior to the articular margin of the glenoid and has been labeled a depressor of the humeral head, especially with external rotation of the humerus [44]. In this position the tendon lies directly over the top of the humeral head. After exiting the joint through a capsule defect, the biceps tendon enters the bicipital groove where it is retained by the transverse humeral ligament.

Scapulothoracic motion

Overhead activities require an optimal balance between mobility and stability of the shoulder, and normal scapulothoracic muscle function is required for coordinated arm elevation. The serratus anterior and the trapezius are the most important muscles for scapular stabilization during arm elevation [7,12], and are more prone to fatigue during repetitive overhead activities such as swimming and throwing [45]. The motion that occurs between the scapulothoracic and the glenohumeral joint during abduction is the most extensively studied shoulder motion and has been termed the 'scapulothoracic rhythm' [7,46]. For the first 30° of abduction glenohumeral motion is much greater than scapulothoracic motion. This ratio has been reported to range between 4:1 and 7:1. Afterwards, both joints move approximately the same amount.

Neuromuscular coordination

The normal shoulder is dependent on the muscles and capsuloligamentous structures that comprise this complex. Since it is usually lax and functions at the extremes of motion, the glenohumeral capsule may provide feedback information regarding joint position sense and provide reflex muscle stabilization around the joint. Studies have suggested that sensory afferent feedback systems exist that transmit information from receptors in the skin, joint and muscles to the brain and spinal pathways to produce motion that is appropriate for a given situation [47].

Proprioception has been defined as a specialized variation of the sensory modality of touch that includes the sensation of joint motion (kinesthesia) and joint position (sense). Relatively little information has been published on proprioception at the glenohumeral joint, with a vast majority of the concepts extrapolated from basic science and clinical studies performed at the knee. Some authors believe that a neurologic feedback mechanism exists that coordinates the actions of the shoulder muscles and protects the glenohumeral capsule from excessive strain [47]. In animals a ligamento-

muscular reflex has been demonstrated [48], and in humans an inhibition of the shoulder muscles is elicited when the anterior capsule is electrically stimulated [49]. Therefore, the risk for joint injury is increased whenever a proprioceptive deficit exists and disrupts this feedback mechanism.

Shoulder proprioception is mediated by peripheral receptors in articular, muscular and cutaneous structures [47]. The glenoid labrum and the glenohumeral ligaments have been found to contain nociceptive free nerve endings and mechanoreceptors such as Ruffini endings, Pacinian corpuscles and Golgi tendon endings. Muscle and joint receptors are probably complementary to each other as they play a role in shoulder stability. The ligaments, capsule and synovial membrane of the shoulder are innervated by the axillary, suprascapular and musculocutaneous nerves as they cross the joint [50].

Clinically proprioception is measured by determining the threshold for detection of passive motion (kinesthesia) and joint position sense. At slow angular velocities (0.5–2°/s) the threshold to detection of passive motion, as well as the reproduction of passive positioning, is thought to selectively stimulate Ruffini or Golgi-type mechanoreceptors in the articular structures [51]. Reproduction of active positioning is believed to involve the stimulation of both joint and muscle receptors and provides a more functional assessment of the afferent pathways.

A number of studies have been performed using a proprioception testing device developed at the University of Pittsburgh [47,51]. In college-age individuals without any history of shoulder injury, no differences were found between dominant and nondominant shoulders, with a minimal variation in proprioception. Groups containing subjects with anterior instability as well as those who had received surgical stabilization procedures were also examined. Significant differences were found between the stable and involved shoulders for subjects with instability. However, no differences could be demonstrated between the surgically reconstructed and contralateral shoulders for any given test.

Proprioception and joint kinematics

A number of biomechanical and electromyographic studies suggest that coordination and synergism of the rotator cuff and biceps muscles are required for normal shoulder function. According to Gowan and his associates [52], two groups of muscles control the shoulder during the pitching motion in professional baseball pitchers. The first group of muscles demonstrates increased electromyographic activity during the early and late cocking phase and decreased activity during the acceleration phase. This group of muscles positions the arm for the delivery of the pitch. The second group of muscles demonstrates increased electromyographic activity during the acceleration phase of the pitch. Using the same measurement technique, Glousman and coworkers [45] showed changes in the electromyographic pattern in baseball pitchers with chronic anterior instability of the glenohumeral joint. Alteration of the normal neuromuscular balance in patients with anterior instability can cause changes in joint kinematics that can lead to repetitive microtrauma of the glenohumeral joint.

History and physical examination

History

When a shoulder patient steps into the consulting room for the first time, it is always exciting to wonder whether this is going to be an easy case or one that will cause a headache. Shoulder problems can be just as difficult to diagnose as abdominal problems, and therefore a thorough patient history is mandatory and can save many speculations and investigations.

Start at the beginning: Is this a traumatic or a non-traumatic disorder?

If traumatic, how did it happen? A precise description of the incident should follow, including the direction and magnitude of the external force that was transferred to the arm and the position and motion of the arm. What were the immediate consequences (pain, fatigue, dislocation, none)? Was it possible to continue activity? What did the patient do then — which treatment was given?

If non-traumatic, how did it start: suddenly or gradually? Were there any changes in normal activities, including sport and work, right before the onset of symptoms (change of technique, increase in the amount of training or workload, etc.)?

Next, how has the course of the disease been? Are symptoms increasing, decreasing, constant or inter-

mittent? Has the disease influenced work or athletic activities? What is the complaint? Pain, tenderness, fatigue, loss of motion, instability?

If there is pain: where is it located? Pain from the subacromial space is projected to the lateral upper arm, and pain from the infraspinatus is projected to the posterior upper arm. Bankart lesions cause pain anteriorly in the shoulder. Acromioclavicular pain is located to the joint and is only projected if the joint impinges on the supraspinatus tendon. Pain from the thoracoscapular bursa is located posteriorly around the upper half of scapula.

As pain from the cervical spine can project to the shoulder girdle and arm, any history of trauma to the cervical spine and pain in the neck itself must be described. In that case the location of pain is often much more diffuse than pain from the shoulder, and in the case of cervical root compression, there will often be neurologic symptoms (numbness, paresthesia, etc.). If such symptoms are present, a detailed description of the nature of the symptoms, any variation and provocative factors, the precise location and information about fatigue of the arm are essential (see pp. 658–62, Chapter 6.5). Some patients with longstanding shoulder problems have diffuse feelings of intermittent numbness in the arm and hand without any pattern specific for a cervical root. These problems are often secondary to muscular tension in the shoulder girdle and will disappear when the primary shoulder problem is solved.

Shoulder dislocation is the ultimate degree of instability, and often it is well documented whether it is anterior or posterior. Subluxations and feelings of instability following traumatic dislocations or multidirectional instability can usually be described by the patient: When does it happen? And how often? On the other hand, anterior instability without a primary dislocation is often unrecognized by the patient but becomes symptomatic because of secondary impingement. Clicks and lockings are indicative of labral lesions.

Physical examination

A basic examination should always be performed. Additional tests can be added depending on the patient history. Both shoulders must be exposed during examination.

Basic examination

The general impression of the shoulder contours gives valuable information: Is this a muscular or a slight individual? Is there atrophy on the affected side of the deltoid (as in axillary nerve palsy), the supraspinatus (as in rotator cuff rupture) or the infraspinatus muscles (as in suprascapular nerve palsy in volleyball players)? Is the humeral head in joint? (An epulet shoulder is characteristic of acute dislocation.) Is the acromioclavicular joint intact or is the clavicle protruding?

Ask the patient to perform active motions: flexion, abduction in the thoracal and scapular planes (the latter 30° anterior to the thoracal plane), outwards rotation with the elbows fixed to the side, inwards rotation in horizontal abduction, hand to neck and hand to the back (optimally reaching as high as the opposite scapula). If any of the motions are reduced compared to the other side (or to normal range of motion), the passive motion is tested by the examiner. With supraspinatus/infraspinatus rupture the active abduction and outward rotation is usually greatly reduced, while passive motion is normal.

In joint stiffness both active and passive motion is reduced. The true motion of the humeroscapular joint can be measured when the scapula is fixed by the examiner's hand on top of the shoulder.

Test strength of the rotator cuff muscles: abduction (in the scapular plane) (Fig. 6.6.6), inwards and outwards rotation (Fig. 6.6.7). A reduced strength can be due to either rotator cuff rupture, muscle fatigue (as in suprascapular nerve palsy with infraspinatus atrophy) or pain (which can eventually be eliminated by injection of local analgetics).

The movements of the scapula are visualized by watching the patient from behind. Asymmetric movements of scapula during the first sequences of abduction, flexion and outwards rotation are indicative of tightness (reduced motion) of the humeroscapular joint or severe dysfunction of the rotator cuff, due to either tendon rupture or very painful conditions. Increased motion of the scapula may indicate muscle pathology in serratus and rhomboid muscles.

Dysfunction of the rotator cuff may not show in scapular movement until a load is applied to the arm in abduction, flexion and rotation (Figs 6.6.6 & 6.6.7), but will of course be demonstrated with the normal

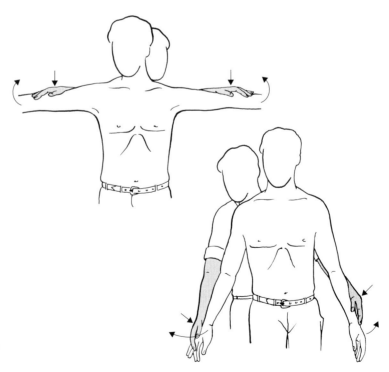

Fig. 6.6.6 Test of abduction power in 30 and 90° of abduction.

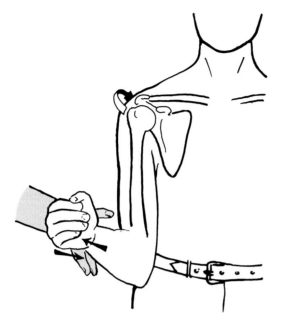

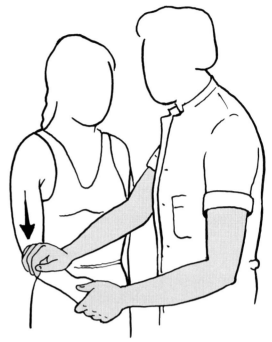

Fig. 6.6.7 Power test for infraspinatus muscle: outwards rotation without abduction.

rotator cuff power tests. Dysfunction of the scapular stabilizers can be demonstrated by asking the patient to perform repeated arm abductions. Fatigue in scapular stabilizers, in particular the anterior serratus and lower trapezius muscles, will show after 10, 20 or more abductions as asymmetric movements or winging of the scapula.

Examination for tenderness is performed in the shoulder muscles, the acromioclavicular joint, the biceptical groove and immediately subacromially.

Bilateral sulcus signs are indicative of multidirectional laxity, and a unilateral sulcus sign for acquired, inferior instability. It is tested for by pulling down on the relaxed arm, and it is positive when a sulcus appears between the acromion and the humeral head (Fig. 6.6.8). The anterior/posterior stability can be graded by holding the humeral head with one hand and moving it anterior–posterior while fixing the glenoid (scapula) with the other hand (drawer test), or using the humerus as a lever for the same maneuver (axial load test, Fig. 6.6.9).

Instability of the acromioclavicular joint can be tested by holding the clavicle down with one hand while applying longitudinal pressure upwards in the

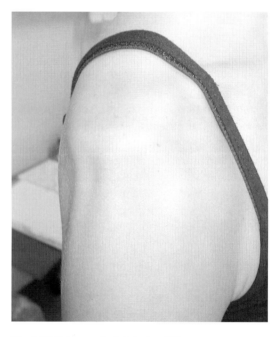

Fig. 6.6.8 Sulcus test for inferior instability.

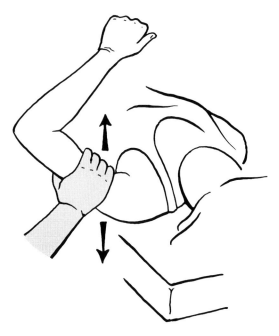

Fig. 6.6.9 Axial load test for anterior–posterior instability.

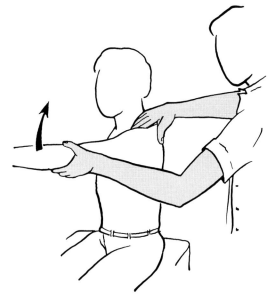

Fig. 6.6.10 Neer's test. The examiner uses one hand to prevent rotation of the scapula and the other to passively raise the patient's arm in a position between flexion and abduction, thereby reducing the space between the anteroinferior acromion and the greater tuberosity and provoking impingement. The test is positive if the patient — usually when the arm is approximately horizontal — experiences the well-known pain [75].

humerus with the other (grabbing around the elbow). If the joint is very loose, moving the arm into the hurra position and back to neutral will often result in painful clicking and locking.

In athletes, it will always be relevant in addition to this basic examination to test for impingement and apprehension, described below.

How good is a shoulder test?

Shoulder tests are tools used to obtain the correct diagnosis and to quantify the results of treatments. Ideally, each test should be specific for one pathologic condition, i.e. precise and specific, and also be sufficiently easy to perform that it leads to the same result when performed by many examiners.

For a number of tests the results have been compared to the diagnoses which were made during arthroscopy. Tests with nearly 100% specificity and sensitivity are reported (the active compression test) [32], but most have a much lower validity [53,54]. Unfortunately the intra- and interobserver variation of many tests—i.e. the degree of agreement regarding the results of a test between several examiners or by repeated testings by the same examiner—seems to

be quite unsatisfactory [55–57]. The tests should therefore be used as an aid in the diagnostic process and not as gold standards for the diagnosis.

Shoulder tests

There are a large number of tests available in shoulder examination, but not all can be described here, and some are overlapping. The following is a selection of those most commonly used.

Tests for primary impingement

Neer's and Hawkins' tests (Figs 6.6.10 & 6.6.11) were designed for primary impingement, for which both have a high sensitivity (nearly 90%) and a reasonably good specificity [53,54], but can also be used for secondary impingement. If any of the tests come out positive, an impingement release test can be performed as follows: while flexing the patient's arm with one hand, the examiner puts a downward pressure on the upper

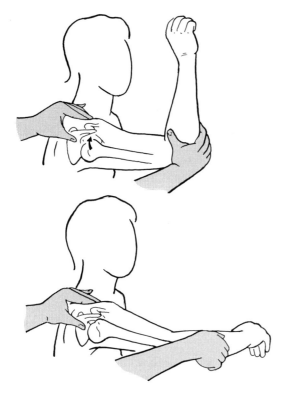

Fig. 6.6.11 Hawkins' test. To provoke subacromial impingement, the arm is passively flexed to horizontal with the elbow in 90° flexion, followed by maximum inwards rotation, reducing the space between the greater tuberosity and the anteroinferior undersurface of the acromion. The test is positive if the well-known pain is provoked [77a].

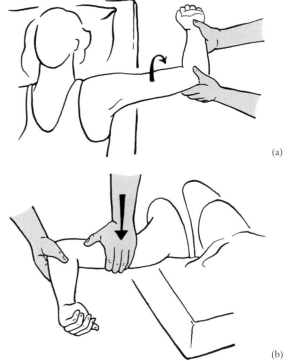

Fig. 6.6.12 (a) Apprehension test for anterior instability of the humeral head is performed with the patient supine and the shoulder just beyond the edge of the examination table. The examiner moves the patient's arm in 90° abduction and lets gravity help to externally rotate the arm as much as possible (often with the patient's hand under the level of the examination table). The test is positive if the patient feels pain or great discomfort (fear of dislocation) in this position. The examiner can eventually augment the test by pushing the humeral head anteriorly from behind [206]. The degree of abduction can be varied, if the examiner wishes to stress different parts of the anterior capsule. (b) Relocation test. If the apprehension test is positive, the examiner applies an anterior force with the free hand to the humeral head, reducing the stress on the anterior structures. The test is positive if the patient is relieved from the discomfort of the apprehension test [206].

arm with the other hand, so that the humeral head is moved down. The release test is positive if it reduces the pain elicited by the impingement test. Further confirmation of a subacromial reason for the pain can be produced if a local analgesic is injected subacromially and the test can be repeated without pain.

Tests for instability
Anterior instability is demonstrated with the apprehension test, which is most easily performed with the patient lying on the examination table (Fig. 6.6.12a). If positive, it should be followed by a relocation test (Fig. 6.6.12b). The anterior slide test is a reversed apprehension test, as it starts with relocation (the examiner applies backwards pressure on the humeral head with the arm in the hurra position) and is positive if the

patient feels pain or discomfort when the pressure is suddenly relieved.

Anterior–posterior instability can be demonstrated with a drawer test or the load-and-shift test (Fig. 6.6.9).

Inferior instability is demonstrated with the sulcus test (Fig. 6.6.8). Many individuals have bilateral sulcus signs without any symptoms from the shoulders.

Test for internal impingement

Pain from internal impingement can be elicited with the patient in the upright position by bringing the arm into maximal external rotation and abduction (hurra position), while the examiner's thumb exerts an anterior pressure on the humeral head at the posterior joint line. Pain is felt posteriorly in the shoulder, and there is soreness where the thumb presses on the joint line. The maneuver resembles the apprehension test, but in the latter pain and discomfort is felt anteriorly.

Tests for labral lesions

The anterior slide test is one of many tests for labral lesions. The basic principle is to apply pressure on the labrum while moving the humeral head. The patient positions the hands on the hips with the thumbs pointing backwards. The examiner is behind the patient and places one hand across the top of the shoulder with the index finger resting on the anterior glenohumeral joint line. The other hand is placed under the elbow, and the examiner applies a forward and superior force to the elbow and upper arm. The patient must push back against this force. An anterior–superior slide of the humeral head appears, which is usually resisted by the superior labrum. The test is positive if it results in pain or clicking in the anterior upper part of the shoulder (under the examiner's index finger), or if it reproduces the patient's symptoms [58].

A sensitivity of 78% and a specificity of 92% for detection of superior labral lesions has been reported for the anterior slide test compared to the result of arthroscopy [58].

A very high sensitivity and specificity for labral lesion has been reported for a recent modification of the active compression test which was originally described in 1936 for detection of biceps tendon problems. The test provokes pain or clicking inside the shoulder in the case of labral lesions [32] (Fig. 6.6.13).

Test of the biceps tendon

A quite specific test for biceps tendon problems (tendinitis, partial tears and instability) is the supination test [53] (Fig. 6.6.14).

Tests for rotator cuff tears

In addition to abduction strength tests (Fig. 6.6.6), an indication of a supraspinatus tear is the lag sign, i.e. the

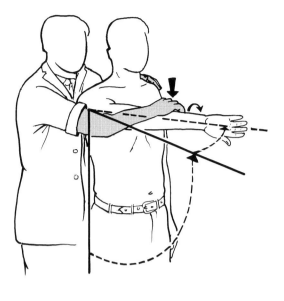

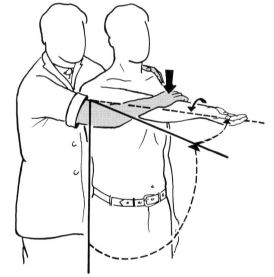

Fig. 6.6.13 Active compression test. This consists of two steps. First the patient flexes the arm to horizontal with the elbow extended, adducts the arm 15° and inwardly rotates it so the thumb points downward. The examiner then applies a downward force to the arm, which the patient must resist. During step 2, the arm is in the same position, but the hand is fully supinated. The examiner again applies a downward force to the arm. The test is positive if pain is elicited during step 1 and reduced or eliminated during step 2. If pain (or painful clicking) is localized inside the shoulder joint, the test indicates labral abnormality. If pain is localized to the acromioclavicular joint or on top of the shoulder, it indicates abnormality of the acromioclavicular joint [32].

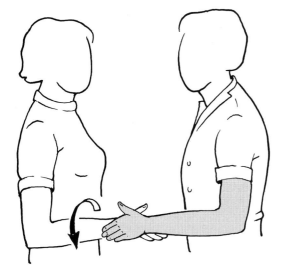

Fig. 6.6.14 Yergason's test. The patient flexes the elbow 90° and pronates the forearm. The examiner holds the patient's wrist to block rotation. The patient then supinates the forearm with maximal power against resistance. The test is positive if the patient feels pain in the bicipital groove.

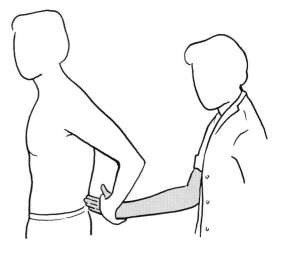

Fig. 6.6.15 Lift-off test. The subscapularis is the only muscle used for this maneuver, which if positive indicates a significant subscapularis tear. The patient internally rotates the arm and rests the dorsum of the hand on the lower back. The patient actively lifts the hand away from the back, eventually against resistance. The test is positive if the hand cannot be lifted from the back, or if power in doing so is reduced [66a].

inability to hold the arm when the examiner has brought it into horizontal abduction [59].

Neer's dropping sign is a very specific and sensitive test for tears of the infraspinatus: with the arm along the body and the elbow flexed 90°, the arm is outwards rotated by the examiner. The patient is unable to hold the arm in outwards rotation when the examiner lets go [60].

A positive lift-off test is indicative of a subscapularis tear (Fig. 6.6.15).

Teres minor is also an external rotator, but mainly when the arm is in 90° abduction. The hornblower's sign is the inability to actively outwards rotate the arm when it is brought into 90° abduction by the examiner, and is very specific and sensitive for teres minor tears (Fig. 6.6.16) [60].

Tests for acromioclavicular disease
Pain can be provoked by compression of the joint, i.e. when the flexed, inwards rotated arm is brought into maximum adduction by the examiner.

The active compression test has been reported to

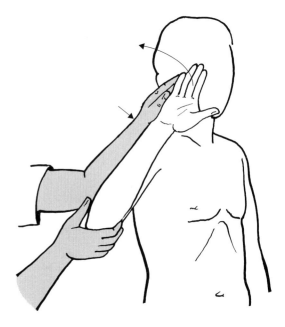

Fig. 6.6.16 Hornblower's sign. The teres minor is the muscle used for this movement. With the arm passively abducted to horizontal, the patient is unable to outwardly rotate the arm [60].

be very specific and sensitive for acromioclavicular joint disease, when the pain provoked by the test is located at the joint on top of the shoulder (Fig. 6.6.13) [32].

Imaging of the shoulder

Shoulder imaging is valuable in the diagnostic process, which in many cases can be refined in detail. The accuracy of MRI and ultrasonography is, however, very dependent on the technical equipment and the examiner. The decision as to which modalities the examiner should use in shoulder diagnostics is therefore often dependent more on the local possibilities than on scientifically based guidelines.

X-ray

A number of projections are available. The physician must select the projections which are most informative in each case.

The two standard projections of the glenohumeral joint are the *anteroposterior* (AP) and *lateral oblique* views. As the scapula with the glenoid is rotated 30° anterior, the joint space is not visible on a true AP view. Therefore, in the standard AP projection the body of the patient is rotated 30° toward the involved side. This projection shows the glenohumeral joint space and the subacromial space. A reduction of the subacromial space is indicative of a large supraspinatus tear. The AP view is usually shot with the arm in slight internal rotation. Additional X-rays with the arm externally rotated highlight the greater tuberosity and can show e.g. cystic changes at the insertion of the supraspinatus tendon and calcifications in the tendon. The lateral view is usually also shot with 30° rotation toward the affected side, and is indispensable for the diagnosis of shoulder dislocations and humeral head fractures. The arch formed by the inferior rim of the scapular neck and the posterior aspect of the humerus is usually unbroken — when it is broken, there is a dislocation of the humeral head, either anteriorly or posteriorly. This may be the only indication of a posterior dislocation, as this is often not visible on the AP view.

The *axillary* view, which is a true inferosuperior X-ray of the glenohumeral joint, is valuable in shoulder instability, where it will show the size of a Hill–Sachs lesion of the humeral head and the amount of bone loss from the anterior rim of the glenoid. This information

is necessary for preoperative planning. In humeral head fractures and in glenoid fractures it gives information about the bone fragments.

The shape of the acromial arch can be revealed with the *supraspinatus outlet* view. The X-ray beam is tangential to the scapular body and is directed 20–30° caudally. It reveals subacromial and acromioclavicular spurring and is used to characterize the shape of the acromion as flat, curved or hooked. A curved or hooked acromion is related to rotator cuff disease, but the outlet view is technically difficult to reproduce, and the information about acromial shape obtained from this projection is not very valid [61].

Anterior spurs of the acromion can be revealed with an AP projection with a 30° *caudal tilt*.

The *acromioclavicular* joint is visualized in an AP view with a 10° cephalic tilt of the X-ray beam. With this projection spurs from the undersurface of the joint as well as degenerative changes of the acromioclavicular joint and the distal clavicle can be visualized. If the patient is standing up, stress can be applied to the joint, either from gravity or a weight, pulling the arm down, revealing dislocation of the acromioclavicular joint.

Computed tomography scan

Computed tomography (CT) is useful for visualizing the bony structures of the shoulder.

Defects of the glenoid in traumatic dislocations of the humeroscapular joint can be measured precisely, which is valuable in preoperative planing; a soft tissue reconstruction of the anterior capsule and ligament attachment to the glenoid is not able to prevent dislocations if a substantial portion of the anterior glenoid is missing. This is also the case if there is a large Hill–Sachs lesion (Fig. 6.6.17). In these situations an Eden–Hybbinette type of operation with a bone block transplanted to the anterior glenoid rim may be preferred.

Coracoid impingement can be demonstrated with CT, either as a protrusion of the coracoid process or as an anterior subluxation of the humeral head [62]. Os acromiale (an unfused epiphysis of the acromion) is demonstrated excellently [63]. Reconstruction in three dimensions can visualize fracture fragments, osteophytes and spurs. The anteversion of the glenoid and the retroversion of the humeral head can be

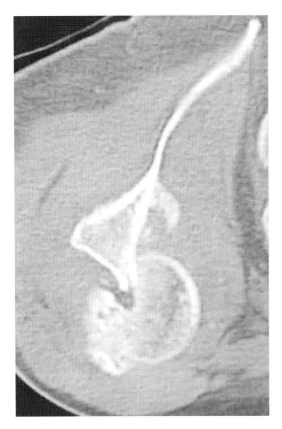

Fig. 6.6.17 CT scan of an anteriorly dislocated shoulder with a huge Hill–Sachs lesion on the posterior aspect of the humerus.

measured precisely with CT, which may be of value in the decision as to treatment of internal impingement in individual cases [64].

Bony spurs in the scapulothoracic space can be demonstrated with CT. In many cases of incongruity between scapula and the thoracic wall, this can only be demonstrated with three-dimensional CT reconstruction [65].

Magnetic resonance imaging

The technical development of magnetic resonance imaging (MRI) is still ongoing, and the introduction of cine MRI has brought about great expectations as to shoulder diagnostics in the future. As there are so many sequences to choose from in MRI, the value of shoulder MRI is very dependent on the available scanner and the expertise employed in operating it and interpreting the pictures.

Subacromial impingement may not be directly visible on MRI, as the arm is usually in few degrees of abduction and slight external rotation during scanning—and this is not the position in which the humeral head impinges on the coracoacromial arch, but the causes of subacromial impingement are detected with great accuracy: osteophytes on the acromion, hypertrophy of the acromioclavicular joint bulging into the supraspinatus muscle, degenerative disease of the acromioclavicular joint, and the type of acromion (flat, curved or hooked) (Fig. 6.6.18). The consequences of impingement are also visible: degenerative or inflammatory changes of the supraspinatus tendon with edema, subacromial bursitis, and fluid around the tendon and in the bursa. With cine MRI the changes in the width of the subacromial space can be measured during motion, and the impingement can be directly visualized [66].

Internal impingement is characteristic on MRI: degenerative changes in the supraspinatus near the insertion on the greater tuberosity, often small cysts in the greater tuberosity, hypertrophy and degeneration of the superior and posterior labrum, and sometimes bone bruise in the greater tuberosity and the superior glenoid [67].

Rotator cuff tears show as disruption and sometimes retraction of the tendon fibers. Full-thickness tears are detected with high accuracy [68]. Partial-thickness tears show as disruptions in the tendon fibers on the bursal or the articular surface of the cuff. Fibrotic or inflammatory changes within the tendon show as abnormal signal inside the tendon with a normal signal on the bursal and articular sides. The accuracy of MRI for partial tears is lower than for full-thickness tears (Fig. 6.6.19).

With MRI it is possible to image the degree of atrophy, fatty degeneration and fibrosis of the rotator cuff muscles, which is useful in the planning of repair of older complete rotator cuff tears. If more than 50% of the matching muscle is fat degenerated or fibrotic, the likelihood of an increase in active motion after repair of the tendon is very small, and the risk for retearing is increased [69].

The labrum and the glenohumeral ligaments are normally clearly visible on MRI, including the biceps tendon anchoring on the superior glenoid. In most persons the superior and middle glenohumeral ligaments

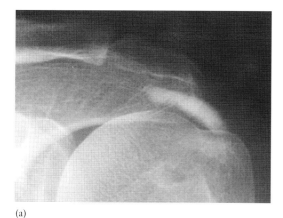

(a)

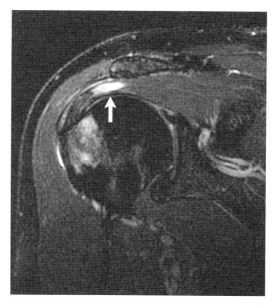

Fig. 6.6.19 MR scan of a complete supraspinatus tear, showing as a light area in the dark tendon (arrow). (From Department of Radiology and MRI, Bispebjerg University Hospital, Copenhagen, Denmark.)

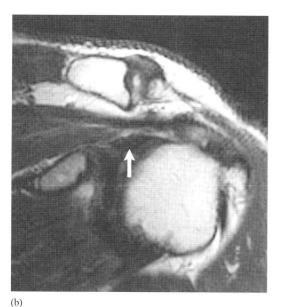

(b)

Fig. 6.6.18 Causes of primary subacromial impingement. (a) X-ray of a huge calcification in the supraspinatus. (b) MRI of a protruding lateral clavicle, impinging the subacromial fat pad and the supraspinatus (arrow). (From Department of Radiology and MRI, Bispebjerg University Hospital, Copenhagen, Denmark.)

are well defined on MRI, whereas the inferior ligament is not regularly seen. Tears of these structures are best seen if there is fluid in the joint, or if contrast is injected intra-articularly. Under optimal conditions SLAP lesions may be detected. With cine MRI the anterior labrum is normally very mobile, whereas the posterior labrum hardly moves during abduction [66].

Biceps tendon inflammation is easily spotted because there is fluid around the tendon. Dislocation of the tendon from the sulcus and disruption is also easily demonstrated, while partial tears are seen with less accuracy.

The suprascapular fossa with the suprascapular nerve and artery is clearly visible, and cysts or ganglia compressing the nerve will be seen (Fig. 6.6.20).

In the bony structures intraosseous changes in the form of bone bruise or compression fractures are easily seen. These may be the result of heavy overload to the bone, e.g. during sports, or trauma. If MRI were used generally in acute shoulder trauma, a lot of changes would show, but for many of these findings, e.g. bone bruise, the clinical implications are unknown.

MRI is not only able to show acute changes in muscles like disruption, hemorrhage and edema, but in conditions with muscular atrophy, it can distinguish between primary muscular changes and atrophy caused by denervation of the muscle [70].

Theoretically, scapulothoracic bursitis should show on MRI, but this has not been reported.

Table 6.6.1 Characteristics of the three types of impingement.

	Primary subacromial impingement	Secondary impingement	Internal impingement
Pain	Subacromial and lateral upper arm	Subacromial and lateral upper arm	Posterior and posterolateral upper arm
Impingement tests	+	(+)	−
Apprehension/relocation test	−	+	(+)
Hurra test	−	−	+
X-ray findings	+	−	+
Ultrasound/MRI findings	+	−	+
Subacromial corticosteroid effective	+	(+)	−

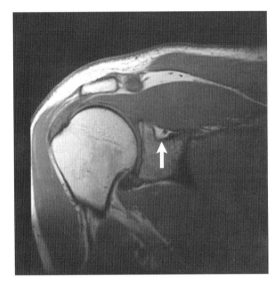

Fig. 6.6.20 MR scan of the glenoid neck with the suprascapular fossa containing the suprascapular nerve and artery. (From Department of Radiology and MRI, Bispebjerg University Hospital, Copenhagen, Denmark.)

Ultrasound

Ultrasonography is non-invasive and fast, and can be performed under dynamic circumstances, allowing visualization of the structures in the shoulder during motion. If experience in shoulder ultrasound investigation is available, it is a very sensitive and specific method for diagnosis of full-thickness tears of the rotator cuff [71,72] (Fig. 6.6.19). Partial tears, in which the pathologic changes extend to only one surface of the tendon, are more difficult to diagnose. With regard to biceps tendon pathology, dislocation of the tendon is recognized with high accuracy, whereas full or partial rupture of the long head of the biceps is diagnosed with less sensitivity [72] and the SLAP lesion is usually invisible with ultrasound. Subacromial fibrosis, edema of the rotator cuff and impingement are diagnosed with reasonably high accuracy. Anterior or posterior labral tears and Bankart lesions are best diagnosed during motion, showing a plump, hypermobile labrum [73].

In many cases the choice between MRI and ultrasonography in the diagnostic process depends on the availability of expertise and the technical standard.

Shoulder impingement

Impingement means collision. Basically there are three forms of impingement in the shoulder:
1 primary impingement, in which the subacromial space is overcrowded and there is too little space for the supraspinatus and biceps tendons;
2 secondary impingement, in which the rotator cuff is subject to microtrauma or overuse during motion, because of glenohumeral instability; and
3 internal impingement, in which the undersurface of the rotator cuff collides with the superior rim of the glenoid. This is probably a natural phenomenon, but becomes symptomatic in the athlete, because the collision happens repetitively and with great force.

Primary impingement occurs mainly in athletes over 40 years of age, whereas secondary impingement is common in younger athletes.

These three forms of shoulder impingement all involve the supraspinatus tendon, but differ in pathophysiology and in the way in which they are diagnosed and treated (Table 6.6.1).

Primary impingement

Pathophysiology

A breakthrough in understanding the pathophysiology of the primary, subacromial impingement came in 1972, when Neer published his article about acromioplasty as treatment of this condition [74]. He recognized that many cases of primary impingement are caused by compression of the supraspinatus tendon between the anterior undersurface of the acromion, the coracoacromial ligament and the acromioclavicular joint on one side, and the humeral head and the greater tuberosity on the other.

It is important to realize that the symptoms of primary impingement originate from the rotator cuff, in particular the supraspinatus tendon, even though in most cases it is caused by structures next to the tendon. Neer's classification of primary impingement depends primarily on the condition of the rotator cuff (Table 6.6.2)[75].

There are several reasons why the anterior part of the subacromial space can get overcrowded. Neer divided these into outlet and non-outlet causes, the first being changes in the coracoacromial arch impinging on the rotator cuff, and the latter being changes in the subacromial bursa or the tendon itself.

The *acromion* can be anteriorly hooked. The acromion can be divided into three categories according to shape: flat, bent and hooked (Fig. 6.6.20). Persons with a hooked acromion have a much higher risk than persons with a flat acromion for developing impingement, simply because the hook reduces the subacromial space. Instead of a hook, the acromion can host an osteophyte on the anterior undersurface. In rare cases the distal acromial epiphysis (in the anterolateral corner of acromion) does not fuse, giving rise to

an *os acromiale*, which can be dragged into the subacromial space by the coracoacromial ligament if the epiphysis is mobile. In some persons, the *coracoacromial ligament* is degenerated and calcified or has a sharp lateral edge [76]. The ligament is subject to some anatomic variation, and can be in three parts, of which one extends very medially from the acromion and can give rise to impingement [76]. The ligament normally stretches when the greater tuberosity passes under it [77], so a decrease in elasticity may result in a reduction of the subacromial space during motion. After trauma or repetitive overload (e.g. from swimming) or as a result of degenerative disease, the *acromioclavicular joint* can be thickened, with either an osteophyte or soft tissue, bulging into the subacromial space and compressing the supraspinatus. Enlargement of the *greater tuberosity* after trauma (fracture) is another reason for impingement.

Acute inflammation of the *subacromial bursa* is very painful and the most dramatic form of primary impingement. This can be a result of either increase in activity (e.g. the number of training hours) or a change—sometimes only a small change—in the nature of the activity (e.g. introduction of a new technique). If the inflammation becomes chronic, the bursa turns into fibrotic tissue, which occupies the subacromial space. The bursa can eventually calcify. Finally, the *supraspinatus tendon and muscle* itself can be subject to exercise-induced hypertrophy, degenerative disease, chronic tendinosis or a partial or full-thickness rupture, and calcium deposits can also develop in the tendon (Fig. 6.6.18a).

A rare form of primary impingement—coracoid impingement—was described as early as 1909. The pathophysiology can be a lateral projection of the *coracoid process*, a subscapular ganglion, calcification of the

Table 6.6.2 Neer's staging of primary impingement (from [75]).

Stage	Pathology	Age of patient	Clinical course	Treatment
1	Edema and hemorrhage	<25 years	Reversible	Conservative
2	Fibrosis and tendinitis	25–40 years	Recurrent	Bursectomy, resection of coracoacromial ligament
3	Bone spurs and tendon rupture	>40 years	Progressive	Acromioplasty, cuff repair

bursa in front of the subscapularis or bony projections from humeral head fractures. It can also result from *anterior instability* of the humeral head. Any of these factors will reduce the space between the coracoid and the subscapularis/rotator interval, introducing compression on the latter [62].

Symptoms — clinical picture

The primary symptom is pain with gradual onset. Pain spreads from the anterior and lateral part of the subacromion to the lateral part of the upper arm, but never below the elbow. Sometimes there is an intermittent feeling of numbness in the radial part of the forearm and the radial fingers. In the early stages of the disease, pain is induced only when the arm is in the horizontal position and particularly in inwards rotation, and the symptoms decrease or disappear during rest. If the cause of the impingement is not treated and the athlete continues activities unrestricted, pain may progress so that it is induced by all movements of the shoulder and present during rest and at night.

When the disease becomes chronic there is often restriction in motion, particularly flexion, inwards rotation and abduction.

At examination, Neer's and Hawkins' impingement tests are usually positive, with a significant reduction in pain when the tests are repeated after injection of a local analgesic in the subacromial space, or during the impingement release test. The joint is stable. Often there is tenderness of the subacromion anteriorly and laterally, and the acromioclavicular joint may be tender. There may be a reduction in supraspinatus strength caused by pain, but strength is normalized after subacromial injection of a local analgesic. X-rays, including an outlet view, will very often be normal, but may show a curved or hooked acromion, spurs at the anterior acromion or under the acromioclavicular joint and calcifications of the subacromial bursa or the supraspinatus tendon. MRI will typically show a reduction of the subacromial fat layer, fluid over the supraspinatus tendon, a compression in the supraspinatus tendon/muscle from spurs, acromion or a hypertrophic acromioclavicular joint, and degenerative changes in the supraspinatus tendon. Ultrasound investigation will typically show subacromial fluid and fibrosis and a slightly inhomogeneous supraspinatus tendon.

In coracoid impingement, flexion combined with adduction and inwards rotation is painful. X-rays, including an axillary view, or CT scan may show protrusion of the coracoid process or bony projections from the humeral head, and MRI will show reduced space between the tip of the coracoid and the rotator cuff [62].

Treatment and prognosis

There are only few randomized studies as to which treatment option is the best.

Stage I impingement — which is the most common form among athletes — is usually reversible during conservative treatment, and rarely requires arthroscopy. Stage II and III are rare in younger athletes, but operative treatment is frequently necessary.

Conservative treatment includes reduction of sports activities, a non-specific anti-inflammatory drug (NSAID) or subacromial injections of corticosteroid [78], and a rehabilitation program which in most cases will include muscle strengthening exercises (primarily of the scapular stabilizers until pain has decreased, and then of the rotator cuff muscles) and range-of-motion exercises to avoid loss of motion and reduce tightness of the posterior capsule.

Conservative treatment for 6–18 months has given good or excellent results in 50–80% of patients with stage I–III impingement [79,80]. Therefore, it is generally agreed that surgical treatment should not be offered before conservative treatment has been given for at least 6 months without satisfactory effect. Six months is somewhat arbitrary, as the proportion of patients with a satisfactory outcome during conservative treatment increases the longer the treatment period is [79]. In older patients with longstanding impingement, acromioplasty is a more successful treatment option than exercises [81].

Operative treatment is acromioplasty, which can be performed as an open or arthroscopic procedure.

In Neer's classic description from 1972, the anterior 5 mm of the acromial edge and enough of the anterior undersurface to make the acromion flat is removed in addition to the coracoacromial ligament. If there is protrusion of the acromioclavicular joint, this is flattened as well. The subacromial bursa or fibrous tissue which has replaced it is removed. Frays and tears in the rotator cuff are trimmed.

It has been questioned whether this standard procedure should be performed in athletes and younger individuals as resection of the coracoacromial ligament may result in anterosuperior instability of the joint, and resection of the undersurface of the acromioclavicular joint will reduce the stability of that joint. Many surgeons choose not to operate on the acromioclavicular joint unless the main part of the patient's symptoms can be attributed to it. In some overhead athletes with primary impingement seemingly caused by the coracoacromial ligament, good results have been reported following resection of the ligament without an acromioplasty [82]. Repair of full-thickness rotator cuff tears seems to give better long-term results than trimming [83], and may be preferable in athletes.

In athletes, up to 80% have a satisfactory pain reduction after acromioplasty for impingement stage II–III, but only half are able to return to their previous level of sports [84]. Undoubtedly, some of the patients with unsatisfactory results have misdiagnosed secondary impingements [85].

If an os acromiale is present, it should be resected or the epiphysis should be fused, as acromioplasty is not sufficient to relieve symptoms [63].

Secondary impingement

Pathophysiology

In secondary impingement, there is nothing 'in the way' in the subacromial space, nothing that the humeral head naturally can collide with. The humeral head is brought into a position where it can collide with the acromion because of hypermobility of the head.

The pathogenesis of secondary impingement seems to be glenohumeral instability with insufficiency of both the passive and dynamic stabilizers (lengthening of the glenohumeral ligaments and the anterior capsule, and dyscoordination and fatigue of the rotator cuff muscles), but the interrelationship between these conditions and impingement is poorly understood.

The instability, which is usually anterior–inferior, can be either constitutional as a part of hyperlaxity, or acquired. Overhead athletic activities, e.g. swimming

and throwing, put enormous strain on the passive stabilizers of the glenohumeral joint: the glenohumeral ligaments and the joint capsule. As a consequence, these passive stabilizers may be physically stretched by the overhead activities, leading to anterior–inferior instability, in particular if the dynamic stabilizers — of which the rotator cuff muscles are the most important — fail to center the humeral head in the glenoid during motion.

There are several hypotheses as to how instability can lead to symptoms from the rotator cuff (impingement).

Mechanically the humeral head is subluxed anteriorly and inferiorly to the glenoid during overhead activities in these patients. Because of the anterior glide, the rotator cuff may impinge on the anterior part of the acromion and the coracoacromial ligament. A tight posterior capsule is often found and may increase the anterior glide.

The supraspinatus and deltoid muscles apply superior shear force to the humeral head [86]. In instability, the supraspinatus muscle will be hyperactive during overhead activities, trying to center the humeral head in the glenoid. This may either lead to a superior glide of the head, compressing the supraspinatus tendon against the acromion, or lead to overuse tendinitis in the supraspinatus tendon.

Fatigue of the scapular rotator muscles (in particular serratus anterior) has been reported in patients with secondary impingement. This may reduce scapular and thereby acromial rotation during overhead sports and bring the acromion into closer contact with the humeral head [87].

It is reported that the coordination of muscle activity in the rotator cuff and the scapular stabilizers in swimmers and throwers is different in athletes with shoulder pain compared to asymptomatic athletes [87,88]. This may be a failure of some muscles to fulfil the demands that the overhead activity places on them.

On the other hand, in athletes with pain in only one shoulder, the muscle coordination is also altered in the symptom-free shoulder, indicating that the dyscoordination of muscles may in some cases be constitutional or caused by an inappropriate technique [89]. In some throwing athletes, signs of instability are found in both shoulders, indicating that laxity of the passive stabilizers in some cases may be constitutional.

Symptoms — clinical picture

The main symptom is pain, often anteriorly in the glenohumeral joint and subacromially, and sometimes extending to the anterior and lateral part of the upper arm. Onset is gradual—if symptoms started after a trauma, one must suspect a primary traumatic instability (a Bankart lesion) and not a typical secondary impingement. At first symptoms are only present during overhead sports activity, but may progress to a more chronic stage with pain during daily activities and at night. In some cases instability is felt as a glide or a click during overhead activities, in particular during maximal abduction and external rotation.

At examination muscular atrophy of the supraspinatus is sometimes seen. Neer's and Hawkins' impingement tests may be positive, but this is not optional as in primary impingement, as the secondary impingement only happens during dynamic activity. The apprehension test is positive as either an unpleasant feeling or pain anteriorly in the glenohumeral joint, with relief during relocation. If there is a significant inferior instability component, a sulcus sign can often be provoked.

X-rays are usually normal. There are no consistent findings described on MRI, but alternative diagnoses can be verified: a Bankart lesion in primary traumatic instability; changes in the lateral parts of the supraspinatus tendon and the superior labrum in internal impingement, labral tears and instability or inflammation of the biceps tendon.

With the patient under anesthesia, the instability can always be demonstrated. During arthroscopy anterior–inferior gliding of the humeral head is present, but there is no avulsion of the anterior capsulolabral complex (including the middle glenohumeral ligament) from the glenoid, as in Bankart instability. There may be frays or tears of the anterior or inferior labrum, due to the gliding of the humeral head over the labrum during overhead activities.

It is probably fair to say that some cases can be a mixture of secondary and internal impingement, it being impossible to say which was first.

Treatment and prognosis

As with primary impingement, pain and inflammation is reduced by decrease in activity, particularly overhead activity, rest, NSAIDs and eventually subacromial corticosteroid injections.

As anterior–inferior instability is a major cause of secondary instability, rehabilitation concentrates on strengthening the dynamic stabilizers (as the passive stabilizers can not be tightened non-operatively), e.g. the rotator cuff and the scapular stabilizers.

When range of motion is full and pain free, the athlete can gradually return to overhead activities. Incorporation of the correct technique is probably very important.

On this conservative program, most overhead athletes have been reported to be able to return to their previous level of sports [90].

Patients who do not respond satisfactorily to the conservative program may be candidates for surgical treatment, which consists of tightening the passive stabilizers. In most cases an arthroscopy will be performed initially to verify the diagnosis and to treat concomitant lesions, such as labral tears. Tightening of the glenohumeral ligaments and the anterior capsule can be performed either as an open capsular shift, originally described by Neer in 1980 and modified by Warren, or as an arthroscopic procedure, where the anterior capsule and the glenohumeral ligaments are sewn to the labrum with internal sutures (Fig. 6.6.21). Both procedures show good results with 75% of patients being able to return to sports [85,91], but the long-term effect of internal suture has not been reported yet. The introduction of capsular shrinkage by burning with laser or electrically was introduced in the early 1990s. Short-term results look promising, but some still regard this procedure as experimental, as the long-term results are unknown.

Prevention

Just as hypermobile individuals have a much greater risk for rupture of the anterior cruciate ligament during sports, so they probably also have a much higher risk for secondary impingement of the shoulder, if they perform overhead sports. Hypermobile individuals may therefore be advised not to choose overhead sports.

Theoretically, strengthening of the dynamic stabilizers should reduce glenohumeral instability, but there are no clinical reports to support the view that if this program is emphasized generally in overhead

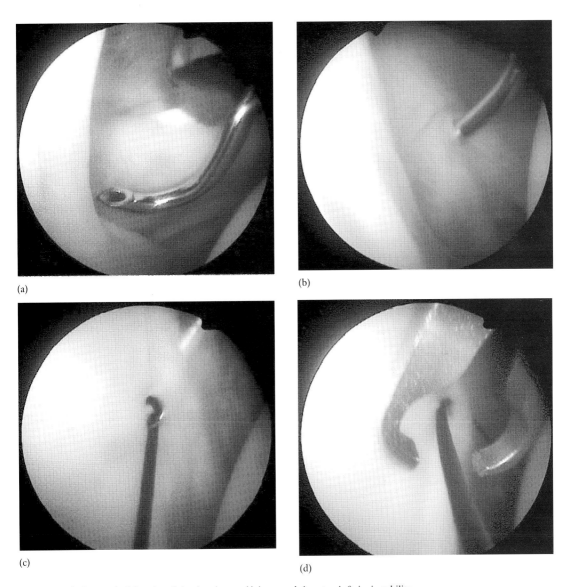

Fig. 6.6.21 Arthroscopic tightening of the glenohumeral joint capsule in anteroinferior instability.

athletes, the risk for secondary impingement is reduced.

Internal impingement

Pathophysiology

Internal or superior glenoid impingement was first described in 1991 by Walch [92]. The collision between the undersurface of the supraspinatus tendon at its insertion and the superior part of the glenoid rim is a natural phenomenon, responsible for the maximal range of motion in abduction and external rotation in most humans [93–95]. Most people only occasionally use these extremes of motion (Figs 6.6.22 & 6.6.23).

Why this collision becomes symptomatic in some athletes, mainly those performing overhead sports (handball, baseball, volleyball, etc.), has been subject to speculation. Walch suggested that the repetitive, forceful way in which the collision theoretically may occur in overhead sports, and which is unphysiologic,

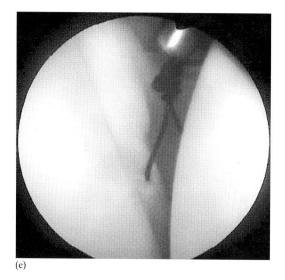

(e)

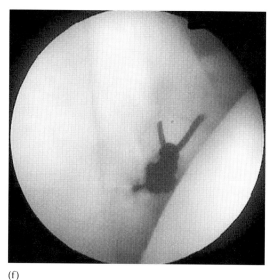

(f)

Fig. 6.6.21 *Continued.*

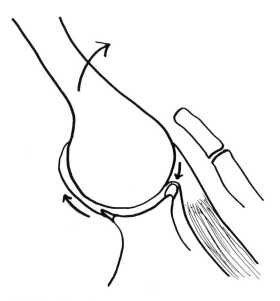

Fig. 6.6.22 The pathophysiology of internal impingement. In throwing, the undersurface of the supraspinatus tendon impinges on the superior labrum and glenoid. The inferior glenohumeral ligament is stretched, resulting in anterior–inferior laxity.

explains why these athletes develop clinical symptoms. He also suggested that too small a retroversion of the humeral head will dispose to internal impingement, because the smaller the retroversion, the smaller the degree of external rotation at which the insertion of the supraspinatus tendon collides with the glenoid [92].

In one series a high percentage of anteroinferior glenohumeral instability among athletes with internal impingement [94] was reported, indicating that instability may be a pathophysiologic factor. If the humeral head glides anteriorly and downwards during throwing (when the arm is in abduction and maximal external rotation), the undersurface of the supraspinatus will be brought closer to the superior glenoid rim, which may induce internal impingement. On the other hand, clear MRI signs of internal impingement in asymptomatic, throwing athletes have been reported to be unrelated to instability [96].

The disease has only been described in overhead athletes [96].

Symptoms—clinical picture

Three stages of the internal impingement are described (Table 6.6.3). The first symptom is pain in the back of the shoulder, perhaps extending down into the lateral and posterior part of the upper arm. Pain is only present with the arm in maximal abduction and external rotation. As the disease progresses, pain in the acceleration phase of throwing increases and the ability to throw is reduced. Clicking and locking may occur.

Table 6.6.3 The three stages of internal impingement.

Stage I	Stiffness of the joint during activity, no pain
Stage II	Pain during activity (in particular throwing), but not during rest
Stage III	Irreversible constant pain

Examination usually reveals normal range of motion and normal strength of the rotator cuff muscles. Neer's and Hawkins' impingement tests are usually negative. Maximal abduction and external rotation (an extreme apprehension test) results in pain posterior in the glenohumeral joint, not to be confused with a positive apprehension test, in which the discomfort is felt anteriorly. Instability tests may be positive. SLAP tests may be positive.

X-rays can show small bone cysts in the top of the greater tuberosity and glenoid [67], but are usually normal. MRI will show degeneration of the supraspinatus at the insertion on humerus, often slight bone bruise in the back and top of the greater tuberosity and the superior glenoid, and in some cases also degeneration of the superior labrum [67]. The subacromial space is usually normal. Ultrasound investigation will show degeneration of the lateral supraspinatus tendon, perhaps small impressions in the greater tuberosity, and sometimes it is possible to see that the posterosuperior labrum is enlarged.

Internal impingement has a typical appearance at arthroscopy [94] (Fig. 6.6.23). There is fraying of the undersurface of the supraspinatus tendon close to the insertion on the humeral head, but usually no inflammation of the tendon. Often there are small lesions in the greater tuberosity just behind the insertion of the supraspinatus. The superior labrum is always frayed and often hypertrophic. The lesion may extend somewhat posteriorly. In some patients, the changes in the superior labrum has the form of a SLAP lesion.

Treatment and prognosis

The treatment of internal impingement is still subject to debate.

The results after debridement of the frayed tendon and labrum seemed to be satisfactory in one series, as 80% were able to return to sports [64].

Riand *et al.* believe that internal impingement is a physiologic phenomenon, and that it becomes symptomatic in some people because they are built with less retroversion (that is <20–30° of retroversion) of their humeral head. So they performed a rotating osteotomy of the humerus with shortening of the subscapularis tendon in 20 patients who had arthroscopically verified internal impingement, and who had persistent pain despite arthroscopic debridement. Sixteen of these patients became pain free and 11 could return to sports at preinjury level [64]. Three of their patients also had multidirectional instability and in these, the operation failed.

Jobe and Paley regard glenohumeral instability as the most likely pathogenesis for internal impingement [94] and advocate surgical correction of the instability as the primary treatment in most cases.

As this disease is not rare, larger treatment series or even randomized studies will hopefully be available in the near future to help in choosing the best treatment option.

Prevention

Theoretically it should be possible to prevent internal impingement by changing technique in overhead sports, reducing the degree of external rotation and abduction during shooting/throwing. But it is doubtful if this is possible, as it would reduce the shooting force, and it is also not documented to be beneficial.

Shoulder instability

When assessing different athletes with shoulder instability you will find a variety of symptoms, signs and also lesions in the shoulder.

Instability itself is a symptom, with which the athlete will present. As the examiner you will assess laxity.

Symptoms

Instability may present in various ways, usually depending on how much the joint is translated during activity. When translation is marked, even frank dislocation is presented. In minor translation pain may be the only symptom (Fig. 6.6.24).

Signs

The sign of laxity must always be evaluated. Manual testing under anesthesia is often very helpful because it

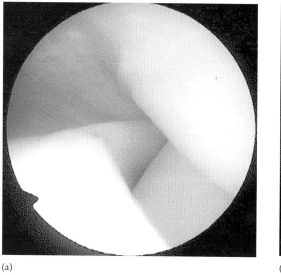

(a)

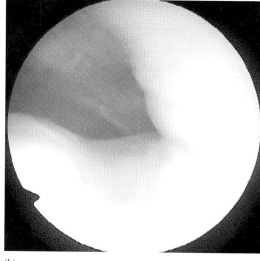

(b)

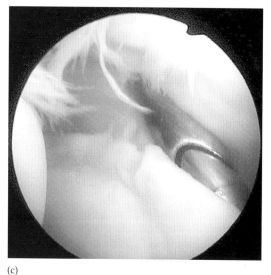

(c)

Fig. 6.6.23 Arthroscopic posterior view of the shoulder with superior labrum to the left, and the undersurface of the supraspinatus tendon to the right. When the arm is elevated into maximum abduction/external rotation, there is impingement between the superior labrum and the supraspinatus (b), which is not occurring when the arm is elevated a few degrees less (a). With repeated forceful impingement, the superior labrum is damaged and the lateral undersurface of the supraspinatus is fraying (c), anterior view.

| Symptoms: | Pain | Apprehension | Dead arm | Subluxation | Dislocation |
| Degree of translation: | Minor | | | | Major |

Fig. 6.6.24 Symptoms in shoulder instability related to the degree of translation.

is more easily assessed. In the normal person, some degree of laxity is always present. As the examiner you must assess whether laxity is increased and in which direction(s) (Fig. 6.6.25) [97].

Anatomic lesions

A number of anatomic factors and structures attribute to stability and changes in these may lead to increased laxity and instability (Table 6.6.4).

Careful assessment of these structures must be performed, usually using clinical testing and radiology. Electromyography, neurography and/or arthroscopy are helpful.

Purely functional factors may also be important. Scapulothoracic motion may be disturbed due to muscle imbalance, muscle fatigue or even palsy (long

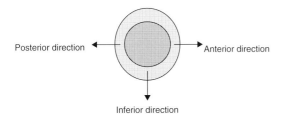

Fig. 6.6.25 Directions of shoulder instability.

Table 6.6.4 Pathoanatomic conditions leading to laxity.

Structure	Change which may lead to instability
Joint conformity	Abnormal version of either the glenoid or the humeral head Fracture
Labrum	Rupture Avulsion from glenoid Fraying secondary to hyperelasticity of the ligaments
Ligaments	Rupture Cumulative microtrauma with plastic deformation Avulsion from glenoid or humeral head Generalized joint laxity Loss of proprioceptive feedback
Muscles	Tendon rupture, SLAP lesion Cumulative microtrauma Paresis due to nerve damage

thoracic nerve). This dyskinesis may lead to the development of instability symptoms.

Only when the patient history (description of instability, traumatic events, activity) is matched with your clinical examination, manual assessment of the laxity and knowledge of anatomic factors (radiology, arthroscopy) can a clear diagnosis be established.

Classification of instability

Instability is usually classified based on three different concepts:
1 volition;
2 direction; and
3 trauma.

Volition

Voluntary dislocators perform the dislocation for a purpose. They are rarely found within the athletic community. They should be treated using other modalities than the ones to be discussed below. Voluntary dislocators will not be discussed further.

Direction

Knowledge of the direction of the instability is crucial. Therefore it is very important to document in which direction the shoulder dislocates. X-rays when the shoulder is dislocated may seem difficult to obtain but are very valuable when assessing recurrent instability.

Trauma

It may seem easy to establish whether a trauma has caused the instability or not, but in clinical practice this may be difficult. When repeated microtrauma is included in this group, the assessment becomes even harder. Throwers accelerate the shoulder up to angular velocities exceeding 7000°/s. Also, in the athletic population, trauma to various parts of the body is included in daily activities.

Involuntary instability may be subdivided and classified in several ways. From a routine, clinical point of view the TUBS and AMBRI classification [98,99] may still be helpful (TUBS = *t*raumatic *u*nilateral *b*ankart lesion *s*urgical treatment; AMBRI = *a*traumatic *m*ultidirectional *b*ilateral *r*ehabilitation first, *i*nferior capsular shift if necessary). Most cases of shoulder instability may be classified as either traumatic, anterior instability or atraumatic, multidirectional instability. With increasing understanding the term 'atraumatic' is being modified and its classification also. We now prefer to differ between atraumatic, overuse-induced instability and atraumatic, hyperlaxity-induced instability. The overuse type is the result of repeated microtrauma, as seen in throwers and swimmers. The hyperlaxity type is often associated with generalized joint laxity and usually also findings and symptoms from other joints (wrist, knee, ankle, etc.).

A summarized classification of recurrent instability is shown in Fig. 6.6.26 [100].

Anterior post-traumatic instability

This is the most common type of shoulder instability. It is the result of a shoulder trauma which causes

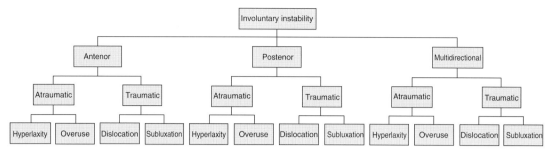

Fig. 6.6.26 Classification of recurrent shoulder instability.

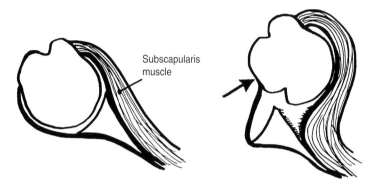

Subscapularis muscle

Fig. 6.6.27 The pathoanatomy of the Bankart lesion (stripping of the labrum and glenohumeral ligaments off the anterior glenoid) in traumatic shoulder dislocation. An impression fracture (the Hill–Sachs lesion) develops on the posterior aspect of the humeral head.

disruption of the anterior glenohumeral ligaments; most often the anterior band and anterior parts of the inferior glenohumeral ligament (IGHL) are detached from the glenoid rim (Fig. 6.6.27). This lesion has been named after Sir Blundell Bankart who described this lesion in his classic paper in 1923 [101]. The IGHL may also rupture in midsubstance or on the humeral side (HAGL lesion) but these injury patterns are less common. A concomitant bony lesion is the compression fracture on the posterosuperior aspect of the humeral head described by several authors and most often named after Hill and Sachs [102].

The trauma is sometimes difficult to assess adequately. The patient may have forgotten the trauma or disregard a minor trauma. The initial trauma may not have provoked a dislocation. In many cases the trauma only results in clinical pain and maybe some swelling. The ligament injury becomes apparent only when the patient dislocates or subluxates the shoulder, sometimes several weeks after the initial trauma.

Diagnosis is established from history (trauma, symptoms) and manual testing (anterior drawer test/ load-and-shift test, apprehension sign, relocation

test). Radiology may be very helpful, showing a Hill–Sachs lesion or even a bony Bankart lesion (avulsion fracture from the anterior–inferior rim of the glenoid).

Post-traumatic anterior instability is seen most commonly in athletes involved in contact sports (ice hockey, soccer, handball, rugby, American football).

Treatment of post-traumatic, recurrent, anterior instability is surgical. No other treatment can restore the lacking ligamentous function. Bankart described this procedure which includes reattachment of the torn ligaments to the glenoid rim. Over the years a number of other authors have proposed different techniques for anterior stabilization (Ricard, Putti–Platt, Magnuson–Stack, Bristow, Eden–Hybbinette and many others) but none of these procedures has been able to produce the same highly satisfactory and reproducible postoperative results as the Bankart procedure. Today, most shoulder surgeons use the Bankart procedure but, on the other hand, there are many variations. Both open and arthroscopic procedures are called 'Bankart'. The common denominating factor is that the IGHL is reattached to the glenoid rim. Variations are use of the labrum, degree of shift, fixating devices, additional lateral procedure, incision in the subscapularis muscle and skin incision used.

The 'standard open Bankart' usually includes:
- straight, anterior, vertical skin incision;
- deltopectoral split;
- subscapularis division of the subscapular tendon;
- medial reattachment of IGHL and superior shifting of the inferior capsule using suture anchors;
- subscapularis tendon repair; and
- skin closure.

Arthroscopic techniques are still developing but are quite often used. In the hands of some skilled surgeons results may be good (less than 10% recurrence) [103–105]. But judging from the literature open techniques still produce results superior to those following arthroscopic techniques [25,99,106] (Fig. 6.6.28).

The postoperative regimen usually includes a short period of immobilization (maximum 3 weeks) followed by increasing physical therapy including range of motion training and strengthening. After 3–6 months full athletic activity is allowed. Up to 95% regain a stable shoulder and usually most of the athletes resume their athletic activity at the preinjury level

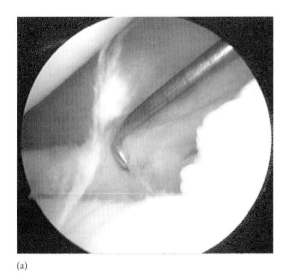

(a)

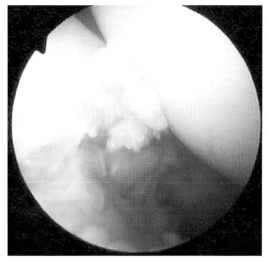

(b)

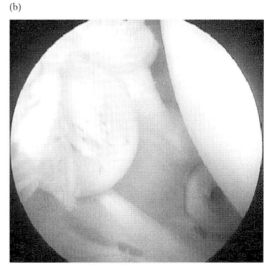

(c)

Fig. 6.6.28 Arthroscopic appearance of a Bankart lesion (a,b) and repair of the lesion with SureTac (c).

[107]. Throwers have the most difficulty in regaining full capacity. Only 50–64% return to the same competition level [108,109].

Acute, first-time anterior dislocation

Initial treatment is of course atraumatic reduction. Injection of local anesthetics may be very effective in reducing pain. Reduction may be achieved using traction or using the Milch technique with the arm in abduction and direct manipulation of the humeral head. Immobilization does not lower the risk for recurrence, neither does any other treatment. The athlete is usually restricted due to pain for 2–4 weeks after the injury.

The first-time dislocation may be a golden opportunity to surgically treat shoulder instability. In these circumstances (fresh wound surfaces, absence of chronic changes) an arthroscopic procedure may suffice. But if an acute repair is considered, the problem is selection of patients suitable for surgery. Since the recurrence rate following initial dislocation is high (60–95%) in the young, athletic population [110,111], it is probable that acute stabilization will become more attractive as our knowledge increases and the arthroscopic procedures become more reproducible [112].

Arthroscopic stabilization in post-traumatic instability

Today, the most controversial discussion is whether stabilization should be open or arthroscopic.

It might seem obvious that the arthroscopic technique would be superior to the open technique since soft tissue damage is less when going through the skin, muscles and tendons. The reattachment of the capsuloligamentous complex looks very convincing when performed by a trained surgeon. However, with the arthroscopic technique the results are still inferior to those following open stabilization (open Bankart procedure) [25,99,106].

Posterior instability

Posterior instability is, as the name indicates, only a directional diagnosis. It may either result from trauma or be atraumatic. The atraumatic cases usually start at the age of 10–12 years without pain or other discomfort. This type of posterior instability may be an expression of a multidirectional instability (see below).

Post-traumatic, posterior instability

The initial accident is usually a fall when the patient holds the arm in flexion, quite often with the elbow flexed. The indirect trauma to the shoulder is usually experienced immediately even though true dislocation does not usually occur. Weeks after the trauma the shoulder is painful in flexion. The instability may present itself either with pain in flexion or a true feeling of instability, or (more rarely) even frank dislocation.

Soft tissue lesions in the shoulder joint usually include disruption of the posterior part of the labrum and detachment of the posterior capsule, most frequently the posterior band of the IGHL.

Athletes engaged in contact sports present with posterior instability: soccer players, wrestlers, American footballers, etc.

The diagnosis is established, as in anterior instability, from the history (trauma, symptoms) and by manual testing (positive posterior drawer test and posterior stress test). Radiology may be very helpful.

Treatment of post-traumatic instability is directed towards repair of the injured structures. Hence, repair of the labrum if possible and reattachment of the posterior capsular ligament complex is indicated. Often this is referred to as a 'posterior Bankart'. The surgical procedure is very much like the original Bankart procedure, but performed from the back. It includes posterior skin incision, deltoid split and division of the infraspinatus muscle. The capsulotomy is performed and the labrum and ligament complex is reattached using suture anchors. Postoperative treatment includes immobilization in neutral rotation in order to avoid stretching the posterior capsule.

Multidirectional instability

The term multidirectional instability (MDI) strictly implies that the athlete suffers from instability symptoms in two or more directions. This strict case is rarely present. The most common problem is that the athlete presents with pain in the shoulder and the examiner finds hyperlaxity in more than one direction (multidirectional hyperlaxity, MDH). Occasionally the patient has problems with instability in several directions, such as inferior gliding of the humeral head when holding the arm at the side and a feeling of posterior subluxation when raising the arm.

In sports medicine the major problem is athletes with shoulder pain during and after activity. Some of these cases may be misinterpreted as having impingement syndrome. And indeed, some of them do have secondary impingement symptoms. As the head lacks stability, it will move superiorly in the joint during motion. This will excessively load the subacromial bursa leading to bursitis and impingement symptoms. Yet the basic problem is the instability and hyperlaxity! Signs which are helpful in establishing the correct diagnosis are, apart from manual laxity testing, external rotation of 90° or more, bilateral symptoms or symptoms of instability from other joints (usually wrist, ankle, femoropatellar joint).

Swimmers are a group of athletes well known to have problems with shoulder pain. Their problems are sometimes referred to as 'swimmer's shoulder'. It is shown that many of them suffer from MDI [4,113]. Among throwing athletes also, both pure MDI and secondary impingement are common; usually, however, only in the dominant arm.

Jobe *et al.* [114] have suggested a classification which may be helpful in assessing athletes with shoulder pain:
• athletes with pure impingement;
• athletes with instability due to anterior labral and ligament injury (post-traumatic instability) with secondary impingement;
• athletes with instability due to hyperelastic ligaments with secondary impingement; and
• athletes with pure instability.

The diagnosis is not easily established. Apart from history and radiology (normal plain X-ray, wide capsule on MRI), manual testing is crucial (anterior and posterior drawer, sulcus sign, etc.).

The treatment of MDI is currently changing. The initial strategy is still to start active physiotherapy with emphasis on balancing the shoulder, strengthening the rotator muscles and improving proprioception. Surgical treatment has largely been based on inferior capsular shift techniques, performed from both the anterior and posterior. Today thermal-induced shrinkage of the capsule is used more widely. Both laser and bi- and monopolar radiofrequency devices are used. Postoperative treatment varies widely as far as immobilization is concerned. Some use up to 6 weeks of immobilization, whereas others start active range of motion exercises immediately. Most reports on human subjects have so far been presented at various symposia. Only a limited number of articles have been published showing results from thermally treated shoulder instability [115,116]. Since long-term results are lacking, this treatment modality is still at the experimental level.

'Golden rule'
A young athlete with shoulder pain usually suffers from instability.

Rotator cuff lesions and tendon trauma

Rotator cuff lesions
The rotator cuff muscles and their respective tendinous insertions to the humerus are considered the primary dynamic stabilizers of the glenohumeral joint and are extensively loaded during overhead and contact sports [117]. The rotator cuff of well-conditioned athletes stabilizes the joint successfully without injury. However, where the demands placed on the rotator cuff are increased beyond its capabilities, injury may result. These injuries can progress from inflammation to microtears to partial and full-thickness tears. Improper throwing mechanics, muscle fatigue and glenohumeral instability increase the loads on the rotator cuff and can result in a cycle of degeneration that causes mechanical impingement, collagen tensile failure, and further rotator cuff dysfunction [118,119].

Athletes involved in overhead sports commonly experience injury to the rotator cuff through repetitive microtrauma, while the mechanism of injury in those participating in contact sports includes blunt force or macrotrauma. Injury to the rotator cuff in athletes involved in overhead sports can be classified into three categories: primary impingement, primary tensile overload, and secondary impingement with tensile overload resulting from glenohumeral instability. A broad spectrum of clinical conditions can result from repetitive microtrauma or acute macrotrauma to the rotator cuff tendons. A thorough history and physical examination are critical for the correct diagnosis and treatment of athletes with rotator cuff pathology.

Two of the most common conditions associated with these types of injuries include partial-thickness and full-thickness rotator cuff tears, which may be identified using simple criteria.

Partial-thickness lesions are associated with pain and weakness during resisted isometric contraction of the involved muscles. The posterior capsule may also be tight and imaging studies can reveal rotator cuff thinning. However, the lesions do not extend through the full thickness of the tendon (Fig. 6.6.29).

The lesions most often involve the supraspinatus tendon near its anterior insertion but may also include the infraspinatus or subscapularis tendons. Symptoms that usually result from these lesions include joint stiffness during passive motion that stretches the tendon, as well as pain and weakness. Partial-thickness tears can be more painful than full-thickness tears due

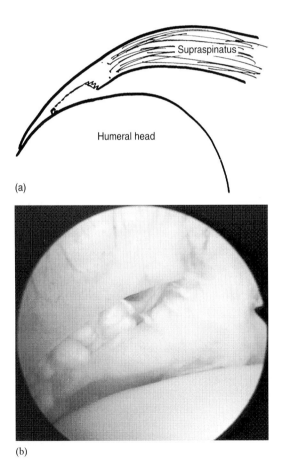

(a)

(b)

Fig. 6.6.29 Partial supraspinatus tear. (a) Schematic pathology. (b) Arthroscopic view from joint side.

to abnormal stiffness and tension in the remaining fibers of the tendon.

The non-operative treatment of partial-thickness rotator cuff tears is quite similar to the management of subacromial impingement and centers on reducing acute pain and inflammation. Initially, rest and ice are used to reduce inflammation. Based on deficits in range of motion, rehabilitation programs must then emphasize stretching in all directions of joint stiffness, including internal and external rotation as well as cross-body adduction and elevation. Scapular mobilization should also be included. Positions that stretch the capsule or cause impingement should be avoided in patients with anterior instability.

As the normal range of passive motion is reestablished, a slowly progressing muscle strengthening program of the rotator cuff and scapular stabilizers should be initiated. The overall goal of these exercises is to promote scar tissue development in the defect that eventually reorganizes in a similar manner to normal tendon. Based on functional deficits, specific muscles can be targeted. However, exercises should begin with the arm adducted using rubber bands to strengthen the internal and external rotators. The scapular stabilizers are incorporated as pain and inflammation decrease followed by resisted exercises with the arm abducted. It is a common fear that subacromial injections of cortisone could damage tendons in the younger athletic population; however, they are commonly used in athletes over 40 years of age with primary impingement.

Those athletes that have experienced acute macrotrauma to the rotator cuff receive treatment based on the suspected degree of injury. A physical examination and diagnostic imaging can reveal rotator cuff contusion or a partial-thickness tear. Following a period of rest and anti-inflammatory medication, the full range of motion should be regained as described previously. Finally, strengthening exercises are begun and the athlete is allowed to return to sport once normal strength has been regained.

Partial-thickness tears can be associated with concomitant pathology such as primary impingement or anterior instability. Therefore, repair of these tears could also benefit from treatment of the associated pathology using subacromial decompression, rotator cuff debridement, or capsular procedures. However, some individuals with rotator cuff pathology may be asymptomatic and surgeons are cautioned not to repair defects merely because they exist. In addition, some defects cannot be repaired because they offer only 'rotten cloth to sew' [23].

Many surgical approaches exist for treatment of rotator cuff tears, including open and arthroscopic procedures. Open techniques include a posterior approach [120], an anterior approach through the acromioclavicular joint as well as the anterior acromioplasty approach [74,121] that preserves the deltoid insertion and acromial lever arm. Arthroscopic techniques are now being used routinely. Conversion of a partial-thickness cuff defect to a full-thickness lesion and subsequent repair should be based on the preoperative evaluation and surgical findings. The thickness of the rotator cuff and percentage of tendon that remains intact should guide the surgeon in considering a repair.

Depending on the location of the tear, an excision is made until a flap of the cuff can be turned back, exposing normal tendon. Any retracted tissue or split layers of tissue are then consolidated. Releasing the coracohumeral ligament and the capsule in the rotator interval from the base of the coracoid can help minimize the tension on the repair. The tissue is then reattached to the humerus, making sure that all fibers are loaded evenly and its superior surface is smooth.

The shoulder should then be moved through its full range of motion to ensure that the repair does not restrict motion and eliminates any subacromial impingement. Postoperatively, rehabilitation should emphasize continuous passive motion and the restoration of a full range of motion. These exercises will prevent stiffness and adhesions at the joint.

Full-thickness rotator cuff tears also present with pain and weakness during resisted isometric contractions of the involved rotator cuff muscles. This type of defect is usually demonstrated on ultrasonography, MRI or arthrography, or during arthroscopy (Fig. 6.6.30). The program for non-operative management of full-thickness rotator cuff tears usually includes rest, non-steroidal anti-inflammatory medications, physical therapy and the avoidance of aggravating activities. Several studies have shown improvement in 33–90% of patients [122,123] with non-operative management. Steroid injections seem to offer little benefit

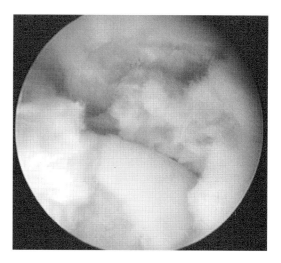

Fig. 6.6.30 Posterior arthroscopic view of a large supra/infraspinatus tear. The acromion is at the top and the humeral head at the bottom. The tendon stump is inserting on the greater tuberosity to the left.

to patients with this type of rotator cuff tear [124]. Even though conservative treatment in some cases results in satisfactory outcomes with patients displaying preserved motion and strength function may deteriorate [125] and in athletes full function is usually not possible to re-establish through non-operative treatment.

The potential for repair of a full-thickness rotator cuff tear is obtained from the physical examination, history, plain radiographs and MRI. Younger, healthy individuals in the athletic population with acute tears seem more likely to have a successful outcome [126]. The degree of fatty degeneration of the muscle, which can be measured on MRI, also influences the outcome, and if more than 50% of the corresponding muscle has degenerated to fat or scar tissue, repair of the rupture has a bad functional outcome [69]. Repair of a massive tear should probably be performed early to avoid irreversible degeneration of the muscle. Two general categories of surgical techniques exist for repairing full-thickness rotator cuff tears: tendon to tendon and advancement of the tendon to bone. In the past, the identification of the tear pattern and the use of direct repair and flaps has been emphasized as indicated by the tear pattern [121]. Others have utilized a side-to-side repair for small tears and tendon-to-bone repair for larger defects [127]. Finally, as the size of the tear progresses, these surgeons have described tendon mobilization or advancement of tendon flaps to restore joint integrity. Repair of full-thickness rotator cuff tears is now often performed arthroscopically.

Post-operatively, some surgeons believe the shoulder should be immobilized in an abduction splint [128]; however, others do not concur [129]. Continued exercises have been found to be important through the postoperative measurement of the isokinetic strength of the shoulder following surgical treatment.

The athlete with an acute episode of macrotrauma to the shoulder that results in rotator cuff pathology usually presents with pain, limited active elevation and a positive 'shrug' sign. Arthroscopy is recommended for patients that have not improved with rehabilitation. The decision to perform surgery depends on the response to non-operative treatment, the severity of the symptoms, and the goals of the athlete. Thickened, inflamed or fibrotic tissue can be excised [130]. On the other hand, partial-thickness tears that involve less than 50% of the cuff thickness should be debrided.

Biceps tendon ruptures

Many authors have described *isolated ruptures* of the tendon from the long head of the biceps muscle, though most ruptures of the biceps tendon have been found with supraspinatus tendon tears [7,131,132]. Studies that document isolated tears using arthroscopic techniques show these lesions to be rare (2.2%). Osteophytes in the bicipital groove may cause these isolated ruptures of the biceps tendon [7].

Treatment of isolated ruptures of the biceps tendon has been separated into two groups based on age. In young and active patients that are particularly involved in overhead sport, weight-lifting or jobs requiring forceful supination, a sudden overload of this tendon may result in an isolated rupture. Physical examination and ultrasonography of the biceps can isolate the rupture site while MRI should be used to examine the status of the rotator cuff. An early repair is recommended [133] for patients with high functional expectations.

Rupture may occur within the musculotendinous junction, within the bicipital groove, or at the attachment of the tendon to the superior glenoid. The most common complaint with rupture of the biceps tendon is anterior shoulder pain in the region of the biceps. Simple inspection of the involved extremity may demonstrate tears evidenced by migration of the muscle belly. Weakness during forearm flexion and supination is also a strong sign of this injury. In the latter two cases, a primary tenodesis has been recommended as giving the best chance of returning to activity and restoration of normal cosmesis. The technique for this procedure involves abrading the groove and tenodesing the tendon with a single staple. Treatment for rupture at the musculotendinous junction includes primary repair of the soft tissue and extended protection of the healing site. Most patients with either repair procedure are restricted from active elbow flexion for 4 weeks, after which rehabilitation may begin for 2 months.

Combined biceps tendon and rotator cuff tears. Patients over the age of 50 and physically inactive usually have a prior history of shoulder problems and treatment. Ruptures in this group usually occur within the bicipital groove and are caused by attrition. In addition, they will have signs of rotator cuff tears or impingement. Therefore, simple observation for 4 weeks may be the treatment of choice resulting in the immediate pain resolving, almost normal strength of the extremity returning, and only minimal deformity. A strong history of shoulder problems indicates that diagnostic studies should be performed to evaluate the integrity of the rotator cuff. Based on the pathologic findings, the rotator cuff tear should be addressed first, followed by the impingement process, and the biceps tendon [133]. Patients with a full-thickness rotator cuff tear that have failed prior treatment must undergo either an arthrotomy, acromioplasty, cuff repair or biceps tenodesis.

Biceps tendon instability

Even though several studies have addressed the issue of biceps tendon subluxation, the definition of instability of this tendon is poorly standardized and controversial [134,135]. Walch defines subluxation of the long head of the biceps tendon as partial or incomplete loss of contact between the tendon and its bony groove [136].

Dislocation is a complete loss of contact between the tendon and its bony groove.

Three types of subluxation have been classified [136]:

Type I—Superior subluxation. The superior glenohumeral and coracohumeral ligaments are partially or completely torn, resulting in a biceps tendon that is subluxed superiorly at the entrance to the bicipital groove.

Type II—Subluxation in the groove. The biceps tendon slips over the medial rim of the bicipital groove and rides on the border of the lesser tuberosity. The main cause of this instability is the tearing of the outermost fibers of the subscapularis.

Type III—Malunion and non-union of the lesser tuberosity. The biceps tendon may slip in and out of its groove following a proximal humerus fracture that included dislocation of the lesser tuberosity with malunion or non-union. Patients with this instability have pain with internal rotation of the humerus.

In the past, some thought that the transverse ligament was the primary stabilizer and that, if lax, the biceps tendon would sublux with the arm in abduction and external rotation. However, three studies have shown that the tendons of the rotator cuff in close proximity to the rotator interval are the primary restraint to tendon subluxation. A cadaveric study found that subluxation only occurred when the supraspinatus and subscapularis tendons were torn [135].

Clinically, most patients that are diagnosed with biceps tendon subluxation could also have a concomitant rotator cuff lesion that allows medial subluxation. This is a common finding in the population over 50 years of age but occasionally occurs in a young athlete [137]. Therefore, the goal of treatment should be to repair the rotator interval defect and thereby eliminate the source of the instability.

Sporadically, an isolated subscapularis tear will be present due to excessive external rotation at the joint [137]. The biceps tendon can also sublux under these conditions with the medial restraint to subluxation disrupted. During a diagnostic arthroscopy, the biceps would be intact but will exit the joint at a much lower position (3–4 o'clock) instead of the typical position (2 o'clock). Surgical treatment usually includes repair of the subscapularis to its normal insertion on the lesser tuberosity. The biceps tendon may be stable following this procedure; however, if instability persists, a biceps tenodesis is warranted.

SLAP lesions

In the late 1980s and early 1990s, Synder and coworkers began to describe a lesion of the superior labral complex that included the biceps tendon [6]. This pathologic finding was called a SLAP (*superior labrum anterior to posterior*) lesion. Following review of over 700 shoulder arthroscopies, 20 patients had varying degrees of this SLAP lesion. The most common mechanism of injury was a fall on an outstretched arm that was forward and elevated, similar to the injury mechanism in posterior instability cases. Other lesions appear to be due to a sudden contraction of the biceps tendon that avulses the superior labrum from the glenoid.

The injuries have been classified into four categories [6] (Fig. 6.6.31).

1 Type I lesion. Superior labrum appears frayed and degenerated. The biceps tendon anchor is normal.

2 Type II lesion. Pathologic detachment of the superior labrum and biceps anchor. The superior labrum may also be frayed.

3 Type III lesion. Vertical tear through a meniscoid-like superior labrum, producing a bucket-handle lesion that may displace into the glenohumeral joint. The biceps anchor and remaining labrum are intact.

4 Type IV lesion. Vertical tear of the superior meniscoid-like labrum that extends into the biceps tendon. The biceps anchor and the remainder of the superior labrum are well attached.

Although uncommon, these lesions may be a source of significant disability since they are difficult to diagnose. Labral tears are frequently associated with other pathology such as instability and rotator cuff tears; therefore these entities need to be ruled out [138]. The most common complaint from patients is overhead pain and a 'popping or clicking' sensation. These symptoms are non-specific and the history may be more consistent with a diagnosis of impingement syndrome, biceps tendinitis or glenohumeral instability. However, patients may also complain of pain while attempting forward flexion with the arm supinated.

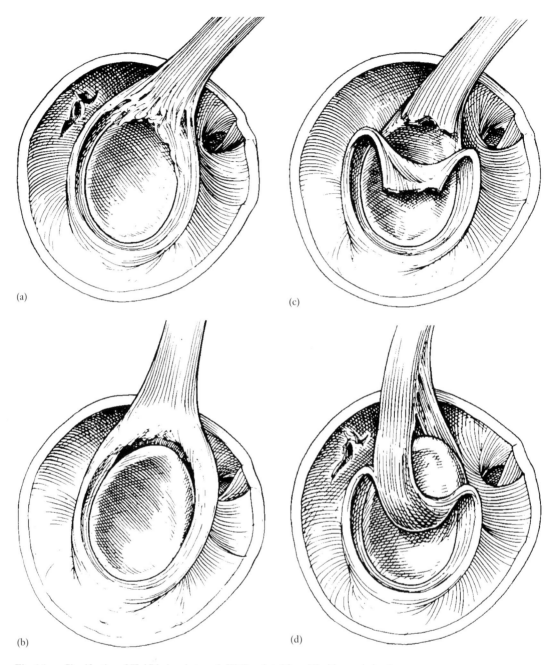

(a)

(b)

(c)

(d)

Fig. 6.6.31 Classification of SLAP lesions in types I–IV. (Reprinted from [6] with permission.)

Physical examination findings and diagnostic imaging techniques are also typically non-specific, with plain radiographic films providing no evidence of these lesions. On MRI the lesion is usually only visible if an arthrography is performed. Therefore, the ultimate diagnosis of labral pathology usually depends on performing an accurate diagnostic arthroscopy.

The treatment of SLAP lesions depends on the type

of labral pathology as previously described. The treatment of a type I lesion in a younger individual includes arthroscopic debridement of the degenerative tissue [138]. This procedure is usually performed with a shaver through the standard anterior and posterior arthroscopic portals. The ultimate goal of the treatment is to obtain an intact stable labrum and remove any source of joint irritation and possible 'catching' of loose tissue.

Surgical treatment of type II SLAP lesions must consider not only the torn labral tissue but reattachment of the biceps anchor to the neck of the superior glenoid. Management of these lesions has progressed over the years as surgical techniques and instrumentation have improved. Initially, simple debridement of the fibrous tissue and decortication of the superior glenoid neck were performed to induce an inflammatory response to restore the biceps anchor [138]. Several studies have reported successful results for the repair of type II SLAP lesions using various arthroscopic repair techniques. A transglenoid suture fixation technique was performed on 20 patients using absorbable monofilament sutures with good or excellent results at 21 months follow-up [139]. Yoneda and coworkers managed these lesions in 10 young athletes arthroscopically with abrasion and staple fixation and demonstrated that all lesions had healed. Others [140] have used titanium cannulated screws and absorbable tacks with the majority of patients showing improvements or returning to sports.

A type III SLAP lesion represents a bucket-handle tear with a meniscoid-type superior labrum and the biceps tendon is not involved. Therefore, the loose labral fragment must simply be excised to prevent pain and the 'popping or clicking' sensation. Debridement is usually performed using standard arthroscopic basket punches and shavers that access the region with the standard anterior and posterior portals. After resection of the loose labral tissue, the labrum and biceps anchor should be examined to verify that it is stable.

A type IV SLAP lesion is a type III lesion as well as a partially torn biceps tendon that can displace with the labral flap into the joint. The biceps anchor is usually firmly attached to the superior glenoid; however, the anchor may also become detached. Therefore this type of lesion becomes difficult to treat, especially in younger patients. If the segment of damaged biceps tendon is less than 10–15% of the tendon, then resection of the torn tissue should be sufficient to restore normal function [138]. When the tear of the biceps tendon is greater than 30% of the diameter, suture repair of the torn segment should be considered.

Acromioclavicular disease

The clavicle is the bony link between the arm and the rest of the body. Therefore, the clavicular joints are exposed to high loads during activity, especially during athletic activity. The acromioclavicular (AC) joint allows the scapula, together with the arm, to move in relation to the clavicle (Fig. 6.6.32). It is obvious that the scapula rotates in both the sagittal and the coronal (frontal) plane. However, knowledge is lacking with regard to the exact range of motion and loads on the AC joint.

Instability

Instability is usually a result of an acute injury. This type of trauma is not uncommon among e.g. skiers, cyclists, ice hockey players and wrestlers (Fig. 6.6.32). In cases with extreme hyperlaxity, AC (as well as sternoclavicular) instability may occur without trauma.

The classic trauma is a fall when the athlete is holding the arm in adduction. This will induce a force acting to push the shoulder downward. Since the clavicle is medially fixed to the sternum and rests on the rib cage, the clavicle cannot move downwards. Hence, the force will end up being a shear force over the AC joint and the adjacent coracoclavicular ligaments. If the force is strong enough, injury will occur in the joint and in the ligaments, the degree of injury being relative to the magnitude of the force. When dislocation is marked, the muscles normally attached onto the lateral clavicle may become injured and even detached.

AC dislocations are classified into at least three types. In rare cases the third type may be extremely dislocated. Therefore, a classification using six types is presented. In this classification type III is subdivided into types III–VI.

Type I

This is a distortion type of injury. It includes only partial injury to the joint and ligaments. Clinically there may be some swelling and always pain and tenderness

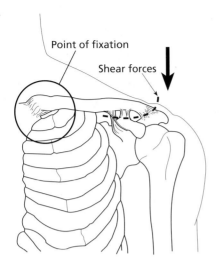

Fig. 6.6.32 The uninjured acromioclavicular joint with intact capsule, joint ligaments and coracoclavicular ligaments.

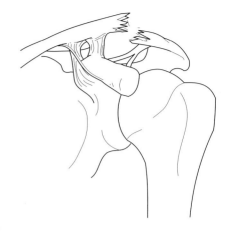

Fig. 6.6.33 Acromioclavicular dislocation type II: the coracoclavicular ligaments are intact.

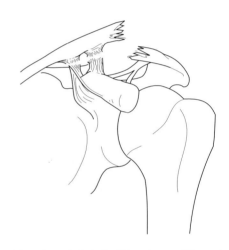

Fig. 6.6.34 Acromioclavicular dislocation type III: complete tearing of coracoclavicular ligaments.

over the AC joint. X-ray is normal. This injury usually heals uneventfully, even though residual symptoms (post-traumatic arthritis) may rarely ensue [141].

Type II (Fig. 6.6.33)
This subluxation includes disruption of the AC joint capsule and ligaments but intact coracoclavicular ligaments. The slight upwards migration of the distal clavicle may be obvious visually. X-ray confirms the upwards subluxation. Primary treatment is again purely symptomatic. Residual symptoms may indicate post-traumatic arthritis.

Type III (Fig. 6.6.34)
Complete rupture of both the AC joint and the coracoclavicular ligaments will result in a clear dislocation and upward migration of the clavicle, accompanied by a slight lowering of the rest of the shoulder. This is quite obvious on the exterior but X-rays must be taken in order to differentiate this from a lateral clavicular fracture.

Treatment of this injury is under constant debate. Most of these patients do well on conservative treatment [142–144] and the few who suffer from residual symptoms (pain, instability) are easy to treat surgically at some later time. Some consider doing only a lateral clavicular resection (a Mumford procedure) [144],

but if the patient suffers from an injury resulting in clavicular instability, then a stabilization should be performed. A lateral resection and reconstruction of the ligaments, a Weaver–Dunn procedure, usually works very well [145].

Type IV–IV injuries are basically a type III dislocation, but the degree of dislocation is much higher. These injuries are rare.

Type IV
The clavicle is displaced more cranially than normal.

Both clinically and on X-ray the displacement is marked. This indicates that the clavicular origin of the deltoid muscle is disrupted. Surgical repair is necessary.

Type V

Here the dislocation is obvious and the lateral end of the clavicle is displaced posteriorly. It may even penetrate the trapezius muscle belly. Usually also the deltoid is detached. Open reduction and repair is necessary.

Type VI

Rare displacement of the clavicle. It is hooked under the coracoid process. Surgery with open reduction is indicated [146].

Overload injuries and degenerative changes

Athletes who include a large portion of weight-lifting in their strengthening exercises may trigger pain in the AC joint. This type of pain and AC problem appears under various names: weight lifter's shoulder, lateral osteolysis of the clavicle and AC arthritis (Fig. 6.6.35).

Overload problems in the AC joint have been described by several authors and not only in weight lifters [147–150]. When athletes other than lifters suffer from AC arthritis, this could simply be due to overambitious training programs. Clinical experience and scientific evaluation indicate that bench press is one of the most pain provoking exercises [151].

The clinical presentation of this problem is pain located to the superior aspect of the shoulder, quite often strictly around the AC joint. Sometimes swelling may be present. In the early stages of the disease X-ray is normal. Later, normal signs of degeneration are evident including subchondral bone cysts or demineralization of the lateral clavicle. MR imaging may reveal early changes, such as edema of the distal clavicle [152]. Pain relief following intra-articular injection of local anesthetics is typical.

Treatment of AC degeneration may be divided into three steps.

1 *Initial and moderate symptoms*: local or systemic use of non-steroidal anti-inflammatory medication and modification of training program.

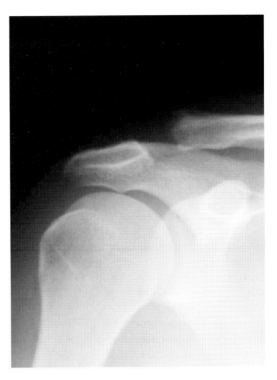

Fig. 6.6.35 X-ray showing osteolysis of the lateral end of the clavicle.

2 *Severe symptoms, normal X-ray*: local injection of corticosteroids and discontinuation of lifting.

3 *Failure of conservative treatment, X-ray changes*: surgical resection of the distal clavicle.

Surgical treatment consists of resection of the lateral end of the clavicle. This procedure may be performed both open or arthroscopically. This procedure is very rewarding, with the majority of the patients able to return to their preinjury level of lifting [153–156].

Soft tissue injuries

Muscle ruptures

Muscle injuries can be caused by strain or by a direct blow [157].

Muscle strain can be caused by excessive stretching or by violent contraction. Three types of response to injury exist: (i) delayed-onset muscle soreness; (ii) acute muscle soreness; and (iii) injury-related soreness [158]. Delayed-onset muscle soreness appears 12–48 h after exercise and results in tenderness on palpation, increased muscle stiffness and a reduction in range of motion. Acute muscle soreness is associated with a rapid onset of pain sensation within a minute of contraction followed by pain relief within 2–3 min after relaxation. Discoordination of antagonistic and agonist functions about a joint during rapid movement result from injury-related muscle soreness. These tendon and muscle strains can induce significant muscle fiber disruption and may produce a true inflammatory response.

Most of these injuries are not well identified and do not cause long-term disability unless a complete rupture of the muscle occurs. Loss of function, especially diminution of strength, has been the primary means of confirming muscular injury as well as palpable deficiencies and atrophy of the muscle substance [159]. The exact pathologic process has not been defined, since muscle strains rarely require surgical exposure for documentation of the process.

Muscle ruptures may be caused by: active contraction of the muscle; contraction of an antagonist; increase of tearing over cohesive power; asynchronic contraction; or additional muscle force provided by another muscle [160]. However, the most common cause of muscle rupture is an overload of an actively contracting muscle group due to the application of a resisting load or external force that exceeds tissue tolerance. The injury usually results in tearing of muscle fiber and the muscle sheath as well as a palpable defect in the muscle. These muscle defects can only heal by the formation of scar tissue with effective surgical repair being difficult to achieve.

Rupture of muscles at the shoulder is uncommon. However, lesions of the pectoralis major, deltoid, triceps, biceps, serratus anterior coracobrachialis and subscapularis have been described [161–166]. In general, the principles of treatment include repair in the acute phase whenever possible, that can be assisted by immobilization of the joint in a position that approximates the edges of the torn muscle. Protected exercise programs can then ensure optimal rehabilitation. Minor strains and partial lesions can be handled conservatively. The application of ice in the acute phase should be followed by heat and mobilization of the shoulder. Finally, stretching and mild strengthening exercises over 6 weeks will return the shoulder to normal function.

Tendinitis

Due to their prevalence in sports, injuries to tendons and their insertions have received considerable attention. These tissues commonly become inflamed due to overuse, leading to tendinitis. Their high strength allows them to withstand the forces placed upon them when muscles contract. However, they can fatigue with repetitive loading. Fatigue occurs most often at the tendon's attachment to bone where the blood supply is usually poor [167].

Rotator cuff tendinitis

Rotator cuff tendinitis is one of the most common injuries at all activity levels in sports with repetitive overhead motions [168]. The classical signs and symptoms of this pathology include crepitus and point tender pain at the anterior and lateral aspects of the shoulder with overhead motion and are relieved with the arm at the side. Two separate etiologies exist for these symptoms.

Symptoms in athletes under 35 years of age are usually due to subclinical or mildly overt instability of the glenohumeral joint due to anteroinferior or anterosuperior capsular and labral deficiencies [169]. These rotator cuff injuries have been termed 'secondary tensile overload injuries' since muscular weakness and imbalance lead to capsular and labral deficiencies [170,171]. Treatment should therefore begin with evaluation of flexibility and strength deficits and proceed to evaluation of the directional instability and include tests for competence of all rotator cuff muscles. Conservative treatment involves decreasing the activity level, range of motion exercises, and gradual strengthening of each muscle group, starting with the scapula and proceeding to the glenohumeral joint. The treatment regimen should be based on the complete analysis of all identified deficiencies [172] that involve tissue overload, tissue injury, clinical symptoms, functional biomechanical deficits, and subclinical adaptations.

Following 6–8 weeks of unsuccessful conservative

treatment, further evaluation may be required to determine whether it is a surgical case. CT arthrogram, MRI or ultrasonography could be used to find pathology in the glenohumeral joint and on the undersurface of the rotator cuff. Most of these cases do not involve the superior surface of the rotator cuff and subacromial space [172].

Older athletes commonly have joint pathology associated with rotator cuff impingement and degeneration. At X-ray many patients show changes in the acromioclavicular joint, subacromial area or greater tuberosity consistent with chronic wear. A pattern of strength imbalances may also be present even though tests for instability may be normal. Conservative treatment can be instituted if there are few indications of muscle tears. A complete diagnosis should be performed early in the treatment process to obtain accurate information regarding diagnosis, prognosis, treatment options and return to sports.

Biceps tendinitis

The long head of the biceps muscle extends intra-articularly under the acromion through the rotator cuff to its insertion on the superior rim of the glenoid. Bicipital tendinitis is produced by the same mechanisms that initiate impingement symptoms in rotator cuff injuries and can inflame the tendon in its subacromial location [158]. This condition can also be caused by subluxation of the tendon out of the bicipital groove on the proximal humerus due to rupture of the transverse ligament (see section on 'Biceps tendon instability', p. 716).

Symptoms of bicipital tendinitis are essentially the same whether due to impingement or tendon subluxation. Local pain is found at the proximal humerus and shoulder. Pain can occur during manual testing of the elbow flexors and during palpation of the tendon itself. Supination of the forearm may also aggravate pain since this is one of the primary functions of the biceps.

For bicipital tendinitis caused by impingement syndrome, treatment should be directed at the impingement syndrome, which may result in resolution of the tendinitis as well. Conservative treatment for bicipital tendinitis due to subluxation of the tendon includes restriction of activities followed by a slow resumption of activities. Strengthening muscles that assist the biceps in elbow flexion and forearm supination may also be helpful. For those patients whose symptoms persist, tenodesis of the biceps tendon or transplantation of the long head into the short head of the biceps may be considered for the older population [158]. However, full recovery from this procedure is difficult for even the highly competitive athlete.

Nerve entrapment syndromes

Thoracic outlet syndrome

Thoracic outlet syndrome is caused by compression of the nerves and vessels of the upper limb as they pass through the interval between the scalene muscles, over the first rib, and into the axilla. The complex pattern of signs and symptoms is significantly related to the posture of the shoulder girdle. The production of the symptoms was first determined in 1912 [173] and included the measurement of the inclination of the clavicle and first rib in different age groups and sexes as well as the descent of the scapula. The causes of thoracic outlet syndrome are now recognized as any pathology in the region of the shoulder complex that alters the posture of the scapula—traumatic or atraumatic [174]. Nerve compression may be the result of a clavicle fracture that reduces the space between the clavicle and first rib. Disuse of the shoulder due to pain or immobilization may cause atrophy of the trapezius, levator scapulae and rhomboids, thereby resulting in ptosis of the scapula.

Diagnostic criteria must be considered for thoracic outlet syndrome since the symptoms are often vague and subtle to the inexperienced examiner. A history often includes pain and parathesias that extend from the lateral aspect of the neck into the shoulder, down the arm, and into the medial aspect of the forearm as well as the little and ring finger of the hand. Symptoms may be experienced during night while trying to sleep or during activities of daily living that require a positional change such as raising the hand above the head. Other authors have suggested abducting and laterally rotating the arm at the shoulder while palpating the pulses at the wrist to reproduce the patient's symptoms [174]. Rapidly flexing and extending the fingers while holding the arm over the head can also cause symptoms within 20–30 s in a high percentage of cases (overhead exercise test).

Treatment of thoracic outlet syndrome should emphasize the reversal of the pathologic condition that is responsible for the nerve compression [175]. Muscle strengthening exercises and postural education can relieve the symptoms in patients with scapular ptosis and muscle atrophy. Physical expression of emotional depression through scapular ptosis should also be dealt with using psychotherapy or medication. However, the foundation of conservative management remains muscle strengthening and postural education. The rehabilitation program must consider each individual's needs and not provoke any further symptoms. A detailed description of the surgical procedures to relieve the compression of the neurovascular structures for patients with thoracic outlet syndrome is beyond the scope of this text since this is not a common procedure. However, several references exist that detail the techniques [176,177].

Quadrilateral space syndrome

The quadrilateral space lies laterally to the inferior border of the teres minor muscle. The posterior humeral circumflex artery and the axillary nerve travel within this space. The quadrilateral space syndrome was initially described in 1983 [178] and usually compromises axillary nerve function by fibrous bands in the quadrilateral space. In most cases function is limited when the arm is positioned in abduction and external rotation or the cocking phase of throwing. Patients can complain of posterior shoulder pain in the area of the teres minor muscle that is heightened by abduction and external rotation of the arm as well as direct tenderness. Diagnoses are most often confirmed with an arteriogram of the subclavian and axillary arteries. Initially the shoulder is placed in the neutral position and the posterior humeral circumflex artery is visualized. After repeated injections with the arm in abduction and external rotation the artery becomes no longer patent.

Rest and injections of cortisone may also prove to be helpful for athletes with this condition. However, if the problems persist, a surgical decompression of the quadrilateral space is warranted.

Suprascapular nerve entrapment

Suprascapular nerve entrapment is an often overlooked cause of shoulder pain. Proximal entrapment of the suprascapular nerve in the suprascapular notch beneath the transverse scapular ligament results in both supraspinatus and infraspinatus muscle weakness, whereas a more distal entrapment at the spinoglenoid notch involves only the infraspinatus muscle. The most frequent site of injury occurs at the point where the suprascapular nerve crosses the suprascapular notch near the transverse scapular ligament (Fig. 6.6.20).

Since its first description by Kopell in 1959 [179], several authors have reported suprascapular nerve entrapment in association with transverse ligament anomalies [180], trauma [181], fractures of the scapula [182], anterior shoulder dislocations [183] and rotator cuff ruptures [184]. The mechanism of injury occurs at the suprascapular notch secondary to the 'sling' effect [185]. The 'sling effect' involves the kinking of the suprascapular nerve against the suprascapular notch under the transverse scapular ligament during forceful throwing.

Another potential site of suprascapular nerve entrapment has been noted at the spinoglenoid notch, where the suprascapular nerve and artery enter the infraspinatus fossa to innervate the infraspinatus muscle [186]. Entrapment of the suprascapular nerve at the spinoglenoid notch is rare, and much less common than at the suprascapular notch, which has been reported to have an incidence of 0.4% [187]. The inferior transverse scapular ligament or spinoglenoid ligament has been described as acting to entrap the suprascapular nerve in volleyball players [188], throwing athletes including baseball pitchers [189], and weight lifters [190].

In the athletic population, this syndrome may appear to be tendinitis but on closer examination the surgeon notices atrophy of the infraspinatus muscle [191]. Surgical treatment of suprascapular nerve entrapment has been variable and return of muscle function is not always good. If the infraspinatus muscle is not completely denervated, some athletes have been able to return to throwing by using the remaining function of the infraspinatus muscle.

Bursitis

Bursae are sacs formed by two layers of synovial tissue that are located at sites where friction exists between tendon and bone. They normally contain a thin layer of joint fluid and can become inflamed from repetitive friction with the overlying tendon or external pressure. This inflammation, called bursitis, causes swelling from an increase in fluid in the bursa. If the inflammation is prolonged, the walls of the bursae may thicken, and sometimes the adjacent tendon degenerates or becomes calcified, causing a chemical bursitis.

Bursitis of the shoulder refers to inflammation of the subacromial bursa. Inflammation of this bursa is generally secondary to shoulder impingement, and therefore both the signs and symptoms and the treatment are similar [158]. Rotator cuff strengthening and stretching exercises may reduce the symptoms. With return of the cuff's normal function, there is greater room under the acromial arch, and less impingement and irritation occur.

Scapulothoracic problems

The scapula and its muscles—the scapula stabilizing muscles, the rotator cuff and the deltoid—is the most important link between the arm and the body. The energy which is created by the muscles in the lower extremity and the spine during overhead sports is essential for forceful overhead activity. So the scapula and its muscles not only transfer these large amounts of energy from the lower part of the body to the arm, but are also a solid base for the energy created in the shoulder and arm, and at the same time control the dynamic motions in the thoracoscapular junction. This is a very difficult task, with extreme demands on muscular strength and requiring a very fine coordination between muscles.

So it is not surprising that dysfunction of the scapular muscles can be demonstrated in most pathologic conditions of the shoulder. For instance, in primary subacromial impingement, the deltoid muscle has reduced activity during motion of the arm [192]. This seems like a rational change of muscular function, as it reduces the superior motion of the humeral head during abduction, thereby reducing the impingement. On the other hand, in overhead athletes with impingement, a reduced function of the anterior serratus and lower trapezius muscles can be demonstrated

[193,194]. This seems irrational, as these muscles elevate the scapula during overhead activity, consequently creating dynamic impingement if they function with reduced activity (that is that the acromion is not in tune to prevent collision with the humeral head).

It is not known to what extent scapular dysfunction causes shoulder problems. Swimmers with a unilateral breathing technique often have a reduced scapular tilting during strokes on the side on which they breathe, and a higher incidence of impingement in the same shoulder [195]. This is an example of a scapular dysfunction causing shoulder pain. However, many cases of scapular dysfunction are probably secondary to pathologic shoulder conditions.

The most common pathologic finding in an athlete's scapula is instability, which shows clinically as fatigue of some of the scapula stabilizing muscles and thereby as disturbance in the coordination of the muscles during motion. Often this condition is symptom free. It can be demonstrated by asking the athlete to perform repeated elevations of the arm. After a number of elevations fatigue occurs in the weakest muscles, demasking a dyscoordination of muscles which is obvious by examination of the scapular motion from behind.

If this dysfunction is a part of a shoulder problem, it is often treated with scapula stabilizing exercises in addition to specific treatment of the shoulder problem. It is not known whether strengthening of the scapular stabilizers by training can prevent shoulder problems in athletes.

It is strange that pain from the scapulothoracic junction is infrequent among athletes when the high frequency of scapular dysfunction is taken into consideration. A quite rare condition is the snapping scapula, in which the scapulothoracic motion is painful and often even crepitating. It usually starts gradually and may be caused by bony or soft tissue abnormalities. The crepitus is obvious during examination, and in most patients there is tenderness at the superomedial angle of the scapula.

X-rays are usually normal. CT scans may show exostosis or other bony deformities, but a three-dimensional CT scan reconstruction should also be performed, as many cases of incongruency between scapular and the thoracic cage can only be visualized in this way [65]. If no incongruency can be demonstrated, the condition may be caused by acute or chronic bursitis of the scapulothoracic bursa, which theoretically should be visible on MRI, or it could be caused by dynamic impingement in the scapulothoracic junction caused by dyscoordination of the scapular muscles.

The treatment depends on the pathophysiology in each case. If a specific mechanical reason such as a spur after a fracture or an exostosis can be demonstrated, it should be corrected surgically. In the case of bursitis, conservative treatment is often successful, consisting of corticosteroid injections into the bursa, NSAIDs, rest and strengthening of the scapular stabilizers [196].

Surgical treatment has traditionally been performed by open operation, but during the 1990s scopic treatment has taken over as first choice. Scopically the bursa can be cleaned up or bony deformities can be resected. If the superomedial angle of the scapula is protruding, it can be resected by open operation. The prognosis is good, as most athletes are able to return to their sports [196].

Rehabilitation of the shoulder

The goal in rehabilitation is to restore normal function and to prevent new injury. In sports medicine this goal does not only concern everyday functions but also athletic activity, often on a very high level. This makes rehabilitation very demanding. On the other hand, the patient is a highly motivated athlete who is very willing to participate. Sometimes the problem is to guide him or her to follow the protocol and prevent too much training which can lead to overload problems.

The main goal is of course to get the athlete back to the desired sport at the desired level. Before doing this, goals to achieve during successful rehabilitation are:
• pain-free activity;
• full range of motion;
• full strength; and
• neuromuscular control.

The first things to assess are the following:
• activity analysis (by therapist, patient and trainer);
• motion analysis—during sports activity and during examination;
• which demands the athlete must meet during sport activity;

• the patient's technique—should be assessed together with trainer;
• the patient's daily training activities (individual and team activities).

The basic principles of shoulder rehabilitation are the same as in other rehabilitation protocols:
• a stepwise increase in activity;
• initial rest, reduction in pain and inflammation;
• positioning and control of movements of the scapula;
• increase in range of motion exercises and pain-free isometric exercises;
• concentric and eccentric training, endurance and proprioception;
• functional sports exercises.

In sports medicine it is necessary to implement individual protocols in close cooperation with the athlete himself and his athletic trainer or coach.

In the following text, some aspects are supported by scientific studies, whereas other statements are based on clinical experience.

Shoulder-specific considerations (Table 6.6.5)

In almost every overhead activity overloading of tissue occurs during either cocking, acceleration, deceleration or the follow-through phase.

In the early cocking phase external rotation may be 180°. During acceleration the angular velocity of the humerus is up to 7500°/s [197]. This means that limitation in external rotation will drastically reduce throwing capacity. To achieve such high angular velocity, the internal rotators must be plyometrically stretched and then produce a high concentric, rotatory torque.

After ball release (during deceleration and follow-through) the arm must be decelerated to 0°/s without distraction of the shoulder joint. This means that the rotator cuff muscles in particular must produce a high torque and compressive forces on the shoulder joint. Especially during follow-through the scapular stabilizers are highly active, including trapezius and rhomboids. They act eccentrically to slow scapular protraction [198]. If muscle function is insufficient, the arm will still decelerate, but by means of distracting forces on the shoulder joint. These forces will eventually result in overstretching of the capsuloliga-

Table 6.6.5 Basic protocol before designing shoulder rehabilitation program.

Cause	*Assess previous:*	
	repetitive activity	
	end-range loading	
	incorrect technique	
	training plan lacking	
	wrong type of training	
	monotonous loading	
	too high loading	
	injury	
	too early return to sports	
	incorrect equipment	
Goals	*Assess desired level of:*	
	loading	
	technique	
	strength	
	range of motion	
	endurance	
	speed	
Examination	*Assess the following variables:*	
	Range of motion	tightness
		laxity
	Body balance	proximal stability
	Shoulder positioning	head centered throughout range of motion?
		humeroscapular rhythm
		kinetic chain
	Muscle function	tightness
		imbalance
		strength
		endurance

mentous structures and instability may occur. Also, fatigue in rotator muscles has been shown by Wickiewicz *et al.* [199] to result in an inability to prevent the humeral head migrating superiorly even during simple abduction of the arm. This could induce an impingement syndrome.

Rehabilitation after overuse injuries

The main idea during shoulder rehabilitation is to consider active stability and the patient's ability to keep the humeral head centred on the glenoid [200]. It is important for the therapist to keep this in mind [201,202] when designing and testing various exercises, and also important to educate the patient on this matter.

The patient usually suffers from a longstanding painful inflammation. Both range of motion (ROM), muscle strength and other functional qualities (neuromuscular control, endurance, proprioception, etc.) are reduced. Most patients have elongation of anterior structures (capsule and ligaments) with hypermobility in external rotation and posterior tightness with limited internal rotation. Weakening of the rotator cuff and the scapulothoracic muscle is also common. These findings are guidelines for the following rehabilitation program [203,204]. The rate of progression through the following protocol may vary according to the type of injury, sport and individual factors (age, health, tissue response, etc.). During the entire rehabilitation period it is important to keep training the uninjured parts of the body.

Phase I

The rehabilitation during this first phase is guided by the symptoms. Avoidance of pain is one of the major concerns of the program for this phase. Another is aerobic training and keeping close contact with the athletic trainer and the rest of the team.

The goals are to reduce pain by reducing inflammation, to improve ROM, to increase neuromuscular control (scapular positioning, centering of humeral head), to prevent muscular atrophy, and to give patient education, including information about anatomy and biomechanics.

Treatment consists of:
• anti-inflammatory therapy;
• rest from painful activity;

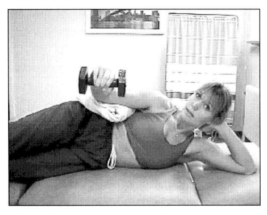

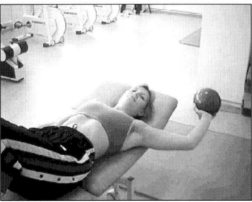

Fig. 6.6.36 External rotation exercise with the patient supine. This can later be expanded to a standing position and with gradual increase in range and abduction.

• guided ROM exercises (Fig. 6.6.36);
• stretching of tight structures (usually posterior capsule); and
• scapulothoracic strengthening.

The rotator cuff and the scapular muscles are critical to shoulder stabilization. Therefore, they must be strengthened first, before other muscle groups. Scapular setting is described as the dynamic orientation of the scapula in a position to optimize the position of the glenoid. This will allow maximal mobility and stability at the glenohumeral joint.

Phase II

Pain should not be a problem, except for truly provocative positions. Therefore, rehabilitation may be more aggressive but still on a much lower level than normal athletic training. Patient education is continued in order to prevent the athlete from increasing the training level too much.

The goals are to gain full pain-free ROM, to increase muscular strength, and to increase neuromuscular control (keeping the scapula positioned and humeral head centred in a greater ROM).

Treatment consists of:
• stretching to end-range;
• concentric and eccentric strengthening with elastic bands or tubing and later light free weights;
• neuromuscular training in everyday situations; and
• strengthening of the kinetic chain.

All muscles of the rotator cuff should be individually strengthened to facilitate optimal recovery. The serratus anterior (Fig. 6.6.37) and trapezius are the most important muscles for providing stability of the scapulothoracic joint. The biceps brachii must not be neglected since it has an important decelerating and stabilizing function on the glenohumeral joint.

Phase III

This phase includes more advanced strengthening exercises. The athlete must have a normal ROM and be able to perform normal activities of daily living without any symptoms. Team work including the trainer is of increasing importance.

The goals are full strength and increased endurance, enabling the athlete to return to low-demand athletic activities, and mastering of adequate technique and coordination in the kinetic chain.

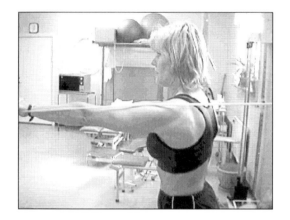

Fig. 6.6.37 Serratus anterior training, standing. This exercise may be started during phase I, but then in the supine position and with minimal load. The patient is instructed to fully protract the scapula by reaching forward.

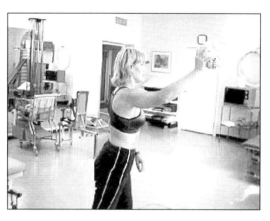

Fig. 6.6.39 Throwing with different types of objects helps to promote technique, power, speed and endurance whilst maintaining full control on the kinetic chain.

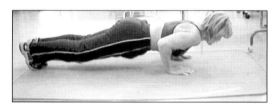

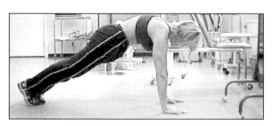

Fig. 6.6.38 Push-ups. The push-ups are performed with an extra push to the ceiling to allow full protraction. This exercise may also be used during phase I but then with much lower loads, practiced against the wall.

Treatment consists of:
• advanced strengthening exercises including eccentric, high-speed, high-energy training and in provocative positions (Fig. 6.6.38);
• submaximal sport activities (e.g. thrower's program);
• plyometric training using different weighted balls; and
• technique exercises.

Phase IV

When this phase is finished the athlete will be in full symptom-free activity. Emphasis must be put on *maintaining* full athletic capacity. This means making the necessary technique modifications and also including prophylactic exercises.

Goals are normal endurance and speed and full return to sports, including preventive training.

Treatment includes:
• continuation of most exercises from phase III but even more aggressively with more repetitions and longer series (Fig. 6.6.39);
• cooperation with the athletic trainer in designing a prophylactic program.

Rehabilitation after traumatic injuries

This protocol may be varied greatly since very different traumatic injuries occur. Therefore, it is important to consider a number of factors before designing the individual rehabilitation program.

Factors to consider include:
• the type of injury, especially if instability may occur;
• the patient's desired activity level and type of sports activity (overhead?); and
• the type of patient: musculature, proprioceptive capacity, dynamic stability, ROM, laxity/hyperlaxity, reaction to previous injuries.

If the injury is a dislocation of the glenohumeral

joint, most reports state that rehabilitation will not reduce the risk for recurrence. Only very few reports suggest the opposite [205].

The stepwise increase in activity is similar to the program following overuse injuries. However, usually the phases are shorter and rehabilitation may progress more rapidly.

Phase I

Immediately it is important to minimize inflammation and pain which may prolong the initial phase. Ice should be used frequently, rest with the arm in neutral rotation and slight abduction.

Goals are to reduce pain and inflammation, to prevent negative effects of rest, an early start of ROM exercises and maintenance of aerobic capacity of uninjured parts.

Treatment includes:
• isometric contractions;
• active-assisted or active ROM exercises below the shoulder, especially in abduction. External rotation should not exceed 30°; and
• scapular stabilizers.

Phase II

Since pain usually is reduced, strengthening and stretching activities may be initiated. Humeroscapular rhythm should be normal.

Goals are normal ROM including external rotation, normalized strength and increasing neuromuscular control.

Treatment includes:
• strengthening using elastic band, tubing or light free weights, including rotations up to 90°;
• rowing; and
• diagonal exercises.

Phase III

Speed and load will be increased in all exercises. Provocative positions may be used but pain or apprehension must be respected. Low-demand athletic activity should be included in cooperation with the trainer.

Goals are full dynamic stability and gradually increased sports activity.

Treatment includes:
• advanced strengthening exercises including eccen-

tric, high-speed, high-energy training and in provocative positions, plyometric exercises; and
• submaximal sports activity.

Phase IV

During this phase the athlete gradually returns to normal activity. This means even closer contact with the trainer. Normal athletic activity is gradually resumed, including a normal strengthening program. Since horizontal abduction and external rotation are the most provocative positions they are slowly progressed to normal.

Summary

Shoulder problems in athletes are mainly seen with overhead sporting activities, e.g. throwing and swimming, in which they are common.

The main problems are *impingement* (subacromial or internal glenohumeral collision with painful squeezing of the supraspinatus tendon), *instability* (either traumatic with dislocation of the glenohumeral ligaments, non-traumatic with stretching of the capsule and glenohumeral ligaments because of chronic overloading, or in athletes with dysfunction of the muscular stabilizers), *rotator cuff overuse or tearing*, and *labral tearing*. Acromioclavicular joint instability or degeneration, and soft tissue overuse or trauma are also regularly seen in athletes.

This chapter has provided a basic introduction to shoulder anatomy, dynamic function, clinical examination and imaging modalities. The clinical pictures of the various shoulder problems in athletes have been presented, including discussions about pathophysiology, diagnosis, treatment and prognosis. In the section on rehabilitation, strengthening exercises for the rotator cuff and scapular muscles were shown, and basic principles for rehabilitation and prevention discussed.

With clinical and experimental observations, arthroscopy and new imaging modalities, we have gained an increasing insight into shoulder problems in athletes over the past decade. This trend will probably continue.

Case story 6.6.1

A 22-year-old female has played handball for more than 10 years, and has developed pain in the back of her right shoulder extending out laterally in the arm during the last year. No trauma. In the beginning, there was no constant pain, but only pain when she was shooting, particularly during maximal outward rotation and abduction (late cocking phase) and when the arm moved foreward with maximal power (acceleration phase). Gradually pain had become constant, waking her at night. She had not been able to play for 6 months. She had normal active and passive movement of the shoulder, no pain during Neer's and Hawkins' impingement tests, pain in the posterior part of the shoulder with maximal abduction and outward rotation but negative apprehension test, and a sulcus sign (which was not found in the other shoulder).

X-rays showed small cysts in the greater tuberosity. These were also found on MRI in addition to degeneration of the supraspinatus close to the insertion on the humeral head.

Arthroscopy showed fraying of the undersurface of the supraspinatus tendon just medial for the insertion, but no inflammation. The superior labrum was torn and had a horizontal lesion behind the biceps tendon, but the tendon was attached to the glenoid. The humeral head was anterior–inferior unstable, but there was no Bankart lesion.

Diagnosis: Interior impingement, stage 3. It is likely, that the right shoulder originally was as stable as the left. As there was no Bankart lesion in the right shoulder, the instability was either present before or secondary to the internal impingement.

Treatment: Debridement of the tendon and the labrum plus a capsular shift to stabilize the glenohumeral joint. After 6 months she was free of symptoms and able to play handball again, but at a lower level.

Case story 6.6.2

A 27-year-old weight lifter gradually developed anterior pain in his left shoulder, extending out anterolateral in the arm. He had pain when weight-lifting, but also in his daily life, lifting shopping bags, during sleep, or working with the arm above horizontal. There were few degrees reduction in flexion, but otherwise normal movements of the shoulder. He had good power in all rotator cuff muscles, but pain when abducting with power against resistance. Neer's and Hawkins' tests were positive, as was the acromioclavicular joint compression test. There was tenderness of the AC-joint. The shoulder was stable.

X-rays of the acromioclavicular joint showed degenerative disease with cysts in the lateral clavicle. On outlet view there was a small spur from the joint, but a flat (type 1) acromion. These findings were also seen on MRI, which also showed a hypertrophic acromioclavicular joint compressing the supraspinatus tendon.

At arthroscopy the humeroscapular joint was normal, except for synovitis on the anterior undersurface of supraspinatus. There was extensive subacromial fibrosis. After cleaning up, the supraspinatus looked intact. The clavicle was hypermobile, protruding 10 mm under the acromion with compression from above, and there was no cartilage at the end of the clavicle.

Diagnosis: Acromioclavicular degeneration complicated with primary impingement.

Treatment: Cleaning up in the subacromial space, flattening of the acromion, leaving the coracoacromial ligament intact. Resection of 15 mm of the lateral clavicle and spurs under the acromioclavicular joint. After 4 months he was free of symptoms and started weightlifting again.

Multiple choice questions

1 *The arm can only abduct actively to 50°. This is seen with (3 out of 5 are correct):*

a a complete supraspinatus tear

b a complete subscapularis tear

c primary subacromial impingement

d acute anterior shoulder dislocation

e acromioclavicular joint dislocation.

2 *In secondary impingement (2 out of 5 are correct):*

a Symptoms are caused by osteophytes on the acromion's undersurface.

b Surgical treatment is often necessary and should be the first choice.

c The apprehension test is usually positive.

d Overhead sporting activity is an important factor for the development of symptoms.

e There are typical findings on MRI.

3 *Which (3 out of 5) are correct:*

a The apprehension and relocation tests are best performed with the patient supine.

b The agreement between several examiners about the result of shoulder testing is usually pretty good.

c Neer's dropping sign, the lift-off test and the hornblower's sign are sensitive for tears of infraspinatus, subscapularis and teres minor.

d In rotator cuff tears ultrasound is valuable to determine the tear, but also to visualize the degree of fatty degeneration in the muscle.

e The anteroposterior X-ray of the shoulder is taken with the other side of the body rotated 30° anterior.

4 *With impingement (2 out of 5 are correct):*

a Pain from primary subacromial impingement is usually felt just around the acromioclavicular joint.

b Subacromial impingement can be caused by extensive rotator cuff activity, e.g. body-building.

c Internal impingement is typical in weight-lifting.

d Reduced activity of the anterior serratus and lower trapezius muscles (scapular elevators) can often be demonstrated during motion in patients with impingement.

e Acromioplasty is the operation of choice in patients with secondary impingement who have not responded to physiotherapy.

References

1 Backx FJG, Erich WBM, Kemper ABA, Verbeek ALM. Sports injuries in school-aged children. *Am J Sports Med* 1989; **17**: 234–40.

2 Collins K, Wagner M, Peterson K, Storey M. Overuse injuries in triathletes. *Am J Sports Med* 1989; **17**: 675–80.

3 Lo YPC, Hsu YCS, Chan KM. Epidemiology of shoulder impingement in upper arm sports events. *Br J Sports Med* 1990; **24**: 173–7.

4 Bak K, Faunl P. Clinical findings in competitive swimmers with shoulder pain. *Am J Sports Med* 1997; **25**: 254–60.

5 McMaster WC, Troup J. A survey of interfering shoulder pain in United States competitive swimmers. *Am J Sports Med* 1993; **21**: 67–70.

6 Snyder SJ, Karzel RP, Del Pizzo W, Ferkel RD, Friedman MJ. SLAP lesions of the shoulder. *Arthroscopy* 1990; **6**: 274–9.

7 Inman VTM, Saunders M, Abbott LC. Observations on the function of the shoulder joint. *J Bone Joint Surg (Am)* 1944; **42-A**: 1–30.

8 Brewer BJ, Wubben RC, Carrera GF. Excessive retroversion of the glenoid cavity. A cause of nontraumatic posterior instability of the shoulder. *J Bone Joint Surg (Am)* 1986; **68-A**: 724–31.

9 Hurley JA, Anderson TE, Dear W, Andrish JT, Bergfeld JA, Weiker GG. Posterior shoulder instability. Surgical versus conservative results with evaluation of glenoid version. *Am J Sports Med* 1992; **20**: 396–400.

10 Saha AK. Dynamic stability of the glenohumeral joint. *Acta Orthop Scand* 1971; **42**: 491–505.

11 Randelli M, Gambrioli PL. Glenohumeral osteometry by computed tomography in normal and unstable. *Clin Orth Rel Res* 1986; **208**: 151–6.

12 Saha AK. Mechanics of elevation of glenohumeral joint. Its application in rehabilitation of flail shoulder in upper brachial plexus injuries and poliomyelitis and in replacement of the upper humerus by prosthesis. *Acta Orthop Scand* 1973; **44**: 668–78.

13 Soslowsky LJ, Flatow EL, Bigliani LU, Mow VC. Articular geometry of the glenohumeral joint. *Clin Orth Rel Res* 1992; **285**: 181–90.

14 Cooper DE, Arnoczky SP, O'Brien SJ, Warren RF, DiCarlo E, Allen AA. Anatomy, histology, and vascularity of the glenoid labrum. An anatomical study. *J Bone Joint Surg (Am)* 1992; **74-A**: 46–52.

15 DePalma AF, Callery G, Bennett GE. Variational anatomy and degenerative lesions of the shoulder joint. American Academy of Orthopaedic Surgeons Instructional Course Lectures. Blount WP. Ann Arbor 1949; 225–281.

16 Bankart AS. The pathology and treatment of recurrent dislocation of the shoulder joint. *Br J Surg* 1938; **26**: 23–9.

17 Bost FC, Inman VT. The pathological changes in recurrent dislocation of the shoulder. *J Bone Joint Surg (Am)* 1942; **24-A**: 595.

18 Lippitt SB, Vanderhooft JE, Harris SL, Sidles JA, Harryman DT, Matsen FA III. Glenohumeral stability from concavity-compression: a quantitative analysis. *J Shoulder Elbow Surg* 1993; **2**: 27–34.

19 Warner JJ, Bowen MK, Deng X, Torzilli PA, Warren RF. Effect of joint compression on inferior stability of the glenohumeral joint. *J Shoulder Elbow Surg* 1999; **8**: 31–6.

20 Warner JJ, Micheli LJ, Arslanian LE, Kennedy J, Kennedy R. Scapulothoracic motion in normal shoulders with glenohumeral instability and impingement syndrome. A study using Moire topographic analysis. *Clin Orth Rel Res* 1992; **285**: 191–9.

21 O'Brien SJ, Neves MC, Arnoczky SP, Rozbruck SR, Dicarlo EF, Warren RF, Schwartz R, Wickiewicz TL. The anatomy and histology of the inferior glenohumeral ligament complex of the shoulder. *Am J Sports Med* 1990; **18**: 449–56.

22 Ferrari DA. Capsular ligaments of the shoulder. Anatomical and functional study of the anterior superior capsule. *Am J Sports Med* 1990; **18**: 20–4.

23 McLaughlin HL. Repair of major cuff ruptures. *Surg Clinics N Am* 1963; **43**: 1535–40.

24 Neer CS II. Unconstrained shoulder arthroplasty. *Instruct Course Lect* 1985; **34**: 278–86.

25 Rowe CR, Zarins B. Recurrent transient subluxation of the shoulder. *J Bone Joint Surg (Am)* 1981; **63-A**: 863–72.

26 Warner JJP, Caborn DNM, Berger R, Fu FH, Seel M. Dynamic capsuloligamentous anatomy of the glenohumeral joint. *J Shoulder Elbow Surg* 1993; **2**: 115–33.

27 Boardman ND, Debski RE, Warner JJ *et al.* Tensile properties of the superior glenohumeral and coracohumeral ligaments. *J Shoulder Elbow Surg* 1996; **5**: 249–54.

28 Neer CS II, Foster CR. Inferior capsular shift for involuntary inferior and multidirectional instability of the shoulder. *J Bone Joint Surg (Am)* 1980; **62-A**: 897–908.

29 Neer CS II, Satterlee CC, Dalsey RM, Flatow EL. The anatomy and potential effects of contracture of the coracohumeral ligament. *Clin Orth Rel Res* 1992; **280**: 182–5.

30 Cooper DE, O'Brien SJ, Arnoczky SP, Warren RF. The structure and function of the coracohumeral ligament: An anatomic and microscopic study. *J Shoulder Elbow Surg* 1993; **2**: 70–7.

31 Patel PR, Imhoff A, Debski RE, Warner JJP, Fu FH, Woo SLY. Anatomy and biomechanics of the coracohumeral and superior glenohumeral ligaments. *Trans Orthopaed Res Soc* 1996; **21**: 702.

32 O'Brien SJ, Pagnani MJ, Fealy S, McGlynn SR, Wilson JB. The active compression test: a new and effective test for diagnosing labral tears and acromioclavicular joint abnormality. *Am J Sports Med* 1998; **26**: 610–3.

33 Turkel SJ, Panio MW, Marshall JL, Girgis FG. Stabilizing mechanisms preventing anterior dislocation of the glenohumeral joint. *J Bone Joint Surg (Am)* 1981; **63-A**: 1208–17.

34 Bigliani LU, Pollock RG, Soslowsky LJ, Flatow EL, Pawluk RJ, Mow VC. Tensile properties of the inferior glenohumeral ligament. *J Orth Res* 1992; **10**: 187–97.

35 Warren RF, Kornblatt IB, Marchand R. Static factors affecting posterior shoulder stability. *Orthop Trans* 1984; **8**: 89.

36 Fronek J, Warren RF, Bowen M. Posterior subluxation of the glenohumeral joint. *J Bone Joint Surg (Am)* 1989; **71-A**: 205–16.

37 Harryman DT, Matsen FA III, Sidles JA. Arthroscopic management of refractory shoulder stiffness. *Arthroscopy* 1997; **13**: 133–47.

38 Clark JM, Sidles JA, Matsen FA. The relationship of the glenohumeral joint capsule to the rotator cuff. *Clin Orth Rel Res* 1990; **254**: 29–34.

39 Colachis SC Jr, Strohm BR, Brechner VL. Effects of axillary nerve block on muscle force in the upper extremity. *Arch Phys Med Rehab* 1969; **50**: 647–54.

40 Howell SM, Imobersteg AM, Seger DH, Marone PJ. Clarification of the role of the supraspinatus muscle in shoulder function. *J Bone Joint Surg (Am)* 1986; **68-A**: 398–404.

41 Colachis SC Jr, Strohm BR. Effect of suprascapular and axillary nerve blocks on muscle force in upper extremity. *Arch Phys Med Rehab* 1971; **52**: 22–9.

42 Saha AK. *Theory of Shoulder Mechanism: Descriptive and Applied.* Springfield, IL: Charles C. Thomas, 1961.

43 Perry J. Biomechanics of the shoulder. In: Rowe CR, ed. *The Shoulder.* New York: Churchill Livingstone, 1988: 1–15.

44 Kumar VP, Satku K, Balasubramaniam P. The role of the long head of biceps brachii in the stabilization of the head of the humerus. *Clin Orth Rel Res* 1989; **244**: 172–5.

45 Glousman RE, Jobe FW, Tibone J, Moynes D, Antonelli DJ, Perry J. Dynamic electromyographic analysis of the throwing shoulder with glenohumeral instability. *J Bone Joint Surg (Am)* 1988; **70-A**: 220–226.

46 Codman EA. *The Shoulder.* Boston, MA: Thomas Todd, 1934.

47 Lephart S, Warner JJP, Borsa P, Fu FH. Proprioception of the shoulder joint in normal, unstable, and surgically repaired individuals. *J Shoulder Elbow Surg* 1994; **3**: 371–80.

48 Guanche C, Knatt T, Solomonow M, Lu Y, Baratta R. The synergistic action of the capsule and the shoulder muscles. *Am J Sports Med* 1995; **23**: 301–6.

49 Voigt M, Jakobsen J, Sinkjær T. Non-noxious stimulation of the glenohumeral joint capsule elicits strong inhibition of active shoulder muscles in conscious human subjects. *Neuroscience Lett* 1998; **254**: 105–8.

50 Gray H, Williams PL, Bannister LH. *Gray's Anatomy.* New York: Churchill Livingstone, 1995.

51 Lephart SM, Pincivero DM, Giraldo JL, Fu FH. The role of proprioception in the management and rehabilitation of athletic injuries. *Am J Sports Med* 1997; **25**: 130–7.

52 Gowan ID, Jobe FW, Tibone JE, Perry J, Moynes DR. A comparative electromyographic analysis of the shoulder during pitching. Professional versus amateur pitchers. *Am J Sports Med* 1987; **15**: 586–90.

53 Calis M, Akgün K, Birtane M, Karacan I, Calis H, Tüzün F. Diagnostic values of clinical diagnostic tests in subacromial impingement syndrome. *Ann Rheumatic Dis* 2000; **59**: 44–7.

54 Ure BM, Tiling T, Kirchner R, Rixen D. The value of clinical shoulder examination in comparison with arthroscopy. *Unfallchirurg* 1993; **96**: 382–6.

55 Bamji AN, Erhardt CC, Price TR, Williams PL. The painful shoulder: Can consultants agree? *Br J Rheum* 1996; **35**: 1172–4.

56 Levy AS, Lintner S, Kenter K, Speer KP. Intra- and interobserver reproducibility of the shoulder laxity examination. *Am J Sports Med* 1999; **27**: 460–3.

57 Nørregard J, Krogsgaard MR, Lorenzen T, Jensen EM. Difficulties in the classification of longstanding or severe shoulder pain. *Ann Rheum Dis* 2002; **61**: 646–9.

58 Kibler WB. Specificity and sensitivity of the anterior slide test in throwing athletes with superior glenoid labral tears. *Arthroscopy* 1995; **3**: 296–300.

59 Hertel R, Ballmer FT, Lambert SM, Gerber C. Lag signs in the diagnosis of rotator cuff rupture. *J Shoulder Elbow Surg* 1996; **5**: 307–13.

60 Walch G, Boulahia A, Calderone S, Robinson AHN. The 'dropping' and 'hornblower's' signs in evaluation of rotator-cuff tears. *J Bone Joint Surg (Brit)* 1998; **80-B**: 624–8.

61 Haygood TM, Langlotz CP, Kneeland JB, Iannotti JP, Williams GR Jr, Dalinka MK. Categorization of acromial shape: interobserver variability with MR imaging and conventional radiography. *Am J Radiol* 1994; **162**: 1377–82.

62 Dumontier C, Sautet A, Gagey O, Apoil A. Rotator interval lesions and their relation to coracoid impingement syndrome. *J Shoulder Elbow Surg* 1999; **8**: 130–5.

63 Hutchinson MR, Veenstra MA. Arthroscopic decompression of shoulder impingement secondary to os acromiale. *Arthroscopy* 1993; **9**: 28–32.

64 Riand N, Levigne C, Renaud E, Walch G. Results of derotational humeral osteotomy in posterosuperior glenoid impingement. *Am J Sports Med* 1998; **26**: 453–9.

65 Mozes G, Bickels J, Ovadia D, Dekel S. The use of three-dimensional computed tomography in evaluating snapping scapula syndrome. *Orthopedics* 1999; **22**: 1029–33.

66 Allmann K-H, Uhl M, Gufler H *et al*. Cine-MR imaging of the shoulder. *Acta Radiol* 1997; **38**: 1043–6.

66a Gerber C, Krushell RJ. Isolated rupture of the tendon of the subscapularis muscle. *J Bone Joint Surg (Brit)* 1991; **73-B**: 389–94.

67 Rossi F, Ternamian PJ, Cerciello G, Walch G. Posterior glenoid rim impingement syndrome in the athlete: diagnostic value of conventional radiology and of magnetic resonance imaging. *Radiol Med* 1994; **87**: 22–7.

68 Quinn SF, Sheley RC, Demlow TA, Szumowski J. Rotator cuff tendon tears: evaluation with fat-suppressed MR imaging with arthroscopic correlation in 100 patients. *Radiology* 1995; **195**: 497–500.

69 Goutallier D, Postel J-M, Bernageau J, Lavau L, Voisin M-C. Fatty muscle degeneration in cuff ruptures. *Clin Orth Rel Res* 1994; **304**: 78–83.

70 Fleckenstein JL, Watumull D, Conner KE *et al*. Denervated human skeletal muscle: MR imaging evaluation. *Radiology* 1993; **187**: 213–8.

71 Read JW, Perko M. Shoulder ultrasound: diagnostic accuracy for impingement syndrome, rotator cuff tear, and biceps tendon pathology. *J Shoulder Elbow Surg* 1998; **7**: 264–71.

72 Teefey SA, Hasan A, Middleton WD, Patel M, Wright RW, Yamaguchi K. Ultrasonography of the rotator cuff. A comparison of ultrasonographic and arthroscopic findings in one hundred consecutive cases. *J Bone Joint Surg (Am)* 2000; **82-A**: 498–504.

73 Schydlowsky P, Strandberg C, Galbo H, Krogsgaard M, Jørgensen U. The value of ultrasonography in the diagnosis of labral lesions in patients with anterior shoulder dislocation. *Eur J Ultrasound* 1998; **8**: 107–13.

74 Neer CS II. Anterior acromioplasty for the chronic impingement syndrome in the shoulder: a preliminary report. *J Bone Joint Surg (Am)* 1972; **54-A**: 41–50.

75 Neer CS II, Welsh RP. The shoulder in sports. *Orthop Clinics N Am* 1977; **8**: 583–91.

76 Pieper H-G, Radas CB, Krahl H, Blank M. Anatomic variation of the coracoacromial ligament: a macroscopic and microscopic cadaveric study. *J Shoulder Elbow Surg* 1997; **6**: 291–6.

77 Burns WC II, Whipple TL. Anatomic relationships in the shoulder impingement syndrome. *Clin Orth Rel Res* 1993; **294**: 96–102.

78 Blair B, Rokito AS, Cuomo F, Jarolem K, Zuckerman JD. Efficacy of injections of corticosteroids for subacromial impingement syndrome. *J Bone Joint Surg (Am)* 1996; **78-A**: 1685–9.

79 Bartolozzi A, Andreychik D, Ahmad S. Determinants of outcome in the treatment of rotator cuff disease. *Clin Orth Rel Res* 1994; **308**: 90–7.

80 Morrison DS, Frogameni AD, Woodworth P. Non-operative treatment of subacromial impingement syndrome. *J Bone Joint Surg (Am)* 1997; **79-A**: 732–7.

81 Brox JI, Gjengedal E, Uppheim G, Bohmer AS, Brevik JI, Ljunggren AE, Staff PH. Arthroscopic surgery versus supervised exercises in patients with rotator cuff disease (stage II impingement syndrome): a prospective, randomized, controlled study in 125 patients with a $2\frac{1}{2}$-year follow-up. *J Shoulder Elbow Surg* 1999; **8**: 102–11.

82 Bigliani LU, Rodosky MW, Newton PM. Arthroscopic coracoacromial ligament resection for impingement in overhead athletes. *J Shoulder Elbow Surg* 1995; **4**: 54.

83 Leroux JL, Mouilleron P, Bonnel F, Herbert P, Thomas E, Blotman F. Postoperative shoulder rotators strength in stages II and III impingement syndrome. *Clin Orth Rel Res* 1995; **320**: 46–54.

84 Ellman H. Arthroscopic subacromial decompression. Analysis of one to three-year results. *Arthroscopy* 1987; **3**: 173–81.

85 Parker RD, Seitz WH Jr. Shoulder impingement/instability overlap syndrome. *J Southern Orthopaedic Assoc* 1997; **6**: 197–203.

86 Payne LZ, Deng XH, Craig EV, Torzilli PA, Warren RF. The combined dynamic and static contributions to subacromial impingement. A biomechanical analysis. *Am J Sports Med* 1997; **25**: 801–8.

87 Glousman RE. Instability versus impingement syndrome in the throwing athlete. *Orthop Clinics N Am* 1993; **24**: 89–99.

88 Ruwe PA, Pink M, Jobe FW, Perry J, Scovazzo ML. The normal and painful shoulders during the breaststroke. Electromyographic and cinematographic analysis of twelve muscles. *Am J Sports Med* 1994; **22**: 789–96.

89 Wadsworth DJS, Bullock-Saxton JE. Recruitment patterns of the scapular rotator muscles in freestyle swimmers with subacromial impingement. *Int J Sports Med* 1997; **18**: 618–24.

90 Jobe FW, Bradley JP. The diagnosis and nonoperative treatment of shoulder injuries in athletes. *Clin Sports Med* 1989; **8**: 419–38.

91 Jobe FW, Giangarra CE, Kvinte RS, Glousman RE. Anterior capsulolabral reconstruction of the shoulder in athletes in overhand sports. *Am J Sports Med* 1991; **19**: 428–34.

92 Walch G, Liotard JP, Boileau P, Noel E. Postero-superior glenoid impingement. Another shoulder impingement. *Rev Chir Orthop Reparatr App Moteur* 1991; **77**: 571–4.

93 McFarland EG, Hsu C-Y, Neira C, O'Neil O. Internal impingement of the shoulder: a clinical and arthroscopic analysis. *J Shoulder Elbow Surg* 1999; **8**: 458–60.

94 Paley KJ, Jobe FW, Pink MM, Kvinte RS, El Attrache NS. Arthroscopic findings in the overhead throwing athlete: evidence for posterior internal impingement of the rotator cuff. *Arthroscopy* 2000; **16**: 35–40.

95 Walch G, Boileau P, Noel E, Donell ST. Impingement of the deep surface of the supraspinatus tendon on the posterosuperior glenoid rim: an arthroscopic study. *J Shoulder Elbow Surg* 1992; **1**: 238–45.

96 Halbrecht JL, Tirman P, Atkin D. Internal impingement of the shoulder: comparison of findings between the throwing and nonthrowing shoulders of college baseball players. *Arthroscopy* 1999; **15**: 253–8.

97 Noyes FR, Grood ES, Torzilli PA. The definitions of terms for motion and position of the knee and injuries of ligaments. *J Bone Joint Surg (Am)* 1989; **71-A**: 465–72.

98 Matsen FA, Thomas SC, Rockwood CA. Anterior glenohumeral instability. In: Rockwood CA, Matsen FA, eds. *The Shoulder*. Philadelphia: W.B. Saunders, 1990: 135–50.

99 Thomas SC, Matsen FA. An approach to the repair of the glenohumeral ligaments in the management of traumatic anterior glenohumeral instability. *J Bone Joint Surg (Am)* 1989; **71-A**: 506–13.

100 Allen AA. Clinical evaluation of the unstable shoulder. In: Warren RF, Craig EV, Altchek DW, eds. *The Unstable Shoulder*. Philadelphia: Lippincott-Raven Publishers, 1999: 93–106.

101 Bankart AS. Recurrent or habitual dislocation of the shoulder-joint. *Br Med J* 1923; **2**: 1132–3 reprinted in *Clin Orth Rel Res* 1993; **291**: 3–6.

102 Hill HA, Sachs MD. The grooved defect of the humeral head. *Radiology* 1940; **35**: 690.

103 Bacilla P, Field LD, Savoie FH. Arthroscopic Bankart repair in a high demand patient population. *Arthroscopy* 1997; **13**: 51–60.

104 Speer KP, Warren RF, Pagnani M, Warner JJP. An arthroscopic technique for anterior stabilization with a bioabsorbable tack. *J Bone Joint Surg (Am)* 1996; **78-A**: 1801–7.

105 Torchia ME, Caspari RB. Arthroscopic transglenoid multiple suture repair: 2–8 years results in 150 shoulders. *Arthroscopy* 1997; **13**: 609–19.

106 Buss DD, Green JR, Meyer RJ. Arthroscopic stabilization. An overview. In: Warren, RF, Craig, EV, Altchek, DW, eds. *The Unstable Shoulder*. Philadelphia: Lippincott-Raven Publishers, 1999: 93–106.

107 Alteck DW, Warren RF, Skybar MJ, Oritz G. T-plasty modification of the Bankart procedure for multidirectional instability of the anterior and inferior types. *J Bone Joint Surg (Am)* 1991; **73**: 105–12.

108 Bigliani LU, Kurzweil PR, Schwartzback CC, Wolfe I, Flatow EL. Inferior capsular shift procedure for anterior–inferior shoulder instability in athletes. *Am J Sports Med* 1994; **22**: 578–84.

109 Kvitne RS, Jobe FW, Jobe CM. Shoulder instability in the overhead or throwing athlete. *Clin Sports Med* 1995; **14**: 917–35.

110 Hovelius L, Eriksson K, Fredin H. Recurrence after initial dislocation of the shoulder. *J Bone Joint Surg (Am)* 1983; **65-A**: 343–9.

111 Simonet WT, Melton LJ, Cofield RH, Ilstrup DM. Incidence of anterior shoulder dislocation in the Olmstedt county, Minn. *Clin Orth Rel Res* 1984; **186**: 186–91.

112 Deberardino TM, Arciero RA, Taylor DC. Arthroscopic stabilization of acute initial shoulder dislocation. *J Southern Orthopaedic Assoc* 1996; **5**: 263–71.

113 Murphy TC. Shoulder injuries in swimming. In: Andrews JR, Wilk KE, eds. *The Athlete's Shoulder*. New York: Churchill Livingstone, 1994: 76–92.

114 Jobe FW, Tibone JE, Jobe CM, Kvitne RS. The shoulder in sports. In: Rockwood CA, Matsen FA, eds. *The Shoulder*. Philadelphia: W.B. Saunders, 1990: 961–90.

115 Hayashi K, Massa KL, Thabit G *et al*. Histological evaluation of the glenohumeral joint capsule after the laser-assisted capsular shift procedure for glenohumeral instability. *Am J Sports Med* 1999; **27**: 162–7.

116 Savoie FH, Field LD. Thermal versus suture treatment of symptomatic capsular laxity. *Clin Sports Med* 2000; **19**: 63–75.

117 Bowen MK, Warren RF. Injuries of the rotator cuff. In: Harries M, ed. *Oxford Textbook of Sports Medicine*. New York: Oxford University Press, 1994: 145–94.

118 Jobe FW, Moynes DR, Tibone JE, Perry J. An EMG

analysis of the shoulder in pitching. A second report. *Am J Sports Med* 1984; **12**: 218–20.

119 Meister K, Andrews JR. Classification and treatment of rotator cuff injuries in the overhand athlete. *J Orth Sports Phys Ther* 1993; **18**: 413–21.

120 Debeyre J, Patte D, Emelik E. Repair of ruptures of the rotator cuff with a note on advancement of the supraspinatus muscle. *J Bone Joint Surg (Brit)* 1965; **47-B**: 36–42.

121 Cofield RH. Rotator cuff disease of the shoulder. *J Bone Joint Surg (Am)* 1985; **67-A**: 974–9.

122 Samilson RL, Binder WF. Symptomatic full thickness tears of rotator cuff. An analysis of 292 shoulders in 276 patients. *Orthop Clinics N Am* 1975; **6**: 449–66.

123 Wolfgang GL. Rupture of the musculotendinous cuff of the shoulder. *Clin Orth Rel Res* 1978; **134**: 230–43.

124 Darlington LG, Coomes EN. The effects of local steroid injection for supraspinatus tears. *Rheumatol Rehabil* 1977; **16**: 172–9.

125 Itoi E, Tabata S. Conservative treatment of rotator cuff tears. *Clin Orth Rel Res* 1992; **275**: 165–73.

126 Matsen FA, Arntz CT, Lippitt SB. Rotator cuff. In: Rockwood CA, Matsen FA, Wirth MA, Harryman DT, eds. *The Shoulder*. Philadelphia: W.B. Saunders, 1998: 755–839.

127 Hawkins RJ, Misamore GW, Hobeika PE. Surgery for full-thickness rotator-cuff tears. *J Bone Joint Surg (Am)* 1985; **67-A**: 1349–55.

128 Bakalim G, Pasila M. Surgical treatment of rupture of the rotator cuff tendon. *Acta Orthop Scand* 1975; **46**: 751–7.

129 Nixon JE, DiStefano V. Ruptures of the rotator cuff. *Orthop Clinics N Am* 1975; **6**: 423–47.

130 Blevins FT, Hayes WM, Warren RF. Rotator cuff injury in contact athletes. *Am J Sports Med* 1996; **24**: 263–7.

131 Neer CS II. Impingement lesions. *Clin Orth Rel Res* 1983; **173**: 70–7.

132 Dejour D, Tayot O. La rupture isolée de la longue portion du biceps. Lyons, France: *Journées Lyonnaises de l'Epaule*, 1993.

133 Burkhead WZ Jr, Arcand MA, Zeman C, Habermeyer P, Walch G. The biceps tendon. In: Rockwood CA, Matsen FA, Wirth MA, Harryman DT, eds. *The Shoulder*. Philadelphia: W.B. Saunders, 1998: 1009–63.

134 O'Donoghue DH. Subluxing biceps tendon in the athlete. *Clin Orth Rel Res* 1982; **164**: 26–9.

135 Petersson CJ. Spontaneous medial dislocation of the tendon of the long biceps brachii. An anatomic study of prevalence and pathomechanics. *Clin Orth Rel Res* 1986; **211**: 224–7.

136 Walch G. Pathologie de la longue portion du biceps. *Conférence d'Enseignement de la SOFCOT*, Paris, 1993.

137 Bell RH, Noble JS. Biceps disorders. In: Hawkins RJ, Misamore GW, Huff TG. *Shoulder Injuries in the Athlete: Surgical Repair and Rehabilitation*. New York: Churchill Livingstone, 1996: 267–82.

138 Williams MM, Karzel RP, Synder SJ. Labral disorders. In: Hawkins RJ, Misamore GW, Huff TG, eds. *Shoulder In-juries in the Athlete: Surgical Repair and Rehabilitation*. New York: Churchill Livingstone, 1996: 291–306.

139 Field LD, Savoie FHD. Arthroscopic suture repair of superior labral detachment lesions of the shoulder. *Am J Sports Med* 1993; **21**: 783–90.

140 Resch H, Golser K, Thoeni H, Spencer G. Arthroscopic repair of superior glenoid labral detachment (the SLAP lesion). *J Shoulder Elbow Surg* 1993; **2**: 147–55.

141 Cox JS. The fate of the acromioclavicular joint in athletic injuries. *Am J Sports Med* 1981; **9**: 50–3.

142 Park JP, Arnold JA, Coker TP, Harris WD, Becker DA. Treatment of acromioclavicular separations. A retrospective study. *Am J Sports Med* 1980; **8**: 251–6.

143 Rawes ML, Dias JJ. Long-term results of conservative treatment for acromioclavicular dislocation. *J Bone Joint Surg (Brit)* 1996; **78-B**: 410–2.

144 Taft TN, Wilson FC, Oglesby JW. Dislocation of the acromioclavicular joint. An end-result study. *J Bone Joint Surg (Am)* 1987; **69-A**: 1045–51.

145 VanFleet TA, Bach B Jr. Injuries to the acromioclavicular joint. *Diagnosis Treatment Orthop Rev* 1994; **23**: 123–9.

146 Post M. Current concepts in the diagnosis and management of acromioclavicular dislocations. *Clin Orth Rel Res* 1985; **200**: 234–47.

147 Brunet ME, Reynolds MC, Cook SD, Brown TW. Atraumatic osteolysis of the distal clavicle: histologic evidence of synovial pathogenesis. A case report. *Orthopedics* 1986; **9**: 557–9.

148 Cahill BR. Osteolysis of the distal part of the clavicle in male athletes. *J Bone Joint Surg* 1982; **64-A**: 1053–8.

149 Stenlund B. Shoulder tendinitis and osteoarthritis of the acromioclavicular joint and their relation to sports. *Br J Sports Med* 1993; **27**: 125–30.

150 Stöhr H, Geyer M, Volle E. Osteolysis of the lateral clavicle after Tossy II injury in ice hockey players. *Sportverletz Sportschaden* 1996; **10**: 70–3.

151 Scavenius M, Iversen BF. Nontraumatic clavicular osteolysis in weight lifters. *Am J Sports Med* 1992; **20**: 463–7.

152 De la Puente R, Boutin RD, Theodorou DJ, Hooper A, Schwietzer M, Resnick D. Post-traumatic and stress-induced osteolysis of the distal clavicle: MR imaging findings in 17 patients. *Skeletal Radiol* 1999; **28**: 202–8.

153 Auge WK, Fischer RA. Arthroscopic distal clavicle resection for isolated atraumatic osteolysis in weight lifters. *Am J Sports Med* 1998; **26**: 189–92.

154 Cook FF, Tibone JE. The Mumford procedure in athletes. An objective analysis of function. *Am J Sports Med* 1988; **16**: 97–100.

155 Flatow EL, Cordasco FA, Bigliani LU. Arthroscopic resection of the outer end of the clavicle from a superior approach: a critical, quantitative, radiographic assessment of bone removal. *Arthroscopy* 1992; **8**: 55–64.

156 Snyder SJ, Banas MP, Karzel RP. The arthroscopic Mumford procedure: an analysis of results. *Arthroscopy* 1995; **11**: 157–64.

157 Solomonow M, D'Ambrosia R. Biomechanics of muscle overuse injuries: a theoretical approach. *Clin Sports Med* 1987; **6**: 241–57.

158 Surgeons, American Academy of Orthopaedic. The shoulder. Athletic training and sports medicine. Surgeons. Park Ridge, IL, American Academy of Orthopaedic Surgeons 1991: 253.

159 Caughey MA, Welsh P. Muscle ruptures affecting the shoulder girdle. In: Rockwood CA, Matsen FA, Wirth MA, Harryman DT, eds. *The Shoulder*. Philadelphia: W.B.Saunders, 1998: 1113–26.

160 Brickner WM, Milch H. Ruptures of muscles and tendons. In: *International Clinics; a Quarterly of Clinical Lectures*. Philadelphia: JB Lippincott, 1997: 106–75.

161 Anzel H, Covey KW, Weiner AD. Disruption of muscles and tendons. An analysis of 1014 cases. *Surgery* 1959; **45**: 406–14.

162 Heckman JD, Levine MI. Traumatic closed transection of the biceps brachii in the military parachutist. *J Bone Joint Surg (Am)* 1978; **60-A**: 369–72.

163 McEntire JE, Hess WE, Coleman SS. Rupture of the pectoralis major muscle. A report of eleven injuries and review of fifty-six. *J Bone Joint Surg (Am)* 1972; **54-A**: 1040–6.

164 Meythaler JM, Reddy NM, Mitz M. Serratus anterior disruption: a complication of rheumatoid arthritis. *Arch Phys Med Rehab* 1986; **67**: 770–2.

165 Symeonides PP. The significance of the subscapularis muscle in the pathogenesis of recurrent anterior dislocation of the shoulder. *J Bone Joint Surg (Brit)* 1972; **54-B**: 476–83.

166 Tarsney FF. Rupture and avulsion of the triceps. *Clin Orth Rel Res* 1972; **83**: 177–83.

167 Leadbetter WB, Buckwalter JA, Gordon SL. *Sports-Induced Inflammation: Clinical and Basic Science Concepts*. Park Ridge, IL: American Academy of Orthopaedic Surgeons, 1990.

168 Curwin S, Stanish WD. *Tendinitis: Its Etiology and Treatment*. Lexington, MA: Collamore Press, 1984.

169 Nirschl RP. Rotator cuff tendinitis: basic concepts of pathoetiology. *Instruct Course Lect* 1989; **38**: 439–45.

170 Jobe FW, Bradley JP. Rotator cuff injuries in baseball. *Prevention Rehabil Sports Med* 1988; **6**: 378–87.

171 Kibler WB. The role of the scapula in the throwing motion. *Contemp Orthop* 1991; **22**: 525–32.

172 Fu FH, Stone DA. *Sports Injuries: Mechanisms, Prevention, Treatment*. Baltimore, MD: Williams & Wilkins, 1994.

173 Todd TW. The descent of the shoulder after birth. *Anatomie* 1912; **14**: 41.

174 Leffert RD. Neurologic problems. In: Rockwood CA, Matsen FA, Wirth MA, Harryman DT, eds. *The Shoulder*. Philadelphia: W.B. Saunders, 1998: 965–88.

175 Jupiter JB, Leffert RD. Non-union of the clavicle. Associated complications and surgical management. *J Bone Joint Surg (Am)* 1987; **69-A**: 753–60.

176 Falconer MA, Li FWP. Resection of the first rib in costo-clavicular compression of the brachial plexus. *Lancet* 1962; **1**: 59.

177 Roos DB. Congenital anomalies associated with thoracic outlet syndrome. Anatomy, symptoms, diagnosis, treatment. *Am J Surg* 1976; **132**: 771–8.

178 Cahill BR, Palmer RE. Quadrilateral space syndrome. *J Hand Surg* 1983; **8**: 65–9.

179 Kopell HP, Walter AL, Thompson MD. Pain and the frozen shoulder. *Surg Gynecol Obstetr* 1959; **109**: 92–6.

180 Alon M, Weiss S, Fishel B, Dekel S. Bilateral suprascapular nerve entrapment syndrome due to an anomalous transverse scapular ligament. *Clin Orth Rel Res* 1988; **234**: 31–3.

181 Yoon TN, Grabois M, Guillen M. Suprascapular nerve injury following trauma to the shoulder. *J Trauma Injury Infect Crit Care* 1981; **21**: 652–5.

182 Solheim LF, Roaas A. Compression of the suprascapular nerve after fracture of the scapular notch. *Acta Orthop Scand* 1978; **49**: 338–40.

183 Zoltan JD. Injury to the suprascapular nerve associated with anterior dislocation of the shoulder: case report and review of the literature. *J Trauma Injury Infect Crit Care* 1979; **19**: 203–6.

184 Drez D Jr. Suprascapular neuropathy in the differential diagnosis of rotator cuff injuries. *Am J Sports Med* 1976; **4**: 43–5.

185 Rengachary SS, Burr D, Lucas S, Hassanein KM, Mohn MP, Matzke H. Suprascapular entrapment neuropathy: a clinical, anatomical, and comparative study. Part 2: anatomical study. *Neurosurgery* 1979; **5**: 447–51.

186 Ringel SP, Treihaft M, Carry M, Fisher R, Jacobs P. Suprascapular neuropathy in pitchers. *Am J Sports Med* 1990; **18**: 80–6.

187 Post M, Mayer J. Suprascapular nerve entrapment: diagnosis and treatment. *Clin Orth Rel Res* 1987; **223**: 126–36.

188 Holzgraefe M, Klingelhofer J, Eggert S, Benecke R. Zur chronischen Neuropathie des N. suprascapularis bei Hochleistungssportlern. *Nervenarzt* 1988; **59**: 545–8.

189 Glennon TP. Isolated injury of the infraspinatus branch of the suprascapular nerve. *Arch Phys Med Rehab* 1992; **73**: 201–2.

190 Black KP, Lombardo JA. Suprascapular nerve injuries with isolated paralysis of the infraspinatus. *Am J Sports Med* 1990; **18**: 225–8.

191 Jobe FW, Tibone JE, Pink MM, Jobe CM, Kvitne RS. The shoulder in sports. In: Rockwood CA, Matsen FA, Wirth MA, Harryman DT, eds. *The Shoulder*. Philadelphia: Saunders, 1998: 1214–38.

192 Michaud M, Arsenault AB, Gravel D, Tremblay G, Simard TG. Muscular compensatory mechanism in the presence of a tendinitis of the supraspinatus. *Am J Phys Med* 1987; **66**: 109–20.

193 Ludewig PM, Cook TM. Alterations in shoulder kinematics and associated muscle activity in people with symp-

toms of shoulder impingement. *Phys Ther* 2000; **80**: 276–91.

194   Warner JJ, Bowen MK, Deng XH, Hannafin JA, Arnoczky SP, Warren RF. Articular contact patterns of the normal glenohumeral joint. *J Shoulder Elbow Surg* 1998; **7**: 381–8.

195   Yani T, Hay JG. Shoulder impingement in front-crawl swimming. II. Analysis of stroking technique. *Med Sci Sports Exerc* 2000; **32**: 30–40.

196   Carlson KL, Haig AJ, Stewart DC. Snapping scapula syndrome: three case reports and an analysis of the literature. *Arch Phys Med Rehab* 1997; **78**: 506–11.

197   Fleisig GS, Escamilla RF, Andrews JR, Matsuo T, Sattershite Y, Barrentine SW. Kinematic and kinetic comparison between baseball pitching and football passing. *J Appl Biomech* 1996; **12**: 207–24.

198   DiGiovine NM, Jobe FW, Pink M, Perry J. An electromyographic analysis of the upper extremity in pitching. *J Shoulder Elbow Surg* 1992; **1**: 15–25.

199   Wickiewicz TH, Chen SK, Otis JC, Warren RF. Glenohumeral kinematics in a muscle fatigue model: a radiographic study. *Orthop Trans* 1995; **18**: 126.

200   Mottram SL. Dynamic stability of the scapula. *Manual Ther* 1997; **2**: 123–31.

201   Moseley JB, Jobe FW, Pink M, Perry J, Tibone J. EMG analysis of the scapular muscles during a shoulder rehabilitation program. *Am J Sports Med* 1992; **2**: 128–34.

202   Townsend H, Jobe FW, Pink M, Perry J. Electromyographic analysis of the glenohumeral muscles during a baseball rehabilitation program. *Am J Sports Med* 1991; **3**: 264–72.

203   Fees M, Decker T, Snyder-Macker L, Axe MJ. Upper extremity weight-training modifications for the injured athlete. *Am J Sports Med* 1998; **5**: 732–42.

204   Wilk KE, Arrigo C. Current concepts in the rehabilitation of the athletic shoulder. *J Orth Sports Phys Ther* 1993; **1**: 365–74.

205   Yoneda B, Welsh RP, Macintosh DL. Conservative treatment of shoulder dislocation in young males. *J Bone Joint Surg (Brit)* 1982; **64-B**: 254–5.

206   Kvinte RS, Jobe FW. The diagnosis and treatment of anterior instability in the throwing athlete. *Clin Orth Rel Res* 1993; **291**: 107–23.

Chapter 6.7
Elbow, Wrist and Hand

NICHOLAS B. BRUGGEMAN,

SCOTT P. STEINMANN, WILLIAM P. COONEY &

MICHAEL R. KROGSGAARD

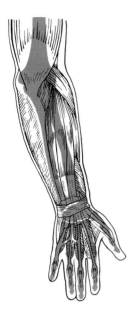

Classical reference

O'Driscoll SW, Bell DF, Morrey BF. Posterolateral
rotatory instability of the elbow. *J Bone Joint Surg
(Am)* 1991; **73**-A: 440–446.

With this article O'Driscoll *et al.* introduced the entity
'posterolateral rotatory instability of the elbow'. They
presented five patients who had all experienced elbow
dislocation, and in whom instability was suspected,
because of recurrent, painful episodes of locking and
snapping. Valgus and varus stress tests could not reveal
any instability, even under anesthesia, but the patients
showed apprehension when the elbow was extended
and the forearm supinated.

O'Driscoll *et al.* introduced the posterolateral rotatory instability test of the elbow, which was positive in
all five patients. While applying axial compression and
valgus stress to the elbow with the forearm supinated,
the semilunar notch of the ulna displaced from the
humeral trochlea, and the radial head could be dislocated or subluxed behind the humeral capitulum when
the arm was moved from extension to slight flexion. At
approximately 40° flexion the dislocation was reduced
(Fig. 6.7.1). They showed a clinical photograph of the

positive test, with a clear osseous prominence of the
dislocated radial head and a dimple in the skin just
proximal to this (Fig. 6.7.2), and X-rays demonstrating the dislocation (Fig. 6.7.3).

O'Driscoll *et al.* hypothesized that this lateral rotatory instability was caused by rupture of the ulnar
portion of the lateral collateral ligament. During
operation this could be confirmed in all five patients,
and in addition they found laxity of the posterolateral
capsule and the radial portion of the radial collateral
ligament. In all patients the annular ligament was
intact, demonstrating that it was not a radioulnar
dislocation.

Two patients had the ulnar portion of the collateral
ligament reattached and three had it reconstructed
with tendon grafts (palmaris longus in two patients) or
triceps fascia (one patient). Of the four patients surviving long-term follow-up, all symptoms had resolved
and the elbows had normal range of motion.

O'Driscoll *et al.* were not the first to describe an
instability in the lateral part of the elbow, but they
explained the anatomic event causing the instability
incidents, and they introduced the test demonstrating
the laxity.

(a)

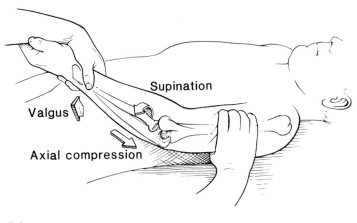

(b)

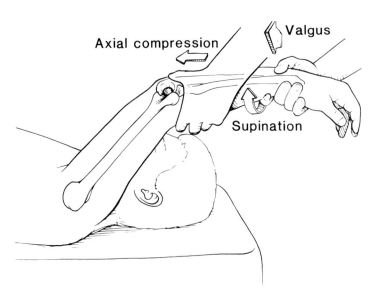

Fig. 6.7.1 The test for posterolateral rotatory instability of the elbow. (a) With the arm at the side and the forearm in supination, supination and valgus moments, as well as axial forces, are applied to the elbow, which is flexed approximately 20–30°. The posterolateral subluxation is visibly and palpably reduced when the elbow is flexed further. (b) The same procedure is performed much more easily with the arm over the patient's head. Full external rotation of the shoulder provides a counterforce for the supination of the forearm and leaves one hand of the examiner free to control valgus movements. Reproduced with permission from [18].

Introduction

Most cases of elbow and wrist problems in sports are related to overuse. This is not because traumatic injuries of the upper extremity are rare, but because overload problems are very common. About half of athletes performing racquet sports experience epicondylitis (mainly lateral) [1].

About 25% of all injuries in sports are related to elbow, forearm and wrist [2].

Sports-related injuries to the upper extremity are caused by one of two basic types: a one-off excessive, uncontrolled force or a persistent controlled cumulative force [3]. These injuries can be caused by trauma, either direct or indirect, or by active outstretching of musculotendinous units [4]. They may involve damage solely to the bony skeleton or to the soft tissues, such as the ligaments or tendons [5]. Single-stress injuries are common in direct contact sports such as foot-

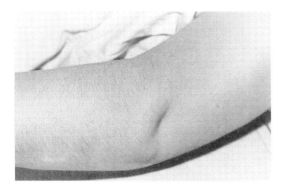

Fig. 6.7.2 Photograph made during a positive test for posterolateral rotatory subluxation of the elbow. The posterolateral dislocation of the radiohumeral joint produces an osseous prominence and an obvious dimple in the skin just proximal to the dislocated radial head. Reproduced with permission from [18].

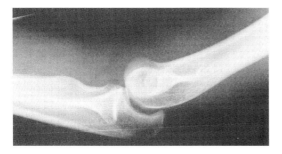

Fig. 6.7.3 Lateral radiograph made simultaneously with Fig. 6.7.2. The radiohumeral joint is dislocated posterolaterally, and there is rotatory subluxation of the ulnohumeral joint. The semilunar notch of the ulna is rotated away from the trochlea. Reproduced with permission from [18].

ball and wrestling, but may also occur in downhill skiers, volleyball, baseball and others [2]. Injuries due to repetitive stresses are common in tennis, bowling, cross-country skiing, rowing, gymnastics and others [6]. These injuries can be seen in non-athletes; however, the approach to the athlete with these conditions differs due to an emphasis on return to a high functional level as soon as possible.

This chapter's intention is to describe the types of elbow, wrist and hand injuries seen in athletes, and to discuss diagnosis and treatment in a concise fashion. Detailed descriptions of splinting techniques and surgical procedures will not be included.

Epidemiology

Hand and wrist injuries are common in all sports. They are more common in children than adults [7]. A study from the Cleveland Clinic showed that 14.8% of all athletic participants under the age of 16 years sustained upper extremity injuries. Of these 16% involved the hand and 9% involved the wrist [8]. Of 113 injuries of the hand and wrist 97 occurred in football, six in soccer, three in wrestling, three in baseball, two in basketball, one in ice hockey and one in rugby. They reported 96 fractures, 35 sprains and four dislocations. Metacarpal fractures accounted for 38 of the 96 fractures. There were 12 distal radius fractures and 11 scaphoid fractures. They reported 12 thumb injuries including 12 ulnar collateral ligament tears [8].

A look at sport-specific injuries is helpful in approaching these problems. A study of a National Football League team over an 8-year period showed the incidence of hand and wrist injuries to be 15.8% [7]. These included wrist and hand fractures in 11% and dislocation in 9%, wrist sprains in 10% and hand sprains in 18%. Fracture of the scaphoid is a common significant injury and an estimated one out of every 100 college football players will sustain this injury [9].

Basketball injuries accounted for 23% of all hand injuries over a 1-year study [10]. Two-thirds were fractures, including scaphoid fractures in 38%, metacarpal fractures in 30%, and phalangeal fractures in 20%. Nineteen per cent of these injuries were sprains and 4% were dislocations. Lacerations and degloving injuries can occur secondary to hitting the hand on the rim or the backboard.

Baseball and softball injuries most often result from direct blows by the ball. One study stated that fractures accounted for 46%, and 33% of these injuries were sprains. One injury that should be noted is a fracture of the hook of the hamate in a baseball or softball player [7].

Hand injuries in golfers are common complaints. Golf injuries are more common in the left wrist and may include de Quervain's tenosynovitis, radial impaction syndrome, and hook of the hamate fractures [7]. Hand and wrist injuries occurred in 20% of all golfers in one study [7].

Injuries in tennis commonly involve the wrist. These often include extensor carpi ulnaris (ECU) tendinitis, subluxation of the ECU, and ulnar carpal impaction syndrome [7].

Gymnastics is a common cause of wrist problems in athletes. It has been estimated that between 46 and 80% of elite gymnasts develop wrist pain at some time in their career [11]. This is due to the conversion of the upper extremity to a weight-bearing limb in gymnasts. The position and mechanism in these types of injuries are dorsiflexion and compression in nearly all gymnastic events [12].

Therefore, the different types of injury are closely associated to the different sports (Table 6.7.1).

The majority of problems in the upper extremity can be treated conservatively; e.g. there is a 90–95% healing rate of epicondylitis with rest, decrease of pain-provoking sports, non-steroidal anti-inflammatory drugs (NSAIDs) and corticosteroid injection [13], even though the mechanism of injury is poorly understood. The conservative and surgical treatments of nerve and muscle syndromes and bony injuries have been well described for several decades, but treatment of ligamentous and intra-articular problems in the elbow and wrist advanced tremendously during the 1990s. Biomechanical studies have led to a better understanding of pathophysiology, and magnetic resonance imaging (MRI) and arthroscopy to a much more detailed diagnosis and specific treatment in individual cases, e.g. regarding elbow instability or lesions to the triangular fibrocartilage complex in the wrist.

Sports-related problems of the elbow, forearm, wrist and hand can therefore to an increasing extent be dealt with on an academic basis, even though there are still many challenges for scientists and clinicians.

Anatomy and biodynamics

Elbow and forearm

The elbow is a hinge joint with two possible motions: flexion and extension. The proximal joint surface consists of the distal end of the humerus, and is divided into the trochlea, to which the semilunar notch of the ulna (olecranon) articulates, and the capitulum, onto which the radial head articulates. The distal joint surface is therefore made up of two bones, and the bony stability of the joint is dependent on both of these; if the radial head is fractured or surgically removed, this reduces the bony stability of the elbow.

The extension is limited by bone contact between

Table 6.7.1 Association between elbow, forearm and wrist problems and sports.

Elbow, forearm or wrist problem	Associated sport
Medial tension overload of elbow	Throwing sports, racquet sports
Posteromedial impingement of elbow	Throwing or racquet sports
Lateral compression of elbow (degenerative cartilaginous disease, osteochondritis)	Throwing or racquet sports, boxing
Lateral epicondylitis	Racquet sports, golf
Medial epicondylitis	Golf, racquet sports, bowling, weight-lifting
Ulnar nerve entrapment (elbow)	Throwing or racquet sports
Ulnar nerve compression, carpal syndrome (wrist)	Cycling
Tenosynovitis (de Quervain, flexor carpi ulnaris)	Golf, cycling
Compartment syndrome	Weight-lifting, body-building
Nerve entrapment (forearm)	Weight-lifting, body-building, racquet sports
Triceps tendonitis	Weight-lifting, gymnastics
Ulnar impaction syndrome, TFCC perforations (wrist)	Gymnastics
Dorsal carpal impingement/ganglia	Gymnastics, golf, racquet sports
Stress fractures, stress epiphysiolysis	Weight-lifting, gymnastics, throwing sports
Carpal fractures	Baseball, contact sports, golf (hook of hamate), cycling
Radius fractures	Cycling, contact sports
Ulnar fractures	Martial arts
Collateral ligament injury (thumb)	Skiing, contact sports

TFCC, triangular fibrocartilage complex.

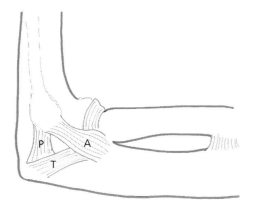

Fig. 6.7.4 Anatomy of the medial collateral ligament complex of the elbow including: the anterior band (A), the posterior band (P) and the transverse band (T).

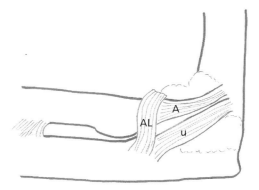

Fig. 6.7.5 Anatomy of the lateral ligament complex of the elbow including the ulnar band (U), the annular band (A) and the annular ligament (AL).

the tip of the olecranon and the humeral olecranon fossa. Maximal extension usually puts the forearm and upper arm in a straight line, but some persons can hyperextend the elbow up to 20°. Flexion is limited by the tip of the coronoid process colliding with the humerus or in muscular individuals by soft tissue contact.

Ligament stability is provided by the medial and lateral collateral ligaments. On the medial side the ligament starts on the anterior and distal parts of the humeral epicondyle and divides into anterior and posterior bands (Fig. 6.7.4). Both insert on the medial border of the ulna, but the anterior band is tight when the elbow moves between 0 and 90°, whereas the posterior band gets tighter the more flexed the elbow is. The anterior band is the thickest and the most important valgus stabilizer [14–17]. The lateral collateral ligament starts on the lateral humeral epicondyle, and divides into an ulnar band, which is the most important varus stabilizer, inserting on the lateral border of the ulna, and an annular band, which fuses with the annular ligament (Fig. 6.7.5). These arrangements ensure that the elbow is stable throughout the full range of motion.

The ulnar nerve is in intimate contact with the elbow as it passes behind the medial humeral condyle in the ulnar groove. The nerve is fixed in the groove by a strong fibrous roof, and because of the rigidity of this system, the nerve can be stretched during valgus stress to the elbow. The nerve can move about 5 mm up and down in the cubital tunnel.

Three muscles flex the elbow: the brachialis, brachioradialis and biceps. Biceps is also a supinator and can only function as a flexor if the forearm is supinated. Only one muscle extends the arm: the triceps, and the medial head is the most powerful.

The extensor muscles of the hand and fingers origin at the lateral humerus epicondyle as a conjoined tendon. The flexors origin as a conjoined tendon at the medial humerus epicondyle.

The two bones of the forearm, the radius and ulna, articulate with each other proximally and distally. Between the joints they are connected by a strong interosseous membrane. Rotation of the forearm (supination and pronation) takes place basically in the proximal radioulnar joint, where the cylindric radial head can rotate freely against the ulna, held in place by a string around the radial neck attached to the ulna: the annular ligament. In the distal radioulnar joint, the radius also rotates, but much less than in the proximal joint, and most of the rotation occurs in the forearm, bringing the hand into supination or pronation.

Wrist and hand

The distal radioulnar and radiocarpal joint complex is quite complicated. The proximal part is made up of the radius and ulna, but most of the ulnar head is covered with a cartilaginous structure: the triangular fibrocartilage complex (TFCC), arising from the ulnar joint rim of the radius, covering the ulnar head and inserting

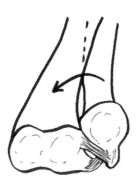
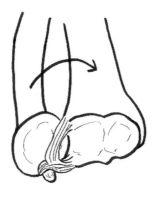

Fig. 6.7.6 Anatomy of the distal radioulnar joint. With the forearm pronated (left) the dorsal radioulnar ligament tightens, whereas during supination (right) the palmar radioulnar ligament is taut. These ligaments control the motion of the ulnar head.

at the base of the styloid process. The complex blends with two strong ligaments, which stabilize the ulna to the radius: the dorsal and palmar radioulnar ligaments (Fig. 6.7.6). In pronation the dorsal radioulnar ligament tightens, whereas in supination it is the palmar ligament. The distal part of the radiocarpal joint is composed of three carpal bones, positioned in a row and held together by rigid ligaments: the scaphoid, the lunate and the triquetrum. This row of carpal bones is stabilized to the radioulnar joint surface by strong ligaments, radially by the dorsal and volar radiocarpal ligaments, and on the ulnar side by the ulnolunate and ulnotriquetral ligaments, which are regarded as part of the triangular fibrocartilage complex and are crucial for the ulnar stability of the wrist.

The distal row of carpal bones articulates with the proximal row of carpal bones on one side and with the second to fifth metacarpal bones on the other. During daily work, about 85% of the energy transversing the wrist is applied through the radiocarpal joint from the second and third metacarpal bones, but this pattern of force transmission is often changed during sports, and a significant load can be applied to the ulnar side of the wrist, e.g. in gymnastics. The first carpometacarpal (CMC) joint is rotated 90° compared to the other CMC joints, allowing the thumb to grip and to be put in opposition to the other four fingers, and proximally the first metacarpal is bound by a very strong ligament to the second metacarpal bone. The thumb has only two phalangeal bones, while the second to fifth fingers have three (proximal, intermediate and distal phalanges). The metacarpophalangeal (MP) joints are stabilized in flexion by strong collateral ligaments, and in particular the ulnar ligament in the thumb is strong,

supporting the grip function. The interphalangeal joints are also stabilized by collateral ligaments. On the volar side of the metacarpophalangeal and interphalangeal joints a triangular cartilage (the volar plate) extends into the joints, bound to the collateral ligaments and the joint capsules, and stabilizing the joints in extension.

The wrist is primarily extended and flexed by radial and ulnar muscles, inserting on the carpal bones (the extensor and flexor carpi muscles), and to a lesser degree by the finger muscles. The second to fifth fingers are moved by the extensor and flexor muscles in the forearm, and by the lumbrical and interosseous muscles in the hand. The forearm extensors are bound in tendon sheaths (compartments) to the dorsal wrist, running dorsally over the MP joints, splitting into a central part inserting on the base of the intermediate phalanx, and two lateral strips, running dorsally along the sides of the proximal interphalangeal joint and inserting on the base of the distal phalanx. The lumbrical and interosseous muscles originate from the metacarpal bones and the flexor tendon sheaths in the palm and blend with the extensor muscles, extending the distal phalanx, but flexing the MP joints. The forearm flexors are held in place by the carpal tunnel as they run on the volar side of the wrist, and by tendon sheets in the palm and on the fingers. The deep flexors insert on the base of the distal phalanges and the superficial on the base of the intermediate phalanges. The thumb is moved by forearm extensors and flexors, and in addition by adductor, abductor and opponens muscles.

Three nerves innervate the hand: The median nerve supplies sensory function to the volar side of the first to the radial half of the fourth fingers and motor function to the thumb muscles. It runs with the flexor tendons in the carpal tunnel. The ulnar nerve supplies sensory function to the volar side of the ulnar half of the fourth and the fifth fingers and motor function to the lumbrical and interosseous muscles. It runs in a separate tunnel, Guyon's canal, between the hook of the hamate and the pisiform carpal bones. The radial nerve supplies sensory function to the dorsal portion of the hand but has no motor innervation in the hand.

Arterial supply is by the radial and ulnar arteries, which unite to form the arterial arcade in the palm. The ulnar artery runs with the ulnar nerve in Guyon's canal. As long as the arcade is intact the hand can be sufficiently supplied by one of the two arteries.

Clinical examination

The patient history should include information about how the problem started. Overuse problems have a gradual onset, and are often connected to repetitive load or increase in load, during either sports activities or work. The throwing activity should be mapped. If a trauma started the problem, the trauma mechanism and the primary findings should be clarified.

Elbow and forearm

The most common elbow symptom is pain. Details of precise location, provoking factors and when the pain is most intense are good clues to the correct diagnosis. Locking is symptomatic for loose bodies, and pseudolocking (sudden pain, which stops motion of the joint, but does not completely lock it) for degenerative changes of the cartilage, but can also be the only symptom of lateral rotatory instability. Reduction in range of motion is usually a sign of degenerative joint disease.

A basic joint examination compared to the opposite elbow (valgus or varus deformity, range of motion in extension, flexion, supination and pronation, crepitation from the joint during motion, swelling and effusion) should be supplemented with specific tests.

Careful recording of tenderness is important. With *epicondylitis* the tenderness is usually located to the medial epicondyle, and with overloading of the *ulnar collateral ligament* 1–2 cm distal to the epicondyle. Laterally tenderness of the epicondyle points at *epi-*

condylitis, pain at the joint line at *degenerative joint disease*, and tenderness distal to the radial head at *pronator syndrome*. Pain along the posterior tip of the olecranon is indicative of *posterior impingement*, and tenderness of the ulnar nerve in its fossa of *overloading to the nerve*. Indirect tenderness is found at the lateral epicondyle during resisted extension of the hand, and at the medial epicondyle during resisted flexion of the hand in *epicondylitis*.

With the valgus extension overload test collision is provoked between the posteromedial olecranon and the humerus by bringing the elbow in full extension while applying valgus stress across the joint. In patients with posterior impingement (typically throwers) this creates posterior pain. In case of overload injury to the ulnar collateral ligament (often seen in throwers), the test elicits pain from this ligament.

Collateral elbow stability is tested with at least 25–30° of flexion, as the tip of the olecranon in the olecranon fossa ensures stability of the extended elbow. Medial stability is tested with the upper arm maximally rotated outwards, and lateral stability during inward rotation of the upper arm. In both cases the hand is supinated. Stability should be compared to the opposite side, as individual variations occur. If instability is detected with a supinated forearm, the test should be repeated with a pronated forearm. Pronation tightens the lateral structures, and instability in pronation is indicative of ulnar collateral ligament insufficiency [18].

Elbow dislocation may result in chronic posterolateral rotatory instability, in which the radial head dislocates posterior to the lateral humerus capitulum during near-extension and valgus stress. This can be misinterpreted as a dislocation of the radial head in the radioulnar joint, but this is not the case. Posterolateral rotatory instability can be demonstrated with the pivot-shift test [18], in which maximal supination, valgus stress and axial load is applied to the nearly extended elbow (Fig. 6.7.1). This dislocates the radial head posterior to the humeral capitulum. While flexing the elbow, at first dislocation is increased (up to 40° of flexion) and then (over 40° of flexion) the dislocation is obviously reduced. The test is best performed during anesthesia, and in the awake patient only discomfort or apprehension may be demonstrated. It is easiest to perform with the arm overhead (Fig. 6.7.1b).

Wrist and hand

As in the elbow, the main symptom with wrist problems is pain. The localization of the pain and information about provoking activities are important indicators for the diagnosis.

The basic examination should include range of active and passive motion of all relevant joints, recording of swelling or crepitation, and precise mapping of tenderness. Decreased rotation is usually caused by problems in the distal or proximal radioulnar joints, and localization of pain when rotation is stressed is indicative of whether the problem is distal or proximal. Even a small reduction in rotation or wrist extension can be a serious problem for athletes. With finger trauma, flexion and extension in all joints should be carefully examined. The sensory function of the three nerves is tested (median nerve: volar side of first to radial part of fourth fingers; ulnar nerve: volar side of ulnar half of fourth plus fifth fingers; and radial nerve: dorsal side of hand), as well as motor function of the median (thumb adduction) and ulnar (spreading fingers) nerves.

Depending on the history and basic examination, specific tests can be added. With nerve entrapment there is usually projecting pain and numbness in the sensory area of the nerve when the examiner taps with a finger in the entrapment area (Tinel's sign). With carpal tunnel syndrome, Phalen's sign is usually positive: with the wrist flexed for 60 s, pain and paresthesia in the median nerve area is elicited, and reversed when the wrist is put in the neutral position. Tendon inflammation is painful on direct palpation but also when the tendon is used, especially against resistance. Finkelstein's test is positive with tenosynovitis in the abductor pollicis longus/extensor pollicis brevis at the radial styloid process: the patient is asked to make a fist with the thumb in the palm. The examiner adds passive ulnar deviation of the hand, which is very painful.

Stability is generally tested by comparison with the other side, as there are individual variations in laxity. The MP joints are tested in 45° flexion except in the thumb, where the ulnar collateral ligament is tested in extension and in 30–45° flexion.

Imaging

Standard radiographs of the elbow are taken in two projections and can besides fractures reveal degenerative changes, including arthrosis with narrowing of the joint space and osteophytes, calcifications of ligaments and osteochondrites. Loose bodies can be seen on X-ray, but computed tomography (CT) scan is more sensitive in demonstrating them. These projections can be supplemented with skyline photos of the olecranon to show osteophytes on the olecranon in posterior impingement. Stress radiographs can usually confirm ulnar (medial) instability but are less sensitive for lateral instability.

Bony pathology in the distal forearm and the fingers can usually be visualized on standard X-rays in two planes. Changes in the carpal bones are often only visible on oblique views, e.g. fractures of the scaphoid or the hook of hamate, and CT scan can be helpful mapping carpal injuries. Instability can by visualized by applying stress (e.g. to the carpal joints) during screening.

MRI scan is useful to demonstrate pathology of the collateral ligaments of the elbow, in particular on the medial side. In some cases it is not possible to distinguish between degenerative changes in the ligament and traumatic rupture. Osteochondrites can be visualized with MRI or CT scan, but CT is better for demonstrating loose bodies. Changes with epicondylitis in the soft tissue around the epicondyle can be seen on MRI or ultrasound, and the spectrum of changes can be demonstrated on MRI (tendon degeneration and partial tearing, muscle strain, macroscopic tendon disruption). This may guide the surgeon as to where degenerative tissue for removal is located, but it rarely adds information to the clinical diagnosis. CT scan may reveal spur formation in epicondylitis, invisible on X-rays [19]. In skeletally immature throwers, the medial epicondylar apophysis may be stressed and avulsed—MRI can demonstrate this condition with high sensitivity. The ulnar nerve and compressing structures can be clearly visualized in the cubital tunnel. MRI is very sensitive for stress fractures of the elbow, as well as for visualization of biceps and triceps tendon ruptures.

In the wrist, MRI is very sensitive for avascular necrosis (Kienböck's disease) and fractures (most often relevant with clinical suspicion of scaphoid fracture despite normal X-rays). Tears of the triangular fibrocartilage complex can be demonstrated with a sensitivity of 90–95% [20], and in dorsal impingement of the wrist tearing of the dorsal cartilage and subchondral sclerosis can often be demonstrated. Carpal ligament disruption can be demonstrated with MRI arthrography. MRI is very sensitive for tenosynovitis and soft tissue pathology in the carpal tunnel.

With scintigraphy bone viability can be visualized. Fractures (e.g. of the scaphoid, not visible on X-rays) will show as increased activity, while necrotic bone (e.g. a fragment of the scaphoid) has decreased or no activity. Scintigraphy is extremely sensitive in this respect.

Elbow and forearm

Epicondylitis

Even though lateral epicondylitis is also named 'tennis elbow' and medial 'golfer's elbow', most cases of epicondylitis are related to overload during work. In athletes, epicondylitis is seen most frequently in racquet sports.

Epidemiology

The incidence of lateral epicondylitis is about 50% in recreational tennis players over 30 years of age [1]. It is rarer in younger persons, probably because their tissue is stronger and more elastic, and in elite players, who in many cases have a better technique than recreational players. Besides racquet sports, lateral epicondylitis is also seen in squash and table tennis. The male/female ratio is nearly 1. The most important factors for development of lateral epicondylitis in tennis players are playing time per day and age [21].

Medial epicondylitis is 1/10–1/5 as common as lateral, and 80% occurs in males [22].

Pathogenesis and pathohistology

Epicondylitis is a result of repeated, very high loads on the extensor muscles (in lateral epicondylitis) or flexor muscles (medial epicondylitis) where the conjoined tendons insert onto the humeral epicondyles. When the tennis ball hits the racquet, high impact is transferred to the musculature controlling the hand and wrist. During the one-handed backhand smash, the load is on the extensor muscles in particular, and lateral epicondylitis can develop. During the forehand smash, impact is applied to the flexor muscles, creating the basis for medial epicondylitis. Symptoms often develop in connection with increasing number of training hours, introduction of a new and tightly strung racquet or heavier balls.

Histologic changes are usually not typical of inflammation. They are described in the muscle–tendon junction of the extensor carpi radialis brevis, first as small ruptures of the muscle, and in later stages as granulomatous tissue, rich in fibroblasts, vessels and nerves, and destroying the natural parallel architecture of the collagen fibrils. Later mucoid degeneration is seen. So instead of an inflammatory disease, histology indicates that epicondylitis is a repair process after microtrauma to the tissue [23].

Clinical presentation and findings

With epicondylitis, pain is felt on either the lateral or medial side of the elbow. Pain is intense, and in the beginning is only present during heavy loading of the muscle, e.g. in racquet sports, lifting, and monotonous work with lower loads, e.g. typing. If symptoms increase, the pain becomes more chronic, and is elicited by daily activities like lifting a coffee pot or shaking hands, and finally becomes constant, even during the night.

Examination reveals intense tenderness at the epicondyle in question, directly by palpation, and indirectly by applying stretch on the muscle: with lateral epicondylitis, dorsal flexion of the hand against resistance will provoke the typical pain. In medial epicondylitis, pain is elicited by forced volar flexion of the hand. Pinpointing the tender tissue by palpation is important to rule out other diagnoses: on the lateral side tenderness at the joint line is indicative of degenerative disease or osteochondral injury in the radiohumeral joint, and tenderness 2–3 cm distal of the radial head is seen with the pronator syndrome. On the medial side tenderness 2–3 cm distal to the condyles is indicative of overload or trauma to the ulnar collateral ligament; tenderness 2 cm further distal of the pronator syndrome and tenderness behind the medial condyle is seen with irritation of the ulnar nerve.

X-rays may show calcifications in the soft tissue. Axial CT scan can demonstrate spur formation at the insertion site of the tendon, apparently more often in cases of more than 1 year's duration than in cases of shorter duration [19]. Changes in the muscle and tendon can be demonstrated by MRI (Fig. 6.7.7) or ultrasound scans. As these soft tissue changes have no prognostic implication, MRI and ultrasound scans should be reserved for cases which do not resolve on conservative treatment.

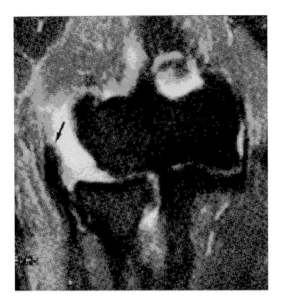

Fig. 6.7.7 Magnetic resonance image of lateral epicondylitis with changes and hypertrophy of the co-joined tendon.

Treatment and prognosis

Most cases of epicondylitis heal on a conservative regimen: decrease in the amount of or avoidance of the activities that elicit the pain [13]. This may mean complete cessation from sports for longer periods, until symptoms have subsided. It is important to minimize the load on the muscles, e.g. by changing to a less tightly strung or lighter racquet or by changing playing technique, e.g. by using two hands instead of one in tennis back hand.

There are a number of conservative treatment options that have some effect on pain, but the long-term effect on the disease process is not well documented. Analgesics, NSAIDs and cryotherapy are first choices. Counterforce bracing reduces the tension on the proximal part of the muscles and can be useful for patients who have symptoms during work [24,25]. Corticosteroid injection under or over the tendon has been shown to shorten the period with pain, but does not affect the long-term cure rate. Injection under the tendon is probably preferable to avoid wasting of the subcutaneous tissue, which may result from direct contact between the tissue and the corticosteroid. It is safest to insert the needle from distal, obliquely, perforating the muscle and positioning the tip between the epicondyle and the tendon. Injection into the tendon must be avoided, as it is very painful and can cause necrosis.

If conservative therapy fails to cure the athlete of the symptoms of epicondylitis or reduce the pain significantly, operative treatment can be considered. Only about 5% of patients with lateral epicondylitis need surgery [26]. At least 6 months' conservative treatment should precede the decision for operation. Failed conservative treatment should always result in re-examination of the patient. Medial instability may be a reason why medial epicondylitis does not respond to therapy. Laterally, instability and degenerative joint disease are important differential diagnoses.

At operation the cojoined tendon is incised longitudinally and released from the epicondyle. All pathologic tissue (tears in the tendon, granulomatous tissue, synovitis in the lateral joint capsule) is removed, the epicondyle is debrided, and the tendon is reattached. The operation can be performed endoscopically. If a spur has been demonstrated, it should be removed. Results after operation are good, as 85–95% of patients can return to their activities without subjective symptoms [27–29], but objectively all have some degree of persistent muscle weakness [26]. There are no randomized studies of the operative treatment.

Posterior impingement

Epidemiology, pathogenesis and pathophysiology

Posterior impingement is caused by bony collision between the humerus and olecranon, most often the humeral trochlea and an osteophyte on the medial facet of the olecranon. This is common in athletes performing overhead activities, in particular throwers, who apply repeated valgus and extension forces over the elbow, gradually creating an osteophyte on the posteromedial facet of the olecranon [30]. It is the most frequent reason for elbow arthroscopy in athletes [31]. Strain of the triceps muscle and small avulsions from the tip of the olecranon are also seen [32].

Posterior impingement may be a solitary entity, but may also appear as an element of thrower's elbow, which besides posterior impingement includes medial (ulnar) instability and degenerative changes in the

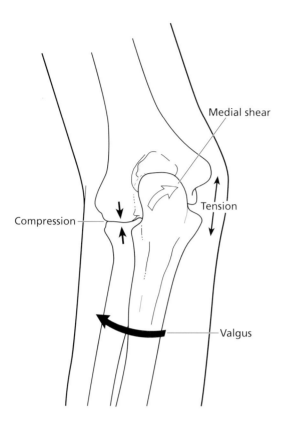

Medial shear

Compression

Tension

Valgus

Fig. 6.7.8 Thrower's elbow. The forces and their region of impact on the elbow during overhand activity include traction of the medial collateral ligament and the ulnar nerve, compression of the lateral compartment and posteromedial impingement.

cartilage of the lateral compartment (Fig. 6.7.8). In baseball players, 25% with posterior impingement also have significant ulnar instability. Thrower's elbow is dealt with in detail on p. 750.

Clinical presentation and findings

The symptom is pain posteromedially in the elbow during throwing, elicited during the late cocking and acceleration stages at the time of ball release, when there is maximum extension and valgus stress on the elbow. In rare cases the osteophyte also impinges on the ulnar nerve, producing local pain in the ulnar tunnel and numbness and paresthesia in the fourth and fifth finger.

Often there is a small extension deficit. There is pain when the valgus extension overload test is performed and tenderness on palpation of the posteromedial facet

of the olecranon. In case of impingement on the ulnar nerve, there is tenderness in the ulnar tunnel and positive Tinel's sign of the ulnar nerve. It is important to test for ulnar stability (see p. 750). Axial X-rays may reveal the olecranon osteophyte, which is usually also visible on MRI scan.

Treatment and prognosis

Except in rare cases with a massive osteophyte, solitary posterior impingement is only symptomatic during throwing and racquet activities. Conservative treatment includes reduction of these activities, and if possible modification of throwing and hitting techniques, if necessary with a brace which prevents full extension. If activities are continued, the prognosis without surgery is poor.

Operative treatment involves resection of the posteromedial osteophyte of the olecranon and debridement of the posterior compartment from fibrous and inflammatory tissue. Fenestration of the olecranon fossa (drilling a hole through the humerus in the fossa) also creates space for a free extension of the olecranon tip. These procedures can be performed arthroscopically, during which chondral defects of the trochlea can also be visualized. If the cartilage is intact, the immediate prognosis after surgery is good, but with continued throwing, there is a high recurrence rate, as the pathogenesis — valgus and extension overload — is not eliminated [31].

Overstress elbow instability (medial instability)

Elbow instability can be a result of trauma (usually elbow dislocation) or ligamentous overload in throwing and racquet sports. Overload instability involves the medial collateral ligament, while traumatic instability is most often lateral. Because of the differences in pathogenesis, these two types of instability are dealt with separately.

Epidemiology

Ulnar ligament instability is almost exclusively related to overhead, throwing sports, in particular baseball and racquet sports. The incidence is unknown, but some symptomatic cases probably remain undiagnosed, combined with or misdiagnosed as medial epicondylitis or posterior impingement. Twenty-five per cent of patients with posterior impingement have significant medial instability.

Pathogenesis and pathophysiology

Medial instability is believed to be a result of repetitive overload to the ulnar collateral ligament [33]. Clinical and electromyographic studies of motions during the baseball pitch form the basis for dividing it into five stages: wind-up, early cocking, late cocking, acceleration and follow-through. In the late cocking stage, the arm is in maximal external rotation and the elbow in full extension and under maximal valgus stress to accumulate as much elastic energy as possible for the pitch. During the acceleration stage, a large valgus stress is still applied to the elbow [34]. In extension, the ulnar collateral ligament is not the only structure securing valgus stability, as the anterior capsule and the lateral joint compartment (the radiohumeral joint) contribute significantly. So during pitching and throwing, intense stretching is applied to the ulnar collateral ligament, and compression to the lateral joint. If the load on the ligament exceeds the rate of repair, it will result in damage to the structure of the ligament, inflammation, chronic changes in the tissue and ultimately ligament instability [35].

In addition to painful medial instability, the fully developed *thrower's elbow* consists of posterior impingement, degeneration of the cartilage in the lateral compartment, posterior impingement and ulnar nerve irritation (Fig. 6.7.8) [36]. Whether there is a progression in the disease from ulnar instability to lateral degeneration or whether all lesions develop at the same time is not known, but there is some variability in the severity of the various lesions between individual patients.

Clinical presentation and findings

Athletes with ulnar ligament overstress experience medial elbow pain of gradual onset, primarily during throwing or serving. Early in the disease, pain is elicited in the late cocking and acceleration stages of throwing, usually when the ball leaves the hand. Later on, all stages of throwing may be painful, and sometimes daily activities as well. A feeling of weakness may develop.

On examination there is tenderness of the ulnar collateral ligament, a couple of cm distal to the epicondyle. By applying valgus stress to the elbow, pain is elicited from the ligament. If medial instability has developed, it will be revealed by stability testing. When the condition is combined with medial epicondylitis, pain from the pronator muscles and ulnar nerve irritation, more than one tender structure can be identified, and clinically the diagnosis can be difficult to make.

X-rays may show calcification of the ulnar collateral ligament, and stress radiographs (compared to the opposite elbow) can document instability. MRI scan will show changes within the ligament, but should primarily be used in clinically difficult cases to confirm or exclude involvement of the ulnar collateral ligament.

Athletes with *thrower's elbow* will also experience posteromedial pain and sometimes lateral pain. They have tenderness of the medial facet of the olecranon and at the lateral joint line, sometimes a small intra-articular effusion, and have a positive valgus extension overload test.

Treatment and prognosis

As with other overload conditions, the primary treatment is conservative: decrease or avoidance of throwing or serving sports and NSAIDs until symptoms have subsided, followed by gradual increase of activities. In most cases this gives good pain relief, and most athletes are able to get back to sporting activities, even in cases of medial instability.

In athletes with a very high activity level, this conservative regimen may fail. With medial instability, operative treatment may be considered, provided that at least 6 months' conservative treatment has been tried.

The aim of surgery is to re-establish medial stability by reconstruction of the ulnar collateral ligament [37]. The ligament is exposed and its laxity is confirmed. Granulomatous and degenerated tissue is removed, and the palmaris longus tendon is harvested from the distal forearm. Both legs of the ligament are reconstructed, as the tendon is fixed to the bone in drill holes. Rehabilitation takes 12 months. After reconstruction more than two-thirds of athletes are able to get back to sports at their previous level [38,39], and two-thirds are able to return to competition [39].

In *thrower's elbow* all symptomatic pathologies should be addressed. In case of posterior impingement, debridement of the posterior compartment should be performed. In case of ulnar nerve irritation, the nerve may be transpositioned anterior to the epicondyle to relieve it from stress. Degenerative changes in the lateral compartment may result in loose bodies or osteophytes, both of which can be removed arthroscopically. Unless there are symptomatic changes in the lateral compartment, the prognosis is good regarding symptom relief and return to sports.

Cartilaginous injuries

Epidemiology

Injuries to the elbow cartilage can be caused by trauma, either a compression injury such as falling on an outstretched arm, or as a concomitant lesion to fracture or dislocation. But most cartilage problems in athletes are non-traumatic, either resulting from repetitive, forceful compression of the lateral compartment in throwing and other sports with valgus stress to the elbow, or taking the form of osteochondritis dissecans. The incidence is unknown, but it is relatively common in throwing, racquet sports and weight-lifting (males), and gymnastics (females) [40,41]. The dominant arm is most often affected.

Pathogenesis and pathophysiology

Cartilaginous overuse lesions most often develop from indirect blows to the cartilage by repetitive valgus stress of the elbow. In addition to a very forceful stretch to the ulnar collateral ligament, the valgus overload creates very strong compressive forces over the lateral and posterior compartments, resulting in degeneration of the cartilage, osteochondral fractures, osteophytes and, in the skeletally immature, perhaps osteochondritis dissecans [40,42]. In most cases the capitulum of the humerus is involved, but the radial head may also reveal cartilaginous changes. Direct injury to the cartilage may be caused by repetitive microtrauma, e.g. in boxing and weight-lifting.

The etiology of osteochondritis dissecans is unknown, but its relationship to throwing and gymnastics in the adolescent makes it likely to be a result of repetitive overload. Sometimes both elbows are affected, and a genetic disposition to develop osteochondritis may exist.

Clinical presentation and findings

Lateral elbow pain during strenuous activities is the key symptom of degenerative disease of the cartilage in the lateral compartment. Locking is experienced in the case of loose bodies, and pseudolocking with large chondral defects.

At examination, there is often a slight reduction in extension and rotation, and tenderness at the lateral joint line. Crepitus may be felt laterally during motion. Supination and pronation on the fully extended elbow may produce lateral pain [42]. It is important to test for instability, either valgus instability in case of ulnar collateral ligament insufficiency, or lateral or posterolateral instability after elbow dislocations. Lateral degeneration may also be an element of *thrower's elbow*.

Standard X-rays usually demonstrate osteochondritis dissecans of the capitulum clearly, and narrowing of the lateral joint line, osteosclerosis and osteophytes can also be seen in degenerative disease. Oblique radiographs may supplement if necessary. Loose bodies are best seen on CT scans. MRI scan is very sensitive in detection of early osteochondritis dissecans changes, and may be indicated in young athletes with lateral elbow pain but no pathologic findings on standard X-rays. If an osteochondritis has been demonstrated, MRI may be able to visualize whether it is loose (in which case it is surrounded by fluid) or covered with cartilage [43]. However, often the status of the cartilage is not determined without arthroscopy.

Treatment and prognosis

The pain related to cartilaginous, degenerative disease often varies with load and is intensified by synovitis. Conservative treatment with rest and eventually a hinged elbow brace reduces symptoms significantly in most cases, and return to sports activity after 3–6 months is often possible, although not documented in the literature.

Surgical treatment is indicated in case of large chondral lesions (either demonstrated on MRI or suspected because of failed conservative treatment), or loose bodies.

Removal of loose bodies and debridement of cartilage flaps can usually be performed arthroscopically. It is debated whether full-thickness lesions to bare subchondral bone should just be debrided [44], or also be drilled or microfractured to initiate the formation of fibrocartilage [45]. Reported results are variable. Young athletes seem to have a good chance of returning to sports [42].

Osteochondritis dissecans represents a special problem. Detached lesions can either be removed and debrided [46] or reattached by fixation. Both procedures are reported to be successful regarding pain, and make return to sports possible in most cases [47]. Successful conservative treatment of early osteochondritis in young baseball players (detected by MRI) has been reported [43]. Two lesions healed after rest and reduction of sports activities, whereas one lesion in a player who did not reduce activities, progressed. Osteochondritis may therefore—at least in the early stages—have a potential for healing.

Elbow dislocation, lateral instability and posterolateral rotatory instability

Epidemiology and pathophysiology

Lateral and posterolateral rotatory instability of the elbow is the late result of a significant trauma, often dislocation of the elbow, and is as such not only a sports injury. Dislocation of the elbow is quite common with an annual incidence of 6/100 000 and representing 10–30% of all injuries to the elbow. It is usually caused by falling on an outstretched hand. In persons under the age of 20, 75% of lateral instabilities are caused by elbow dislocations, whereas in persons older than 20 years, the primary incident is most often a varus trauma without dislocation.

Some cases of lateral instability are complications of surgery for lateral epicondylitis, where the lateral collateral ligament has incidentally been damaged.

In pure lateral instability, the most important lateral stabilizer, the radial ulnohumeral ligament, is torn. In posterolateral rotatory instability the lateral capsule is also lax, which allows the radial head to sublux or even dislocate posteriorly to the humerus [18].

Elbow dislocations

Elbow dislocations without fracture are defined as simple dislocations. The extent of ligament injury is probably variable, but there is always rupture of the capsule, and it is believed that the essential lesion in elbow dislocation is rupture of the lateral ligamentous complex [18]. In addition, in many cases evidence of ulnar collateral ligament rupture can also be found with stabil-

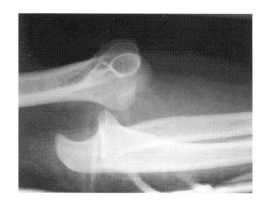

Fig. 6.7.9 Elbow dislocation with fracture of the radial head and the coronoid process.

ity testing straight after reduction of the dislocation [48].

Dislocations with fractures are termed complex (Fig. 6.7.9). The most frequent concomitant fractures are radial head, coronoid process and humeral epicondyle.

In complex dislocations it is regarded essential to surgically re-establish the stability provided by the coronoid process and the collateral ligaments. In simple dislocations, suture or reinsertion of the ligaments is often advocated if the elbow is unstable after reduction, even though no advantage of surgery could be found in a prospective, randomized study comparing conservative treatment with splinting and surgery [49].

Conservative treatment includes reduction, primary immobilization in a 90° splint for about a week followed by gradual mobilization. Splinting for more than 3 weeks results in marked stiffness and reduction in range of motion. The risk for recurrent dislocation after conservative treatment of simple dislocations is 1–2% [49]. Surgical treatment includes reduction and fixation of fractures and suture of ligament ruptures. The risk for redislocation after complex dislocations is up to 17% [50].

For the athlete the most significant complication to elbow dislocation is usually reduction in range of motion, which has dramatic consequences for e.g. throwing. It is unknown how often instability during sports activities is the main late symptom of elbow dislocation.

Lateral and posterolateral rotatory instability

Clinical presentation and findings

The symptoms of lateral and posterolateral rotatory instability are not typical. They vary according to the degree of instability. Redislocations are rare. Most commonly complaints are vague: diffuse elbow pain, clicking, catching, locking and snapping during activity. Posterolateral rotatory instability most often shows as episodes of apprehension when the arm is supinated in extension, or during supination in slight flexion when valgus stress is applied to the arm [18,51].

Demonstration of instability can be difficult. The varus and valgus stress tests should be performed to reveal medial and lateral instability. In the case of instability, the valgus test should be repeated with the forearm in pronation, and if positive, this is indicative of medial instability, which should be addressed. The pivot-shift test should be performed, and if negative should be repeated under anesthesia if history makes posterolateral rotatory instability possible. In some cases instability can only be demonstrated during elbow arthroscopy, in which subluxation of the radial head can be directly visualized during the pivot-shift test.

Instability may be demonstrated on stress X-rays. The radial head subluxation can be shown, if the pivot-shift test is performed during stress X-rays [52]. Ligament disruption can be demonstrated nicely on MRI [52].

Treatment and prognosis

Acute disruption of the lateral ligaments should be treated with a hinged elbow brace in 4–6 weeks with the forearm in pronation [51].

Chronic, symptomatic lateral or posterolateral instability can only be treated operatively. If the radioulnar ligament is detached but intact, it can be reinserted or tightened during open operation, and the lateral capsule tightened as well. Tightening of the lateral structures can also be performed arthroscopically. If the ligamentous tissue is poor, the ligament can be reconstructed with the palmaris longus tendon, placed in drill holes in humerus and ulnar in the anatomic position of the ligament [53]. The results after operative treatment are optimistic, with 85% categorized as excellent or good.

Biceps and triceps tendon rupture

Rupture of the *distal biceps tendon* from its insertion on the radius occurs with forceful flexion of the elbow and supination of the forearm, typically in weight-lifting. In most cases the rupture is complete with retraction of the tendon by a few cm, and the condition is usually recognized in the acute situation. The athlete feels pain in the cubital fossa with aggravation during flexion and supination. At examination there is swelling and hematoma of the cubital fossa and reduced power in flexion and supination. Often a defect at the proximal end of the biceps can be felt — in particular if compared to the contralateral arm. The rupture can be demonstrated with ultrasound or MRI scanning, if not clinically obvious.

Treated conservatively, a complete, distal biceps tendon rupture will result in significantly reduced flexion and supination strength [54]. Surgical treatment with reinsertion of the tendon to the radial tuberosity is therefore recommended, and if treated in the acute phase, results are very satisfactory with restoration of full flexion and supination strength in nearly all cases [55].

Partial tears are rare and can be demonstrated on ultrasound or MRI scans. Usually they can be treated conservatively with rest and gradual return to sports after 3–4 months. Late-diagnosed complete ruptures (> 6 weeks) can be treated surgically, but the complication rate (radial nerve injury and reduced muscle strength) is higher than after primary operation.

Rupture of the *distal triceps tendon* typically occurs after falling on an outstretched arm and complete tears are easily diagnosed, as triceps is the only elbow extensor. There is a defect just proximal to the tip of the olecranon, and extension of the elbow is impossible or only possible with greatly reduced power. X-rays may show an avulsion from the olecranon. If clinically in doubt, the rupture can be demonstrated on ultrasound or MRI scan. Complete tears should be reinserted by operation, as conservative treatment results in greatly reduced extension power in the elbow, which is very disabling. Results after repair are good, as nearly all patients re-establish full extension strength and normal range of motion.

Partial tears are usually located at the muscle–tendon junction and result in pain and reduced strength in extension. The extent of tearing can be evaluated on MRI or ultrasound, and smaller lesions can be treated conservatively.

Nerve entrapment

Entrapment of a nerve occurs when it is compressed or when it is stretched over a point of fixation, e.g. a ligamentous structure. Nerve injuries can be divided into three types. *Neuropraxia* is loss of conduction along an intact nerve, and is the mildest form, being completely reversible. This is the most common type in athletes. *Axonotmesis* is a more chronic condition with degeneration of the nerve distal to the entrapment, but with intact connecting tissue. The prognosis for recovery is reasonably good. In *neuretmesis* there is complete disruption of the nerve, and full recovery is never gained. This is only rarely related to sports.

The symptoms of nerve entrapment are pain located at the point of affection, and dysfunction of the nerve distally to this. A number of nerve entrapment syndromes are caused by repetitive stress over the elbow.

Musculocutaneous nerve overload

The nerve can be compressed between the lateral border of the biceps aponeurosis and the brachial fascia during repetitive elbow extension combined with forearm pronation. Symptoms are burning hyperesthesia in the lateral forearm, and tenderness and weakness of the biceps muscle. Examination reveals atrophy of biceps and reduced sensation on the lateral forearm. Treatment consists of rest and with persisting symptoms decompression with resection of a wedge of the biceps aponeurosis [56].

Ulnar nerve (cubital tunnel syndrome and compression)

The nerve which is most often affected in the arm is the ulnar nerve. Around the elbow it can be entrapped at three sites: 6–8 cm proximal to the elbow at the arcade of Struthers, in the cubital tunnel, and about 4 cm distal to the elbow at the flexor carpi ulnaris and the medial intermuscular septum.

Entrapment in the cubital tunnel (posterior to the medial humeral condyle and roofed by the arcuate ligament) is the most common. The ulnar nerve is elongated about 5 mm in the tunnel during normal flexion, and it is further loaded during throwing, when

a valgus stress is applied to the elbow, and a compression force on the nerve of up to six times resting pressure can be measured. If the cubital tunnel is narrowed and the ulnar nerve cannot glide freely, additional entrapment occurs. Narrowing of the tunnel can be caused by hypertrophy of the medial collateral ligament, fibrosis, osteophytes, etc.

Entrapment at the arcade of Struthers in the upper arm or the flexor carpi ulnaris muscle in the forearm is seen with muscular hypertrophy.

Symptoms are tenderness and pain at the site of entrapment, most often around the medial joint line, and neurologic symptoms, starting with paresthesia and numbness in the fourth and fifth finger, and progressing to decreased strength of the hand muscles. Clinically there is tenderness along the cubital tunnel (or at the arcade of Struthers or the flexor carpi ulnaris muscle) with positive Tinel's sign (radiating pain when tapping on the nerve), reduced sensation on the volar side of the fifth and ulnar half of the fourth finger, and possibly atrophy of the interosseous muscles.

Osteophytes in the cubital tunnel or calcifications of the medial collateral ligament can be demonstrated on X-rays (including axial radiographs), CT scans or MRI scans. Nerve conduction measurements are indicated if there is doubt about the location of entrapment, but usually this is clinically obvious.

The primary treatment is conservative: rest and reduction of the activities which stress the nerve, e.g. throwing or body-building (muscular hypertrophy). With persisting symptoms, surgical treatment is necessary. The nerve is decompressed at the site of entrapment. In the cubital tunnel this can be achieved by either *in situ* decompression or transposition of the nerve anterior to the epicondyle. Osteophytes are removed. If the nerve entrapment is an element of thrower's elbow (medial instability, posterior impingement, lateral cartilagenous degeneration and ulnar nerve entrapment), the medial instability should be addressed, as decompression alone rarely reduces medial pain [38].

Median nerve (pronator syndrome; anterior interosseous nerve palsy)

Distal to the elbow, the median nerve runs between the two heads of the pronator teres muscle and continues under the fibrous tissue of the flexor digitorum muscle. At the distal edge of the pronator, it gives off the anterior interosseous branch, which is a purely motoric nerve to the pronator quadratus, flexor pollicis longus and flexor digitorum profundus to the index finger.

Entrapment of the median nerve (pronator syndrome) can happen with hypertrophy of the pronator teres muscles or by fibrous bands from the pronator or flexor digitorum profundus muscles, but can also be caused by enlarged vessels, a fibroma or other compressing tissues. It is mainly seen in athletes with a very well-developed muscle mass in the upper extremity and provoked by forceful pronation and gripping, e.g. in throwing, weight-lifting, racquet sports, arm wrestling and rowing. Entrapment of the anterior interosseous nerve is usually caused by fibrous bands. Nerve palsy can also be postviral.

The pronator syndrome is by far the most commonly seen. The symptom is pain at the anterior upper forearm during repetitive pronation and wrist flexion, e.g. in racquet sports. There can be paresthesias in the first four and the radial half of the fifth fingers, but usually there are no motor nerve symptoms. Examination reveals tenderness 4–5 cm distal to the medial epicondyle at the pronator teres.

In *anterior interosseous nerve palsy* there is in addition motor symptoms from the three muscles innervated by the interosseous branch: decreased flexion power in the distal phalanx of the thumb and index fingers, and decreased pronation strength with the elbow maximally flexed [57]. At examination there is decreased strength in the three muscles in addition to tenderness at the pronator teres muscle. In cases where the compression is caused by a tumor, it may not be felt by examination, and therefore an MRI scan is often performed in cases with motor deficiency.

Nearly all cases of pronator syndrome resolve with conservative treatment: rest, NSAIDs and decrease in upper-extremity activities. If symptoms have not disappeared within 3–6 months, operative release of the nerve can be performed [57]. With unresolved entrapment of the motor nerve, operative release of the anterior interosseous branch should be performed.

Radial nerve (high radial palsy, radial tunnel syndrome; posterior interosseous nerve syndrome)

High radial palsy is not a specific sports injury, but is seen with trauma or longer compression (e.g. from sleeping on the arm in state of drunkenness). Symptoms are mixed sensory and motoric with numbness on the dorsal side of the hand and reduction of extension force in the wrist and fingers. The triceps muscle may be involved.

The radial nerve can be entrapped in the radial tunnel at five sites (Fig. 6.7.10) [58]: fibrous bands anterior to the radial head, vessels to brachioradialis, the tendon of the extensor carpi radialis brevis, Fröhse's arcade (the fibrous arch at the proximal edge of the supinator muscle) and a fibrous band at the distal edge of the supinator muscle. It may probably also be compressed in the supinator muscle. Entrapment in the radial tunnel or by the supinator muscle is termed *radial tunnel syndrome*, and if motor symptoms are prominent it is termed *posterior interosseous nerve syndrome (PINS)*, after the branch of the radial nerve which supplies the

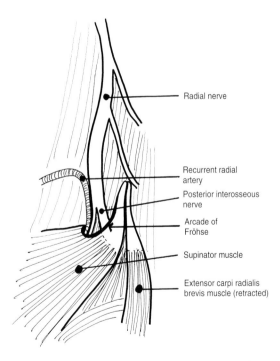

Radial nerve

Recurrent radial artery

Posterior interosseous nerve

Arcade of Fröhse

Supinator muscle

Extensor carpi radialis brevis muscle (retracted)

Fig. 6.7.10 Anatomy of the radial tunnel and compression sites of the radial nerve in the proximal forearm.

extensor muscles [59]. The syndrome is seen with repetitive pronation/supinations, as in racquet sports, and in particular with stressed wrist extension, as in weight-lifting, bowling, rowing and golf.

Symptoms are pain laterally in the forearm during activity, and in the quite rare cases of PINS also decreased strength of the muscles extending the wrist. On examination there is often pain at the supinator muscle, 4–5 cm distally to the elbow, and pain can be provoked by resisted supination with the elbow extended. There is often pain at the proximal part of the extensor muscles, especially with resisted extension of the fingers, in particular the middle finger, but this is also typical of tennis elbow. If there are motor nerve symptoms, extension strength of the fingers and the wrist is decreased. There are no sensory symptoms in this syndrome.

Most cases resolve with conservative treatment, and cure after injection of corticosteroid at the tender point of compression has been described. In unresolved cases after 3–6 months surgical decompression can be performed with 50–80% successful results.

Compartment syndrome

The muscle groups in the forearm are surrounded by fasciae, which are inelastic. A rapid increase in the content of the fasciae, either hematoma, edema or hypertrophy of the musculature, therefore leads to increased compartmental pressure. With small or intermittent increases, a reversible ischemia of the muscle occurs, but the pressure may be so high that it leads to irreversible ischemia and necrosis of the muscle. A compartment pressure of 30 mmHg or more for more than 8 h leads to muscle death.

Compartment syndrome of the forearm is in most cases post-traumatic, caused by hematoma or edema, and not particularly a sports injury. Very often the person has been lying on the arm for several hours during intoxication by alcohol or medicine. Direct trauma or muscle tears during sports can lead to edema and intracompartmental bleeding and a fulminant compartment syndrome. The symptoms are constant pain and fatigue of the involved muscle group. Clinically the involved muscle group is swollen, hard and very tender, and active function exerts extreme pain. The person should be admitted to hospital as fast as possible for surgical decompression by splitting the

muscle fascia. It is essential that this is done quickly, as irreversible changes in the muscle are induced after a few hours.

Repeated heavy work with the forearm muscles, e.g. in weight-lifting, gradually increases muscle mass, which can cause compartment syndrome, as can acute edema of the muscle after excessive training [60,61]. In the exertional compartment syndrome symptoms appear during activity, e.g. weight-lifting or racquet sports, and they resolve quickly after activity, leaving tenderness of the muscles for some hours. Examination during activity reveals tenderness and fatigue of the muscle. Measurement of the intracompartmental pressure during activity is useful [61], and with increased pressures or strong clinical evidence of compartment syndrome, fasciotomy can be performed with good results.

Wrist

Tendon problems

Any tendon that crosses the wrist can become inflamed with stress-related sports activities [62–64]. The cause can be a sudden initiation of motion or a chronic loading mechanism. The symptoms are usually pain which runs along the tendon, and is provoked by resisted activation. Treatment always starts with nonoperative means such as splinting, ice, NSAIDs and avoidance of aggravating activities. Flexibility and strength programs can be initiated after the acute inflammation has resolved. Modifications of techniques such as poor positioning of the hands on a racquet may be helpful and can be directed by a trainer to avoid future injuries.

Intersection syndrome

This refers to a condition of pain, crepitus, tenderness and swelling where the abductor pollicis longus and extensor pollicis brevis cross the extensor carpi radialis longus and brevis tendons, approximately 6–8 cm proximal to Lister's tubercle. This condition can be seen in sports which require repetitive wrist flexion and extension against resistance such as rowing or gymnastics [64,65], and the etiology is secondary to peritendinous inflammation and bursitis [3].

Non-operative treatment consists of avoiding aggravating activities, splinting of the thumb and

NSAIDs. This is usually effective [3]. The addition of a steroid injection may be indicated if initial measures fail. If these measures fail and symptoms warrant it, surgical exploration with decompression of the second dorsal wrist compartment and debridement of the inflamed bursa should be considered.

de Quervain's tenosynovitis

de Quervain's tenosynovitis is the most common form of stenosing tenosynovitis in the wrist and is seen frequently in racquet-ball players [62] (Fig. 6.7.11). This condition is secondary to inflammation of the first dorsal compartment tendons (abductor pollicis longus and extensor pollicis brevis) as they pass through a tight fibro-osseous tunnel at the level of the radial styloid [3].

Clinically, the patient complains of pain about the first dorsal compartment which can radiate along the tendons and is related to activities, particularly thumb use. Examination reveals tenderness to palpation and swelling along the course of the tendon on the dorso-lateral wrist. Confirmation of the diagnosis is by Finkelstein's test with pain reproduced by ulnar deviation of the hand with the thumb tucked under the fist. Around 80% of patients respond to non-operative treatment [62] of a combination of an injection of steroid into the compartment with attention paid to the superficial radial nerve and immobilization in a thumb spica for 2 weeks. Surgical release can be considered in recalcitrant cases [3].

Extensor insertional tenosynovitis

Extensor insertional tenosynovitis can occur in any of the extensor tendons. Pain along the tendon is the presenting complaint. The second dorsal compartment (extensor carpi radialis longus and brevis) is the most common of the extensor tendons to be affected. It may be associated with bony thickening at the insertion site which is referred to as carpal bossing [66–68]. This condition should be distinguished from a dorsal wrist ganglion where the mass is more proximal and transilluminates. Radiographic examination can

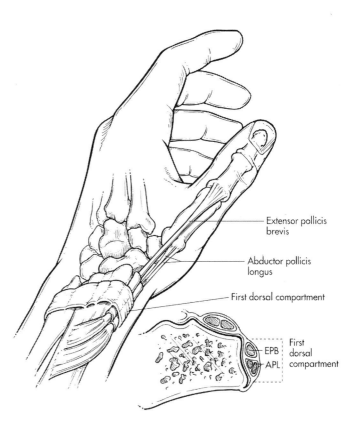

Extensor pollicis brevis

Abductor pollicis longus

First dorsal compartment

EPB

APL

First dorsal compartment

Fig. 6.7.11 De Quervain's anatomy. From Cooney, W. (ed.) *The Wrist: Diagnosis and Operative Treatment.* Mosby, 1998.

confirm the osseous nature of this process. The condition frequently responds to non-operative management [3].

Tenosynovitis of the extensor pollicis longus can occur and is seen after distal radius fractures in squash or tennis players. The tendon is at risk as it crosses around Lister's tubercle. The patient presents with a history of dorsal radial wrist pain which is elicited with resisted thumb extension. Treatment consists of splinting and NSAIDs. An injection of steroid can be added to the regimen if initial methods fail. In cases resistant to non-operative measures, transposition of the tendon radial to Lister's tubercle can be considered.

Extensor carpi ulnaris tenosynovitis

Extensor carpi ulnaris (ECU) tenosynovitis is an uncommon condition seen typically in racquet sports [62,69]. The ECU is notable because of its distinct sheath which crosses the wrist (Fig. 6.7.12) [70]. The ECU is believed to contribute to the stability of the wrist. Patients with ECU tenosynovitis typically present with dorsal ulnar wrist pain and swelling. Examination demonstrates tenderness over the ECU at the wrist with pain provoked by ulnar deviation of the wrist and restricted dorsiflexion in the supinated position [69]. The treatment consists of a steroid injection combined with immobilization for 2 weeks in a long arm splint in the pronated position. If non-operative measures fail, surgical decompression of the radial side of the subsheath may be performed. The repair of the extensor retinaculum should be done in a meticulous fashion to avoid subluxation of the extensor carpi ulnaris.

Recurrent subluxation of the ECU can be caused by a traumatic event in which the ulnar aspect of the ECU fibro-osseous sheath is disrupted [64]. This is due to a sudden supination, ulnar deviation and palmar flexion force. The condition may be seen in golf, tennis and weight-lifting [71–73]. The patient presents with complaints of pain associated with a clicking with forearm rotation. This can be elicited on examination although in some cases reproduction may be difficult. If the condition is detected within the first 6 weeks, immobilization in pronation and radial deviation should be successful. Chronic cases require surgical stabilization [3].

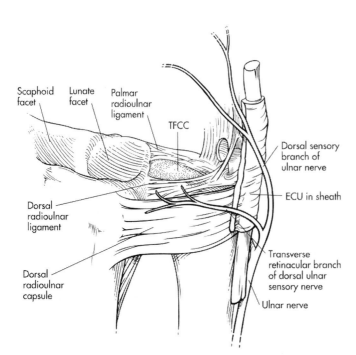

Fig. 6.7.12 Extensor carpi ulnaris (ECU) anatomy. From Cooney, W. (ed.) *The Wrist: Diagnosis and Operative Treatment.* Mosby, 1998.

Nerve disorders

Nerve disorders can be common in certain athletic endeavors such as cycling, baseball, karate, rugby and handball [3]. Problems in these athletes may include carpal tunnel syndrome, cyclist's palsy, gymnast palsy and Wartenberg's syndrome. The cause of these disorders is believed to be mechanical compression secondary to local tissue edema, blunt trauma, adjacent joint synovitis or equipment constraints which results in compression and vascular compromise of the nerve. This mechanical compression causes venous obstruction and subsequent congestion, resulting in anoxia. This anoxia results in greater edema and an inflammatory response, with the end result being fibroblastic proliferation and constriction of the nerve [3].

Cyclist's palsy (ulnar nerve Guyon's canal)

Cyclists can develop numbness and paresthesias in the ulnar nerve-innervated digits secondary to compression of the ulnar nerve in and distal to Guyon's canal. This condition can arise in any sport that involves repeated compression of the ulnar palm. There are three types of compression that have been described [74]. Type 1 involves motor and sensory branches. The site of compression is proximal to the canal. Type 2 involves the canal to the area of the hook of the hamate and involves the motor branch only. The type 3 lesion involves only the sensory branch and occurs in the distal third of the canal. Patients with this condition present with symptoms of paresthesias in the ulnar two digits. There is often a positive Tinel's sign and tenderness over Guyon's canal. Weakness can arise in the chronic cases due to compression of the motor branch [75]. Weakness can occur in the first dorsal interosseous muscle, the thumb adductor muscle which results in a positive Froment's sign, or in the third palmar interosseous muscle which may result in a positive Wartenberg sign. Neurologic examination may note a deficit in two-point discrimination. Allen's test should be performed to rule out vascular injury at the level of the canal [3].

Causative factors such as poor riding conditions or equipment such as unpadded handlebars which contribute to this condition are noted frequently in the history. Treatment includes avoiding direct pressure over the hypothenar eminence until inflammation and symptoms have resolved. Splinting and anti-inflammatory medications may be used. If these methods fail, decompression of Guyon's canal can be considered. A return to sports should be avoided until symptoms have been resolved [3].

Gymnast's palsy

Gymnast's palsy is caused by direct compression of or injury to the posterior interosseous nerve secondary to hyperextension of the wrist [4,76]. On examination wrist extension may cause pain or simply direct compression over the dorsal aspect of the wrist may reproduce symptoms (Fig. 6.7.13). Treatment consists of cessation from hyperextension activities as well as splinting for competition. Posterior interosseous nerve neurectomy may be required if these measures fail and symptoms warrant.

Wartenberg's syndrome

Any sport which requires repetitive forearm rotation and ulnar deviation of the wrist can lead to traction neuropathy of the superficial branch of the radial nerve. This condition is common in non-athletes as well. The nerve can be found located in a subcutaneous position between the extensor carpi radialis longus and the brachioradialis in the mid-distal forearm. As the nerve continues distally to the wrist, the brachioradialis and extensor carpi radialis muscles transition from muscular to tendinous portion and this is where the location of entrapment occurs. Patients complain of pain and numbness over the dorsal radial aspect of the hand and thumb. Physical examination includes Tinel's sign over the nerve with reproduction of symptoms in wrist flexion and ulnar deviation [3]. Treatment includes cessation of aggravating activities, ice, and splinting in a cock-up wrist splint. If these measures are not successful in alleviating symptoms the nerve can be released over the point of maximal Tinel's sign [3].

Carpal tunnel syndrome

Carpal tunnel syndrome is the most common compressive neuropathy at the wrist and may be associated with sporting activities secondary to flexor tenosynovitis or lumbrical muscle hypertrophy as well as an extension injury [3,7]. The signs and symptoms of carpal tunnel have been well described: the patient presents

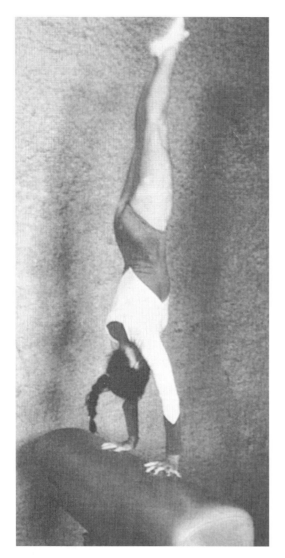

Fig. 6.7.13 Gymnastic dorsiflexion injury mechanism. From Cooney, W. (ed.) *The Wrist: Diagnosis and Operative Treatment.* Mosby, 1998.

with pain and paresthesias in the first, second and third digits of the hand, which can radiate along the course of the nerve. Frequently patients complain of nocturnal awakening, pain and paresthesias. Physical examination includes provocative tests such as Phalen's sign, carpal tunnel compression sign, and Tinel's sign. Electromyography and nerve conduction velocities are helpful in confirming the diagnosis and noting the severity of the condition [3]. It is important to rule out other causes of median nerve compression such as pronator syndrome, anterior interosseous syndrome and cervical radiculopathy. Treatment of carpal tunnel syndrome begins with splinting, especially at night. Causative activities should be avoided and anti-inflammatory medication may help decrease the synovitis in the carpal tunnel. Injection of the carpal tunnel may assist in resolution of the symptoms. If non-operative measures fail, surgical decompression is recommended [3].

Vascular disorders

Hypothenar hammer syndrome

Thrombosis of the ulnar artery in Guyon's canal may occur in sports such as judo, karate, basketball, hockey, handball and lacrosse [3,5,77,78]. It may occur as a result of a single traumatic event or as a repetitive trauma [10]. The ulnar nerve and ulnar artery are susceptible to injury in Guyon's canal. Injury to the ulnar artery may involve only the intima, in which case thrombosis occurs. A true aneurysm results from fusiform swelling of all three areas of the arterial wall, and false aneurysm is the result of a rupture of the vessel with encapsulation of a resulting hematoma [75]. A pseudoaneurysm results if the outer layers are disrupted, allowing a bulge of the vessel [75]. Patients present with pain and coldness of the fingers and palm. In advanced cases distal ulcerations of the skin can develop. When examining patients with these symptoms, Tinel's sign may indicate nerve involvement and if absent, this suggests a primary vascular etiology. Allen's test is the most important examination to evaluate patency of the vessels [75]. Differential diagnoses may include thoracic outlet syndrome, subclavian steal, systemic disease such as Raynaud's or a vasculitis [75]. Beyond physical examination, Doppler studies or an angiogram may be helpful in diagnosis. Treatment initially involves rest from the offending activity. Baseball players should increase padding over the glove which can be helpful. Surgical options include exploration of the thrombosed ulnar artery with ligation and excision or vein grafting to re-establish flow [75].

Bony injuries and disorders

Scaphoid fractures

The scaphoid is the most frequently fractured carpal bone in athletes and occurs commonly in sports such as football, basketball, hockey and boxing [3]. Non-union occurs in approximately 10–15% of patients and key factors in preventing this are early recognition and appropriate management. Most scaphoid fractures heal in an acceptable position with cast treatment [79]. Diagnosis is made by history and examination. Clues from the history include the mechanism of injury and location of pain, and on examination tenderness and swelling in the anatomic snuff box are noted [3]. Radiographs may be diagnostic; however, the absence of fracture on plain films does not rule out this injury. High clinical suspicion warrants a bone scan, CT or MRI. These studies have all been used to diagnose scaphoid fractures [80,81]. Treatment options are determined by displacement and chronicity of the injury. Non-displaced scaphoid fractures can be treated in a long arm thumb spica cast. Displaced fractures should be addressed surgically [3].

Capitate fractures

Injury to the capitate occurs from direct trauma or extreme dorsiflexion of the wrist and is often associated with high-impact velocity sports [3]. The mechanism of injury is extreme wrist dorsiflexion and an axial load [82]. This allows the capitate to come into contact with the dorsal rim of the radius. Radiographs are often difficult to interpret due to superimposition of the other carpal bones; suspicion is therefore high, and tomograms may be helpful [3]. There is a high frequency of non-unions and avascular necrosis in capitate fractures therefore anatomic reduction is required [3]. Rigid anatomic reduction can be accomplished by internal fixation.

Hook of the hamate fractures

Hook of the hamate fractures can occur in direct contact sports or racquet-sport injuries as well as golf [3]. The hamate hook projects into the palm in the area of the hypothenar eminence and is vulnerable at this position. Due to the proximity of Guyon's canal any hook of the hamate fracture can be associated with neurovascular injury [3]. Patients present with complaints of pain in the palm aggravated by grasp. There is often loss of grip strength, and symptoms of ulnar nerve paresthesias and weakness of ulnar nerve-innervated muscles in the hand may be present [3]. On examination there is pain with direct palpation over the hook of the hamate. Standard X-rays should be obtained and if there is a possibility of fracture a CT scan may aid in the diagnosis [3] (Figs 6.7.14 & 6.7.15). Prognosis is determined by expedient diagnosis. A short arm cast is the initial treatment of choice. A delayed diagnosis may not allow for return to competition [83]. If non-union occurs excision of the hook of the hamate may be done [3]. Open reduction and internal fixation can

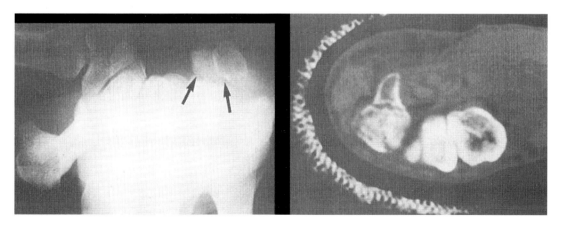

Fig. 6.7.14 CT scan of the hamate fracture. From Cooney, W. (ed.) *The Wrist: Diagnosis and Operative Treatment.* Mosby, 1998.

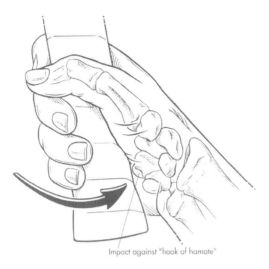

Impact against "hook of hamate"

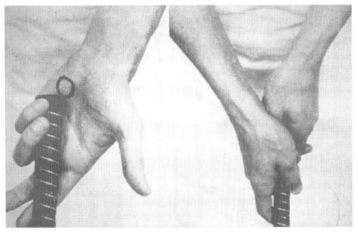

Fig. 6.7.15 Hook of hamate fracture. From Cooney, W. (ed.) *The Wrist: Diagnosis and Operative Treatment.* Mosby, 1998.

be considered in both acute or delayed fractures. If the fracture is displaced or diagnosed late (more than 2 weeks) open reduction and internal fixation is recommended [3].

Triquetrum impaction fractures

Fractures of the triquetrum are seen in athletes; however, there is no consistent association with any particular sport [3]. They tend to happen as a result of a fall or blunt trauma to the dorsum of the hand. Others have suggested impaction of the triquetrum against the ulnar styloid [3,84]. Patients present with dorsal ulnar wrist pain. Placement of the wrist in the position of dorsiflexion and ulnar deviation will reproduce the pain. Another consideration with this injury is associated carpal instability, which should be addressed on examination. The triangular fibrocartilage complex (TFCC) may be injured in association with this mechanism of injury. Diagnoses made on radiographs, however, may be missed. Treatment is with immobilization in a short arm cast [3].

Carpometacarpal (CMC) fractures and dislocations

Injuries to the CMC joints are relatively rare due to the intrinsic stability of these joints. The most frequent mechanism of injury is axial load applied to a clenched fist. The key to treating this injury is early diagnosis, and a 45° pronation oblique view is the most effective method of diagnosis on radiographs [3]. Recommended treatment is closed reduction and stabilization by percutaneous pin fixation. If closed reduction is unsuccessful, the fracture or dislocation should be opened [3,85,86].

Gymnast's wrist

The popularity of gymnastics has increased over the past two decades. There are often overuse injuries at the level of the wrist associated with gymnastics [12]. Chronic repetitive compressive forces on the distal radius have adverse effects on enchondral ossification. Repeated microtrauma may disrupt the metaphyseal vascular network. This may result in a wide and irregular physis [3]. Patients will present with a prolonged history of dorsal wrist pain that is exacerbated by activities and may also have local swelling over the wrist. X-rays in this condition will show widening of the distal radial physis and cystic changes and irregularity of the metaphyseal margin of the physis and palmar radial beaking adjacent to the physis and haziness of the physis [3,87]. This process is thought to be a result of extreme dorsiflexion. The treatment consists of cessation of aggravating activities and weight-bearing on the affected extremity should not be resumed until the patient is asymptomatic [3].

Impaction syndromes

There have been several impaction syndromes associated with repeated hyperextension injuries including ulnar carpal impaction syndrome, scaphoid impaction syndrome and triquetrolunate impaction syndrome. These are all commonly seen in gymnasts but may be seen in other sports [3]. The general approach to these types of injuries includes rest and splinting (Fig. 6.7.16).

Triangular fibrocartilage complex (TFCC) injuries

Injuries to the TFCC can occur in athletes and are a result of a fall on the pronated outstretched hand. They may also occur secondary to a rotational force or traction to the ulnar border of the hand. These lesions may be classified by the Palmer classification [52]. The TFCC is thought to contribute to the stability of the ulnar side of the wrist as well as serving as an origin for

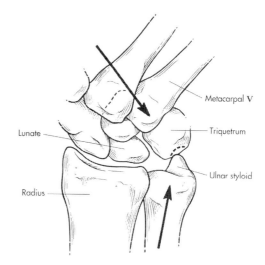

Fig. 6.7.16 Ulnar–triquetral impaction. From Cooney, W. (ed.) *The Wrist: Diagnosis and Operative Treatment.* Mosby, 1998.

palmar ulnocarpal ligaments [3]. Patients present with complaints of ill-defined, poorly localized pain in the ulnar aspect of the wrist, and diagnosis by wrist arthroscopy has been recommended by some [88]. Treatment depends on the classification and involves a combination of wrist arthroscopy with debridement or repair and immobilization [3].

Instability

Dislocation of the distal radioulnar joint. Distal ulnar dislocation can be either dorsal (in extreme pronation) or volar (in extreme supination by a direct blow on the ulna). Often the TFCC is torn, and rotation is very painful. This condition can be a cause of ulnar pain in athletes. Acute cases can be treated conservatively with a plaster, but in chronic cases operative repair of the TFCC is often necessary.

Carpal instability is seen with rupture of the intercarpal ligaments (in most cases between the scaphoid and lunate, but sometimes between lunate and triquetrum) after a trauma to the extended, pronated wrist, e.g. during motor sport or football. The instability can be shown clinically. X-rays may be normal without stress, and the condition is sometimes overlooked. Symptoms are pain and locking. Treatment is often operative.

Hand

Fractures

Subungual hematomas and tuft fracture

Direct trauma to the distal aspect of the fingertip can cause a painful hematoma deep to the nail. This can often be associated with a fracture of the distal phalanx. Evacuation of the hematoma may decrease the symptoms of pain and if the hematoma occupies greater than 50% of the exposed nail there is a high likelihood of a significant nailbed laceration which should be surgically repaired [89].

Fractures of the phalanges and metacarpals

Fractures in the hand encountered in sports are often a result of low-energy injuries and are frequently stable [89]. Diagnosis is often easily made by an X-ray. On physical examination it is important to assess rotation of the ray by asking the patient to flex the fingertips and touch the palm (Fig. 6.7.17). Fractures of the distal phalanx may be divided into tuft, shaft and base or physeal fractures in children [90]. Most closed shaft and tuft fractures are stable and these may be associated with nailbed injuries. Stable fractures may be immobilized with a stack splint. Base fractures of the distal phalanx will be discussed in mallet finger deformities. Proximal and middle phalanx fractures are very common, especially in the index and small fingers [91]. Fractures are classified according to their anatomic location and include condylar neck and subcondylar shaft and base or epiphyseal fractures [92–94]. Condylar fractures are either uni- or bicondylar and displaced fractures should be treated surgically in an attempt to prevent articular incongruity [89]. Non-displaced fractures treated in cast immobilization should be followed closely due to the inherent instability of the injury. Subcondylar neck fractures are uncommon in adults but can be seen in the proximal phalanx in children [89]. An important injury to assess for is the fracture of the proximal phalanx that involves 90° rotation of the condylar fragment and entrapment of the volar plate in the joint [90]. These injuries should be treated surgically. Shaft fractures are more common in adults and are stable if not displaced and are amenable to cast immobilization for 3–4 weeks. It is important again to note on

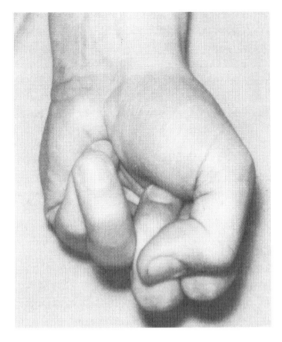

Fig. 6.7.17 Rotational deformity secondary to a metacarpal or phalangeal fracture as best demonstrated with the fingers flexed. The malrotated ring finger overlaps the little finger. From Sports related injuries of the hand and wrist. *Clinics in Sports Medicine* 1990; 9.

examination any rotational displacement of these fractures.

Base fractures in adults may be associated with joint dislocations. A significant injury that is sometimes overlooked is one that involves fracture of the volar base of the middle phalanx with dorsal subluxation of the joint [95]. The subluxation should be reduced and is accomplished by gentle longitudinal traction and flexion of the joint; however, if the patient extends the finger, the joint will tend to resubluxate due to soft tissue disruption. The patient should be immobilized in an extension block splint which prevents extension beyond 45–60°. This fracture should be closely followed due to the possibility of resubluxation [95]. Surgical treatment has been recommended for treatment of fractures which involve more than 40% of the articular surface [86,96,97].

Boxer's fracture

Fractures of the neck of the fifth metacarpal are common in sports, especially in boxing. It has been

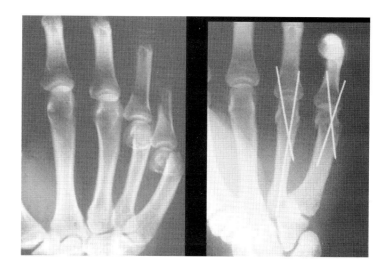

Fig. 6.7.18 Boxer's fracture and 4th metacarpal fracture. From *Green's Operative Hand Surgery*, 3rd edn. Churchill & Livingstone, 1993.

reported that the angulation of a fifth metacarpal fracture up to 60° can be accepted; however, 30° or less is preferable [95,98]. These fractures are often easily reduced, but may, however, be unstable and should be followed closely (Fig. 6.7.18). As with other fractures in the hand, malrotation should be assessed and corrected. Splinting in a well-molded plaster splint will be helpful in maintaining any reduction. If reduction cannot be maintained with plaster, percutaneous K-wire fixation should be performed [95].

Metacarpal shaft fractures

Fractures of the metacarpal shaft can be transverse, oblique or comminuted. Non-displaced stable fractures can be treated by cast immobilization; however, any displacement, difficulty with reduction or shortening should be addressed operatively. Transverse fractures may be treated by percutaneous fixation with a K-wire. More rigid internal fixation can be provided with a plate and screws for any type of metacarpal shaft fracture [95].

Special attention has been paid to the thumb metacarpal fractures and these have been divided into Bennett's and Rolando fractures as well as epibasal fractures (Fig. 6.7.19). Epibasal thumb fractures are extra-articular fractures and are amenable to thumb spica casting. Bennett's fractures are two-part inter-articular fractures at the metacarpal base and the small fragment is held in place by a volar oblique ligament while the larger portion is distracted by the

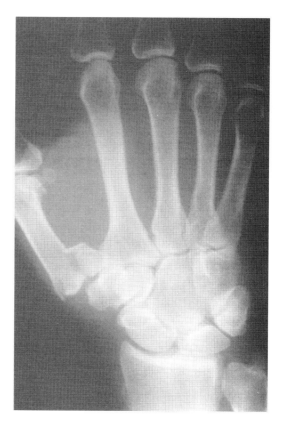

Fig. 6.7.19 Rolando fracture. From *Campbell's Operative Orthopedics*, 9th edn. Mosby, 1998.

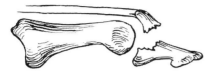

Fig. 6.7.20 Mallet finger originating from bone injury. From *Rockwood and Green's Fractures in Adults*, 4th edn. Lippincott-Raven, 1996.

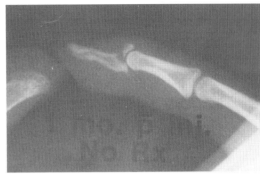

(a)

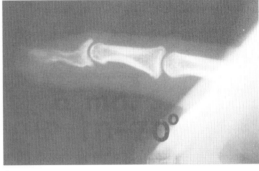

(b)

Fig. 6.7.21 Mallet fractures that are moderately displaced (a) usually heal with reasonably good congruity (b). From *Rockwood and Green's Fractures in Adults*, 4th edn. Lippincott-Raven, 1996.

attachment of the abductor pollicis longus [89]. Closed reduction and cast immobilization has been effective; however, closed reduction and percutaneous pinning for less than 3 mm of fracture displacement and open reduction and fixation for larger displacements has been effective in treating these injuries [99]. Rolando fractures are three-part interarticular fractures of the thumb metacarpal that should be treated surgically.

Tendon injuries

Mallet finger

Mallet finger injuries are a result of disruption of the extensor tendon or a fracture of the distal phalangeal dorsal base which results in extension lag at the distal interphalangeal joint and possibly volar subluxation of the distal phalanx [89]. In children the fracture occurs through the physis. Open mallet fingers should include surgical debridement as well as a repair of the nailbed. Closed mallet and bony mallet fingers should be splinted for 6–8 weeks and large interarticular fragments can be treated with percutaneous pinning [89] (Figs 6.7.20 & 6.7.21).

Boutonnière deformity

Disruption of the extensor mechanism as it inserts to the base of the middle phalanx may present as a pure ligamentous or a bony avulsion. Boutonnière deformities do not immediately present but develop over the course of 2–3 weeks, as the lateral bands migrate volarly producing flexion at the proximal interphalangeal joint (PIP) and extension at the distal interphalangeal joint [89].

Acutely, the diagnosis can be made with PIP joint tenderness and weak PIP extension against resistance as well as loss of greater than 20° of active extension

with the wrist and metacarpophalangeal joints fully flexed [89]. This injury should be immediately splinted in extension. If initial non-operative treatments fail, surgical repair of the extensor tendon can be considered after adequate range of motion is obtained.

Avulsions of the flexor digitorum profundus

Avulsion of the flexor digitorum profundus tendon is similar to a mallet deformity and is diagnosed as inability to actively flex the distal interphalangeal joint, associated with pain and swelling. Radiographs may show avulsion of the volar base of the distal phalanx. The ring finger is most often involved and is seen in football injuries as the finger is caught in the opponent's jersey. Surgical treatment of the tendon should be performed within 7–10 days to avoid retraction of the flexor tendon.

Dislocations/sprains

Proximal interphalangeal joint (PIP)

Dorsal dislocations of the PIP are very common and are typically reduced prior to presentation. Reduction can be accomplished by longitudinal traction of a digit. Dorsal dislocations may involve the volar plate and it is important to differentiate pure dislocation from fracture-dislocations where a fracture fragment or soft tissue is located in the joint space. Treatment of simple dislocations involves buddy taping for 6 weeks [100]. Complex dislocations may be difficult to reduce by closed methods.

Sprain of the collateral ligaments are extremely common in sports, especially basketball. If gross instability is not present, the injury can be managed with buddy taping during activities for approximately 1 month. Resolution of this injury usually takes 4–6 months and residual swelling may be present [89,101].

Metacarpophalangeal joint

Dorsal dislocation of the metacarpophalangeal joint can be simple or complex. Simple dislocations often appear to be hyperextended and they are reduced by flexing the first phalangeal base while maintaining dorsal pressure on the metacarpal head. Traction alone should not be used, in order to avoid converting a simple dislocation to a complex dislocation. Complex dislocations involve the flexor tendon and lumbrical muscle as well as an injury to the volar plate which is trapped in the joint. These injuries often require operative treatment if not reduced by closed means [102]. Simple dislocations can be addressed with reduction and buddy taping and return to activities as tolerated.

Skiier's thumb

Injuries to the ulnar collateral ligament of the thumb are frequent in sporting activities. Occasionally the ulnar collateral ligament is completely avulsed, allow-ing the adductor epineurosis to become interposed between it and its distal insertion site. This is referred to as a Stenner lesion [102,103]. This injury can often be palpated on the ulnar aspect of the thumb metacarpophalangeal joint and it prevents normal healing. This results in chronic instability. Stability of the joint to adduction stress is performed with the MP joint held in the extended position as well as flexion at 30°. Comparison to the non-injured side is mandatory to assess laxity. Injuries with increased laxity of less than 30° that have firm or minimally soft end points are considered to be grade I or II sprains and they are best treated in a thumb spica for 3–6 weeks. Surgery is indicated for: (i) irreducible injuries due to soft tissue interposition; (ii) interarticular fractures that are displaced or rotated; (iii) grossly unstable injuries; or (iv) the presence of a Stenner lesion [89].

Summary

Overuse problems in elbow and wrist are very common in sports, but most cases can be treated conservatively with a good outcome.

In the elbow, throwing and racquet sports cause epicondylitis, tension overload of the medial ligament, posteromedial impingement and degenerative disease of the lateral compartment. Elbow instability, either from medial overload or after traumatic dislocations, can often be treated surgically.

In the wrist, tendon problems are common in golf, racquet sports and cycling. Impaction and impingement problems are common in gymnastics. Nerve entrapment is an overload problem in both elbow, forearm and wrist.

Hand problems in sports are mainly traumatic. A precise diagnosis of fractures, ligament or tendon ruptures and dislocations is important for an optimal outcome.

This chapter has dealt with the pathogenesis, trauma mechanisms, diagnosis, imaging, treatment, outcome and prevention of these conditions.

Case story 6.7.1

A 45-year-old-man has played tennis for 30 years. He had never experienced problems until last year, when he had to stop playing 2 months before the end of the season, because of medial pain in the elbow during serving and smashes. Symptoms resolved. Two weeks into the new season he developed medial and lateral elbow pain during serving and slashing. The medial pain resolved after the matches, but the lateral pain is constant, and gets worse during daily activities. With continued playing he now also experiences paresthesia in the ulnar fingers.

At examination, there is tenderness laterally, on the epicondyle and on the joint line, as well as medially some cm distal to the joint line. There is a slight extension defect and posteromedial pain with forced extension.

1 Which specific clinical tests should be performed?
2 Which diagnoses are possible?
3 What is the treatment and prognosis?

1–Specific tests

Forced extension and flexion of the fingers and wrist to unmask lateral or medial epicondylitis. Palpation of the ulnar nerve in the cubital tunnel and Tinel's test for entrapment of the ulnar nerve. Test for medial stability, noting if valgus stress elicits medial pain. The valgus extension overload test should be performed for posteromedial impingement.

2–Diagnoses

Lateral epicondylitis is the most common problem in middle-aged tennis players, and will also be symptomatic during daily activities. The forced extension test will be positive, and the other specific tests will come out normal.

But the history and basic findings (including a small extension deficiency) are suggestive of medial overload syndrome with tearing of the medial collateral ligament, medial instability, posterior impingement, ulnar nerve overload and lateral joint degeneration. The valgus stress test will elicit pain medially, and there may or may not be

instability. The valgus extension over load test will elicit posteromedial pain in posterior impingement, and X-rays may show osteophytes on the olecranon. There may be osteophytes in the cubital tunnel and a positive Tinel's sign, but entrapment of the ulnar nerve at other locations is of course also possible. Lateral joint degeneration may show on X-rays as decreased joint space and eventually osteophytes or osteochondritis.

The history should be supplemented with information about the racquet, playing intensity, and technique. If he has changed to harder strings or a heavier racquet or increased his training hours, it may explain why he gets overload symptoms, and these factors should be corrected. If he uses a one-hand technique, he could reduce the load on the elbow by changing to a two-hand technique.

3–Treatment

Primary treatment is conservative: a break from tennis, rest, NSAIDs and if necessary a corticosteroid injection laterally. Gradually as symptoms resolve he can return to tennis. If activities can be modified, the prognosis is good.

With recurrent, chronic symptoms despite at least 6 months conservative treatment, surgery can be considered. For lateral epicondylitis the cojoined tendon can be cleaned up. In posterior impingement the osteophyte on the olecranon can be removed, but in the case of medial instability, symptoms will probably develop again. With medial collateral ligament tearing without instability, the ligament can be cleaned up, but the ligament should be visualized by MRI before operation is planned. With instability, reconstruction of the ligament is the ultimate operative option, but it may be reserved for younger athletes. Degenerative changes in the lateral compartment can be cleaned up arthroscopically. Ulnar nerve transposition or cleaning up in the cubital tunnel can be performed in case of nerve entrapment. The chance of returning to recreational tennis after surgical intervention is best in cases of epicondylitis (85%) and lower in the other conditions (50–75%).

Cse story 6.7.2

A 20-year-old telemark skier falls onto his wrist while skiing above the Arctic Circle. He is unable to seek medical attention until many months later. At that time he complains of chronic pain in his wrist. Plain radiographs demonstrate a scaphoid fracture (Fig. 6.7.22a). What tests are relevant for a scaphoid fracture?

A patient with a scaphoid fracture will complain of pain on the radial aspect of the wrist. Pressure over the volar tubercle on the scaphoid will result in pain. Also, palpation of the snuff box area between the first and third dorsal compartments will result in discomfort. Radiographs will usually demonstrate a displaced fracture, however, many scaphoid fractures are initially non-displaced. Suspicion should be raised if an athlete falls onto the wrist and he presents with chronic wrist pain. A bone scan, tomogram, or CT scan may demonstrate a fracture of the scaphoid, even if the plain radiographs are nor-mal. MRI is also very sensitive to demonstrate the fracture and the possibility of an avascular proximal segment. Most non-displaced scaphoid fractures respond well to cast immobilization for 6 to 8 weeks. In those athletes who desire greater mobility during the healing period, operative reduction with a screw is possible, using a variety of techniques including a percutaneous approach, arthroscopy, or traditional open exposure. Approximately 10% of scaphoid fractures may not heal, even with adequate cast immobilization. In such cases, open reduction and internal fixation with a bone graft is required. The bone graft can be obtained from either the iliac crest or as a vascular graft from the distal radius. In the case presented here (Fig. 6.7.22b) the young skier underwent a vascularized bone graft from the distal radius with screw fixation. His fracture healed at 12 weeks and he was able to return to telemark skiing.

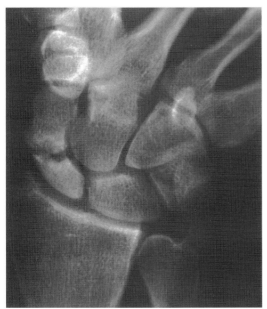

(a)

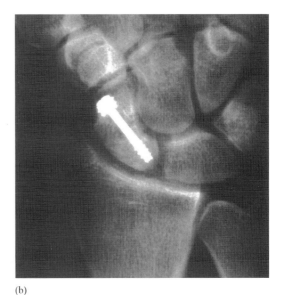

(b)

Fig. 6.7.22 An old scaphoid fracture (a), treated with a bone graft and screw fixation (b).

Multiple choice questions

1 Medial elbow pain in throwing athletes:

a is usually caused by tennis elbow

b can be caused by elbow instability

c in most cases develops after a traumatic elbow injury, e.g. dislocation

d combined with distinct tenderness of the medial humeral epicondyle and pain during restricted wrist flexion is most likely a golfer's elbow.

e can never be treated surgically, but should be treated with corticosteroid injections.

2 Posterior elbow pain during sports activity:

a is often caused by posterolateral rotatory elbow instability

b is often seen in athletes with medial elbow instability

c is usually caused by collision (impingement) between the ulnar nerve and olecranon

d can be treated by arthroscopic operation

e often resolves with conservative treatment in active throwing athletes.

3 Lateral elbow pain:

a elicited in the late cocking phase of throwing can be a symptom of posterolateral rotatory elbow instability

b elicited in the late cocking phase of throwing can be a symptom of medial elbow instability

c elicited during racquet sports in the middle-aged, recreational athlete is most likely lateral epicondylitis

d caused by nerve entrapment is usually not combined with muscle fatigue

e caused by tennis elbow usually resolves with rest, NSAIDs and eventually corticosteroid injection.

References

1   Nirschl RP. Soft-tissue injuries about the elbow. *Clin Sports Med* 1986; **5**: 637–52.

2   Amadio PS. Epidemiology of hand and wrist injuries in sports. *Hand Clinics* 1990; **6**: 379–81.

3   Topper S, Wood MB, Cooney WP. Athletic injuries of the wrist. In: Cooney WP, Linscheid RL, Dobyns JH, eds. *The Wrist: Diagnosis and Operative Treatment.* St. Louis: Mosby, 1998: 1031–74.

4   Dobyns JH, Sim FH, Linscheid RL. Sports stress syndromes of the hand and wrist. *Am J Sports Med* 1978; **6**: 236–54.

5   Conn J Jr, Bergan JJ, Bell JL. Hypothenar hammer syndrome: Post-traumatic digital ischemia. *Surgery* 1970; **68**: 1122–8.

6   Cooney WP. Sports injuries to the upper extremity. *Post Grad Med* 1984; **76**: 45–50.

7   Rettig AC. Epidemiology of hand and wrist injuries in sports. *Clin Sports Med* 1998; **17**: 401–6.

8   Bergfeld JA, Wieker GG, Andrish JT *et al.* Soft plain splint for protection of significant hand and wrist injuries in sports. *Am J Sports Med* 1982; **10**: 293–6.

9   Riester JN, Baker BE, Mosher JF *et al.* A review of scaphoid fracture healing in competitive athletes. *Am J Sports Med* 1985; **13**: 154–61.

10 Rettig AC, Ryan RO, Stone JA. Epidemiology of hand injuries in sports. In: Strickland JW, Rettig AC, eds. *Hand Injuries in Athletes.* Philadelphia: W.B. Saunders, 1992: 37–44.

11 Caine D, Roy S, Singer KM *et al.* Stress changes of the distal radial growth plate: a radiographic survey and review of the literature. *Am J Sports Med* 1992; **20**: 290–8.

12 Dobyns JH, Gabel GT. Gymnast's wrist. *Hand Clinics* 1990; **6**: 493–505.

13 Binder AI, Hazleman BL. Lateral humeral epicondylitis — a study of natural history and the effect of conservative therapy. *Br J Rheum* 1983; **22**: 73–6.

14 Davidson PA, Pink M, Perry J, Jobe FW. Functional anatomy of the flexor pronator muscle group in relation to the medial collateral ligament of the elbow. *Am J Sports Med* 1995; **23**: 245–50.

15 Field LD, Callaway GH, O'Brien SJ, Altcheck DW. Arthroscopic assessment of the medial collateral ligament complex of the elbow. *Am J Sports Med* 1995; **23**: 396–400.

16 Morrey BF, An KN. Functional anatomy of the ligaments of the elbow. *Clin Orth Rel Res* 1985; **201**: 84–90.

17 Schwab GH, Bennett JB, Woods GW, Tullos HS. Biomechanics of elbow instability: the role of the medial collateral ligament. *Clin Orth Rel Res* 1980; **146**: 42–52.

18 O'Driscoll SW, Bell DF, Morrey BF. Posterolateral rotatory instability of the elbow. *J Bone Joint Surg (Am)* 1991; **73**: 440–6.

19 Edelson G, Kunos CA, Vigder F, Obed E. Bony changes at the lateral epicondyle of possible significance in tennis elbow syndrome. *J Shoulder Elbow Surg* 2001; **10**: 158–63.

20 Kang HS, Kindynis P, Brahme SK, Resnick D, Haghighi P, Haller J, Sartoris DJ. Triangular fibrocartilage and intercarpal ligaments of the wrist: MR imaging. Cadaveric study with gross pathologic and histologic correlation. *Radiology* 1991; **181**: 401–4.

21 Gruchow HW, Pelletier D. An epidemiologic study of tennis elbow. Incidence, recurrence, and effectiveness of prevention strategies. *Am J Sports Med* 1979; **7**: 234–8.

22 Nirschl RP. Tennis elbow. *Orthop Clinics N Am* 1973; **4**: 787–800.

23 Kibler WB. Pathophysiology of overload injuries around the elbow. *Clin Sports Med* 1995; **14**: 447–57.

24 Froimson AI. Treatment of tennis elbow with forearm support band. *J Bone Joint Surg (Am)* 1971; **53-A**: 183–4.

25 Groppel JL, Nirschl RP. A mechanical and electromyographic analysis of the effects of various joint counterforce braces on the tennis player. *Am J Sports Med* 1986; **14**: 195–200.

26 Ciccotti MG, Lombardo SJ. Lateral and medial epicondylitis of the elbow. In: Jobe FW, ed. *Operative Techniques in Upper Extremity Sports Injuries*. St. Louis: Mosby, 1996: 431.

27 Leach RE, Miller JK. Lateral and medial epicondylitis of the elbow. *Clin Sports Med* 1987; **6**: 259–72.

28 Nirschl RP, Pettrone FA. Tennis elbow. The surgical treatment of lateral epicondylitis. *J Bone Joint Surg (Am)*, 1979; **61**: 832–9.

29 Vangness CT Jr, Jobe FW. Surgical treatment of medial epicondylitis. Result in 35 elbows. *J Bone Joint Surg (Brit)* 1991; **73-B**: 409–11.

30 Slocum DB. Classification of elbow injuries from baseball pitching. *Texas Med* 1968; **64**: 48–53.

31 Andrews JR, Timmerman LA. Outcome of elbow surgery in professional baseball players. *Am J Sports Med* 1995; **23**: 404.

32 Andrews JR, Craven WM. Lesions of the posterior compartment of the elbow. *Clin Sports Med* 1991; **10**: 637–51.

33 Jobe FW, Kvinte RS. Elbow instability in the athlete. *Instruct Course Lect* 1991; **40**: 17.

34 Glousman RE, Barron J, Jobe FW, Perry J, Pink M. A electromyographic analysis of the elbow in normal and injured pitchers with medial collateral ligament insufficiency. *Am J Sports Med* 1992; **20**: 311–7.

35 Andrews JR. Bony injuries about the elbow in the throwing athlete. *Instruct Course Lect* 1985; **34**: 323–31.

36 Glousman RE. Ulnar nerve problems in the athlete's elbow. *Clin Sports Med* 1990; **9**: 365–77.

37 Jobe FW, Stark H, Lombardo SJ. Reconstruction of the ulnar collateral ligament in athletes. *J Bone Joint Surg (Am)* 1986; **68**: 1158–63.

38 Conway JE, Jobe FW, Glousman RE, Pink M. Medial instability of the elbow in the throwing athlete. Treatment by repair or reconstruction of the ulnar collateral ligament. *J Bone Joint Surg (Am)* 1992; **74-A**: 67–83.

39 Thompson WH, Jobe FW, Yocum LA, Pink MM. Ulnar collateral ligament reconstruction in athletes: Muscle-splitting approach without transposition of the ulnar nerve. *J Shoulder Elbow Surg* 2001; **10**: 152–7.

40 Jackson DW, Silvino N, Reiman P. Osteochondritis in the female gymnast's elbow. *Arthroscopy* 1989; **5**: 129–36.

41 Tullos HS, King JW. Lesions of the pitching arm in adolescents. *J Am Med Assoc* 1972; **220**: 264–71.

42 Baumgarten TE, Andrews JR, Satterwhite YE. The arthroscopic classification and treatment of osteochondritis dissecans of the capitellum. *Am J Sports Med* 1998; **26**: 520–3.

43 Takahara M, Shundo M, Kondo M *et al*. Early detection of osteochondritis dissecans of the capitellum in young baseball players. Report of three cases. *J Bone Joint Surg (Am)* 1998; **80-A**: 892–7.

44 Bauer M, Jonsson K, Josefsson PO, Linden B. Osteochondritis dissecans of the elbow: a long-term follow-up study. *Clin Orth Rel Res* 1992; **284**: 156–60.

45 Mitsunaga MM, Adishian DA, Bianco AJ Jr. Osteochondritis dissecans of the capitellum. *J Trauma* 1982; **22**: 53–5.

46 Woodward AH, Bianco AJ Jr. Osteochondritis of the elbow. *Clin Orth Rel Res* 1975; **110**: 35–41.

47 McManama GB Jr, Micheli LJ, Berry MV, Sohn RS. The surgical treatment of osteochondritis of the capitellum. *Am J Sports Med* 1985; **13**: 11–21.

48 Josefsson PO, Johnell O, Gentz CF. Long-term sequelae of simple dislocations of the elbow. *J Bone Joint Surg (Am)* 1984; **66**: 927–30.

49 Josefsson PO, Gentz CF, Johnell O, Wendeberg B. Surgical versus non-surgical treatment of ligamentous injuries following dislocation of the elbow joint: a prospective randomized study. *J Bone Joint Surg (Am)* 1987; **69**: 605–8.

50 Josefsson PO, Gentz CF, Johnell O, Wendeberg B. Dislocations of the elbow and intraarticular fractures. *Clin Orth Rel Res* 1989; **246**: 126–30.

51 Cohen MS, Hastings H. Rotatory instability of the elbow: The anatomy and role of the lateral stabilizers. *J Bone Joint Surg (Am)* 1997; **79-A**: 225–33.

52 Rayan GM. Recurrent dislocation of the extensor carpi ulnaris in athletes. *Am J Sports Med* 1983; **11**: 183–4.

53 Nestor BJ, O'Driscoll SW, Morrey BF. Ligamentous reconstruction for posterolateral rotatory instability of the elbow. *J Bone Joint Surg (Am)* 1992; **74-A**: 1235–41.

54 Morrey BF, Askew LJ, An KN, Dobyns JH. Rupture of the distal tendon of the biceps brachii. A biomechanical study. *J Bone Joint Surg (Am)* 1985; **67**: 418–21.

55 D'Alessandro DF, Shields CL Jr, Tibone JE. Repair of distal biceps tendon ruptures in athletes. *Am J Sports Med* 1993; **21**: 114–9.

56 Davidson JJ, Bassett FH, Nunley JA. Musculocutaneous nerve entrapment revisited. *J Shoulder Elbow Surg* 1998; **7**: 250–5.

57 Spinner M. The anterior interosseous-nerve syndrome, with special attention to its variations. *J Bone Joint Surg (Am)* 1970; **52-A**: 84–94.

58 Sponseller PD, Engber WD. Double-entrapment radial tunnel syndrome. *J Hand Surg (Am)* 1983; **8**: 420–3.

59 Potter HG, Weiland AJ, Schatz JA, Paletta GA, Hotchkiss RN. Posterolateral rotatory instability of the elbow. Usefulness of MR imaging in diagnosis. *Radiology* 1997; **204**: 185–9.

60 Jawed S, Jawed AS, Padhiar N, Perry JD. Chronic exertional compartment syndrome of the forearms secondary to weight training. *Rheumatology (Oxf)* 2001; **40**: 344–5.

61 Søderberg TA. Bilateral chronic compartment syndrome in the forearm and the hand. *J Bone Joint Surg (Brit)* 1996; **78-B**: 780–2.

62 Osterman AL, Moskow L, Low DW. Soft tissue injuries of the hand and wrist in racquet sports. *Clin Sports Med* 1998; **7**: 329–48.

63 Stern PJ. Tendinitis, overuse syndromes and tendon injuries. *Hand Clinics* 1990; **6**: 467–76.

64 Wood MB, Dobyns JH. Sports related extra-articular wrist syndromes. *Clin Orth Rel Res* 1986; **202**: 93–102.

65 Wood MB, Linscheid RL. Abductor pollicis longus bursitis. *Clin Orth Rel Res* 1973; **93**: 293–6.

66 Linscheid RL, Dobyns JH. Athletic injuries of the wrists. *Clin Orth Rel Res* 1985; **198**: 141–51.

67 McCune FC III, Baugher WH, Kuland DN. Hand and wrist injuries in the athlete. *Am J Sports Med* 1979; **8**: 275–86.

68 Pettrone FA, Ricciardelli E. Gymnastic injuries: The Virginia experience. *Am J Sports Med* 1987; **15**: 59–62.

69 Hajj AA, Wood MB. Stenosing tenosynovitis of the extensive carpi ulnaris. *Am J Hand Surg* 1986; **11**: 519.

70 Spinner M, Kaplan EB. Extensor carpi ulnaris: Its relationship to the stability of the distal radioulnar joint. *Clin Orth Rel Res* 1970; **68**: 124–9.

71 Burkhart SS, Wood MB, Linscheid RL. Post-traumatic recurrent subluxation of the extensor carpi ulnaris tendon. *Am J Hand Surg* 1982; **7**: 1–3.

72 Plancher KD, Peterson RK, Steichen JB. Compressive neuropathies and tendinopathies in the athletic elbow and wrist. *Clin Sports Med* 1996; **15**: 331–71.

73 Rowland SA. Acute traumatic subluxation of the extensor carpi ulnaris at the wrist. *Am J Hand Surg* 1986; **11**: 809–11.

74 Shea JD, McClain EJ. Ulnar nerve compression syndromes at and below the wrist. *J Bone Joint Surg (Am)* 1969; **51-A**: 1095–1103.

75 Rettig AC. Neurovascular injuries in the wrists and hands of athletes. *Clin Sports Med* 1990; **9**: 389–417.

76 Dellon AL, Seif SS. Anatomic dissections relating the posterior interosseous nerve to the carpus and etiology of dorsal wrist ganglion pain. *Am J Hand Surg* 1978; **3**: 326–32.

77 Aulicino PL. Neurovascular injuries in the hands of athletes. *Hand Clinics* 1990; **6**: 455–66.

78 Ho PK, Dellon AL, Wilgis EF. True aneurysms of the hand resulting from athletic injuries. Report of two cases. *Am J Sports Med* 1985; **13**: 136–8.

79 Cooney WP, Dobyns JH, Linscheid RL. Fractures of the scaphoid: a rational approach to management. *Clin Orth Rel Res* 1980; **149**: 90–7.

80 Perlik PC, Guilford WB. Magnetic resonance imaging to assess the vascularity of scaphoid nonunions. *Am J Hand Surg* 1991; **16**: 479–84.

81 Recht MP, Burk DL Jr, Dalinka MK. Radiology of wrist and hand injuries in athletes. *Clin Sports Med* 1987; **6**: 811–28.

82 Stein F, Seigel MW. Naviculocapitate fracture syndrome: A case report. New thoughts on the mechanism of injury. *J Bone Joint Surg (Am)* 1969; **51-A**: 391–5.

83 Whalen JL, Bishop AT, Linscheid RL. Nonoperative treatment of acute hamate hook fractures. *Am J Hand Surg* 1992; **17**: 507–11.

84 Levy M, Fischel RE, Stern GM *et al.* Chip fractures of the os triquetrum: The mechanism of injury. *J Bone Joint Surg (Am)* 1979; **61-B**: 355–7.

85 Garcia-Elias M, Dobyns JH, Cooney WP III *et al.* Traumatic axial dislocations of the carpus. *Am J Hand Surg* 1989; **14**: 446–57.

86 Garcia-Elias M, Bishop AT, Dobyns JH *et al.* Transcarpal carpometacarpal dislocations excluding the thumb. *Am J Hand Surg* 1990; **15**: 531–40.

87 Read MT. Stress fractures of the distal radius in adolescent gymnasts. *Br J Sports Med* 1981; **15**: 272–6.

88 Cooney WP. Evaluation of chronic wrist pain by arthrography, arthroscopy and arthrotomy. *Am J Hand Surg* 1993; **18**: 815–22.

89 Mastey R, Weiss A, Akelma E. Primary care of hand and wrist athletic injuries. *Clin Sports Med* 1997; **16**: 705–24.

90 Dixon GL, Loon NF. Rotational supracondylar fractures of the proximal phalanx in children. *Clin Orth Rel Res* 1972; **83**: 151–6.

91 Simmons BP, Lavallo JL. Hand and wrist injuries in children. *Clin Sports Med* 1988; **7**: 495–512.

92 Jupiter JB, Belsky MR. Fractures and dislocations in the hand. In: Browner BD, Jupiter JB, Levine AM *et al.*, eds. *Skeletal Trauma*, third edn. Philadelphia: W.B. Saunders, 1992: 925–1024.

93 O'Brien ET. Fractures of the hand and wrist regions. In: Rockwood CA, Wilkins KE, King RE, eds. *Fractures in Children*, third edn. Philadelphia: J P Lippincott, 1991: 319–413.

94 Palmer AK. Triangular fibrocartilage complex lesions: a classification. *Am J Hand Surg* 1989; **14**: 594–606.

95 Culver JE. Sports related fractures of the hand and wrist. *Clin Sports Med* 1990; **9**: 85–109.

96 Agee J. Unstable fracture dislocations of the proximal interphalangeal joint of the fingers: a preliminary report of a new technique. *Am J Hand Surg* 1978; **3**: 386–9.

97 Schenck RR. Dynamic traction and early passive movement for fractures of the proximal interphalangeal joint. *Am J Hand Surg* 1986; **11**: 850–8.

98 Smith RJ, Peimer CA. Injuries to the metacarpal bones and joints. *Adv Surg* 1977; **11**: 341–74.

99 Pelligrini VD Jr. Fractures at the base of the thumb. *Hand Clinics* 1988; **4**: 87–102.

100 Eaton RG, Malerich MM. Volar plate arthroplasty for the proximal interphalangeal joint: a 10-year review. *Am J Hand Surg* 1980; **5**: 260–8.

101 Green DP, Rowland SA. Fractures and dislocations in the hand. In: Rockwood CA, Green DP, Bucholz RW, eds. *Fractures in Adults*, third edn. Philadelphia: JP Lippincott, 1991: 441–561.

102 Becton JL, Christian JD Jr, Goodwin HN, Jackson JG III. A simplified technique for treating the complex dislocation of the index metacarpophalangeal joint. *J Bone Joint Surg (Am)* 1975; **57-A**: 698–700.

103 Stenner B. Displacement of the ruptured ulnar collateral ligament of the metacarpophalangeal joint of the thumb. A clinical and anatomical study. *J Bone Joint Surg (Brit)* 1962; **44-B**: 869–79.

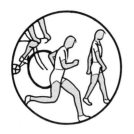

Chapter 6.8
Practical Sports Medicine

SVERRE MÆHLUM, HENNING LANGBERG &
INGGARD LEREIM

The sports medicine team

Sports medicine encompasses many different areas of professional specialization, such as exercise physiologists, sports psychologists, coaches, medical doctors and physical therapists. Needless to say each of these areas of specialization make a significant contribution and it is essential to realize that only a team approach that takes maximal advantage of everyone's talent and expertise can most optimally ensure a rapid and successful return of the athlete to a competition level after injury. Ideally all medical teams should include a medical doctor, a physiotherapist and a sports psychologist. To ensure that the athlete receives the best treatment and care during the rehabilitation process and in the preventive phase it is paramount that medical records be kept, and that all decisions concerning the athlete be communicated to all members of the medical team.

The different members of the Sports Medicine team have to conduct assessments at various times after the injury. Such assessments may have distinct purposes: (i) at the time of injury to determine first aid, emergency care measures and transportation needs; (ii) prior to initial treatment to determine the general and specific course for treatment; (iii) during the treatment phase to determine the effectiveness of the treatment and the need for changes in treatment; and (iv) before returning the athlete to full sport participation to assess the athlete's readiness to return.

It is also important that each member of the medical team has detailed knowledge of the physical and psychological demands of the sport and the type of injuries that are likely to occur, and is familiar with the sport-specific training, conditioning and competition so as to be able to formulate prevention strategies and determine etiology, treatment and the readiness of the athletes to return to play after injury. It is also essential to be familiar with the relevant rules of the sport, including regulations regarding on-field assessment, the use of braces and the doping rules. With respect to assessment and treatment it is important for the sports medical team to have full access to a separate room. An established routine for making appointments and a waiting area is useful. Appropriate medical services will ensure adequate treatment of acute injuries and thus contribute to better and more rapid rehabilitation.

Injury assessment

Before an injury is sustained it is important for the sports medicine team to have an emergency plan in place for management and transportation of the injured athlete. The method of transporting the athlete off the field is based on the type of injury and its severity. The sports medicine team must be able to provide assessment and emergency care of injuries instantaneously, and thus be able to be contacted easily by players and officials. In many team sports the obvious location for the medical personnel is on the bench. At the time of injury, it is essential that a member of the medical team immediately perform an *on-field assessment* to exclude the presence of life-threatening conditions. Hereafter the necessary first aid is carried out and the athlete is safely transported off the field. On the sideline, a second and more detailed *sideline assessment* can be conducted.

On-field assessment

The best handling of an acute injury starts with a good on-field assessment. The purpose of the on-field assessment is to rule out life-threatening and serious injuries, to determine the severity of the injury, to decide on the mode of transportation of the athlete off the field, to make a quick assessment, and to initially treat the injury in order to minimize any secondary injury. This type of assessment is the most important since an incorrect decision can have dire consequences.

Primary examination

The first and foremost aim of any initial on-site examination is to save life, and thereafter to address non-life-threatening injuries. While most sports-related injuries are not life-threatening it still remains incumbent on the medical staff to ensure that such is the case. Thus, first and foremost it is necessary to conduct a primary assessment for life-threatening conditions by checking airways, breathing and circulation. Thereafter an assessment of neurologic status should be performed, including a Glasgow coma scale, and when appropriate issues of exposure should be addressed, e.g. hypothermia in the case of a skiing accident. If the athlete is unconscious, try to arouse him by speaking loudly, or eliciting a pain response. Remember that athletes with severe injuries or severe pain are most susceptible to shock. When signs or symptoms of shock are observed immediate relevant action must be undertaken. If it is not possible to arouse the athlete immediate first aid must be performed.

If the injury is not life-threatening an on-field history should be taken, determining the mechanism, location and severity of the injury. A complete history is not needed during on-field assessment. The goal is to gather the critical information necessary to determine the overall nature and extent of the injury and to decide on the best way of transporting the athlete off the field. The rest of the history-taking can be postponed to the sideline evaluation once the athlete has been safely removed from the playing field. If a spinal injury is suspected from the history of the injury the athlete's head should be stabilized while performing a bilateral peripheral nerve assessment for sensory and motor innervations. For a suspected head injury, proceed by asking questions to find out about the athlete's orientation with respect to time, place and person.

If the injury involves bony structures, palpation for possible fractures or dislocations should be undertaken. In summary, initial screening should give sufficient information to determine the extent and severity of the injury and thus allow for proceeding with the immediate action plan.

Sideline assessment

The sideline assessment either follows an on-field assessment or serves as the initial evaluation of an injured athlete who has been able to walk off the field. If observed, the occurrence of the injury itself often provides information as to the region and type of injury. The purpose of the sideline assessment is to determine more precisely the nature and severity of the injury so that the appropriate initial treatment can be administered. The sideline assessment includes history, observation, palpation, special tests and tests of range of motion and strength, and finally neurologic, circulatory and functional tests depending on the type and severity of the injury. In the following sections the individual parts of the sideline assessment are described in more detail.

History

Once off the field the athlete's subjective impression of the injury should be obtained with regard to the direction and position of the impact, the exact position of the body, the type and timing and location of the pain, whether any sounds were 'heard' and whether previous injuries related to the present injury are present.

Observation

Observation starts during the transportation of the athlete off the field by observing the loading and the position of the injured area, eventual protection of the injured part, and the reaction during removal of shoes or clothing and inspection of the contour and position of the injured area compared to the non-injured side.

Palpation

The goal of palpation is to obtain information regarding the presence or absence of swelling, the texture of the soft tissues, and the contours of the bony structures. In addition, the palpation gives information on pulse and temperature, and the athlete's sensitivity and level of pain. All this information is essential for determining the severity of the injury and for planning the optimal treatment. It is, however, important that the palpation is performed in a systematic fashion including all relevant structures. Preferably the palpation is performed first on the non-injured side in order to familiarize the athlete with the assessment. The results from the non-injured side serve as 'the normal reference' of the athlete. Superficial and outlying structures shoud be palpated first leaving the most painful areas to be palpated last. Remember to obtain the relative severity of the pain by asking the athlete e.g. to rate the pain on a 0–10-point scale.

Special tests, range of motion and strength

The history, observation and palpation of the athlete provide a rough idea of the type and severity of the injury. In order to eliminate or confirm a specific diagnosis a range of special tests must be performed. These tests should allow the investigator to stress the structures sufficiently to distinguish between injured or non-injured structures without aggravating the injury. As for palpation of the extremities, the specific tests should first be performed on the non-injured side. The sum of the results from the tests performed should help in narrowing the possibilities of the diagnosis. When testing the range of motion (ROM) it is recommended to start by allowing the athlete to actively move the injured joint, observing the quantity and quality of the movement. Based on the result further information can be obtained by passively moving the injured joint, making an assessment of the end-feel of the joint possible. Following the determination of ROM, strength testing can provide information on the neuromuscular integrity in the activated contractive structures on the injured area. Preferably first isometric strength with the joint in midposition is tested slowly, building up the resistance with respect to the athlete's pain and the severity of the injury. The result of the strength assessment is strongly influenced by the presence of pain. If no strength can be produced in spite of the absence of pain, nerve injury or musculotendinous rupture may be possible and neurologic examination must be undertaken.

Neurologic, circulatory and functional tests

Neurologic tests include both testing of the innervations of the muscles as well as testing of sensation of the skin and reflexes. In all normal assessments of sports-related injuries a screening of the nerves should be included as a standard. Again, systematic examination is important making the screening quick, easy and reliable. For testing of the circulatory system pulses are palpated in the area of the injury and distally thereafter. The presence, strength and regularity are registered. The color and temperature of the skin also give valuable information on the circulation in the area. If the injury appears to be of minor severity, functional tests related to the specific sport should be performed before permitting the athlete to return to the field. The tests should stress the structures beginning with slow controlled movements progressing in terms of speed and direction towards movements related to the specific sport. These tests make assessment of the quality of the movements possible.

Acute treatment — special emphasis on muscle injury

If an acute trauma has occurred involving joints, muscle or soft tissue injury it is essential to use an aggressive approach in order to stop the bleeding within and around the tissue. To this effect (i) local cooling, (ii) external compression to the injured area, and (iii) elevation of the injured limb is widely recommended (the RICE concept) [1–7].

The pain-relieving effect of cold application is well documented and has also been hypothesized to reduce the activity of inflammatory enzymes [8,9]. Based more on clinical than on experimental evidence, it has been suggested that application of ice decreases local blood flow and thus reduces the tendency of swelling. The reduction in local blood flow is very dependent on the depth of injury tissue [10]. In the event of an acute injury with intratissue bleeding, the delayed reaction of cryotherapy on local blood flow means that cold application should not be the primary treatment unless the main concern is solely to relieve the pain associated with the injury [10,11]. Somewhat in contrast to cold application, external compression has been shown to reduce local blood flow [10,12,13]. Therefore in order to quickly stop intratissue bleeding and effectively reduce the size of the hematoma, instant application of external compression on the injured area should logically be of primary concern [10].

For elevation of the injured limb to be efficient in reducing the local blood flow an elevation of at least 30 cm above heart level is required before significant reduction of blood flow can be expected [14,15]. Medication administered in the acute phase includes analgesics, anesthetics and relaxants to relieve pain and reduce cramping. Often non-steroidal anti-inflammatory drugs (NSAIDs) are recommended not only to relieve pain but also to prevent swelling and excessive inflammatory reaction [2,16,17]. It is not known, however, whether a reduction of the inflammation has any influence on the recovery after injury or whether the inflammation is essential for the repair of the injured tissue [18–20]. For further information on the effect of NSAIDs in relation to sports injury treatment please see Chapters 2.1 (Recovery) and 2.5 (Pharmacology treatment).

In relation to acute treatment of any injury it cannot be emphasized enough that pain relief after the initial treatment may not lead to the conclusion that the athlete can resume the activity.

Off-field assessment

Often it is not possible to evaluate the injury immediately after it occurs. More often, athletes are seen hours or days after an acute trauma, or after a slowly progressing overuse injury. In these cases the history and the assessment alone has to provide the necessary information concerning the severity, irritability and nature of the injury. You have to bear in mind that the symptoms and thus the picture of the injury will often be less clear, as the profile of the injury changes with time and the findings are no longer the same as immediately after the onset of the injury. The off-field assessment is roughly identically to the sideline assessment although no time pressure is present and the facilities during off-field assessment permit more accurate and specific assessment. In addition the off-field assessment can be assisted by diagnostic tests such as laboratory tests, ultrasound scans, MR and radiographic tests, or even arthroscopy investigations, making specific diagnosis possible (see Chapter 5.1).

Sports medicine kit

A list of the most essential equipment and supplies which should be available for assessment and treatment of injuries during training and games is found in the box below. A presence of a large number of the items mentioned for general treatment is not necessarily based on scientific evidence for their effect, but is based on practical experience from team doctors and physiotherapists.

General treatment
Air splint
Cold spray
Instant cold packs
Heat cream
Massage oil
Sun cream
Lip balm
Insect repellent
Safety pins, rubber bands
Thermometer
Scissors
Nail clippers
Disposable gloves
Syringes
Sterile cannulas
Stethoscope

Alcohol swabs
Medical supplies

Current list of permitted and prohibited medication (doping)
Analgesics
Oral steroid (glucocortocoid)
Antihistamines
Antifungal agent
Eye drops
Ear topical treatment
Nasal spray
NSAID
Motion sickness tablets
Antiseptic solution
Local anesthetic, local glucocorticoid

Bandages	Underwrap
Strapping tape 12 mm, 25 mm, 38 mm, 50 mm	Adhesive spray
Waterproof tape 25 mm	Bandage clips
Elastic adhesive tape 50 mm	Triangular bandages
Elastic compression bandages 50 mm, 75 mm, 100 mm	Second skin
	Sterile strips, butterfly closures
Tubular support bandage	Splinting and basic orthotic material

Work during travel

Competitive sport is today recognized on a global scale. Thus athletes at many levels from the elite international stars to the recreational runner have the opportunity to compete all over the world. They accordingly often have to travel to distant places, and they must acclimatize to new environments and times of day in order to perform optimally. Such journeys pose many challenges for the medical team traveling with athletic teams. The task is greater when traveling with a large team to World Championships or Olympic Games, but basically the same problems have to be solved for all athletes who are traveling to an international competition.

The work that needs to be done can for didactic purposes be divided into the following areas:
• Preparatory work prior to departure.
• Work during travel.
• Work during stay at the competition venue.
• Work following the competition and in connection with the return home.

Preparatory work prior to departure

Obtaining information about the competitive site

When the location of the competition is known—as when an Olympic Games or World Championships is awarded to a city—the first thing that has to be done is to obtain information about the location. This can be done through a precompetition visit or through other channels if the place is well known already.

Information regarding climatic conditions (heat or cold, humidity, winds, rain, etc.) should be sought. Usually this information is readily available from the organizers. However, it is important to realize that different nations emphasize different aspects of the information given. Scandinavians for instance would be more interested in details regarding heat and humidity than Africans, since the former have to undergo acclimatization to a hot and humid climate.

It is also important to find out what the health situation is in the country one is about to visit. Are there any specific diseases that are prevalent at the competition site? What are the local hospitals like? Will it be possible to obtain prescription drugs or get qualified help if deemed necessary? Also one has to check what sort of electric current is available—in case it should be necessary to use electric equipment brought from home.

All this information is usually available through the organizers, and in addition it can be obtained through the Internet from, among other sources, the WHO or the Centers for Disease Control (CDC). In some instances vaccination is advocated prior to departure. Thus vaccination against hepatitis A is often recommended for Scandinavians. In addition, vaccination against yellow fever is mandatory upon entering some African countries. It is also necessary to find out whether prophylaxis against malaria is mandated. What needs to be taken will vary from region to region, and information about the drugs of choice can be obtained either through the WHO, through the health authorities at home or sometimes through the ministry of foreign affairs (via an Embassy or Consulate in the region).

It is also important to ascertain the level of hygiene both in general and more specifically in the hotels where the teams will stay. Can the water be drunk? What restrictions will have to be applied regarding eating? The team physician must have answers to these questions.

Making the information known to athletes, coaches and leaders

When all the details about the competition site are known, it is important to make sure that the athletes, coaches and leaders all are briefed about the details important to them. Most effectively this can be done in meetings with the group that is going. However, it has been shown time and time again that it is often necessary to repeat vital information on a one-to-one basis in order to make sure that everything is understood. Too often athletes and coaches arrive at large competitions not optimally prepared because they did not realize the importance of the information given to them. If vaccination is deemed necessary this has to be timed so that it does not interfere with the athletes' competitive schedule. Also if acclimatization is necessary either to the climate or to a new time zone, it should be recognized early so that the athletes may organize their competitive and training schedule around this.

Acclimatization to time zones

When crossing many time zones travelers face problems that are very different in nature from the ordinary travel fatigue felt after flying north–south. These problems are called 'jet lag' and are a familiar experience to the long-distance traveler. It is of particular concern to elite athletes when the competition is to be held at distant places. Thus when there is more than three time zones' difference from home, acclimatization to the new time of day will be necessary in order to perform optimally.

'Jet lag' results from the disruption of a number of physiologic functions in the body which all operate rhythmically during the 24-h day/night period. The regulation of these functions is controlled in part by external factors such as light/dark, sleep/wake cycle and food intake, and in part by internal factors—among those the hormone melatonin. When we travel across many time zones, the external factors are changed immediately upon arrival since we eat, sleep and are active according to the new time zone. However, the internal regulators take longer to adjust. Therefore the delicately balanced control is disrupted

and 'jet lag' occurs. This then results in sleep disturbances, digestive and gastrointestinal problems, general physiologic and mental symptoms of fatigue as well as changes in endocrine secretions and hormone patterns.

In general the problems are greater after eastward travel as compared to westward travel. As a rule of thumb the problems associated with jet lag last, in days, about as long as the number of time zones crossed when going east, and about half the number of days when going west. Younger persons as a rule adjust better than older persons. However, when planning travel for a group of athletes it should also be borne in mind that about 25% adjust much slower than the average. To be sure that everyone is adjusted prior to the competition it is necessary therefore either to know how each individual athlete adjusts, or to travel earlier in order to leave room for even the 'slow adapters'.

Part of the acclimatization to the new time zone (about 3 h) can be performed at home prior to departure. Thus, when traveling in a westward direction, one can 'change the daily schedule' by around 3 h, including going to bed and getting up 3 h later in the week preceding the departure. Most people find this easy, and it is therefore feasible. However, when traveling eastbound one has to get up and go to bed up to 3 h earlier. This is, of course, also theoretically possible, but is very rarely done, since most athletes (and leaders) find it hard to get up at 0300 or 0400 in the morning and go to bed at 1800 or 1900 at night.

Acclimatization to heat

If the competition is to be held in a hot climate, athletes from the more temperate climates (such as the Scandinavians) will have to acclimatize to heat—especially if the event is held in a hot and humid climate. It is generally believed that around 10–12 days of acclimatization is required. It is necessary to train about 100 min in the heat every day for 10 days in order to be optimally acclimatized. If the work intensity is very high a shorter daily training period may be sufficient. The acclimatization effect lasts for around 3 weeks. It is therefore possible to acclimatize to the heat at a hot place, and then go back home for a couple of weeks in order to avoid heat overexposure. If one decides to acclimatize just prior to the competition, the departure date will have to be about 2 weeks earlier than otherwise necessary.

When there is a need to acclimatize both to heat and to a new time zone, these two processes can, of course, run in parallel.

Planning the travel

When all the relevant information regarding the need for acclimatization to heat and time zone has been obtained, the travel plans can be finalized. For long travels across many time zones it is an advantage to arrive at the destination at night so that the athletes can go to bed almost immediately upon arrival. This will improve the adjustment to the new time zone. However, such a scheme is often not possible with the flights available with commercial airlines.

It is also important to make sure that the aircraft carry enough liquids, especially when travelling far and with a large team. Most airlines will provide more water when asked to do so. The alternative is to ask the athletes to bring water bottles in their carry-on luggage. Likewise, a member from the medical team or the dietician should talk to the airlines regarding the food they serve. Often athletes are used to foods other than those provided by most airlines. Sometimes it is possible to make the airlines change their menus when they carry a large athletic team. Again, the alternative is to ask the athletes to bring their own food. One must bear in mind, though, that many countries have very strict rules about what foodstuffs can be imported.

Obtaining equipment

If one travels with only a few athletes, bringing an ordinary doctor's bag will be sufficient. However, when a large team is going, it will be necessary to bring more equipment and in addition more prescription drugs.

All of this must be organized prior to departure. When bringing prescription medicines out of the country it will in some countries — as in Scandinavia — be necessary to obtain an export license for the drugs. Also an import license to the destination country may be necessary. Both documents should be in the carry-on luggage ready to be presented to the custom official if demanded. However, it has been the experience of the present authors through 25 years of international travel with sports teams that these documents are re-

quired very rarely. However, they should be in order. Otherwise the medical team may be stopped at the border, and will not be able to accompany the team.

Work during the actual travel

The duties of the medical team during the actual travel — i.e. during the flight — will basically be to make sure that the athletes optimize the acclimatization procedures. The air on board is very dry. Dehydration is detrimental for acclimatization to both time zones and heat, and should therefore be avoided. This can be done by:
- Making sure that the athletes drink enough while on the plane. Also it is important that they do not drink alcohol, tea or coffee since all these beverages have a diuretic effect. They should drink water. As mentioned above either one should have made the airline provide extra water or the athletes should bring their own — or both.
- Making sure that the athletes set their watches to the time of the destination immediately upon starting the journey. If possible they should eat and sleep according to the new time.
- Making sure that the athletes get some exercise while flying. They should be encouraged to take frequent walks about the cabin.

Work during stay at the competition venue

The main work will of course be the diagnosis and treatment of injuries and diseases. This is covered in the rest of the book, and will not be discussed here. However, in addition the medical team will have to perform some other tasks during the competitions.

Control of residential area

The food, water and general hygiene of the place where the athletes stay should be controlled. Obviously the physician is not able to perform a complete hygienic check on everything, but he/she should nonetheless inspect the dining hall, the kitchen and the rooms including the bathrooms. This should preferably be done prior to arrival, but sometimes it has to be done upon arrival. If hygiene is found to be below the desired standard, it is the responsibility of the medical team to try to improve it. If this is not possible they must ensure that the athletes take this into consideration. They may for instance have to avoid eating or drinking certain food or drinks or be extremely careful with personal hygiene.

Assistance in doping controls

A member of the medical team should accompany any athlete picked for doping controls. He/she should therefore know the doping regulations and ensure that the control is being performed 'according to the book'.

Ensuring that the regimens for acclimatization are being followed

When a team has traveled across more than three time zones or to a hot and humid climate that they are not used to, there are certain regimes to be followed upon arrival. The medical team must make sure that these regimes are followed, including:

Acclimatization to a new time zone

It is known that acclimatization to a new time zone is more rapid when athletes do it as a group. Also athletes must be prevented from sleeping in the middle of the day and thus prolonging the acclimatization period.

During the first couple of days after arrival the athletes should train only lightly. Since concentration is one of the factors which is affected during these first days, athletes should refrain from technical training or training that demands a lot of concentration. They should gradually get back into normal training over a period of 3–4 days—all depending upon how many times zones they have crossed.

Acclimatization to heat

Athletes have to train in the heat to acclimatize to a hot and humid climate. Daily training of about $1–1\frac{1}{2}$ h is sufficient. However, it is important that the total heat exposure is not too great. The medical team must therefore make sure that the athletes do not stay out in the hot sun for hours following training. They should be in the shade or indoors in air conditioning—even though for Scandinavians staying in the sun may seem very attractive. Athletes who have to train and compete many times in the sun—such as for instance football players—have to be particularly careful as to their total heat exposure. Too much heat will in the long run wear the athletes down, and their performance may drop as the tournament proceeds.

Work following the competition

The medical team should plan the trip home just as they planned the trip to the competition. Usually the athletes still have many important competitions to participate in after the trip, and it is therefore important to be as well rested as possible when one comes home. There is, of course, usually no need for acclimatization to the home climate, but there may be a need for a readjustment to the time zone at home. This should be done the same way as it was done when going to the competition only that the time has to be switched the other way.

After very important tournaments/events such as the Olympic Games or World Championships there is always the question as to when the athlete should start competing again. Such large tournaments will—especially for athletes in team events who may have to go through many matches—be a severe stress on key players. If they then go home and start playing in their home series directly without being allowed a short rest, these players often experience a fall in performance as the season progresses. Thus, the medical team should in cooperation with the trainers try to assess the load the athletes have gone through and, on the basis of this advice, the players, the teams and the federation as to when he/she feels that the players may start playing regular games again. This may sometimes be a difficult decision, but the problem should nonetheless be addressed since it could be very important for some players.

References

1 Baker BE. Current concepts in the diagnosis and treatment of musculotendinous injuries. *Med Sci Sports Exerc* 1984; **16**: 323–7.
2 Garret WE Jr. Muscle strain injuries: clinical and basic aspects. *Med Sci Sports Exerc* 1990; **22**: 436–43.
3 Glick JM. Muscle strains: prevention and *treatment*. *Physician Sportsmed* 1980; **8**: 73–7.
4 Herring SA. Rehabilitation of muscle injuries. *Med Sci Sports Exerc* 1990; **22**: 453–6.
5 Järvinen TA, Kaariainen M, Järvinen M, Kalimo H. Muscle strain injuries. *Curr Opin Rheumatol* 2000; **12**: 155–61.
6 Kellet. J. Acute soft tissue injuries—a review of the literature. *Med Sci Sports Exerc* 1986; **18**: 489–500.
7 Swenson C, Swärd L, Karlsson J. Cryotherapy in sports medicine. *Scand J Med Sci Sports* 1996; **6**: 193–200.
8 Dorwart BB, Hansell JR, Schumacher HR. Effects of heat, cold and mechanical agitation on crystal-induced arthritis in the dog. *Arthritis Rheum* 1973; **16**: 540–56.

9 Harris ED Jr, McCroskery PA. The influence of temperature and fibril stability on degradation of cartilage collagen by rheumatoid synovial collagenase. *N Engl J Med* 1974; **290**: 1–6.

10 Thorsson O, Hemdal B, Lilja B, Westlin N. *Med Sci Sports Exerc* 1987; **19**: 469–73.

11 Thorsson O, Lilja B, Ashgren L, Hemdal B, Westlin N. *Med Sci Sports Exerc* 1985; **17**: 710–3.

12 Ashton H. The effect of increased tissue pressure on blood flow. *Clin Orth* 1975; **113**: 15–26.

13 Nielsen HV. External pressure–blood flow relations during limb compression in man. *Acta Physiol Scand* 1983; **119**: 253–60.

14 Aronen JG, Chronister RD. Quariceps contusions. Hastening the return to play. *Physician Sportsmed* 1992; **20**: 130–6.

15 Nielsen HV. Arterial pressure-blood relations during limb compression in man. *Acta Physiol Scand* 1983; **188**: 405–13.

16 Agerskov Andersen L, Götzshe PC. Naprowen and aspirin in acute musculoskeletal disorders: a double-blind, parallel study in patients with sports injuries. *Pharmatherapeutica* 1984; **3**: 531–7.

17 Lehto M, Järvinen MJ. Muscle injuries, their healing process and treatment. *Ann Chir Gynaecol* 1991; **80**: 102–8.

18 Almekinders LC, Gilbert JA, Healing of experimental muscle strains and the effects of nonsteroidal antiinflammatory medication. *Am J Sports Med* 1986; **14**: 303–8.

19 Almekinders LC. The efficacy of nonsteroidal anti-inflammatory drugs in the treatment of ligament injuries. *Sports Med* 1990; **9**: 137–42.

20 Järvinen M, Lehto M, Sorvari T, Mikola A. Effects of anti-inflammatory agents on the healing of ruptured muscle. An experimental study in rats. *J Sports Traumatol* 1992; **14**: 19–28.

Chapter 7.1
Multiple Choice Answers

Chapter 1.1
1 *d* and *f*
2 *a*, *e* and *f*
3 *e*
4 *a*, *d* and *e*
5 *c*, *a* and *e*

Chapter 1.2
1 *c*
2 *a*
3 *c* and *d*
4 *b*, *c* and *d*
5 *c* and *e*

Chapter 1.3
1 *c*
2 *c*
3 *c*
4 *c*

Chapter 1.4
1 *b*
2 *e*
3 *e*
4 *e*
5 *a*

Chapter 1.5
1 *c*
2 *a*
3 *c*
4 *a*
5 *b*

Chapter 1.6
1 *b*
2 *a*
3 *d*

4 *d*
5 *d*

Chapter 1.7
1 *b*
2 *c*
3 *c*
4 *a*, *d* and *e*
5 *a*, *b*, *d* and *e*
6 *a* and *c*
7 *b* and *c*

Chapter 1.8
1 *e*
2 *g*
3 *e*
4 *e*
5 *a*

Chapter 2.1
1 *a*
2 *c*
3 *a*
4 *e*
5 *d* and *e*

Chapter 2.2
1 *e*
2 *e*
3 *c*
4 *e*
5 *e*

Chapter 2.3
1 *b* and *c*
2 *a*, *c* and *f*
3 *b*, *d* and *f*
4 *b* and *e*

5 *b, d* and *e*
6 *a, b* and *e*
7 *d* and *e*
8 *a*
9 *b, c* and *d*
10 *a* and *d*
11 *a, c* and *e*
12 *c* and *d*
13 *a, b, d* and *e*

Chapter 2.4
1 *c* and *d* (*d* is only correct if energy needs are met.)
2 *d* (only if energy needs are met)
3 *b*
4 *d*

Chapter 2.5
1 *d* and *e*
2 *d* and *e*
3 *a, b, c* and *e*
4 *a, d* and *e*
5 *a, b, c, d* and *e*

Chapter 3.1
1 *a*
2 *e*
3 *d*
4 *a*
5 *b*

Chapter 3.2
1 *c*
2 *d*
3 *a* and *b*
4 none

Chapter 3.3
1 *d*
2 *c*
3 *a*
4 *c*

Chapter 3.4
1 *c*
2 none
3 *a, b, c* and *d*
4 *b* and *c*
5 *b*

Chapter 3.5
1 *c*
2 *d*
3 *b*
4 *a*
5 *c*

Chapter 4.1
1 *c*
2 *a, b, c* and *d*
3 *c*
4 *b* and *d*
5 *b, c* and *d*

Chapter 4.2
1 *a, b, c, d* and *e*
2 *a* and *c*
3 *a* and *c*
4 *a, b, c* and *d*

Chapter 4.3
1 *b* and *c*
2 *c* and *d*

Chapter 4.4
1 *a*
2 *b*
3 *b*
4 *b*
5 *a*

Chapter 4.5
1 *b*
2 *b*
3 *a*
4 *a*
5 *b*
6 *c*

Chapter 4.6
1 *b*
2 *a*
3 *a, b, d* and *e*
4 *a, c, d* and *e*
5 *a, b* and *e*

Chapter 4.7
1 *c*
2 *c*
3 *d*

4 *a*

5 *a*

Chapter 4.8

1 *c*

2 *b*

3 *a, b, d* and *e*

4 *a, b, c* and *e*

5 *a, b, d* and *e*

Chapter 5.1

1 *b, d* and *e*. Stress fractures can be demonstrated after few days by bone scintigraphy as a point of heavy activity. CT is not very sensitive. Diffuse activity in the tibia is typical of medial stress syndrome and not stress fracture.

2 *d*. Narrowing of joint space is seen in osteoarthritis and not after cartilage injuries. Cartilage does not show very well on standard MRI sequences, but can be visualized on special cartilage sequences. Bone bruise is closely connected to cartilage injury, but often diffuse injury and not necessarily solitary cartilage defects. MRI is not able to distinguish between fibrocartilage and hyaline cartilage.

3 *a, c* and *e*. In healed meniscus lesions MRI will show a compete tear, as scar tissue looks like a lesion. Healing can be demonstrated because there is no inflow of fluid into the scar tissue. There is not necessarily an association between a ligament tear and instability.

4 *a, c, d* and *e*. There is not a very good association between the changes in tendons seen by ultrasound and symptoms (pain).

5 *d*. X-rays can in addition to a Hill–Sachs lesion demonstrate a bony Bankart lesion, but not a soft tissue Bankart lesion (which is the most common injury), and cannot usually discriminate between traumatic and non-traumatic instability. Standard MRI can sometimes demonstrate soft tissue Bankart lesions, but SLAP lesions and labral lesions are best demonstrated by MRI arthrography. CT cannot be used for tendon diagnoses; ultrasound or MRI can demonstrate rotator cuff lesions with good sensitivity. In rotator cuff tendinitis ultrasound can demonstrate intratendinous changes, also visible on MRI. Arthrography is used regularly in shoulder MRI and CT.

Chapter 6.1

1 *d*

2 *b*

3 *b*

4 *e*

5 *b*

Chapter 6.2

1 *d*

2 *c*

3 *c*

4 *e*

5 *c*

6 *a*

7 *c*

8 *d*

9 *b*

10 *e*

Chapter 6.3

1 *c*

2 *a* and *e*

3 *b* and *e*

4 *d*

5 *a* and *c*

Chapter 6.4

1 *c*

2 *e*

3 *e*

4 *e*

5 *b*

Case story 6.4.1

1 It is essential for his brain to recover from the concussion by taking it easy. If he has a baseline neuropsychological assessment registered, this investigation should be repeated, and he will be ready to return to any sports activity when he has returned to his baseline. In the period following the concussion he should avoid head injuries, as the damage is cumulative and there is a risk of second impact syndrome. If no baseline assessment exists, he can probably return to his sports 2 weeks after he feels subjectively well.

2 A CT scan should be performed immediately. It will probably show an epidural hematoma, which should be acutely evacuated to prevent impingement of the brainstem. If neurologic deficit appears, the prognosis is dubious.

Chapter 6.5

1 *b*

2 *d*

3 *c*

4 *e*

5 *e*

Chapter 6.6

1 *a, c* and *d.*

With a complete supraspinatus tear active abduction is reduced, but passive abduction is usually normal.

In subacromial impingement the reduced abduction is caused by fibrous tissue and is present with active as well as passive abduction.

In acute anterior dislocation the humeral head is locked in front of the glenoid and can move only very little.

With a complete subscapularis tear the internal rotation force is reduced, but abduction is usually normal.

With acromioclavicular joint dislocation the range of motion in the shoulder joint is usually normal.

2 *c* and *d.*

As shoulder instability is often the reason for the secondary impingement, the apprehension and relocation tests are usually positive.

Overhead sporting activities can only be performed with great demands on stability in the shoulder joint. Instability will therefore be symptomatic (secondary impingement) in overhead activities. In addition the enormous strain throwing puts on the anterior–inferior shoulder capsule may stretch the capsule and ligaments and create instability.

Secondary impingement is usually not (contrary to primary subacromial impingement) caused by changes to the subacromial arch (osteophytes) but by a dynamic impingement caused by the instability (and not fully understood).

As secondary impingement is caused by instability, the dynamic stabilizers should be trained first—which is sufficient in most cases. With persisting symptoms, surgical stabilization of the passive stabilizers (capsule and glenohumeral ligaments) can be performed.

There are no typical findings on MRI.

3 *a, c* and *e.*

The apprehension test can be performed on the standing patient, but the relocation test can only be performed on the supine patient.

In addition to the three tests mentioned the lag-test is sensitive for supraspinatus rupture (the inability to hold the arm over horizontal when the examiner has lifted it passively).

It is necessary to rotate the person 30° to visualize the glenohumeral joint line, as the glenoid rotates 30° anterior (because the scapula rotates).

Unfortunately, the interobserver agreement in shoulder testing is quite poor.

Ultrasound is very good at visualizing a tear in the rotator cuff, but only MRI can grade the fatty degeneration in the corresponding muscle. This is important in chronic tears, as a fatty degeneration of more than 50% of the muscle makes it unlikely that the muscle will ever function again, even if the tendon tear is repaired.

4 *b* and *d.*

During extensive rotator cuff activity, two conditions can elicit subacromial impingement: acute inflammation of the subacromial bursa, and hypertrophy of the supraspinatus muscle. Both will reduce the subacromial space and create overcrowding.

In patients with impingement, these two scapular elevators dysfunction. It is not known whether this is the reason for the impingement (as the acromion is not lifted sufficiently during overhead activity and therefore will impinge with the humeral head) or a consequence of the impingement. Strengthening of these muscles is a key point in rehabilitation of impingement patients.

Pain from primary subacromial impingement is felt on the lateral side of the upper arm. Pain is felt at the acromioclavicular joint with degenerative disease in that joint (which can of course also create a subacromial impingement if the joint is bulging into the supraspinatus tendon).

In wrestling, primary subacromial impingement and acromioclavicular joint degeneration is typical in addition to tendinitis. Internal impingement is only seen in overhead sports with repetitive, forceful abduction and external rotation.

As secondary impingement is caused by instability, acromiplasty will have no effect. The surgical treatment of choice is capsular shifting.

Chapter 6.7

1 *a* No. Tennis elbow is lateral epicondylitis. Lateral

pain caused by degenerative cartilage disease can be seen in combination with medial pain in the case of thrower's elbow, and will show with tenderness of the lateral joint line and not tenderness at the lateral epicondyle, as typical for tennis elbow.

b Yes. Valgus overload of the elbow during throwing applies stress to the medial collateral ligament, at first causing degenerative changes of the ligament and gradually loss of tension and instability. Pain is elicited from the ligament during valgus loading.

c No. It is seen as a complication to elbow dislocation with injury to the medial collateral ligament and capsule, but most cases in throwing athletes are caused by repetitive valgus overload during the throwing motion.

d Yes. Pain from the medial collateral ligament shows a couple of cm below the epicondyle and is not typically provoked by restricted flexion of the wrist, but by application of valgus stress to the elbow.

e No. If medial pain is caused by golfer's elbow, conservative treatment with rest and eventually corticosteroid injections under the cojoined flexor tendon attatchment at the medial humeral epicondyle is the first choice, but with continuous symptoms, surgical intervention can be necessary. If medial pain is caused by overload of the medial collateral ligament, conservative treatment is also the first choice, but corticosteroid injections should not be used, as they may weaken the ligament further. Continuous medial pain with medial instability should be treated operatively with tensioning or reconstruction of the medial collateral ligament.

2 *a* No. Symptoms of posterolateral rotatory elbow instability are lateral elbow pain and locking/clicking.

b Yes. It is caused by posteromedial impingement between the olecranon and the humerus and is an element of thrower's elbow: medial instability, posteromedial impingement, lateral cartilagenous degeneration and eventually ulnar nerve compression.

c No. Collision takes place between the tip of olecranon and the olecranon fossa (in cases without

medial instability, e.g. in boxing), or the posteromedial facet of the olecranon and humerus. Pain can also be caused by partial tears of the triceps tendon.

d Yes. In posterior or posteromedial impingement an osteophyte in gradually formed on the olecranon, and this as well as fibrous tissue can be removed arthroscopically.

e No. Often an osteophyte will have formed on the olecranon as a reaction to the forced extension and valgus stress on the elbow during throwing. Even if the osteophyte is surgically removed, the posterior impingement has a high recurrence rate, as long as the underlying mechanism of injury continues.

3 *a* Yes, it can, in particular if supination plus extension also elicits clicking or locking. In posterolateral rotatory elbow instability the radial head subluxes or dislocates posterior to the humeral capitulum during extension plus supination. As posterolateral rotatory instability is usually caused by elbow dislocation, it is quite rare compared to medial instability, which can also be a cause of lateral elbow pain.

b Yes, it can. Medial elbow instability is most often an overuse injury caused by repeated valgus stress to the elbow, including powerful compressive forces of the lateral compartment, resulting in degenerative cartilagenous changes, which can be painful during throwing. Tenderness is found on the lateral joint line.

c Yes. Up to 50% of recreational racquet athletes experience lateral epicondylitis regularly.

d Yes. Radial nerve entrapment causes lateral forearm pain during activity, but only rarely motor symptoms (fatigue of the hand extensors). Median nerve entrapment (pronator syndrome) causes anterior forearm pain (which may also be felt laterally), but only with entrapment of the anterior interosseus branch also motor symptoms (decreased power with flexion of the first and second distal finger joint and pronation during flexion).

e Yes, nearly all cases of tennis elbow resolve with conservative treatment. Only about 5% with continuous symptoms for 6–12 months despite conservative treatment are candidates for operative treatment.

Index

low back pain *see* back pain, low
lower leg   529–58
  injuries
    frequency   529–30
    overuse soft tissue   529–34
  muscles   *530*
  stress fractures   530
  see also ankle; foot
Ludloff's sign   625
lumbar radiculopathy   664, *669*, 671–2
lumbrical muscles   744
lunate   744
lung function
  in asthma   452, 454, 456
  in cerebral palsy   379
luteinizing hormone (LH)   464
lymphocytes   410
lymphokine-activated killer (LAK) cells   413

macrophages, in muscle injury   190
macrotrauma   203
magnesium   270–1
magnetic resonance imaging (MRI)   4, **503**,
      509–15
  in ankle injuries   544
  classical reference   501, **501**
  in groin injuries   620–1
  in knee injuries   501, **501**, 510–13, 579–81
  in low back pain   669
  principles   509–10
  in shoulder problems   513, *514*, 698–9, *700*
  in soft tissue injury   510–15
  in spinal injuries   656
  strength training-induced changes   91–2
  upper extremity   746–7
magnetic resonance (MR) arthrography   580–1
magnetic stimulation, transcutaneous   209
maintenance training   216
malaria prophylaxis   777
mallet finger   766
maltodextrin   266
manual therapy, back pain   678
marathon, wheelchair   387
marathon runners, gastrointestinal symptoms
      490–1, *492*
march fracture   554
Marfan's syndrome   365
masters athletes
  aerobic power   348–9
  bone changes   349
  connective tissue changes   349
  performance   341
  strength and power   348
  see also veteran athletes
matrix metalloproteinases (MMPs)   136, 137,
      138
maxillofacial injuries   641
maximal aerobic power (oxygen uptake) *see*
      $\dot{V}O_{2max}$
maximal voluntary contraction (MVC)   61
maximum achievable ventilation (MAV, maximal
      breathing capacity, MBC)   17, 18
M-band   51, *52*
McArdle's disease   379
McIntosh test   571
McMurray meniscal test   575
meals
  energy sources after   40, 41–2
  hormonal changes after   43
mechanocoupling   174

mechanotransduction
  in bone   173–8
  in muscle   60
medial collateral ligament (MCL) (complex)
      of the knee   565–6
  components   566
  injuries   146–50, 586–7
    combined with ACL injuries   149–50, 167
    factors affecting healing   149–50
    magnetic resonance imaging   511, *512*
    natural history   147
    non-surgical treatment   148–9, 587
    physical examination   571, 586
    surgical treatment   148–9, 587
    tissue engineering approaches   150
  mechanical properties   147
medial collateral ligament (MCL) of the elbow
      743
  instability   749, 750
  magnetic resonance imaging   513, *514*
medial patellofemoral ligament   567
medial patellotibial ligament   567
medial suprapatellar plica   567–8, *569*
medial tibial stress syndrome   518, *521*, 530–1,
      536
median nerve   744–5, 746
  entrapments   754–5, 759–60
medical problems, pre-existing   389–90
medicines *see* drugs
men, bone mass and physical activity   181–2
menarche, age at   361, 362
meniscal cysts   579, 586
meniscectomy   585–6
  knee joint changes   168, 422, 426
  magnetic resonance imaging after   510–12,
      580–1
  rehabilitation   608
meniscus
  allografts   586
  anatomy   564
  discoid   606
  injuries   585–6, 597
    in adolescents   602, 606
    articular cartilage changes   168
    clinical tests   575
    diagnosis   585
    incidence   562
    magnetic resonance imaging   501, **501**,
      510–12, 580
    osteoarthritis after   425–6, 585, 586
    repair   585, 586
    rehabilitation   608
    scintigraphy   519, *522*
    treatment   426, 585–6
    ultrasound imaging   579
menopause   346, 347
  see also postmenopausal women
menstrual dysfunction
  in athletes   462, 463
  see also amenorrhea
mental handicap   381, 382–3, 390
mental health   330–1
meralgia paresthetica   634
mesenchymal stem cells (MSC), in ligament
      injury   150
metabolic myopathies   379
metabolic rate
  basal *see* basal metabolic rate
  in cold conditions   230
  resting (RMR), in athletic amenorrhea   465

metabolism   1, **2**, 30–46
  aerobic   31, 35–6, 37
  anaerobic   31–3, 36–7
  classical references   30
  effects of infections   414–15
  energy expenditure and   38–9
  exercise   38–9
  in recovery from training   192–3
metacarpals   744
  boxer's fracture   764–5
  fractures   764
  shaft fractures   765–6
metacarpophalangeal (MP) joints   744
  dislocations/sprains   767
  stability testing   746
metatarsals
  fractures   553
  stress fractures   516, *517*, 554–5
methylprednisolone   657
MET values   255
MHC *see* myosin heavy chain
microfracture technique   583
microtrauma   203
middle glenohumeral ligament (MGHL)
      687
minerals   262, 268–71
  excessive intake   268
  supplements   267, 268–71
mitochondria   51
  proteins and enzymes   **54**, 56, 61, 213
mitogen-activated protein kinases (MAPKs)
      175
mitral valve prolapse   403
modulus, bone–ligament–bone complex   147
moment
  net joint   *107*, 118
  support   118
moment of force   72
  peak   72
moment–velocity relationship   72
MONICA project   328
mononucleosis, infectious   417, 418
montelukast   367, 457, 458
mood
  effects of exercise   330–1
  in overtraining syndrome   194
morphine, detection   285
mortality, physical activity and   339, 401
Morton's metatarsalgia   555–6
mosaicplasty   584
motion segment, spine   647–8, *649*
motivation   **5**, 6, 486
motoneuron diseases   378
motoneurons   50
  α-   55
  in bilateral vs. unilateral muscle contraction
      82–3
  discharge doublets   76, 95, *96*
  in eccentric contraction   79–82
  evoked reflex responses   74, 77–9
  firing frequency   76–7
  high-frequency firing pattern   95
  inhibitory mechanisms   84–6
  in muscle injury   67
  synchronization in firing   77
motor endplate (neuromuscular junction)   50,
      55
motor nerves   49, 50
  intramuscular rupture, in muscle injury   67
  see also motoneurons